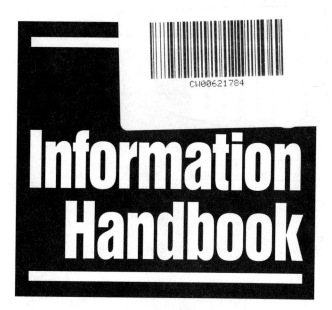

Information Handbook

for the
Allied Health Professional
with
Indication/Therapeutic Category Index

7th Edition 2000-2001

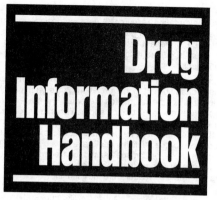

Drug Information Handbook

— for the —
Allied Health Professional
with
Indication/Therapeutic Category Index

7th Edition **2000-2001**

Leonard L. Lance, RPh, BSPharm
Senior Editor
Pharmacist
Lexi-Comp Inc.
Hudson, Ohio

Charles F. Lacy, PharmD, FCSHP
Editor
Clinical Coordinator and
Drug Information Specialist
Cedars-Sinai Health System
Los Angeles, California

Morton P. Goldman, PharmD, BCPS
Associate Editor
Assistant Director, Pharmacotherapy Services
Department of Pharmacy
Cleveland Clinic Foundation
Cleveland, Ohio

Lora L. Armstrong, RPh, BSPharm, BCPS
Associate Editor
Clinical Pharmacist
Caremark Pharmaceutical Group
Northbrook, Illinois

LEXI-COMP INC
Hudson (Cleveland)

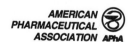

AMERICAN PHARMACEUTICAL ASSOCIATION APhA

NOTICE

This handbook is intended to serve the user as a handy quick reference and not as a complete drug information resource. It does not include information on every therapeutic agent available. The publication covers commonly used drugs and is specifically designed to present certain important aspects of drug data in a more concise format than is generally found in medical literature or product material supplied by manufacturers.

Drug information is constantly evolving because of ongoing research and clinical experience and is often subject to interpretation. While great care has been taken to ensure the accuracy of the information presented, the reader is advised that the authors, editors, reviewers, contributors, and publishers cannot be responsible for the continued currency of the information or for any errors, omissions, or the application of this information, or for any consequences arising therefrom. Therefore, the author(s) and/or the publisher shall have no liability to any person or entity with regard to claims, loss, or damage caused, or alleged to be caused, directly or indirectly, by the use of information contained herein. Because of the dynamic nature of drug information, readers are advised that decisions regarding drug therapy must be based on the independent judgment of the clinician, changing information about a drug (eg, as reflected in the literature and manufacturer's most current product information), and changing medical practices. The editors are not responsible for any inaccuracy of quotation or for any false or misleading implication that may arise due to the text or formulas as used or due to the quotation of revisions no longer official. Further, the *Drug Information Handbook for the Allied Health Professional* is not offered as a guide to dosing. The reader, herewith, is advised that information shown under the heading **Usual Dosage** is provided only as an indication of the amount of the drug typically given or taken during therapy. Actual dosing amount for any specific drug should be based on an in-depth evaluation of the individual patient's therapy requirement and strong consideration given to such issues as contraindications, warnings, precautions, adverse reactions, along with the interaction of other drugs. The manufacturers most current product information or other standard recognized references should always be consulted for such detailed information prior to drug use.

The editors and contributors have written this book in their private capacities. No official support or endorsement by any federal agency or pharmaceutical company is intended or inferred.

If you have any suggestions or questions regarding any information presented in this handbook, please contact our drug information pharmacist at

1-800-837-LEXI (5394)

This manual was produced using the FormuLex™ Program — a complete publishing service of Lexi-Comp Inc.

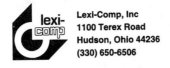

Lexi-Comp, Inc
1100 Terex Road
Hudson, Ohio 44236
(330) 650-6506

ISBN 0-916589-96-X

TABLE OF CONTENTS

ABOUT THE AUTHORS

Leonard L. Lance, RPh, BSPharm

Leonard L. (Bud) Lance has been directly involved in the pharmaceutical industry since receiving his bachelor's degree in pharmacy from Ohio Northern University in 1970. Upon graduation from ONU, Mr Lance spent four years as a navy pharmacist in various military assignments and was instrumental in the development and operation of the first whole hospital I.V. admixture program in a military (Portsmouth Naval Hospital) facility.

After completing his military service, he entered the retail pharmacy field and has managed both an independent and a home I.V. franchise pharmacy operation. Since the late 1970s, Mr Lance has focused much of his interest on using computers to improve pharmacy service and to advance the dissemination of drug information to practitioners and other health care professionals.

As a result of his strong publishing interest, he serves in the capacity of pharmacy editor and technical advisor as well as pharmacy (information) database coordinator for Lexi-Comp. Along with the *Drug Information Handbook for the Allied Health Professional*, he provides technical support to Lexi-Comp's Clinical Reference Library™ publications. Mr Lance has also assisted approximately 120 major hospitals in producing their own formulary (pharmacy) publications through Lexi-Comp's custom publishing service.

Mr Lance is a member and past president (1984) of the Summit Pharmaceutical Association (SPA). He is also a member of the Ohio Pharmacists Association (OPA), the American Pharmaceutical Association (APhA), and the American Society of Health-System Pharmacists (ASHP).

Charles F. Lacy, PharmD, FCSHP

Dr Lacy received his doctorate from the University of Southern California School of Pharmacy. With over 18 years of clinical experience at one of the nation's largest teaching hospitals, he has developed a reputation as an acknowledged expert in drug information and critical care drug therapy.

In his current capacity as Coordinator of Clinical Pharmacy Services and Drug Information Services at Cedar-Sinai Health System in Los Angeles, Dr Lacy plays an active role in the education and training of the medical, pharmacy, and nursing staff. He coordinates the Drug Information Center, clinical pathways development, the Medical Center's Intern Pharmacist Clinical Training Program, clinical pharmacy staff development, the Department's Continuing Education Program for Pharmacists, and Pharmacy Residency Clinical Assessment and Training Program. He maintains the Medical Center formulary program and coordinates all pharmacy clerkship programs at the Medical Center. He also supervises the activities of clinical specialists in medication use evaluation, antibiotic use review, infectious disease control, investigational drug protocols, pain management programs, Adverse Drug Reaction Monitoring Program, the Medical Center's Medication Error Detection and Remedy Program, and is editor of the Medical Center's *Drug Formulary Handbook* and the drug information newsletter *Prescription*.

Presently, Dr Lacy holds teaching affiliations with the University of Southern California School of Pharmacy, the University of California at San Francisco School of Pharmacy, the University of the Pacific School of Pharmacy, the University of Alberta at Edmonton, School of Pharmacy and Health Sciences, and Southern Nevada School of Pharmacy in Las Vegas. Additionally, Dr Lacy is the current Director of the Center for International Health Care Practitioners at Western University of Health Sciences, where he plays a leading role in the advanced training of postgraduate pharmacists from areas throughout the Pacific rim, including Japan, Hong Kong, New Zealand, and Korea.

Dr Lacy is an active member of numerous professional associations including the American Society of Health-System Pharmacists (ASHP), the California Society of Hospital Pharmacists (CSHP), the American Society of Consultant Pharmacists (ASCP), American Pharmaceutical Association (APhA), and the American College of Clinical Pharmacy (ACCP).

Morton P. Goldman, PharmD, BCPS

Dr Goldman received his bachelor's degree in pharmacy from the University of Pittsburgh, College of Pharmacy and his Doctor of Pharmacy degree from the University of Cincinnati, Division of Graduate Studies and Research. He completed his concurrent 2-year hospital pharmacy residency at the VA Medical Center in Cincinnati. Dr Goldman is presently the Assistant Director of Pharmacotherapy Services for the Department of Pharmacy at the Cleveland Clinic Foundation (CCF) after having spent over 3 years at CCF as an Infectious Disease pharmacist and 4 years as Clinical Manager. He holds faculty appointments from Case Western Reserve University, College of Medicine; The University of Toledo, College of Pharmacy; and The University of Cincinnati, College of Pharmacy. Dr Goldman is a board-certified Pharmacotherapy Specialist.

In his capacity as Assistant Director of Pharmacotherapy Services at CCF, Dr Goldman remains actively involved in patient care and clinical research with the Department of Infectious Disease, as well as the continuing education of the medical and pharmacy staff. He is an editor of CCF's *Guidelines for Antibiotic Use* and coordinates their annual Antimicrobial Review retreat. He is a member of the Pharmacy and Therapeutics Committee and many of its subcommittees. Dr Goldman has authored numerous journal articles and lectures locally and nationally on infectious diseases topics and current drug therapies. He is currently a reviewer for the *Annals of Pharmacotherapy* and the *Journal of the American Medical Association*, an editorial board member of the *Journal of Infectious Disease Pharmacotherapy*, and coauthor of the *Drug Information Handbook* produced by Lexi-Comp, Inc. He also provides technical support to Lexi-Comp's Clinical Reference Library™ publications.

Dr Goldman is an active member of Cleveland's local clinical pharmacy society, the Ohio College of Clinical Pharmacy, the Society of Infectious Disease Pharmacists, the American College of Clinical Pharmacy, and the American Society of Health-Systems Pharmacy.

Lora L. Armstrong, RPh, BSPharm, BCPS

Lora L. Armstrong received her bachelor's degree in pharmacy from Ferris State University. She has been a Board Certified Pharmacotherapy Specialist (BCPS) since 1994.

During her 17 years of clinical experience at one of the nation's most prominent teaching institutions, Ms Armstrong has developed a reputation as an acknowledged expert in drug information. Ms Armstrong served as the Director of Drug Information Services at the University of Chicago Hospitals. Her interests included the areas of critical care, hematology, oncology, infectious disease, and pharmacokinetics. Ms Armstrong also played an active role in the education and training of medical, pharmacy, and nursing staff. She coordinated the Drug Information Center, the medical center's Adverse Drug Reaction Monitoring Program, and the Continuing Education Program for pharmacists. Ms Armstrong maintained the hospital's strict formulary program and was editor of the University of Chicago Hospitals *Formulary of Accepted Drugs* and the drug information monthly newsletter *Topics in Drug Therapy.*

In her current position, Ms Armstrong serves as clinical pharmacist in Clinical Development and Information Resources at Caremark Rx, Inc, Prescription Services Division. Ms Armstrong is responsible for development and enhancement of clinical management programs, physician and staff education, and formulary management. She participates in the development and evaluation of clinical programs that include Formulary Management, Concurrent Interventions, Retrospective Case Management, Physician Profiling, and Utilization Review Pharmacy Management. Ms Armstrong also provides support for Caremark Rx, Inc's National Pharmacy and Therapeutics Committee activities.

Ms Armstrong is an active member of the Academy of Managed Care Pharmacy (AMCP), the American Society of Health-System Pharmacists (ASHP), the American Pharmaceutical Association (APhA), the American College of Clinical Pharmacy (ACCP), and the Society of Critical Care Medicine (SCCM). Ms Armstrong also serves on the Editorial Advisory Board of the Journal of the American Pharmaceutical Association.

EDITORIAL ADVISORY PANEL

Matthew A. Fuller, PharmD, BCPS, BCPP, FASHP
Clinical Pharmacy Specialist
Psychiatry
Cleveland Department of Veterans Affairs Medical Center
Brecksville, Ohio

Mark Geraci, PharmD
Department of Pharmacy Practice
University of Illinois
Chicago, Illinois

Harold J. Grady, PhD
Director of Clinical Chemistry
Truman Medical Center
Kansas City, Missouri

Larry D. Gray, PhD
Director of Microbiology
Bethesda Hospitals
Cincinnati, Ohio

Martin D. Higbee, PharmD
Associate Professor
Department of Pharmacy Practice
The University of Arizona
Tucson, Arizona

Jane Hurlburt Hodding, PharmD
Supervisor, Children's Pharmacy
Memorial Miller Children's Hospital
Long Beach, California

Rebecca T. Horvat, PhD
Assistant Professor of Pathology and Laboratory Medicine
University of Kansas Medical Center
Kansas City, Kansas

Carlos M. Isada, MD
Department of Infectious Disease
Cleveland Clinic Foundation
Cleveland, Ohio

David S. Jacobs, MD
President, Pathologists Chartered
Overland Park, Kansas

Bernard L. Kasten, Jr, MD
Vice-President/Medical Director
Corning Clinical Laboratories
Teterboro, New Jersey

Polly E. Kintzel, PharmD
Clinical Pharmacy Specialist
Bone Marrow Transplantation, Detroit Medical Center
Harper Hospital
Detroit, Michigan

Donna M. Kraus, PharmD
Associate Professor of Pharmacy Practice
Departments of Pharmacy Practice and Pediatrics
Pediatric Clinical Pharmacist
University of Illinois at Chicago
Chicago, Illinois

Brenda R. Lance, RN, MSN
Nurse Coordinator
Ritzman Infusion Services
Akron, Ohio

Jerrold B. Leikin, MD
Associate Director
Emergency Services
Rush Presbyterian-St Luke's Medical Center
Chicago, Illinois

5

EDITORIAL ADVISORY PANEL *(Continued)*

PREFACE

Working with clinical pharmacists, hospital pharmacy and therapeutics committees, and hospital drug information centers, the editors of this handbook have directly assisted in the development and production of hospital-specific formulary documentation for several hundred major medical institutions in the United States and Canada. The resultant documentation provides pertinent detail concerning use of medications within the hospital and other clinical settings. The most current information on medications has been extracted, reviewed, coalesced, and cross-referenced by the editors to create this *Drug Information Handbook for the Allied Health Professional*.

Thus, this handbook gives the user quick access to data on 1573 medications with cross referencing to 5284 U.S., Canadian, and Mexican brand or trade names. Selection of the included medications was based on the analysis of those medications offered in a wide range of hospital formularies. The concise standardized format for data used in this handbook was developed to ensure a consistent presentation of information for all medications.

All generic drug names and synonyms appear in lower case, whereas brand or trade names appear in upper/lower case with the proper trademark information. These three items appear as individual entries in the alphabetical listing of drugs and, thus, there is no requirement for an alphabetical index of drugs names.

Two new features for this edition of the *Drug Information Handbook for the Allied Health Professional* are the inclusion of Canadian only drug names and a listing of Pharmaceutical Manufacturers and Drug Distributors with their mailing and WEB site addresses.

The Indication/Therapeutic Category Index is an expedient mechanism for locating the medication of choice along with its classification. This index will help the user, with knowledge of the disease state, to identify medications which are most commonly used in treatment. All disease states are cross-referenced to a varying number of medications with the most frequently used medication(s) noted.

— L.L. Lance

ACKNOWLEDGMENTS

The *Drug Information Handbook for the Allied Health Professional* exists in its present form as the result of the concerted efforts of the following individuals: Robert D. Kerscher, publisher and president of Lexi-Comp Inc; Lynn D. Coppinger, managing editor; Barbara F. Kerscher, production manager; David C. Marcus, director of information systems; and Julian I. Graubart, American Pharmaceutical Association (APhA), Director of Books and Electronic Products.

Other members of the Lexi-Comp staff whose contributions deserve special mention include Jeanne E. Wilson, production/systems liaison; Ginger S. Conner, Leslie J. Ruggles, and Kathleen E. Schleicher, reference publishing project managers; Stacey L. Hurd, Tonya Parsley, Jennifer L. Rocky, and Linda L. Taylor, custom project managers; Alexandra J. Hart, composition specialist; Kathy Smith and Stacy Robinson, production assistants; Tracey J. Reinecke, graphic designer; Mark F. Bonfiglio, BS, PharmD, RPh, director of pharmacotherapy resources; Leonard L. Lance, BSPharm, RPh, pharmaceutical database specialist; Liz Tomsik, PharmD, pharmacotherapy specialist; Cynthia A. Bell, CPhT, drug identification database manager; Edmund A. Harbart, vice-president, custom publishing division; Jack L. Stones, vice-president, reference publishing division; Jay L. Katzen, director of marketing and business development; Jerry M. Reeves, Marc L. Long, and Patrick T. Grubb, regional sales managers; Brad F. Bolinski, Kristin M. Thompson, Matthew C. Kerscher, Tina L. Collins, and Kelene A. Gluntz, sales and marketing representatives; Paul A. Rhine and Jason M. Buchwald, academic account managers; Kenneth J. Hughes, manager of authoring systems; Sean M. Conrad, James M. Stacey, and Matthew J. Houser, system analysts; Thury L. O'Connor, vice-president of technology; David J. Wasserbauer, vice-president, finance and administration; Elizabeth M. Conlon, Rebecca A. Dryhurst, and Leslie G. Rodia, accounting; Marta Pacur and Mary Jane Podesta, receptionists; and Frederick C. Kerscher, inventory and fulfillment manager.

Special thanks goes to Chris Lomax, PharmD, director of pharmacy, Children's Hospital, Los Angeles, who played a significant role in bringing APhA and Lexi-Comp together.

Much of the material contained in this book was a result of pharmacy contributors throughout the United States and Canada. Lexi-Comp has assisted many medical institutions to develop hospital-specific formulary manuals that contains clinical drug information as well as dosing. Working with these clinical pharmacists, hospital pharmacy and therapeutics committees, and hospital drug information centers, Lexi-Comp has developed an evolutionary drug database that reflects the practice of pharmacy in these major institutions.

In addition, the authors wish to thank their families, friends, and colleagues who supported them in their efforts to complete this handbook.

DESCRIPTION OF SECTIONS AND FIELDS USED IN THIS HANDBOOK

The *Drug Information Handbook for the Allied Health Professional* is organized into a drug information section, an appendix, and an indication/therapeutic category index.

The drug information section of the handbook, wherein all drugs are listed alphabetically, details information pertinent to each drug. Extensive cross referencing is provided by brand name and synonyms.

Drug Information is presented in a consistent format and for quick reference will provide the following:

Generic Name	U.S. Adopted Name (USAN) or International Nonproprietary Name (INN)
	If a drug product is only available in Canada, a *(Canada only)* will be attached to that product and will appear with every occurrence of that drug throughout the book
Pronunciation Guide	Subjective aid for pronouncing drug names
U.S. Brand Names	Common trade names used in the United States
Canadian Brand Names	Unique trade names found in Canada (if brand name is the same as U.S. the entry has not been duplicated)
Mexican Brand Names	Trade names found in Mexico
Synonyms	Official names and some slang
Generic Available	Informs the user if there is a generic and the available form
Therapeutic Category	Lexi-Comp's own system of logical medication classification
Use	Information pertaining to appropriate use of the drug
Controlled Substance	According to DEA classification (see descriptions in appendix)
Usual Dosage	The amount of the drug to be typically given or taken during therapy
Dietary Considerations	Explains how medication should be taken concerning meals or food
Nursing/Pharmacy Information	Information "Pearls" for all healthcare practitioners, including monitoring parameters and stability
Dosage Forms	Information with regard to form, strength, and availability of the drug

Appendix

The appendix offers a compilation of tables, guidelines, and conversion information that can often be helpful when considering patient care.

Indication/Therapeutic Category Index

This index provides a listing of accepted drugs for various disease states thus focusing attention on selection of medications most frequently prescribed in relation to a clinical diagnosis. Diseases may have other nonofficial drugs for their treatment and this indication/therapeutic category index should not be used by itself to determine the appropriateness of a particular therapy. The listed indications may encompass varying degrees of severity and, since certain medications may not be appropriate for a given degree of severity, it should not be assumed that the agents listed for specific indications are interchangeable. Also included as a valuable reference is each medication's therapeutic category.

SAFE WRITING PRACTICES

Health professionals and their support personnel frequently produce handwritten copies of information they see in print; therefore, such information is subjected to even greater possibilities for error or misinterpretation on the part of others. Thus, particular care must be given to how drug names and strengths are expressed when creating written healthcare documents.

The following are a few examples of safe writing rules suggested by the Institute for Safe Medication Practices, Inc.*

1. There should be a space between a number and its units as it is easier to read. There should be no periods after the abbreviations mg or mL.

Correct	Incorrect
10 mg	10mg
100 mg	100mg

2. Never place a decimal and a zero after a whole number (2 mg is correct and 2.0 mg is **incorrect**). If the decimal point is not seen because it falls on a line or because individuals are working from copies where the decimal point is not seen, this causes a tenfold overdose.

3. Just the opposite is true for numbers less than one. Always place a zero before a naked decimal (0.5 mL is correct, .5 mL is **incorrect**).

4. Never abbreviate the word unit. The handwritten U or u, looks like a 0 (zero), and may cause a tenfold overdose error to be made.

5. IU is not a safe abbreviation for international units. The handwritten IU looks like IV. Write out international units or use int. units.

6. Q.D. is not a safe abbreviation for once daily, as when the Q is followed by a sloppy dot, it looks like QID which means four times daily.

7. O.D. is not a safe abbreviation for once daily, as it is properly interpreted as meaning "right eye" and has caused liquid medications such as saturated solution of potassium iodide and Lugol's solution to be administered incorrectly. There is no safe abbreviation for once daily. It must be written out in full.

8. Do not use chemical names such as 6-mercaptopurine or 6-thioguanine, as sixfold overdoses have been given when these were not recognized as chemical names. The proper names of these drugs are mercaptopurine or thioguanine.

9. Do not abbreviate drug names (5FC, 6MP, 5-ASA, MTX, HCTZ, CPZ, PBZ, etc) as they are misinterpreted and cause error.

10. Do not use the apothecary system or symbols.

11. Do not abbreviate microgram as µg; instead use mcg as there is less likelihood of misinterpretation.

12. When writing an outpatient prescription, write a complete prescription. A complete prescription can prevent the prescriber, the pharmacist, and/or the patient from making a mistake and can eliminate the need for further clarification. The legible prescriptions should contain:

    a. patient's full name

    b. for pediatric or geriatric patients: their age (or weight where applicable)

    c. drug name, dosage form and strength; if a drug is new or rarely prescribed, print this information

    d. number or amount to be dispensed

    e. complete instructions for the patient, including the purpose of the medication

    f. when there are recognized contraindications for a prescribed drug, indicate to the pharmacist that you are aware of this fact (ie, when prescribing a potassium salt for a patient receiving an ACE inhibitor, write "K serum leveling being monitored")

*From "Safe Writing" by Davis NM, PharmD and Cohen MR, MS, Lecturers and Consultants for Safe Medication Practices, 1143 Wright Drive, Huntington Valley, PA 19006. Phone: (215) 947-7566.

ALPHABETICAL LISTING OF DRUGS

- **642®** *see* propoxyphene *on page 526*
- **A-200™ Shampoo [OTC]** *see* pyrethrins and piperonyl butoxide *on page 533*
- **A and D™ Ointment [OTC]** *see* vitamin A and vitamin D *on page 651*

abacavir *New Drug* (a BAK a veer)
U.S. Brand Names Ziagen™
Generic Available No
Therapeutic Category Nucleoside Analog Reverse Transcriptase Inhibitor
Use Treatment of HIV infections in combination with other antiretroviral agents
Usual Dosage Oral:
Children: 3 months to 16 years: 8 mg/kg body weight twice daily (maximum: 300 mg twice daily) in combination with other antiretroviral agents
Adults: 300 mg twice daily in combination with other antiretroviral agents
Dosage Forms
Solution, oral: 20 mg/mL (240 mL)
Tablet: 300 mg

- **Abbokinase®** *see* urokinase *on page 639*
- **ABCD** *see* amphotericin B cholesteryl sulfate complex *on page 44*

abciximab (ab SIK si mab)
Synonyms c7E3
U.S. Brand Names ReoPro®
Generic Available No
Therapeutic Category Platelet Aggregation Inhibitor
Use Adjunct to percutaneous transluminal coronary angioplasty or atherectomy (PTCA) for the prevention of acute cardiac ischemic complications; prevent cardiac ischemic complications in a wider range of percutaneous coronary interventions (PCIs), including balloon angioplasty and stent placement, and without qualification of high risk for abrupt vessel closure; unstable angina that does not respond to conventional therapy when PCI is planned with 24 hours
Usual Dosage I.V.: 0.25 mg/kg bolus followed by an infusion of 10 mcg/minute for 12 hours
Nursing/Pharmacy Information Do not shake the vial. Maintain bleeding precautions, avoid unnecessary arterial and venous punctures, use saline or heparin lock for blood drawing; assess sheath insertion site and distal pulses of affected leg every 15 minutes for the first hour and then every 1 hour for the next 6 hours. Observe patient for mental status changes, hemorrhage, assess nose and mouth mucous membranes, puncture sites for oozing, ecchymosis and hematoma formation, and examine urine, stool, and emesis for presence of occult or frank blood. Gentle care should be provided when removing dressings.
Dosage Forms Injection: 2 mg/mL (5 mL)

- **Abelcet™** *see* amphotericin B lipid complex *on page 45*
- **Abenol®** *see* acetaminophen *on page 13*
- **Abitrate®** *see* clofibrate *on page 158*
- **ABLC** *see* amphotericin B lipid complex *on page 45*
- **absorbable cotton** *see* cellulose, oxidized *on page 127*
- **absorbable gelatin sponge** *see* gelatin, absorbable *on page 288*
- **Absorbine® Antifungal [OTC]** *see* tolnaftate *on page 618*
- **Absorbine® Antifungal Foot Powder [OTC]** *see* miconazole *on page 413*
- **Absorbine® Jock Itch [OTC]** *see* tolnaftate *on page 618*
- **Absorbine Jr.® Antifungal [OTC]** *see* tolnaftate *on page 618*
- **Acanol** *see* loperamide *on page 374*

acarbose (AY car bose)
U.S. Brand Names Precose®
Generic Available No
Therapeutic Category Antidiabetic Agent, Oral
Use Treatment of noninsulin-dependent diabetes mellitus (NIDDM); as monotherapy or in combination with a sulfonylurea when diet plus acarbose or a sulfonylurea does not result in adequate glycemic control; also used with insulin or metformin in patients with noninsulin-dependent diabetes mellitus (NIDDM)
Usual Dosage Adults: Oral: Dosage must be individualized on the basis of effectiveness and tolerance while not exceeding the maximum recommended dose of 100 mg 3 times/day
Initial dose: 25 mg 3 times/day with the first bite of each main meal

Maintenance dose: Should be adjusted at 4- to 8-week intervals based on 1-hour postprandial glucose levels and tolerance. Dosage may be increased from 25 mg 3 times/day to 50 mg 3 times/day; some patients may benefit from increasing the dose to 100 mg 3 times/day; maintenance dose ranges: 50-100 mg 3 times/day.

Maximum dose:
≤60 kg: 50 mg 3 times/day
>60 kg: 100 mg 3 times/day

Nursing/Pharmacy Information Administer acarbose 3 times/day at the start (with the first bite) of each main meal. It is important to continue to adhere to dietary instructions, a regular exercise program, and regular testing of urine and/or blood glucose. The risk of hypoglycemia, its symptoms and treatment, and conditions that predispose to its development should be well understood by patients and responsible family members. A source of glucose (dextrose) should be readily available to treat symptoms of low blood glucose when taking acarbose in combination with a sulfonylurea or insulin. If side effects occur, they usually develop during the first few weeks of therapy and are most often mild to moderate gastrointestinal effects, such as flatulence, diarrhea, or abdominal discomfort and generally diminish in frequency and intensity with time.

Dosage Forms Tablet: 25 mg, 50 mg, 100 mg

♦ **Accolate**® see zafirlukast on page 657
♦ **Accupril**® see quinapril on page 536
♦ **Accuretic**® see quinapril and hydrochlorothiazide (Canada only) on page 536
♦ **Accutane**® see isotretinoin on page 350

acebutolol (a se BYOO toe lole)
U.S. Brand Names Sectral®
Canadian Brand Names Monitan®; Rhotral®
Generic Available Yes
Therapeutic Category Antiarrhythmic Agent, Class II; Beta-Adrenergic Blocker
Use Treatment of hypertension; ventricular arrhythmias; angina
Usual Dosage Adults: Oral: 400-800 mg/day in 2 divided doses
Dietary Considerations May be administered without regard to meals
Nursing/Pharmacy Information Advise against abrupt withdrawal; monitor blood pressure, orthostatic hypotension, heart rate, CNS effects, EKG, and CVP
Dosage Forms Capsule, as hydrochloride: 200 mg, 400 mg

♦ **Acel-Imune**® see diphtheria, tetanus toxoids, and acellular pertussis vaccine on page 210
♦ **Aceon**® see perindopril erbumine on page 481
♦ **Acephen**® [OTC] see acetaminophen on page 13
♦ **Aceta**® [OTC] see acetaminophen on page 13

acetaminophen (a seet a MIN oh fen)
Synonyms APAP; n-acetyl-p-aminophenol; paracetamol
U.S. Brand Names Acephen® [OTC]; Aceta® [OTC]; Apacet® [OTC]; Dapa® [OTC]; Dapacin® [OTC]; Dorcol® [OTC]; Feverall™ [OTC]; Genapap® [OTC]; Genebs® [OTC]; Liquiprin® [OTC]; Mapap® [OTC]; Maranox® [OTC]; Meda-Cap® [OTC]; Meda® Tab [OTC]; Myapap® [OTC]; Neopap® [OTC]; Panadol® [OTC]; Redutemp® [OTC]; Ridenol® [OTC]; Silapap® [OTC]; Snaplets-FR® Granules [OTC]; Tapanol® [OTC]; Tempra® [OTC]; Tylenol® [OTC]; Ty-Pap [OTC]; Uni-Ace® [OTC]
Canadian Brand Names Abenol®; AF®; Atasol®; Pediatrix®; Tantaphen®
Mexican Brand Names Algitrin®; Analphen; Cilag®; Febrin®; Minofen®; Neodol; Sinedol; Sinedol 500; Temperal; Tylex 750; Winasorb
Generic Available Yes
Therapeutic Category Analgesic, Non-narcotic; Antipyretic
Use Treatment of mild to moderate pain and fever; does not have antirheumatic or systemic anti-inflammatory effects
Usual Dosage Oral, rectal (if fever not controlled with acetaminophen alone, administer with full doses of aspirin on an every 4- to 6-hour schedule, if aspirin is not otherwise contraindicated):

Children <12 years: 10-15 mg/kg/dose every 4-6 hours as needed; do **not** exceed 5 doses (2.6 g) in 24 hours
Adults: 325-650 mg every 4-6 hours or 1000 mg 3-4 times/day; do **not** exceed 4 g/day
(Continued)

acetaminophen *(Continued)*

Dietary Considerations May be administered with food if needed; rate of absorption may be decreased when administered with food high in carbohydrates; food may slightly delay absorption of extended-release preparations; excessive intake of alcohol may increase the risk of acetaminophen-induced hepatotoxicity; avoid or limit alcohol intake

Nursing/Pharmacy Information Do not freeze suppositories; before pouring a dose, shake oral suspension well

Dosage Forms
Caplet: 160 mg, 325 mg, 500 mg
Caplet, extended: 650 mg
Capsule: 80 mg
Drops: 48 mg/mL (15 mL); 60 mg/0.6 mL (15 mL); 80 mg/0.8 mL (15 mL); 100 mg/mL (15 mL, 30 mL)
Elixir: 80 mg/5 mL, 120 mg/5 mL, 160 mg/5 mL, 167 mg/5 mL, 325 mg/5 mL
Liquid, oral: 160 mg/5 mL, 500 mg/15 mL
Solution: 100 mg/mL (15 mL); 120 mg/2.5 mL
Suppository, rectal: 80 mg, 120 mg, 125 mg, 300 mg, 325 mg, 650 mg
Suspension, oral: 160 mg/5 mL
Suspension, oral drops: 80 mg/0.8 mL
Tablet: 325 mg, 500 mg, 650 mg
Tablet, chewable: 80 mg, 160 mg

♦ **acetaminophen and butalbital compound** *see* butalbital compound and acetaminophen *on page 99*

acetaminophen and codeine (a seet a MIN oh fen & KOE deen)

Synonyms codeine and acetaminophen

U.S. Brand Names Capital® and Codeine; Tylenol® With Codeine

Canadian Brand Names Atasol® 8, 15, 30 W/ Caffeine; Empracet®-30, -60; Emtec-30®; Lenoltec® No.1, 2, 3, 4; Novo-Gesic-C8®; Novo-Gesic-C15®; Novo-Gesic-C30®

Mexican Brand Names Tylex CD

Generic Available Yes

Therapeutic Category Analgesic, Narcotic

Controlled Substance C-III; C-V

Use Relief of mild to moderate pain

Usual Dosage Doses should be adjusted according to severity of pain and response of the patient. Adult doses ≥60 mg codeine fail to give commensurate relief of pain but merely prolong analgesia and are associated with an appreciably increased incidence of side effects. Oral:

Children:
Analgesic: 0.5-1 mg codeine/kg/dose every 4-6 hours
Acetaminophen: 10-15 mg/kg/dose every 4 hours up to a maximum of 2.6 g/ 24 hours for children <12 years
3-6 years: 5 mL 3-4 times/day as needed of elixir
7-12 years: 10 mL 3-4 times/day as needed of elixir
>12 years: 15 mL every 4 hours as needed of elixir
Adults:
Antitussive: Based on codeine (15-30 mg/dose) every 4-6 hours
Analgesic: Based on codeine (30-60 mg/dose) every 4-6 hours
1-2 tablets every 4 hours to a maximum of 12 tablets/24 hours

Dietary Considerations Rate of absorption of acetaminophen may be decreased when administered with food high in carbohydrates

Nursing/Pharmacy Information Observe patient for excessive sedation or confusion, respiratory depression, constipation, relief of pain, blood pressure

Dosage Forms
Capsule:
#2: Acetaminophen 325 mg and codeine phosphate 15 mg (C-III)
#3: Acetaminophen 325 mg and codeine phosphate 30 mg (C-III)
#4: Acetaminophen 325 mg and codeine phosphate 60 mg (C-III)
Elixir: Acetaminophen 120 mg and codeine phosphate 12 mg per 5 mL with alcohol 7% (C-V)
Suspension, oral, alcohol free: Acetaminophen 120 mg and codeine phosphate 12 mg per 5 mL (C-V)
Tablet: Acetaminophen 500 mg and codeine phosphate 30 mg (C-III); acetaminophen 650 mg and codeine phosphate 30 mg (C-III)
Tablet:
#1: Acetaminophen 300 mg and codeine phosphate 7.5 mg (C-III)
#2: Acetaminophen 300 mg and codeine phosphate 15 mg (C-III)

#3: Acetaminophen 300 mg and codeine phosphate 30 mg (C-III)
#4: Acetaminophen 300 mg and codeine phosphate 60 mg (C-III)

acetaminophen and dextromethorphan
(a seet a MIN oh fen & dex troe meth OR fan)

U.S. Brand Names Bayer® Select® Chest Cold Caplets [OTC]; Drixoral® Cough & Sore Throat Liquid Caps [OTC]

Generic Available Yes

Therapeutic Category Antitussive/Analgesic

Use Treatment of mild to moderate pain; symptomatic relief of coughs caused by minor viral upper respiratory tract infections or inhaled irritants; most effective for a chronic nonproductive cough

Usual Dosage Oral:
Children: 10-15 mg/kg/dose every 4-6 hours as needed; do **not** exceed 5 doses in 24 hours
Adults: 325-650 mg every 4-6 hours or 1000 mg 3-4 times/day; do **not** exceed 4 g/day

Dosage Forms
Caplet: Acetaminophen 500 and dextromethorphan hydrobromide 15 mg
Capsule: Acetaminophen 325 and dextromethorphan hydrobromide 15 mg

acetaminophen and diphenhydramine
(a seet a MIN oh fen & dye fen HYE dra meen)

U.S. Brand Names Excedrin® P.M. [OTC]; Midol® PM [OTC]

Generic Available Yes

Therapeutic Category Analgesic, Non-narcotic

Use Relief of mild to moderate pain or sinus headache

Usual Dosage Oral:
Children <12 years: Not recommended
Adults: 2 caplets or 5 mL of liquid at bedtime or as directed by physician; do not exceed recommended dosage

Dosage Forms
Caplet:
Excedrin® P.M.: Acetaminophen 500 mg and diphenhydramine citrate 30 mg
Arthritis Foundation® Nighttime, Midol® PM: Acetaminophen 500 mg and diphenhydramine 25 mg
Liquid (wild berry flavor) (Excedrin® P.M.): Acetaminophen 1000 mg and diphenhydramine hydrochloride 50 mg per 30 mL (180 mL)

♦ **acetaminophen and hydrocodone** *see* hydrocodone and acetaminophen *on page 319*

♦ **acetaminophen and oxycodone** *see* oxycodone and acetaminophen *on page 462*

acetaminophen and phenyltoloxamine
(a seet a MIN oh fen & fen il to LOKS a meen)

U.S. Brand Names Percogesic® [OTC]

Generic Available Yes

Therapeutic Category Analgesic, Non-narcotic

Use Relief of mild to moderate pain

Usual Dosage Adults: Oral: 1-2 tablets every 4 hours

Dosage Forms Tablet: Acetaminophen 325 mg and phenyltoloxamine citrate 30 mg

♦ **acetaminophen and propoxyphene** *see* propoxyphene and acetaminophen *on page 526*

acetaminophen and pseudoephedrine
(a seet a MIN oh fen & soo doe e FED rin)

Synonyms pseudoephedrine and acetaminophen

U.S. Brand Names Allerest® No Drowsiness [OTC]; Bayer® Select® Head Cold Caplets [OTC]; Coldrine® [OTC]; Dristan® Cold Caplets [OTC]; Dynafed®, Maximum Strength [OTC]; Ornex® No Drowsiness [OTC]; Sinarest®, No Drowsiness [OTC]; Sine-Aid®, Maximum Strength [OTC]; Sine-Off® Maximum Strength No Drowsiness Formula [OTC]; Sinus Excedrin® Extra Strength [OTC]; Sinus-Relief® [OTC]; Sinutab® Without Drowsiness [OTC]; Tylenol® Sinus, Maximum Strength [OTC]

Generic Available Yes

Therapeutic Category Decongestant/Analgesic

Use Symptomatic relief of congestion, fever, and aches/pain of colds/flu

Usual Dosage Adults: Oral: 2 tablets every 4-6 hours
(Continued)

acetaminophen and pseudoephedrine *(Continued)*

Dosage Forms Tablet:
Allerest® No Drowsiness; Coldrine®, Tylenol® Sinus, Maximum Strength; Ornex® No Drowsiness, Sinus-Relief®: Acetaminophen 325 mg and pseudoephedrine hydrochloride 30 mg

Bayer® Select Head Cold; Dristan® Cold; Dynafed®, Maximum Strength; Sinarest®, No Drowsiness; Sine-Aid®, Maximum Strength; Sine-Off® Maximum Strength No Drowsiness Formula; Sinus Excedrin® Extra Strength; Sinutab® Without Drowsiness; Tylenol® Sinus, Maximum Strength: Acetaminophen 500 mg and pseudoephedrine hydrochloride 30 mg

acetaminophen, aspirin, and caffeine

(a seet a MIN oh fen, AS pir in, & KAF een)

U.S. Brand Names Excedrin®, Extra Strength [OTC]; Gelpirin® [OTC]; Goody's® Headache Powders

Generic Available Yes

Therapeutic Category Analgesic, Non-narcotic

Use Relief of mild to moderate pain or fever

Usual Dosage Adults: Oral: 1-2 tablets or powders every 2-6 hours as needed for pain

Dosage Forms
Geltab: Acetaminophen 250 mg, aspirin 250 mg, and caffeine 65 mg
Powder: Acetaminophen 250 mg, aspirin 520 mg, and caffeine 32.5 mg per dose
Tablet: Acetaminophen 125 mg, aspirin 240 mg, and caffeine 32 mg; acetaminophen 250 mg, aspirin 250 mg, and caffeine 65 mg

♦ **acetaminophen, caffeine, hydrocodone, chlorpheniramine, and phenylephrine** *see* hydrocodone, chlorpheniramine, phenylephrine, acetaminophen, and caffeine *on page 321*

acetaminophen, chlorpheniramine, and pseudoephedrine

(a seet a MIN oh fen, klor fen IR a meen, & soo doe e FED rin)

U.S. Brand Names Alka-Seltzer® Plus Cold Liqui-Gels® [OTC]; Aspirin-Free Bayer® Select® Allergy Sinus Caplets [OTC]; Co-Hist® [OTC]; Sinutab® Tablets [OTC]

Generic Available Yes

Therapeutic Category Antihistamine/Decongestant/Analgesic

Use Temporary relief of sinus symptoms

Usual Dosage Adults: Oral: 2 caplets/capsules/tablets every 6 hours

Dosage Forms
Caplet: Acetaminophen 500 mg, chlorpheniramine maleate 2 mg, and pseudoephedrine hydrochloride 30 mg
Capsule: Acetaminophen 250 mg, chlorpheniramine maleate 2 mg, and pseudoephedrine hydrochloride 30 mg
Tablet: Acetaminophen 325 mg, chlorpheniramine maleate 2 mg, and pseudoephedrine hydrochloride 30 mg

acetaminophen, dextromethorphan, and pseudoephedrine

(a seet a MIN oh fen, deks troe meth OR fan, & soo doe e FED rin)

Synonyms dextromethorphan, acetaminophen, and pseudoephedrine; pseudoephedrine, acetaminophen, and dextromethorphan; pseudoephedrine, dextromethorphan, and acetaminophen

U.S. Brand Names Alka-Seltzer® Plus Flu & Body Aches Non-Drowsy Liqui-Gels® [OTC]; Comtrex® Maximum Strength Non-Drowsy [OTC]; Sudafed® Severe Cold [OTC]; Theraflu® Non-Drowsy Formula Maximum Strength [OTC]; Tylenol® Cold No Drowsiness [OTC]; Tylenol® Flu Maximum Strength [OTC]

Generic Available Yes

Therapeutic Category Cold Preparation

Use Symptomatic relief of congestion, fever, cough, and aches/pain of colds/flu

Usual Dosage Adults: Oral: 2 tablets every 6 hours

Dosage Forms Tablet:
Alka-Seltzer® Plus Flu & Body Aches Non-Drowsy: Acetaminophen 500 mg, dextromethorphan hydrobromide 10 mg, and pseudoephedrine hydrochloride 30 mg
Comtrex® Maximum Strength Non-Drowsy; Sudafed® Severe Cold; Theraflu® Non-Drowsy Formula Maximum Strength; Tylenol® Flu Maximum Strength:

Acetaminophen 500 mg, dextromethorphan hydrobromide 15 mg, and pseudoephedrine hydrochloride 30 mg

Tylenol® Cold No Drowsiness: Acetaminophen 325 mg, dextromethorphan hydrobromide 15 mg, and pseudoephedrine hydrochloride 30 mg

acetaminophen, isotheptene, and dichloralphenazone

(a seet a MIN oh fen, eye soe me THEP teen, & dye KLOR al FEN a zone)

U.S. Brand Names Isocom®; Isopap®; Midchlor®; Midrin®; Migratine®

Generic Available Yes

Therapeutic Category Analgesic, Non-narcotic

Use Relief of migraine and tension headache

Usual Dosage Adults: Oral: 2 capsules at first sign of headache, followed by 1 capsule every 60 minutes until relieved, up to 5 capsules in a 12-hour period

Dosage Forms Capsule: Acetaminophen 325 mg, isometheptene mucate 65 mg, dichloralphenazone 100 mg

♦ **Acetasol® HC Otic** see acetic acid, propylene glycol diacetate, and hydrocortisone on page 18

♦ **Acetazolam®** see acetazolamide on page 17

acetazolamide (a set a ZOLE a mide)

U.S. Brand Names Diamox®; Diamox Sequels®

Canadian Brand Names Acetazolam®; Apo®-Acetazolamide; Novo-Zolamide®

Generic Available Yes

Therapeutic Category Anticonvulsant; Carbonic Anhydrase Inhibitor

Use Reduce elevated intraocular pressure in glaucoma, a diuretic, an adjunct to the treatment of refractory seizures and acute altitude sickness; centrencephalic epilepsies

Usual Dosage

Children:

Glaucoma:

Oral: 8-30 mg/kg/day divided every 6-8 hours

I.M., I.V.: 20-40 mg/kg/day divided every 6 hours

Edema: Oral, I.M., I.V.: 5 mg/kg or 150 mg/m^2 once every day or every other day

Epilepsy: Oral: 8-30 mg/kg/day in 2-4 divided doses, not to exceed 1 g/day

Adults:

Glaucoma:

Oral: 250 mg 1-4 times/day or 500 mg sustained release capsule twice daily

I.M., I.V.: 250-500 mg, may repeat in 2-4 hours

Edema: Oral, I.M., I.V.: 250-375 mg once daily

Epilepsy: Oral: 8-30 mg/kg/day in 1-4 divided doses

Altitude sickness: Oral: 250 mg every 8-12 hours

Dietary Considerations May be administered with food to decrease GI upset

Nursing/Pharmacy Information

Oral: Tablet may be crushed and suspended in cherry or chocolate syrup to disguise the bitter taste of the drug

Parenteral: Reconstitute with at least 5 mL sterile water to provide an I.V. solution containing not more than 100 mg/mL; maximum concentration: 100 mg/mL; maximum rate of I.V. infusion: 500 mg/minute

Monitor intraocular pressure, potassium, serum bicarbonate; serum electrolytes, periodic CBC with differential

Stability: Reconstituted solution may be stored under refrigeration (2°C to 8°C) for 24 hours (the product contains no preservative); discard unused solutions after 24 hours

Dosage Forms

Capsule, sustained release: 500 mg

Injection, as sodium: 500 mg

Tablet: 125 mg, 250 mg

acetic acid (a SEE tik AS id)

Synonyms ethanoic acid

U.S. Brand Names Aci-jel® Vaginal; VōSol® Otic

Generic Available Yes

Therapeutic Category Antibacterial, Otic; Antibacterial, Topical

Use Continuous or intermittent irrigation of the bladder; treatment of superficial bacterial infections of the external auditory canal and vagina

(Continued)

acetic acid *(Continued)*

Usual Dosage

Irrigation: For continuous irrigation of the urinary bladder with 0.25% acetic acid irrigation, the rate of administration will approximate the rate of urine flow; usually 500-1500 mL/24 hours; for periodic irrigation of an indwelling urinary catheter to maintain patency, approximately 50 mL of 0.25% acetic acid irrigation is required. (Note: Dosage of an irrigating solution depends on the capacity or surface area of the structure being irrigated.)

Otic: Insert saturated wick, keep moist 24 hours; remove wick and instill 5 drops 3-4 times/day

Vaginal: One applicatorful morning and evening

Nursing/Pharmacy Information

For continuous or intermittent irrigation of the urinary bladder, urine pH should be checked at least 4 times/day and the irrigation rate adjusted to maintain a pH of 4.5-5; not for internal intake or I.V. infusion; topical use or irrigation use only

Obtain chest x-ray, respiratory status

Dosage Forms

Jelly, vaginal (Aci-jel®): 0.921% with oxyquinolone sulfate 0.025%, ricinoleic acid 0.7%, and glycerin 5% (85 g)

Solution:
Irrigation: 0.25% (1000 mL)
Otic (VōSol®): Acetic acid 2% in propylene glycol (15 mL, 30 mL, 60 mL)

♦ **acetic acid and aluminum acetate otic** *see* aluminum acetate and acetic acid on page 32

acetic acid, propylene glycol diacetate, and hydrocortisone

(a SEE tik AS id, PRO pa leen GLY kole dye AS e tate, & hye droe KOR ti sone)

U.S. Brand Names Acetasol® HC Otic; VōSol® HC Otic

Generic Available Yes

Therapeutic Category Antibiotic/Corticosteroid, Otic

Use Treatment of superficial infections of the external auditory canal caused by organisms susceptible to the action of the antimicrobial, complicated by inflammation

Usual Dosage Adults: Otic: Instill 4 drops in ear(s) 3-4 times/day

Dosage Forms Solution, otic: Acetic acid 2%, propylene glycol diacetate 3%, and hydrocortisone 1% (10 mL)

acetohexamide (a set oh HEKS a mide)

U.S. Brand Names Dymelor®

Generic Available Yes

Therapeutic Category Antidiabetic Agent, Oral

Use Adjunct to diet for the management of mild to moderately severe, stable, noninsulin-dependent (type II) diabetes mellitus

Usual Dosage Adults: Oral: 250 mg to 1.5 g/day in 1-2 divided doses

Dietary Considerations May be administered with food

Nursing/Pharmacy Information

Patients who are anorexic or NPO may need to have their dose held to avoid hypoglycemia

Blood (preferred) and urine glucose concentrations should be monitored when therapy is started; normally takes 7 days to determine therapeutic response

Dosage Forms Tablet: 250 mg, 500 mg

acetohydroxamic acid (a SEE toe hye droks am ik AS id)

Synonyms AHA

U.S. Brand Names Lithostat®

Generic Available No

Therapeutic Category Urinary Tract Product

Use Adjunctive therapy in chronic urea-splitting urinary infection

Usual Dosage Oral:
Children: Initial: 10 mg/kg/day
Adults: 250 mg 3-4 times/day for a total daily dose of 10-15 mg/kg/day

Dietary Considerations Should be administered 1 hour before or 2 hours after meals

Dosage Forms Tablet: 250 mg

♦ **Acetoxyl®** *see* benzoyl peroxide on page 81

♦ **acetoxymethylprogesterone** *see* medroxyprogesterone acetate *on page 389*

acetylcholine (a se teel KOE leen)
U.S. Brand Names Miochol-E®
Generic Available No
Therapeutic Category Cholinergic Agent
Use Produces complete miosis in cataract surgery, keratoplasty, iridectomy and other anterior segment surgery where rapid miosis is required
Usual Dosage Adults: Intraocular: 0.5-2 mL of 1% injection (5-20 mg) instilled into anterior chamber before or after securing one or more sutures
Nursing/Pharmacy Information
  Discard any solution that is not used; open under aseptic conditions only
  Stability: Prepare solution immediately before use; acetylcholine solutions are unstable
Dosage Forms Powder, intraocular, as chloride: 1:100 [10 mg/mL] (2 mL)

acetylcysteine (a se teel SIS teen)
Synonyms mercapturic acid; NAC; *N*-acetylcysteine; *N*-acetyl-L-cysteine
U.S. Brand Names Mucomyst®; Mucosil™
Canadian Brand Names Parvolex®
Generic Available Yes
Therapeutic Category Mucolytic Agent
Use Adjunctive therapy in patients with abnormal or viscid mucous secretions in bronchopulmonary diseases, pulmonary complications of surgery, and cystic fibrosis; diagnostic bronchial studies; antidote for acute acetaminophen toxicity; enema to treat bowel obstruction due to meconium ileus or its equivalent
Usual Dosage
  Acetaminophen poisoning: Children and Adults: Oral: 140 mg/kg; followed by 17 doses of 70 mg/kg every 4 hours; repeat dose if emesis occurs within 1 hour of administration; therapy should continue until all doses are administered even though the acetaminophen plasma level has dropped below the toxic range
  Inhalation: Acetylcysteine 10% and 20% solution (Mucomyst®) (dilute 20% solution with sodium chloride or sterile water for inhalation); 10% solution may be used undiluted
    Infants: 1-2 mL of 20% solution or 2-4 mL 10% solution until nebulized administered 3-4 times/day
    Children: 3-5 mL of 20% solution or 6-10 mL of 10% solution until nebulized administered 3-4 times/day
    Adolescents: 5-10 mL of 10% to 20% solution until nebulized administered 3-4 times/day
    Note: Patients should receive an aerosolized bronchodilator 10-15 minutes prior to acetylcysteine
  Meconium ileus equivalent: Children and Adults: 100-300 mL of 4% to 10% solution by irrigation or orally
Nursing/Pharmacy Information
  Assess patient for nausea, vomiting, and skin rash following oral administration for treatment of acetaminophen poisoning; intermittent aerosol treatments are commonly administered when patient arises, before meals, and just before retiring at bedtime
  Stability: Store opened vials in the refrigerator, use within 96 hours; dilutions should be freshly prepared and used within 1 hour; light purple color of solution does **not** affect its mucolytic activity
Dosage Forms Solution, as sodium: 10% [100 mg/mL] (4 mL, 10 mL, 30 mL); 20% [200 mg/mL] (4 mL, 10 mL, 30 mL, 100 mL)

♦ **acetylsalicylic acid** *see* aspirin *on page 61*
♦ **Aches-N-Pain® [OTC]** *see* ibuprofen *on page 332*
♦ **Achromycin® Ophthalmic** *see* tetracycline *on page 601*
♦ **Achromycin® Parenteral (Discontinued)** *see page 743*
♦ **Achromycin® Topical** *see* tetracycline *on page 601*
♦ **Achromycin® V Capsule (Discontinued)** *see page 743*
♦ **Achromycin® V Oral Suspension (Discontinued)** *see page 743*
♦ **aciclovir** *see* acyclovir *on page 21*
♦ **Acifur** *see* acyclovir *on page 21*
♦ **Aci-jel® Vaginal** *see* acetic acid *on page 17*
♦ **Acilac** *see* lactulose *on page 359*
♦ **Acimox** *see* amoxicillin *on page 43*

♦ **Aciphex™** see rabeprazole *New Drug on page 538*

acitretin (a si TRE tin)
U.S. Brand Names Soriatane™
Generic Available No
Therapeutic Category Retinoid-like Compound
Use Treatment of severe psoriasis (includes erythrodermic and pustular types) and other disorders of keratinization
Usual Dosage Adults: Oral: Individualization of dosage is required to achieve maximum therapeutic response while minimizing side effects

Initial: Therapy should be initiated at 25 mg/day, given as a single dose with the main meal; if by 4 weeks the response is unsatisfactory, and in the absence of toxicity, the daily dose may be gradually increased to a maximum of 75 mg/day; the dose may be reduced if necessary to minimize side effects
Maintenance: Doses of 25 to 50 mg/day may be given after initial response to treatment; the maintenance dose should be based on clinical efficacy and tolerability; it may be necessary in some cases to increase the dose to a maximum of 75 mg/day

Dosage Forms Capsule: 10 mg, 25 mg

♦ **Acloral®** see ranitidine hydrochloride *on page 541*
♦ **Aclovate® Topical** see alclometasone *on page 26*
♦ **Acnex®** see salicylic acid *on page 557*
♦ **Acnomel®** see salicylic acid *on page 557*
♦ **Acnomel® B.P.5** see benzoyl peroxide *on page 81*

acrivastine and pseudoephedrine
(AK ri vas teen & soo doe e FED rin)
Synonyms pseudoephedrine and acrivastine
U.S. Brand Names Semprex®-D
Generic Available No
Therapeutic Category Antihistamine/Decongestant Combination
Use Temporary relief of nasal congestion, decongest sinus openings, running nose, itching of nose or throat, and itchy, watery eyes due to hay fever or other upper respiratory allergies
Usual Dosage Adults: 1 capsule 3-4 times/day
Dosage Forms Capsule: Acrivastine 8 mg and pseudoephedrine hydrochloride 60 mg

♦ **Acromicina** see tetracycline *on page 601*
♦ **ACT** see dactinomycin *on page 180*
♦ **ACT® [OTC]** see fluoride *on page 274*
♦ **Actagen-C®** see triprolidine, pseudoephedrine, and codeine *on page 632*
♦ **Actagen® Syrup [OTC]** see triprolidine and pseudoephedrine *on page 632*
♦ **Actagen® Tablet [OTC]** see triprolidine and pseudoephedrine *on page 632*
♦ **ACTH** see corticotropin *on page 169*
♦ **ACTH-40® (Discontinued)** see page 743
♦ **Acthar®** see corticotropin *on page 169*
♦ **Acti-B₁₂®** see hydroxocobalamin *on page 326*
♦ **Acticin® Cream** see permethrin *on page 482*
♦ **Acticort® Topical** see hydrocortisone (topical) *on page 324*
♦ **Actidil® (Discontinued)** see page 743
♦ **Actidose-Aqua® [OTC]** see charcoal *on page 131*
♦ **Actidose® With Sorbitol [OTC]** see charcoal *on page 131*
♦ **Actifed® Allergy Tablet (Day) [OTC]** see pseudoephedrine *on page 530*
♦ **Actifed® Allergy Tablet (Night) [OTC]** see diphenhydramine and pseudoephedrine *on page 209*
♦ **Actifed® Syrup (Discontinued)** see page 743
♦ **Actifed® With Codeine (Discontinued)** see page 743
♦ **Actigall™** see ursodiol *on page 640*
♦ **Actimmune®** see interferon gamma-1b *on page 343*
♦ **Actinex® Topical** see masoprocol *on page 385*
♦ **actinomycin D** see dactinomycin *on page 180*
♦ **Actiq® Oral Transmucosal** see fentanyl *on page 263*
♦ **Activase®** see alteplase *on page 31*
♦ **activated carbon** see charcoal *on page 131*
♦ **activated dimethicone** see simethicone *on page 566*
♦ **activated ergosterol** see ergocalciferol *on page 237*

- **activated methylpolysiloxane** *see* simethicone *on page 566*
- **Activelle™** *see* estradiol and norethindrone *on page 243*
- **Actonel®** *see* risedronate *on page 551*
- **Actos™** *see* pioglitazone *New Drug on page 495*
- **Actron® [OTC]** *see* ketoprofen *on page 355*
- **ACU-dyne® [OTC]** *see* povidone-iodine *on page 510*
- **Acular® Ophthalmic** *see* ketorolac tromethamine *on page 355*
- **Acupril** *see* quinapril *on page 536*
- **Acutrim® 16 Hours [OTC]** *see* phenylpropanolamine *on page 489*
- **Acutrim® II, Maximum Strength [OTC]** *see* phenylpropanolamine *on page 489*
- **Acutrim® Late Day [OTC]** *see* phenylpropanolamine *on page 489*
- **ACV** *see* acyclovir *on page 21*
- **acycloguanosine** *see* acyclovir *on page 21*

acyclovir (ay SYE kloe veer)

Synonyms aciclovir; ACV; acycloguanosine
U.S. Brand Names Zovirax®
Canadian Brand Names Avirax™
Mexican Brand Names Acifur
Generic Available Yes
Therapeutic Category Antiviral Agent
Use Treatment of initial and prophylaxis of recurrent mucosal and cutaneous herpes simplex (HSV-1 and HSV-2) infections; herpes simplex encephalitis; herpes zoster infections; varicella-zoster infections in healthy, nonpregnant persons >13 years of age, children >12 months of age who have a chronic skin or lung disorder or are receiving long-term aspirin therapy, and immunocompromised patients

Usual Dosage
Children and Adults: I.V.:
  Mucocutaneous HSV infection: 750 mg/m^2/day divided every 8 hours or 15 mg/kg/day divided every 8 hours for 5-10 days
  HSV encephalitis: 1500 mg/m^2/day divided every 8 hours or 30 mg/kg/day divided every 8 hours for 10 days
  Varicella-zoster virus infection: 1500 mg/m^2/day divided every 8 hours or 30 mg/kg/day divided every 8 hours for 5-10 days
Adults:
  Oral: Initial: 200 mg every 4 hours while awake (5 times/day); prophylaxis: 200 mg 3-4 times/day or 400 mg twice daily. Prophylaxis of varicella or herpes zoster in HIV positive patients: 400 mg 5 times/day
  Topical: ½" ribbon of ointment every 3 hours (6 times/day)

Herpes zoster in immunocompromised patients:
  Children: Oral: 250-600 mg/m^2/dose 4-5 times/day
  Adults: Oral: 800 mg every 4 hours (5 times/day) for 7-10 days
  Children and Adults: I.V.: 7.5 mg/kg/dose every 8 hours
Varicella-zoster infections: Oral:
  Children: 10-20 mg/kg/dose (up to 800 mg) 4 times/day
  Adults: 600-800 mg/dose 5 times/day for 7-10 days or 1000 mg every 6 hours for 5 days
Prophylaxis of bone marrow transplant recipients: Children and Adults: I.V.:
  Autologous patients who are HSV seropositive: 150 mg/m^2/dose every 12 hours; with clinical symptoms of herpes simplex: 150 mg/m^2/dose every 8 hours
  Autologous patients who are CMV seropositive: 500 mg/m^2/dose every 8 hours; for clinically symptomatic CMV infection, ganciclovir should be used in place of acyclovir

Dietary Considerations May be administered with food
Nursing/Pharmacy Information
Parenteral: Reconstitute vial for injection with paraben-free sterile water; administer by slow I.V. infusion over at least 1 hour at a final concentration not to exceed 7 mg/mL since rapid infusions can cause nephrotoxicity with crystalluria and renal tubular damage; in patients who require fluid restriction, a concentration of up to 10 mg/mL has been infused; concentration >10 mg/mL increases the risk of phlebitis
Monitor urinalysis, BUN, serum creatinine, liver enzymes, CBC
Stability: **Incompatible** with blood products and protein-containing solutions; reconstituted solutions remain stable for 24 hours at room temperature; do not refrigerate reconstituted solutions as they may precipitate
(Continued)

acyclovir *(Continued)*

Dosage Forms
Capsule: 200 mg
Powder for Injection: 500 mg (10 mL); 1000 mg (20 mL)
Ointment, topical: 5% [50 mg/g] (3 g, 15 g)
Suspension, oral (banana flavor): 200 mg/5 mL (480 mL)
Tablet: 400 mg, 800 mg

- ♦ **Adagen™** *see* pegademase (bovine) *on page 472*
- ♦ **Adalat®** *see* nifedipine *on page 442*
- ♦ **Adalat® CC** *see* nifedipine *on page 442*
- ♦ **Adalat® Oros** *see* nifedipine *on page 442*
- ♦ **Adalat PA®** *see* nifedipine *on page 442*
- ♦ **Adalat® Retard** *see* nifedipine *on page 442*
- ♦ **Adalken®** *see* penicillamine *on page 473*
- ♦ **adamantanamine** *see* amantadine *on page 35*

adapalene *(a DAP a leen)*

U.S. Brand Names Differin®
Generic Available No
Therapeutic Category Acne Products
Use Topical treatment of acne vulgaris
Usual Dosage Adults: Topical: Apply once daily, before retiring, in a thin film to affected areas after washing; not recommended in children
Dosage Forms
Gel, topical (alcohol free): 0.1% (15 g, 45 g)
Solution, topical: 0.1% (30 mL)

- ♦ **Adapin® Oral** *see* doxepin *on page 219*
- ♦ **Adderall®** *see* dextroamphetamine and amphetamine *on page 194*
- ♦ **Adeflor®** *see* vitamin, multiple (pediatric) *on page 654*

adefovir *New Drug* *(a DEF o veer)*

U.S. Brand Names Preveon®
Generic Available No
Therapeutic Category Reverse Transcriptase Inhibitor
Use Treatment of HIV infections in combination with at least two other antiretroviral agents; also has some activity against hepatitis B virus and herpes viruses
Usual Dosage Oral:
HIV: 125 mg once daily
Hepatitis B: 125 mg once daily

- ♦ **ADEKs® Pediatric Drops** *see* vitamin, multiple (pediatric) *on page 654*
- ♦ **Adena a Ungena** *see* vidarabine *on page 648*
- ♦ **adenine arabinoside** *see* vidarabine *on page 648*
- ♦ **Adenocard®** *see* adenosine *on page 22*

adenosine *(a DEN oh seen)*

Synonyms 9-beta-D-ribofuranosyladenine
U.S. Brand Names Adenocard®
Generic Available No
Therapeutic Category Antiarrhythmic Agent, Miscellaneous
Use Treatment of paroxysmal supraventricular tachycardia (PSVT)
Usual Dosage
Children: Initial: Rapid I.V.: 0.05 mg/kg; if not effective within 2 minutes, increase dose in 0.05 mg/kg increments every 2 minutes to a maximum dose of 0.25 mg/kg or until termination of PSVT; median dose required: 0.15 mg/kg; do not exceed adult doses
Adults: Rapid I.V. push: 6 mg, if the dose is not effective within 1-2 minutes, a rapid I.V. dose of 12 mg may be administered; may repeat 12 mg bolus if needed
Dietary Considerations Avoid food or drugs with caffeine
Nursing/Pharmacy Information
Be alert for possible exacerbation of asthma in asthmatic patients; for rapid bolus I.V. use only, administer over 1-2 seconds; administer at I.V. site closest to patient; follow each bolus with normal saline flush
Monitor EKG, heart rate, blood pressure, respirations
Stability: Do **not** refrigerate, precipitation may occur (may dissolve by warming to room temperature)

Dosage Forms Injection, preservative free: 3 mg/mL (2 mL, 5 mL, 20 mL, 30 mL)

- **Adipex-P®** *(Discontinued)* see page 743
- **Adipost®** *(Discontinued)* see page 743
- **Adlone® Injection** see methylprednisolone on page 407
- **Adphen®** *(Discontinued)* see page 743
- **ADR** see doxorubicin on page 220
- **Adrenalin® Chloride** see epinephrine on page 234
- **adrenaline** see epinephrine on page 234
- **adrenocorticotropic hormone** see corticotropin on page 169
- **Adriamycin PFS™** see doxorubicin on page 220
- **Adriamycin RDF®** see doxorubicin on page 220
- **Adrin®** *(Discontinued)* see page 743
- **Adrucil® Injection** see fluorouracil on page 275
- **Adsorbocarpine® Ophthalmic** see pilocarpine on page 493
- **Adsorbonac® Ophthalmic [OTC]** see sodium chloride on page 571
- **Adsorbotear® Ophthalmic Solution [OTC]** see artificial tears on page 59
- **Advanced Formula Oxy® Sensitive Gel [OTC]** see benzoyl peroxide on page 81
- **Advil® [OTC]** see ibuprofen on page 332
- **Advil® Cold & Sinus Caplets [OTC]** see pseudoephedrine and ibuprofen on page 531
- **Aeroaid® [OTC]** see thimerosal on page 607
- **Aerobec** see beclomethasone on page 75
- **AeroBid®-M Oral Aerosol Inhaler** see flunisolide on page 272
- **AeroBid® Oral Aerosol Inhaler** see flunisolide on page 272
- **Aerodine® [OTC]** see povidone-iodine on page 510
- **Aerolate III®** see theophylline on page 603
- **Aerolate JR®** see theophylline on page 603
- **Aerolate® Oral Solution** *(Discontinued)* see page 743
- **Aerolate SR®** see theophylline on page 603
- **Aeroseb-Dex®** see dexamethasone (topical) on page 191
- **Aeroseb-HC® Topical** see hydrocortisone (topical) on page 324
- **Aerosporin® Injection** *(Discontinued)* see page 743
- **AeroZoin® [OTC]** see benzoin on page 80
- **AF®** see acetaminophen on page 13
- **Afrin® Children's Nose Drops [OTC]** see oxymetazoline on page 463
- **Afrin® Nasal Solution [OTC]** see oxymetazoline on page 463
- **Afrinol® [OTC]** see pseudoephedrine on page 530
- **Afrin® Saline Mist [OTC]** see sodium chloride on page 571
- **Aftate® [OTC]** see tolnaftate on page 618
- **A.F. Valdecasas®** see folic acid on page 281
- **Agenerase™** see amprenavir New Drug on page 47
- **Aggrastat®** see tirofiban on page 614
- **Aggrenox®** see dipyridamole and aspirin New Drug on page 212
- **AgNO₃** see silver nitrate on page 565
- **Agoral® Plain** *(Discontinued)* see page 743
- **Agrylin™** see anagrelide on page 48
- **AHA** see acetohydroxamic acid on page 18
- **AHF** see antihemophilic factor (human) on page 51
- **A-hydroCort®** see hydrocortisone (systemic) on page 323
- **Airet®** see albuterol on page 25
- **Akarpine® Ophthalmic** see pilocarpine on page 493
- **AKBeta® Ophthalmic** see levobunolol on page 364
- **AK-Chlor® Ophthalmic** see chloramphenicol on page 133
- **AK-Cide® Ophthalmic** see sulfacetamide and prednisolone on page 585
- **AK-Con® Ophthalmic** see naphazoline on page 431
- **AK-Dex® Ophthalmic** see dexamethasone (ophthalmic) on page 189
- **AK-Dilate® Ophthalmic Solution** see phenylephrine on page 487
- **AK-Fluor Injection** see fluorescein sodium on page 273
- **AK-Homatropine® Ophthalmic** see homatropine on page 314
- **Akineton®** see biperiden on page 87
- **AK-Mycin®** see erythromycin (systemic) on page 240
- **AK-NaCl® [OTC]** see sodium chloride on page 571

- **AK-Nefrin® Ophthalmic Solution** *see* phenylephrine *on page 487*
- **Akne-Mycin® Topical** *see* erythromycin (ophthalmic/topical) *on page 239*
- **AK-Neo-Dex® Ophthalmic** *see* neomycin and dexamethasone *on page 435*
- **Akoline® C.B. Tablet** *(Discontinued) see page 743*
- **Akorazol** *see* ketoconazole *on page 354*
- **AK-Pentolate®** *see* cyclopentolate *on page 174*
- **AK-Poly-Bac® Ophthalmic** *see* bacitracin and polymyxin B *on page 71*
- **AK-Pred® Ophthalmic** *see* prednisolone (ophthalmic) *on page 514*
- **AK-Spore® H.C. Ophthalmic Ointment** *see* bacitracin, neomycin, polymyxin B, and hydrocortisone *on page 72*
- **AK-Spore® H.C. Ophthalmic Suspension** *see* neomycin, polymyxin B, and hydrocortisone *on page 437*
- **AK-Spore® H.C. Otic** *see* neomycin, polymyxin B, and hydrocortisone *on page 437*
- **AK-Spore® Ophthalmic Ointment** *see* bacitracin, neomycin, and polymyxin B *on page 71*
- **AK-Spore® Ophthalmic Solution** *see* neomycin, polymyxin B, and gramicidin *on page 437*
- **AK-Sulf®** *see* sulfacetamide *on page 584*
- **AK-Taine®** *see* proparacaine *on page 524*
- **AKTob® Ophthalmic** *see* tobramycin *on page 615*
- **AK-Tracin® Ophthalmic** *see* bacitracin *on page 70*
- **AK-Trol®** *see* neomycin, polymyxin B, and dexamethasone *on page 436*
- **Akwa Tears® Solution [OTC]** *see* artificial tears *on page 59*
- **AK-Zol® Tablet** *(Discontinued) see page 743*
- **Ala-Cort® Topical** *see* hydrocortisone (topical) *on page 324*
- **Ala-Scalp® Topical** *see* hydrocortisone (topical) *on page 324*
- **Ala-Tet®** *(Discontinued) see page 743*
- **alatrofloxacin** *see* trovafloxacin *on page 634*
- **Alazide®** *see* hydrochlorothiazide and spironolactone *on page 318*
- **Albalon-A® Ophthalmic** *see* naphazoline and antazoline *on page 431*
- **Albalon® Liquifilm® Ophthalmic** *see* naphazoline *on page 431*

albendazole (al BEN da zole)

U.S. Brand Names Albenza®
Mexican Brand Names Entoplus; Eskazole; Lurdex
Generic Available No
Therapeutic Category Anthelmintic
Use Treatment of parenchymal neurocysticercosis and cystic hydatid disease of the liver, lung, and peritoneum; albendazole may also be useful in the treatment of ascariasis, trichuriasis, enterobiasis, hook worm, strongyloidiasis, giardiasis, and microsporidiosis in AIDS
Usual Dosage Oral:
Children ≤2 years:
Neurocysticercosis: 15 mg/kg for 8 days; repeat as necessary
Hookworm, pinworm, roundworm: 200 mg as a single dose; may be repeated in 3 weeks
Strongyloidiasis and tapeworm: 200 mg/day for 3 days; may repeat in 3 weeks
Children >2 years and Adults:
Hydatid cyst: 400 mg twice daily with meals for 3 cycles (each cycle consists of 28 days of dosing followed by a 14-day albendazole-free interval)
Neurocysticercosis: 400 mg twice daily for 8-30 days
Roundworm, pinworm, hookworm: 400 mg as a single dose; treatment may be repeated in 3 weeks
Giardiasis: Strongyloidiasis and tapeworm: 400 mg/day for 3 days; treatment may be repeated in 3 weeks (giardiasis is a single course)
Dietary Considerations Administer with a high fatty diet
Dosage Forms Tablet: 200 mg

- **Albenza®** *see* albendazole *on page 24*
- **Albert® Docusate** *see* docusate *on page 214*
- **Albert® Glyburide** *see* glyburide *on page 294*

albumin (al BYOO min)

Synonyms albumin (human)
U.S. Brand Names Albuminar®; Albumisol®; Albunex®; Albutein®; Buminate®; Plasbumin®
Generic Available Yes

Therapeutic Category Blood Product Derivative

Use Treatment of hypovolemia; plasma volume expansion and maintenance of cardiac output in the treatment of certain types of shock or impending shock; hypoproteinemia resulting in generalized edema or decreased intravascular volume (eg, hypoproteinemia associated with acute nephrotic syndrome, premature infants)

Usual Dosage 5% should be used in hypovolemic patients; 25% should be used in patients in whom fluid and sodium intake must be minimized

Children:

Emergency initial dose: 25 g

Nonemergencies: 25% to 50% of the adult dose

Adults: Dosage depends on the condition of patient, usual adult dose is 25 g; no more than 250 g should be administered within 48 hours

Hypoproteinemia: I.V.: 0.5-1 g/kg/dose; repeat every 1-2 days as calculated to replace ongoing losses

Hypovolemia: I.V.: 0.5-1 g/kg/dose; repeat as needed; maximum dose: 6 g/kg/day

Nursing/Pharmacy Information

Albumin administration must be completed within 4 hours after entering container, provided that administration is begun within 4 hours of entering the container; use 5 micron filter or larger, do **not** administer through 0.22 micron filter

Parenteral: I.V. after initial volume replacement:

5%: Do not exceed 2-4 mL/minute

25%: Do not exceed 1 mL/minute

Observe for signs of hypervolemia, pulmonary edema, and cardiac failure

Stability: Do not use solution if it is turbid or contains a deposit; use within 4 hours after entering container

Dosage Forms Injection, as human: 5% [50 mg/mL] (50 mL, 250 mL, 500 mL, 1000 mL); 25% [250 mg/mL] (10 mL, 20 mL, 50 mL, 100 mL)

♦ **Albuminar**® *see albumin on page 24*

♦ **albumin (human)** *see albumin on page 24*

♦ **Albumisol**® *see albumin on page 24*

♦ **Albunex**® *see albumin on page 24*

♦ **Albutein**® *see albumin on page 24*

albuterol (al BYOO ter ole)

Synonyms salbutamol

U.S. Brand Names Airet®; Proventil®; Proventil® HFA; Ventolin®; Ventolin® Rotocaps®

Canadian Brand Names Apo®-Salvent; Novo-Salmol®; Sabulin®; Volmax®

Mexican Brand Names Salbulin; Salbutalan

Generic Available Yes

Therapeutic Category Adrenergic Agonist Agent

Use Bronchodilator in reversible airway obstruction due to asthma or COPD

Usual Dosage

Oral:

2-6 years: 0.1-0.2 mg/kg/dose 3 times/day; maximum dose not to exceed 12 mg/day (divided doses)

6-12 years: 2 mg/dose 3-4 times/day; maximum dose not to exceed 24 mg/day (divided doses)

>12 years: 2-4 mg/dose 3-4 times/day; maximum dose not to exceed 32 mg/day (divided doses)

Inhalation:

MDI: 90 mcg/spray:

<12 years: 1-2 inhalations 4 times/day using a tube spacer

≥12 years: 1-2 inhalations every 4-6 hours

Exercise-induced bronchospasm: 2 inhalations 15 minutes before exercising

Nebulization: 2.5 mg = 0.5 mL of the 0.5% inhalation solution to be diluted in 1-2.5 mL of NS

<5 years: 1.25-2.5 mg every 4-6 hours as needed

>5 years: 2.5-5 mg every 4-6 hours

Dietary Considerations Limit caffeine intake; should be administered with water 1 hour before or 2 hours after meals

Nursing/Pharmacy Information Before using, the inhaler must be shaken well; assess lung sounds, pulse, and blood pressure before administration and during peak of medication; observe patient for wheezing after administration, if this occurs, call physician

(Continued)

albuterol *(Continued)*

Dosage Forms
Aerosol: 90 mcg/dose (17 g) [200 doses]
  Proventil®, Ventolin®: 90 mcg/dose (17 g) [200 doses]
Aerosol, as sulfate, chlorofluorocarbon free (Proventil® HFA): 90 mcg/dose (17 g)
Capsule, as sulfate, for oral inhalation (Ventolin® Rotocaps®): 200 mcg [to be used with Rotahaler® inhalation device]
Solution, as sulfate, inhalation: 0.083% (3 mL); 0.5% (20 mL)
  Airet®: 0.083%
  Proventil®: 0.083% (3 mL); 0.5% (20 mL)
  Ventolin®: 0.5% (20 mL)
Syrup, as sulfate: 2 mg/5 mL (90 mL, 120 mL, 240 mL, 480 mL)
  Proventil®, Ventolin®: 2 mg/5 mL (480 mL)
Tablet, as sulfate: 2 mg, 4 mg
  Proventil®, Ventolin®: 2 mg, 4 mg
Tablet, as sulfate, extended release:
  Proventil® Repetabs®: 4 mg
  Volmax®: 4 mg, 8 mg

♦ **Alcaine®** *see* proparacaine *on page 524*

alclometasone *(al kloe MET a sone)*
U.S. Brand Names Aclovate® Topical
Generic Available No
Therapeutic Category Corticosteroid, Topical
Use Inflammation of corticosteroid-responsive dermatosis
Usual Dosage Topical: Apply a thin film to the affected area 2-3 times/day
Nursing/Pharmacy Information For external use only; do not use on open wounds; apply sparingly to occlusive dressings; should not be used in the presence of open or weeping lesions
Dosage Forms
Cream, as dipropionate: 0.05% (15 g, 45 g, 60 g)
Ointment, topical, as dipropionate: 0.05% (15 g, 45 g, 60 g)

alcohol, ethyl *(AL koe hol, ETH il)*
Synonyms ethanol
U.S. Brand Names Lavacol® [OTC]
Generic Available Yes
Therapeutic Category Intravenous Nutritional Therapy; Pharmaceutical Aid
Use Topical anti-infective; pharmaceutical aid; an antidote for ethylene glycol overdose; an antidote for methanol overdose
Usual Dosage
I.V.: Doses of 100-125 mg/kg/hour to maintain blood levels of 100 mg/dL are recommended after a loading dose of 0.6 g/kg; maximum dose: 400 mL of a 5% solution within 1 hour
Topical: Use as needed
Nursing/Pharmacy Information Caution must be taken to avoid extravasation; administer only by slow I.V. infusion
Dosage Forms
Injection, absolute: 2 mL
Liquid, topical, denatured: 70% (473 mL)
Solution, inhalation: 20%, 40%

♦ **Alconefrin® Nasal Solution [OTC]** *see* phenylephrine *on page 487*
♦ **Aldactazide®** *see* hydrochlorothiazide and spironolactone *on page 318*
♦ **Aldactone®** *see* spironolactone *on page 578*
♦ **Aldara™** *see* imiquimod *on page 335*

aldesleukin *(al des LOO kin)*
Synonyms interleukin-2
U.S. Brand Names Proleukin®
Generic Available No
Therapeutic Category Biological Response Modulator
Use Primarily investigated in tumors known to have a response to immunotherapy, such as melanoma and renal cell carcinoma; has been used in conjunction with LAK cells, TIL cells, IL-1, and interferon
Usual Dosage All orders should be written in million International units (million int. units) (refer to individual protocols)

Adults: Metastatic renal cell carcinoma:

Treatment consists of two 5-day treatment cycles separated by a rest period. 600,000 int. units/kg (0.037 mg/kg)/dose administered every 8 hours for a 15-minute I.V. infusion for a total of 14 doses; following 9 days of rest, the schedule is repeated for another 14 doses, for a maximum of 28 doses per course.

Investigational regimen: I.V. continuous infusion: 4.5 million int. units/m²/day in 250-1000 mL of D_5W for 5 days

Dose modification: Hold or interrupt a dose rather than reducing dose; refer to protocol

Retreatment: Patients should be evaluated for response ~4 weeks after completion of a course of therapy and again immediately prior to the scheduled start of the next treatment course. Additional courses of treatment may be administered to patients only if there is some tumor shrinkage following the last course and retreatment is not contraindicated. Each treatment course should be separated by a rest period of at least 7 weeks from the date of hospital discharge. Tumors have continued to regress up to 12 months following the initiation of therapy.

Nursing/Pharmacy Information

Prior to treatment: Standard hematologic tests, blood chemistries, chest x-rays

During treatment: Pulmonary function, assessment of vital signs and pulse oximetry. Patients with dyspnea or clinical signs of respiratory impairment: Arterial blood gas determination

Stability: Dilutions in D_5W: Concentrations of 100-500 mcg/mL are stable 6 days at room temperature, concentrations of 5-60 mcg/mL are only stable if 0.1% serum albumin is added prior to dilution, concentrations of 60-100 mcg/mL are unstable

Dosage Forms Powder for injection, lyophilized: 22 x 10⁶ IU [18 million IU/mL = 1.1 mg/mL when reconstituted]

♦ **Aldoclor®** *see* chlorothiazide and methyldopa *on page 137*

♦ **Aldomet®** *see* methyldopa *on page 406*

♦ **Aldoril®** *see* methyldopa and hydrochlorothiazide *on page 406*

alendronate (a LEN droe nate)

U.S. Brand Names Fosamax®

Generic Available No

Therapeutic Category Bisphosphonate Derivative

Use Treatment of osteoporosis in postmenopausal women, Paget's disease of the bone; treatment of glucocorticoid-induced osteoporosis in males and females with low bone mineral density who are receiving a daily dosage ≥7.5 mg of prednisone (or equivalent)

Usual Dosage Oral:

Adults: Patients with osteoporosis or Paget's disease should receive supplemental calcium and vitamin D if dietary intake is inadequate

Osteoporosis in postmenopausal women: 10 mg once daily. Safety of treatment for >4 years has not been studied (extension studies are ongoing).

Paget's disease of bone: 40 mg once daily for 6 months

Retreatment: Relapses during the 12 months following therapy occurred in 9% of patients who responded to treatment. Specific retreatment data are not available. Retreatment with alendronate may be considered, following a 6-month post-treatment evaluation period, in patients who have relapsed based on increases in serum alkaline phosphatase, which should be measured periodically. Retreatment may also be considered in those who failed to normalize their serum alkaline phosphatase.

Treatment of glucocorticoid-induced osteoporosis: 5 mg once daily. A dose of 10 mg once daily should be used in postmenopausal women who are not receiving estrogen. Patients treated with glucocorticoids should receive adequate amounts of calcium and vitamin D.

Elderly: No dosage adjustment is necessary

Nursing/Pharmacy Information

Patients should be instructed that the expected benefits of alendronate may only be obtained when each tablet is administered with plain water the first thing in the morning and at least 30 minutes before the first food, beverage, or medication of the day. Also instruct them that waiting >30 minutes will improve alendronate absorption. Even dosing with orange juice or coffee markedly reduces the absorption of alendronate.

Patients should be instructed to take alendronate with a full glass of water (6-8 oz 180-240 mL) and not to lie down (stay fully upright sitting or standing) for (Continued)

alendronate *(Continued)*

at least 30 minutes following administration to facilitate delivery to the stomach and reduce the potential for esophageal irritation.

Patients should be instructed to take supplemental calcium and vitamin D if dietary intake is inadequate. Consider weight-bearing exercise along with the modification of certain behavioral factors, such as excessive cigarette smoking or alcohol consumption if these factors exist.

Dosage Forms Tablet, as sodium: 5 mg, 10 mg, 40 mg

♦ **Alepsal** *see* phenobarbital *on page 485*
♦ **Alesse™** *see* ethinyl estradiol and levonorgestrel *on page 250*
♦ **Aleve® [OTC]** *see* naproxen *on page 432*
♦ **Alfenta®** *see* alfentanil *on page 28*

alfentanil *(al FEN ta nil)*

U.S. Brand Names Alfenta®
Generic Available No
Therapeutic Category Analgesic, Narcotic; General Anesthetic
Controlled Substance C-II
Use Analgesia; analgesia adjunct; anesthetic agent
Usual Dosage Doses should be titrated to appropriate effects; wide range of doses is dependent upon desired degree of analgesia/anesthesia

Children <12 years: Dose not established
Adults: Anesthesia of ≤30 minutes: Initial (induction): 8-20 mcg/kg, then 3-5 mcg/kg/dose or 0.5-1 mcg/kg/minute for maintenance; total dose: 8-40 mcg/kg; higher doses used for longer anesthesia required procedures

Nursing/Pharmacy Information
Monitor respiratory rate, blood pressure, heart rate
Stability: Dilute in D_5W, normal saline, or lactated Ringer's

Dosage Forms Injection, preservative free, as hydrochloride: 500 mcg/mL (2 mL, 5 mL, 10 mL, 20 mL)

♦ **Alferon® N** *see* interferon alfa-n3 *on page 342*
♦ **Alfotax** *see* cefotaxime *on page 122*
♦ **Algitrin®** *see* acetaminophen *on page 13*

alglucerase *(al GLOO ser ase)*

Synonyms glucocerebrosidase
U.S. Brand Names Ceredase®
Generic Available No
Therapeutic Category Enzyme
Use Long-term enzyme replacement in patients with confirmed Type I Gaucher's disease who exhibit one or more of the following conditions: Moderate to severe anemia; thrombocytopenia and bleeding tendencies; bone disease; hepatomegaly or splenomegaly
Usual Dosage I.V. infusion: Administer 20-60 units/kg with a frequency ranging from 3 times/week to once every 2 weeks
Nursing/Pharmacy Information
Parenteral: Dilute to a final volume of 100 mL or less of normal saline and infuse I.V. over 1-2 hours; an in-line filter should be used; do not shake solution as it denatures the enzyme
Monitor CBC, platelets, liver function tests
Stability: Refrigerate (4°C), do not shake

Dosage Forms Injection: 10 units/mL (5 mL); 80 units/mL (5 mL)

♦ **Alidol** *see* ketorolac tromethamine *on page 355*
♦ **Alin** *see* dexamethasone (systemic) *on page 190*
♦ **Alin Depot** *see* dexamethasone (systemic) *on page 190*

alitretinoin *New Drug* *(a li TRET i noyn)*

U.S. Brand Names Panretin™
Generic Available No
Therapeutic Category Antineoplastic Agent, Miscellaneous; Retinoic Acid Derivative
Use Topical treatment of cutaneous lesions in AIDS-related Kaposi's sarcoma; not indicated when systemic therapy for Kaposi's sarcoma is indicated
Usual Dosage Topical: Apply gel twice daily to cutaneous Kaposi's sarcoma lesions
Dosage Forms Gel: 0.1% (60 g)

♦ **Alkaban-AQ®** *see* vinblastine *on page 648*

- **Alka-Mints®** [OTC] *see* calcium carbonate *on page 103*
- **Alka-Seltzer® Plus Cold Liqui-Gels®** [OTC] *see* acetaminophen, chlorpheniramine, and pseudoephedrine *on page 16*
- **Alka-Seltzer® Plus Flu & Body Aches Non-Drowsy Liqui-Gels®** [OTC] *see* acetaminophen, dextromethorphan, and pseudoephedrine *on page 16*
- **Alkeran®** *see* melphalan *on page 390*
- **Allbee® With C** [OTC] *see* vitamin B complex with vitamin C *on page 651*
- **Allegra®** *see* fexofenadine *on page 267*
- **Allegra-D™** *see* fexofenadine and pseudoephedrine *on page 267*
- **Aller-Chlor® Oral** [OTC] *see* chlorpheniramine *on page 138*
- **Allercon® Tablet** [OTC] *see* triprolidine and pseudoephedrine *on page 632*
- **Allerdryl®** *see* diphenhydramine *on page 208*
- **Allerest® 12 Hour Capsule** [OTC] *see* chlorpheniramine and phenylpropanolamine *on page 139*
- **Allerest® 12 Hour Nasal Solution** [OTC] *see* oxymetazoline *on page 463*
- **Allerest® Eye Drops** [OTC] *see* naphazoline *on page 431*
- **Allerest® Maximum Strength** [OTC] *see* chlorpheniramine and pseudoephedrine *on page 140*
- **Allerest® No Drowsiness** [OTC] *see* acetaminophen and pseudoephedrine *on page 15*
- **Allerfrin® Syrup** [OTC] *see* triprolidine and pseudoephedrine *on page 632*
- **Allerfrin® Tablet** [OTC] *see* triprolidine and pseudoephedrine *on page 632*
- **Allerfrin® w/Codeine** *see* triprolidine, pseudoephedrine, and codeine *on page 632*
- **Allergan® Ear Drops** *see* antipyrine and benzocaine *on page 53*
- **AllerMax® Oral** [OTC] *see* diphenhydramine *on page 208*
- **Allernix®** *see* diphenhydramine *on page 208*
- **Allerphed® Syrup** [OTC] *see* triprolidine and pseudoephedrine *on page 632*

allopurinol (al oh PURE i nole)

U.S. Brand Names Zyloprim®
Canadian Brand Names Apo®-Allopurinol; Novo-purol®; Purinol®
Mexican Brand Names Atisuril®; Unizuric 300
Generic Available Yes
Therapeutic Category Xanthine Oxidase Inhibitor
Use Prevention of attacks of gouty arthritis and nephropathy; also used to treat secondary hyperuricemia which may occur during treatment of tumors or leukemia; prevent recurrent calcium oxalate calculi
Usual Dosage
Oral:
Children: 10 mg/kg/day in 2-3 divided doses or 200-300 mg/m^2/day in 2-4 divided doses, maximum: 600 mg/24 hours
Alternative:
<6 years: 150 mg/day in 3 divided doses
6-10 years: 300 mg/day in 2-3 divided doses
Children >10 years and Adults: Daily doses >300 mg should be administered in divided doses
Myeloproliferative neoplastic disorders: 600-800 mg/day in 2-3 divided doses for prevention of acute uric acid nephropathy for 2-3 days starting 1-2 days before chemotherapy
Gout: 200-300 mg/day (mild); 400-600 mg/day (severe)
Maximum dose: 800 mg/day
I.V.: Intravenous daily dose can be given as a single infusion or in equally divided doses at 6-, 8-, or 12-hour intervals. A fluid intake sufficient to yield a daily urinary output of at least 2 L in adults and the maintenance of a neutral or, preferably, slightly alkaline urine are desirable.
Children: Starting dose: 200 mg/m^2/day
Adults: 200-400 mg/m^2/day (max: 600 mg/day)
Dosing adjustment in renal impairment: I.V.:
Cl$_{cr}$ 10-20 mL/minute: 200 mg/day
Cl$_{cr}$ 3-10 mL/minute: 100 mg/day
Cl$_{cr}$ <3 mL/minute: 100 mg/day at extended intervals
Dietary Considerations Should be administered after meals with plenty of fluid
Nursing/Pharmacy Information Monitor CBC, serum uric acid levels, I & O, hepatic and renal function, especially at start of therapy
Dosage Forms
Injection, as sodium: 500 mg
Tablet: 100 mg, 300 mg

- **all-*trans*-retinoic acid** *see* tretinoin (oral) *on page 622*
- **Alocril™** *see* nedocromil (ophthalmic) *New Drug on page 434*
- **Aloid** *see* miconazole *on page 413*
- **Alomide® Ophthalmic** *see* lodoxamide tromethamine *on page 373*
- **Alor® 5/500** *see* hydrocodone and aspirin *on page 319*
- **Alora® Transdermal** *see* estradiol *on page 242*
- **alpha₁-PI** *see* alpha₁-proteinase inhibitor *on page 30*

alpha₁-proteinase inhibitor (al fa won PRO tee in ase in HI bi tor)
Synonyms alpha₁-PI
U.S. Brand Names Prolastin®
Generic Available No
Therapeutic Category Antitrypsin Deficiency Agent
Use Congenital alpha₁-antitrypsin deficiency
Usual Dosage Adults: I.V.: 60 mg/kg once weekly
Nursing/Pharmacy Information
Sodium content of 1 L after reconstitution: 100-210 mEq
Stability: Store in refrigerator, do not freeze; administer within 3 hours of reconstitution; do not refrigerate after reconstitution; may administer without further dilution or after further dilution with normal saline
Dosage Forms Injection (human): 500 mg alpha₁-PI (20 mL diluent); 1000 mg alpha ₁-PI (40 mL diluent)

- **Alpha-Baclofen®** *see* baclofen *on page 72*
- **Alpha-Dextrano"40"** *see* dextran *on page 192*
- **Alphagan®** *see* brimonidine *on page 92*
- **Alphamul® [OTC]** *see* castor oil *on page 118*
- **Alphanate®** *see* antihemophilic factor (human) *on page 51*
- **AlphaNine® SD** *see* factor IX complex (human) *on page 257*
- **Alpha-Tamoxifen®** *see* tamoxifen *on page 592*
- **Alphatrex® Topical** *see* betamethasone (topical) *on page 85*

alprazolam (al PRAY zoe lam)
U.S. Brand Names Xanax®
Canadian Brand Names Apo®-Alpraz; Novo-Aloprazol®; Nu-Alprax®
Mexican Brand Names Tafil
Generic Available Yes
Therapeutic Category Benzodiazepine
Controlled Substance C-IV
Use Treatment of anxiety; adjunct in the treatment of depression; management of panic attacks
Usual Dosage Oral:
Children <18 years: Dose not established
Adults: 0.25-0.5 mg 2-3 times/day, titrate dose upward; maximum: 4 mg/day (anxiety); 10 mg/day (panic attacks)
Dietary Considerations May be administered with food or water to avoid upset
Nursing/Pharmacy Information
Assist with ambulation during beginning of therapy; allow patient to rise slowly to avoid fainting
Monitor respiratory and cardiovascular status
Dosage Forms Tablet: 0.25 mg, 0.5 mg, 1 mg, 2 mg

alprostadil (al PROS ta dill)
Synonyms PGE₁; prostaglandin E₁
U.S. Brand Names Caverject® Injection; Edex® Injection; Muse® Pellet; Prostin VR Pediatric® Injection
Generic Available Yes
Therapeutic Category Prostaglandin
Use Temporary maintenance of patency of ductus arteriosus in neonates with ductal-dependent congenital cyanotic or acyanotic heart disease until surgery can be performed; these defects include cyanotic (eg, pulmonary atresia, pulmonary stenosis, tricuspid atresia, Fallot's tetralogy, transposition of the great vessels) and acyanotic (eg, interruption of aortic arch, coarctation of aorta, hypoplastic left ventricle) heart disease. Alprostadil has also been used investigationally for the treatment of pulmonary hypertension in infants and children with congenital heart defects with left-to-right shunts and primary graft nonfunction following liver transplant. Used in penile erectile dysfunction

Usual Dosage

Patent ductus arteriosus (Prostin VR Pediatric®):

I.V. continuous infusion into a large vein, or alternatively through an umbilical artery catheter placed at the ductal opening: 0.05-0.1 mcg/kg/minute with therapeutic response, rate is reduced to lowest effective dosage; with unsatisfactory response, rate is increased gradually; maintenance: 0.01-0.4 mcg/kg/minute

PGE_1 is usually given at an infusion rate of 0.1 mcg/kg/minute, but it is often possible to reduce the dosage to $\frac{1}{2}$ or even $\frac{1}{10}$ without losing the therapeutic effect. The mixing schedule is shown in the table.

Add 1 Ampul (500 mcg) to:	Concentration (mcg/mL)	Infusion Rate	
		mL/min/kg Needed to Infuse 0.1 mcg/kg/min	mL/kg/24 h
250 mL	2	0.05	72
100 mL	5	0.02	28.8
50 mL	10	0.01	14.4
25 mL	20	0.005	7.2

Therapeutic response is indicated by increased pH in those with acidosis or by an increase in oxygenation (pO_2) usually evident within 30 minutes

Erectile dysfunction:

Caverject®:

Vasculogenic, psychogenic, or mixed etiology: Individualize dose by careful titration; usual dose: 2.5-60 mcg (doses >60 mcg are not recommended); initiate dosage titration at 2.5 mcg, increasing by 2.5 mcg to a dose of 5 mcg and then in increments of 5-10 mcg depending on the erectile response until the dose produces an erection suitable for intercourse, not lasting >1 hour; if there is absolutely no response to initial 2.5 mcg dose, the second dose may increased to 7.5 mcg, followed by increments of 5-10 mcg

Neurogenic etiology (eg, spinal cord injury): Initiate dosage titration at 1.25 mcg, increasing to a doses of 2.5 mcg and then 5 mcg; increase further in increments 5 mcg until the dose is reached that produces an erection suitable for intercourse, not lasting >1 hour

Note: Patient must stay in the physician's office until complete detumescence occurs; if there is no response, then the next higher dose may be given within 1 hour; if there is still no response, a 1-day interval before giving the next dose is recommended; increasing the dose or concentration in the treatment of impotence results in increasing pain and discomfort

Muse® Pellet: Intraurethral: Administer as needed to achieve an erection; duration of action: ~30-60 minutes; use only two systems per 24-hour period

Nursing/Pharmacy Information

Ductus arteriosus: Monitor arterial pressure; assess all vital functions; apnea and bradycardia may indicate overdose, stop infusion if occurring; infuse for the shortest time and at the lowest dose that will produce the desired effects. Flushing is usually a result of catheter malposition; central line preferred for I.V. administration.

Erectile dysfunction: Use a $\frac{1}{2}$", 27- to 30-gauge needle; inject into the dorsolateral aspect of the proximal third of the penis, avoiding visible veins; alternate side of the penis for injections. If the patient is going to be self-injecting at home, carefully assess their aseptic technique for injection and knowledge of proper disposal of the syringe, needle and vial. Observe for signs of infection, penile fibrosis, and significant pain or priapism,

Dosage Forms

Injection:

Caverject®: 5 mcg, 10 mcg, 20 mcg

Edex® Injection: 10 mcg, 20 mcg, 40 mcg

Prostin VR Pediatric®: 500 mcg/mL (1 mL)

Pellet, urethral (Muse®): 125 mcg, 250 mcg, 500 mcg, 1000 mcg

- ◆ **Alrex™** *see* loteprednol *on page 377*
- ◆ **AL-Rr® Oral [OTC]** *see* chlorpheniramine *on page 138*
- ◆ **Altace™** *see* ramipril *on page 541*

alteplase (AL te plase)

Synonyms alteplase, recombinant; tissue plasminogen activator, recombinant; t-PA

(Continued)

alteplase *(Continued)*

U.S. Brand Names Activase®
Canadian Brand Names Lysatec-rt-PA®
Generic Available No
Therapeutic Category Thrombolytic Agent
Use Management of acute myocardial infarction for the lysis of thrombi in coronary arteries; management of acute massive pulmonary embolism (PE) in adults
Usual Dosage
   Coronary artery thrombi: I.V.: Front loading dose: Total dose is 100 mg over 1.5 hours (for patients who weigh <65 kg, use 1.25 mg/kg/total dose). Add this dose to a 100 mL bag of 0.9% sodium chloride for a total volume of 200 mL. Infuse 15 mg (30 mL) over 1-2 minutes; infuse 50 mg (100 mL) over 30 minutes. Begin heparin 5000-10,000 unit bolus followed by continuous infusion of 1000 units/hour. Infuse 35 mg/hour (70 mL) for next 2 hours.
   Acute pulmonary embolism: 100 mg over 2 hours
Nursing/Pharmacy Information
   Assess for hemorrhage during first hour of treatment
   Stability: Refrigerate; must be used within 8 hours of reconstitution; alteplase is **incompatible** with dobutamine, dopamine, heparin, and nitroglycerin infusions; physically **compatible** with lidocaine, metoprolol, propranolol when administered via Y site
Dosage Forms Powder for injection, lyophilized (recombinant): 50 mg [29 million units] (50 mL); 100 mg [58 million units] (100 mL)

♦ **alteplase, recombinant** *see* alteplase *on page 31*
♦ **Alter-H₂®** *see* ranitidine hydrochloride *on page 541*
♦ **ALternaGEL® [OTC]** *see* aluminum hydroxide *on page 33*

altretamine (al TRET a meen)

Synonyms hexamethylmelamine
U.S. Brand Names Hexalen®
Generic Available No
Therapeutic Category Antineoplastic Agent
Use Palliative treatment of persistent or recurrent ovarian cancer
Usual Dosage Adults: Oral (refer to protocol): 4-12 mg/kg/day in 3-4 divided doses for 21-90 days
   Alternatively: 240-320 mg/m²/day in 3-4 divided doses for 21 days, repeated every 6 weeks
   Alternatively: 260 mg/m²/day for 14-21 days of a 28-day cycle in 4 divided doses
Dietary Considerations Should be administered after meals
Nursing/Pharmacy Information Advise patient to report any numbness or tingling in extremities to physician; nausea and vomiting may occur and even begin up to weeks after therapy is stopped
Dosage Forms Capsule: 50 mg

♦ **Alu-Cap® [OTC]** *see* aluminum hydroxide *on page 33*
♦ **Aludrox® [OTC]** *see* aluminum hydroxide and magnesium hydroxide *on page 34*

aluminum acetate and acetic acid

   (a LOO mi num AS e tate & a SEE tik AS id)
Synonyms acetic acid and aluminum acetate otic; Burow's otic
U.S. Brand Names Otic Domeboro®
Generic Available Yes
Therapeutic Category Otic Agent, Anti-infective
Use Treatment of superficial infections of the external auditory canal
Usual Dosage Otic: Instill 4-6 drops in ear(s) every 2-3 hours
Dosage Forms Solution, otic: Aluminum acetate 10% and acetic acid 2% (60 mL)

aluminum acetate and calcium acetate

   (a LOO mi num SUL fate & KAL see um AS e tate)
U.S. Brand Names Bluboro® [OTC]; Boropak® [OTC]; Domeboro® Topical [OTC]; Pedi-Boro® [OTC]
Generic Available Yes
Therapeutic Category Topical Skin Product
Use Astringent wet dressing for relief of inflammatory conditions of the skin and to reduce weeping that may occur in dermatitis

Usual Dosage Topical: Soak affected area in the solution 2-4 times/day for 15-30 minutes or apply wet dressing soaked in the solution 2-4 times/day for 30-minute treatment periods; rewet dressing with solution every few minutes to keep it moist

Dosage Forms

Powder, to make topical solution: 1 packet/pint of water [1:40 solution]
Tablet, effervescent: 1 tablet/pint [1:40 dilution]

aluminum carbonate (a LOO mi num KAR bun ate)

U.S. Brand Names Basaljel® [OTC]
Generic Available Yes
Therapeutic Category Antacid
Use Hyperacidity; hyperphosphatemia
Usual Dosage Adults: Oral:

Antacid: 2 tablets/capsules or 10 mL of suspension every 2 hours, up to 12 times/day

Hyperphosphatemia: 2 tablets/capsules or 12 mL of suspension with meals

Dietary Considerations Should be administered with meals
Nursing/Pharmacy Information Dilute dose in water or juice, shake well
Dosage Forms

Capsule: Equivalent to 500 mg aluminum hydroxide
Suspension: Equivalent to 400 mg/5 mL aluminum hydroxide
Tablet: Equivalent to 500 mg aluminum hydroxide

aluminum chloride hexahydrate

(a LOO mi num KLOR ide heks a HYE drate)
U.S. Brand Names Drysol™
Generic Available Yes
Therapeutic Category Topical Skin Product
Use Astringent in the management of hyperhidrosis
Usual Dosage Adults: Topical: Apply at bedtime
Nursing/Pharmacy Information For external use only
Dosage Forms Solution, topical: 20% in SD alcohol 40 (35 mL, 37.5 mL)

aluminum hydroxide (a LOO mi num hye DROKS ide)

U.S. Brand Names ALternaGEL® [OTC]; Alu-Cap® [OTC]; Alu-Tab® [OTC]; Amphojel® [OTC]; Dialume® [OTC]; Nephrox Suspension [OTC]
Generic Available Yes
Therapeutic Category Antacid
Use Hyperacidity; hyperphosphatemia
Usual Dosage Oral:

Peptic ulcer disease:
Children: 5-15 mL/dose every 3-6 hours or 1 and 3 hours after meals and at bedtime
Adults: 15-45 mL every 3-6 hours or 1 and 3 hours after meals and at bedtime

Prophylaxis against gastrointestinal bleeding:
Infants: 2-5 mL/dose every 1-2 hours
Children: 5-15 mL/dose every 1-2 hours
Adults: 30-60 mL/dose every hour
Titrate to maintain the gastric pH >5

Hyperphosphatemia:
Children: 50 mg to 150 mg/kg/24 hours in divided doses every 4-6 hours, titrate dosage to maintain serum phosphorus within normal range
Adults: 500-1800 mg, 3-6 times/day, between meals and at bedtime

Antacid: Adults: 30 mL 1 and 3 hours postprandial and at bedtime

Dietary Considerations Should be administered 1-3 hours after meals
Nursing/Pharmacy Information Monitor phosphorous levels periodically when patient is on chronic therapy (observe for constipation, fecal impaction, diarrhea)

Dosage Forms

Capsule:
Alu-Cap®: 400 mg
Dialume®: 500 mg
Liquid: 600 mg/5 mL
ALternaGEL®: 600 mg/5 mL
Suspension, oral: 320 mg/5 mL; 450 mg/5 mL; 675 mg/5 mL
Amphojel®: 320 mg/5 mL
Tablet:
Amphojel®: 300 mg, 600 mg
Alu-Tab®: 500 mg

(Continued)

aluminum hydroxide and magnesium carbonate

(a LOO mi num hye DROKS ide & mag NEE zhum KAR bun nate)

U.S. Brand Names Gaviscon® Liquid [OTC]

Generic Available Yes

Therapeutic Category Antacid

Use Temporary relief of symptoms associated with gastric acidity

Usual Dosage Adults: Oral: 15-30 mL 4 times/day after meals and at bedtime

Dietary Considerations Should be administered 1-3 hours after meals with water, milk or juice

Nursing/Pharmacy Information Monitor stool frequency

Dosage Forms Liquid: Aluminum hydroxide 95 mg and magnesium carbonate 358 mg per 15 mL

aluminum hydroxide and magnesium hydroxide

(a LOO mi num hye DROKS ide & mag NEE zhum hye DROK side)

Synonyms magnesium hydroxide and aluminum hydroxide

U.S. Brand Names Aludrox® [OTC]; Maalox® [OTC]; Maalox® Therapeutic Concentrate [OTC]

Generic Available Yes

Therapeutic Category Antacid

Use Antacid, hyperphosphatemia in renal failure

Usual Dosage Adults: Oral: 5-10 mL or 1-2 tablets 4-6 times/day, between meals and at bedtime; may be used every hour for severe symptoms

Dietary Considerations Should be administered 1-3 hours after meals

Nursing/Pharmacy Information

Administer 1-2 hours apart from oral drugs; shake suspensions well

Observe for constipation, fecal impaction, diarrhea, and hypophosphatemia

Dosage Forms

Suspension:

Aludrox®: Aluminum hydroxide 307 mg and magnesium hydroxide 103 mg per 5 mL

Maalox®: Aluminum hydroxide 225 mg and magnesium hydroxide 200 mg per 5 mL

High potency (Maalox® TC): Aluminum hydroxide 600 mg and magnesium hydroxide 300 mg per 5 mL

Tablet, chewable (Maalox®): Aluminum hydroxide 600 mg and magnesium hydroxide 300 mg

aluminum hydroxide and magnesium trisilicate

(a LOO mi num hye DROKS ide & mag NEE zhum trye SIL i kate)

U.S. Brand Names Gaviscon®-2 Tablet [OTC]; Gaviscon® Tablet [OTC]

Generic Available Yes

Therapeutic Category Antacid

Use Temporary relief of hyperacidity

Usual Dosage Adults: Oral: Chew 2-4 tablets 4 times/day or as directed by physician

Dietary Considerations Should be administered 1-3 hours after meals with water, milk, or juice

Nursing/Pharmacy Information Tablets should be chewed and not swallowed whole; can dilute liquid in water or juice

Dosage Forms Tablet, chewable:

Gaviscon®: Aluminum hydroxide 80 mg and magnesium trisilicate 20 mg

Gaviscon®-2: Aluminum hydroxide 160 mg and magnesium trisilicate 40 mg

aluminum hydroxide, magnesium hydroxide, and simethicone

(a LOO mi num hye DROKS ide, mag NEE zhum hye DROKS ide, & sye METH i kone)

U.S. Brand Names Di-Gel® [OTC]; Gas-Ban DS® [OTC]; Maalox® Plus [OTC]; Magalox Plus® [OTC]; Mylanta® [OTC]; Mylanta®-II [OTC]

Generic Available Yes

Therapeutic Category Antacid; Antiflatulent

Use Temporary relief of hyperacidity associated with gas; may also be used for indications associated with other antacids

Usual Dosage Adults: Oral: 15-30 mL or 2-4 tablets 4-6 times/day between meals and at bedtime; may be used every hour for severe symptoms

Dietary Considerations Should be administered 1-3 hours after meals
Nursing/Pharmacy Information Administer 1-2 hours apart from oral drugs
Dosage Forms
Liquid:
Mylanta®: Aluminum hydroxide 200 mg, magnesium hydroxide, 200 mg, and simethicone 20 mg per 5 mL
Maalox® Plus: Aluminum hydroxide 225 mg, magnesium hydroxide 200 mg, and simethicone 25 mg per 5 mL (30 mL, 180 mL)
Mylanta®-II: Aluminum hydroxide 400 mg, magnesium hydroxide 400 mg, and simethicone 40 mg per 5 mL (150 mL, 360 mL)
Tablet, chewable:
Magalox Plus®: Aluminum hydroxide 200 mg, magnesium hydroxide 200 mg, and simethicone 25 mg
Mylanta®: Aluminum hydroxide 200 mg, magnesium hydroxide 200 mg, and simethicone 20 mg
Gas-Ban DS®, Mylanta®-II: Aluminum hydroxide 400 mg, magnesium hydroxide 400 mg, and simethicone 40 mg

♦ **aluminum sucrose sulfate, basic** *see* sucralfate *on page 583*
♦ **Alupent®** *see* metaproterenol *on page 397*
♦ **Alu-Tab® [OTC]** *see* aluminum hydroxide *on page 33*
♦ **Alvidina** *see* ranitidine hydrochloride *on page 541*

amantadine (a MAN ta deen)
Synonyms adamantanamine
U.S. Brand Names Symadine®; Symmetrel® Syrup
Canadian Brand Names Endantadine™; PMS-Amantadine
Generic Available Yes
Therapeutic Category Anti-Parkinson's Agent; Antiviral Agent
Use Prophylaxis and treatment of influenza A viral infection; symptomatic and adjunct treatment of parkinsonism
Usual Dosage Oral:
Children:
1-9 years: 4.4-8.8 mg/kg/day in 1-2 divided doses to a maximum of 150 mg/day
9-12 years: 100-200 mg/day in 1-2 divided doses
After first influenza A virus vaccine dose, amantadine prophylaxis may be administered for up to 6 weeks or until 2 weeks after the second dose of vaccine
Adults:
Parkinson's disease: 100 mg twice daily
Influenza A viral infection: 200 mg/day in 1-2 divided doses
Prophylaxis: Minimum 10-day course of therapy following exposure or continue for 2-3 weeks after influenza A virus vaccine is administered
Elderly patients should administer the drug in 2 daily doses rather than a single dose to avoid adverse neurologic reactions
Dietary Considerations Avoid alcohol
Nursing/Pharmacy Information
If insomnia occurs, the last daily dose should be administered several hours before retiring
Monitor renal function
Stability: Protect from freezing
Dosage Forms
Capsule, as hydrochloride: 100 mg
Syrup, as hydrochloride: 50 mg/5 mL (120 mL, 480 mL)
Tablet, as hydrochloride: 100 mg

♦ **Amaphen®** *see* butalbital compound and acetaminophen *on page 99*
♦ **Amaryl®** *see* glimepiride *on page 292*

ambenonium (am be NOE nee um)
U.S. Brand Names Mytelase® Caplets®
Generic Available No
Therapeutic Category Cholinergic Agent
Use Treatment of myasthenia gravis
Usual Dosage Adults: Oral: 5-25 mg 3-4 times/day
Nursing/Pharmacy Information Have atropine ready to combat hypercholinergic response; have epinephrine ready to combat anaphylaxis
Dosage Forms Tablet, as chloride: 10 mg

♦ **Ambenyl® Cough Syrup** *see* bromodiphenhydramine and codeine *on page 93*

♦ **Ambi 10®** [OTC] *see* benzoyl peroxide *on page 81*
♦ **Ambien**™ *see* zolpidem *on page 661*
♦ **Ambi® Skin Tone** [OTC] *see* hydroquinone *on page 325*
♦ **AmBisome®** *see* amphotericin B liposomal *on page 46*
♦ **Ambotetra** *see* tetracycline *on page 601*

amcinonide (am SIN oh nide)
U.S. Brand Names Cyclocort® Topical
Generic Available No
Therapeutic Category Corticosteroid, Topical
Use Relief of the inflammatory and pruritic manifestations of corticosteroid-responsive dermatoses
Usual Dosage Adults: Topical: Apply in a thin film 2-3 times/day
Nursing/Pharmacy Information Assess for worsening of rash or fever
Dosage Forms
Cream: 0.1% (15 g, 30 g, 60 g)
Lotion: 0.1% (20 mL, 60 mL)
Ointment, topical: 0.1% (15 g, 30 g, 60 g)

♦ **Amcort® Injection** *see* triamcinolone (systemic) *on page 624*
♦ **Ameblin** *see* metronidazole *on page 411*
♦ **Amen® Oral** *see* medroxyprogesterone acetate *on page 389*
♦ **Amerge®** *see* naratriptan *on page 433*
♦ **Americaine®** [OTC] *see* benzocaine *on page 79*
♦ **A-methaPred® Injection** *see* methylprednisolone *on page 407*
♦ **amethocaine** *see* tetracaine *on page 600*
♦ **amethopterin** *see* methotrexate *on page 402*
♦ **amfepramone** *see* diethylpropion *on page 201*
♦ **Amgenal® Cough Syrup** *see* bromodiphenhydramine and codeine *on page 93*
♦ **Amicar®** *see* aminocaproic acid *on page 37*
♦ **Amidate®** *see* etomidate *on page 255*

amifostine (am i FOS teen)
Synonyms ethiofos; gammaphos
U.S. Brand Names Ethyol®
Generic Available No
Therapeutic Category Antidote
Use Reduce the incidence of moderate to severe xerostomia in patients undergoing postoperative radiation treatment for head and neck cancer, where the radiation port includes a substantial portion of the parotid glands. Protection against cisplatin-induced nephrotoxicity in advanced ovarian cancer patients; it may also provide protection from cisplatin-induced peripheral neuropathy
Usual Dosage I.V.: 910 mg/m² beginning 30 minutes before starting chemotherapy; reduction of xerostomia from head and neck radiation: 200 mg/m² I.V. (as a 3-minute infusion) once daily, starting 15-30 minutes before standard fraction radiation therapy; dose adjustment is recommended for subsequent doses if the previous dose was interrupted, and not able to be resumed; secondary to hypotension, the recommended dose for subsequent administration is 740 mg/m²
Dosage Forms Injection: 500 mg

amikacin (am i KAY sin)
U.S. Brand Names Amikin®
Mexican Brand Names Amikafur®; Amikayect; Amikin®; Biclin; Gamikal; Yectamid
Generic Available Yes
Therapeutic Category Aminoglycoside (Antibiotic)
Use Treatment of documented gram-negative enteric infection resistant to gentamicin and tobramycin; documented infection of mycobacterial organisms susceptible to amikacin
Usual Dosage I.M., I.V.:
Infants and Children: 15-20 mg/kg/day divided every 8 hours
Adults: 15 mg/kg/day divided every 8-12 hours
Nursing/Pharmacy Information
Aminoglycoside levels measured from blood taken from Silastic® central catheters can sometimes give falsely elevated readings; peak serum levels should be drawn 30 minutes after the end of a 30-minute infusion; trough levels are

drawn within 30 minutes before the next dose; provide optimal patient hydration

Monitor urinalysis, BUN, serum creatinine, and be alert to ototoxicity

Stability: 24 hours at room temperature when mixed in D_5W, $D_5^{1}/_4NS$, $D_5^{1}/_2NS$, normal saline, or lactated Ringer's

Dosage Forms Injection, as sulfate: 5 mg/mL (100 mL); 50 mg/mL (2 mL); 62.5 mg/mL (8 mL); 250 mg/mL (2 mL, 3 mL, 4 mL, 50 mL)

♦ **Amikafur**® *see amikacin on page 36*
♦ **Amikayect** *see amikacin on page 36*
♦ **Amikin**® *see amikacin on page 36*

amiloride (a MIL oh ride)
U.S. Brand Names Midamor®
Generic Available Yes
Therapeutic Category Diuretic, Potassium Sparing
Use Counteract potassium loss induced by other diuretics in the treatment of hypertension or edematous conditions including CHF, hepatic cirrhosis and hypoaldosteronism; usually used in conjunction with a more potent diuretic such as thiazides or loop diuretics
Usual Dosage Oral:
Children: Although safety and efficacy have not been established by the FDA in children, a dosage of 0.625 mg/kg/day has been used in children weighing 6-20 kg
Adults: 5-10 mg/day (up to 20 mg)
Dietary Considerations This diuretic does not cause you to lose potassium; because salt substitutes and low-salt milk may contain potassium, do not use these products without checking with your physician; too much potassium can be as harmful as too little
Nursing/Pharmacy Information Monitor blood pressure, serum electrolytes, renal function, I & O ratios, and daily weight throughout therapy
Dosage Forms Tablet, as hydrochloride: 5 mg

amiloride and hydrochlorothiazide
(a MIL oh ride & hye droe klor oh THYE a zide)
Synonyms hydrochlorothiazide and amiloride
U.S. Brand Names Moduretic®
Generic Available Yes
Therapeutic Category Diuretic, Combination
Use Antikaliuretic diuretic, antihypertensive
Usual Dosage Adults: Oral: Start with 1 tablet/day, then may be increased to 2 tablets/day if needed; usually administered in a single dose
Dietary Considerations May be administered with food
Nursing/Pharmacy Information Monitor blood pressure, serum electrolytes, renal function
Dosage Forms Tablet: Amiloride hydrochloride 5 mg and hydrochlorothiazide 50 mg

♦ **Amin-Aid**® *(Discontinued) see page 743*
♦ **2-amino-6-mercaptopurine** *see thioguanine on page 607*
♦ **2-amino-6-trifluoromethoxy-benzothiazole** *see riluzole on page 550*
♦ **aminobenzylpenicillin** *see ampicillin on page 46*

aminocaproic acid (a mee noe ka PROE ik AS id)
U.S. Brand Names Amicar®
Generic Available Yes
Therapeutic Category Hemostatic Agent
Use Treatment of excessive bleeding resulting from systemic hyperfibrinolysis and urinary fibrinolysis
Usual Dosage In the management of acute bleeding syndromes, oral dosage regimens are the same as the I.V. dosage regimens in adults and children

Chronic bleeding: Oral, I.V.: 5-30 g/day in divided doses at 3- to 6-hour intervals
Acute bleeding syndrome:
Children: Oral, I.V.: 100 mg/kg or 3 g/m^2 during the first hour, followed by continuous infusion at the rate of 33.3 mg/kg/hour or 1 g/m^2/hour; total dosage should not exceed 18 g/m^2/24 hours
Adults:
Oral: For elevated fibrinolytic activity, administer 5 g during first hour, followed by 1-1.25 g/hour for approximately 8 hours or until bleeding stops
(Continued)

aminocaproic acid *(Continued)*

I.V.: Administer 4-5 g in 250 mL of diluent during first hour followed by continuous infusion at the rate of 1-1.25 g/hour in 50 mL of diluent, continue for 8 hours or until bleeding stops

Nursing/Pharmacy Information Administration by infusion using appropriate I.V. solution (dextrose 5% or sodium chloride 0.9%); rapid I.V. injection (IVP) should be avoided since hypotension, bradycardia, and arrhythmia may result. Aminocaproic acid may accumulate in patients with decreased renal function.

Dosage Forms
Injection: 250 mg/mL (20 mL)
Syrup: 1.25 g/5 mL (480 mL)
Tablet: 500 mg

♦ **Amino-Cerv™ Vaginal Cream** *see* urea *on page 638*

aminoglutethimide *(a mee noe gloo TETH i mide)*

U.S. Brand Names Cytadren®
Generic Available No
Therapeutic Category Antineoplastic Agent
Use Suppression of adrenal function in selected patients with Cushing's syndrome; also used successfully in postmenopausal patients with advanced breast carcinoma and in patients with metastatic prostate carcinoma
Usual Dosage Adults: Oral: 250 mg every 6 hours, may be increased at 1- to 2-week intervals to a total of 2 g/day; administer in divided doses 2-3 times/day to reduce incidence of nausea and vomiting
Nursing/Pharmacy Information Administer in divided doses, 2-3 times/day, to reduce incidence of nausea and vomiting
Dosage Forms Tablet, scored: 250 mg

♦ **Amino-Opti-E® [OTC]** *see* vitamin E *on page 652*

aminophylline *(am in OFF i lin)*

Synonyms theophylline ethylenediamine
U.S. Brand Names Phyllocontin®; Truphylline®
Generic Available Yes
Therapeutic Category Theophylline Derivative
Use Bronchodilator in reversible airway obstruction due to asthma or COPD; increase diaphragmatic contractility; neonatal idiopathic apnea of prematurity
Usual Dosage
Neonates: Apnea of prematurity:
Loading dose: 5 mg/kg for one dose
Maintenance: I.V.:
0-24 days: Begin at 2 mg/kg/day divided every 12 hours and titrate to desired levels and effects
>24 days: 3 mg/kg/day divided every 12 hours; increased dosages may be indicated as liver metabolism matures (usually >30 days of life); monitor serum levels to determine appropriate dosages
Theophylline levels should be initially drawn after 3 days of therapy; repeat levels are indicated 3 days after each increase in dosage or weekly if on a stabilized dosage

Treatment of acute bronchospasm:
Loading dose (in patients not currently receiving aminophylline or theophylline): 6 mg/kg (based on aminophylline) administered I.V. over 20-30 minutes; administration rate should not exceed 25 mg/minute (aminophylline)

Approximate I.V. maintenance dosages are based upon **continuous infusions**; bolus dosing (often used in children <6 months of age) may be determined by multiplying the hourly infusion rate by 24 hours and dividing by the desired number of doses/day
6 weeks to 6 months: 0.5 mg/kg/hour
6 months to 1 year: 0.6-0.7 mg/kg/hour
1-9 years: 1-1.2 mg/kg/hour
9-12 years and young adult smokers: 0.9 mg/kg/hour
12-16 years: 0.7 mg/kg/hour
Adults (healthy, nonsmoking): 0.7 mg/kg/hour
Older patients and patients with cor pulmonale, patients with congestive heart failure or liver failure: 0.25 mg/kg/hour
Dosage should be adjusted according to serum level measurements during the first 12- to 24-hour period; avoid using suppositories due to erratic, unreliable absorption.

Rectal: Adults: 500 mg 3 times/day

Dietary Considerations Food does not appreciably affect absorption; avoid extremes of dietary protein and carbohydrate intake; limit charcoal-broiled foods

Nursing/Pharmacy Information

Avoid I.M. injection, too painful; do not inject I.V. solution faster than 25 mg/minute; oral and I.V. should be administered around-the-clock rather than 4 times/day, 3 times/day, etc, (ie, 12-6-12-6, not 9-1-5-9) to promote less variation in peak and trough serum levels; do not crush sustained release drug products; do not crush enteric coated drug product; encourage patient to drink adequate fluids (2 L/day) to decrease mucous viscosity in airways

Monitor vital signs, I & O, serum concentrations, and CNS effects (insomnia, irritability)

Stability: Do not use solutions if discolored or if crystals are present

Dosage Forms

Injection: 25 mg/mL (10 mL, 20 mL)

Liquid, oral: 105 mg/5 mL (10 mL, 240 mL, 500 mL)

Suppository, rectal: 250 mg, 500 mg

Tablet: 100 mg, 200 mg

aminophylline, amobarbital, and ephedrine
(am in OFF i lin, am oh BAR bi tal, & e FED rin)

Generic Available Yes

Therapeutic Category Theophylline Derivative

Use Symptomatic relief of asthma

Usual Dosage Adults: Oral: 1 capsule every 6 hours

Dietary Considerations Should be administered with water 1 hour before or 2 hours after meals

Dosage Forms Capsule: Aminophylline 130 mg, amobarbital 24 mg, and ephedrine sulfate 24 mg

aminosalicylate sodium (a MEE noe sa LIS i late SOW dee um)

Synonyms PAS

Canadian Brand Names Tubasal®

Mexican Brand Names Salofalk

Generic Available Yes

Therapeutic Category Nonsteroidal Anti-inflammatory Drug (NSAID)

Use Treatment of tuberculosis with combination drugs

Usual Dosage Oral:

Children: 150-300 mg/kg/day in 3-4 equally divided doses

Adults: 150 mg/kg/day in 2-3 equally divided doses (usually 12-14 g/day)

Dietary Considerations May be administered with food

Nursing/Pharmacy Information Store in dry place; do not administer tablets if discolored

Dosage Forms Tablet: 500 mg

♦ **5-aminosalicylic acid** *see* mesalamine *on page 395*

amiodarone (a MEE oh da rone)

U.S. Brand Names Cordarone®; Pacerone®

Mexican Brand Names Braxan; Cardiorona

Generic Available Yes

Therapeutic Category Antiarrhythmic Agent, Class III

Use Management of resistant, life-threatening ventricular arrhythmias unresponsive to conventional therapy with less toxic agents; also used for treatment of supraventricular arrhythmias unresponsive to conventional therapy; injectable available from manufacturer via orphan drug status or compassionate use for acute treatment and prophylaxis of life-threatening ventricular tachycardia or ventricular fibrillation (see Dosage Forms)

Usual Dosage Children <1 year should be dosed as calculated by body surface area

Children: Loading dose: 10-15 mg/kg/day or 600-800 mg/1.73 m²/day for 4-14 days or until adequate control of arrhythmia or prominent adverse effects occur (this loading dose may be administered in 1-2 divided doses/day); dosage should then be reduced to 5 mg/kg/day or 200-400 mg/1.73 m²/day administered once daily for several weeks; if arrhythmia does not recur reduce to lowest effective dosage possible; usual daily minimal dose: 2.5 mg/kg; maintenance doses may be administered for 5 of 7 days/week

Adults: Ventricular arrhythmias: 800-1600 mg/day in 1-2 doses for 1-3 weeks, then 600-800 mg/day in 1-2 doses for 1 month; maintenance: 400 mg/day; (Continued)

amiodarone (Continued)

lower doses are recommended for supraventricular arrhythmias, usually 100-400 mg/day

Dietary Considerations May be administered with food

Nursing/Pharmacy Information

Avoid exposure of patient to sunlight; use sunscreen, sunglasses; intoxication with amiodarone necessitates EKG monitoring; bradycardia may be atropine resistant, I.V. isoproterenol or cardiac pacemaker may be required; hypotension, heart block and Q-T prolongation may also be seen

Monitor EKG, baseline pulmonary function tests, thyroid function tests, and liver enzymes; patients should be monitored for several days following ingestion due to long half-life

Dosage Forms

Injection, as hydrochloride: 50 mg/mL with benzyl alcohol (3 mL)

Tablet, scored, as hydrochloride: 200 mg

♦ **Amipaque®** see radiological/contrast media (non-ionic) on page 540

♦ **Ami-Tex LA®** see guaifenesin and phenylpropanolamine on page 301

♦ **Amitone® [OTC]** see calcium carbonate on page 103

amitriptyline (a mee TRIP ti leen)

U.S. Brand Names Elavil®; Emitrip®; Enovil® ·

Canadian Brand Names Apo®-Amitriptyline; Levate®; Novo-Tryptin®

Mexican Brand Names Anapsique; Tryptanol®

Generic Available Yes

Therapeutic Category Antidepressant, Tricyclic (Tertiary Amine)

Use Treatment of various forms of depression, often in conjunction with psychotherapy; analgesic for certain chronic and neuropathic pain; migraine prophylaxis

Usual Dosage

Children <12 years: Not recommended

Adolescents: Oral: Initial: 25-50 mg/day; may administer in divided doses; increase gradually to 100 mg/day in divided doses

Adults:

Oral: 30-100 mg/day single dose at bedtime or in divided doses; dose may be gradually increased up to 300 mg/day; once symptoms are controlled, decrease gradually to lowest effective dose

I.M.: 20-30 mg 4 times/day

Dietary Considerations Limit caffeine; may be administered with food to decrease GI distress; riboflavin dietary requirements may be increased

Nursing/Pharmacy Information

Do not administer I.V.

Monitor blood pressure and pulse rate prior to and during initial therapy, evaluate mental status; monitor weight

Stability: Protect injection and Elavil® 10 mg tablets from light

Dosage Forms

Injection, as hydrochloride: 10 mg/mL (10 mL)

Tablet, as hydrochloride: 10 mg, 25 mg, 50 mg, 75 mg, 100 mg, 150 mg

amitriptyline and chlordiazepoxide

(a mee TRIP ti leen & klor dye az e POKS ide)

Synonyms chlordiazepoxide and amitriptyline

U.S. Brand Names Limbitrol® DS 10-25

Generic Available Yes

Therapeutic Category Antidepressant, Tricyclic (Tertiary Amine)

Controlled Substance C-IV

Use Treatment of moderate to severe anxiety and/or agitation and depression

Usual Dosage Oral: Initial: 3-4 tablets in divided doses; this may be increased to 6 tablets/day as required; some patients respond to smaller doses and can be maintained on 2 tablets

Dosage Forms Tablet:

5-12.5: Amitriptyline hydrochloride 12.5 mg and chlordiazepoxide 5 mg

10-25: Amitriptyline hydrochloride 25 mg and chlordiazepoxide 10 mg

amitriptyline and perphenazine

(a mee TRIP ti leen & per FEN a zeen)

Synonyms perphenazine and amitriptyline

U.S. Brand Names Etrafon®; Triavil®

Generic Available Yes

Therapeutic Category Antidepressant/Phenothiazine

Use Treatment of patients with moderate to severe anxiety and depression

Usual Dosage Oral: 1 tablet 2-4 times/day

Nursing/Pharmacy Information Monitor blood pressure and pulse rate prior to and during initial therapy; evaluate mental status; monitor weight; may increase appetite and possibly a craving for sweets; offer patient sugarless hard candy for dry mouth

Dosage Forms Tablet:
2-10: Amitriptyline hydrochloride 10 mg and perphenazine 2 mg
4-10: Amitriptyline hydrochloride 10 mg and perphenazine 4 mg
2-25: Amitriptyline hydrochloride 25 mg and perphenazine 2 mg
4-25: Amitriptyline hydrochloride 25 mg and perphenazine 4 mg
4-50: Amitriptyline hydrochloride 50 mg and perphenazine 4 mg

amlexanox (am LEKS an oks)

U.S. Brand Names Aphthasol™
Generic Available No
Therapeutic Category Anti-inflammatory Agent, Locally Applied
Use Treating signs and symptoms of canker sores (minor aphthous ulcers)
Usual Dosage Administer directly on ulcers 4 times/day following oral hygiene, after meals, and before going to bed
Dosage Forms Cream: 5% (5 g)

amlodipine (am LOE di peen)

U.S. Brand Names Norvasc®
Mexican Brand Names Norvas
Generic Available No
Therapeutic Category Calcium Channel Blocker
Use Treatment of hypertension alone or in combination with antihypertensives; chronic stable angina alone or with other antianginal agents; vasospastic angina alone or in combination with other agents
Usual Dosage Oral:
Adults: 2.5-10 mg once daily
Elderly: 2.5 mg once daily; increase by 2.5 mg increments at 7- to 14-day intervals; maximum recommended dose: 10 mg/day
Nursing/Pharmacy Information Do not discontinue abruptly; report any dizziness, shortness of breath, palpitations, or edema
Dosage Forms Tablet: 2.5 mg, 5 mg, 10 mg

amlodipine and benazepril (am LOE di peen & ben AY ze pril)

Synonyms benazepril and amlodipine
U.S. Brand Names Lotrel®
Generic Available No
Therapeutic Category Antihypertensive Agent, Combination
Use Treatment of hypertension
Usual Dosage Adults: Oral: 1 capsule daily
Dosage Forms Capsule:
Amlodipine 2.5 mg and benazepril hydrochloride 10 mg
Amlodipine 5 mg and benazepril hydrochloride 10 mg
Amlodipine 5 mg and benazepril hydrochloride 20 mg

♦ **ammonapse** see sodium phenylbutyrate on page 573

ammonia spirit, aromatic (a MOE nee ah SPEAR it, air oh MAT ik)

Synonyms smelling salts
U.S. Brand Names Aromatic Ammonia Aspirols®
Generic Available Yes
Therapeutic Category Respiratory Stimulant
Use Respiratory and circulatory stimulant; treatment of fainting
Usual Dosage "Smelling salts" to treat or prevent fainting
Nursing/Pharmacy Information Aromatic ammonia spirit should be protected from light and stored at a temperature not exceeding 30°C
Dosage Forms
Inhalant, crushable glass perles: 0.33 mL, 0.4 mL
Solution: 30 mL, 60 mL, 120 mL

ammonium chloride (a MOE nee um KLOR ide)

Generic Available Yes
Therapeutic Category Electrolyte Supplement, Oral
Use Diuretic or systemic and urinary acidifying agent; treatment of hypochloremic states
(Continued)

ammonium chloride *(Continued)*

Usual Dosage
Children: Oral, I.V.: 75 mg/kg/day in 4 divided doses for urinary acidification; maximum daily dose: 6 g

Adults:
Oral: 2-3 g every 6 hours
I.V.: 1.5 g/dose every 6 hours

Nursing/Pharmacy Information
Rapid I.V. injection may increase the likelihood of ammonia toxicity; dilute to 0.2 mEq/mL and infuse I.V. over 3 hours; maximum concentration: 0.4 mEq/mL; maximum rate of infusion: 1 mEq/kg/hour

Monitor serum electrolytes, serum ammonia

Dosage Forms Injection: 26.75% [5 mEq/mL] (20 mL)

♦ **ammonium lactate** *see* lactic acid with ammonium hydroxide *on page 358*

♦ **Amobarbital®** *see* amobarbital *on page 42*

amobarbital (am oh BAR bi tal)

Synonyms amylobarbitone
U.S. Brand Names Amytal®
Canadian Brand Names Amobarbital®
Generic Available Yes: Capsule
Therapeutic Category Barbiturate
Controlled Substance C-II
Use Used to control status epilepticus or acute seizure episodes; also used in catatonic, negativistic, or manic reactions and in "Amytal® Interviewing" for narcoanalysis

Usual Dosage Hypnotic: Adults:
I.M.: 65-500 mg, should not exceed 500 mg
I.V.: 65-500 mg, should not exceed 1000 mg

Nursing/Pharmacy Information Monitor vital signs; drug should be injected within 30 minutes after opening vial because of hydrolysis

Dosage Forms Injection, as sodium: 500 mg

amobarbital and secobarbital
(am oh BAR bi tal & see koe BAR bi tal)

Synonyms secobarbital and amobarbital
U.S. Brand Names Tuinal®
Generic Available No
Therapeutic Category Barbiturate
Controlled Substance C-II
Use Short-term treatment of insomnia
Usual Dosage Adults: Oral: 1-2 capsules at bedtime
Dosage Forms Capsule: 100: Amobarbital 50 mg and secobarbital 50 mg

♦ **Amonidrin® Tablet** *(Discontinued)* *see page 743*

♦ **AMO Vitrax®** *see* sodium hyaluronate *on page 572*

amoxapine (a MOKS a peen)

U.S. Brand Names Asendin®
Mexican Brand Names Demolox
Generic Available Yes
Therapeutic Category Antidepressant, Tricyclic (Secondary Amine)
Use Treatment of neurotic and endogenous depression and mixed symptoms of anxiety and depression

Usual Dosage Oral (once symptoms are controlled, decrease gradually to lowest effective dose):

Children <16 years: Dose not established
Adolescents: Initial: 25-50 mg/day; increase gradually to 100 mg/day; may administer as divided doses or as a single dose at bedtime
Adults: Initial: 25 mg 2-3 times/day, if tolerated, dosage may be increased to 100 mg 2-3 times/day; may be administered in a single bedtime dose when dosage <300 mg/day
Maximum daily dose:
Outpatient: 400 mg
Inpatient: 600 mg

Dietary Considerations May be administered with food to decrease GI distress

Nursing/Pharmacy Information Monitor blood pressure and pulse rate prior to a during initial therapy; evaluate mental status; monitor weight, may increase appetite and possibly a craving for sweets; recognize signs of neuro-leptic malignant syndrome and tardive dyskinesia

Dosage Forms Tablet: 25 mg, 50 mg, 100 mg, 150 mg

amoxicillin (a moks i SIL in)

Synonyms amoxicillin; *p*-hydroxyampicillin

U.S. Brand Names Amoxil®; Trimox®; Wymox®

Canadian Brand Names Apo-Amoxi®; Novamoxin®; Nu-Amoxi; Pro-Amox®

Mexican Brand Names Acimox; Amoxifur; Amoxisol; Amoxivet; Flemoxon; Gimalxina; Grunicina; Hidramox®

Generic Available Yes

Therapeutic Category Penicillin

Use Treatment of otitis media, sinusitis, and infections involving the respiratory tract, skin, and urinary tract due to susceptible *H. influenzae, N. gonorrhoeae, E. coli, P. mirabilis, E. faecalis,* streptococci, and nonpenicillinase-producing staphylococci; prophylaxis of bacterial endocarditis

Usual Dosage Oral:

Children: 25-50 mg/kg/day in divided doses every 8 hours

Uncomplicated gonorrhea: ≥2 years: 50 mg/kg plus probenecid 25 mg/kg in a single dose; do not use this regimen in children <2 years of age, proben-ecid is contraindicated in this age group

SBE prophylaxis: 50 mg/kg 1 hour before procedure and 25 mg/kg 6 hours later; not to exceed adult dosage

Adults: 250-500 mg every 8 hours or 500-875 mg twice daily; maximum dose: 2-3 g/day

Uncomplicated gonorrhea: 3 g plus probenecid 1 g in a single dose

Endocarditis prophylaxis: 3 g 1 hour before procedure and 1.5 g 6 hours later

Dietary Considerations May be mixed with formula, milk, or juice; may be administered with food, however, peak concentrations may be delayed

Nursing/Pharmacy Information

Assess patient at beginning and throughout therapy for infection; observe for signs and symptoms of anaphylaxis; obtain specimens for C&S before the first dose; administer around-the-clock rather than 3 times/day, etc, (ie, 8-4-12, not 9-1-5) to promote less variation in peak and trough serum levels

With prolonged therapy, monitor renal, hepatic, and hematologic function peri-odically

Stability: Oral suspension and pediatric drops remain stable for 7 days at room temperature or 14 days if refrigerated

Dosage Forms

Capsule, as trihydrate: 250 mg, 500 mg

Powder for oral suspension, as trihydrate: 125 mg/5 mL (80 mL, 100 mL, 150 mL); 250 mg/5 mL (80 mL, 100 mL, 150 mL)

Powder for oral suspension, drops, as trihydrate: 50 mg/mL (15 mL, 30 mL)

Tablet, chewable, as trihydrate: 125 mg, 250 mg, 400 mg

Tablet, film coated: 500 mg, 875 mg

amoxicillin and clavulanate potassium

(a moks i SIL in & klav yoo LAN ate poe TASS ee um)

Synonyms amoxicillin and clavulanic acid; clavulanate potassium and amoxi-cillin

U.S. Brand Names Augmentin®

Canadian Brand Names Clavulin®

Mexican Brand Names Clavulin®; Eumetinex

Generic Available No

Therapeutic Category Penicillin

Use Infections caused by susceptible organisms involving the lower respiratory tract, otitis media, sinusitis, skin and skin structure, and urinary tract; spectrum same as amoxicillin in addition to beta-lactamase-producing *B. catarrhalis, H. influenzae, N. gonorrhoeae,* and *S. aureus* (not MRSA)

Usual Dosage Oral:

Children ≤40 kg: 20-40 mg (amoxicillin)/kg/day in divided doses every 8 hours

Children >40 kg and Adults: 250-500 mg every 8 hours or 875 mg every 12 hours

Dietary Considerations May be administered with meals or on an empty stomach; may mix with milk, formula, or juice

Nursing/Pharmacy Information

Assess patient at beginning and throughout therapy for infection; observe for signs and symptoms of anaphylaxis; obtain specimens for C&S before the first dose; administer around-the-clock rather than 3 times/day to promote

(Continued)

amoxicillin and clavulanate potassium *(Continued)*

less variation in peak and trough serum levels; do not administer two 250 mg tablets as substitute for a 500 mg tablet

With prolonged therapy, monitor renal, hepatic, and hematologic function periodically

Stability: Reconstituted oral suspension should be kept in refrigerator; discard unused suspension after 10 days

Dosage Forms

Suspension, oral:

125 (banana flavor): Amoxicillin trihydrate 125 mg and clavulanate potassium 31.25 mg per 5 mL (75 mL, 100 mL, 150 mL)

200: Amoxicillin 200 mg and clavulanate potassium 28.5 mg per 5 mL (50 mL, 75 mL, 100 mL, 150 mL)

250 (orange flavor): Amoxicillin trihydrate 250 mg and clavulanate potassium 62.5 mg per 5 mL (75 mL, 100 mL, 150 mL)

400: Amoxicillin 400 mg and clavulanate potassium 57 mg per 5 mL (50 mL, 75 mL, 100 mL)

Tablet:

250: Amoxicillin trihydrate 250 mg and clavulanate potassium 125 mg

500: Amoxicillin trihydrate 500 mg and clavulanate potassium 125 mg

875: Amoxicillin trihydrate 875 mg and clavulanate potassium 125 mg

Tablet, chewable:

125: Amoxicillin trihydrate 125 mg and clavulanate potassium 31.25 mg

200: Amoxicillin trihydrate 200 mg and clavulanate potassium 28.5 mg

250: Amoxicillin trihydrate 250 mg and clavulanate potassium 62.5 mg

400: Amoxicillin trihydrate 400 mg and clavulanate potassium 57 mg

- ♦ **amoxicillin and clavulanic acid** *see* amoxicillin and clavulanate potassium *on page 43*
- ♦ **Amoxifur** *see* amoxicillin *on page 43*
- ♦ **Amoxil®** *see* amoxicillin *on page 43*
- ♦ **Amoxisol** *see* amoxicillin *on page 43*
- ♦ **Amoxivet** *see* amoxicillin *on page 43*
- ♦ **amoxycillin** *see* amoxicillin *on page 43*
- ♦ **Amphojel® [OTC]** *see* aluminum hydroxide *on page 33*
- ♦ **Amphotec®** *see* amphotericin B cholesteryl sulfate complex *on page 44*

amphotericin B cholesteryl sulfate complex

(am foe TER i sin bee kole LES te ril SUL fate KOM plecks)

Synonyms ABCD; amphotericin B colloidal dispersion

U.S. Brand Names Amphotec®

Generic Available No

Therapeutic Category Antifungal Agent

Use Effective in the treatment of invasive mycoses in patient refractory to or intolerant of conventional amphotericin B

Usual Dosage Children and Adults: 3-4 mg/kg/day I.V. (infusion of 1 mg/kg/hour); maximum: 7.5 mg/kg/day; duration of therapy is often <6 weeks

Nursing/Pharmacy Information May premedicate with acetaminophen and diphenhydramine 30 minutes prior to infusion; meperidine may help reduce rigors; avoid injection faster than 1 mg/kg/hour

Dosage Forms Suspension for injection: 50 mg, 100 mg

- ♦ **amphotericin B colloidal dispersion** *see* amphotericin B cholesteryl sulfate complex *on page 44*

amphotericin B (conventional) (am foe TER i sin bee)

U.S. Brand Names Fungizone®

Generic Available Yes

Therapeutic Category Antifungal Agent

Use Treatment of severe systemic infections and meningitis caused by susceptible fungi such as *Candida* species, *Histoplasma capsulatum*, *Cryptococcus neoformans*, *Aspergillus* species, *Blastomyces dermatitidis*, *Torulopsis glabrata*, and *Coccidioides immitis*; fungal peritonitis; irrigant for bladder fungal infections; and topically for cutaneous and mucocutaneous candidal infections

Usual Dosage

I.V.:

Infants and Children:

Test dose (not required): I.V.: 0.1 mg/kg/dose to a maximum of 1 mg; infuse over 30-60 minutes

Initial therapeutic dose: 0.25 mg/kg gradually increased, usually in 0.25 mg/kg increments on each subsequent day, until the desired daily dose is reached

Maintenance dose: 0.25-1 mg/kg/day given once daily; infuse over 2-6 hours. Once therapy has been established, amphotericin B can be administered on an every other day basis at 1-1.5 mg/kg/dose; cumulative dose: 1.5-2 g over 6-10 week

Adults:

Test dose (not required): 1 mg infused over 20-30 minutes

Initial dose: 0.25 mg/kg administered over 2-6 hours, gradually increased on subsequent days to the desired level by 0.25 mg/kg increments per day; in critically ill patients, may initiate with 1-1.5 mg/kg/day with close observation

Maintenance dose: 0.25-1 mg/kg/day or 1.5 mg/kg over 4-6 hours every other day; do not exceed 1.5 mg/kg/day; cumulative dose: 1-4 g over 4-10 weeks

Duration of therapy varies with nature of infection: histoplasmosis, *Cryptococcus*, or blastomycosis may be treated with total dose of 2-4 g

I.T.:

Children.: 25-100 mcg every 48-72 hours; increase to 500 mcg as tolerated

Adults: 25-300 mcg every 48-72 hours; increase to 500 mcg to 1 mg as tolerated

Oral: 1 mL (100 mg) 4 times daily

Topical: Apply to affected areas 2-4 times/day for 1-4 weeks of therapy depending on nature and severity of infection

Administration in dialysate: Children and Adults: 1-2 mg/L of peritoneal dialysis fluid either with or without low-dose I.V. amphotericin B (a total dose of 2-10 mg/kg given over 7-14 days)

Administration via bladder irrigation: Children and Adults: 50 mg/day in 1 L of sterile water irrigation solution instilled over 24 hours for 2-7 days or until cultures are clear

Nursing/Pharmacy Information

Cardiovascular collapse has been reported after rapid amphotericin injection; may premedicate patients who experience mild adverse reactions with acetaminophen and diphenhydramine 30 minutes prior to the amphotericin infusion. Meperidine may help to reduce rigors. Amphotericin is administered by I.V. infusion over 2-6 hours at a final concentration not to exceed 0.1 mg/mL; in patients unable to tolerate a large fluid volume, amphotericin B 0.25 mg/mL in D_5W administered through a central venous catheter is the highest concentration reported to have been administered

Monitor electrolytes, BUN, serum creatinine, hematocrit, liver function tests, CBC regularly; monitor I & O; monitor for signs of hypokalemia (muscle weakness, cramping, drowsiness, EKG changes, etc)

Stability: Reconstitute only with sterile water without preservatives, not bacteriostatic water; benzyl alcohol, sodium chloride, or other electrolyte solutions may cause precipitation; for I.V. infusion, an in-line filter (>1 micron mean pore diameter) may be used; short-term exposure (<24 hours) to light during I.V. infusion does **not** appreciably affect potency

Dosage Forms

Cream: 3% (20 g)

Lotion: 3% (30 mL)

Powder for injection, lyophilized, as deoxycholate: 50 mg

Suspension, oral: 100 mg/mL (24 mL with dropper)

amphotericin B lipid complex

(am foe TER i sin bee LIP id KOM pleks)

Synonyms ABLC

U.S. Brand Names Abelcet™

Generic Available No

Therapeutic Category Antifungal Agent

Use Treatment of aspergillosis in patients who are refractory to or intolerant of conventional amphotericin B therapy. This indication is based on results obtained primarily from emergency use studies for the treatment of aspergillosis; orphan drug status for cryptococcal meningitis

Usual Dosage Children and Adults: I.V.: 2.5-5 mg/kg/day as a single infusion

Note: Significantly higher dose of ABLC are tolerated; it appears that attaining higher doses with ABLC produce more rapid fungicidal activity *in vivo* than standard amphotericin B preparations

(Continued)

amphotericin B lipid complex *(Continued)*

Nursing/Pharmacy Information I.V. therapy may take several months; personal hygiene is very important to help reduce the spread and recurrence of lesions; most skin lesions require 1-3 weeks of therapy; report any hearing loss

Dosage Forms Injection: 5 mg/mL (20 mL)

amphotericin B liposomal *(am foe TER i sin bee lye po SO mal)*

Synonyms L-AmB

U.S. Brand Names AmBisome®

Generic Available No

Therapeutic Category Antifungal Agent, Systemic

Use Empirical therapy for presumed fungal infection in febrile, neutropenic patients. Treatment of patients with *Aspergillus* species, *Candida* species and/or *Cryptococcus* species infections refractory to amphotericin B deoxycholate, or in patients where renal impairment or unacceptable toxicity precludes the use of amphotericin B deoxycholate. Treatment of visceral leishmaniasis. In immunocompromised patients with visceral leishmaniasis treated with AmBisome, relapse rates were high following initial clearance of parasites

Usual Dosage Children and Adults: I.V.:

Empirical therapy: Recommended initial dose of 3 mg/kg/day

Systemic fungal infections (*Aspergillus*, *Candida*, *Cryptococcus*): Recommended initial dose of 3-5 mg/kg/day

Treatment of visceral leishmaniasis: AmBisome® achieved high rates of acute parasite clearance in immunocompetent patients when total doses of 12-30 mg/kg were administered. Most of these immunocompetent patients remained relapse-free during follow-up periods of 6 months or longer. While acute parasite clearance was achieved in most of the immunocompromised patients who received total doses of 30-40 mg/kg, the majority of these patients were observed to relapse in the 6 months following the completion of therapy.

Dosage Forms Injection: 50 mg

ampicillin *(am pi SIL in)*

Synonyms aminobenzylpenicillin

U.S. Brand Names Marcillin®; Omnipen®; Omnipen®-N; Principen®; Totacillin®

Canadian Brand Names Ampicin®; Apo-Ampi®; Jaa Amp®; Nu-Ampi; Pro-Ampi®; Taro-Ampicillin®

Mexican Brand Names Anglopen; Binotal; Dibacilina; Flamicina; Lampicin; Marovilina®; Pentrexyl; Sinaplin

Generic Available Yes

Therapeutic Category Penicillin

Use Treatment of susceptible bacterial infections caused by streptococci, pneumococci, nonpenicillinase-producing staphylococci, *Listeria*, meningococci; some strains of *H. influenzae*, *Salmonella*, *Shigella*, *E. coli*, *Enterobacter*, and *Klebsiella*

Usual Dosage

Infants and Children:

Oral: 50-100 mg/kg/day divided every 6 hours; maximum dose: 2-3 g/day

I.M., I.V.: 100-200 mg/kg/day in 4-6 divided doses; meningitis: 200-400 mg/kg/day in 4-6 divided doses; maximum dose: 12 g/day

Adults:

Oral: 250-500 mg every 6 hours

I.M., I.V.: 8-12 g/day in 4-6 divided doses

Dietary Considerations Should be administered on an empty stomach (at least 1 hour before or 2 hours after eating) with a full glass of water (8 oz) unless otherwise directed; food decreases rate and extent of absorption

Nursing/Pharmacy Information

Ampicillin and gentamicin should not be mixed in the same I.V. tubing or administered concurrently; ampicillin can be administered IVP over 3-5 minutes at a rate not to exceed 100 mg/minute or I.V. intermittent infusion over 15-30 minutes; final concentration for I.V. administration should not exceed 100 mg/mL (IVP) or 30 mg/mL (I.V. intermittent infusion)

With prolonged therapy, monitor renal, hepatic, and hematologic function periodically

Stability: Oral suspension is stable for 7 days at room temperature or for 14 days under refrigeration; solutions for I.M. or direct I.V. should be used within 1 hour; solutions for I.V. infusion will be inactivated by dextrose at room temperature; if dextrose-containing solutions are to be used, the resultant solution will only be stable for 2 hours versus 8 hours in the 0.9% sodium chloride injection. D_5W has limited stability.

Minimum volume: Concentration should not exceed 30 mg/mL; manufacturer may supply as either the anhydrous or the trihydrate form

Dosage Forms
Capsule, as anhydrous: 250 mg, 500 mg
Capsule, as trihydrate: 250 mg, 500 mg
Powder for injection, as sodium: 125 mg, 250 mg, 500 mg, 1 g, 2 g, 10 g
Powder for oral suspension, as trihydrate: 125 mg/5 mL (100 mL, 150 mL, 200 mL); 250 mg/5 mL (100 mL, 150 mL, 200 mL)

ampicillin and sulbactam (am pi SIL in & SUL bak tam)

Synonyms sulbactam and ampicillin
U.S. Brand Names Unasyn®
Mexican Brand Names Unasyna; Unasyna Oral
Generic Available No
Therapeutic Category Penicillin
Use Treatment of susceptible bacterial infections involved with skin and skin structure, intra-abdominal infections, gynecological infections; spectrum is that of ampicillin plus organisms producing beta-lactamases such as *S. aureus, H. influenzae, E. coli, Klebsiella, Acinetobacter, Enterobacter* and anaerobes
Usual Dosage Unasyn® (ampicillin/sulbactam) is a combination product. Each 3 g vial contains 2 g of ampicillin and 1 g of sulbactam. Sulbactam has very little antibacterial activity by itself, but effectively extends the spectrum of ampicillin to include beta-lactamase producing strains that are resistant to ampicillin alone. Therefore, dosage recommendations for Unasyn® are based on the ampicillin component.

I.M., I.V.:
Children: 100-200 mg ampicillin/kg/day (150-300 mg Unasyn®) divided every 6 hours; maximum dose: 8 g ampicillin/day (12 g Unasyn®)
Adults: 1-2 g ampicillin (1.5-3 g Unasyn®) every 6-8 hours; maximum dose: 8 g ampicillin/day (12 g Unasyn®)

Nursing/Pharmacy Information
Do culture and sensitivity (C&S) before starting therapy; keep resuscitation equipment, epinephrine, and antihistamine close by in the event of an anaphylactic reaction; observe for superinfection; for I.M. injection reconstitute with sterile water or 0.5% or 2% lidocaine hydrochloride. Reduce dose with decreased renal function. Can be administered by slow I.V. injection over 10-15 minutes at a final concentration for administration not to exceed 45 mg Unasyn® (30 mg ampicillin and 15 mg sulbactam)/mL

Observe patient for signs and symptoms of hypersensitivity; with prolonged therapy, monitor hematologic, renal, and hepatic function

Stability: I.M. and direct I.V. administration: Use within 1 hour after preparation; reconstitute with sterile water for injection or 0.5% or 2% lidocaine hydrochloride injection (I.M.); sodium chloride 0.9% (NS) is the diluent of choice for I.V. piggyback use, solutions made in normal saline are stable up to 72 hours when refrigerated whereas dextrose solutions (same concentration) are stable for only 4 hours

Dosage Forms Powder for injection: 1.5 g [ampicillin sodium 1 g and sulbactam sodium 0.5 g]; 3 g [ampicillin sodium 2 g and sulbactam sodium 1 g]; 15 g [ampicillin sodium 10 g and sulbactam sodium 5 g]

♦ **Ampicin®** see ampicillin on page 46

amprenavir *New Drug* (am PRE na veer)
U.S. Brand Names Agenerase™
Generic Available No
Therapeutic Category Protease Inhibitor
Use Treatment of HIV infections in combination with at least two other antiretroviral agents
Usual Dosage Adults: Oral: 1200 mg twice daily
Dosage Forms
Capsule: 50 mg, 150 mg
Solution, oral: 15 mg/mL (240 mL)

♦ **AMPT** see metyrosine on page 412

amrinone (AM ri none)
U.S. Brand Names Inocor®
Generic Available Yes
Therapeutic Category Adrenergic Agonist Agent
Use Treatment of low cardiac output states (sepsis, congestive heart failure); adjunctive therapy of pulmonary hypertension
(Continued)

amrinone *(Continued)*

Usual Dosage Dosage is based on clinical response. **Note:** Dose should not exceed 10 mg/kg/24 hours.

Children: 0.75 mg/kg I.V. bolus over 2-3 minutes followed by maintenance infusion 5-10 mcg/kg/minute; I.V. bolus may need to be repeated in 30 minutes

Adults: 0.75 mg/kg I.V. bolus over 2-3 minutes followed by maintenance infusion of 5-10 mcg/kg/minute

Nursing/Pharmacy Information

Do **not** "Y" furosemide IVP into amrinone solutions; may be administered undiluted for I.V. bolus doses. For continuous infusion: Dilute with 0.45% or 0.9% sodium chloride to final concentration of 1-3 mg/mL use within 24 hours.

Monitor cardiac index, stroke volume, systemic vascular resistance, and pulmonary vascular resistance (if Swan-Ganz catheter available); CVP, SBP, DBP, heart rate, platelet count, CBC, liver function and renal function tests

Stability: May be administered undiluted for I.V. bolus doses. For continuous infusion: Dilute with 0.45% or 0.9% sodium chloride to final concentration of 1-3 mg/mL; use within 24 hours; do not directly dilute with dextrose-containing solutions, chemical interaction occurs; may be administered I.V. into running dextrose infusions. Furosemide forms a precipitate when injected in I.V. lines containing amrinone.

Dosage Forms Injection, as lactate: 5 mg/mL (20 mL)

- **Amvisc®** *see* sodium hyaluronate *on page 572*
- **Amvisc® Plus** *see* sodium hyaluronate *on page 572*
- **Amyl Nitrate Vaporole®** *see* amyl nitrite *on page 48*

amyl nitrite *(AM il NYE trite)*

Synonyms isoamyl nitrite
U.S. Brand Names Amyl Nitrate Vaporole®; Amyl Nitrite Aspirols®
Generic Available Yes
Therapeutic Category Vasodilator
Use Coronary vasodilator in angina pectoris; an adjunct in treatment of cyanide poisoning; also used to produce changes in the intensity of heart murmurs
Usual Dosage 1-6 inhalations from 1 capsule are usually sufficient to produce the desired effect
Nursing/Pharmacy Information
Monitor blood pressure during therapy
Stability: Store in cool place; protect from light
Dosage Forms Inhalant, crushable glass perles: 0.3 mL

- **Amyl Nitrite Aspirols®** *see* amyl nitrite *on page 48*
- **amylobarbitone** *see* amobarbital *on page 42*
- **Amytal®** *see* amobarbital *on page 42*
- **Anabolin®** *see* nandrolone *on page 431*
- **Anacin® [OTC]** *see* aspirin *on page 61*
- **Anacin-3® (all Products) *(Discontinued)*** *see page 743*
- **Anadrol®** *see* oxymetholone *on page 464*
- **Anafranil®** *see* clomipramine *on page 159*

anagrelide *(an AG gre lide)*

U.S. Brand Names Agrylin™
Generic Available No
Therapeutic Category Platelet Aggregation Inhibitor
Use Agent for essential thrombocythemia (ET)
Usual Dosage Adults: Oral: 0.5 mg 4 times/day or 1 mg twice daily, maintain for ≥1 week, then adjust to the lowest effective dose to reduce and maintain platelet count <600,000 μL ideally to the normal range
Dosage Forms Capsule, as hydrochloride: 0.5 mg

- **Anaids® Tablet *(Discontinued)*** *see page 743*
- **Ana-Kit®** *see* insect sting kit *on page 339*
- **Analphen** *see* acetaminophen *on page 13*
- **Anamine® Syrup [OTC]** *see* chlorpheniramine and pseudoephedrine *on page 140*
- **Anandron®** *see* nilutamide *on page 443*
- **Anapenil** *see* penicillin V potassium *on page 476*
- **Anaplex® Liquid [OTC]** *see* chlorpheniramine and pseudoephedrine *on page 140*

- **Anapolon®** *see* oxymetholone *on page 464*
- **Anaprox®** *see* naproxen *on page 432*
- **Anapsique** *see* amitriptyline *on page 40*
- **Anaspaz®** *see* hyoscyamine *on page 329*

anastrozole (an AS troe zole)

U.S. Brand Names Arimidex®
Generic Available No
Therapeutic Category Antineoplastic Agent
Use Treatment of advanced breast cancer in postmenopausal women with disease progression following tamoxifen therapy. Patients with ER-negative disease and patients who did not respond to tamoxifen therapy rarely responded to anastrozole.
Usual Dosage Breast cancer: Adults: Oral (refer to individual protocols): 1 mg once daily
Nursing/Pharmacy Information Use with caution in patients with hyperlipidemias; mean serum total cholesterol and LDL cholesterol occurs in patients receiving anastrozole
Dosage Forms Tablet: 1 mg

- **Anatrast®** *see* radiological/contrast media (ionic) *on page 539*
- **Anatuss® [OTC]** *see* guaifenesin, phenylpropanolamine, and dextromethorphan *on page 303*
- **Anatuss® DM [OTC]** *see* guaifenesin, pseudoephedrine, and dextromethorphan *on page 304*
- **Anbesol® [OTC]** *see* benzocaine *on page 79*
- **Anbesol® Maximum Strength [OTC]** *see* benzocaine *on page 79*
- **Ancef®** *see* cefazolin *on page 120*
- **Ancobon®** *see* flucytosine *on page 271*
- **Ancotil®** *see* flucytosine *on page 271*

ancrod (AN krod)

Canadian Brand Names Viprinex®
Generic Available No
Therapeutic Category Anticoagulant
Use Safe for anticoagulation of patients with heparin induced thrombocytopenia (HIT syndrome); to establish and maintain anticoagulation in herparin-intolerant patients undergoing cardiopulmonary bypass; drug derived from the venom of Malaysian pit vipers that appears to be effective in increasing recovery rates from stroke (U.S. orphan drug)
Usual Dosage Adults: I.V.:
Bolus: 1-2 int. units/kg over 8-12 hours
Maintenance dose: 0.5-1 int. units/kg over 6-24 hours to maintain fibrinogen levels 0.2-0.7 g/L; may be given as intermittent I.V. injections every 12 hours or as continuous infusion; should not be given I.M. as it may induce antibody formation
Dosage Forms Injection: 70 int. units/mL (1 mL)

- **Androcur®** *see* cyproterone *(Canada only) on page 177*
- **Androcur® Depot** *see* cyproterone *(Canada only) on page 177*
- **Androderm® Transdermal System** *see* testosterone *on page 598*
- **Andro/Fem®** *see* estradiol and testosterone *on page 243*
- **Android®** *see* methyltestosterone *on page 408*
- **Andro-L.A.® Injection** *see* testosterone *on page 598*
- **Androlone®** *see* nandrolone *on page 431*
- **Androlone®-D** *see* nandrolone *on page 431*
- **Andropository® Injection** *see* testosterone *on page 598*
- **Anectine® Chloride** *see* succinylcholine *on page 582*
- **Anectine® Flo-Pack®** *see* succinylcholine *on page 582*
- **Anergan® 25 Injection *(Discontinued)*** *see page 743*
- **Anestacon® Topical Solution** *see* lidocaine *on page 368*
- **aneurine** *see* thiamine *on page 606*
- **Anexate®** *see* flumazenil *on page 272*
- **Anexsia®** *see* hydrocodone and acetaminophen *on page 319*
- **Angio Conray®** *see* radiological/contrast media (ionic) *on page 539*
- **Angiotrofin** *see* diltiazem *on page 205*
- **Angiotrofin A.P.** *see* diltiazem *on page 205*
- **Angiotrofin Retard** *see* diltiazem *on page 205*
- **Angiovist®** *see* radiological/contrast media (ionic) *on page 539*

♦ **Anglix** *see* nitroglycerin *on page 444*
♦ **Anglopen** *see* ampicillin *on page 46*

anisotropine (an iss oh TROE peen)
Canadian Brand Names Miradon®
Generic Available Yes
Therapeutic Category Anticholinergic Agent
Use Adjunctive treatment of peptic ulcer
Usual Dosage Adults: Oral: 50 mg 3 times/day
Nursing/Pharmacy Information Monitor vital signs and I & O
Dosage Forms Tablet, as methylbromide: 50 mg

♦ **anisoylated plasminogen streptokinase activator complex** *see* anistreplase *on page 50*
♦ **Anistal** *see* ranitidine hydrochloride *on page 541*

anistreplase (a NISS tre plase)
Synonyms anisoylated plasminogen streptokinase activator complex; APSAC
U.S. Brand Names Eminase®
Generic Available No
Therapeutic Category Thrombolytic Agent
Use Management of acute myocardial infarction (AMI) in adults; lysis of thrombi obstructing coronary arteries, reduction of infarct size; and reduction of mortality associated with AMI
Usual Dosage Adults: I.V.: 30 units injected over 2-5 minutes as soon as possible after onset of symptoms
Nursing/Pharmacy Information
   Can be administered as a bolus and does not require a slow I.V. administration like t-PA or streptokinase; avoid I.M. injections and nonessential handling of patient after administration of drug; drug should not be used for any condition in which bleeding constitutes a significant hazard or would be particularly difficult to manage
   Stability: Discard solution 30 minutes after reconstitution if not administered; do not shake solution
Dosage Forms Powder for injection, lyophilized: 30 units

♦ **Anitrim** *see* co-trimoxazole *on page 170*
♦ **Anodynos-DHC®** *see* hydrocodone and acetaminophen *on page 319*
♦ **Anoquan®** *see* butalbital compound and acetaminophen *on page 99*
♦ **Anoxine-AM® Capsule** *(Discontinued) see page 743*
♦ **Ansaid® Oral** *see* flurbiprofen *on page 278*
♦ **ansamycin** *see* rifabutin *on page 548*
♦ **Antabuse®** *see* disulfiram *on page 213*
♦ **Antagon™** *see* ganirelix *New Drug on page 288*
♦ **Antalgin® Dialicels** *see* indomethacin *on page 337*
♦ **Antazoline-V® Ophthalmic** *see* naphazoline and antazoline *on page 431*
♦ **Antazone®** *see* sulfinpyrazone *on page 588*
♦ **Antepsin** *see* sucralfate *on page 583*
♦ **Anthra-Derm®** *see* anthralin *on page 50*
♦ **Anthraforte®** *see* anthralin *on page 50*

anthralin (AN thra lin)
Synonyms dithranol
U.S. Brand Names Anthra-Derm®; Drithocreme®; Drithocreme® HP 1%; Dritho-Scalp®; Micanol® Cream
Canadian Brand Names Anthraforte®; Anthranol®; Anthrascalp®
Mexican Brand Names Anthranol®
Generic Available Yes
Therapeutic Category Keratolytic Agent
Use Treatment of psoriasis
Usual Dosage Adults: Topical: Generally, apply once daily or as directed. The irritant potential of anthralin is directly related to the strength being used and each patient's individual tolerance. Always commence treatment for at least one week using the lowest strength possible.

   Skin application: Apply sparingly only to psoriatic lesions and rub gently and carefully into the skin until absorbed. Avoid applying an excessive quantity which may cause unnecessary soiling and staining of the clothing or bed linen.

Scalp application: Comb hair to remove scalar debris and, after suitably parting, rub cream well into the lesions, taking care to prevent the cream from spreading onto the forehead

Remove by washing or showering; optimal period of contact will vary according to the strength used and the patient's response to treatment. Continue treatment until the skin is entirely clear (ie, when there is nothing to feel with the fingers and the texture is normal)

Nursing/Pharmacy Information Wear gloves; can discolor skin, hair, or clothes

Dosage Forms Cream: 0.1% (50 g); 0.5% (50 g); 1% (50 g)

♦ **Anthranol®** *see* anthralin *on page 50*
♦ **Anthrascalp®** *see* anthralin *on page 50*

anthrax vaccine, adsorbed *New Drug*

(AN thraks vak SEEN ad SORBED)

Generic Available No

Therapeutic Category Vaccine

Use Recommended for individuals who may come in contact with animal products which come from anthrax endemic areas and may be contaminated with *Bacillus anthracis* spores; recommended for high-risk persons such as veterinarians and other handling potentially infected animals. Routine immunization for the general population is not recommended.

The Department of Defense is implementing an anthrax vaccination program against the biological warfare agent anthrax, which will be administered to all active duty and reserve personnel.

Usual Dosage

Primary immunization: S.C.: Three injections of 0.5 mL each given 2 weeks apart followed by three additional S.C. injections given at 6, 12, and 18 months

Subsequent booster injections: 0.5 mL at 1-year intervals are recommended for immunity to be maintained

Dosage Forms Injection: 5 mL (10 doses each)

♦ **Antiben®** *see* antipyrine and benzocaine *on page 53*
♦ **AntibiOtic® Otic** *see* neomycin, polymyxin B, and hydrocortisone *on page 437*
♦ **anti-CD20 monoclonal antibodies** *see* rituximab *on page 552*
♦ **antidigoxin Fab fragments** *see* digoxin immune Fab *on page 203*
♦ **antidiuretic hormone (ADH)** *see* vasopressin *on page 645*

antihemophilic factor (human)

(an tee hee moe FIL ik FAK tor HYU man)

Synonyms AHF; factor VIII

U.S. Brand Names Alphanate®; Hemofil® M; Koāte®-DVI; Koāte®-HP

Generic Available Yes

Therapeutic Category Blood Product Derivative

Use Management of hemophilia A in patients whom a deficiency in factor VIII has been demonstrated

Usual Dosage I.V.: Individualize dosage based on coagulation studies performed prior to and during treatment at regular intervals. One AHF unit is the activity present in 1 mL of normal pooled human plasma; dosage should be adjusted to actual vial size currently stocked in the pharmacy.

Hospitalized patients: 20-50 units/kg/dose; may be higher for special circumstances; dose can be administered every 12-24 hours and more frequently in special circumstances

Nursing/Pharmacy Information

Parenteral: I.V. administration only; maximum rate of administration is product dependent: Monoclate-P® 2 mL/minute; Humate-P® 4 mL/minute; administration of other products should not exceed 10 mL/minute; use filter needle to draw product into syringe; reduce rate of administration or temporarily discontinue if patient becomes tachycardiac

Monitor heart rate (before and during I.V. administration), antihemophilic factor levels

Stability: Dried concentrate should be refrigerated, but may be stored at room temperature for up to 6 months depending upon specific product; if refrigerated, the dried concentrate and diluent should be warmed to room temperature before reconstitution; gently agitate or rotate vial after adding diluent, do not shake vigorously; do **not** refrigerate after reconstitution, a precipitation

(Continued)

antihemophilic factor (human) *(Continued)*

may occur; administer within 3 hours after reconstitution; reconstituted solution is stable for 24 hours at room temperature; Method M, monoclonal purified products should be administered within 1 hour after reconstitution

Dosage Forms Injection: Dried concentrate of Factor VIII: 1 unit

antihemophilic factor (porcine)

(an tee hee moe FIL ik FAK ter POR seen)

U.S. Brand Names Hyate®:C

Generic Available No

Therapeutic Category Antihemophilic Agent

Use Treatment of congenital hemophiliacs with antibodies to human factor VIII:C and also for previously nonhemophiliac patients with spontaneously acquired inhibitors to human factor VIII:C; patients with inhibitors who are bleeding or who are to undergo surgery

Usual Dosage Clinical response should be used to assess efficacy rather than relying upon a particular laboratory value for recovery of factor VIII:C.

Initial dose:
Antibody level to human factor VIII:C <50 Bethesda units/mL: 100-150 porcine units/kg (body weight) is recommended
Antibody level to human factor VIII:C >50 Bethesda units/mL: Activity of the antibody to porcine factor VIII:C should be determined; **an antiporcine antibody level** >20 Bethesda units/mL indicates that the patient is unlikely to benefit from treatment; for lower titers, a dose of 100-150 porcine units/kg is recommended
If a patient has previously been treated with Hyate®:C, this may provide a guide to his likely response and, therefore, assist in estimation of the preliminary dose
Subsequent doses: Following administration of the initial dose, if the recovery of factor VIII:C in the patient's plasma is not sufficient, a further higher dose should be administered; if recovery after the second dose is still insufficient, a third and higher dose may prove effective

Nursing/Pharmacy Information
Sodium ion concentration is not more than 200 mmol/L; the assayed amount of activity is stated on the label, but may vary depending on the type of assay and hemophilic substrate plasma used
Stability: Store at temperature of -15°C to <20°C; use before expiration date; reconstituted Hyate®:C must not be stored, stable for 24 hours at room temperature

Dosage Forms Powder for injection, lyophilized: 400-700 porcine units to be reconstituted with 20 mL sterile water

antihemophilic factor (recombinant)

(an tee hee moe FIL ik FAK tor ree KOM be nant)

Synonyms factor VIII recombinant

U.S. Brand Names Bioclate®; Helixate®; Kogenate®; Recombinate®

Generic Available No

Therapeutic Category Blood Product Derivative

Use Management of hemophilia A in patients whom a deficiency in factor VIII has been demonstrated

Usual Dosage I.V.: Individualize dosage based on coagulation studies performed prior to and during treatment at regular intervals. One AHF unit is the activity present in 1 mL of normal pooled human plasma; dosage should be adjusted to actual vial size currently stocked in the pharmacy.

Hospitalized patients: 20-50 units/kg/dose; may be higher for special circumstances; dose can be administered every 12-24 hours and more frequently in special circumstances

Nursing/Pharmacy Information Monitor heart rate (before and during I.V. administration); plasma antihemophilic factor levels prior to and during treatment

Dosage Forms Injection: 250 units, 500 units, 1000 units

♦ **Antihist-1®** [OTC] *see* clemastine *on page 155*
♦ **Antihist-D®** *see* clemastine and phenylpropanolamine *on page 156*

anti-inhibitor coagulant complex

(an tee-in HI bi tor coe AG yoo lant KOM pleks)

Synonyms coagulant complex inhibitor

U.S. Brand Names Autoplex® T; Feiba VH Immuno®

Generic Available No

Therapeutic Category Hemophilic Agent

Use Patients with factor VIII inhibitors who are to undergo surgery or those who are bleeding

Usual Dosage Dosage range: I.V.: 25-100 factor VIII correctional units per kg depending on the severity of hemorrhage

Nursing/Pharmacy Information
Monitor hypotension
Stability: Store at 2°C to 8°C (36°F to 46°F); use within 1-3 hours after reconstitution

Dosage Forms Injection:
Autoplex® T, with heparin 2 units: Each bottle is labeled with correctional units of Factor VIII
Feiba VH Immuno®, heparin free: Each bottle is labeled with correctional units of Factor VIII

- ♦ **Antilirium®** *see* physostigmine *on page 492*
- ♦ **Antiminth® [OTC]** *see* pyrantel pamoate *on page 532*
- ♦ **Antinea® Cream** *(Discontinued) see page 743*

antipyrine and benzocaine (an tee PYE reen & BEN zoe kane)

Synonyms benzocaine and antipyrine

U.S. Brand Names Allergan® Ear Drops; Antiben®; Auralgan®; Aurodex®; Auroto®; Dolotic®

Generic Available Yes

Therapeutic Category Otic Agent, Analgesic; Otic Agent, Cerumenolytic

Use Temporary relief of pain and reduction of inflammation associated with acute congestive and serous otitis media, swimmer's ear, otitis externa; facilitates ear wax removal

Usual Dosage Otic: Fill ear canal; moisten cotton pledget, place in external ear, repeat every 1-2 hours until pain and congestion is relieved; for ear wax removal instill drops 3-4 times/day for 2-3 days

Nursing/Pharmacy Information Use of otic anesthetics may mask symptoms of a fulminating middle ear infection (acute otitis media); not intended for prolonged use

Dosage Forms Solution, otic: Antipyrine 5.4% and benzocaine 1.4% (10 mL, 15 mL)

antirabies serum (equine) (an tee RAY beez SEER um EE kwine)

Synonyms ARS

Generic Available No

Therapeutic Category Serum

Use Rabies prophylaxis

Usual Dosage I.M.: 1000 units/55 lb in a single dose, infiltrate up to 50% of dose around the wound

Nursing/Pharmacy Information Because of a significantly lower incidence of adverse reactions, Rabies Immune Globulin, Human is preferred over Antirabies Serum Equine; take careful history of asthma, angioneurotic edema, or other allergies

Dosage Forms Injection: 125 units/mL (8 mL)

- ♦ **Antispas® Injection** *see* dicyclomine *on page 199*

antithrombin III (an tee THROM bin three)

Synonyms ATIII; heparin cofactor I

U.S. Brand Names Thrombate III™

Generic Available No

Therapeutic Category Blood Product Derivative

Use Agent for hereditary antithrombin III deficiency

Usual Dosage After first dose of antithrombin III, level should increase to 120% of normal; thereafter maintain at levels >80%. Generally, achieved by administration of maintenance doses once every 24 hours; initially and until patient is stabilized, measure antithrombin III level at least twice daily, thereafter once daily and always immediately before next infusion.

Initial dosage (units) = [desired AT-III level % - baseline AT-III level %] x body weight (kg) divided by 1%/units/kg

Measure antithrombin III preceding and 30 minutes after dose to calculate *in vivo* recovery rate; maintain level within normal range for 2-8 days depending on type of surgery or procedure

Nursing/Pharmacy Information
Infuse over 5-10 minutes; rate of infusion: 50 units/minute (1 mL/minute) not to exceed 100 units/minute (2 mL/minute)
(Continued)

antithrombin III *(Continued)*

Stability: Reconstitute with 10 mL sterile water for injection, normal saline or D_5W; do not shake; I.V. admixture is stable for 24 hours at room temperature; do not refrigerate

Dosage Forms Powder for injection: 500 units (50 mL)

♦ **antithymocyte globulin (equine)** see lymphocyte immune globulin *on page 378*

antithymocyte globulin (rabbit) *New Drug*

(an te THY moe site GLOB yu lin RAB bit)

Generic Available No

Therapeutic Category Immunosuppressant Agent

Use Treatment of acute moderate-to-severe renal allograft rejection

Usual Dosage Adults: I.V.: Treatment of acute renal allograft rejection: 1.5 mg/kg/day for 7-14 days.

Dosage Forms Each package contains two 7 mL vials:
Vial 1: antithymocyte globulin (rabbit) 25 mg
Vial 2: Diluent (sterile water for injection) >5 mL

♦ **Anti-Tuss® Expectorant [OTC]** see guaifenesin *on page 299*

antivenin (*Crotalidae*) polyvalent

(an tee VEN in (kroe TAL ih die) pol i VAY lent)

Synonyms crotaline antivenin, polyvalent; North and South American antisnake-bite serum; pit vipers antivenin; snake (pit vipers) antivenin

Generic Available No

Therapeutic Category Antivenin

Use Neutralization of venoms of North and South American crotalids: rattlesnake, copperhead, cottonmouth, tropical moccasins, fer-de-lance, bushmaster

Usual Dosage Initial intradermal sensitivity test. The entire initial dose of antivenin should be administered as soon as possible to be most effective (within 4 hours after the bite).

Children and Adults: I.V.: Minimal envenomation: 20-40 mL; moderate envenomation: 50-90 mL; severe envenomation: 100-150 mL

Additional doses of antivenin is based on clinical response to the initial dose. If swelling continues to progress, symptoms increase in severity, hypotension occurs, or decrease in hematocrit appears, an additional 10-50 mL should be administered.

For I.V. infusion: 1:1-1:10 dilution of reconstituted antivenin in normal saline or D_5W should be prepared. Infuse the initial 5-10 mL of diluted antivenin over 3-5 minutes monitoring closely for signs of sensitivity reactions.

Nursing/Pharmacy Information

Do not inject into a finger or toe; epinephrine should be available. Antivenin may be administered I.M. for minimal envenomation. I.V. administration of antivenin is preferred for moderate to severe envenomation or in the presence of shock; for I.V. infusion, prepare a 1:1 to 1:10 dilution of reconstituted antivenin in normal saline or D_5W; infuse the initial 5-10 mL dilution over 3-5 minutes while carefully observing the patient for signs and symptoms of sensitivity reactions. If no reaction occurs, continue infusion at a safe I.V. fluid delivery rate.

Monitor vital signs, hematocrit

Stability: Store in refrigerator, avoid temperatures >37°C; reconstituted solutions should be used within 48 hours

Dosage Forms Injection: Lyophilized serum, diluent (10 mL); one vacuum vial to yield 10 mL of serum

antivenin (*Latrodectus mactans*)

(an tee VEN in lak tro DUK tus MAK tans)

Synonyms black widow spider antivenin (*Latrodectus mactans*); *Latrodectus mactans* antivenin

Generic Available No

Therapeutic Category Antivenin

Use Treat patients with symptoms of black widow spider bites

Usual Dosage

Children <12 years (severe or shock): I.V.: 2.5 mL in 10-50 mL over 15 minutes

Children and Adults: I.M.: 2.5 mL

Nursing/Pharmacy Information

Do not inject into a finger or toe; epinephrine should be available. Desensitization may need to be performed on patients with positive skin test reaction or history of sensitivity to equine serum; 1% of patients with negative skin test may still react when antivenin is administered; skin test should not be done in patients with mild reactions to the spider bite.

Stability: Refrigerate

Dosage Forms Powder for injection: 6000 antivenin units (2.5 mL)

antivenin (*Micrurus fulvius*)
(an tee VEN in mye KRU rus FUL vee us)

Synonyms North American coral snake antivenin

Generic Available No

Therapeutic Category Antivenin

Use Neutralize the venom of Eastern coral snake and Texas coral snake but does not neutralize venom of Arizona or Sonoran coral snake

Usual Dosage I.V.: 3-5 vials by slow injection

Nursing/Pharmacy Information

Supportive therapy: Appropriate tetanus prophylaxis is indicated; morphine or other narcotics that depress respiration are contraindicated; use sedatives with extreme caution

Stability: Avoid temperatures >37°C; reconstituted solutions should be used within 48 hours

Dosage Forms Injection: One vial antivenin and one vial diluent

♦ **Antivert®** see meclizine *on page 387*
♦ **Antivert® Chewable Tablet** *(Discontinued)* see page 743
♦ **Antizol™** see fomepizole *on page 282*
♦ **Antrizine®** see meclizine *on page 387*
♦ **Antrocol® Capsule & Tablet** *(Discontinued)* see page 743
♦ **Anturan®** see sulfinpyrazone *on page 588*
♦ **Anturane®** see sulfinpyrazone *on page 588*
♦ **Anusol® HC-1 Topical [OTC]** see hydrocortisone (topical) *on page 324*
♦ **Anusol® HC-2.5% Topical [OTC]** see hydrocortisone (topical) *on page 324*
♦ **Anusol-HC® Suppository** see hydrocortisone (rectal) *on page 322*
♦ **Anusol® Ointment [OTC]** see pramoxine *on page 512*
♦ **Anxanil® Oral** see hydroxyzine *on page 328*
♦ **Anzemet®** see dolasetron *on page 216*
♦ **Apacet® [OTC]** see acetaminophen *on page 13*
♦ **APAP** see acetaminophen *on page 13*
♦ **Apatate® [OTC]** see vitamin B complex *on page 651*
♦ **Aphrodyne™** see yohimbine *on page 657*
♦ **Aphthasol™** see amlexanox *on page 41*
♦ **A.P.L.®** see chorionic gonadotropin *on page 149*
♦ **Aplisol®** see tuberculin tests *on page 635*
♦ **Aplitest®** see tuberculin tests *on page 635*
♦ **Apo®-Acetazolamide** see acetazolamide *on page 17*
♦ **Apo®-Allopurinol** see allopurinol *on page 29*
♦ **Apo®-Alpraz** see alprazolam *on page 30*
♦ **Apo®-Amitriptyline** see amitriptyline *on page 40*
♦ **Apo-Amoxi®** see amoxicillin *on page 43*
♦ **Apo-Ampi®** see ampicillin *on page 46*
♦ **Apo®-ASA** see aspirin *on page 61*
♦ **Apo®-Atenol** see atenolol *on page 63*
♦ **Apo®-Bisacodyl** see bisacodyl *on page 88*
♦ **Apo® Bromocriptine** see bromocriptine *on page 93*
♦ **Apo®-C** see ascorbic acid *on page 60*
♦ **Apo-Cal®** see calcium carbonate *on page 103*
♦ **Apo®-Capto** see captopril *on page 110*
♦ **Apo®-Carbamazepine** see carbamazepine *on page 112*
♦ **Apo®-Cephalex** see cephalexin *on page 128*
♦ **Apo®-Chlordiazepoxide** see chlordiazepoxide *on page 134*
♦ **Apo®-Chlorpromazine** see chlorpromazine *on page 144*
♦ **Apo-Chlorpropamide®** see chlorpropamide *on page 145*
♦ **Apo-Chlorthalidone®** see chlorthalidone *on page 146*
♦ **Apo®-Cimetidine** see cimetidine *on page 150*
♦ **Apo-Clomipramine®** see clomipramine *on page 159*
♦ **Apo®-Clonidine** see clonidine *on page 159*
♦ **Apo®-Clorazepate** see clorazepate *on page 160*

- **Apo®-Cloxi** *see* cloxacillin *on page 161*
- **Apo®-Diazepam** *see* diazepam *on page 196*
- **Apo®-Diclo** *see* diclofenac *on page 198*
- **Apo-Diflunisal®** *see* diflunisal *on page 202*
- **Apo®-Diltiaz** *see* diltiazem *on page 205*
- **Apo®-Dimenhydrinate** *see* dimenhydrinate *on page 206*
- **Apo®-Dipyridamole FC** *see* dipyridamole *on page 212*
- **Apo®-Dipyridamole SC** *see* dipyridamole *on page 212*
- **Apo®-Doxepin** *see* doxepin *on page 219*
- **Apo®-Doxy** *see* doxycycline *on page 222*
- **Apo®-Doxy Tabs** *see* doxycycline *on page 222*
- **Apo®-Enalapril** *see* enalapril *on page 230*
- **Apo®-Erythro E-C** *see* erythromycin (systemic) *on page 240*
- **Apo-Famotidine** *see* famotidine *on page 259*
- **Apo-Ferrous® Gluconate** *see* ferrous gluconate *on page 265*
- **Apo-Ferrous® Sulfate** *see* ferrous sulfate *on page 265*
- **Apo®-Fluphenazine** *see* fluphenazine *on page 277*
- **Apo®-Flurazepam** *see* flurazepam *on page 278*
- **Apo®-Folic** *see* folic acid *on page 281*
- **Apo®-Furosemide** *see* furosemide *on page 285*
- **Apo®-Gain** *see* minoxidil *on page 417*
- **Apo-Gemfibrozil®** *see* gemfibrozil *on page 289*
- **Apo-Glyburide®** *see* glyburide *on page 294*
- **Apo-Guanethidine®** *see* guanethidine *on page 305*
- **Apo®-Hydralazine** *see* hydralazine *on page 316*
- **Apo®-Hydro** *see* hydrochlorothiazide *on page 317*
- **Apo®-Hydroxyzine** *see* hydroxyzine *on page 328*
- **Apo®-Imipramine** *see* imipramine *on page 334*
- **Apo®-Indomethacin** *see* indomethacin *on page 337*
- **Apo-ISDN®** *see* isosorbide dinitrate *on page 349*
- **Apo-Keto-E®** *see* ketoprofen *on page 355*
- **Apo®-Lorazepam** *see* lorazepam *on page 375*
- **Apo-Meprobamate®** *see* meprobamate *on page 394*
- **Apo®-Methyldopa** *see* methyldopa *on page 406*
- **Apo®-Metoclop** *see* metoclopramide *on page 409*
- **Apo-Metoprolol®** *see* metoprolol *on page 410*
- **Apo®-Metronidazole** *see* metronidazole *on page 411*
- **Apo-Minocycline®** *see* minocycline *on page 416*
- **Apomorphine *(Discontinued)*** *see page 743*
- **Apo®-Nadol** *see* nadolol *on page 427*
- **Apo®-Naproxen** *see* naproxen *on page 432*
- **Apo®-Nifed** *see* nifedipine *on page 442*
- **Apo®-Nitrofurantoin** *see* nitrofurantoin *on page 444*
- **Apo-Oxazepam®** *see* oxazepam *on page 460*
- **Apo-Pen VK** *see* penicillin V potassium *on page 476*
- **Apo-Pindol®** *see* pindolol *on page 495*
- **Apo®-Piroxicam** *see* piroxicam *on page 497*
- **Apo®-Prazo** *see* prazosin *on page 513*
- **Apo®-Prednisone** *see* prednisone *on page 515*
- **Apo®-Primidone** *see* primidone *on page 517*
- **Apo®-Procainamide** *see* procainamide *on page 518*
- **Apo®-Propranolol** *see* propranolol *on page 527*
- **Apo®-Ranitidine** *see* ranitidine hydrochloride *on page 541*
- **Apo®-Salvent** *see* albuterol *on page 25*
- **Apo®-Sulfamethoxazole** *see* sulfamethoxazole *on page 587*
- **Apo®-Sulfasalazine** *see* sulfasalazine *on page 587*
- **Apo®-Sulfatrim** *see* co-trimoxazole *on page 170*
- **Apo-Sulfinpyrazone®** *see* sulfinpyrazone *on page 588*
- **Apo®-Sulin** *see* sulindac *on page 589*
- **Apo-Tamox®** *see* tamoxifen *on page 592*
- **Apo®-Terfenadine** *see* terfenadine *on page 597*
- **Apo®-Tetra** *see* tetracycline *on page 601*
- **Apo®-Thioridazine** *see* thioridazine *on page 608*
- **Apo®-Timol** *see* timolol *on page 613*

- ◆ **Apo®-Timop** *see* timolol *on page 613*
- ◆ **Apo-Tolbutamide®** *see* tolbutamide *on page 617*
- ◆ **Apo-Triazide®** *see* hydrochlorothiazide and triamterene *on page 318*
- ◆ **Apo®-Triazo** *see* triazolam *on page 625*
- ◆ **Apo®-Trihex** *see* trihexyphenidyl *on page 628*
- ◆ **Apo-Trimip®** *see* trimipramine *on page 630*
- ◆ **Apo®-Verap** *see* verapamil *on page 646*
- ◆ **Apo®-Zidovudine** *see* zidovudine *on page 658*
- ◆ **APPG** *see* penicillin G procaine *on page 476*

apraclonidine (a pra KLOE ni deen)
U.S. Brand Names Iopidine®
Generic Available Yes
Therapeutic Category Alpha₂-Adrenergic Agonist Agent, Ophthalmic
Use 1%: Prevention and treatment of postsurgical intraocular pressure elevation; 0.5%: Short-term adjunctive therapy in patients on maximally tolerated medical therapy who require additional redirection of intraocular pressure
Usual Dosage Adults: Ophthalmic: Instill 1 drop in operative eye 1 hour prior to laser surgery, second drop in eye upon completion of procedure
Nursing/Pharmacy Information
Wait 5 minutes between instillation of other ophthalmic agents to avoid washout of previous dose; after topical instillation, finger pressure should be applied to lacrimal sac to decrease drainage into the nose and throat and minimize possible systemic absorption
Stability: Store in tight, light-resistant containers
Dosage Forms Solution, ophthalmic, as hydrochloride: 0.5% (5 mL, 10 mL); 1% (0.1 mL)

- ◆ **Apresazide®** *see* hydralazine and hydrochlorothiazide *on page 317*
- ◆ **Apresolina** *see* hydralazine *on page 316*
- ◆ **Apresoline®** *see* hydralazine *on page 316*
- ◆ **Aprodine® Syrup [OTC]** *see* triprolidine and pseudoephedrine *on page 632*
- ◆ **Aprodine® Tablet [OTC]** *see* triprolidine and pseudoephedrine *on page 632*
- ◆ **Aprodine® w/C** *see* triprolidine, pseudoephedrine, and codeine *on page 632*
- ◆ **Apro-Flurbiprofen®** *see* flurbiprofen *on page 278*

aprotinin (a proe TYE nin)
U.S. Brand Names Trasylol®
Generic Available No
Therapeutic Category Hemostatic Agent
Use Reduction or prevention of blood loss in patients undergoing coronary artery bypass surgery when a high index of suspicion of excessive bleeding potential exists; this includes open heart reoperation, pre-existing coagulopathy, operations on the great vessels, and patients whose religious beliefs prohibit blood transfusions
Usual Dosage Test dose: **All** patients should receive a 1 mL I.V. test dose at least 10 minutes prior to the loading dose to assess the potential for allergic reactions

Regimen A (standard dose):
2 million units (280 mg) loading dose I.V. over 20-30 minutes
2 million units (280 mg) into pump prime volume
500,000 units/hour (70 mg/hour) I.V. during operation
Regimen B (low dose):
1 million units (140 mg) loading dose I.V. over 20-30 minutes
1 million units (140 mg) into pump prime volume
250,000 units/hour (35 mg/hour) I.V. during operation
Nursing/Pharmacy Information All intravenous doses should be administered through a central line
Dosage Forms Injection: 1.4 mg/mL [10,000 units/mL] (100 mL, 200 mL)

- ◆ **Aprovel** *see* irbesartan *on page 345*
- ◆ **APSAC** *see* anistreplase *on page 50*
- ◆ **Aquacare® Topical [OTC]** *see* urea *on page 638*
- ◆ **Aquachloral® Supprettes®** *see* chloral hydrate *on page 132*
- ◆ **Aquacort®** *see* hydrocortisone (topical) *on page 324*
- ◆ **AquaMEPHYTON® Injection** *see* phytonadione *on page 493*
- ◆ **Aquaphyllin®** *see* theophylline *on page 603*
- ◆ **AquaSite® Ophthalmic Solution [OTC]** *see* artificial tears *on page 59*
- ◆ **Aquasol A®** *see* vitamin A *on page 650*

- **Aquasol E®** [OTC] *see* vitamin E *on page 652*
- **AquaTar®** [OTC] *see* coal tar *on page 162*
- **Aquatensen®** *see* methyclothiazide *on page 405*
- **aqueous procaine penicillin G** *see* penicillin G procaine *on page 476*
- **aqueous testosterone** *see* testosterone *on page 598*
- **Aquest®** *see* estrone *on page 246*
- **ARA-A** *see* vidarabine *on page 648*
- **arabinofuranosyladenine** *see* vidarabine *on page 648*
- **arabinosylcytosine** *see* cytarabine *on page 178*
- **ARA-C** *see* cytarabine *on page 178*
- **Aralen® Phosphate** *see* chloroquine phosphate *on page 136*
- **Aralen® Phosphate With Primaquine Phosphate** *see* chloroquine and primaquine *on page 136*
- **Aramine®** *see* metaraminol *on page 397*
- **Arava™** *see* leflunomide *on page 361*
- **Arcotinic® Tablet** *(Discontinued) see page 743*

ardeparin (ar dee PA rin)

U.S. Brand Names Normiflo®
Generic Available No
Therapeutic Category Anticoagulant
Use Prevention of deep vein thrombosis (DVT) which may lead to pulmonary embolism following knee replacement surgery
Usual Dosage Adults: S.C.: 50 anti-Xa units every 12 hours
Nursing/Pharmacy Information Administer by deep subcutaneous injection; do not give I.M.; patient should be sitting or lying down; may be injected into abdomen (avoid the navel), the anterior aspect of the thighs, or the outer aspect of the upper arms
Dosage Forms Injection, as sodium: Anti-Xa units 5000 (0.5 mL); Anti-Xa units 10,000 (0.5 mL)

- **Arduan®** *see* pipecuronium *on page 496*
- **Aredia™** *see* pamidronate *on page 466*
- **Argesic®-SA** *see* salsalate *on page 559*

arginine (AR ji neen)

U.S. Brand Names R-Gene®
Generic Available Yes
Therapeutic Category Diagnostic Agent
Use Pituitary function test (growth hormone); management of severe, uncompensated, metabolic alkalosis (pH $\geq$7.55) **after** optimizing therapy with sodium, potassium, or ammonium chloride supplements
Usual Dosage I.V.:
  Growth hormone (pituitary function) reserve test:
    Children: 500 mg (5 mL) kg/dose administered over 30 minutes
    Adults: 30 g (300 mL) administered over 30 minutes
  Metabolic alkalosis: Children and Adults: Usual dose: 10 g/hour
    Acid required (mEq) =
      [1] 0.2 (L/kg) x wt (kg) x [103 - serum chloride] (mEq/L) **or**
      [2] 0.3 (L/kg) x wt (kg) x base excess (mEq/L) **or**
      [3] 0.5 (L/kg) x wt (kg) x [serum HCO_3 - 24] (mEq/L)
    Administer 1/2 to 2/3 of calculated dose and re-evaluate

Note: Arginine hydrochloride should never be used as an alternative to chloride supplementation but used in the patient who is unresponsive to sodium chloride or potassium chloride supplementation
Nursing/Pharmacy Information
  I.V. infiltration of arginine may cause necrosis and phlebitis; may be infused without further dilution; maximum rate of I.V. infusion: 1 g/kg/hour (maximum: 60 g/hour)
  Monitor acid-base status (arterial or capillary blood gases), serum electrolytes (sodium, potassium, chloride, HCO_3^-), BUN, glucose
  Stability: Store at room temperature
Dosage Forms Injection, as hydrochloride: 10% [100 mg/mL = 950 mOsm/L] (500 mL)

- **8-arginine vasopressin** *see* vasopressin *on page 645*
- **Argyrol® S.S.** *(Discontinued) see page 743*
- **Aricept®** *see* donepezil *on page 217*
- **Arimidex®** *see* anastrozole *on page 49*

- **Aristocort® A Topical** *see* triamcinolone (topical) *on page 624*
- **Aristocort® Forte Injection** *see* triamcinolone (systemic) *on page 624*
- **Aristocort® Intralesional Injection** *see* triamcinolone (systemic) *on page 624*
- **Aristocort® Oral** *see* triamcinolone (systemic) *on page 624*
- **Aristocort® Topical** *see* triamcinolone (topical) *on page 624*
- **Aristospan® Intra-articular Injection** *see* triamcinolone (systemic) *on page 624*
- **Aristospan® Intralesional Injection** *see* triamcinolone (systemic) *on page 624*
- **Arlidin® *(Discontinued)*** *see page 743*
- **Arm-a-Med® Isoetharine** *see* isoetharine *on page 346*
- **Arm-a-Med® Isoproterenol** *see* isoproterenol *on page 348*
- **Arm-a-Med® Metaproterenol** *see* metaproterenol *on page 397*
- **A.R.M.® Caplet [OTC]** *see* chlorpheniramine and phenylpropanolamine *on page 139*
- **Armour® Thyroid** *see* thyroid *on page 610*
- **Aromasin®** *see* exemestane *New Drug on page 257*
- **Aromatic Ammonia Aspirols®** *see* ammonia spirit, aromatic *on page 41*
- **Arovit** *see* vitamin A *on page 650*
- **Arrestin®** *see* trimethobenzamide *on page 629*
- **ARS** *see* antirabies serum (equine) *on page 53*
- **Artane®** *see* trihexyphenidyl *on page 628*
- **Artha-G®** *see* salsalate *on page 559*
- **Arthritis Foundation® Ibuprofen *(Discontinued)*** *see page 743*
- **Arthritis Foundation® Nighttime *(Discontinued)*** *see page 743*
- **Arthritis Foundation® Pain Reliever, Aspirin Free *(Discontinued)*** *see page 743*
- **Arthritis Strength Bufferin® *(Discontinued)*** *see page 743*
- **Arthropan® [OTC]** *see* choline salicylate *on page 148*
- **Arthrotec®** *see* diclofenac and misoprostol *on page 199*
- **Articulose-50® Injection *(Discontinued)*** *see page 743*

artificial tears (ar ti FISH il tears)

Synonyms polyvinyl alcohol

U.S. Brand Names Adsorbotear® Ophthalmic Solution [OTC]; Akwa Tears® Solution [OTC]; AquaSite® Ophthalmic Solution [OTC]; Bion® Tears Solution [OTC]; Comfort® Tears Solution [OTC]; Dakrina® Ophthalmic Solution [OTC]; Dry Eye® Therapy Solution [OTC]; Dry Eyes® Solution [OTC]; Dwelle® Ophthalmic Solution [OTC]; Eye-Lube-A® Solution [OTC]; HypoTears PF Solution [OTC]; HypoTears Solution [OTC]; Isopto® Plain Solution [OTC]; Isopto® Tears Solution [OTC]; Just Tears® Solution [OTC]; Lacril® Ophthalmic Solution [OTC]; Liquifilm® Tears Solution [OTC]; Liquifilm® Forte Solution [OTC]; LubriTears® Solution [OTC]; Moisture® Ophthalmic Drops [OTC]; Murine® Solution [OTC]; Murocel® Ophthalmic Solution [OTC]; Nature's Tears® Solution [OTC]; Nu-Tears® Solution [OTC]; Nu-Tears® II Solution [OTC]; OcuCoat® Ophthalmic Solution [OTC]; OcuCoat® PF Ophthalmic Solution [OTC]; Puralube® Tears Solution [OTC]; Refresh® Ophthalmic Solution [OTC]; Refresh® Plus Ophthalmic Solution [OTC]; Tear Drop® Solution [OTC]; Tear-Gard® Ophthalmic Solution [OTC]; Teargen® Ophthalmic Solution [OTC]; Tearisol® Solution [OTC]; Tears Naturale® Free Solution [OTC]; Tears Naturale® II Solution [OTC]; Tears Naturale® Solution [OTC]; Tears Plus® Solution [OTC]; Tears Renewed® Solution [OTC]; Ultra Tears® Solution [OTC]; Viva-Drops® Solution [OTC]

Generic Available Yes

Therapeutic Category Ophthalmic Agent, Miscellaneous

Use Ophthalmic lubricant; relief of dry eyes and eye irritation

Usual Dosage Ophthalmic: Use as needed to relieve symptoms, 1-2 drops into eye(s) 3-4 times/day

Nursing/Pharmacy Information Not for use with soft contact lenses

Dosage Forms Solution, ophthalmic: 15 mL and 30 mL with dropper

- **Artosin** *see* tolbutamide *on page 617*
- **Artrenac** *see* diclofenac *on page 198*
- **Artron** *see* naproxen *on page 432*
- **Artyflam** *see* piroxicam *on page 497*
- **A.S.A. [OTC]** *see* aspirin *on page 61*
- **5-ASA** *see* mesalamine *on page 395*

- **Asacol®** **Oral** *see* mesalamine *on page 395*
- **Asaphen** *see* aspirin *on page 61*
- **Asasantine®** **[with Aspirin also]** *see* dipyridamole *on page 212*
- **Asasantine®** *see* dipyridamole and aspirin *New Drug on page 212*
- **Asbron-G®** **Elixir** *(Discontinued)* *see page 743*
- **Asbron-G®** **Tablet** *(Discontinued)* *see page 743*
- **Ascorbic®** **500** *see* ascorbic acid *on page 60*

ascorbic acid (a SKOR bik AS id)

Synonyms vitamin C
U.S. Brand Names Ascorbicap® [OTC]; C-Crystals® [OTC]; Cebid®; Cecon® [OTC]; Cevalin® [OTC]; Cevi-bid® [OTC]; Ce-Vi-Sol® [OTC]; Dull-C® [OTC]; Flavorcee® [OTC]; N'ice®; Timecelles® [OTC]; Vita-C® [OTC]; Vitamin C Drops [OTC]
Canadian Brand Names Apo®-C; Ascorbic® 500; Duo-CVP®; Redoxon®; Revitalose C-1000®
Mexican Brand Names Ce-Vi-Sol®; Redoxon® Forte
Generic Available Yes
Therapeutic Category Vitamin, Water Soluble
Use Prevention and treatment of scurvy; urinary acidification; dietary supplementation; prevention and reduction in the severity of colds
Usual Dosage Oral, I.M., I.V., S.C.:
Recommended daily allowance (RDA):
<6 months: 30 mg
6 months to 1 year: 35 mg
1-3 years: 40 mg
4-10 years: 45 mg
11-14 years: 50 mg
>14 years and Adults: 60 mg

Children:
Scurvy: 100-300 mg/day in divided doses for at least 2 weeks
Urinary acidification: 500 mg every 6-8 hours
Dietary supplement: 35-100 mg/day
Adults:
Scurvy: 100-250 mg 1-2 times/day for at least 2 weeks
Urinary acidification: 4-12 g/day in 3-4 divided doses
Prevention and treatment of colds: 1-3 g/day
Dietary supplement: 50-200 mg/day
Nursing/Pharmacy Information
Avoid rapid I.V. injection
Monitor urine pH when using as an acidifying agent
Stability: Injectable form should be stored under refrigeration (2°C to 8°C); protect oral dosage forms from light; is rapidly oxidized when in solution in air and alkaline media
Dosage Forms
Capsule, timed release: 500 mg
Crystals: 4 g/teaspoonful (100 g, 500 g); 5 g/teaspoonful (180 g)
Injection: 250 mg/mL (2 mL, 30 mL); 500 mg/mL (2 mL, 50 mL)
Liquid, oral: 35 mg/0.6 mL (50 mL)
Lozenges: 60 mg
Powder: 4 g/teaspoonful (100 g, 500 g)
Solution, oral: 100 mg/mL (50 mL)
Syrup: 500 mg/5 mL (5 mL, 10 mL, 120 mL, 480 mL)
Tablet: 25 mg, 50 mg, 100 mg, 250 mg, 500 mg, 1000 mg
Tablet:
Chewable: 100 mg, 250 mg, 500 mg
Timed release: 500 mg, 1000 mg, 1500 mg

- **ascorbic acid and ferrous sulfate** *see* ferrous salt and ascorbic acid *on page 265*
- **Ascorbicap®** **[OTC]** *see* ascorbic acid *on page 60*
- **Ascriptin®** **[OTC]** *see* aspirin *on page 61*
- **Asendin®** *see* amoxapine *on page 42*
- **Asmalix®** *see* theophylline *on page 603*

asparaginase (a SPIR a ji nase)

Synonyms colaspase
U.S. Brand Names Elspar®
Canadian Brand Names Kidrolase®
Mexican Brand Names Leunase

Generic Available No

Therapeutic Category Antineoplastic Agent

Use Treatment of acute lymphocytic leukemia, lymphoma; used for induction therapy

Usual Dosage Refer to individual protocols; the manufacturer recommends performing intradermal sensitivity testing before the initial dose

Children and Adults:

I.M. (preferred route): 6000 units/m^2 3 times/week for 3 weeks for combination therapy

I.V.: 1000 units/kg/day for 10 days for combination therapy or 200 units/kg/day for 28 days if combination therapy is inappropriate

Nursing/Pharmacy Information

Use two injection sites for I.M. doses >2 mL; appropriate agents for maintenance of an adequate airway and treatment of a hypersensitivity reaction (antihistamine, epinephrine, oxygen, I.V. corticosteroids) should be readily available; I.V. must be infused over a minimum of 30 minutes

Monitor vital signs during administration, CBC, urinalysis, amylase, liver enzymes, prothrombin time, renal function tests, urine dipstick for glucose, blood glucose

Stability: Powder should be refrigerated (<8°C); lyophilized powder should be reconstituted with sterile water for I.V. administration or normal saline for I.M. use; reconstituted solutions and those further diluted for I.V. infusion should be stored at 2°C to 8°C and should be discarded after 24 hours; shake well but not too vigorously; use of a 5-micron in-line filter is recommended to remove fiber-like particles in the solution (not 0.2 micron)

Dosage Forms Injection: 10,000 units/vial

♦ **A-Spas® S/L** see hyoscyamine on page 329
♦ **Aspergum® [OTC]** see aspirin on page 61

aspirin (AS pir in)

Synonyms acetylsalicylic acid; ASA

U.S. Brand Names Anacin® [OTC]; A.S.A. [OTC]; Ascriptin® [OTC]; Aspergum® [OTC]; Bayer® Aspirin [OTC]; Bufferin® [OTC]; Easprin®; Ecotrin® [OTC]; Empirin® [OTC]; Halfprin® [OTC]; Measurin® [OTC]; ZORprin®

Canadian Brand Names Apo®-ASA; ASA®; Asaphen; Entrophen®; MSD® Enteric Coated ASA; Novasen

Generic Available Yes

Therapeutic Category Analgesic, Non-narcotic; Antiplatelet Agent; Antipyretic; Nonsteroidal Anti-inflammatory Drug (NSAID)

Use Treatment of mild to moderate pain, inflammation and fever; adjunctive treatment of Kawasaki disease; may be used for prophylaxis of myocardial infarction and transient ischemic attacks (TIA)

Usual Dosage

Children:

Analgesic and antipyretic: Oral, rectal: 10-15 mg/kg/dose every 4-6 hours

Anti-inflammatory: Oral: Initial: 60-90 mg/kg/day in divided doses; usual maintenance: 80-100 mg/kg/day divided every 6-8 hours; monitor serum concentrations

Kawasaki disease: Oral: 100 mg/kg/day divided every 6 hours; after fever resolves: 8-10 mg/kg/day once daily; monitor serum concentrations

Adults:

Analgesic and antipyretic: Oral, rectal: 325-1000 mg every 4-6 hours up to 4 g/day

Anti-inflammatory: Oral: Initial: 2.4-3.6 g/day in divided doses; usual maintenance: 3.6-5.4 g/day; monitor serum concentrations

Transient ischemic attack: Oral: 1.3 g/day in 2-4 divided doses

Myocardial infarction prophylaxis: 160-325 mg/day

Dietary Considerations

Alcohol: Combination causes GI irritation, possible bleeding; avoid or limit alcohol; patients at increased risk include those prone to hypoprothrombinemia, vitamin K deficiency, thrombocytopenia, thrombotic thrombocytopenia purpura, severe hepatic impairment, and those receiving anticoagulants

Food: May decrease the rate but not the extent of oral absorption; may cause GI upset, bleeding, ulceration, perforation; administer with food or or large volume of water or milk to minimize GI upset

Folic Acid: Hyperexcretion of folate; folic acid deficiency may result, leading to macrocytic anemia; supplement with folic acid if necessary

Iron: With chronic use and at doses of 3-4 g/day, iron deficiency anemia may result; supplement with iron if necessary

(Continued)

aspirin *(Continued)*

Sodium: Hypernatremia resulting from buffered aspirin solutions or sodium salicylate containing high sodium content; avoid or use with caution in CHF or any condition where hypernatremia would be detrimental

Curry powder, paprika, licorice, Benedictine liqueur, prunes, raisins, tea and gherkins: Potential salicylate salicylate accumulation; these foods contain 6 mg salicylate/100 g; an ordinarily American diet contains 10-200 mg/day of salicylate; foods containing salicylates may contribute to aspirin hypersensitivity; patients at greatest risk for aspirin hypersensitivity include those with asthma, nasal polyposis or chronic urticaria

Fresh fruits containing vitamin C: Displaces drug from binding sites, resulting in increased urinary excretion of aspirin; educate patients regarding the potential for a decreased analgesic effect of aspirin with consumption of foods high in vitamin C

Nursing/Pharmacy Information

Monitor serum concentrations

Stability: Keep suppositories in refrigerator, do not freeze; hydrolysis of aspirin occurs upon exposure to water or moist air, resulting in salicylate and acetate, which possess a vinegar-like odor; do not use if a strong odor is present

Dosage Forms

Capsule: 356.4 mg and caffeine 30 mg

Suppository, rectal: 60 mg, 120 mg, 125 mg, 130 mg, 195 mg, 200 mg, 300 mg, 325 mg, 600 mg, 650 mg, 1.2 g

Tablet: 65 mg, 75 mg, 81 mg, 325 mg, 500 mg

Tablet: 400 mg and caffeine 32 mg

Tablet:

Buffered: 325 mg and magnesium-aluminum hydroxide 150 mg; 325 mg, magnesium hydroxide 75 mg, aluminum hydroxide 75 mg, buffered with calcium carbonate; 325 mg and magnesium-aluminum hydroxide 75 mg

Chewable: 81 mg

Controlled release: 800 mg

Delayed release: 81 mg

Enteric coated: 81 mg, 325 mg, 500 mg, 650 mg, 975 mg

Gum: 227.5 mg

Timed release: 650 mg

♦ **aspirin and butalbital compound** *see* butalbital compound and aspirin *on page 99*

aspirin and codeine (AS pir in & KOE deen)

Synonyms codeine and aspirin

U.S. Brand Names Empirin® With Codeine

Canadian Brand Names Coryphen® Codeine

Generic Available Yes

Therapeutic Category Analgesic, Narcotic

Controlled Substance C-III

Use Relief of mild to moderate pain

Usual Dosage Oral:

Children:

Aspirin: 10 mg/kg/dose every 4 hours

Codeine: 0.5-1 mg/kg/dose every 4 hours

Adults: 1-2 tablets every 4-6 hours as needed for pain

Nursing/Pharmacy Information

Administer with food or a full glass of water to minimize GI distress

Observe patient for excessive sedation, respiratory depression

Dosage Forms Tablet:

#2: Aspirin 325 mg and codeine phosphate 15 mg

#3: Aspirin 325 mg and codeine phosphate 30 mg

#4: Aspirin 325 mg and codeine phosphate 60 mg

♦ **aspirin and hydrocodone** *see* hydrocodone and aspirin *on page 319*

aspirin and meprobamate (AS pir in & me proe BA mate)

Synonyms meprobamate and aspirin

U.S. Brand Names Equagesic®

Generic Available Yes

Therapeutic Category Skeletal Muscle Relaxant

Controlled Substance C-IV

Use Adjunct to treatment of skeletal muscular disease in patients exhibiting tension and/or anxiety

Usual Dosage Oral: 1 tablet 3-4 times/day
Dietary Considerations May be administered with food to minimize GI upset
Dosage Forms Tablet: Aspirin 325 mg and meprobamate 200 mg

- ◆ **aspirin and methocarbamol** *see* methocarbamol and aspirin *on page 402*
- ◆ **aspirin and oxycodone** *see* oxycodone and aspirin *on page 463*
- ◆ **aspirin and propoxyphene** *see* propoxyphene and aspirin *on page 526*
- ◆ **Aspirin-Free Bayer® Select® Allergy Sinus Caplets [OTC]** *see* acetaminophen, chlorpheniramine, and pseudoephedrine *on page 16*
- ◆ **aspirin, orphenadrine, and caffeine** *see* orphenadrine, aspirin, and caffeine *on page 458*
- ◆ **Asproject®** *(Discontinued) see page 743*
- ◆ **Astelin® Nasal Spray** *see* azelastine *on page 68*
- ◆ **AsthmaHaler® Mist [OTC]** *see* epinephrine *on page 234*
- ◆ **AsthmaNefrin® [OTC]** *see* epinephrine *on page 234*
- ◆ **Astramorph™ PF Injection** *see* morphine sulfate *on page 422*
- ◆ **Atabrine® Tablet** *(Discontinued) see page 743*
- ◆ **Atacand™** *see* candesartan *on page 109*
- ◆ **Atarax® Oral** *see* hydroxyzine *on page 328*
- ◆ **Atasol®** *see* acetaminophen *on page 13*
- ◆ **Atasol® 8, 15, 30 W/ Caffeine** *see* acetaminophen and codeine *on page 14*
- ◆ **Atemperator-S®** *see* valproic acid and derivatives *on page 641*

atenolol (a TEN oh lole)

U.S. Brand Names Tenormin®
Canadian Brand Names Apo®-Atenol; Novo-Atenol®; Nu-Atenol®; Taro-Atenol®
Generic Available Yes
Therapeutic Category Beta-Adrenergic Blocker
Use Treatment of hypertension, alone or in combination with other agents; management of angina pectoris; antiarrhythmic; postmyocardial infarction patients; acute alcohol withdrawal
Usual Dosage
Oral:
Children: 1-2 mg/kg/dose administered daily
Adults:
Hypertension: 50 mg once daily, may increase to 100 mg/day; doses >100 mg are unlikely to produce any further benefit
Angina pectoris: 50 mg once daily, may increase to 100 mg/day; some patients may require 200 mg/day
Postmyocardial infarction: Follow I.V. dose with 100 mg/day or 50 mg twice daily for 6-9 days postmyocardial infarction
I.V.: Postmyocardial infarction: Early treatment: 5 mg slow I.V. over 5 minutes; may repeat in 10 minutes; if both doses are tolerated, may start oral atenolol 50 mg every 12 hours or 100 mg/day for 6-9 days postmyocardial infarction
Dietary Considerations May be administered without regard to meals
Nursing/Pharmacy Information
Modify dosage in patients with renal insufficiency; administer by slow I.V. injection at a rate not to exceed 1 mg/minute; the injection can be administered undiluted or diluted with a compatible I.V. solution
Monitor blood pressure, heart rate, fluid I & O, daily weight, respiratory rate
Dosage Forms
Injection: 0.5 mg/mL (10 mL)
Tablet: 25 mg, 50 mg, 100 mg

atenolol and chlorthalidone (a TEN oh lole & klor THAL i done)

Synonyms chlorthalidone and atenolol
U.S. Brand Names Tenoretic®
Generic Available Yes
Therapeutic Category Antihypertensive Agent, Combination
Use Treatment of hypertension with a cardioselective beta-blocker and a diuretic
Usual Dosage Adults: Oral: Initial: 1 tablet (50) once daily, then individualize dose until optimal dose is achieved
Dietary Considerations Should be administered on empty stomach
Nursing/Pharmacy Information May contain povidone as inactive ingredient
Dosage Forms Tablet:
50: Atenolol 50 mg and chlorthalidone 25 mg
100: Atenolol 100 mg and chlorthalidone 25 mg

- ◆ **ATG** *see* lymphocyte immune globulin *on page 378*
- ◆ **Atgam**® *see* lymphocyte immune globulin *on page 378*
- ◆ **Atiflan** *see* naproxen *on page 432*
- ◆ **ATIII** *see* antithrombin III *on page 53*
- ◆ **Atiquim**® *see* naproxen *on page 432*
- ◆ **Atisuril**® *see* allopurinol *on page 29*
- ◆ **Ativan**® *see* lorazepam *on page 375*
- ◆ **Atolone**® **Oral** *see* triamcinolone (systemic) *on page 624*

atorvastatin (a TORE va sta tin)
U.S. Brand Names Lipitor®
Generic Available No
Therapeutic Category HMG-CoA Reductase Inhibitor
Use Adjunct to diet for the reduction of elevated total and LDL-cholesterol levels in patients with hypercholesterolemia (Type IIa, IIb, and IIc); used in hypercholesterolemic patients without clinically evident heart disease to reduce the risk of myocardial infarction, to reduce the risk for revascularization, and reduce the risk of death due to cardiovascular causes with no increase in death from noncardiovascular diseases
Usual Dosage Adults: Oral: Initial: 10 mg/day, with a range of 10-80 mg/day, administered as a single dose at any time of day, with or without food
Dosage Forms Tablet: 10 mg, 20 mg, 40 mg

atovaquone (a TOE va kwone)
U.S. Brand Names Mepron™
Generic Available No
Therapeutic Category Antiprotozoal
Use Acute oral treatment of mild to moderate *Pneumocystis carinii* pneumonia (PCP) in patients who are intolerant to co-trimoxazole
Usual Dosage Adults: Oral: 750 mg twice daily with food for 21 days
Dietary Considerations Administer with a high-fat meal
Nursing/Pharmacy Information Notify physician if patient is unable to eat significant amounts of food on an ongoing basis
Dosage Forms Suspension, oral (citrus flavor): 750 mg/5 mL (210 mL)

- ◆ **Atozine**® **Oral** *see* hydroxyzine *on page 328*

atracurium (a tra KYOO ree um)
U.S. Brand Names Tracrium®
Generic Available Yes
Therapeutic Category Skeletal Muscle Relaxant
Use Eases endotracheal intubation as an adjunct to general anesthesia and relaxes skeletal muscle during surgery or mechanical ventilation
Usual Dosage I.V.:
  Children 1 month to 2 years: Initial: 0.3-0.4 mg/kg followed by maintenance doses of 0.08-0.1 mg/kg as needed to maintain neuromuscular blockade
  Children >2 years to Adults: Initial: 0.4-0.5 mg/kg then 0.08-0.1 mg/kg every 20-45 minutes after initial dose to maintain neuromuscular block
  Continuous infusion: 0.4-0.8 mg/kg/hour
Nursing/Pharmacy Information
  Not for I.M. injection due to tissue irritation; may be administered without further dilution by rapid I.V. injection; for continuous infusions, dilute to a maximum concentration of 0.5 mg/mL (more concentrated solutions when diluted with I.V. fluids have reduced stability, ie, <24 hours at room temperature)
  Monitor vital signs (heart rate, blood pressure, respiratory rate)
  Stability: Refrigerate; unstable in alkaline solutions; **compatible** with D_5W, D_5NS, and normal saline; do not dilute in lactated Ringer's
Dosage Forms
  Injection, as besylate: 10 mg/mL (5 mL, 10 mL)
  Injection, preservative-free, as besylate: 10 mg/mL (5 mL)

- ◆ **Atrohist**® **Plus** *see* chlorpheniramine, phenylephrine, phenylpropanolamine, and belladonna alkaloids *on page 142*
- ◆ **Atromid-S**® *see* clofibrate *on page 158*
- ◆ **Atropair**® *see* atropine *on page 64*

atropine (A troe peen)
U.S. Brand Names Atropair®; Atropine-Care®; Atropisol®; Isopto® Atropine; I-Tropine®
Mexican Brand Names Tropyn Z

Generic Available Yes

Therapeutic Category Anticholinergic Agent

Use Preoperative medication to inhibit salivation and secretions; treatment of sinus bradycardia; management of peptic ulcer; treatment of exercise-induced bronchospasm; antidote for organophosphate pesticide poisoning; used to produce mydriasis and cycloplegia for examination of the retina and optic disk and accurate measurement of refractive errors; treatment of uveitis

Usual Dosage

Preanesthesia: I.M., I.V., S.C.:

Infants:

<5 kg: 0.04 mg/kg/dose repeated every 4-6 hours as needed

>5 kg: 0.03 mg/kg/dose repeated every 4-6 hours as needed

Children: 0.01 mg/kg/dose up to a maximum of 0.4 mg/dose; repeat every 4-6 hours as needed

Adults: 0.5 mg/dose repeated every 4-6 hours as needed

Bronchodilation:

Children:

Oral: 0.02 mg/kg/dose 3 times/day

Inhalation: 0.03-0.05 mg/kg/dose 3-4 times/day

Adults: Inhalation: 0.025-0.05 mg/kg/dose over 10 minutes, repeated every 4-5 hours as needed

Cardiopulmonary resuscitation (bradycardia): I.T., I.V.:

Infants: 0.02-0.04 mg/kg/dose; repeat every 2-5 minutes, if needed, up to 2-3 times

Children: 0.01-0.02 mg/kg/dose; repeat every 2-5 minutes, if needed, up to 2-3 times; minimum dose should be 0.1 mg (smaller doses may cause paradoxic bradycardia); maximum total dose is 1 mg (2 mg for adolescents)

Adults: 0.5 mg/dose; repeat every 5 minutes, if needed, up to 2-3 times for a maximum total dose of 2 mg

Organophosphate or carbamate poisoning: I.V.:

Children: 0.02-0.05 mg/kg/dose every 10-20 minutes until atropine effect (dry flushed skin, tachycardia, mydriasis, fever) is observed, then every 1-4 hours to maintain atropine effect for at least 24 hours

Children >12 years and Adults: 1-2 mg/dose every 10-20 minutes until atropine effect (see above) is observed, then 1-3 mg/dose every 1-4 hours, as needed to maintain atropine effect for at least 24 hours

Neuromuscular blockade reversal: I.V.:

Before neostigmine: Administer 25-30 mcg/kg (0.025-0.03 mg/kg) 30 seconds before neostigmine (0.07-0.08 mg/kg)

Before edrophonium: 10 mcg/kg (0.01 mg/kg) 30 seconds before edrophonium (1 mg/kg)

Note: May contain benzyl alcohol as a preservative; administration of benzyl alcohol in doses ranging from 99-234 mg/kg has been associated with a fatal gasping syndrome in neonates; clinical signs of this syndrome include metabolic acidosis, hypotension, CNS depression, and cardiovascular collapse

Nursing/Pharmacy Information

Observe for tachycardia if patient has cardiac problems; lack of saliva may increase chance of cavities, therefore, good oral hygiene should be promoted; administer undiluted by rapid I.V. injection; slow injection may result in paradoxical bradycardia

Monitor heart rate

Stability: Store injection below 40°C, avoid freezing

Dosage Forms

Injection, as sulfate: 0.1 mg/mL (5 mL, 10 mL); 0.3 mg/mL (1 mL, 30 mL); 0.4 mg/mL (1 mL, 20 mL, 30 mL); 0.5 mg/mL (1 mL, 5 mL, 30 mL); 0.8 mg/mL (0.5 mL, 1 mL); 1 mg/mL (1 mL, 10 mL)

Ointment, ophthalmic, as sulfate: 0.5%, 1% (3.5 g)

Solution, ophthalmic, as sulfate: 0.5% (1 mL, 5 mL); 1% (1 mL, 2 mL, 5 mL, 15 mL); 2% (1 mL, 2 mL); 3% (5 mL)

♦ **atropine and difenoxin** *see* difenoxin and atropine *on page 201*

♦ **atropine and diphenoxylate** *see* diphenoxylate and atropine *on page 209*

♦ **Atropine-Care®** *see* atropine *on page 64*

♦ **atropine, hyoscyamine, scopolamine, and phenobarbital** *see* hyoscyamine, atropine, scopolamine, and phenobarbital *on page 330*

♦ **Atropine Soluble Tablet** *(Discontinued) see page 743*

♦ **Atropisol®** *see* atropine *on page 64*

♦ **Atrovent®** *see* ipratropium *on page 345*

♦ **A/T/S® Topical** *see* erythromycin (ophthalmic/topical) *on page 239*

attapulgite (at a PULL gite)

U.S. Brand Names Children's Kaopectate® [OTC]; Diasorb® [OTC]; Kaopectate® Advanced Formula [OTC]; Kaopectate® Maximum Strength Caplets; Rheaban® [OTC]

Generic Available Yes

Therapeutic Category Antidiarrheal

Use Treatment of uncomplicated diarrhea

Usual Dosage Oral:

Children:

<3 years: Not recommended

3-6 years: 750 mg/dose up to 2250 mg/24 hours

6-12 years: 1200-1500 mg/dose up to 4500 mg/24 hours

Adults: 1200-1500 mg after each loose bowel movement or every 2 hours; 15-30 mL up to 8 times/day, up to 9000 mg/24 hours

Nursing/Pharmacy Information

Shake well before administering; re-evaluate cause of diarrhea if not controlled in 48 hours; diarrhea should also be treated by diet, ie, clear liquids, bland foods, and no dairy products for first 24-48 hours

Monitor for signs of fluid and electrolyte loss

Dosage Forms

Liquid, oral concentrate: 600 mg/15 mL (180 mL, 240 mL, 360 mL, 480 mL); 750 mg/15 mL (120 mL)

Tablet: 750 mg

Tablet, chewable: 300 mg, 600 mg

♦ **Attenuvax®** *see* measles virus vaccine, live *on page 386*

♦ **Augmentin®** *see* amoxicillin and clavulanate potassium *on page 43*

♦ **Auralgan®** *see* antipyrine and benzocaine *on page 53*

auranofin (au RANE oh fin)

U.S. Brand Names Ridaura®

Generic Available No

Therapeutic Category Gold Compound

Use Management of active stage of classic or definite rheumatoid or psoriatic arthritis in patients that do not respond to or tolerate other agents

Usual Dosage Oral:

Children: Initial: 0.1 mg/kg/day divided daily; usual maintenance: 0.15 mg/kg/day in 1-2 divided doses; maximum: 0.2 mg/kg/day in 1-2 divided doses

Adults: 6 mg/day in 1-2 divided doses; after 3 months may be increased to 9 mg/day in 3 divided doses; if still no response after 3 months at 9 mg/day, discontinue drug

Nursing/Pharmacy Information

Therapy should be discontinued if platelet count falls below 100,000/mm³

Monitor CBC with differential, platelet count, urinalysis, baseline renal and liver function tests; metallic taste may indicate stomatitis

Stability: Store in tight, light-resistant containers at 15°C to 30°C

Dosage Forms Capsule: 3 mg [gold 29%]

♦ **Aureomycin®** *(Discontinued)* see page 743

♦ **Aurodex®** *see* antipyrine and benzocaine *on page 53*

♦ **Auro® Ear Drops [OTC]** *see* carbamide peroxide *on page 112*

♦ **Aurolate®** *see* gold sodium thiomalate *on page 296*

aurothioglucose (aur oh thye oh GLOO kose)

U.S. Brand Names Solganal®

Generic Available No

Therapeutic Category Gold Compound

Use Management of active stage of classic or definite rheumatoid or psoriatic arthritis in patients that do not respond to or tolerate other agents

Usual Dosage I.M. (doses should initially be administered at weekly intervals):

Children 6-12 years: Initial: 0.25 mg/kg/dose first week; increment at 0.25 mg/kg/dose increasing with each weekly dose; maintenance: 0.75-1 mg/kg/dose weekly not to exceed 25 mg/dose to a total of 20 doses, then every 2-4 weeks

Adults: 10 mg first week; 25 mg second and third week; then 50 mg/week until 800 mg to 1 g cumulative dose has been administered - if improvement occurs without adverse reactions, administer 25-50 mg every 2-3 weeks, then every 3-4 weeks

Nursing/Pharmacy Information

Deep I.M. injection into the upper outer quadrant of the gluteal region; vial should be thoroughly shaken before withdrawing a dose. Do not administer I.V.

Monitor CBC with differential, platelet count, urinalysis, baseline renal and liver function tests

Stability: Protect from light and store at 15°C to 30°C

Dosage Forms Injection, suspension: 50 mg/mL [gold 50%] (10 mL)

- ◆ **Auroto**® *see antipyrine and benzocaine on page 53*
- ◆ **Autoplex**® **T** *see anti-inhibitor coagulant complex on page 52*
- ◆ **Avandia**® *see rosiglitazone New Drug on page 554*
- ◆ **Avapro**® *see irbesartan on page 345*
- ◆ **Avapro**® **HCT** *see irbesartan and hydrochlorothiazide New Drug on page 345*
- ◆ **AVC**™ **Cream** *see sulfanilamide on page 587*
- ◆ **AVC**™ **Suppository** *see sulfanilamide on page 587*
- ◆ **Aveeno**® **Cleansing Bar [OTC]** *see sulfur and salicylic acid on page 589*
- ◆ **Aventyl**® **Hydrochloride** *see nortriptyline on page 449*
- ◆ **A-Vicon** *see vitamin A on page 650*
- ◆ **Avirax**™ *see acyclovir on page 21*
- ◆ **Avitene**® *see microfibrillar collagen hemostat on page 414*
- ◆ **A-Vitex** *see vitamin A on page 650*
- ◆ **Avlosulfon**® *see dapsone on page 182*
- ◆ **Avonex**™ *see interferon beta-1a on page 343*
- ◆ **Axid**® *see nizatidine on page 446*
- ◆ **Axid**® **AR [OTC]** *see nizatidine on page 446*
- ◆ **Axocet**® *see butalbital compound and acetaminophen on page 99*
- ◆ **Axotal**® *(Discontinued) see page 743*
- ◆ **Ayercillin**® *see penicillin G procaine on page 476*
- ◆ **Aygestin**® *see norethindrone on page 447*
- ◆ **Ayr**® **Nasal [OTC]** *see sodium chloride on page 571*

azacitidine (ay za SYE ti deen)

Synonyms AZA-CR; 5-azacytidine; 5-AZC; ladakamycin
U.S. Brand Names Mylosar®
Generic Available No
Therapeutic Category Antineoplastic Agent
Use Refractory acute lymphocytic and myelogenous leukemia
Usual Dosage Children and Adults: I.V.: 200-300 mg/m²/day for 5-10 days, repeated at 2- to 3-week intervals
Nursing/Pharmacy Information

Administer by slow infusion over <3 hours; may be administered S.C.
Stability: Refrigerate

Dosage Forms Injection: 100 mg

- ◆ **AZA-CR** *see azacitidine on page 67*
- ◆ **Azactam**® *see aztreonam on page 69*
- ◆ **5-azacytidine** *see azacitidine on page 67*
- ◆ **Azantac** *see ranitidine hydrochloride on page 541*

azatadine (a ZA ta deen)

U.S. Brand Names Optimine®
Mexican Brand Names Idulamine®
Generic Available No
Therapeutic Category Antihistamine
Use Treatment of perennial and seasonal allergic rhinitis and chronic urticaria
Usual Dosage Children >12 years and Adults: Oral: 1-2 mg twice daily
Dietary Considerations May be administered with food
Nursing/Pharmacy Information Assist with ambulation
Dosage Forms Tablet, as maleate: 1 mg

azatadine and pseudoephedrine

(a ZA ta deen & soo doe e FED rin)
Synonyms pseudoephedrine and azatadine
U.S. Brand Names Rynatan®; Trinalin®
Generic Available No
Therapeutic Category Antihistamine/Decongestant Combination
Use Perennial and seasonal allergic rhinitis and other allergic symptoms including urticaria

(Continued)

azatadine and pseudoephedrine *(Continued)*
Usual Dosage Adults: 1 tablet twice daily
Dietary Considerations May be administered with food, milk, or water
Dosage Forms Tablet: Azatadine maleate 1 mg and pseudoephedrine sulfate 120 mg

azathioprine (ay za THYE oh preen)
U.S. Brand Names Imuran®
Mexican Brand Names Azatrilem
Generic Available No
Therapeutic Category Immunosuppressant Agent
Use Adjunct with other agents in prevention of transplant rejection; also used as an immunosuppressant in a variety of autoimmune diseases such as systemic lupus erythematosus, severe rheumatoid arthritis unresponsive to other agents, and nephrotic syndrome
Usual Dosage
  Children and Adults: Renal transplantation: Oral, I.V.: Initial: 3-5 mg/kg/day; maintenance: 1-3 mg/kg/day
  Adults: Rheumatoid arthritis: Oral: 1 mg/kg/day for 6-8 weeks; increase by 0.5 mg/kg every 4 weeks until response or up to 2.5 mg/kg/day I.V. dose is equivalent to oral dose
Dietary Considerations May be administered with food
Nursing/Pharmacy Information
  Can be administered IVP over 5 minutes at a concentration not to exceed 10 mg/mL; or azathioprine can be further diluted with normal saline or D_5W and administered by intermittent infusion over 15-60 minutes
  Monitor CBC, platelet counts, total bilirubin, alkaline phosphatase; hematologic status should be monitored during therapy
  Stability: Parenteral admixture is stable at temperatures of 4°C to 25°C for 24 hours; stable in neutral or acid solutions, but is hydrolyzed to mercaptopurine in alkaline solutions
Dosage Forms
  Injection, as sodium: 100 mg (20 mL)
  Tablet (scored): 50 mg

♦ **Azatrilem** *see azathioprine on page 68*
♦ **5-AZC** *see azacitidine on page 67*
♦ **Azdone®** *see hydrocodone and aspirin on page 319*

azelaic acid (a zeh LAY ik AS id)
U.S. Brand Names Azelex®
Generic Available No
Therapeutic Category Topical Skin Product
Use Treatment of mild to moderate acne vulgaris
Usual Dosage Adults: Topical: After skin is thoroughly washed and patted dry, gently but thoroughly massage a thin film of azelaic acid cream into the affected areas twice daily, in the morning and evening. The duration of use can vary and depends on the severity of the acne. In the majority of patients with inflammatory lesions, improvement of the condition occurs within 4 weeks.
Nursing/Pharmacy Information Wash hands following application
Dosage Forms Cream: 20% (30 g)

azelastine (a ZEL as teen)
U.S. Brand Names Astelin® Nasal Spray
Generic Available No
Therapeutic Category Antihistamine
Use Seasonal allergic rhinitis
Usual Dosage Children ≥12 years and Adults: Nasal: 2 sprays in each nostril twice daily
Dosage Forms Spray, nasal: 137 mcg/actuation [100 actuations/bottle]

♦ **Azelex®** *see azelaic acid on page 68*
♦ **azidothymidine** *see zidovudine on page 658*

azithromycin (az ith roe MYE sin)
U.S. Brand Names Zithromax™
Generic Available No
Therapeutic Category Macrolide (Antibiotic)

Use

Children: Treatment of acute otitis media due to *H. influenzae*, *M. catarrhalis* or *S. pneumoniae*; pharyngitis/tonsillitis due to *S. pyogenes*

Adults:

Treatment of mild to moderate upper and lower respiratory tract infections, infections of the skin and skin structure, and sexually transmitted diseases due to susceptible strains of *C. trachomatis*, *M. catarrhalis*, *H. influenzae*, *S. aureus*, *S. pneumoniae*, *Mycoplasma pneumoniae*, and *C. psittaci*; community-acquired pneumonia, pelvic inflammatory disease (PID)

For preventing or delaying the onset of infection with *Mycobacterium avium* complex (MAC)

Usual Dosage Oral:

Children:

Acute otitis media: 10 mg/kg on day 1 (not to exceed 500 mg/day) followed by 5 mg/kg/day once daily on days 2-5 (not to exceed 250 mg/day)

Pharyngitis/tonsillitis: 12 mg/kg/day for 5 days (not to exceed 500 mg/day)

Adolescents ≥16 years and Adults:

Mild to moderate respiratory tract, skin, and soft tissue infections: 500 mg in a single dose on day 1; 250 mg in a single dose on days 2-5

Nongonococcal urethritis and cervicitis: 1 g in a single dose

Chancroid and *Chlamydia*: 1 g in a single dose

I.V.: Adults:

Community-acquired pneumonia: 500 mg as a single dose for at least 2 days, follow I.V. therapy by the oral route with a single daily dose of 500 mg to complete a 7- to 10-day course of therapy

Pelvic inflammatory disease (PID): 500 mg as a single dose for 1-2 days, follow I.V. therapy by the oral route with a single daily dose of 250 mg to complete a 7-day course of therapy

Dietary Considerations Should be administered at least 1 hour prior to a meal or 2 hours after a meal; should not be administered with food; presence of food decrease bioavailability by up to 50%

Nursing/Pharmacy Information

Do not administer concurrently with aluminum or magnesium antacids

Monitor liver function tests; tolerance to medication; respiratory, cardiac, and fluid status of nursing home patients being treated for pneumonia

Parenteral: Infusate concentration and rate of infusion for azithromycin for injection should be either 1 mg/mL over 3 hours or 2 mg/mL over 1 hour

Dosage Forms

Capsule, as dihydrate: 250 mg

Powder for injection: 500 mg

Powder for oral suspension, as dihydrate: 100 mg/5 mL (15 mL); 200 mg/5 mL (15 mL, 22.5 mL); 1 g (single-dose packet)

Tablet, as dihydrate: 250 mg, 600 mg

♦ **Azlin® Injection** *(Discontinued) see page 743*

♦ **Azmacort™ Oral Inhaler** *see* triamcinolone (inhalation, oral) *on page 623*

♦ **Azo Gantanol®** *(Discontinued) see page 743*

♦ **Azo Gantrisin®** *(Discontinued) see page 743*

♦ **Azopt®** *see* brinzolamide *on page 92*

♦ **Azo-Standard®** *see* phenazopyridine *on page 483*

♦ **Azo Wintomylon** *see* phenazopyridine *on page 483*

♦ **AZT** *see* zidovudine *on page 658*

♦ **AZT + 3TC** *see* zidovudine and lamivudine *on page 659*

♦ **azthreonam** *see* aztreonam *on page 69*

aztreonam (AZ tree oh nam)

Synonyms azthreonam

U.S. Brand Names Azactam®

Generic Available No

Therapeutic Category Antibiotic, Miscellaneous

Use Treatment of patients with documented multidrug resistant aerobic gram-negative infection in which beta-lactam therapy is contraindicated; used for urinary tract infection, lower respiratory tract infections, septicemia, skin/skin structure infections, intra-abdominal infections and gynecological infections caused by susceptible *Enterobacteriaceae*, *H. influenzae*, and *P. aeruginosa*

Usual Dosage

Children >1 month: I.M., I.V.: 90-120 mg/kg/day divided every 6-8 hours

Cystic fibrosis: 50 mg/kg/dose every 6-8 hours (ie, up to 200 mg/kg/day); maximum: 6-8 g/day

Adults:

Urinary tract infection: I.M., I.V.: 500 mg to 1 g every 8-12 hours

(Continued)

aztreonam *(Continued)*

Moderately severe systemic infections: 1 g I.V. or I.M. or 2 g I.V. every 8-12 hours

Severe systemic or life-threatening infections (especially caused by *Pseudomonas aeruginosa*): I.V.: 2 g every 6-8 hours; maximum: 8 g/day

Nursing/Pharmacy Information

Administer by IVP over 3-5 minutes at a maximum concentration of 66 mg/mL or by intermittent infusion over 20-60 minutes at a final concentration not to exceed 20 mg/mL

Monitor periodic liver function test

Stability: Reconstituted solutions are colorless to light yellow straw and may turn pink upon standing without affecting potency; use reconstituted solutions and I.V. solutions (in normal saline and D_5W) within 48 hours if kept at room temperature or 7 days if kept in refrigerator; reconstituted solutions are **not** for multiple-dose use; **incompatible** when mixed with nafcillin, metronidazole

Dosage Forms Powder for injection: 500 mg (15 mL, 100 mL); 1 g (15 mL, 100 mL); 2 g (15 mL, 100 mL)

- **Azulfidine®** *see* sulfasalazine *on page 587*
- **Azulfidine® EN-tabs®** *see* sulfasalazine *on page 587*
- **Azulfidine® Suspension** *(Discontinued) see page 743*
- **Babee® Teething® [OTC]** *see* benzocaine *on page 79*
- **BAC** *see* benzalkonium chloride *on page 78*

bacampicillin (ba kam pi SIL in)

Synonyms carampicillin

U.S. Brand Names Spectrobid® Tablet

Generic Available No

Therapeutic Category Penicillin

Use Treatment of susceptible bacterial infections involving the urinary tract, skin structure, upper and lower respiratory tract; activity is identical to that of ampicillin

Usual Dosage Oral:

Children: 25-50 mg/kg/day in divided doses every 12 hours

Adults: 400-800 mg every 12 hours

Dietary Considerations May be administered with meals or on an empty stomach; may mix with milk, formula, or juice

Nursing/Pharmacy Information

Assess patient at beginning and throughout therapy for infection; observe for signs and symptoms of anaphylaxis

Monitor renal, hepatic, and hematologic function tests

Stability: Reconstituted suspension is stable for 10 days when stored in the refrigerator

Dosage Forms

Powder for oral suspension, as hydrochloride: 125 mg/5 mL [chemically equivalent to ampicillin 87.5 mg per 5 mL] (70 mL)

Tablet, as hydrochloride: 400 mg [chemically equivalent to ampicillin 280 mg]

- **B-A-C®** *(Discontinued) see page 743*
- **Bacid® [OTC]** *see* Lactobacillus *on page 358*
- **Baciguent® Topical [OTC]** *see* bacitracin *on page 70*
- **Baci-IM® Injection** *see* bacitracin *on page 70*
- **Bacillus Calmette-Guérin (BCG) Live** *see* BCG vaccine *on page 74*
- **Bacimyxin** *see* bacitracin and polymyxin B *on page 71*
- **Bacitin** *see* bacitracin *on page 70*

bacitracin (bas i TRAY sin)

U.S. Brand Names AK-Tracin® Ophthalmic; Baciguent® Topical [OTC]; Baci-IM® Injection

Canadian Brand Names Bacitin

Generic Available Yes

Therapeutic Category Antibiotic, Ophthalmic; Antibiotic, Topical; Antibiotic, Miscellaneous

Use Treatment of pneumonia and emphysema caused by susceptible staphylococci; prevention or treatment of superficial skin infections or infections of the eye caused by susceptible organisms; due to its toxicity, use of bacitracin systemically or as an irrigant should be limited to situations where less toxic alternatives would not be effective; treatment of antibiotic-associated colitis

Usual Dosage I.M. recommended; **do not administer I.V.:**

Infants:

<2.5 kg: 900 units/kg/day in 2-3 divided doses

>2.5 kg: 1000 units/kg/day in 2-3 divided doses

Children: 800-1200 units/kg/day divided every 8 hours

Adults: 10,000-25,000 units/dose every 6 hours; not to exceed 100,000 units/day

Topical: Apply 1-5 times/day

Ophthalmic ointment: $1/4$" to $1/2$" ribbon every 3-4 hours to conjunctival sac for acute infections or 2-3 times/day for mild to moderate infections for 7-10 days

Irrigation, solution: 50-100 units/mL in normal saline, lactated Ringer's, or sterile water for irrigation; soak sponges in solution for topical compresses 1-5 times/day or as needed during surgical procedures

Nursing/Pharmacy Information

For I.M. administration, pH of urine should be kept above 6 by using sodium bicarbonate

Monitor urinalysis, renal function tests

Stability: Sterile powder should be stored in the refrigerator; once reconstituted, bacitracin is stable for 1 week under refrigeration (2°C to 8°C); bacitracin sterile powder should be dissolved in 0.9% sodium chloride injection containing 2% procaine hydrochloride for I.M. use; do not use diluents containing parabens

Dosage Forms

Injection: 50,000 units

Ointment:

Ophthalmic: 500 units/g (3.5 g, 3.75 g)

AK-Tracin®: 500 units/g (3.5 g)

Topical: 500 units/g (1.5 g, 3.75 g, 15 g, 30 g, 120 g, 454 g)

bacitracin and polymyxin B (bas i TRAY sin & pol i MIKS in bee)

Synonyms polymyxin B and bacitracin

U.S. Brand Names AK-Poly-Bac® Ophthalmic; Betadine® First Aid Antibiotics + Moisturizer [OTC]; Polysporin® Ophthalmic; Polysporin® Topical

Canadian Brand Names Bacimyxin; Bioderm; Polytopic®; Polytracin®

Generic Available Yes

Therapeutic Category Antibiotic, Ophthalmic; Antibiotic, Topical

Use Treatment of superficial infections involving the conjunctiva and/or cornea caused by susceptible organisms; prevent infection in minor cuts, scrapes and burns

Usual Dosage

Ophthalmic: Apply $1/2$" ribbon to the affected eye(s) every 3-4 hours

Topical: Apply to affected area 1-3 times/day; may cover with sterile bandage if needed

Nursing/Pharmacy Information

Ophthalmic ointment may cause blurred vision; do not share eye medications with others

Ophthalmic administration: Tilt head back, place medication in conjunctival sac and close eyes; apply light finger pressure on lacrimal sac for 1 minute following instillation

Dosage Forms

Ointment:

Ophthalmic: Bacitracin 500 units and polymyxin B sulfate 10,000 units per g (3.5 g)

Topical: Bacitracin 500 units and polymyxin B sulfate 10,000 units per g in white petrolatum (15 g, 30 g)

Powder: Bacitracin 500 units and polymyxin B sulfate 10,000 units per g (10 g)

bacitracin, neomycin, and polymyxin B

(bas i TRAY sin, nee oh MYE sin & pol i MIKS in bee)

Synonyms neomycin, bacitracin, and polymyxin B; polymyxin B, bacitracin, and neomycin

U.S. Brand Names AK-Spore® Ophthalmic Ointment; Medi-Quick® Topical Ointment [OTC]; Mycitracin® Topical [OTC]; Neomixin® Topical; Neosporin® Ophthalmic Ointment; Neosporin® Topical Ointment [OTC]; Ocutricin® Topical Ointment; Septa® Topical Ointment [OTC]; Triple Antibiotic® Topical

Canadian Brand Names Neotopic®

Generic Available Yes

Therapeutic Category Antibiotic, Ophthalmic; Antibiotic, Topical

Use Help prevent infection in minor cuts, scrapes and burns; short-term treatment of superficial external ocular infections caused by susceptible organisms

(Continued)

bacitracin, neomycin, and polymyxin B *(Continued)*

Usual Dosage Children and Adults:
Ophthalmic ointment: Instill into the conjunctival sac one or more times/day every 3-4 hours for 7-10 days
Topical: Apply 1-3 times/day
Nursing/Pharmacy Information Symptoms of neomycin sensitization include itching, reddening, edema, failure to heal; ophthalmic ointments may retard corneal healing
Dosage Forms Ointment:
Ophthalmic: Bacitracin 400 units, neomycin sulfate 3.5 mg, and polymyxin B sulfate 10,000 units and per g
Topical: Bacitracin 400 units, neomycin sulfate 3.5 mg, and polymyxin B sulfate 5000 units per g

bacitracin, neomycin, polymyxin B, and hydrocortisone

(bas i TRAY sin, nee oh MYE sin, pol i MIKS in bee & hye droe KOR ti sone)
Synonyms hydrocortisone, bacitracin, neomycin, and polymyxin B; neomycin, bacitracin, polymyxin B, and hydrocortisone; polymyxin B, bacitracin, neomycin, and hydrocortisone
U.S. Brand Names AK-Spore® H.C. Ophthalmic Ointment; Cortisporin® Ophthalmic Ointment; Cortisporin® Topical Ointment; Neotricin HC® Ophthalmic Ointment
Generic Available Yes
Therapeutic Category Antibiotic/Corticosteroid, Ophthalmic; Antibiotic/Corticosteroid, Topical
Use Prevention and treatment of susceptible superficial topical infections
Usual Dosage
Ophthalmic ointment: Apply ½" ribbon to inside of lower lid every 3-4 hours until improvement occurs
Topical: Apply sparingly 2-4 times/day
Dosage Forms Ointment:
Ophthalmic: Bacitracin 400 units, neomycin sulfate 3.5 mg, polymyxin B sulfate 10,000 units, and hydrocortisone 10 mg per g (3.5 g)
Topical: Bacitracin 400 units, neomycin sulfate 3.5 mg, polymyxin B sulfate 10,000 units, and hydrocortisone 10 mg per g (15 g)

bacitracin, neomycin, polymyxin B, and lidocaine

(bas i TRAY sin, nee oh MYE sin, pol i MIKS in bee & LYE doe kane)
U.S. Brand Names Clomycin® [OTC]
Generic Available No
Therapeutic Category Antibiotic, Topical
Use Prevention and treatment of susceptible superficial topical infections
Usual Dosage Adults: Topical: Apply 1-4 times/day to infected areas; cover with sterile bandage if needed
Dosage Forms Ointment, topical: Bacitracin 500 units, neomycin base 3.5 g, polymyxin B sulfate 5000 units, and lidocaine 40 mg per g (28.35 g)

baclofen (BAK loe fen)

U.S. Brand Names Lioresal®
Canadian Brand Names Alpha-Baclofen®; PMS-Baclofen
Generic Available Yes: Tablets only
Therapeutic Category Skeletal Muscle Relaxant
Use Treatment of reversible spasticity associated with multiple sclerosis or spinal cord lesions; intrathecal use for the management of spasticity in patients who are unresponsive to oral baclofen or experience intolerable CNS side effects; treatment of trigeminal neuralgia; adjunctive treatment of tardive dyskinesia
Usual Dosage
Oral:
Children:
2-7 years: Initial: 10-15 mg/24 hours divided every 8 hours; titrate dose every 3 days in increments of 5-15 mg/day to a maximum of 40 mg/day
≥8 years: Maximum: 60 mg/day in 3 divided doses
Adults: 5 mg 3 times/day, may increase 5 mg/dose every 3 days to a maximum of 80 mg/day

Intrathecal:

Test dose: 50-100 mcg, doses >50 mcg should be administered in 25 mcg increments, separated by 24 hours

Maintenance: After positive response to test dose, a maintenance intrathecal infusion can be administered via an implanted intrathecal pump. Initial dose via pump: Infusion at a 24-hourly rate dosed at twice the test dose.

Nursing/Pharmacy Information

Epileptic patients should be closely monitored; supervise ambulation; avoid abrupt withdrawal of the drug

Monitor muscle rigidity, spasticity (decrease in number and severity of spasms)

Dosage Forms

Injection, intrathecal, preservative free: 500 mcg/mL (20 mL); 2000 mcg/mL (5 mL)

Tablet: 10 mg, 20 mg

- ◆ **Bactelan** see co-trimoxazole on page 170
- ◆ **Bactigras®** see chlorhexidine gluconate on page 134
- ◆ **Bactine® Hydrocortisone [OTC]** see hydrocortisone (topical) on page 324
- ◆ **Bactocill® (Discontinued)** see page 743
- ◆ **Bactocin** see ofloxacin on page 454
- ◆ **BactoShield® [OTC]** see chlorhexidine gluconate on page 134
- ◆ **Bactrim™** see co-trimoxazole on page 170
- ◆ **Bactrim™ DS** see co-trimoxazole on page 170
- ◆ **Bactroban®** see mupirocin on page 424
- ◆ **Bactroban® Nasal** see mupirocin on page 424
- ◆ **Baker's P&S Topical [OTC]** see phenol on page 486
- ◆ **baking soda** see sodium bicarbonate on page 570
- ◆ **BAL** see dimercaprol on page 206

balanced salt solution (BAL anced salt soe LOO shun)

U.S. Brand Names BSS® Ophthalmic

Generic Available Yes

Therapeutic Category Ophthalmic Agent, Miscellaneous

Use Intraocular irrigating solution; also used to soothe and cleanse the eye in conjunction with hard contact lenses

Usual Dosage Use as needed for foreign body removal, gonioscopy, and other general ophthalmic office procedures

Nursing/Pharmacy Information Contains sodium 0.49%, potassium 0.075%, magnesium 0.03%, calcium chloride 0.04%, sodium acetate 0.39%, and sodium citrate 0.17%; mix aseptically just prior to use

Dosage Forms Ophthalmic:

Drops: 15 mL

Solution, sterile: 500 mL

- ◆ **Balcoran** see vancomycin on page 642
- ◆ **Baldex®** see dexamethasone (ophthalmic) on page 189
- ◆ **BAL in Oil®** see dimercaprol on page 206
- ◆ **Balminil® Decongestant** see pseudoephedrine on page 530
- ◆ **Balminil®-DM, -DM Children** see dextromethorphan on page 194
- ◆ **Balminil® Expectorant** see guaifenesin on page 299
- ◆ **Balnetar®** see coal tar on page 162
- ◆ **Balnetar® [OTC]** see coal tar, lanolin, and mineral oil on page 163
- ◆ **Bancap® (Discontinued)** see page 743
- ◆ **Bancap HC®** see hydrocodone and acetaminophen on page 319
- ◆ **Banesin® (Discontinued)** see page 743
- ◆ **Banophen® Decongestant Capsule [OTC]** see diphenhydramine and pseudoephedrine on page 209
- ◆ **Banophen® Oral [OTC]** see diphenhydramine on page 208
- ◆ **Banthine®** see methantheline on page 400
- ◆ **Bantron® (Discontinued)** see page 743
- ◆ **Bapadin®** see bepridil on page 83
- ◆ **Barbidonna®** see hyoscyamine, atropine, scopolamine, and phenobarbital on page 330
- ◆ **Barbilixir®** see phenobarbital on page 485
- ◆ **Barbita®** see phenobarbital on page 485
- ◆ **Barc™ Liquid [OTC]** see pyrethrins and piperonyl butoxide on page 533
- ◆ **Baricon®** see radiological/contrast media (ionic) on page 539
- ◆ **Baridium®** see phenazopyridine on page 483

- **Barobag**® *see* radiological/contrast media (ionic) *on page 539*
- **Baro-CAT**® *see* radiological/contrast media (ionic) *on page 539*
- **Baroflave**® *see* radiological/contrast media (ionic) *on page 539*
- **Barosperse**® *see* radiological/contrast media (ionic) *on page 539*
- **Bar-Test**® *see* radiological/contrast media (ionic) *on page 539*
- **Basaljel**® **[OTC]** *see* aluminum carbonate *on page 33*

basiliximab (ba si LIKS i mab)

U.S. Brand Names Simulect®
Generic Available No
Therapeutic Category Immunosuppressant Agent
Use Prophylaxis of acute organ rejection in renal transplantation
Usual Dosage I.V.:

Children: 12 mg/m² (maximum: 20 mg) within 2 hours prior to transplant surgery, followed by a second dose of 12 mg/m² (maximum: 20 mg) 4 days after transplantation

Adults: 20 mg within 2 hours prior to transplant surgery, followed by a second 20 mg dose 4 days after transplantation

Dosage Forms Powder for injection: 20 mg

- **Batrizol** *see* co-trimoxazole *on page 170*
- **Baycol**™ *see* cerivastatin *on page 130*
- **Bayer**® **Aspirin [OTC]** *see* aspirin *on page 61*
- **Bayer**® **Select**® **Chest Cold Caplets [OTC]** *see* acetaminophen and dextromethorphan *on page 15*
- **Bayer**® **Select**® **Head Cold Caplets [OTC]** *see* acetaminophen and pseudoephedrine *on page 15*
- **Baypress**® *(Discontinued) see page 743*
- **Bayrab**® *see* rabies immune globulin (human) *on page 538*

BCG vaccine (bee see jee vak SEEN)

Synonyms Bacillus Calmette-Guérin (BCG) Live
U.S. Brand Names TheraCys®; TICE® BCG
Canadian Brand Names ImmuCyst®; Pacis™
Generic Available No
Therapeutic Category Biological Response Modulator
Use BCG vaccine is no longer recommended for adults at high risk for tuberculosis in the United States. BCG vaccination may be considered for infants and children who are skin test-negative to 5 tuberculin units of tuberculin and who cannot be given isoniazid preventive therapy but have close contact with untreated or ineffectively treated active tuberculosis patients or who belong to groups which other control measures have not been successful.

In the United States, tuberculosis control efforts are directed toward early identification, treatment of cases, and preventive therapy with isoniazid.

Usual Dosage Intravesical treatment and prophylaxis for carcinoma *in situ* of the urinary bladder: Begin between 7-14 days after biopsy or transurethral resection. Administer a dose of 3 vials of BCG live intravesically under aseptic conditions once weekly for 6 weeks (induction therapy). Each dose (3 reconstituted vials) is further diluted in an additional 50 mL sterile, preservative free saline for a total of 53 mL. A urethral catheter is inserted into the bladder under aseptic conditions, the bladder is drained, and then the 53 mL suspension is instilled slowly by gravity, following which the catheter is withdrawn. If the bladder catheterization has been traumatic, BCG live should not be administered, and there must be a treatment delay of at least 1 week. Resume subsequent treatment; follow the induction therapy by one treatment administered 3, 6, 12, 18 and 24 months following the initial treatment.

Nursing/Pharmacy Information
Should only be administered intradermally; **do not administer I.V.**
Stability: Refrigerate, protect from light, use within 2 (TICE® BCG) hours of mixing

Dosage Forms Freeze-dried suspension for reconstitution
Injection: 50 mg (2 mL)
Injection, intravesical: 27 mg (3 vials)

- **BCNU** *see* carmustine *on page 116*
- **B-D Glucose**® **[OTC]** *see* glucose, instant *on page 293*
- **Beben**® *see* betamethasone (topical) *on page 85*

becaplermin (be KAP ler min)

U.S. Brand Names Regranex®
Generic Available No
Therapeutic Category Topical Skin Product
Use Treatment of diabetic ulcers that occur on the lower limbs and feet
Usual Dosage Adults: Topical: Apply once daily; applied with a cotton swab or similar tool, as a coating over the ulcer
Dosage Forms Gel, topical: 0.01%

♦ **Because® [OTC]** *see* nonoxynol 9 *on page 446*
♦ **Beclodisk® Diskhaler®** *see* beclomethasone *on page 75*
♦ **Becloforte®** *see* beclomethasone *on page 75*

beclomethasone (be kloe METH a sone)

U.S. Brand Names Beclovent® Oral Inhaler; Beconase AQ® Nasal Inhaler; Beconase® Nasal Inhaler; Vancenase® AQ 84 mcg; Vancenase® AQ Inhaler; Vancenase® Nasal Inhaler; Vanceril® 84 mcg Double Strength; Vanceril® Oral Inhaler
Canadian Brand Names Beclodisk® Diskhaler®; Becloforte®; Propaderm®
Mexican Brand Names Aerobec; Beconase Aqua; Becotide 100; Becotide 250; Becotide Aerosol
Generic Available No
Therapeutic Category Adrenal Corticosteroid
Use
Oral inhalation: Treatment of bronchial asthma in patients who require chronic administration of corticosteroids
Nasal aerosol: Symptomatic treatment of seasonal or perennial rhinitis and nasal polyposis
Usual Dosage
Inhalation:
Children 6-12 years: 1-2 inhalations 3-4 times/day, not to exceed 10 inhalations/day
Adults: 2-4 inhalations twice daily, not to exceed 20 inhalations/day
Aerosol inhalation (nasal):
Children 6-12 years: 1 spray each nostril 3 times/day
Adults: 2-4 sprays each nostril twice daily
Aqueous inhalation (nasal): 1-2 sprays each nostril twice daily
Nursing/Pharmacy Information
Shake thoroughly before using; for asthmatics (to reduce chance of coughing): inhale drug slowly or use prescribed inhaled bronchodilator 5 minutes before beclomethasone
Stability: Do not store near heat or open flame
Dosage Forms
Nasal, as dipropionate:
Inhalation: (Beconase®, Vancenase®): 42 mcg/inhalation [200 metered doses] (16.8 g)
Spray, as dipropionate (Vancenase® AQ Nasal): 0.084% [120 actuations] (19 g)
Spray, aqueous, nasal, as dipropionate (Beconase AQ®, Vancenase® AQ): 42 mcg/inhalation [≥200 metered doses] (25 g); 84 mcg/inhalation [≥200 metered doses] (25 g)
Oral: Inhalation, as dipropionate:
Beclovent®, Vanceril®: 42 mcg/inhalation [200 metered doses] (16.8 g)
Vanceril® Double Strength: 84 mcg/inhalation (5.4 g - 40 metered doses, 12.2 g - 120 metered doses)

♦ **Beclovent® Oral Inhaler** *see* beclomethasone *on page 75*
♦ **Becomject-100® (Discontinued)** *see page 743*
♦ **Beconase AQ® Nasal Inhaler** *see* beclomethasone *on page 75*
♦ **Beconase Aqua** *see* beclomethasone *on page 75*
♦ **Beconase® Nasal Inhaler** *see* beclomethasone *on page 75*
♦ **Becotide 100** *see* beclomethasone *on page 75*
♦ **Becotide 250** *see* beclomethasone *on page 75*
♦ **Becotide Aerosol** *see* beclomethasone *on page 75*
♦ **Becotin® Pulvules®** *see* vitamin, multiple (oral) *on page 654*
♦ **Beepen-VK®** *see* penicillin V potassium *on page 476*
♦ **Beesix® (Discontinued)** *see page 743*
♦ **Beknol** *see* benzonatate *on page 80*
♦ **Belix® Oral [OTC]** *see* diphenhydramine *on page 208*

belladonna (bel a DON a)
Generic Available Yes
Therapeutic Category Anticholinergic Agent
Use Decrease gastrointestinal activity in functional bowel disorders and to delay gastric emptying as well as decrease gastric secretion
Usual Dosage Tincture: Oral:
Children: 0.03 mL/kg 3 times/day
Adults: 0.6-1 mL 3-4 times/day
Nursing/Pharmacy Information
Monitor CNS depression; assist patient with ambulation
Stability: Store in tight, light-resistant container at 15°C to 30°C
Dosage Forms Tincture: Belladonna alkaloids (principally hyoscyamine and atropine) 0.3 mg/mL with alcohol 65% to 70% (120 mL, 480 mL, 3780 mL)

belladonna and opium (bel a DON a & OH pee um)
Synonyms opium and belladonna
U.S. Brand Names B&O Supprettes®
Canadian Brand Names PMS-Opium & Beladonna
Generic Available Yes
Therapeutic Category Analgesic, Narcotic
Controlled Substance C-II
Use Relief of moderate to severe pain associated with rectal or bladder tenesmus that may occur in postoperative states and neoplastic situations; pain associated with ureteral spasms not responsive to non-narcotic analgesics and to space intervals between injections of opiates
Usual Dosage Rectal:
Children: Dose not established
Adults: 1 suppository 1-2 times/day, up to 4 doses/day
Nursing/Pharmacy Information
Monitor CNS depression
Stability: Store at 15°C to 30°C (avoid freezing)
Dosage Forms Suppository:
#15 A: Belladonna extract 15 mg and opium 30 mg
#16 A: Belladonna extract 15 mg and opium 60 mg

belladonna, phenobarbital, and ergotamine tartrate
(bel a DON a, fee noe BAR bi tal, & er GOT a meen TAR trate)
Synonyms ergotamine tartrate, belladonna, and phenobarbital; phenobarbital, belladonna, and ergotamine tartrate
U.S. Brand Names Bellergal-S®; Bel-Phen-Ergot S®; Phenerbel-S®
Generic Available Yes
Therapeutic Category Ergot Alkaloid and Derivative
Use Management and treatment of menopausal disorders, gastrointestinal disorders and recurrent throbbing headache
Usual Dosage Oral: 1 tablet each morning and evening
Nursing/Pharmacy Information May cause drowsiness
Dosage Forms Tablet, sustained release: l-alkaloids of belladonna 0.2 mg, phenobarbital 40 mg, and ergotamine tartrate 0.6 mg

♦ Bellafoline® *(Discontinued)* see page 743
♦ Bellatal® see hyoscyamine, atropine, scopolamine, and phenobarbital on page 330
♦ Bellergal-S® see belladonna, phenobarbital, and ergotamine tartrate on page 76
♦ Bel-Phen-Ergot S® see belladonna, phenobarbital, and ergotamine tartrate on page 76
♦ Bemote® *(Discontinued)* see page 743
♦ Bena-D® *(Discontinued)* see page 743
♦ Benadon see pyridoxine on page 534
♦ Benadryl® 50 mg Capsule *(Discontinued)* see page 743
♦ Benadryl® Cold/Flu *(Discontinued)* see page 743
♦ Benadryl® Decongestant Allergy Tablet [OTC] see diphenhydramine and pseudoephedrine on page 209
♦ Benadryl® Injection see diphenhydramine on page 208
♦ Benadryl® Oral [OTC] see diphenhydramine on page 208
♦ Benadryl® Topical see diphenhydramine on page 208
♦ Benahist® Injection *(Discontinued)* see page 743
♦ Ben-Allergin-50® Injection see diphenhydramine on page 208
♦ Ben-Aqua® [OTC] see benzoyl peroxide on page 81

♦ **Benaxima** *see cefotaxime on page 122*
♦ **Benaxona** *see ceftriaxone on page 126*

benazepril (ben AY ze pril)
U.S. Brand Names Lotensin®
Generic Available No
Therapeutic Category Angiotensin-Converting Enzyme (ACE) Inhibitor
Use Treatment of hypertension, either alone or in combination with other antihypertensive agents
Usual Dosage Adults: Oral: 20-40 mg/day as a single dose or 2 divided doses
Nursing/Pharmacy Information
May cause depression in some patients; discontinue if angioedema of the face, extremities, lips, tongue, or glottis occurs; watch for hypotensive effect within 1-3 hours of first dose or new higher dose
Monitor BUN, serum creatinine, renal function; nausea, headache, diarrhea, change in taste, cough
Dosage Forms Tablet, as hydrochloride: 5 mg, 10 mg, 20 mg, 40 mg

♦ **benazepril and amlodipine** *see amlodipine and benazepril on page 41*

benazepril and hydrochlorothiazide
(ben AY ze pril & hye droe klor oh THYE a zide)
Synonyms hydrochlorothiazide and benazepril
U.S. Brand Names Lotensin® HCT
Generic Available No
Therapeutic Category Antihypertensive Agent, Combination
Use Treatment of hypertension
Usual Dosage Dose is individualized
Dosage Forms Tablet: Benazepril 5 mg and hydrochlorothiazide 6.25 mg; benazepril 10 mg and hydrochlorothiazide 12.5 mg; benazepril 20 mg and hydrochlorothiazide 12.5 mg; benazepril 20 mg and hydrochlorothiazide 25 mg

bendroflumethiazide (ben droe floo meth EYE a zide)
U.S. Brand Names Naturetin®
Generic Available Yes
Therapeutic Category Diuretic, Thiazide
Use Management of mild to moderate hypertension, edema associated with congestive heart failure, pregnancy, or nephrotic syndrome; reportedly does not alter serum electrolyte concentrations appreciably at recommended doses
Usual Dosage Oral:
Children: Initial: 0.1-0.4 mg/kg in 1-2 doses; maintenance dose: 0.05-0.1 mg/kg/day in 1-2 doses
Adults: 2.5-20 mg/day or twice daily in divided doses
Nursing/Pharmacy Information Assess weight, I & O reports daily to determine fluid loss
Dosage Forms Tablet: 5 mg, 10 mg

♦ **Benecid Probenecida Valdecasas** *see probenecid on page 517*
♦ **BeneFix™** *see factor IX complex (human) on page 257*
♦ **Benemid®** *see probenecid on page 517*
♦ **Benoject®** *(Discontinued) see page 743*
♦ **Benoquin®** *see monobenzone on page 421*
♦ **Benoxyl®** *see benzoyl peroxide on page 81*

benserazide and levodopa *(Canada only)*
(ben SER a zide & lee voe DOE pa)
Canadian Brand Names Prolopa®
Generic Available No
Therapeutic Category Anti-Parkinson's Agent
Use Treatment of Parkinson's syndrome with exception of drug-induced parkinsonism
Usual Dosage Adult: Oral: The optimal dose for most patients is usually 4-8 capsules of 100-25 daily (400-800 mg levodopa) divided into 4-6 doses
Dosage Forms Capsule:
50-12.5: Levodopa 50 and benserazide 12.5 mg
100-25: Levodopa 100 mg and benserazide 25 mg
200-50: Levodopa 200 mg and benserazide 50 mg

bentoquatam (ben to KWA tam)
U.S. Brand Names IvyBlock®
Generic Available No
(Continued)

bentoquatam *(Continued)*

Therapeutic Category Protectant, Topical

Use To protect the skin from rash due to exposure to poison sumac, poison ivy or poison oak

Usual Dosage Topical: Apply to exposed skin at least 15 minutes before potential contact and reapply every 4 hours

Dosage Forms Lotion: 5% (120 mL)

♦ **Bentyl® Hydrochloride Injection** *see* dicyclomine *on page 199*

♦ **Bentyl® Hydrochloride Oral** *see* dicyclomine *on page 199*

♦ **Bentylol®** *see* dicyclomine *on page 199*

♦ **Benuryl™** *see* probenecid *on page 517*

♦ **Benylin® Cough Syrup [OTC]** *see* diphenhydramine *on page 208*

♦ **Benylin DM® [OTC]** *see* dextromethorphan *on page 194*

♦ **Benylin® Expectorant [OTC]** *see* guaifenesin and dextromethorphan *on page 300*

♦ **Benylin® Pediatric [OTC]** *see* dextromethorphan *on page 194*

♦ **Benza® [OTC]** *see* benzalkonium chloride *on page 78*

♦ **Benzac AC® Gel** *see* benzoyl peroxide *on page 81*

♦ **Benzac AC® Wash** *see* benzoyl peroxide *on page 81*

♦ **Benzac W® Gel** *see* benzoyl peroxide *on page 81*

♦ **Benzac W® Wash** *see* benzoyl peroxide *on page 81*

♦ **5-Benzagel®** *see* benzoyl peroxide *on page 81*

♦ **10-Benzagel®** *see* benzoyl peroxide *on page 81*

♦ **Benzagel® Gel** *see* benzoyl peroxide *on page 81*

♦ **Benzagel® Lotion** *see* benzoyl peroxide *on page 81*

♦ **Benzagel® Wash** *see* benzoyl peroxide *on page 81*

benzalkonium chloride *(benz al KOE nee um KLOR ide)*

Synonyms BAC

U.S. Brand Names Benza® [OTC]; Zephiran® [OTC]

Generic Available Yes

Therapeutic Category Antibacterial, Topical

Use Surface antiseptic and germicidal preservative

Usual Dosage Thoroughly rinse anionic detergents and soaps from the skin or other areas prior to use of solutions because they reduce the antibacterial activity of BAC; to protect metal instruments stored in BAC solution, add crushed Anti-Rust Tablets, 4 tablets per quart, to antiseptic solution, change solution at least once weekly; not to be used for storage of aluminum or zinc instruments, instruments with lenses fastened by cement, lacquered catheters or some synthetic rubber goods

Nursing/Pharmacy Information The following substances are **incompatible** with BAC solutions: Iodine, silver nitrate, fluorescein, nitrates, peroxide, lanolin, potassium permanganate, aluminum, caramel, kaolin, pine oil, zinc sulfate, zinc oxide and yellow mercuric oxide

Dosage Forms

Concentrate, topical: 17% (500 mL, 4000 mL)

Solution, aqueous: 1:750 (60 mL, 120 mL, 240 mL)

Tincture: 1:750 (30 mL, 960 mL)

Tincture, spray: 1:750 (30 g, 180 g)

Tissue: 1:750 (packets)

♦ **benzalkonium chloride, benzocaine, butyl aminobenzoate, tetracaine** *see* benzocaine, butyl aminobenzoate, tetracaine, and benzalkonium chloride *on page 79*

♦ **Benzamycin®** *see* erythromycin and benzoyl peroxide *on page 239*

♦ **Benzanil** *see* penicillin G, parenteral, aqueous *on page 475*

♦ **Benzashave® Cream** *see* benzoyl peroxide *on page 81*

♦ **benzathine benzylpenicillin** *see* penicillin G benzathine *on page 474*

♦ **benzathine penicillin g** *see* penicillin G benzathine *on page 474*

♦ **benzazoline** *see* tolazoline *on page 617*

♦ **Benzedrex® [OTC]** *see* propylhexedrine *on page 528*

♦ **benzene hexachloride** *see* lindane *on page 370*

♦ **Benzetacil** *see* penicillin G benzathine *on page 474*

♦ **benzhexol** *see* trihexyphenidyl *on page 628*

♦ **Benzilfan** *see* penicillin G benzathine *on page 474*

benzocaine (BEN zoe kane)

Synonyms ethyl aminobenzoate

U.S. Brand Names Americaine® [OTC]; Anbesol® [OTC]; Anbesol® Maximum Strength [OTC]; Babee® Teething® [OTC]; Benzocol® [OTC]; Benzodent® [OTC]; Chiggertox® [OTC]; Cylex® [OTC]; Dermoplast® [OTC]; Foille® [OTC]; Foille® Medicated First Aid [OTC]; Hurricaine®; Lanacane® [OTC]; Maximum Strength Anbesol® [OTC]; Maximum Strength Orajel® [OTC]; Mycinettes® [OTC]; Numzitdent® [OTC]; Numzit Teething® [OTC]; Orabase®-B [OTC]; Orabase®-O [OTC]; Orajel® Brace-Aid Oral Anesthetic [OTC]; Orajel® Maximum Strength [OTC]; Orajel® Mouth-Aid [OTC]; Orasept® [OTC]; Orasol® [OTC]; Rhulicaine® [OTC]; Rid-A-Pain® [OTC]; Slim-Mint® [OTC]; Solarcaine® [OTC]; Spec-T® [OTC]; Tanac® [OTC]; Trocaine® [OTC]; Unguentine® [OTC]; Vicks Children's Chloraseptic® [OTC]; Vicks Chloraseptic® Sore Throat [OTC]; Zilactin-B® Medicated [OTC]

Mexican Brand Names Graneodin-B

Generic Available Yes

Therapeutic Category Local Anesthetic

Use Temporary relief of pain associated with pruritic dermatosis, pruritus, minor burns, toothache, minor sore throat pain, canker sores, hemorrhoids, rectal fissures; anesthetic lubricant for passage of catheters and endoscopic tubes

Usual Dosage

Children and Adults:

Mucous membranes: Dosage varies depending on area to be anesthetized and vascularity of tissues

Oral mouth/throat preparations: Do not administer for >2 days or in children <2 years of age, unless directed by a physician; refer to specific package labeling

Topical: Apply to affected area as needed

Adults: Nonprescription diet aid: 6-15 mg just prior to food consumption, not to exceed 45 mg/day

Dietary Considerations Administer nonprescription diet aid just prior to food consumption

Nursing/Pharmacy Information Patient should not eat within 1 hour after application to oral mucosa

Dosage Forms

Topical for mucous membranes:

Gel: 6% (7.5 g); 20% (2.5 g, 3.75 g, 7.5 g, 30 g)

Liquid: 20% (3.75 mL, 9 mL, 13.3 mL, 30 mL)

Topical for skin disorders:

Aerosol, external use: 5% (92 mL, 105 g); 20% (82.5 mL, 90 mL, 92 mL, 150 mL)

Cream: (30 g, 60 g); 5% (30 g, 1 lb); 6% (28.4 g)

Lotion: (120 mL); 8% (90 mL)

Ointment: 5% (3.5 g, 28 g)

Spray: 5% (97.5 mL); 20% (20 g, 60 g, 120 g, 13.3 mL, 120 mL)

Mouth/throat preparations:

Cream: 5% (10 g)

Gel: 6.3% (7.5 g); 7.5% (7.2 g, 9.45 g, 14.1 g); 10% (6 g, 9.45 g, 10 g, 15 g); 15% (10.5 g); 20% (9.45 g, 14.1 g)

Liquid: (3.7 mL); 5% (8.8 mL); 6.3% (9 mL, 22 mL, 14.79 mL); 10% (13 mL); 20% (13.3 mL)

Lotion: 0.2% (15 mL); 2.5% (15 mL)

Lozenges: 5 mg, 6 mg, 10 mg, 15 mg

Ointment: 20% (30 g)

Paste: 20% (5 g, 15 g)

Nonprescription diet aid:

Candy: 6 mg

Gum: 6 mg

♦ **benzocaine and antipyrine** see antipyrine and benzocaine on page 53

♦ **benzocaine and cetylpyridinium chloride** see cetylpyridinium and benzocaine on page 130

benzocaine, butyl aminobenzoate, tetracaine, and benzalkonium chloride

(BEN zoe kane, BYOO til a meen oh BENZ oh ate, TET ra kane, & benz al KOE nee um KLOR ide)

Synonyms benzalkonium chloride, benzocaine, butyl aminobenzoate, tetracaine; butyl aminobenzoate, benzocaine, tetracaine, and benzalkonium chloride; tetracaine hydrochloride, benzocaine, butyl aminobenzoate, and benzalkonium chloride

(Continued)

benzocaine, butyl aminobenzoate, tetracaine, and benzalkonium chloride *(Continued)*

U.S. Brand Names Cetacaine®
Generic Available No
Therapeutic Category Local Anesthetic
Use Topical anesthetic to control pain or gagging
Usual Dosage Topical: Apply to affected area for approximately 1 second or less
Nursing/Pharmacy Information Only topical anesthetic which comes in an easy to spray bottle, however, sensitization may result from any one of the ingredients
Dosage Forms Aerosol: Benzocaine 14%, butyl aminobenzoate 2%, tetracaine 2%, and benzalkonium chloride 0.5% (56 g)

benzocaine, gelatin, pectin, and sodium carboxymethylcellulose

(BEN zoe kane, JEL a tin, PEK tin, & SOW dee um kar box ee meth il SEL yoo lose)
U.S. Brand Names Orabase® With Benzocaine [OTC]
Generic Available No
Therapeutic Category Local Anesthetic
Use Topical anesthetic and emollient for oral lesions
Usual Dosage Topical: Apply 2-4 times/day
Dosage Forms Paste: Benzocaine 20%, gelatin, pectin, and sodium carboxymethylcellulose (15 g, 5 g)

♦ **Benzocol® [OTC]** *see* benzocaine *on page 79*
♦ **Benzodent® [OTC]** *see* benzocaine *on page 79*

benzoic acid and salicylic acid

(ben ZOE ik AS id & sal i SIL ik AS id)
Synonyms salicylic acid and benzoic acid
U.S. Brand Names Whitfield's Ointment [OTC]
Generic Available Yes
Therapeutic Category Antifungal Agent
Use Treatment of athlete's foot and ringworm of the scalp
Usual Dosage Topical: Apply 1-4 times/day
Nursing/Pharmacy Information For external use only
Dosage Forms
Lotion, topical:
Full strength: Benzoic acid 12% and salicylic acid 6% with isopropyl alcohol 70% (240 mL)
Half strength: Benzoic acid 6% and salicylic acid 3% with isopropyl alcohol 70% (240 mL)
Ointment, topical: Benzoic acid 12% and salicylic acid 6% in anhydrous lanolin and petrolatum (30 g, 454 g)

benzoin (BEN zoyn)

Synonyms gum benjamin
U.S. Brand Names AeroZoin® [OTC]; TinBen® [OTC]; TinCoBen® [OTC]
Generic Available Yes
Therapeutic Category Pharmaceutical Aid; Protectant, Topical
Use Protective application for irritations of the skin; sometimes used in boiling water as steam inhalants for their expectorant and soothing action
Usual Dosage Topical: Apply 1-2 times/day
Nursing/Pharmacy Information For external use only
Dosage Forms
Spray, as compound tincture: 40% (105 mL)
Tincture: 79% (480 mL)
Tincture, as compound tincture: 20% (60 mL); 25% (120 mL)

benzonatate (ben ZOE na tate)

U.S. Brand Names Tessalon® Perles
Mexican Brand Names Beknol; Pebegal; Tesalon
Generic Available Yes
Therapeutic Category Antitussive
Use Symptomatic relief of nonproductive cough
Usual Dosage Oral:
Children <10 years: 8 mg/kg in 3-6 divided doses

Children >10 years and Adults: 100 mg 3 times/day up to 600 mg/day
Nursing/Pharmacy Information
Change patient position every 2 hours to prevent pooling of secretions in lung; capsules are not to be crushed
Monitor patient's chest sounds and respiratory pattern
Dosage Forms Capsule: 100 mg

benzoyl peroxide (BEN zoe il peer OKS ide)
U.S. Brand Names Advanced Formula Oxy® Sensitive Gel [OTC]; Ambi 10® [OTC]; Ben-Aqua® [OTC]; Benoxyl®; Benzac AC® Gel; Benzac AC® Wash; Benzac W® Gel; Benzac W® Wash; 5-Benzagel®; 10-Benzagel®; Benzashave® Cream; BlemErase® Lotion [OTC]; Brevoxyl® Gel; Clear By Design® Gel [OTC]; Clearsil® Maximum Strength [OTC]; Del Aqua-5® Gel; Del Aqua-10® Gel; Desquam-E™ Gel; Desquam-X® Gel; Desquam-X® Wash; Dryox® Gel [OTC]; Dryox® Wash [OTC]; Exact® Cream [OTC]; Fostex® 10% BPO Gel [OTC]; Fostex® 10% Wash [OTC]; Fostex® Bar [OTC]; Loroxide® [OTC]; Neutrogena® Acne Mask [OTC]; Oxy-5® Advanced Formula for Sensitive Skin [OTC]; Oxy-5® Tinted [OTC]; Oxy-10® Advanced Formula for Sensitive Skin [OTC]; Oxy 10® Wash [OTC]; PanOxyl®-AQ; PanOxyl® Bar [OTC]; Perfectoderm® Gel [OTC]; Peroxin A5®; Peroxin A10®; Persa-Gel®; Theroxide® Wash [OTC]; Vanoxide® [OTC]
Canadian Brand Names Acetoxyl®; Acnomel® B.P.5; Benzagel® Gel; Benzagel® Lotion; Benzagel® Wash; H₂Oxyl®; Oxyderm™ 5%, 10%, 20%; Solugel® 4, 8
Generic Available Yes
Therapeutic Category Acne Products
Use Adjunctive treatment of mild to moderate acne vulgaris
Usual Dosage Children and Adults:
Cleansers: Wash once or twice daily; control amount of drying or peeling by modifying dose frequency or concentration
Topical: Apply sparingly once daily; gradually increase to 2-3 times/day if needed. If excessive dryness or peeling occurs, reduce dose frequency or concentration; if excessive stinging or burning occurs, remove with mild soap and water; resume use the next day.
Nursing/Pharmacy Information Watch for signs of systemic infection; granulation may indicate effectiveness
Dosage Forms
Bar: 5% (113 g); 10% (106 g, 113 g)
Cream: 5% (18 g, 113.4 g); 10% (18 g, 28 g, 113.4 g)
Gel: 2.5% (30 g, 42.5 g, 45 g, 57 g, 60 g, 90 g, 113 g); 5% (42.5 g, 45 g, 60 g, 80 g, 90 g, 113.4 g); 10% (30 g, 42.5 g, 45 g, 56.7 g, 60 g, 90 g, 113.4 g, 120 g); 20% (30 g, 60 g)
Liquid: 5% (120 mL, 150 mL, 240 mL); 10% (120 mL, 150 mL, 240 mL)
Lotion: 5% (25 mL, 30 mL); 5.5% (25 mL); 10% (12 mL, 29 mL, 30 mL, 60 mL)
Mask: 5% (30 mL, 60 mL, 60 g)

♦ **benzoyl peroxide and erythromycin** see erythromycin and benzoyl peroxide on page 239

benzoyl peroxide and hydrocortisone
(BEN zoe il peer OKS ide & hye droe KOR ti sone)
Synonyms hydrocortisone and benzoyl peroxide
U.S. Brand Names Vanoxide-HC®
Generic Available No
Therapeutic Category Acne Products
Use Treatment of acne vulgaris and oily skin
Usual Dosage Topical: Shake well; apply thin film 1-3 times/day, gently massage into skin
Dosage Forms Lotion: Benzoyl peroxide 5% and hydrocortisone alcohol 0.5% (25 mL)

benzphetamine (benz FET a meen)
U.S. Brand Names Didrex®
Generic Available No
Therapeutic Category Anorexiant
Controlled Substance C-III
Use Short-term adjunct in exogenous obesity
Usual Dosage Adults: Oral: 25-50 mg 2-3 times/day, preferably twice daily, midmorning and midafternoon
Nursing/Pharmacy Information Monitor CNS
Dosage Forms Tablet, as hydrochloride: 25 mg, 50 mg

benzthiazide (benz THYE a zide)
U.S. Brand Names Exna®
Generic Available Yes
Therapeutic Category Diuretic, Thiazide
Use Management of mild to moderate hypertension; treatment of edema in congestive heart failure and nephrotic syndrome
Usual Dosage Adults: Oral: 50-200 mg/day
Nursing/Pharmacy Information Monitor blood pressure, serum electrolytes, BUN, creatinine; assess weight, I & O reports daily to determine fluid loss; take blood pressure with patient lying down and standing
Dosage Forms Tablet: 50 mg

benztropine (BENZ troe peen)
U.S. Brand Names Cogentin®
Canadian Brand Names PMS-Benztropine
Generic Available Yes: Tablet
Therapeutic Category Anticholinergic Agent; Anti-Parkinson's Agent
Use Adjunctive treatment of parkinsonism; also used in treatment of drug-induced extrapyramidal effects (except tardive dyskinesia) and acute dystonic reactions
Usual Dosage Titrate dose in 0.5 mg increments at 5- to 6-day intervals
Extrapyramidal reaction, drug induced: Oral, I.M., I.V.:
Children >3 years: 0.02-0.05 mg/kg/dose 1-2 times/day
Adults: 1-4 mg/dose 1-2 times/day
Parkinsonism: Oral: 0.5-6 mg/day in 1-2 divided doses; if one dose is greater, administer at bedtime
Dietary Considerations May be administered with food
Nursing/Pharmacy Information No significant difference in onset of I.M. or I.V. injection, therefore, there is usually no need to use the I.V. route; improvement is sometimes noticeable a few minutes after injection. Do not discontinue drug abruptly
Dosage Forms
Injection, as mesylate: 1 mg/mL (2 mL)
Tablet, as mesylate: 0.5 mg, 1 mg, 2 mg

♦ **benzylpenicillin** *see* penicillin G, parenteral, aqueous *on page 475*
♦ **benzylpenicillin benzathine** *see* penicillin G benzathine *on page 474*

benzylpenicilloyl-polylysine (BEN zil pen i SIL oyl pol i LIE seen)
Synonyms penicilloyl-polylysine; PPL
U.S. Brand Names Pre-Pen®
Generic Available No
Therapeutic Category Diagnostic Agent
Use As an adjunct in assessing the risk of administering penicillin (penicillin or benzylpenicillin) in patients with a history of clinical penicillin hypersensitivity
Usual Dosage
Use scratch technique with a 20-gauge needle to make 3-5 mm scratch on epidermis, apply a small drop of solution to scratch, rub in gently with applicator or toothpick
A positive reaction consists of a pale wheal surrounding the scratch site which develops within 10 minutes and ranges from 5-15 mm or more in diameter
If the scratch test is negative an intradermal test may be performed
Intradermal test: Use intradermal test with a tuberculin syringe with a 26- to 30-gauge short bevel needle; a dose of 0.01-0.02 mL is injected intradermally. A control of 0.9% sodium chloride should be injected at least 1½" from the PPL test site. Most skin responses to the intradermal test will develop within 5-15 minutes.
(-) = no reaction or increase in size compared to control
(±) = wheal slightly larger with or without erythematous flare and larger than control site
(+) = itching and increase in size of original bleb may exceed 20 mm in diameter
Nursing/Pharmacy Information
PPL is administered by a scratch technique or by intradermal injection. For initial testing, PPL should always be applied via the scratch technique. Do not administer intradermally to patients who have positive reactions to a scratch test.
Stability: Store in refrigerator; discard if left at room temperature >1 day
Dosage Forms Solution: 0.25 mL

bepridil (BE pri dil)

U.S. Brand Names Vascor®

Canadian Brand Names Bapadin®

Generic Available No

Therapeutic Category Calcium Channel Blocker

Use Treatment of chronic stable angina; only approved indication is hypertension, but may be used for congestive heart failure; doses should not be adjusted for at least 10 days after beginning therapy

Usual Dosage Adults: Oral: Initial: 200 mg/day, then adjust dose until optimal response is achieved; maximum daily dose: 400 mg

Nursing/Pharmacy Information
May cause cardiac arrhythmias if potassium is low
Monitor EKG and serum electrolytes

Dosage Forms Tablet, as hydrochloride: 200 mg, 300 mg, 400 mg

beractant (ber AKT ant)

Synonyms bovine lung surfactant; natural lung surfactant

U.S. Brand Names Survanta®

Generic Available No

Therapeutic Category Lung Surfactant

Use Prevention and treatment of respiratory distress syndrome (RDS) in premature infants

Prophylactic therapy: Infants with body weight <1250 g who are at risk for developing or with evidence of surfactant deficiency

Rescue therapy: Treatment of infants with RDS confirmed by x-ray and requiring mechanical ventilation

Usual Dosage Intratracheal:

Prophylactic treatment: Administer 4 mL/kg as soon as possible; as many as 4 doses may be administered during the first 48 hours of life, no more frequently than 6 hours apart. The need for additional doses is determined by evidence of continuing respiratory distress; if the infant is still intubated and requiring at least 30% inspired oxygen to maintain a PaO$_2$ ≤80 torr.

Rescue treatment: Administer 4 mL/kg as soon as the diagnosis of RDS is made

Nursing/Pharmacy Information

For intratracheal administration only. Suction infant prior to administration; inspect solution to verify complete mixing of the suspension. Administer intratracheally by instillation through a 5-French end-hole catheter inserted into the infant's endotracheal tube. Administer the dose in four 1 mL/kg aliquots. Each quarter-dose is instilled over 2-3 seconds; each quarter-dose is administered with the infant in a different position; slightly downward inclination with head turned to the right, then repeat with head turned to the left; then slightly upward inclination with head turned to the right, then repeat with head turned to the left. Do not shake; if settling occurs during storage, swirl gently.

Continuous EKG and transcutaneous O$_2$ saturation should be monitored during administration; frequent ABG sampling is necessary to prevent postdosing hyperoxia and hypocarbia

Stability: Refrigerate; protect from light, prior to administration warm by standing at room temperature for 20 minutes or held in hand for 8 minutes; artificial warming methods should **not** be used; unused, unopened vials warmed to room temperature may be returned to the refrigerator within 8 hours of warming only once

Dosage Forms Suspension: 200 mg (8 mL)

♦ **Berocca®** see vitamin B complex with vitamin C and folic acid *on page 652*

♦ **Berotec® Forte Inhalation Aerosol** see fenoterol *(Canada only) on page 262*

♦ **Berotec® Inhalation Aerosol** see fenoterol *(Canada only) on page 262*

♦ **Berotec® Solution** see fenoterol *(Canada only) on page 262*

♦ **Berubigen®** see cyanocobalamin *on page 173*

♦ **Beta-2®** see isoetharine *on page 346*

beta-carotene (BAY tah KARE oh teen)

Generic Available Yes

Therapeutic Category Vitamin, Fat Soluble

Use Reduce the severity of photosensitivity reactions in patients with erythropoietic protoporphyria (EPP)

Usual Dosage Oral:
Children <14 years: 30-150 mg/day
(Continued)

beta-carotene *(Continued)*

Adults: 30-300 mg/day

Dietary Considerations May be administered with meals

Nursing/Pharmacy Information Skin may appear slightly yellow-orange; not a proven sunscreen

Dosage Forms Capsule: 15 mg, 30 mg

- ♦ **Betachron®** *see* propranolol *on page 527*
- ♦ **Betacort™** *see* betamethasone (topical) *on page 85*
- ♦ **Betaderm** *see* betamethasone (topical) *on page 85*
- ♦ **Betadine® [OTC]** *see* povidone-iodine *on page 510*
- ♦ **Betadine® 5% Sterile Ophthalmic Prep Solution** *see* povidone-iodine *on page 510*
- ♦ **Betadine® First Aid Antibiotics + Moisturizer [OTC]** *see* bacitracin and polymyxin B *on page 71*
- ♦ **9-beta-D-ribofuranosyladenine** *see* adenosine *on page 22*
- ♦ **Betaferon®** *see* interferon beta-1b *on page 343*
- ♦ **Betagan® [OTC]** *see* povidone-iodine *on page 510*
- ♦ **Betagan® Liquifilm® Ophthalmic** *see* levobunolol *on page 364*

betahistine *(Canada only)* (bay ta HISS teen)

Canadian Brand Names Serc®

Generic Available No

Therapeutic Category Antihistamine

Use May be of value in the treatment of Ménière's disease

Usual Dosage Adult: Oral: 4-8 mg 3 times/day

Dosage Forms Tablet, as hydrochloride: 4 mg

betaine anhydrous (BAY tayne an HY drus)

U.S. Brand Names Cystadane®

Generic Available No

Therapeutic Category Urinary Tract Product

Use Treatment of homocystinuria

Usual Dosage Oral: 6 g/day, usually given in two 3 g doses

Dosage Forms Powder: 1 g/1.7 mL (180 g)

- ♦ **Betalene® Topical** *see* betamethasone (topical) *on page 85*
- ♦ **Betalin®S** *see* thiamine *on page 606*
- ♦ **Betaloc®** *see* metoprolol *on page 410*
- ♦ **Betaloc Durules®** *see* metoprolol *on page 410*

betamethasone and clotrimazole

(bay ta METH a sone & kloe TRIM a zole)

Synonyms clotrimazole and betamethasone

U.S. Brand Names Lotrisone®

Generic Available No

Therapeutic Category Antifungal/Corticosteroid

Use Topical treatment of various dermal fungal infections

Usual Dosage Topical: Apply twice daily

Nursing/Pharmacy Information For external use only; do not use on open wounds

Dosage Forms Cream: Betamethasone dipropionate 0.05% and clotrimazole 1% (15 g, 45 g)

betamethasone (systemic) (bay ta METH a sone)

U.S. Brand Names Celestone® Oral; Celestone® Phosphate Injection; Celestone® Soluspan®; Cel-U-Jec® Injection

Canadian Brand Names Selestoject®

Generic Available Yes

Therapeutic Category Adrenal Corticosteroid

Use Anti-inflammatory; immunosuppressant agent; corticosteroid replacement therapy

Usual Dosage Children and Adults:

I.M.: Betamethasone sodium phosphate and betamethasone acetate: 0.5-9 mg/day (1/3 to 1/2 of oral dose)

Intrabursal, intra-articular: 0.5-2 mL

Oral: 0.6-7.2 mg/day

Dietary Considerations May be administered with food to decrease GI distress; systemic use of corticosteroids may require a diet with increased potassium, vitamins A, B$_6$, C, D, folate, calcium, zinc, and phosphorus and decreased sodium

Nursing/Pharmacy Information Not for alternate-day therapy; once daily doses should be administered in the morning; do not administer injectable sodium phosphate/acetate suspension I.V.

Dosage Forms
Base (Celestone®), Oral:
  Syrup: 0.6 mg/5 mL (118 mL)
  Tablet: 0.6 mg
Dipropionate (Diprosone®)
  Aerosol: 0.1% (85 g)
  Cream: 0.05% (15 g, 45 g)
  Lotion: 0.05% (20 mL, 30 mL, 60 mL)
  Ointment: 0.05% (15 g, 45 g)
Dipropionate augmented (Diprolene®)
  Cream: 0.05% (15 g, 45 g)
  Gel: 0.05% (15 g, 45 g)
  Lotion: 0.05% (30 mL, 60 mL)
  Ointment, topical: 0.05% (15 g, 45 g)
Valerate (Betatrex®, Valisone®)
  Cream: 0.01% (15 g, 60 g); 0.1% (15 g, 45 g, 110 g, 430 g)
  Lotion: 0.1% (20 mL, 60 mL)
  Ointment: 0.1% (15 g, 45 g)
Valerate (Beta-Val®)
  Cream: 0.01% (15 g, 60 g); 0.1% (15 g, 45 g, 110 g, 430 g)
  Lotion: 0.1% (20 mL, 60 mL)
Injection: Sodium phosphate (Celestone Phosphate®, Cel-U-Jec®): 4 mg betamethasone phosphate/mL (equivalent to 3 mg betamethasone/mL) (5 mL)
Injection, suspension: Sodium phosphate and acetate (Celestone® Soluspan®): 6 mg/mL (3 mg of betamethasone sodium phosphate and 3 mg of betamethasone acetate per mL) (5 mL)

betamethasone (topical) (bay ta METH a sone)

Synonyms flubenisolone
U.S. Brand Names Alphatrex® Topical; Betalene® Topical; Betatrex® Topical; Beta-Val® Topical; Diprolene® AF Topical; Diprolene® Topical; Diprosone® Topical; Maxivate® Topical; Psorion® Topical; Teladar® Topical; Valisone® Topical
Canadian Brand Names Beben®; Betacort™; Betaderm; Betnesol®; Betnovate®; Celestoderm®-V, -EV/2; Diprolene® Glycol; Ectosone; Occlucort®; Rhoprolene®; Rhoprosone®; Taro-Sone®; Topilene®; Topisone®
Generic Available Yes
Therapeutic Category Corticosteroid, Topical
Use Inflammatory dermatoses such as psoriasis, seborrheic or atopic dermatitis, neurodermatitis, inflammatory phase of xerosis, late phase of allergic dermatitis or irritant dermatitis
Usual Dosage Topical: Adults: Apply thin film 2-4 times/day
Dietary Considerations May be administered with food to decrease GI distress; systemic use of corticosteroids may require a diet with increased potassium, vitamins A, B$_6$, C, D, folate, calcium, zinc, and phosphorus and decreased sodium

Nursing/Pharmacy Information
Apply topical sparingly to areas; not for use on broken skin or in areas of infection; do not apply to wet skin unless directed; do not apply to face or inguinal area
Not for alternate-day therapy; once daily doses should be administered in the morning; do not administer injectable sodium phosphate/acetate suspension I.V.

Dosage Forms
Betamethasone dipropionate
  Aerosol: 0.1% (85 g)
  Cream: 0.05% (15 g, 45 g)
  Lotion: 0.05% (20 mL, 30 mL, 60 mL)
  Ointment: 0.05% (15 g, 45 g)
Betamethasone dipropionate augmented
  Cream: 0.05% (15 g, 45 g)
  Gel: 0.05% (15 g, 45 g)
  Lotion: 0.05% (30 mL, 60 mL)
  Ointment, topical: 0.05% (15 g, 45 g)
Betamethasone valerate
  Cream: 0.01% (15 g, 60 g); 0.1% (15 g, 45 g, 110 g, 430 g)
(Continued)

betamethasone (topical) *(Continued)*

    Lotion: 0.1% (20 mL, 60 mL)
    Ointment: 0.1% (15 g, 45 g)

- **Betapace®** *see* sotalol *on page 577*
- **Betapen-VK®** *(Discontinued) see page 743*
- **Betasept® [OTC]** *see* chlorhexidine gluconate *on page 134*
- **Betaseron®** *see* interferon beta-1b *on page 343*
- **Beta-Tim®** *see* timolol *on page 613*
- **Betatrex® Topical** *see* betamethasone (topical) *on page 85*
- **Beta-Val® Ointment** *(Discontinued) see page 743*
- **Beta-Val® Topical** *see* betamethasone (topical) *on page 85*
- **Betaxin®** *see* thiamine *on page 606*

betaxolol (be TAKS oh lol)

U.S. Brand Names Betoptic® Ophthalmic; Betoptic® S Ophthalmic; Kerlone® Oral

Generic Available No

Therapeutic Category Beta-Adrenergic Blocker

Use Treatment of chronic open-angle glaucoma, ocular hypertension; management of hypertension

Usual Dosage Adults:

    Ophthalmic: Instill 1 drop twice daily

    Oral: 10 mg/day; may increase dose to 20 mg/day after 7-14 days if desired response is not achieved; initial dose in elderly patients: 5 mg/day

Nursing/Pharmacy Information

    Use cautiously in diabetics receiving hypoglycemic agents; teach proper instillation of eye drops

    Monitor intraocular pressure (ophthalmic); blood pressure, pulse, respiratory difficulty (bronchospasm)

    Stability: Avoid freezing

Dosage Forms

    Solution, ophthalmic, as hydrochloride (Betoptic®): 0.5% (2.5 mL, 5 mL, 10 mL)

    Suspension, ophthalmic, as hydrochloride (Betoptic® S): 0.25% (2.5 mL, 10 mL, 15 mL)

    Tablet, as hydrochloride (Kerlone®): 10 mg, 20 mg

bethanechol (be THAN e kole)

U.S. Brand Names Duvoid®; Myotonachol™; Urabeth®; Urecholine®

Canadian Brand Names PMS-Bethanechol Chloride

Generic Available Yes: Tablet

Therapeutic Category Cholinergic Agent

Use Treatment of nonobstructive urinary retention and retention due to neurogenic bladder; gastroesophageal reflux

Usual Dosage

    Children:

        Oral:

            Abdominal distention or urinary retention: 0.6 mg/kg/day divided 3-4 times/day

            Gastroesophageal reflux: 0.1-0.2 mg/kg/dose administered 30 minutes to 1 hour before each meal to a maximum of 4 times/day

        S.C.: 0.15-0.2 mg/kg/day divided 3-4 times/day

    Adults:

        Oral: 10-50 mg 2-4 times/day

        S.C.: 2.5-5 mg 3-4 times/day, up to 7.5-10 mg every 4 hours for neurogenic bladder

Dietary Considerations Should be administered 1 hour before meals or 2 hours after meals

Nursing/Pharmacy Information Contraindicated for I.M. or I.V. use due to a likely severe cholinergic reaction; for S.C. injection only; observe closely for side effects; have bedpan readily available if administered for urinary retention

Dosage Forms

    Injection, as chloride: 5 mg/mL (1 mL)

    Tablet, as chloride: 5 mg, 10 mg, 25 mg, 50 mg

- **Betnesol®** *see* betamethasone (topical) *on page 85*
- **Betnovate®** *see* betamethasone (topical) *on page 85*
- **Betoptic® Ophthalmic** *see* betaxolol *on page 86*
- **Betoptic® S Ophthalmic** *see* betaxolol *on page 86*
- **Bewon®** *see* thiamine *on page 606*

♦ **Bexophene**® *see* propoxyphene and aspirin *on page 526*

bezafibrate *(Canada only)* (be za FYE brate)
Canadian Brand Names Bezalip®
Generic Available No
Therapeutic Category Antilipemic Agent
Use Adjunct to dietary therapy in the management of hyperlipidemias associated with high triglyceride levels (types III, IV, V); primarily lowers triglycerides and very low density lipoprotein
Usual Dosage Adult: Oral: 200 mg 3 times/day
Dosage Forms Tablet: 200 mg, 400 mg

♦ **Bezalip**® *see* bezafibrate *(Canada only) on page 87*
♦ **Biamine**® **Injection** *(Discontinued) see page 743*
♦ **Biavax**® II *see* rubella and mumps vaccines, combined *on page 555*
♦ **Biaxin**™ *see* clarithromycin *on page 155*

bicalutamide (bye ka LOO ta mide)
U.S. Brand Names Casodex®
Generic Available No
Therapeutic Category Androgen
Use Combination therapy with a luteinizing hormone-releasing hormone (LHRH) analog for the treatment of advanced prostate cancer
Usual Dosage Adults: Oral: 50 mg once daily (morning or evening), with or without food, in combination with a LHRH analog
Dietary Considerations May be administered with or without food
Nursing/Pharmacy Information Administer at the same time as treatment with LHRH analog
Dosage Forms Tablet: 50 mg

♦ **Bicillin**® **C-R** *see* penicillin G benzathine and procaine combined *on page 475*
♦ **Bicillin**® **C-R 900/300** *see* penicillin G benzathine and procaine combined *on page 475*
♦ **Bicillin**® **L-A** *see* penicillin G benzathine *on page 474*
♦ **Biclin** *see* amikacin *on page 36*
♦ **BiCNU**® *see* carmustine *on page 116*
♦ **Bilem** *see* tamoxifen *on page 592*
♦ **Bilezyme**® **Tablet** *(Discontinued) see page 743*
♦ **Bilopaque**® *see* radiological/contrast media (ionic) *on page 539*
♦ **Biltricide**® *see* praziquantel *on page 512*
♦ **Binotal** *see* ampicillin *on page 46*
♦ **Biocef**® *see* cephalexin *on page 128*
♦ **Bioclate**® *see* antihemophilic factor (recombinant) *on page 52*
♦ **Bioderm** *see* bacitracin and polymyxin B *on page 71*
♦ **Biodine [OTC]** *see* povidone-iodine *on page 510*
♦ **Biohist-LA**® *see* carbinoxamine and pseudoephedrine *on page 113*
♦ **Biomox**® *(Discontinued) see page 743*
♦ **Bion**® **Tears Solution [OTC]** *see* artificial tears *on page 59*
♦ **Biosint**® *see* cefotaxime *on page 122*
♦ **Bio-Tab**® *see* doxycycline *on page 222*
♦ **Biozyme-C**® *see* collagenase *on page 167*

biperiden (bye PER i den)
U.S. Brand Names Akineton®
Generic Available No
Therapeutic Category Anticholinergic Agent; Anti-Parkinson's Agent
Use Treatment of all forms of Parkinsonism including drug-induced type (extrapyramidal symptoms)
Usual Dosage Adults:
Parkinsonism: Oral: 2 mg 3-4 times/day
Extrapyramidal:
Oral: 2-6 mg 2-3 times/day
I.M., I.V.: 2 mg every 30 minutes up to 4 doses or 8 mg/day
Nursing/Pharmacy Information No significant difference in onset of I.M. or I.V. injection, therefore, there is usually no need to use the I.V. route. Improvement is sometimes noticeable a few minutes after injection. Do not discontinue drug abruptly.
(Continued)

biperiden *(Continued)*

Dosage Forms
Injection, as lactate: 5 mg/mL (1 mL)
Tablet, as hydrochloride: 2 mg

♦ **Biphetamine®** *(Discontinued)* see page 743
♦ **Biquin® Durules®** see quinidine on page 536
♦ **Bisac-Evac® [OTC]** see bisacodyl on page 88

bisacodyl (bis a KOE dil)
U.S. Brand Names Bisac-Evac® [OTC]; Bisacodyl Uniserts®; Bisco-Lax® [OTC]; Carter's Little Pills® [OTC]; Clysodrast®; Dacodyl® [OTC]; Deficol® [OTC]; Dulcolax® [OTC]; Fleet® Laxative [OTC]
Canadian Brand Names Apo®-Bisacodyl; PMS-Bisacodyl
Generic Available Yes
Therapeutic Category Laxative
Use Treatment of constipation; colonic evacuation prior to procedures or examination
Usual Dosage
Children:
Oral: >6 years: 5-10 mg (0.3 mg/kg) at bedtime or before breakfast
Rectal suppository:
<2 years: 5 mg as a single dose
>2 years: 10 mg
Adults:
Oral: 5-15 mg as single dose (up to 30 mg when complete evacuation of bowel is required)
Rectal suppository: 10 mg as single dose
Tannex:
Enema: 2.5 g in 1000 mL warm water
Barium enema: 2.5-5 g in 1000 mL barium suspension
Do not administer >10 g within a 72-hour period
Dietary Considerations Should not be administered within 1 hour of milk, any dairy products, or taking an antacid, to protect the coating; should be administered with glass of water on empty stomach for rapid effect
Nursing/Pharmacy Information Administer tablets 2 hours prior to or 4 hours after antacids; increased pH may dissolve the enteric coating leading to GI distress; do not crush enteric coated drug product
Dosage Forms
Powder, as tannex: 2.5 g packets (50 packet/box)
Suppository, rectal: 5 mg, 10 mg
Tablet, enteric coated: 5 mg

♦ **Bisacodyl Uniserts®** see bisacodyl on page 88
♦ **Bisco-Lax® [OTC]** see bisacodyl on page 88
♦ **bishydroxycoumarin** see dicumarol on page 199
♦ **Bismatrol® [OTC]** see bismuth subsalicylate on page 88

bismuth subgallate (BIZ muth sub GAL ate)
U.S. Brand Names Devrom® [OTC]
Generic Available Yes
Therapeutic Category Gastrointestinal Agent, Miscellaneous
Use Symptomatic treatment of mild, nonspecific diarrhea
Usual Dosage Oral: 1-2 tablets 3 times/day with meals
Dietary Considerations May be administered with meals
Nursing/Pharmacy Information Seek causes for diarrhea
Dosage Forms Tablet, chewable: 200 mg

bismuth subsalicylate (BIZ muth sub sa LIS i late)
U.S. Brand Names Bismatrol® [OTC]; Pepto-Bismol® [OTC]
Generic Available Yes
Therapeutic Category Gastrointestinal Agent, Miscellaneous
Use Symptomatic treatment of mild, nonspecific diarrhea including traveler's diarrhea; chronic infantile diarrhea
Usual Dosage Oral:
Nonspecific diarrhea:
Children: Up to 8 doses/24 hours:
3-6 years: 1/3 tablet or 5 mL every 30 minutes to 1 hour as needed
6-9 years: 2/3 tablet or 10 mL every 30 minutes to 1 hour as needed
9-12 years: 1 tablet or 15 mL every 30 minutes to 1 hour as needed

Adults: 2 tablets or 30 mL every 30 minutes to 1 hour as needed up to 8 doses/24 hours

Prevention of traveler's diarrhea: 2.1 g/day or 2 tablets 4 times/day before meals and at bedtime

Dietary Considerations Should be administered before meals

Nursing/Pharmacy Information Seek causes for diarrhea; may aggravate or cause gout attack; may enhance bleeding if used with anticoagulants

Dosage Forms

Caplet, swallowable: 262 mg

Liquid: 262 mg/15 mL (120 mL, 240 mL, 360 mL, 480 mL); 524 mg/15 mL (120 mL, 240 mL, 360 mL)

Tablet, chewable: 262 mg

bismuth subsalicylate, metronidazole, and tetracycline

(BIZ muth sub sa LIS i late, me troe NI da zole, & tet ra SYE kleen)

U.S. Brand Names Helidac™

Generic Available No

Therapeutic Category Antidiarrheal

Use In combination with an H_2 antagonist, used to treat and decrease rate of recurrence of active duodenal ulcer associated with *H. pylori* infection

Usual Dosage Adults: Chew 2 bismuth subsalicylate 262.4 mg tablets, swallow 1 metronidazole 250 mg tablet, and swallow 1 tetracycline 500 mg capsule plus an H_2 antagonist 4 times/day at meals and bedtime for 14 days; follow with 8 oz of water

Dosage Forms

Tablet:

Bismuth subsalicylate: Chewable: 262.4 mg

Metronidazole: 250 mg

Capsule: Tetracycline: 500 mg

bisoprolol (bis OH proe lol)

U.S. Brand Names Zebeta®

Generic Available No

Therapeutic Category Beta-Adrenergic Blocker

Use Treatment of hypertension, alone or in combination with other agents

Usual Dosage Adults: Oral: 5 mg once daily, may be increased to 10 mg, and then up to 20 mg once daily, if necessary

Dietary Considerations May be administered without regard to meals

Nursing/Pharmacy Information

Modify dosage in patients with renal insufficiency

Patient's therapeutic response may be evaluated by looking at blood pressure, apical and radial pulses, fluid I & O, daily weight, respirations, and circulation in extremities before and during therapy; monitor for CNS side effects

Dosage Forms Tablet, as fumarate: 5 mg, 10 mg

bisoprolol and hydrochlorothiazide

(bis OH proe lol & hye droe klor oh THYE a zide)

Synonyms hydrochlorothiazide and bisoprolol

U.S. Brand Names Ziac™

Generic Available No

Therapeutic Category Antihypertensive Agent, Combination

Use Treatment of hypertension

Usual Dosage Adults: Oral: Dose is individualized, administered once daily

Nursing/Pharmacy Information Monitor blood pressure, EKG

Dosage Forms Tablet: Bisoprolol fumarate 2.5 mg and hydrochlorothiazide 6.25 mg; bisoprolol fumarate 5 mg and hydrochlorothiazide 6.25 mg; bisoprolol fumarate 10 mg and hydrochlorothiazide 6.25 mg

♦ **bistropamide** *see* tropicamide *on page 634*

bitolterol (bye TOLE ter ole)

U.S. Brand Names Tornalate®

Generic Available No

Therapeutic Category Adrenergic Agonist Agent

Use Prevent and treat bronchial asthma and bronchospasm

Usual Dosage Children >12 years and Adults:

Bronchospasm: 2 inhalations at an interval of at least 1-3 minutes, followed by a third inhalation if needed

Prevention of bronchospasm: 2 inhalations every 8 hours

(Continued)

bitolterol *(Continued)*

Nursing/Pharmacy Information Before using, the inhaler must be shaken well; assess lung sounds, pulse, and blood pressure before administration and during peak of medication; observe patient for wheezing after administration, if this occurs, call physician

Dosage Forms

Aerosol, oral, as mesylate: 0.8% [370 mcg/metered spray, 300 inhalations] (15 mL)

Solution, inhalation, as mesylate: 0.2% (10 mL, 30 mL, 60 mL)

- ◆ **Black Draught® [OTC]** *see* senna *on page 563*
- ◆ **black widow spider antivenin (*Latrodectus mactans*)** *see* antivenin (*Latrodectus mactans*) *on page 54*
- ◆ **Blanex® Capsule *(Discontinued)*** *see page 743*
- ◆ **Blastocarb** *see* carboplatin *on page 114*
- ◆ **Blastolem** *see* cisplatin *on page 153*
- ◆ **BlemErase® Lotion [OTC]** *see* benzoyl peroxide *on page 81*
- ◆ **Blenoxane®** *see* bleomycin *on page 90*
- ◆ **Bleolem** *see* bleomycin *on page 90*

bleomycin *(blee oh MYE sin)*

Synonyms BLM

U.S. Brand Names Blenoxane®

Mexican Brand Names Bleolem

Generic Available No

Therapeutic Category Antineoplastic Agent

Use Palliative treatment of squamous cell carcinoma, testicular carcinoma, germ cell tumors, and the following lymphomas: Hodgkin's, lymphosarcoma and reticulum cell sarcoma; sclerosing agent to control malignant effusions

Usual Dosage Refer to individual protocol

Children and Adults:

Test dose for lymphoma patients: I.M., I.V., S.C.: 1-2 units of bleomycin for the first 2 doses; monitor vital signs every 15 minutes; wait a minimum of 1 hour before administering remainder of dose

I.M., I.V., S.C.: 10-20 units/m² (0.25-0.5 units/kg) 1-2 times/week in combination regimens

I.V. continuous infusion: 15-20 units/m²/day for 4-5 days

Adults: Intracavitary injection for pleural effusion: 15-240 units have been administered

Nursing/Pharmacy Information

Parenteral: Administer I.V. slowly over at least 10 minutes (no greater than 1 unit/minute) at a concentration not to exceed 3 units/mL; bleomycin for I.V. continuous infusion can be further diluted in normal saline (preferred) or D₅W

Monitor pulmonary function tests (total lung volume, forced vital capacity, carbon monoxide diffusion), renal function, chest x-ray, temperature initially, CBC with differential and platelet count

Stability: Refrigerate powder, reconstituted at room temperature is stable for 28 days in refrigerator or for 14 days at room temperature; stability decreases in PVC bags; **incompatible** with amino acid solutions, ascorbic acid, cefazolin, furosemide, diazepam, hydrocortisone, mitomycin, nafcillin, penicillin G, aminophylline; prolonged infusions in PVC containers should be avoided and glass bottles should be used; **compatible** with cyclophosphamide, doxorubicin, mesna, vinblastine, vincristine

Dosage Forms Powder for injection, as sulfate: 15 units

- ◆ **Bleph®-10** *see* sulfacetamide *on page 584*
- ◆ **Blephamide® Ophthalmic** *see* sulfacetamide and prednisolone *on page 585*
- ◆ **BLM** *see* bleomycin *on page 90*
- ◆ **Blocadren® Oral** *see* timolol *on page 613*
- ◆ **Blocan** *see* cimetidine *on page 150*
- ◆ **Bluboro® [OTC]** *see* aluminum acetate and calcium acetate *on page 32*
- ◆ **Bonamine®** *see* meclizine *on page 387*
- ◆ **Bonine® [OTC]** *see* meclizine *on page 387*
- ◆ **Bontril PDM®** *see* phendimetrazine *on page 484*
- ◆ **Bontril® Slow-Release** *see* phendimetrazine *on page 484*

boric acid *(BOR ik AS id)*

U.S. Brand Names Borofax® Topical [OTC]; Dri-Ear® Otic [OTC]; Swim-Ear® Otic [OTC]

Generic Available Yes

Therapeutic Category Pharmaceutical Aid

Use

Ophthalmic: Mild antiseptic used for inflamed eyelids

Otic: Prophylaxis of swimmer's ear

Topical ointment: Temporary relief of chapped, chafed, or dry skin, diaper rash, abrasions, minor burns, sunburn, insect bites, and other skin irritations

Usual Dosage

Ophthalmic: Apply to lower eyelid 1-2 times/day

Otic: Place 2-4 drops in ears

Topical: Apply as needed

Nursing/Pharmacy Information Application to abraded skin or open wounds has caused fatal poisonings in infants

Dosage Forms

Ointment:

Ophthalmic: 5% (3.5 g); 10% (3.5 g)

Topical: 5% (52.5 g); 10% (28 g)

Topical (Borofax®): 5% boric acid and lanolin (1¾ oz)

Solution, otic: 2.75% with isopropyl alcohol (30 mL)

♦ **Borofax® Topical [OTC]** see boric acid on page 90

♦ **Boropak® [OTC]** see aluminum acetate and calcium acetate on page 32

♦ **B&O Supprettes®** see belladonna and opium on page 76

♦ **Botox®** see botulinum toxin type A on page 91

botulinum toxin type A (BOT yoo lin num TOKS in type aye)

U.S. Brand Names Botox®

Generic Available No

Therapeutic Category Ophthalmic Agent, Toxin

Use Treatment of strabismus and blepharospasm

Usual Dosage

Strabismus: 1.25-5 units (0.05-0.15 mL) injected into any one muscle

Subsequent doses for residual/recurrent strabismus: Re-examine patients 7-14 days after each injection to assess the effect of that dose. Subsequent doses for patients experiencing incomplete paralysis of the target may be increased up to two fold the previously administered dose. Maximum recommended dose as a single injection for any one muscle is 25 units.

Blepharospasm: 1.25-2.5 units (0.05-0.10 mL) injected into the orbicularis oculi muscle

Subsequent doses: Each treatment lasts approximately 3 months. At repeat treatment sessions, the dose may be increased up to twofold if the response from the initial treatment is considered insufficient (usually defined as an effect that does not last >2 months). There appears to be little benefit obtainable from injecting >5 units per site. Some tolerance may be found if treatments are administered any more frequently than every 3 months.

The cumulative dose should not exceed 200 units in a 30-day period

Nursing/Pharmacy Information

One unit corresponds to the calculated median lethal intraperitoneal dose (LD_{50}) in mice

Stability: Keep in undiluted vials in freezer; refrigerate reconstituted solution; administer within 4 hours after vial is removed from the freezer and reconstituted

Dosage Forms Injection: 100 units Clostridium botulinum toxin type A

♦ **bovine lung surfactant** see beractant on page 83

♦ **Braccoprial®** see pyrazinamide on page 532

♦ **Braxan** see amiodarone on page 39

♦ **Breathe Free® [OTC]** see sodium chloride on page 571

♦ **Breezee® Mist Antifungal [OTC]** see miconazole on page 413

♦ **Breonesin® [OTC]** see guaifenesin on page 299

♦ **Brethaire®** see terbutaline on page 596

♦ **Brethine®** see terbutaline on page 596

♦ **Bretylate®** see bretylium on page 91

bretylium (bre TIL ee um)

Canadian Brand Names Bretylate®

Generic Available Yes

Therapeutic Category Antiarrhythmic Agent, Class III

Use Ventricular tachycardia or ventricular fibrillation; other serious ventricular arrhythmias resistant to lidocaine

(Continued)

bretylium *(Continued)*

Usual Dosage

Children:

I.M.: 2-5 mg/kg as a single dose

I.V.: Initial: 5 mg/kg, then attempt electrical defibrillation; repeat with 10 mg/kg if ventricular fibrillation persists

Maintenance dose: I.M., I.V.: 5 mg/kg every 6-8 hours

Adults:

Immediate life-threatening ventricular arrhythmias; ventricular fibrillation; unstable ventricular tachycardia. **Note:** Patients should undergo defibrillation/cardioversion before and after bretylium doses as necessary:

Initial dose: I.V.: 5 mg/kg (undiluted) over 1 minute; if arrhythmia persists, administer 10 mg/kg (undiluted) over 1 minute and repeat as necessary (usually at 15- to 30-minute intervals) up to a total dose of 30 mg/kg

Other life-threatening ventricular arrhythmias:

Initial dose: I.M., I.V.: 5-10 mg/kg, may repeat every 1-2 hours if arrhythmia persist; administer I.V. dose (diluted) over 10-30 minutes

Maintenance dose: I.M.: 5-10 mg/kg every 6-8 hours; I.V. (diluted): 5-10 mg/kg every 6 hours; I.V. infusion (diluted): 1-2 mg/minute (little experience with doses >40 mg/kg/day)

Nursing/Pharmacy Information

I.M. route not recommended for ventricular fibrillation; may administer undiluted I.V. push over <30 seconds for life-threatening situations; dilute to 10 mg/mL for nonlife-threatening situations and administer slow I.V. push over at least 8 minutes

Monitor EKG, heart rate, blood pressure

Stability: The premix infusion should be stored at room temperature and protected from freezing

Dosage Forms

Injection, as tosylate: 50 mg/mL (10 mL, 20 mL)

Injection, as tosylate, premixed in D_5W: 1 mg/mL (500 mL); 2 mg/mL (250 mL); 4 mg/mL (250 mL, 500 mL)

- **Bretylol®** *(Discontinued) see page 743*
- **Brevibloc®** *see esmolol on page 241*
- **Brevicon®** *see ethinyl estradiol and norethindrone on page 250*
- **Brevital® Sodium** *see methohexital on page 402*
- **Brevoxyl® Gel** *see benzoyl peroxide on page 81*
- **Bricanyl®** *see terbutaline on page 596*
- **Brietal Sodium®** *see methohexital on page 402*

brimonidine *(bri MOE ni deen)*

U.S. Brand Names Alphagan®

Generic Available No

Therapeutic Category Alpha$_2$-Adrenergic Agonist Agent, Ophthalmic

Use Lowering of intraocular pressure in patients with open-angle glaucoma or ocular hypertension

Usual Dosage Adults: Ophthalmic: 1 drop in affected eye(s) 3 times/day (approximately every 8 hours)

Dosage Forms Solution, ophthalmic, as tartrate: 0.2% (5 mL, 10 mL)

brinzolamide *(brin ZOH la mide)*

U.S. Brand Names Azopt®

Generic Available No

Therapeutic Category Carbonic Anhydrase Inhibitor

Use Lowers intraocular pressure to treat glaucoma in patients with ocular hypertension or open-angle glaucoma

Usual Dosage Adults: Ophthalmic: Instill 1 drop in eye(s) 3 times/day

Dosage Forms Suspension, ophthalmic: 1% (2.5 mL, 5 mL, 10 mL, 15 mL)

- **Brispen** *see dicloxacillin on page 199*
- **British anti-lewisite** *see dimercaprol on page 206*
- **Brofed® Elixir [OTC]** *see brompheniramine and pseudoephedrine on page 95*
- **Bromaline® Elixir [OTC]** *see brompheniramine and phenylpropanolamine on page 94*
- **Bromanate® DC** *see brompheniramine, phenylpropanolamine, and codeine on page 95*
- **Bromanate® Elixir [OTC]** *see brompheniramine and phenylpropanolamine on page 94*

♦ **Bromanyl® Cough Syrup** see bromodiphenhydramine and codeine *on page 93*

♦ **Bromarest® [OTC]** see brompheniramine *on page 94*

♦ **Bromatapp® [OTC]** see brompheniramine and phenylpropanolamine *on page 94*

bromazepam *(Canada only)* (broe MA ze pam)
Canadian Brand Names Lectopam®
Generic Available No
Therapeutic Category Benzodiazepine; Sedative
Use Short-term, symptomatic relief of manifestations of excessive anxiety in patients with anxiety nerosis
Usual Dosage Adults: Oral: 6-18 mg/day in equally divided doses. depending on the severity of symptoms and response of the patient
Dosage Forms Tablet: 1.5 mg, 3 mg, 6 mg

♦ **Brombay® [OTC]** see brompheniramine *on page 94*

♦ **Bromfed® Syrup [OTC]** see brompheniramine and pseudoephedrine *on page 95*

♦ **Bromfed® Tablet [OTC]** see brompheniramine and pseudoephedrine *on page 95*

♦ **Bromfenex®** see brompheniramine and pseudoephedrine *on page 95*

♦ **Bromfenex® PD** see brompheniramine and pseudoephedrine *on page 95*

bromocriptine (broe moe KRIP teen)
U.S. Brand Names Parlodel®
Canadian Brand Names Apo® Bromocriptine
Mexican Brand Names Cryocriptina; Serocryptin®
Generic Available Yes
Therapeutic Category Anti-Parkinson's Agent; Ergot Alkaloid and Derivative
Use Treatment of parkinsonism in patients unresponsive or allergic to levodopa; also used in conditions associated with hyperprolactinemia and to suppress lactation
Usual Dosage Oral:
  Parkinsonism: 1.25 mg twice daily, increased by 2.5 mg/day in 2- to 4-week intervals (usual dose range: 30-90 mg/day in 3 divided doses)
  Hyperprolactinemia and postpartum lactation: 2.5 mg 2-3 times/day
Dietary Considerations May be administered with food to decrease GI distress
Nursing/Pharmacy Information
  Raise bed rails and institute safety measures; aid patient with ambulation; may cause postural hypotension and drowsiness
  Monitor blood pressure closely as well as hepatic, hematopoietic, and cardiovascular function
Dosage Forms
  Capsule, as mesylate: 5 mg
  Tablet, as mesylate: 2.5 mg

bromodiphenhydramine and codeine
(brome oh dye fen HYE dra meen & KOE deen)
Synonyms codeine and bromodiphenhydramine
U.S. Brand Names Ambenyl® Cough Syrup; Amgenal® Cough Syrup; Bromanyl® Cough Syrup; Bromotuss® w/Codeine Cough Syrup
Generic Available Yes
Therapeutic Category Antihistamine/Antitussive
Controlled Substance C-V
Use Relief of upper respiratory symptoms and cough associated with allergies or common cold
Usual Dosage Oral: 5-10 mL every 4-6 hours
Dosage Forms Liquid: Bromodiphenhydramine hydrochloride 12.5 mg and codeine phosphate 10 mg per 5 mL

♦ **Bromotuss® w/Codeine Cough Syrup** see bromodiphenhydramine and codeine *on page 93*

♦ **Bromphen® [OTC]** see brompheniramine *on page 94*

♦ **Bromphen® DC w/Codeine** see brompheniramine, phenylpropanolamine, and codeine *on page 95*

brompheniramine (brome fen IR a meen)

Synonyms parabromdylamine

U.S. Brand Names Bromarest® [OTC]; Brombay® [OTC]; Bromphen® [OTC]; Brotane® [OTC]; Chlorphed® [OTC]; Cophene-B®; Diamine T.D.® [OTC]; Dimetane® Extentabs® [OTC]; Nasahist B®; ND-Stat®

Generic Available Yes

Therapeutic Category Antihistamine

Use Perennial and seasonal allergic rhinitis and other allergic symptoms including urticaria

Usual Dosage

Oral:

Children:

<6 years: 0.125 mg/kg/dose administered every 6 hours; maximum: 6-8 mg/day

6-12 years: 2-4 mg every 6-8 hours; maximum: 12-16 mg/day

Adults: 4 mg every 4-6 hours or 8 mg of sustained release form every 8-12 hours or 12 mg of sustained release every 12 hours; maximum: 24 mg/day

I.M., I.V., S.C.:

Children <12 years: 0.5 mg/kg/24 hours divided every 6-8 hours

Adults: 5-50 mg every 4-12 hours, maximum: 40 mg/24 hours

Dietary Considerations May be administered with food, milk, or water

Nursing/Pharmacy Information

Dilute in 1-10 mL D_5W or normal saline and infuse over several minutes; the patient should be in a recumbent position during the infusion; sustained release tablets should be swallowed whole, do not crush or chew

Stability: Solutions may crystallize if stored below 0°C, crystals will dissolve when warmed

Dosage Forms

Elixir, as maleate: 2 mg/5 mL with 3% alcohol (120 mL, 480 mL, 4000 mL)

Injection, as maleate: 10 mg/mL (10 mL)

Tablet, as maleate: 4 mg, 8 mg, 12 mg

Tablet, sustained release, as maleate: 8 mg, 12 mg

brompheniramine and phenylephrine

(brome fen IR a meen & fen il EF rin)

U.S. Brand Names Dimetane® Decongestant Elixir [OTC]

Generic Available Yes

Therapeutic Category Antihistamine/Decongestant Combination

Use Temporary relief of symptoms of seasonal and perennial allergic rhinitis, and vasomotor rhinitis, including nasal obstruction

Usual Dosage Children >12 years and Adults: Oral: 10 mL every 4 hours

Dosage Forms Elixir: Brompheniramine maleate 4 mg and phenylephrine hydrochloride 5 mg per 5 mL

brompheniramine and phenylpropanolamine

(brome fen IR a meen & fen il proe pa NOLE a meen)

Synonyms phenylpropanolamine and brompheniramine

U.S. Brand Names Bromaline® Elixir [OTC]; Bromanate® Elixir [OTC]; Bromatapp® [OTC]; Bromphen® Tablet [OTC]; Cold & Allergy® Elixir [OTC]; Dimaphen® Elixir [OTC]; Dimaphen® Tablets [OTC]; Dimetapp® 4-Hour Liqui-Gel Capsule [OTC]; Dimetapp® Elixir [OTC]; Dimetapp® Extentabs® [OTC]; Dimetapp® Tablet [OTC]; Genatap® Elixir [OTC]; Tamine® [OTC]; Vicks® DayQuil® Allergy Relief 4 Hour Tablet [OTC]

Generic Available Yes

Therapeutic Category Antihistamine/Decongestant Combination

Use Temporary relief of nasal congestion, running nose, sneezing, and itchy, watery eyes

Usual Dosage Oral:

Children:

1-6 months: 1.25 mL 3-4 times/day

7-24 months: 2.5 mL 3-4 times/day

2-4 years: 3.75 mL 3-4 times/day

4-12 years: 5 mL 3-4 times/day

Adults: 5-10 mL 3-4 times/day or regular capsule or tablet 3-4 times daily or 1 sustained release tablet twice daily

Nursing/Pharmacy Information Swallow tablet whole, do not crush or chew

Dosage Forms

Capsule (Dimetapp® 4-Hour Liqui-Gel): Brompheniramine maleate 4 mg and phenylpropanolamine hydrochloride 25 mg

Liquid (Bromaline®, Bromanate®, Cold & Allergy®, Dimaphen®, Dimetapp®, Genatap®): Brompheniramine maleate 2 mg and phenylpropanolamine hydrochloride 12.5 mg per 5 mL

Tablet (Dimaphen®, Dimetapp®, Vicks® DayQuil® Allergy Relief 4 Hour): Brompheniramine maleate 4 mg and phenylpropanolamine hydrochloride 25 mg

Tablet, sustained release: Brompheniramine maleate 12 mg and phenylpropanolamine hydrochloride 75 mg

brompheniramine and pseudoephedrine
(brome fen IR a meen & soo doe e FED rin)

U.S. Brand Names Brofed® Elixir [OTC]; Bromfed® Syrup [OTC]; Bromfed® Tablet [OTC]; Bromfenex®; Bromfenex® PD; Drixoral® Syrup [OTC]; Iofed®; Iofed® PD

Generic Available Yes

Therapeutic Category Antihistamine/Decongestant Combination

Use Temporary relief of symptoms of seasonal and perennial allergic rhinitis, and vasomotor rhinitis, including nasal obstruction

Usual Dosage Oral:
Children 6-12 years: 5-10 mL 3-4 times/day
Children >12 years and Adults: 1 or 2 capsules every 12 hours or 1 or 2 tablets 3-4 times/day or 5-10 mL 3-4 times/day

Dosage Forms
Capsule, extended release:
Bromfenex® PD, Iofed® PD: Brompheniramine maleate 6 mg and pseudoephedrine hydrochloride 60 mg
Bromfenex®, Iofed®: Brompheniramine maleate 12 mg and pseudoephedrine hydrochloride 120 mg
Elixir:
Brofed®: Brompheniramine maleate 4 mg and pseudoephedrine hydrochloride 30 mg per 5 mL
Bromfed®: Brompheniramine maleate 2 mg and pseudoephedrine hydrochloride 30 mg per 5 mL
Drixoral®: Brompheniramine maleate 2 mg and pseudoephedrine sulfate 30 mg per 5 mL
Tablet (Bromfed®): Brompheniramine maleate 4 mg and pseudoephedrine hydrochloride 60 mg

brompheniramine, phenylpropanolamine, and codeine
(brome fen IR a meen, fen il proe pa NOLE a meen, & KOE deen)

Synonyms codeine, brompheniramine, and phenylpropanolamine; phenylpropanolamine, brompheniramine, and codeine

U.S. Brand Names Bromanate® DC; Bromphen® DC w/Codeine; Dimetane®-DC; Myphetane DC®; Poly-Histine CS®

Generic Available Yes

Therapeutic Category Antihistamine/Decongestant/Antitussive

Controlled Substance C-V

Use Relief of coughs and upper respiratory symptoms, including nasal congestion, associated with allergy or the common cold

Usual Dosage Oral:
Children:
2-6 years: 2.5 mL every 4 hours
6-12 years: 5 mL every 4 hours
Children >12 years and Adults: 10 mL every 4 hours

Dosage Forms Liquid: Brompheniramine maleate 2 mg, phenylpropanolamine hydrochloride 12.5 mg, and codeine phosphate 10 mg per 5 mL with alcohol 0.95% (480 mL)

♦ **Bromphen® Tablet [OTC]** see brompheniramine and phenylpropanolamine on page 94
♦ **Bronalide®** see flunisolide on page 272
♦ **Bronchial®** see theophylline and guaifenesin on page 604
♦ **Bronitin® Mist [OTC]** see epinephrine on page 234
♦ **Bronkaid® Mist [OTC]** see epinephrine on page 234
♦ **Bronkephrine®** *(Discontinued)* see page 743
♦ **Bronkometer®** see isoetharine on page 346
♦ **Bronkosol®** see isoetharine on page 346
♦ **Brontex® Liquid** see guaifenesin and codeine on page 300
♦ **Brontex® Tablet** see guaifenesin and codeine on page 300
♦ **Brotane® [OTC]** see brompheniramine on page 94
♦ **BSS® Ophthalmic** see balanced salt solution on page 73

budesonide (byoo DES oh nide)
U.S. Brand Names Pulmicort® Turbuhaler®; Rhinocort®
Canadian Brand Names Entocort®; Rhinocort® Turbuhaler®
Generic Available No
Therapeutic Category Adrenal Corticosteroid
Use
Children and Adults: Management of symptoms of seasonal or perennial rhinitis
Adults: Nonallergic perennial rhinitis
Usual Dosage
Children ≥6 years and Adults: 256 mcg/day, administered as either 2 sprays in each nostril in the morning and evening or as 4 sprays in each nostril in the morning
Rhinocort® Aqua™: 64 mcg/day as a single 32 mcg spray in each nostril. Some patients who do not achieve adequate control may benefit from increased dosage. A reduced dosage may be effective after initial control is achieved. Maximum dose: Children <12 years: 129 mcg/day; Adults: 256 mcg/day
Nursing/Pharmacy Information Inhaler should be shaken well immediately prior to use; while activating inhaler, deep breathe for 3-5 seconds, hold breath for ~10 seconds and allow ≥1 minute between inhalations
Dosage Forms
Aerosol, nasal: 32 mcg per actuation (7 g)
Powder (dry) for inhalation: 200 mcg per metered dose (200 doses)

♦ **Buffered®, Tri-buffered** *(Discontinued) see page 743*
♦ **Bufferin® [OTC]** *see aspirin on page 61*
♦ **Bufferin® Arthritis Strength** *(Discontinued) see page 743*
♦ **Bufferin® Extra Strength** *(Discontinued) see page 743*
♦ **Bufigen** *see nalbuphine on page 429*
♦ **Buf-Puf® Acne Cleansing Bar** *(Discontinued) see page 743*
♦ **Bumedyl®** *see bumetanide on page 96*

bumetanide (byoo MET a nide)
U.S. Brand Names Bumex®
Canadian Brand Names Burinex®
Mexican Brand Names Bumedyl®
Generic Available Yes
Therapeutic Category Diuretic, Loop
Use Management of edema secondary to congestive heart failure or hepatic or renal disease including nephrotic syndrome; may also be used alone or in combination with antihypertensives in the treatment of hypertension
Usual Dosage
Children:
<6 months: Dose not established
>6 months:
Oral: Initial: 0.015 mg/kg/dose once daily or every other day; maximum dose: 0.1 mg/kg/day
I.M., I.V.: Dose not established
Adults:
Oral: 0.5-2 mg/dose (maximum: 10 mg/day) 1-2 times/day
I.M., I.V.: 0.5-1 mg/dose (maximum: 10 mg/day)
Dietary Considerations This product may cause a potassium loss; your physician may prescribe a potassium supplement, another medication to help prevent the potassium loss, or recommend that you eat foods high in potassium, especially citrus fruits; do not change your diet on your own while taking this medication, especially if you are taking potassium supplements or medications to reduce potassium loss; too much potassium can be as harmful as too little
Nursing/Pharmacy Information
Administer I.V. slowly, over 1-2 minutes; be alert to complaints about hearing difficulty; check patient for orthostasis
Monitor blood pressure, serum electrolytes, renal function
Stability: I.V. infusion solutions should be used within 24 hours after preparation
Dosage Forms
Injection: 0.25 mg/mL (2 mL, 4 mL, 10 mL)
Tablet: 0.5 mg, 1 mg, 2 mg

♦ **Bumex®** *see bumetanide on page 96*
♦ **Buminate®** *see albumin on page 24*

♦ **Bupap®** *see* butalbital compound and acetaminophen *on page 99*

♦ **Buphenyl®** *see* sodium phenylbutyrate *on page 573*

bupivacaine (byoo PIV a kane)
U.S. Brand Names Marcaine®; Sensorcaine®; Sensorcaine®-MPF
Mexican Brand Names Buvacaina
Generic Available Yes
Therapeutic Category Local Anesthetic
Use Local anesthetic (injectable) for peripheral nerve block, infiltration, sympa-thetic block, caudal or epidural block, retrobulbar block
Usual Dosage Dose varies with procedure, depth of anesthesia, vascularity of tissues, duration of anesthesia and condition of patient

Caudal block (with or without epinephrine):
Children: 1-3.7 mg/kg
Adults: 15-30 mL of 0.25% or 0.5%
Epidural block (other than caudal block):
Children: 1.25 mg/kg/dose
Adults: 10-20 mL of 0.25% or 0.5%
Peripheral nerve block: 5 mL dose of 0.25% or 0.5% (12.5-25 mg); maximum: 2.5 mg/kg (plain); 3 mg/kg (with epinephrine); up to a maximum of 400 mg/day
Sympathetic nerve block: 20-50 mL of 0.25% (no epinephrine) solution
Nursing/Pharmacy Information
Monitor fetal heart rate during paracervical anesthesia
Stability: Solutions with epinephrine should be protected from light
Dosage Forms
Injection, as hydrochloride: 0.25% (10 mL, 20 mL, 30 mL, 50 mL); 0.5% (10 mL, 20 mL, 30 mL, 50 mL); 0.75% (2 mL, 10 mL, 20 mL, 30 mL)
Injection, as hydrochloride, with epinephrine (1:200,000): 0.25% (10 mL, 30 mL, 50 mL); 0.5% (1.8 mL, 3 mL, 5 mL, 10 mL, 30 mL, 50 mL); 0.75% (30 mL)

♦ **Buprenex®** *see* buprenorphine *on page 97*

buprenorphine (byoo pre NOR feen)
U.S. Brand Names Buprenex®
Mexican Brand Names Temgesic®
Generic Available Yes
Therapeutic Category Analgesic, Narcotic
Controlled Substance C-V
Use Management of moderate to severe pain
Usual Dosage Adults: I.M., slow I.V.: 0.3-0.6 mg every 6 hours as needed
Nursing/Pharmacy Information
Gradual withdrawal of drug is necessary to avoid withdrawal symptoms
Monitor pain relief, respiratory and mental status, blood pressure
Stability: Protect from excessive heat or light
Dosage Forms Injection, as hydrochloride: 0.3 mg/mL (1 mL)

bupropion (byoo PROE pee on)
U.S. Brand Names Wellbutrin®; Wellbutrin® SR; Zyban™
Generic Available No
Therapeutic Category Antidepressant, Aminoketone
Use Treatment of depression; as an aid to smoking cessation treatment
Usual Dosage Oral:
Adults:
Depression: 100 mg 3 times/day; begin at 100 mg twice daily; may increase to a maximum dose of 450 mg/day
Smoking cessation: Initiate with 150 mg once daily for 3 days; increase to 150 mg twice daily; treatment should continue for 7-12 weeks
Elderly: Depression: 50-100 mg/day, increase by 50-100 mg every 3-4 days as tolerated; there is evidence that the elderly respond at 150 mg/day in divided doses, but some may require a higher dose
Nursing/Pharmacy Information
Be aware that drug may cause seizures
Monitor body weight
Dose should not be increased by more than 50 mg/day once weekly
Dosage Forms
Tablet (Wellbutrin®): 75 mg, 100 mg
Tablet, sustained release (Wellbutrin® SR, Zyban®): 100 mg, 150 mg

♦ **Burinex®** *see* bumetanide *on page 96*

♦ **Burow's otic** *see* aluminum acetate and acetic acid *on page 32*
♦ **BuSpar®** *see* buspirone *on page 98*

buspirone (byoo SPYE rone)
U.S. Brand Names BuSpar®
Mexican Brand Names Neurosine
Generic Available Yes
Therapeutic Category Antianxiety Agent
Use Management of anxiety
Usual Dosage Adults: Oral: 15 mg/day (5 mg 3 times/day); may increase to a maximum of 60 mg/day
Dietary Considerations Food may decrease the absorption of buspirone, but it may also decrease the first-pass metabolism, thereby increasing the bioavailability of buspirone
Nursing/Pharmacy Information Monitor mental status
Dosage Forms Tablet, as hydrochloride: 5 mg, 10 mg

busulfan (byoo SUL fan)
U.S. Brand Names Busulfex®; Myleran®
Generic Available No
Therapeutic Category Antineoplastic Agent
Use
Injection: Use in combination with cyclophosphamide as a conditioning regimen prior to allogeneic hematopoietic progenitor cell transplantation for chronic myelogenous leukemia
Oral: Chronic myelogenous leukemia and bone marrow disorders, such as polycythemia vera and myeloid metaplasia, conditioning regimens for bone marrow transplantation
Usual Dosage
I.V.: Adult: As a component of a conditioning regimen prior to bone marrow or peripheral blood progenitor cell replacement support is 0.8 mg/kg of ideal body weight or actual body weight, whichever is lower, administered every 6 hours for 4 days (a total of 16 doses)
Oral (**refer to individual protocols**):
Children:
For remission induction of CML: 0.06-0.12 mg/kg/day **or** 1.8-4.6 mg/m^2/day; titrate dosage to maintain leukocyte count above 40,000/mm^3; reduce dosage by 50% if the leukocyte count reaches 30,000-40,000/mm^3; discontinue drug if counts fall to ≤20,000/mm^3
BMT marrow-ablative conditioning regimen: 1 mg/kg/dose (ideal body weight) every 6 hours for 16 doses

Adults:
BMT marrow-ablative conditioning regimen: 1 mg/kg/dose (ideal body weight) every 6 hours for 16 doses
Dietary Considerations No clear or firm data on the effect of food on busulfan bioavailability
Nursing/Pharmacy Information
Avoid I.M. injection if platelet count falls <100,000/mm^3
Monitor CBC with differential and platelet count, hemoglobin, liver function tests
Dosage Forms
Injection: 6 mg/mL (10 mL)
Tablet: 2 mg

♦ **Busulfex®** *see* busulfan *on page 98*

butabarbital sodium (byoo ta BAR bi tal SOW dee um)
U.S. Brand Names Butalan®; Buticaps®; Butisol Sodium®
Generic Available Yes
Therapeutic Category Barbiturate
Controlled Substance C-III
Use Sedative, hypnotic
Usual Dosage
Children: Preop: 2-6 mg/kg/dose; maximum: 100 mg
Adults:
Sedative: 15-30 mg 3-4 times/day
Hypnotic: 50-100 mg
Preop: 50-100 mg 1-1½ hours before surgery
Nursing/Pharmacy Information
Raise bed rails; initiate safety measures; aid with ambulation
Monitor CNS depression

Dosage Forms
Capsule: 15 mg, 30 mg
Elixir, with alcohol 7%: 30 mg/5 mL (480 mL, 3780 mL); 33.3 mg/5 mL (480 mL, 3780 mL)
Tablet: 15 mg, 30 mg, 50 mg, 100 mg

♦ **Butace®** *(Discontinued) see page 743*
♦ **Butacortelone** *see ibuprofen on page 332*
♦ **Butalan®** *see butabarbital sodium on page 98*

butalbital compound and acetaminophen
(byoo TAL bi tal KOM pound & a seet a MIN oh fen)
Synonyms acetaminophen and butalbital compound
U.S. Brand Names Amaphen®; Anoquan®; Axocet®; Bupap®; Endolor®; Esgic®; Esgic-Plus®; Femcet®; Fioricet®; G-1®; Medigesic®; Phrenilin®; Phrenilin® Forte; Repan®; Sedapap-10®; Triapin®; Two-Dyne®
Generic Available Yes
Therapeutic Category Barbiturate/Analgesic
Controlled Substance C-III
Use Relief of the symptomatic complex of tension or muscle contraction headache
Usual Dosage Adults: Oral: 1-2 tablets or capsules every 4 hours; not to exceed 6/day
Nursing/Pharmacy Information
Raise bed rails; initiate safety measures; aid with ambulation
Monitor for CNS depression
Dosage Forms
Capsule:
Amaphen®, Anoquan®, Butace®, Endolor®, Esgic®, Femcet®, G-1®, Medigesic®, Repan®, Two-Dyne®: Butalbital 50 mg, caffeine 40 mg, and acetaminophen 325 mg
Axocet®, Phrenilin® Forte: Butalbital 50 mg and acetaminophen 650 mg
Bancap®, Triapin®: Butalbital 50 mg and acetaminophen 325 mg
Tablet:
Bupap®: Butalbital 50 mg and acetaminophen 650 mg
Esgic®, Fioricet®, Repan®: Butalbital 50 mg, caffeine 40 mg, and acetaminophen 325 mg
Phrenilin®: Butalbital 50 mg and acetaminophen 325 mg
Sedapap-10®: Butalbital 50 mg and acetaminophen 650 mg

butalbital compound and aspirin
(byoo TAL bi tal KOM pound & AS pir in)
Synonyms aspirin and butalbital compound
U.S. Brand Names Fiorgen PF®; Fiorinal®; Isollyl® Improved; Lanorinal®
Generic Available Yes
Therapeutic Category Barbiturate/Analgesic
Controlled Substance C-III (Fiorinal®)
Use Relief of the symptomatic complex of tension or muscle contraction headache
Usual Dosage Adults: Oral: 1-2 tablets or capsules every 4 hours; not to exceed 6/day
Nursing/Pharmacy Information
Raise bed rails; initiate safety measures; aid with ambulation; children and teenagers should not use for chickenpox or flu symptoms before a physician is consulted about Reye's syndrome (Fiorinal®)
Monitor for CNS depression
Dosage Forms
Capsule: (Fiorgen PF®, Fiorinal®, Isollyl® Improved, Lanorinal®, Marnal®): Butalbital 50 mg, caffeine 40 mg, and aspirin 325 mg
Tablet: (Fiorinal®, Isollyl® Improved, Lanorinal®, Marnal®): Butalbital 50 mg, caffeine 40 mg, and aspirin 325 mg

butalbital compound and codeine
(byoo TAL bi tal KOM pound & KOE deen)
Synonyms codeine and butalbital compound
U.S. Brand Names Fiorinal® With Codeine
Generic Available Yes
Therapeutic Category Analgesic, Narcotic; Barbiturate
Controlled Substance C-III
Use Mild to moderate pain when sedation is needed
(Continued)

butalbital compound and codeine *(Continued)*

Usual Dosage Adults: Oral: 1-2 capsules every 4 hours as needed for pain; up to 6/day

Nursing/Pharmacy Information Abrupt discontinuation after sustained use (generally >10 days) may cause withdrawal symptoms

Dosage Forms Capsule: Butalbital 50 mg, caffeine 40 mg, aspirin 325 mg and codeine phosphate 30 mg

butenafine (byoo TEN a fine)

U.S. Brand Names Mentax®

Generic Available No

Therapeutic Category Antifungal Agent

Use Topical treatment of interdigital tinea pedis (athlete's foot) due to *Epidermophyton floccosum*, *Trichophyton mentagrophytes*, or *Trichophyton rubrum*

Usual Dosage Adults: Topical: Apply cream to the affected area and surrounding skin once daily for 4 weeks

Dosage Forms Cream, as hydrochloride: 1% (2 g, 15 g, 30 g)

♦ **Buticaps®** *see* butabarbital sodium *on page 98*

♦ **Butisol Sodium®** *see* butabarbital sodium *on page 98*

butoconazole (byoo toe KOE na zole)

Generic Available No

Therapeutic Category Antifungal Agent

Use Local treatment of vulvovaginal candidiasis

Usual Dosage Adults:

Nonpregnant: Insert 1 applicatorful (~5 g) intravaginally at bedtime for 3 days, may extend for up to 6 days if necessary

Pregnant: **Use only during second or third trimesters**

Nursing/Pharmacy Information May cause burning or stinging on application; if symptoms of vaginitis persist, contact physician

Dosage Forms Cream, vaginal, as nitrate: 2% with applicator (28 g)

butorphanol (byoo TOR fa nole)

U.S. Brand Names Stadol®; Stadol® NS

Generic Available Yes

Therapeutic Category Analgesic, Narcotic

Controlled Substance C-IV

Use Management of moderate to severe pain

Usual Dosage Adults:

I.M.: 1-4 mg every 3-4 hours as needed

I.V.: 0.5-2 mg every 3-4 hours as needed

Nasal: Initial: 1 mg (1 spray in one nostril), allow 60-90 minutes to elapse before deciding whether a second 1 mg dose is needed; this 2-dose sequence may be repeated in 3-4 hours if needed

Dietary Considerations Alcohol: Additive CNS effects; avoid or limit alcohol; watch for sedation

Nursing/Pharmacy Information

Raise bed rails, aid with ambulation

Monitor pain relief, respiratory and mental status, blood pressure

Stability: Store at room temperature, protect from freezing; **incompatible** when mixed in the same syringe with diazepam, dimenhydrinate, methohexital, pentobarbital, secobarbital, thiopental

Dosage Forms Butorphanol tartrate:

Injection: 1 mg/mL (1 mL); 2 mg/mL (1 mL, 2 mL, 10 mL)

Spray, nasal: 10 mg/mL [14-15 doses] (2.5 mL)

♦ **butyl aminobenzoate, benzocaine, tetracaine, and benzalkonium chloride** *see* benzocaine, butyl aminobenzoate, tetracaine, and benzalkonium chloride *on page 79*

♦ **Buvacaina** *see* bupivacaine *on page 97*

♦ **Byclomine® Injection** *see* dicyclomine *on page 199*

♦ **Bydramine® Cough Syrup [OTC]** *see* diphenhydramine *on page 208*

♦ **C2B8 monoclonal antibody** *see* rituximab *on page 552*

♦ **c7E3** *see* abciximab *on page 12*

♦ **C8-CCK** *see* sincalide *on page 567*

♦ **311C90** *see* zolmitriptan *on page 661*

cabergoline (ca BER go leen)
U.S. Brand Names Dostinex®
Generic Available No
Therapeutic Category Ergot-like Derivative
Use Treatment of hyperprolactinemia
Usual Dosage Adults: Oral: 0.25 mg twice weekly; dosage may be increased by 0.25 mg twice weekly to a dose of up to 1 mg twice weekly (according to the patient's prolactin level)
Dosage Forms Tablet: 0.5 mg

♦ **Cafatine-PB®** see ergotamine on page 238
♦ **Cafergot®** see ergotamine on page 238
♦ **Cafetrate®** see ergotamine on page 238

caffeine and sodium benzoate
(KAF een & SOW dee um BEN zoe ate)
Synonyms sodium benzoate and caffeine
Generic Available Yes
Therapeutic Category Diuretic, Miscellaneous
Use Emergency stimulant in acute circulatory failure; as a diuretic; and to relieve spinal puncture headache
Usual Dosage
Children: I.M., I.V., S.C.: 8 mg/kg every 4 hours as needed
Adults: I.M., I.V.: 500 mg, maximum single dose: 1 g
Nursing/Pharmacy Information Monitor CNS, GI, and cardiac reactions
Dosage Forms Injection: Caffeine 125 mg and sodium benzoate 125 mg per mL (2 mL)

caffeine, citrated (KAF een, SIT rated)
Generic Available Yes
Therapeutic Category Respiratory Stimulant
Use Central nervous system stimulant; used in the treatment of idiopathic apnea of prematurity
Usual Dosage Apnea of prematurity: Oral:
Loading dose: 10-20 mg/kg as caffeine citrate (5-10 mg/kg as caffeine base). If theophylline has been administered to the patient within the previous 5 days, a full or modified loading dose (50% to 75% of a loading dose) may be administered at the discretion of the physician.
Maintenance dose: 5-10 mg/kg/day as caffeine citrate (2.5-5 mg/kg/day as caffeine base) once daily starting 24 hours after the loading dose. Maintenance dose is adjusted based on patient's response, (efficacy and adverse effects), and serum caffeine concentrations.
Nursing/Pharmacy Information Monitor serum caffeine concentrations, blood pressure, heart rate
Dosage Forms
Solution, oral: 20 mg/mL [anhydrous caffeine 10 mg/mL]
Tablet: 65 mg [anhydrous caffeine 32.5 mg]

♦ **caffeine, hydrocodone, chlorpheniramine, phenylephrine, and acetaminophen** see hydrocodone, chlorpheniramine, phenylephrine, acetaminophen, and caffeine on page 321
♦ **caffeine, orphenadrine, and aspirin** see orphenadrine, aspirin, and caffeine on page 458
♦ **Caladryl® Spray (Discontinued)** see page 743
♦ **Calan®** see verapamil on page 646
♦ **Calan® SR** see verapamil on page 646
♦ **Cal Carb-HD®** [OTC] see calcium carbonate on page 103
♦ **Calcibind®** see cellulose sodium phosphate on page 127
♦ **Calci-Chew™** [OTC] see calcium carbonate on page 103
♦ **Calciday-667®** [OTC] see calcium carbonate on page 103

calcifediol (kal si fe DYE ole)
Synonyms 25-D$_3$; 25-hydroxycholecalciferol; 25-hydroxyvitamin D$_3$
U.S. Brand Names Calderol®
Generic Available No
Therapeutic Category Vitamin D Analog
Use Treatment and management of metabolic bone disease associated with chronic renal failure
Usual Dosage Hepatic osteodystrophy: Oral:
Infants: 5-7 mcg/kg/day
(Continued)

calcifediol *(Continued)*

Children and Adults: 20-100 mcg/day or every other day; titrate to obtain normal serum calcium/phosphate levels

Nursing/Pharmacy Information Monitor calcium and phosphate levels closely; monitor symptoms of hypercalcemia

Dosage Forms Capsule: 20 mcg, 50 mcg

♦ **Calciferol™** *see* ergocalciferol *on page 237*
♦ **Calcijex™** *see* calcitriol *on page 103*
♦ **Calcilean® [HepCalium]** *see* heparin *on page 310*
♦ **Calcimar®** *see* calcitonin *on page 102*
♦ **Calci-Mix™ [OTC]** *see* calcium carbonate *on page 103*
♦ **Calciparine® Injection *(Discontinued)*** *see page 743*

calcipotriene (kal si POE try een)

U.S. Brand Names Dovonex®
Generic Available No
Therapeutic Category Antipsoriatic Agent
Use Treatment of plaque psoriasis
Usual Dosage Topical: Apply to skin lesions twice daily
Nursing/Pharmacy Information Apply only to affected areas; do not exceed the ordered dose
Dosage Forms
Cream: 0.005% (30 g, 60 g, 100 g)
Ointment, topical: 0.005% (30 g, 60 g, 100 g)
Solution, topical: 0.005%

♦ **Calcite-500** *see* calcium carbonate *on page 103*

calcitonin (kal si TOE nin)

Synonyms calcitonin (human); calcitonin (salmon)
U.S. Brand Names Calcimar®; Cibacalcin®; Miacalcin®; Miacalcin® Nasal Spray; Osteocalcin®; Salmonine®
Canadian Brand Names Caltine®
Generic Available No
Therapeutic Category Polypeptide Hormone
Use
Calcitonin (salmon): Treatment of Paget's disease of bone and as adjunctive therapy for hypercalcemia; also used in postmenopausal osteoporosis and osteogenesis imperfecta
Calcitonin (human): Treatment of Paget's disease of bone
Usual Dosage
Children: Dosage not established
Adults:
Paget's disease: Salmon calcitonin:
I.M., S.C.: 100 units/day to start, 50 units/day or 50-100 units every 1-3 days maintenance dose
Human calcitonin: S.C.: Initial: 0.5 mg/day (maximum: 0.5 mg twice daily); maintenance: 0.5 mg 2-3 times/week or 0.25 mg/day
Hypercalcemia: Initial: Salmon calcitonin: I.M., S.C.: 4 units/kg every 12 hours; may increase up to 8 units/kg every 12 hours to a maximum of every 6 hours
Osteogenesis imperfecta: Salmon calcitonin: I.M., S.C.: 2 units/kg 3 times/week
Postmenopausal osteoporosis: Salmon calcitonin:
I.M., S.C.: 100 units/day
Intranasal: 200 units (1 spray)/day
Dietary Considerations Adequate vitamin D and calcium intake essential
Nursing/Pharmacy Information
Skin test should be performed prior to administration of salmon calcitonin; I.M. route is preferred
Monitor serum calcium and electrolytes
Stability: Refrigeration is recommended for calcitonin salmon, stable for up to 2 weeks at room temperature; normal saline has been recommended for the dilution to prepare a skin test; protect from light; calcitonin human may be stored at room temperature; store in refrigerator when volume exceeds 2 mL
Dosage Forms
Injection:
Human (Cibacalcin®): 0.5 mg/vial
Salmon: 200 units/mL (2 mL)

Spray, nasal: 200 units/activation (0.09 mL/dose) (2 mL glass bottle with pump)

♦ **calcitonin (human)** *see* calcitonin *on page 102*
♦ **calcitonin (salmon)** *see* calcitonin *on page 102*

calcitriol (kal si TRYE ole)

Synonyms 1,25 dihydroxycholecalciferol
U.S. Brand Names Calcijex™; Rocaltrol®
Generic Available No
Therapeutic Category Vitamin D Analog
Use Management of hypocalcemia in patients on chronic renal dialysis; reduce elevated parathyroid hormone levels
Usual Dosage Individualize dosage to maintain calcium levels of 9-10 mg/dL
Renal failure: Oral:
Children: Initial: 15 ng/kg/day; maintenance: 30-60 ng/kg/day
Adults: 0.25 mcg/day or every other day (may require 0.5-1 mcg/day)
Unlabeled dose:
Renal failure: I.V.: Adults: 0.5 mcg (0.01 mcg/kg) 3 times/week; most doses in the range of 0.5-3 mcg (0.01-0.05 mcg/kg) 3 times/week
Hypoparathyroidism/pseudohypoparathyroidism: Oral:
Children 1-5 years: 0.25-0.75 mcg/day
Children >6 years and Adults: 0.5-2 mcg/day
Nursing/Pharmacy Information
May be administered as a bolus dose I.V. through the catheter at the end of hemodialysis
Monitor serum calcium and phosphate levels during therapy
Stability: Store in tight, light-resistant container; calcitriol degrades upon prolonged exposure to light
Dosage Forms
Capsule: 0.25 mcg, 0.5 mcg
Injection: 1 mcg/mL (1 mL); 2 mcg/mL (1 mL)

calcium acetate (KAL see um AS e tate)

U.S. Brand Names Calphron®; PhosLo®
Generic Available No
Therapeutic Category Electrolyte Supplement, Oral
Use Control of hyperphosphatemia in end-stage renal failure and does not promote aluminum absorption
Usual Dosage Adults: Oral: 2 tablets with each meal; dosage may be increased to bring serum phosphate value to <6 mg/dL; most patients require 3-4 tablets with each meal
Dietary Considerations Tablets must be administered with meals to be effective
Nursing/Pharmacy Information 12.7 mEq/g; 250 mg/g elemental calcium (25% elemental calcium)
Dosage Forms Elemental calcium listed in brackets
Capsule (Phos-Ex® 125): 500 mg [125 mg]
Tablet:
Calphron®: 667 mg [169 mg]
PhosLo®: 667 mg [169 mg]

calcium carbonate (KAL see um KAR bun ate)

U.S. Brand Names Alka-Mints® [OTC]; Amitone® [OTC]; Cal Carb-HD® [OTC]; Calci-Chew™ [OTC]; Calciday-667® [OTC]; Calci-Mix™ [OTC]; Cal-Plus® [OTC]; Caltrate® 600 [OTC]; Caltrate, Jr.® [OTC]; Chooz® [OTC]; Dicarbosil® [OTC]; Equilet® [OTC]; Florical® [OTC]; Gencalc® 600 [OTC]; Mallamint® [OTC]; Nephro-Calci® [OTC]; Os-Cal® 500 [OTC]; Oyst-Cal 500 [OTC]; Oystercal® 500; Rolaids® Calcium Rich [OTC]; Tums® [OTC]; Tums® E-X Extra Strength Tablet [OTC]; Tums® Extra Strength Liquid [OTC]
Canadian Brand Names Apo-Cal®; Calcite-500; Calsan®; Pharmacal®
Generic Available Yes
Therapeutic Category Antacid; Electrolyte Supplement, Oral
Use Treatment and prevention of calcium depletion; relief of acid indigestion, heartburn
Usual Dosage Dosage is in terms of elemental calcium
Recommended daily allowance (RDA): Oral:
<6 months: 360 mg/day
6-12 months: 540 mg/day
1-10 years: 800 mg/day
10-18 years: 1200 mg/day
(Continued)

calcium carbonate *(Continued)*

Adults: 800 mg/day
Hypocalcemia (dose depends on clinical condition and serum calcium level):
Children: 20-65 mg/kg/day in 4 divided doses
Adults: 1-2 g or more per day

Dietary Considerations Should be administered 1-3 hours after meals; may decrease iron absorption so should be administered 1-2 hours before or after iron supplementation; should not be administered with bran, foods high in oxalates or whole grain cereals which may decrease calcium absorption

Nursing/Pharmacy Information
Monitor serum calcium levels
Stability: Admixture **incompatibilities** include carbonates, phosphates, sulfates, tartrates

Dosage Forms Elemental calcium listed in brackets
Capsule: 1500 mg [600 mg]
Calci-Mix™: 1250 mg [500 mg]
Florical®: 364 mg [145.6 mg] with sodium fluoride 8.3 mg
Liquid (Tums® Extra Strength): 1000 mg/5 mL (360 mL)
Lozenge (Mylanta® Soothing Antacids): 600 mg [240 mg]
Powder (Cal Carb-HD®): 6.5 g/packet [2.6 g]
Suspension, oral: 1250 mg/5 mL [500 mg]
Tablet: 650 mg [260 mg], 1500 mg [600 mg]
Calciday-667®: 667 mg [267 mg]
Os-Cal® 500, Oyst-Cal 500, Oystercal® 500: 1250 mg [500 mg]
Cal-Plus®, Caltrate® 600, Gencalc® 600, Nephro-Calci®: 1500 mg [600 mg]
Chewable:
Alka-Mints®: 850 mg [340 mg]
Amitone®: 350 mg [140 mg]
Caltrate, Jr.®: 750 mg [300 mg]
Calci-Chew™, Os-Cal®: 750 mg [300 mg]
Chooz®, Dicarbosil®, Equilet®, Tums®: 500 mg [200 mg]
Mallamint®: 420 mg [168 mg]
Rolaids® Calcium Rich: 550 mg [220 mg]
Tums® E-X Extra Strength: 750 mg [300 mg]
Tums® Ultra®: 1000 mg [400 mg]
Florical®: 364 mg [145.6 mg]with sodium fluoride 8.3 mg

calcium carbonate and magnesium carbonate

(KAL see um KAR bun ate & mag NEE zhum KAR bun ate)

U.S. Brand Names Mylanta® Gelcaps®
Generic Available No
Therapeutic Category Antacid
Use Hyperacidity
Usual Dosage Adults: Oral: 2-4 Gelcaps® as needed
Dosage Forms Capsule: Calcium carbonate 311 mg and magnesium carbonate 232 mg

calcium carbonate and simethicone

(KAL see um KAR bun ate & sye METH i kone)

Synonyms simethicone and calcium carbonate
U.S. Brand Names Titralac® Plus Liquid [OTC]
Generic Available Yes
Therapeutic Category Antacid; Antiflatulent
Use Relief of acid indigestion, heartburn, peptic esophagitis, hiatal hernia, and gas
Usual Dosage Oral: 0.5-2 g 4-6 times/day
Nursing/Pharmacy Information 40% of calcium carbonate is elemental calcium
Dosage Forms Elemental calcium listed in brackets
Liquid: Calcium carbonate 500 mg [200 mg] and simethicone 20 mg per 5 mL

calcium chloride (KAL see um KLOR ide)

Generic Available Yes
Therapeutic Category Electrolyte Supplement, Oral
Use Emergency treatment of hypocalcemic tetany; treatment of hypermagnesemia; cardiac disturbances of hyperkalemia, hypocalcemia or calcium channel blocking agent toxicity

Usual Dosage I.V.:
Cardiac arrest in the presence of hyperkalemia or hypocalcemia, magnesium toxicity, or calcium antagonist toxicity:
Infants and Children: 10-20 mg/kg; may repeat in 10 minutes if necessary
Adults: 1.5-4 mg/kg/dose or 2.5-5 mL/dose every 10 minutes
Hypocalcemia:
Infants and Children: 10-20 mg/kg/dose, repeat every 4-6 hours if needed
Adults: 500 mg to 1 g at 1- to 3-day intervals
Exchange transfusion: 0.45 mEq after each 100 mL of blood exchanged I.V.
Hypocalcemia secondary to citrated blood transfusion: Administer 0.45 mEq **elemental** calcium for each 100 mL citrated blood infused
Tetany:
Infants and Children: 10 mg/kg over 5-10 minutes; may repeat after 6 hours or follow with an infusion with a maximum dose of 200 mg/kg/day
Adults: 1 g over 10-30 minutes; may repeat after 6 hours

Nursing/Pharmacy Information
Do not inject calcium chloride I.M. or administer subcutaneously since severe necrosis and sloughing may occur. Extravasation of calcium chloride can also result in severe necrosis and sloughing. Do not use scalp vein or small hand or foot veins for I.V. administration; rapid I.V. injection at a maximum rate of 50 mg/minute; for I.V. infusion, dilute to a maximum concentration of 20 mg/mL and infuse over 1 hour or no greater than 45-90 mg/kg/hour (0.6-1.2 mEq/kg/hour).
Monitor EKG
Stability: Admixture **incompatibilities** include carbonates, phosphates, sulfates, tartrates

Dosage Forms Elemental calcium listed in brackets
Injection: 10% = 100 mg/mL [27.2 mg/mL] (10 mL)

calcium citrate (KAL see um SIT rate)

U.S. Brand Names Citracal® [OTC]
Generic Available No
Therapeutic Category Electrolyte Supplement, Oral
Use Adjunct in prevention of postmenopausal osteoporosis, treatment and prevention of calcium depletion
Usual Dosage Oral (dosage is in terms of elemental calcium): Adults: Oral: 1-2 g/day

Recommended daily allowance (RDA):
<6 months: 360 mg/day
6-12 months: 540 mg/day
1-10 years: 800 mg/day
10-18 years: 1200 mg/day
Adults: 800 mg/day

Nursing/Pharmacy Information Monitor serum calcium
Dosage Forms Elemental calcium listed in brackets
Tablet: 950 mg [200 mg]
Effervescent: 2376 mg [500 mg]

♦ **Calcium Disodium Versenate®** *see* edetate calcium disodium *on page 227*
♦ **calcium edta** *see* edetate calcium disodium *on page 227*

calcium glubionate (KAL see um gloo BYE oh nate)

U.S. Brand Names Neo-Calglucon® [OTC]
Generic Available No
Therapeutic Category Electrolyte Supplement, Oral
Use Treatment and prevention of calcium depletion
Usual Dosage Oral (syrup is a hyperosmolar solution; dosage is in terms of calcium glubionate):

Neonatal hypocalcemia: 1200 mg/kg/day in 4-6 divided doses
Maintenance: Infants and Children: 600-2000 mg/kg/day in 4 divided doses up to a maximum of 9 g/day
Adults: 6-18 g/day in divided doses

Recommended daily allowance (RDA):
<6 months: 360 mg/day
6-12 months: 540 mg/day
1-10 years: 800 mg/day
10-18 years: 1200 mg/day
Adults: 800 mg/day

Dietary Considerations Should be administered 1-3 hours after meals; may decrease iron absorption so should be administered 1-2 hours before or after
(Continued)

calcium glubionate *(Continued)*

iron supplementation; should not be administered with bran, foods high in oxalates or whole grain cereals which may decrease calcium absorption

Nursing/Pharmacy Information Monitor serum calcium, magnesium, phosphate

Dosage Forms Elemental calcium listed in brackets
Syrup: 1.8 g/5 mL [115 mg/5 mL] (480 mL)

calcium gluceptate (KAL see um gloo SEP tate)

Generic Available Yes

Therapeutic Category Electrolyte Supplement, Oral

Use Emergency treatment of hypocalcemia; treatment of hypermagnesemia; cardiac disturbances of hyperkalemia, hypocalcemia, or calcium channel blocker toxicity

Usual Dosage I.V.:
Cardiac resuscitation in the presence of hypocalcemia, hyperkalemia, or calcium channel blocker toxicity:
Children: 110 mg/kg/dose or 0.5 mL/kg/dose every 10 minutes
Adults: 5 mL every 10 minutes
Hypocalcemia:
Children: 200-500 mg/kg/day divided every 6 hours
Adults: 500 mg to 1.1 g/dose as needed
Exchange transfusion: 0.45 mEq (0.5 mL) after each 100 mL of blood exchanged
After citrated blood administration: Children and Adults: 0.4 mEq/100 mL blood infused

Nursing/Pharmacy Information
Parenteral: Rapid I.V. injection at a maximum rate of 50 mg/minute; for I.V. infusion, dilute to a maximum concentration of 55 mg/mL and infuse over 1 hour or no greater than 150-300 mg/kg/hour (0.6-1.2 mEq calcium/kg/hour)
Monitor serum calcium
Stability: Admixture **incompatibilities** include carbonates, phosphates, sulfates, tartrates

Dosage Forms Elemental calcium listed in brackets
Injection: 220 mg/mL [18 mg/mL] (5 mL, 50 mL)

calcium gluconate (KAL see um GLOO koe nate)

U.S. Brand Names Kalcinate®

Generic Available Yes

Therapeutic Category Electrolyte Supplement, Oral

Use Treatment and prevention of hypocalcemia, hypermagnesemia, cardiac disturbances of hyperkalemia, hypocalcemia, or calcium channel blocker toxicity

Usual Dosage Dosage is in terms of elemental calcium
Recommended daily allowance (RDA):
<6 months: 360 mg/day
6-12 months: 540 mg/day
1-10 years: 800 mg/day
10-18 years: 1200 mg/day
Adults: 800 mg/day
Calcium gluconate electrolyte requirement in newborn period:
Premature: 200-1000 mg/kg/24 hours
Term:
0-24 hours: 0-500 mg/kg/24 hours
24-48 hours: 200-500 mg/kg/24 hours
48-72 hours: 200-600 mg/kg/24 hours
>3 days: 200-800 mg/kg/24 hours
Hypocalcemia:
I.V.:
Infants and Children: 200-1000 mg/kg/day as a continuous infusion or in 4 divided doses
Adults: 2-15 g/24 hours as a continuous infusion or in divided doses
Oral:
Children: 200-500 mg/kg/day divided every 6 hours
Adults: 500 mg to 2 g 2-4 times/day
Calcium antagonist toxicity, magnesium intoxication; cardiac arrest in the presence of hyperkalemia or hypocalcemia: I.V.:
Infants and Children: 100 mg/kg/dose
Adults: 1-3 g
Tetany: I.V.: doses or as an infusion

Infants and Children: 100-200 mg/kg/dose over 5-10 minutes; may repeat after 6 hours or follow with an infusion of 500 mg/kg/day

Adults: 1-3 g may be administered until therapeutic response occurs

Cardiac resuscitation: I.V.:

Infants and Children: 100 mg/kg/dose (1 mL/kg/dose) every 10 minutes

Adults: 500-800 mg/dose (5-8 mL) every 10 minutes

Hypocalcemia secondary to citrated blood infusion; administer 0.45 mEq **elemental** calcium for each 100 mL citrated blood infused

Exchange transfusion:

Adults: 300 mg/100 mL of citrated blood exchanged

Maintenance electrolyte requirements for total parenteral nutrition: I.V.: Daily requirements: Adults: 10-20 mEq/1000 kcals/24 hours

Dietary Considerations Do not administer orally with bran, foods high in oxalates, or whole grain cereals which may decrease calcium absorption

Nursing/Pharmacy Information

Do not administer I.M. or S.C.; for I.V. infusion, dilute to a maximum concentration of 50 mg/mL and infuse over 1 hour or no greater than 120-240 mg/kg/hour (0.6-1.2 mEq calcium/kg/hour)

Monitor serum calcium

Stability: Admixture **incompatibilities** include carbonates, phosphates, sulfates, tartrates; store at room temperature; do not use if precipitate occurs

Dosage Forms Elemental calcium listed in brackets

Injection: 10% = 100 mg/mL [9 mg/mL] (10 mL, 50 mL, 100 mL, 200 mL)

Tablet: 500 mg [45 mg], 650 mg [58.5 mg], 975 mg [87.75 mg], 1 g [90 mg]

calcium lactate (KAL see um LAK tate)

Generic Available Yes

Therapeutic Category Electrolyte Supplement, Oral

Use Treatment and prevention of calcium depletion

Usual Dosage Oral:

Infants: 400-500 mg/kg/day divided every 4-6 hours

Children: 500 mg/kg/day divided every 6-8 hours; maximum daily dose: 9 g

Adults: 1.5-3 g divided every 8 hours

Dietary Considerations Do not administer with bran, foods high in oxalates, or whole grain cereals which may decrease calcium absorption

Nursing/Pharmacy Information Monitor serum calcium

Dosage Forms Elemental calcium listed in brackets

Tablet: 325 mg [42.25 mg], 650 mg [84.5 mg]

♦ **calcium pantothenate** see pantothenic acid on page 469

calcium phosphate, dibasic (KAL see um FOS fate dye BAY sik)

Synonyms dicalcium phosphate

U.S. Brand Names Posture® [OTC]

Generic Available Yes

Therapeutic Category Electrolyte Supplement, Oral

Use Adjunct in prevention of postmenopausal osteoporosis, treatment and prevention of calcium depletion

Usual Dosage Oral:

Children: 45-65 mg/kg/day

Adults: 1-2 g/day (doses in g of elemental calcium)

Nursing/Pharmacy Information 19.3 mEq/g; 390 mg elemental calcium/g (39% elemental calcium)

Dosage Forms Elemental calcium listed in brackets

Tablet, sugar free: 1565.2 mg [600 mg]

calcium polycarbophil (KAL see um pol i KAR boe fil)

U.S. Brand Names Equalactin® Chewable Tablet [OTC]; Fiberall® Chewable Tablet [OTC]; FiberCon® Tablet [OTC]; Fiber-Lax® Tablet [OTC]; Mitrolan® Chewable Tablet [OTC]

Generic Available Yes

Therapeutic Category Gastrointestinal Agent, Miscellaneous; Laxative

Use Treatment of constipation or diarrhea by restoring a more normal moisture level and providing bulk in the patient's intestinal tract; calcium polycarbophil is supplied as the approved substitute whenever a bulk-forming laxative is ordered in a tablet, capsule, wafer, or other oral solid dosage form

Usual Dosage Oral:

Children:

2-6 years: 500 mg 1-2 times/day, up to 1.5 g/day

6-12 years: 500 mg 1-3 times/day, up to 3 g/day

Adults: 1 g 4 times/day, up to 6 g/day

(Continued)

calcium polycarbophil *(Continued)*

Nursing/Pharmacy Information Bulk laxatives increase stool frequency; watch for signs of fluid/electrolyte loss, patient should drink adequate fluids (8 oz of water or other fluids) with each dose

Dosage Forms Tablet:
Sodium free:
Fiber-Lax®: 625 mg
FiberCon®: 500 mg
Chewable:
Equalactin®, Mitrolan®: 500 mg
Equalactin®: 650 mg
Fiberall®: 1250 mg

♦ **CaldeCort® Anti-Itch Topical Spray** *see* hydrocortisone (topical) *on page 324*

♦ **CaldeCort® Topical [OTC]** *see* hydrocortisone (topical) *on page 324*

♦ **Calderol®** *see* calcifediol *on page 101*

♦ **Caldesene® Topical [OTC]** *see* undecylenic acid and derivatives *on page 637*

calfactant *(cal FAC tant)*

U.S. Brand Names Infasurf®
Generic Available No
Therapeutic Category Lung Surfactant
Use Prevention of respiratory distress syndrome (RDS) in premature infants at high risk for RDS and for the treatment ("rescue") of premature infants who develop RDS; decreases the incidence of RDS, mortality due to RDS, and air leaks associated with RDS
Usual Dosage Should be administered intratracheally through a side-port adapter into the endotracheal tube; two attendants, one to instill the suspension, the other to monitor the patient and assist in positioning, facilitate the dosing; the dose (3 mL/kg) should be administered in two aliquots of 1.5 mL/kg each; after each aliquot is instilled, the infant should be positioned with either the right or the left side dependent; administration is made while ventilation is continued over 20-30 breaths for each aliquot, with small bursts timed only during the inspiratory cycles; a pause followed by evaluation of the respiratory status and repositioning should separate the two aliquots
Dosage Forms Suspension, intratracheal: 6 mL

♦ **Calm-X® Oral [OTC]** *see* dimenhydrinate *on page 206*

♦ **Calmylin Expectorant** *see* guaifenesin *on page 299*

♦ **Calphron®** *see* calcium acetate *on page 103*

♦ **Cal-Plus® [OTC]** *see* calcium carbonate *on page 103*

♦ **Calsan®** *see* calcium carbonate *on page 103*

♦ **Caltine®** *see* calcitonin *on page 102*

♦ **Caltrate® 600 [OTC]** *see* calcium carbonate *on page 103*

♦ **Caltrate, Jr.® [OTC]** *see* calcium carbonate *on page 103*

♦ **Camalox® Suspension & Tablet *(Discontinued)* *see page 743*

♦ **Campho-Phenique® [OTC]** *see* camphor and phenol *on page 108*

camphor and phenol *(KAM for & FEE nole)*

U.S. Brand Names Campho-Phenique® [OTC]
Generic Available Yes
Therapeutic Category Topical Skin Product
Use Relief of pain and for minor infections
Usual Dosage Topical: Apply as needed
Dosage Forms Liquid: Camphor 10.8% and phenol 4.7%

♦ **camphorated tincture of opium** *see* paregoric *on page 470*

camphor, menthol, and phenol *(KAM for, MEN thol, & FEE nole)*

U.S. Brand Names Sarna [OTC]
Generic Available Yes
Therapeutic Category Topical Skin Product
Use Relief of dry, itching skin
Usual Dosage Topical: Apply as needed for dry skin
Nursing/Pharmacy Information Usual formulation involves about 4% to 10% camphor and 2% to 5% phenol
Dosage Forms Lotion, topical: Camphor 0.5%, menthol 0.5%, and phenol 0.5% in emollient base (240 mL)

♦ **Camptosar**® *see* irinotecan *on page 346*

candesartan (kan de SAR tan)
U.S. Brand Names Atacand™
Generic Available No
Therapeutic Category Angiotensin II Antagonist
Use Treatment of hypertension; may be used alone or in combination with other antihypertensive agents
Usual Dosage Adults: Oral: Dosage must be individualized; blood pressure response is dose-related over the range of 2-32 mg; the usual recommended starting dose of 16 mg once daily when it is used as monotherapy in patients who are not volume depleted; it can be administered once or twice daily with total daily doses ranging from 8-32 mg; larger doses do not appear to have a greater effect and there is relatively little experience with such doses; most of the antihypertensive effect is present within 2 weeks and maximal blood pressure reduction is generally obtained within 4-6 weeks of treatment
Dosage Forms Tablet, as cilexetil: 4 mg, 8 mg, 16 mg, 32 mg

Candida albicans (Monilia) (KAN dee da AL bi kans mo NIL ya)
Synonyms *Monilia* skin test
U.S. Brand Names Dermatophytin-O
Generic Available No
Therapeutic Category Diagnostic Agent
Use Screen for detection of nonresponsiveness to antigens in immunocompromised individuals
Usual Dosage Intradermal: 0.1 mL, examine reaction site in 24-48 hours; induration of ≥5 mm in diameter is a positive reaction
Nursing/Pharmacy Information
Shallow S.C. injection is a less painful alternate method that may be used
Stability: Refrigerate
Dosage Forms Injection:
Intradermal: 1:100 (5 mL)
Scratch: 1:10 (5 mL)

♦ **Candistatin**® *see* nystatin *on page 452*
♦ **Canesten**® **Topical** *see* clotrimazole *on page 161*
♦ **Canesten**® **Vaginal** *see* clotrimazole *on page 161*
♦ **Cantharone**® *(Discontinued) see page 743*
♦ **Cantharone Plus**® *(Discontinued) see page 743*
♦ **Cantil**® *see* mepenzolate *on page 392*
♦ **Capastat**® **Sulfate** *see* capreomycin *on page 109*

capecitabine (kap eh SITE a bean)
U.S. Brand Names Xeloda™
Generic Available No
Therapeutic Category Antineoplastic Agent, Antimetabolite
Use Treatment of patients with metastatic breast cancer resistant to both paclitaxel and an anthracycline-containing chemotherapy regimen or resistant to paclitaxel and for whom further anthracycline therapy is not indicated (eg, patients who have received cumulative doses of 400 mg/m^2 of doxorubicin or doxorubicin equivalents). Resistance is defined as progressive disease while on treatment, with or without an initial response, or relapse within 6 months of completing treatment with an anthracycline-containing adjuvant regimen.
Usual Dosage Refer to individual protocols.
2510 mg/m^2 days 1-14 every 3 weeks
1657 mg/m^2 days 1-14 every 3 weeks
1331 mg/m^2/day
Dosage Forms Tablet: 150 mg, 500 mg

♦ **Capital**® **and Codeine** *see* acetaminophen and codeine *on page 14*
♦ **Capitral**® *see* captopril *on page 110*
♦ **Capitrol**® *see* chloroxine *on page 138*
♦ **Capoten**® *see* captopril *on page 110*
♦ **Capotena** *see* captopril *on page 110*
♦ **Capozide**® *see* captopril and hydrochlorothiazide *on page 111*

capreomycin (kap ree oh MYE sin)
U.S. Brand Names Capastat® Sulfate
Generic Available No
Therapeutic Category Antibiotic, Miscellaneous
(Continued)

capreomycin *(Continued)*

Use In conjunction with at least one other antituberculosis agent in the treatment of tuberculosis

Usual Dosage Adults: I.M.: 15 mg/kg/day up to 1 g/day for 60-120 days

Nursing/Pharmacy Information Administer by deep I.M. injection into large muscle mass; the solution for injection may acquire a pale straw color and darken with time; this is not associated with a loss of potency or development of toxicity

Dosage Forms Injection, as sulfate: 100 mg/mL (10 mL)

capsaicin *(kap SAY sin)*

U.S. Brand Names Capsin® [OTC]; Capzasin-P® [OTC]; Dolorac™ [OTC]; No Pain-HP® [OTC]; R-Gel® [OTC]; Zostrix® [OTC]; Zostrix®-HP [OTC]

Generic Available No

Therapeutic Category Analgesic, Topical

Use FDA approved for the topical treatment of pain associated with postherpetic neuralgia, rheumatoid arthritis, osteoarthritis, diabetic neuropathy, and postsurgical pain

Unlabeled uses: Treatment of pain associated with psoriasis, chronic neuralgias unresponsive to other forms of therapy, and intractable pruritus

Usual Dosage Children >2 years and Adults: Topical: Apply to area up to 3-4 times/day only

Nursing/Pharmacy Information Wash hands with soap and water after applying to avoid spreading cream to eyes or other sensitive areas of the body

Dosage Forms

Cream:

Capzasin-P®, Zostrix®: 0.025% (45 g, 90 g)

Dolorac™: 0.25% (28 g)

Zostrix®-HP: 0.075% (30 g, 60 g)

Gel (R-Gel®): 0.025% (15 g, 30 g)

Lotion (Capsin®): 0.025% (59 mL); 0.075% (59 mL)

Roll-on (No Pain-HP®): 0.075% (60 mL)

♦ **Capsin® [OTC]** *see* capsaicin *on page 110*

captopril *(KAP toe pril)*

U.S. Brand Names Capoten®

Canadian Brand Names Apo®-Capto; Novo-Captopril®; Nu-Capto®; Syn-Captopril®

Mexican Brand Names Capitral®; Capotena; Cardipril®; Cryopril; Ecapresan; Ecaten; Kenolan; Lenpryl; Precaptil; Romir

Generic Available Yes

Therapeutic Category Angiotensin-Converting Enzyme (ACE) Inhibitor

Use Management of hypertension and treatment of congestive heart failure; in postmyocardial infarction, improves survival in clinically stable patients with left ventricular dysfunction

Usual Dosage Note: Dosage must be titrated according to patient's response; use lowest effective dose. Oral:

Infants: Initial: 0.15-0.3 mg/kg/dose; titrate dose upward to maximum of 6 mg/kg/day in 1-4 divided doses; usual required dose: 2.5-6 mg/kg/day

Children: Initial: 0.5 mg/kg/dose; titrate upward to maximum of 6 mg/kg/day in 2-4 divided doses

Older Children: Initial: 6.25-12.5 mg/dose every 12-24 hours; titrate upward to maximum of 6 mg/kg/day

Adolescents and Adults: Initial: 12.5-25 mg/dose administered every 8-12 hours; increase by 25 mg/dose to maximum of 450 mg/day

Note: Smaller dosages administered every 8-12 hours are indicated in patients with renal dysfunction. Renal function and leukocyte count should be carefully monitored during therapy.

Dietary Considerations Should be administered at least 1 hour before or 2 hours after eating; absorption of captopril may be reduced by food; long-term use of captopril may result in a zinc deficiency which can result in a decrease in taste perception; zinc supplements may be used

Nursing/Pharmacy Information

Watch for hypotensive effect within 1-3 hours of first dose or new higher dose; tablets may be used to make a solution of captopril

Monitor BUN, serum creatinine, urine dipstick for protein, complete leukocyte count, and blood pressure

Stability: Unstable in aqueous solutions; to prepare solution for oral administration, mix prior to administration and use within 10 minutes

Dosage Forms Tablet: 12.5 mg, 25 mg, 50 mg, 100 mg

captopril and hydrochlorothiazide
(KAP toe pril & hye droe klor oh THYE a zide)
Synonyms hydrochlorothiazide and captopril
U.S. Brand Names Capozide®
Generic Available Yes
Therapeutic Category Antihypertensive Agent, Combination
Use Management of hypertension and treatment of congestive heart failure
Usual Dosage Adults: Oral:
Hypertension: Initial: 25 mg 2-3 times/day; may increase at 1- to 2-week intervals up to 150 mg 3 times/day (captopril dosages)
Congestive heart failure: 6.25-25 mg 3 times/day (maximum: 450 mg/day) (captopril dosages)
Dosage Forms Tablet:
25/15: Captopril 25 mg and hydrochlorothiazide 15 mg
25/25: Captopril 25 mg and hydrochlorothiazide 25 mg
50/15: Captopril 50 mg and hydrochlorothiazide 15 mg
50/25: Captopril 50 mg and hydrochlorothiazide 25 mg

♦ **Capzasin-P® [OTC]** *see* capsaicin *on page 110*
♦ **Carafate®** *see* sucralfate *on page 583*

caramiphen and phenylpropanolamine
(kar AM i fen & fen il proe pa NOLE a meen)
Synonyms phenylpropanolamine and caramiphen
U.S. Brand Names Ordrine AT® Extended Release Capsule; Rescaps-D® S.R. Capsule; Tuss-Allergine® Modified T.D. Capsule; Tussogest® Extended Release Capsule
Generic Available Yes
Therapeutic Category Antihistamine/Decongestant Combination
Use Symptomatic relief of cough and nasal congestion associated with the common cold
Usual Dosage Oral:
Children:
2-6 years: ¹/₂ teaspoonful every 4 hours
6-12 years: 1 teaspoonful every 4 hours
Children >12 years and Adults: 1 capsule every 12 hours or 2 teaspoonfuls every 4 hours
Dosage Forms
Capsule, timed release: Caramiphen edisylate 40 mg and phenylpropanolamine hydrochloride 75 mg
Liquid: Caramiphen edisylate 6.7 mg and phenylpropanolamine hydrochloride 12.5 mg per 5 mL

♦ **carampicillin** *see* bacampicillin *on page 70*
♦ **Carbac** *see* loracarbef *on page 375*

carbachol (KAR ba kole)
Synonyms carbacholine; carbamylcholine chloride
U.S. Brand Names Carbastat® Ophthalmic; Carboptic® Ophthalmic; Isopto® Carbachol Ophthalmic; Miostat® Intraocular
Generic Available No
Therapeutic Category Cholinergic Agent
Use Lower intraocular pressure in the treatment of glaucoma; to cause miosis during surgery
Usual Dosage Adults:
Intraocular: 0.5 mL instilled into anterior chamber before or after securing sutures
Ophthalmic: Instill 1-2 drops up to 4 times/day
Nursing/Pharmacy Information
Instillation for miosis prior to eye surgery should be gentle and parallel to the iris face and tangential to the pupil border; discard unused portion; finger pressure should be applied on the lacrimal sac for 1-2 minutes following topical instillation; remove excess around the eye with a tissue
Stability: Store at 8°C to 27°C (46°F to 80°F)
Dosage Forms Solution:
Intraocular (Carbastat®, Miostat®): 0.01% (1.5 mL);
Topical, ophthalmic:
Carboptic®: 3% (15 mL)
Isopto® Carbachol: 0.75% (15 mL, 30 mL); 1.5% (15 mL, 30 mL); 2.25% (15 mL); 3% (15 mL, 30 mL)

♦ **carbacholine** *see* carbachol *on page 111*

carbamazepine (kar ba MAZ e peen)

U.S. Brand Names Carbatrol®; Epitol®; Tegretol®; Tegretol-XR®

Canadian Brand Names Apo®-Carbamazepine; Mazepine®; Novo-Carbamaz®; Nu-Carbamazepine®; PMS-Carbamazepine

Mexican Brand Names Carbazep; Carbazina; Neugeron

Generic Available Yes: Tablet

Therapeutic Category Anticonvulsant

Use Prophylaxis of generalized tonic-clonic, partial (especially complex partial), and mixed partial or generalized seizure disorder; may be used to relieve pain in trigeminal neuralgia or diabetic neuropathy; has been used to treat bipolar disorders

Usual Dosage Oral (dosage must be adjusted according to patient's response and serum concentrations):

Children:

<6 years: Initial: 5 mg/kg/day; dosage may be increased every 5-7 days to 10 mg/kg/day; then up to 20 mg/kg/day if necessary; administer in 2-4 divided doses/day

6-12 years: Initial: 100 mg twice daily or 10 mg/kg/day in 2 divided doses; increase by 100 mg/day depending upon response; usual maintenance: 15-30 mg/kg/day in 2-4 divided doses/day; maximum: 1000 mg/24 hours

Children >12 years and Adults: 200 mg twice daily to start, increase by 200 mg/day at weekly intervals until therapeutic levels achieved; usual dose: 800-1200 mg/day in 3-4 divided doses; some patients have required up to 1.6-2.4 g/day

Dietary Considerations

Food: May cause GI upset; administer with large amount of water or food to decrease GI upset; may need to split doses to avoid GI upset

Sodium: SIADH and water intoxication; monitor fluid status; may need to restrict fluid

Nursing/Pharmacy Information

Shake suspension well before use

Monitor CBC with platelet count, liver function tests, serum drug concentration; observe patient for excessive sedation especially when instituting or increasing therapy

Dosage Forms

Capsule, extended release: 200 mg, 300 mg

Suspension, oral (citrus-vanilla flavor): 100 mg/5 mL (450 mL)

Tablet: 200 mg

Tablet, chewable: 100 mg

Tablet, extended release: 100 mg, 200 mg, 400 mg

♦ **carbamide** *see* urea *on page 638*

carbamide peroxide (KAR ba mide per OKS ide)

Synonyms urea peroxide

U.S. Brand Names Auro® Ear Drops [OTC]; Debrox® Otic [OTC]; E•R•O Ear [OTC]; Gly-Oxide® Oral [OTC]; Mollifene® Ear Wax Removing Formula [OTC]; Murine® Ear Drops [OTC]; Orajel® Perioseptic® [OTC]; Proxigel® Oral [OTC]

Canadian Brand Names Clamurid®

Generic Available Yes

Therapeutic Category Anti-infective Agent, Oral; Otic Agent, Cerumenolytic

Use

Oral: Relief of minor inflammation of gums, oral mucosal surfaces and lips including canker sores and dental irritation; adjunct in oral hygiene

Otic: Emulsify and disperse ear wax

Usual Dosage Children >12 years and Adults:

Oral: Apply several drops undiluted to affected area of the mouth 4 times/day and at bedtime for up to 7 days, expectorate after 2-3 minutes; as an adjunct to oral hygiene after brushing, swish 10 drops for 2-3 minutes, then expectorate; gel: massage on affected area 4 times/day

Otic: Instill 5-10 drops twice daily for up to 4 days; keep drops in ear for several minutes by keeping head tilted or placing cotton in ear

Nursing/Pharmacy Information

Drops foam on contact with ear wax

Stability: Store in tight, light-resistant containers; oral gel should be stored under refrigeration

Dosage Forms

Gel, oral (Proxigel®): 10% (34 g)

Solution:
Oral:
Gly-Oxide®: 10% in glycerin (15 mL, 60 mL)
Orajel® Perioseptic®: 15% in glycerin (13.3 mL)
Otic (Auro® Ear Drops, Debrox®, Mollifene® Ear Wax Removing, Murine® Ear Drops): 6.5% in glycerin (15 mL, 30 mL)

- ♦ **carbamylcholine chloride** *see* carbachol *on page 111*
- ♦ **Carbastat® Ophthalmic** *see* carbachol *on page 111*
- ♦ **Carbatrol®** *see* carbamazepine *on page 112*
- ♦ **Carbazep** *see* carbamazepine *on page 112*
- ♦ **Carbazina** *see* carbamazepine *on page 112*
- ♦ **Carbecin Inyectable** *see* carbenicillin *on page 113*

carbenicillin (kar ben i SIL in)
Synonyms carindacillin
U.S. Brand Names Geocillin®
Canadian Brand Names Geopen®
Mexican Brand Names Carbecin Inyectable
Generic Available No
Therapeutic Category Penicillin
Use Treatment of urinary tract infections, asymptomatic bacteriuria, or prostatitis caused by susceptible strains of *Pseudomonas aeruginosa*, *E. coli*, indole-positive *Proteus*, and *Enterobacter*
Usual Dosage Oral:
Children: 30-50 mg/kg/day divided every 6 hours; maximum dose: 2-3 g/day
Adults: 1-2 tablets every 6 hours
Dietary Considerations Should be administered with water on empty stomach
Nursing/Pharmacy Information
Administer around-the-clock to promote less variation in peak and trough serum levels
Watch for increased edema, rales, or signs of congestion, bruising, or bleeding; monitor renal, hepatic, and hematologic function tests
Dosage Forms Tablet, film coated, as indanyl sodium ester: 382 mg [base]

carbidopa (kar bi DOE pa)
U.S. Brand Names Lodosyn®
Generic Available No
Therapeutic Category Anti-Parkinson's Agent; Dopaminergic Agent (Anti-Parkinson's)
Use With levodopa in the treatment of parkinsonism to enable a lower dosage of the latter to be used and a more rapid response to be obtained, and to decrease side-effects; for details of administration and dosage
Usual Dosage Adults: Oral: 70-100 mg/day; maximum daily dose: 200 mg
Dietary Considerations May be administered with meals to decrease GI upset
Dosage Forms Tablet: 25 mg

- ♦ **carbidopa and levodopa** *see* levodopa and carbidopa *on page 365*

carbinoxamine and pseudoephedrine
(kar bi NOKS a meen & soo doe e FED rin)
Synonyms pseudoephedrine and carbinoxamine
U.S. Brand Names Biohist-LA®; Carbiset® Tablet; Carbiset-TR® Tablet; Carbodec® Syrup; Carbodec® Tablet; Carbodec® TR Tablet; Cardec-S® Syrup; Rondec® Drops; Rondec® Filmtab®; Rondec® Syrup; Rondec-TR®
Generic Available Yes
Therapeutic Category Antihistamine/Decongestant Combination
Use Temporary relief of nasal congestion, running nose, sneezing, itching of nose or throat, and itchy, watery eyes due to the common cold, hay fever, or other respiratory allergies
Usual Dosage Oral:
Children:
Drops: 1-18 months: 0.25-1 mL 4 times/day
Syrup:
18 months to 6 years: 2.5 mL 3-4 times/day
>6 years: 5 mL 2-4 times/day
Adults:
Liquid: 5 mL 4 times/day
Tablet: 1 tablet 4 times/day
(Continued)

carbinoxamine and pseudoephedrine *(Continued)*

Nursing/Pharmacy Information Raise bed rails; institute safety measures; assist with ambulation

Dosage Forms

Drops: Carbinoxamine maleate 2 mg and pseudoephedrine hydrochloride 25 mg per mL (30 mL with dropper)

Syrup: Carbinoxamine maleate 4 mg and pseudoephedrine hydrochloride 60 mg per 5 mL (120 mL, 480 mL)

Tablet:

Film-coated: Carbinoxamine maleate 4 mg and pseudoephedrine hydrochloride 60 mg

Sustained release: Carbinoxamine maleate 8 mg and pseudoephedrine hydrochloride 120 mg

carbinoxamine, pseudoephedrine, and dextromethorphan

(kar bi NOKS a meen, soo doe e FED rin, & deks troe meth OR fan)

U.S. Brand Names Carbodec DM®; Cardec DM®; Pseudo-Car® DM; Rondamine-DM® Drops; Rondec®-DM; Tussafed® Drops

Generic Available Yes

Therapeutic Category Antihistamine/Decongestant/Antitussive

Use Relief of coughs and upper respiratory symptoms, including nasal congestion, associated with allergy or the common cold

Usual Dosage

Infants: Drops:

1-3 months: $1/4$ mL 4 times/day

3-6 months: $1/2$ mL 4 times/day

6-9 months: $3/4$ mL 4 times/day

9-18 months: 1 mL 4 times/day

Children $1\frac{1}{2}$ to 6 years: Syrup: 2.5 mL 4 times/day

Children >6 years and Adults: Syrup: 5 mL 4 times/day

Dosage Forms

Drops: Carbinoxamine maleate 2 mg, pseudoephedrine hydrochloride 25 mg, and dextromethorphan hydrobromide 4 mg per mL (30 mL)

Syrup: Carbinoxamine maleate 4 mg, pseudoephedrine hydrochloride 60 mg, and dextromethorphan hydrobromide 15 mg per 5 mL (120 mL, 480 mL, 4000 mL)

♦ **Carbiset® Tablet** *see* carbinoxamine and pseudoephedrine *on page 113*

♦ **Carbiset-TR® Tablet** *see* carbinoxamine and pseudoephedrine *on page 113*

♦ **Carbocaine®** *see* mepivacaine *on page 394*

♦ **Carbodec DM®** *see* carbinoxamine, pseudoephedrine, and dextromethorphan *on page 114*

♦ **Carbodec® Syrup** *see* carbinoxamine and pseudoephedrine *on page 113*

♦ **Carbodec® Tablet** *see* carbinoxamine and pseudoephedrine *on page 113*

♦ **Carbodec® TR Tablet** *see* carbinoxamine and pseudoephedrine *on page 113*

carbol-fuchsin solution (kar bol-FOOK sin soe LOO shun)

Synonyms Castellani paint

Generic Available Yes

Therapeutic Category Antifungal Agent

Use Treatment of superficial mycotic infections

Usual Dosage Topical: Apply to affected area 2-4 times/day

Nursing/Pharmacy Information Will stain area unless colorless is used

Dosage Forms Solution: Basic fuchsin 0.3%, boric acid 1%, phenol 4.5%, resorcinol 10%, acetone 5%, and alcohol 10%

♦ **carbolic acid** *see* phenol *on page 486*

♦ **Carbolit®** *see* lithium *on page 372*

♦ **Carbolith™** *see* lithium *on page 372*

♦ **Carboplat** *see* carboplatin *on page 114*

carboplatin (KAR boe pla tin)

Synonyms CBDCA

U.S. Brand Names Paraplatin®

Mexican Brand Names Carboplat; Blastocarb

Generic Available No

Therapeutic Category Antineoplastic Agent

Use Palliative treatment of ovarian carcinoma; also used in the treatment of small cell lung cancer, squamous cell carcinoma of the esophagus; solid tumors of the bladder, cervix and testes; pediatric brain tumor, neuroblastoma

Usual Dosage I.V. (refer to individual protocols):

Children:

Solid tumor: 560 mg/m^2 once every 4 weeks

Brain tumor: 175 mg/m^2 once weekly for 4 weeks with a 2-week recovery period between courses; dose is then adjusted on platelet count and neutrophil count values

Adults: Single agent: 360 mg/m^2 once every 4 weeks; dose is then adjusted on platelet count and neutrophil count values

Nursing/Pharmacy Information

Needle or intravenous administration sets containing aluminum parts should not be used in the administration or preparation of carboplatin (aluminum can interact with carboplatin resulting in precipitate formation and loss of potency); administer by I.V. intermittent infusion over 15 minutes to 1 hour, or by continuous infusion (continuous infusion regimens may be less toxic than the bolus route); reconstituted carboplatin 10 mg/mL should be further diluted to a final concentration of 0.5-2 mg/mL with D$_5$W or NS for administration

Monitor CBC with differential and platelet count, serum electrolytes, urinalysis, creatinine clearance, liver function tests

Stability: Store unopened vials at room temperature; after preparation, solutions are stable for 8 hours; dilute dose to concentrations as low as 0.5-2 mg/mL in D$_5$W or normal saline; aluminum needles should not be used for administration due to binding with the platinum ion; protect from light; **compatible** with etoposide

Dosage Forms Powder for injection, lyophilized: 50 mg, 150 mg, 450 mg

carboprost tromethamine (KAR boe prost tro METH a meen)

U.S. Brand Names Hemabate™

Generic Available No

Therapeutic Category Prostaglandin

Use Termination of pregnancy

Usual Dosage I.M.: Initial: 250 mcg, then 250 mcg at 1½-hour to 3½-hour intervals depending on uterine response; a 500 mcg dose may be administered if uterine response is not adequate after several 250 mcg doses

Nursing/Pharmacy Information

Do not inject I.V. (may result in bronchospasm, hypertension, vomiting and anaphylaxis)

Stability: Refrigerate ampuls

Dosage Forms Injection: Carboprost 250 mcg and tromethamine 83 mcg per mL (1 mL)

♦ **Carboptic® Ophthalmic** see carbachol on page 111

♦ **carbose d** see carboxymethylcellulose on page 115

carboxymethylcellulose (kar boks ee meth il SEL yoo lose)

Synonyms carbose d; carboxymethylcellulose sodium

U.S. Brand Names Cellufresh® [OTC]; Celluvisc® [OTC]

Generic Available Yes

Therapeutic Category Ophthalmic Agent, Miscellaneous

Use Preservative-free artificial tear substitute

Usual Dosage Adults: Ophthalmic: Instill 1-2 drops into eye(s) 3-4 times/day

Dosage Forms Solution, ophthalmic, as sodium, preservative free: 0.5% (0.3 mL); 1% (0.3 mL)

♦ **carboxymethylcellulose sodium** see carboxymethylcellulose on page 115

♦ **Cardec DM®** see carbinoxamine, pseudoephedrine, and dextromethorphan on page 114

♦ **Cardec-S® Syrup** see carbinoxamine and pseudoephedrine on page 113

♦ **Cardene®** see nicardipine on page 440

♦ **Cardene® SR** see nicardipine on page 440

♦ **Cardilate®** see erythrityl tetranitrate on page 239

♦ **Cardinit** see nitroglycerin on page 444

♦ **Cardio-Green®** see indocyanine green on page 337

♦ **Cardioquin®** see quinidine on page 536

♦ **Cardiorona** see amiodarone on page 39

♦ **Cardipril®** see captopril on page 110

♦ **Cardizem® CD** see diltiazem on page 205

- ◆ **Cardizem® Injectable** *see* diltiazem *on page 205*
- ◆ **Cardizem® SR** *see* diltiazem *on page 205*
- ◆ **Cardizem® Tablet** *see* diltiazem *on page 205*
- ◆ **Cardura®** *see* doxazosin *on page 219*
- ◆ **Carexan** *see* itraconazole *on page 351*
- ◆ **carindacillin** *see* carbenicillin *on page 113*
- ◆ **carisoprodate** *see* carisoprodol *on page 116*

carisoprodol (kar i soe PROE dole)

Synonyms carisoprodate; isobamate
U.S. Brand Names Soma®
Mexican Brand Names Dolaren (Carisoprodol With Diclofenac); Naxodol (Carisoprodol With Naproxen)
Generic Available Yes
Therapeutic Category Skeletal Muscle Relaxant
Use Skeletal muscle relaxant
Usual Dosage Adults: Oral: 350 mg 3-4 times/day; administer last dose at bedtime; compound: 1-2 tablets 4 times/day
Nursing/Pharmacy Information
  Raise bed rails, institute safety measures, assist with ambulation
  Monitor for relief of pain and/or muscle spasm and avoid excessive drowsiness
Dosage Forms Tablet: 350 mg

carisoprodol and aspirin (kar i soe PROE dole & AS pir in)

U.S. Brand Names Soma® Compound
Generic Available Yes
Therapeutic Category Skeletal Muscle Relaxant
Use Skeletal muscle relaxant
Usual Dosage Adults: Oral: 1-2 tablets 4 times/day
Nursing/Pharmacy Information Raise bed rails; institute safety measures; assist with ambulation
Dosage Forms Tablet: Carisoprodol 200 mg and aspirin 325 mg

carisoprodol, aspirin, and codeine

(kar i soe PROE dole, AS pir in, and KOE deen)
U.S. Brand Names Soma® Compound w/Codeine
Generic Available No
Therapeutic Category Skeletal Muscle Relaxant
Controlled Substance C-III
Use Skeletal muscle relaxant
Usual Dosage Adults: Oral: 1-2 tablets 4 times/day
Nursing/Pharmacy Information Raise bed rails; institute safety measures; assist with ambulation
Dosage Forms Tablet: Carisoprodol 200 mg, aspirin 325 mg, and codeine phosphate 16 mg

- ◆ **Carmol-HC® Topical** *see* urea and hydrocortisone *on page 639*
- ◆ **Carmol® Topical [OTC]** *see* urea *on page 638*

carmustine (kar MUS teen)

Synonyms BCNU
U.S. Brand Names BiCNU®
Generic Available No
Therapeutic Category Antineoplastic Agent
Use Brain tumors, multiple myeloma, Hodgkin's disease, and non-Hodgkin's lymphomas; some activity in malignant melanoma; glioblastoma multiforme (wafer)
Usual Dosage Children and Adults:
  I.V. infusion (refer to individual protocols): 75-100 mg/m^2/day for 2 days or 150-200 mg/m^2 every 6 weeks as a single dose or divided into daily injections on 2 successive days; next dose is to be determined based on hematologic response to the previous dose
  Wafer: Implant 8 wafer in resected brain cavity, if size and shape allow
Nursing/Pharmacy Information
  Must administer in glass containers; accidental skin contact may cause transient burning and brown discoloration of the skin
  Monitor CBC with differential and platelet count, pulmonary function, liver function, and renal function tests; monitor blood pressure during administration

Stability: Store in refrigerator, protect from light; stable for 8 hours at room temperature, 48 hours when refrigerated after further dilution in D_5W or normal saline in glass bottle to a concentration of 0.2 mg/mL; **incompatible** with sodium bicarbonate; **compatible** with cisplatin

Dosage Forms
Powder for injection: 100 mg/vial packaged with 3 mL of absolute alcohol for use as a sterile diluent
Wafer: 7.7 mg

- ◆ **Carnation Instant Breakfast®** [OTC] *see* enteral nutritional products *on page 233*
- ◆ **Carnitor® Injection** *see* levocarnitine *on page 365*
- ◆ **Carnitor® Oral** *see* levocarnitine *on page 365*
- ◆ **Carnotprim Primperan®** *see* metoclopramide *on page 409*
- ◆ **Carnotprim Primperan® Retard** *see* metoclopramide *on page 409*
- ◆ **Caroid®** *(Discontinued) see page 743*

carteolol (KAR tee oh lole)
U.S. Brand Names Cartrol® Oral; Ocupress® Ophthalmic
Generic Available No
Therapeutic Category Beta-Adrenergic Blocker
Use Management of hypertension; treatment of increased intraocular pressure
Usual Dosage Adults:
Oral: 2.5 mg as a single daily dose, maintenance dose: 2.5-5 mg once daily
Ophthalmic: 1 drop in eye(s) twice daily
Nursing/Pharmacy Information
Advise against abrupt withdrawal
Monitor intraocular pressure (ophthalmic); monitor orthostatic blood pressures, apical and peripheral pulse and mental status changes (ie, confusion, depression)
Dosage Forms Carteolol hydrochloride:
Solution, ophthalmic (Ocupress®): 1% (5 mL, 10 mL)
Tablet (Cartrol®): 2.5 mg, 5 mg

- ◆ **Carter's Little Pills®** [OTC] *see* bisacodyl *on page 88*
- ◆ **Cartrol® Oral** *see* carteolol *on page 117*

carvedilol (KAR ve dil ole)
U.S. Brand Names Coreg®
Generic Available No
Therapeutic Category Beta-Adrenergic Blocker
Use Management of hypertension, congestive heart failure; can be used alone or in combination with other agents, especially thiazide-type diuretics
Usual Dosage Adults: Oral:
Hypertension: 6.25 mg twice daily; if tolerated, dose should be maintained for 1-2 weeks, then increased to 12.5 mg twice daily; dosage may be increased to a maximum of 25 mg twice daily after 1-2 weeks; reduce dosage if heart rate drops to <55 beats/minute
Congestive heart failure: 3.125 mg twice daily for 2 weeks; if this dose is tolerated, may increase to 6.25 mg twice daily. Double the dose every 2 weeks to the highest dose tolerated by patient. (Prior to initiating therapy, other heart failure medications should be stabilized.)
Maximum recommended dose:
<85 kg: 25 mg twice daily
>85 kg: 50 mg twice daily
Angina pectoris (unlabeled use): 25-50 mg twice daily
Idiopathic cardiomyopathy (unlabeled use): 6.25-25 mg twice daily
Dietary Considerations Should be administered with food to minimize the risk of hypotension
Dosage Forms Tablet: 3.125 mg, 6.25 mg, 12.5 mg, 25 mg

- ◆ **casanthranol and docusate** *see* docusate and casanthranol *on page 215*

cascara sagrada (kas KAR a sah GRAH dah)
Generic Available Yes
Therapeutic Category Laxative
Use Temporary relief of constipation; sometimes used with milk of magnesia ("black and white" mixture)
Usual Dosage Note: Cascara sagrada fluid extract is 5 times more potent than cascara sagrada aromatic fluid extract
Oral (aromatic fluid extract):
Infants: 1.25 mL/day (range: 0.5-1.5 mL) as needed
(Continued)

cascara sagrada *(Continued)*

  Children 2-11 years: 2.5 mL/day (range: 1-3 mL) as needed
  Children ≥12 years and Adults: 5 mL/day (range: 2-6 mL) as needed at
  bedtime (1 tablet as needed at bedtime)
Dietary Considerations Administer on empty stomach for rapid effect
Nursing/Pharmacy Information
  Cascara sagrada fluid extract is 5 times more potent than cascara sagrada
  aromatic fluid extract
  Stability: Protect from light and heat
Dosage Forms
  Aromatic fluid extract: 120 mL, 473 mL
  Tablet: 325 mg

♦ **Casodex®** *see* bicalutamide *on page 87*
♦ **Castellani paint** *see* carbol-fuchsin solution *on page 114*

castor oil *(KAS tor oyl)*

Synonyms oleum ricini
U.S. Brand Names Alphamul® [OTC]; Emulsoil® [OTC]; Fleet® Flavored Castor
  Oil [OTC]; Neoloid® [OTC]; Purge® [OTC]
Generic Available Yes
Therapeutic Category Laxative
Use Preparation for rectal or bowel examination or surgery; rarely used to
  relieve constipation; also applied to skin as emollient and protectant
Usual Dosage Oral:
  Castor oil:
    Infants <2 years: 1-5 mL or 15 mL/m^2/dose as a single dose
    Children 2-11 years: 5-15 mL as a single dose
    Children ≥12 years and Adults: 15-60 mL as a single dose
  Emulsified castor oil:
    Infants: 2.5-7.5 mL/dose
    Children <2 years: 5-15 mL/dose
    Children 2-11 years: 7.5-30 mL/dose
    Children ≥12 years and Adults: 30-60 mL/dose
Dietary Considerations Should be administered on an empty stomach with
  juice or carbonated beverages
Nursing/Pharmacy Information
  Do not administer at bedtime because of rapid onset of action; chill or admin-
  ister with juice or carbonated beverage to improve palatability
  Monitor I & O, serum electrolytes, stool frequency
  Stability: Protect from heat (castor oil emulsion should be protected from
  freezing)
Dosage Forms
  Emulsion, oral:
    Alphamul®: 60% (90 mL, 3780 mL)
    Emulsoil®: 95% (63 mL)
    Fleet® Flavored Castor Oil: 67% (45 mL, 90 mL)
    Neoloid®: 36.4% (118 mL)
  Liquid, oral:
    100% (60 mL, 120 mL, 480 mL)
    Purge®: 95% (30 mL, 60 mL)

♦ **Cataflam® Oral** *see* diclofenac *on page 198*
♦ **Catapresan-100®** *see* clonidine *on page 159*
♦ **Catapres® Oral** *see* clonidine *on page 159*
♦ **Catapres-TTS® Transdermal** *see* clonidine *on page 159*
♦ **Catarase® 1:5000 *(Discontinued)*** *see page 743*
♦ **Cauteridol®** *see* ranitidine hydrochloride *on page 541*
♦ **Caverject® Injection** *see* alprostadil *on page 30*
♦ **CBDCA** *see* carboplatin *on page 114*
♦ **CCNU** *see* lomustine *on page 374*
♦ **C-Crystals® [OTC]** *see* ascorbic acid *on page 60*
♦ **2-CdA** *see* cladribine *on page 154*
♦ **CDDP** *see* cisplatin *on page 153*
♦ **Cebid®** *see* ascorbic acid *on page 60*
♦ **Ceclor®** *see* cefaclor *on page 119*
♦ **Ceclor® CD** *see* cefaclor *on page 119*
♦ **Cecon® [OTC]** *see* ascorbic acid *on page 60*
♦ **Cedax®** *see* ceftibuten *on page 125*

- **Cedilanid-D® Injection** *(Discontinued)* *see page 743*
- **Cedocard-SR®** *see isosorbide dinitrate on page 349*
- **CeeNU®** *see lomustine on page 374*
- **Ceepryn® [OTC]** *see cetylpyridinium on page 130*

cefaclor (SEF a klor)

U.S. Brand Names Ceclor®; Ceclor® CD
Generic Available Yes
Therapeutic Category Cephalosporin (Second Generation)
Use Infections caused by susceptible organisms including *Staph aureus*, *S. pneumoniae*, and *H. influenzae*; treatment of otitis media, sinusitis, and infections involving the respiratory tract, skin and skin structure, bone and joint, and urinary tract
Usual Dosage Oral:
  Children >1 month: 20-40 mg/kg/day divided every 8-12 hours; maximum dose: 2 g/day (twice daily option is for treatment of otitis media or pharyngitis)
  Adults: 250-500 mg every 8 hours or daily dose can be administered in 2 divided doses
Dietary Considerations May be administered with food, however, there is delayed absorption
Nursing/Pharmacy Information
  With prolonged therapy, monitor CBC and stool frequency periodically
  Stability: Refrigerate suspension after reconstitution; discard after 14 days; do not freeze
Dosage Forms
  Capsule: 250 mg, 500 mg
  Powder for oral suspension (strawberry flavor): 125 mg/5 mL (75 mL, 150 mL); 187 mg/5 mL (50 mL, 100 mL); 250 mg/5 mL (75 mL, 150 mL); 375 mg/5 mL (50 mL, 100 mL)
  Tablet, extended release: 375 mg, 500 mg

cefadroxil (sef a DROKS il)

U.S. Brand Names Duricef®
Mexican Brand Names Cefamox; Duracef®
Generic Available Yes
Therapeutic Category Cephalosporin (First Generation)
Use Treatment of susceptible bacterial infections including group A beta-hemolytic streptococcal pharyngitis or tonsillitis; skin and soft tissue infections caused by streptococci or staphylococci; urinary tract infections caused by *Klebsiella*, *E. coli*, and *Proteus mirabilis*
Usual Dosage Oral:
  Children: 30 mg/kg/day divided twice daily up to a maximum of 2 g/day
  Adults: 1-2 g/day in 2 divided doses
Dietary Considerations Concomitant administration with food, infant formula, or cow's milk does **not** significantly affect absorption
Nursing/Pharmacy Information
  Administer around-the-clock to promote less variation in peak and trough serum levels
  Stability: Refrigerate suspension after reconstitution; discard after 14 days
Dosage Forms Cefadroxil monohydrate:
  Capsule: 500 mg
  Suspension, oral: 125 mg/5 mL, 250 mg/5 mL, 500 mg/5 mL (50 mL, 100 mL)
  Tablet: 1 g

- **Cefadyl®** *see cephapirin on page 129*

cefamandole (sef a MAN dole)

U.S. Brand Names Mandol®
Generic Available No
Therapeutic Category Cephalosporin (Second Generation)
Use Treatment of susceptible bacterial infection; mainly respiratory tract, skin and skin structure, bone and joint, urinary tract and gynecologic as well as septicemia, perioperative prophylaxis
Usual Dosage I.M., I.V.:
  Children: 100-150 mg/kg/day in divided doses every 4-6 hours
  Adults: 4-12 g/24 hours divided every 4-6 hours 500-1000 mg every 4-8 hours
Nursing/Pharmacy Information
  Monitor prothrombin time
  Stability: After reconstitution, CO_2 gas is liberated which allows solution to be withdrawn without injecting air; solution is stable for 24 hours at room
  (Continued)

cefamandole *(Continued)*

temperature and 96 hours when refrigerated; for I.V., infusion in normal saline and D_5W is stable for 24 hours at room temperature, 1 week when refrigerated, or 26 weeks when frozen

Dosage Forms Powder for injection, as nafate: 500 mg (10 mL); 1 g (10 mL, 100 mL); 2 g (20 mL, 100 mL); 10 g (100 mL)

- ◆ **Cefamezin** *see* cefazolin *on page 120*
- ◆ **Cefamox** *see* cefadroxil *on page 119*
- ◆ **Cefanex®** *see* cephalexin *on page 128*
- ◆ **Cefaxim** *see* cefotaxime *on page 122*
- ◆ **Cefaxona** *see* ceftriaxone *on page 126*

cefazolin (sef A zoe lin)

U.S. Brand Names Ancef®; Kefzol®; Zolicef®
Mexican Brand Names Cefamezin
Generic Available Yes
Therapeutic Category Cephalosporin (First Generation)
Use Treatment of respiratory tract, skin and skin structure, urinary tract, biliary tract, bone and joint infections and septicemia due to susceptible gram-positive cocci (except enterococcus); some gram-negative bacilli including *E. coli*, *Proteus*, and *Klebsiella* may be susceptible; perioperative prophylaxis
Usual Dosage I.M., I.V.:

Infants and Children: 50-100 mg/kg/day in 3 divided doses; maximum dose: 6 g/day

Adults: 1-2 g every 8 hours
Nursing/Pharmacy Information

Administer around-the-clock rather than 3 times/day (ie, 8-4-12) to promote less variation in peak and trough serum levels; dosage modification required in renal insufficiency; can be administered IVP over 3-5 minutes at a maximum concentration of 100 mg/mL or I.V. intermittent infusion over 10-60 minutes at a final concentration for I.V. administration of 20 mg/mL. In fluid-restricted patients, a concentration of 138 mg/mL can be administered IVP. Monitor renal function periodically when used in combination with other nephrotoxic drugs

Stability: Reconstituted solution is stable for 24 hours at room temperature and 96 hours when refrigerated; for I.V. infusion in normal saline or D_5W solution is stable for 24 hours at room temperature, 96 hours when refrigerated or 12 weeks when frozen; after freezing, thawed solution is stable for 48 hours at room temperature or 10 days when refrigerated
Dosage Forms Cefazolin sodium:

Infusion, premixed in D_5W (frozen) (Ancef®): 500 mg (50 mL); 1 g (50 mL)
Injection (Kefzol®): 500 mg, 1 g
Powder for injection (Ancef®, Zolicef®): 250 mg, 500 mg, 1 g, 5 g, 10 g, 20 g

cefdinir (SEF di ner)

Synonyms CFDN
U.S. Brand Names Omnicef®
Generic Available No
Therapeutic Category Cephalosporin (Third Generation)
Use Treatment of community-acquired pneumonia, acute exacerbations of chronic bronchitis, acute bacterial otitis media, acute maxillary sinusitis, pharyngitis/tonsillitis, and uncomplicated skin and skin structure infections.
Usual Dosage Oral:

Children (otitis media with effusion): 7 mg/kg orally twice daily or 14 mg/kg orally once daily

Adolescents and Adults: 300 mg orally twice daily; an oral dose of 600 mg once daily has been used in streptococcal pharyngitis
Dosage Forms

Capsule: 300 mg
Suspension, oral: 125 mg/5 mL (60 mL, 100 mL)

cefepime (SEF e pim)

U.S. Brand Names Maxipime®
Generic Available No
Therapeutic Category Cephalosporin (Fourth Generation)
Use Treatment of respiratory tract infections (including bronchitis and pneumonia), cellulitis and other skin and soft tissue infections, and urinary tract infections; considered a fourth generation cephalosporin because it has good

gram-negative coverage similar to third generation cephalosporins, but better gram-positive coverage

Usual Dosage I.V.:

Children: Unlabeled: 50 mg/kg every 8 hours; maximum dose: 2 g

Adults:

Most infections: 1-2 g every 12 hours for 5-10 days; higher doses or more frequent administration may be required in pseudomonal infections

Urinary tract infections, uncomplicated: 500 mg every 12 hours

Nursing/Pharmacy Information

Do not admix with aminoglycosides in the same bottle/bag

Observe for signs and symptoms of bacterial infection, including defervescence; observe for anaphylaxis during first dose

Dosage Forms Powder for injection, as hydrochloride: 500 mg, 1 g, 2 g

cefixime (sef IKS eem)

U.S. Brand Names Suprax®

Mexican Brand Names Denvar; Novacef

Generic Available No

Therapeutic Category Cephalosporin (Third Generation)

Use Treatment of urinary tract infections, otitis media, respiratory infections due to susceptible organisms including *S. pneumoniae* and *pyogenes*, *H. influenzae*, *M. catarrhalis*, and many *Enterobacteriaceae*; documented poor compliance with other oral antimicrobials; outpatient therapy of serious soft tissue or skeletal infections due to susceptible organisms; single-dose oral treatment of uncomplicated cervical/urethral gonorrhea due to *N. gonorrhoeae*; treatment of shigellosis in areas with a high rate of resistance to TMP-SMX

Usual Dosage Oral:

Children: 8 mg/kg/day in 1-2 divided doses; maximum dose: 400 mg/day

Children >50 kg or >12 years and Adults: 400 mg/day in 1-2 divided doses

Dietary Considerations May be administered with food, however, there is delayed absorption

Nursing/Pharmacy Information

Modify dosage in patients with renal impairment

Monitor renal and hepatic function periodically, with prolonged therapy

Stability: After mixing, suspension may be kept for 14 days at room temperature

Dosage Forms

Powder for oral suspension (strawberry flavor): 100 mg/5 mL (50 mL, 100 mL)

Tablet, film coated: 200 mg, 400 mg

♦ **Cefizox®** *see* ceftizoxime *on page 125*

cefmetazole (sef MET a zole)

U.S. Brand Names Zefazone®

Generic Available No

Therapeutic Category Cephalosporin (Second Generation)

Use Second generation cephalosporin with an antibacterial spectrum similar to cefoxitin, useful on many aerobic and anaerobic gram-positive and gram-negative bacteria

Usual Dosage Adults: I.V.:

Infections: 2 g every 6-12 hours for 5-14 days

Prophylaxis: 2 g 30-90 minutes before surgery

Nursing/Pharmacy Information

Monitor prothrombin times; observe for signs and symptoms of anaphylaxis

Stability: Reconstituted solution and I.V. infusion in normal saline or D_5W solution are stable for 24 hours at room temperature, 7 days when refrigerated, or 6 weeks when frozen; after freezing, thawed solution is stable for 24 hours at room temperature or 7 days when refrigerated

Dosage Forms Powder for injection, as sodium: 1 g, 2 g

♦ **Cefobid®** *see* cefoperazone *on page 122*

♦ **Cefoclin** *see* cefotaxime *on page 122*

♦ **Cefol® Filmtab®** *see* vitamin, multiple (oral) *on page 654*

cefonicid (se FON i sid)

U.S. Brand Names Monocid®

Mexican Brand Names Monocidur

Generic Available No

Therapeutic Category Cephalosporin (Second Generation)

(Continued)

cefonicid *(Continued)*

Use Treatment of susceptible bacterial infection; mainly respiratory tract, skin and skin structure, bone and joint, urinary tract and gynecologic as well as septicemia; second generation cephalosporin

Usual Dosage Adults: I.M., I.V.: 1 g every 24 hours

Nursing/Pharmacy Information

I.M. injection into relatively large muscle and aspirate; dose of 2 g should be divided in half and administered into two separate sites

Stability: Reconstituted solution and I.V. infusion in normal saline or D_5W solution are stable for 24 hours at room temperature or 72 hours if refrigerated

Dosage Forms Powder for injection, as sodium: 500 mg, 1 g, 10 g

cefoperazone *(sef oh PER a zone)*

U.S. Brand Names Cefobid®

Generic Available No

Therapeutic Category Cephalosporin (Third Generation)

Use Treatment of susceptible bacterial infections, mainly respiratory tract, skin and skin structure, urinary tract and sepsis; as a third generation cephalosporin, cefoperazone has activity against gram-negative bacilli (eg, *E. coli*, *Klebsiella*, and *Haemophilus*) but variable activity against *Streptococcus* and *Staphylococcus* species; it has activity against *Pseudomonas aeruginosa*, but less than ceftazidime

Usual Dosage I.M., I.V.:

Children: 100-150 mg/kg/day divided every 8-12 hours

Adults: 2-4 g/day in divided doses every 12 hours (up to 12 g/day)

Dietary Considerations Cefoperazone may decrease vitamin K synthesis by suppressing GI flora; vitamin K deficiency may occur and result in an increased risk of hemorrhage; patients at risk include those with malabsorption states (eg, cystic fibrosis) or poor nutritional status; monitor prothrombin time and administer vitamin K as needed

Nursing/Pharmacy Information

Administer around-the-clock to promote less variation in peak and trough serum levels

Monitor coagulation abnormalities, diarrhea

Stability: Reconstituted solution and I.V. infusion in normal saline or D_5W solution are stable for 24 hours at room temperature, 5 days when refrigerated or 3 weeks, when frozen; after freezing, thawed solution is stable for 48 hours at room temperature or 10 days when refrigerated

Dosage Forms Cefoperazone sodium:

Injection, premixed (frozen): 1 g (50 mL); 2 g (50 mL)

Powder for injection: 1 g, 2 g

♦ **Cefotan®** *see* cefotetan *on page 123*

cefotaxime *(sef oh TAKS eem)*

U.S. Brand Names Claforan®

Mexican Brand Names Alfotax; Benaxima; Biosint®; Cefaxim; Cefoclin; Fotexina; Taporin; Viken

Generic Available No

Therapeutic Category Cephalosporin (Third Generation)

Use Treatment of susceptible lower respiratory tract, skin and skin structure, bone and joint, intra-abdominal and genitourinary tract infections; treatment of a documented or suspected meningitis due to susceptible organisms such as *H. influenzae* and *N. meningitidis*; nonpseudomonal gram-negative rod infection in a patient at risk of developing aminoglycoside-induced nephrotoxicity and/or ototoxicity; infection due to an organism whose susceptibilities clearly favor cefotaxime over cefuroxime or an aminoglycoside

Usual Dosage I.M., I.V.:

Infants and Children 1 month to 12 years:

<50 kg: 100-200 mg/kg/day in 3-4 divided doses

Meningitis: 200 mg/kg/day in 4 divided doses

>50 kg: Moderate to severe infection: 1-2 g every 6-8 hours; life-threatening infection: 2 g/dose every 4 hours; maximum dose: 12 g/day

Children >12 years and Adults: 1-2 g every 6-8 hours (up to 12 g/day)

Nursing/Pharmacy Information

Parenteral: Can be administered IVP over 3-5 minutes at a maximum concentration of 100 mg/mL or I.V. intermittent infusion over 15-30 minutes at a final concentration for I.V. administration of 20-60 mg/mL; in fluid-restricted patients, a concentration of 150 mg/mL can be administered IVP

With prolonged therapy, monitor renal, hepatic, and hematologic function periodically

Stability: Reconstituted solution is stable for 24 hours at room temperature and 10 days when refrigerated; for I.V. infusion in normal saline or D_5W solution is stable for 24 hours at room temperature, 5 days when refrigerated, or 13 weeks when frozen; after freezing, thawed solution is stable for 24 hours at room temperature or 10 days when refrigerated

Dosage Forms Cefotaxime sodium:

Infusion, premixed in D_5W (frozen): 1 g (50 mL); 2 g (50 mL)

Powder for injection: 500 mg, 1 g, 2 g, 10 g

cefotetan (SEF oh tee tan)

U.S. Brand Names Cefotan®

Generic Available No

Therapeutic Category Cephalosporin (Second Generation)

Use Treatment of susceptible lower respiratory tract, skin and skin structure, bone and joint, genitourinary tract, sepsis, gynecologic, and intra-abdominal infections; active against anaerobes including *Bacteroides* species of gastrointestinal tract, gram-negative enteric bacilli including *E. coli*, *Klebsiella*, and *Proteus*; active against many strains of *N. gonorrhoeae*; perioperative prophylaxis

Usual Dosage I.M., I.V.:

Children: 40-80 mg/kg/day divided every 12 hours

Adults: 1-6 g/day in divided doses every 12 hours, 1-2 g may be administered every 24 hours for urinary tract infection

Nursing/Pharmacy Information

Administer around-the-clock to promote less variation in peak and trough serum levels; monitor for unusual bleeding or bruising; I.M. doses should be administered in a large muscle mass (ie, gluteus maximus)

Monitor for unusual bleeding or bruising

Stability: Reconstituted solution is stable for 24 hours at room temperature and 96 hours when refrigerated; for I.V. infusion in normal saline or D_5W solution and after freezing, thawed solution is stable for 24 hours at room temperature or 96 hours when refrigerated; frozen solution is stable for 12 weeks

Dosage Forms Powder for injection, as disodium: 1 g (10 mL, 100 mL); 2 g (20 mL, 100 mL); 10 g (100 mL)

cefoxitin (se FOKS i tin)

U.S. Brand Names Mefoxin®

Generic Available No

Therapeutic Category Cephalosporin (Second Generation)

Use Treatment of susceptible lower respiratory tract, skin and skin structure, bone and joint, genitourinary tract, sepsis, gynecologic, and intra-abdominal infections; active against anaerobes including *Bacteroides* species of the gastrointestinal tract, gram-negative enteric bacilli including *E. coli*, *Klebsiella*, and *Proteus*; active against many strains of *N. gonorrhoeae*; perioperative prophylaxis

Usual Dosage I.M., I.V.:

Infants >3 months and Children:

Mild-moderate infection: 80-100 mg/kg/day in divided doses every 4-6 hours

Severe infection: 100-160 mg/kg/day in divided doses every 4-6 hours

Maximum dose: 12 g/day

Adults: 1-2 g every 6-8 hours (I.M. injection is painful)

Nursing/Pharmacy Information

Administer around-the-clock rather than 4 times/day, 3 times/day, etc, (ie, 12-6-12-6, not 9-1-5-9) to promote less variation in peak and trough serum levels; modify dosage in patients with renal insufficiency; can be administered IVP over 3-5 minutes at a maximum concentration of 100 mg/mL or I.V. intermittent infusion over 10-60 minutes at a final concentration for I.V. administration not to exceed 40 mg/mL

Monitor renal function periodically when used in combination with other nephrotoxic drugs

Stability: Reconstituted solution is stable for 24 hours at room temperature and 48 hours when refrigerated; I.V. infusion in normal saline or D_5W solution is stable for 24 hours at room temperature, 1 week when refrigerated, or 26 weeks when frozen; after freezing, thawed solution is stable for 24 hours at room temperature or 5 days when refrigerated

Dosage Forms Cefoxitin sodium:

Infusion, premixed in D_5W (frozen): 1 g (50 mL); 2 g (50 mL)

Powder for injection: 1 g, 2 g, 10 g

cefpodoxime (sef pode OKS eem)

U.S. Brand Names Vantin®

Generic Available No

Therapeutic Category Cephalosporin (Second Generation)

Use Treatment of susceptible acute, community-acquired pneumonia caused by *S. pneumoniae* or nonbeta-lactamase producing *H. influenzae*; alternative regimen for acute uncomplicated gonorrhea caused by *N. gonorrhoeae*; uncomplicated skin and skin structure infections caused by *S. aureus* or *S. pyogenes*; acute otitis media caused by *S. pneumoniae*, *H. influenzae*, or *M. catarrhalis*; pharyngitis or tonsillitis; and uncomplicated urinary tract infections caused by *E. coli*, *Klebsiella*, and *Proteus*

Usual Dosage Oral:

Children >6 months to 12 years: 10 mg/kg/day divided every 12 hours for 10 days

Adults: 100-400 mg every 12 hours for 7-14 days

Dietary Considerations May be administered with food, however, there is delayed absorption

Nursing/Pharmacy Information

Assess patient at beginning and throughout therapy for infection; administer around-the-clock to promote less variation in peak and trough serum levels

Observe patient for diarrhea; with prolonged therapy, monitor renal function periodically

Stability: After mixing, keep suspension in refrigerator, shake well before using; discard unused portion after 14 days

Dosage Forms Cefpodoxime proxetil:

Granules for oral suspension (lemon creme flavor): 50 mg/5 mL (100 mL); 100 mg/5 mL (100 mL)

Tablet, film coated: 100 mg, 200 mg

cefprozil (sef PROE zil)

U.S. Brand Names Cefzil®

Generic Available No

Therapeutic Category Cephalosporin (Second Generation)

Use Infections caused by susceptible organisms including *S. pneumoniae*, *H. influenzae*, *M. catarrhalis*, *S. aureus*, *S. pyogenes*; treatment of infections involving the respiratory tract, skin and skin structure, and otitis media

Usual Dosage Oral:

Infants and Children >6 months to 12 years: 15 mg/kg every 12 hours for 10 days

Children >13 years and Adults: 250-500 mg every 12-24 hours for 10 days

Dietary Considerations May be administered with food, however, there is delayed absorption

Nursing/Pharmacy Information

Administer around-the-clock to promote less variation in peak and trough serum levels

Assess patient at beginning and throughout therapy for infection

Dosage Forms

Powder for oral suspension, as anhydrous: 125 mg/5 mL (50 mL, 75 mL, 100 mL); 250 mg/5 mL (50 mL, 75 mL, 100 mL)

Tablet, as anhydrous: 250 mg, 500 mg

ceftazidime (SEF tay zi deem)

U.S. Brand Names Ceptaz™; Fortaz®; Tazicef®; Tazidime®

Mexican Brand Names Ceftazim; Fortum; Tagal; Taloken; Waytrax

Generic Available No

Therapeutic Category Cephalosporin (Third Generation)

Use Treatment of infections of the respiratory tract, urinary tract, skin and skin structure, intra-abdominal, osteomyelitis, sepsis, and meningitis caused by susceptible gram-negative aerobic organisms *Enterobacteriaceae pseudomonas*; pseudomonal infection in patient at risk of developing aminoglycoside-induced nephrotoxicity and/or ototoxicity; empiric therapy for febrile, granulocytopenic patients

Usual Dosage

Infants and Children 1 month to 12 years: 30-50 mg/kg/dose every 8 hours; maximum dose: 6 g/day

Adults: 1-2 g every 8-12 hours (250-500 mg every 12 hours for urinary tract infections)

Nursing/Pharmacy Information

Parenteral: Any carbon dioxide bubbles that may be present in the withdrawn solution should be expelled prior to injection; ceftazidime can be administered IVP over 3-5 minutes at a maximum concentration of 100 mg/mL or I.V. intermittent infusion over 15-30 minutes at a final concentration of ≤40 mg/mL

Monitor serum creatinine with concurrent use of an aminoglycoside; a change in renal function necessitates a change in dose

Stability: Reconstituted solution and I.V. infusion in normal saline or D_5W solution are stable for 24 hours at room temperature, 10 days when refrigerated, or 12 weeks when frozen; after freezing, thawed solution is stable for 24 hours at room temperature or 4 days when refrigerated; 96 hours under refrigeration, after mixing

Dosage Forms

Infusion, premixed (frozen) (Fortaz®): 1 g (50 mL); 2 g (50 mL)

Powder for injection: 500 mg, 1 g, 2 g, 6 g

♦ **Ceftazim** see ceftazidime on page 124

ceftibuten (sef TYE byoo ten)

U.S. Brand Names Cedax®

Generic Available No

Therapeutic Category Cephalosporin (Third Generation)

Use Oral cephalosporin for bronchitis, otitis media, and strep throat

Usual Dosage Oral:

Children: 9 mg/kg/day for 10 days; maximum daily dose: 400 mg

Children ≥12 years and Adults: 400 mg once daily for 10 days

Dietary Considerations Administer without regard to food

Nursing/Pharmacy Information After mixing suspension, may be kept for 14 days if stored in refrigerator; discard any unused portion after 14 days; must be administered at least 2 hours before meals or 1 hour after a meal; shake suspension well before use

Dosage Forms

Capsule: 400 mg

Powder for oral suspension (cherry flavor): 90 mg/5 mL (30 mL, 60 mL, 120 mL); 180 mg/5 mL (30 mL, 60 mL, 120 mL)

♦ **Ceftin® Oral** see cefuroxime on page 126

ceftizoxime (sef ti ZOKS eem)

U.S. Brand Names Cefizox®

Mexican Brand Names Ultracef®

Generic Available No

Therapeutic Category Cephalosporin (Third Generation)

Use Treatment of susceptible bacterial infections, mainly respiratory tract, skin and skin structure, bone and joint, urinary tract and sepsis; as a third generation cephalosporin, ceftizoxime has activity against gram-negative enteric bacilli (eg, *E. coli*, *Klebsiella*), and cocci (eg, *Neisseria*), and variable activity against gram-positive cocci (*Staphylococcus* and *Streptococcus*); it has some anaerobic coverage but is less active against *B. fragilis* than cefoxitin; also indicated for *Neisseria gonorrhoeae* infections (including uncomplicated cervical and urethral gonorrhea and gonorrhea pelvic inflammatory disease), and *Haemophilus influenzae* meningitis

Usual Dosage I.M., I.V.:

Children ≥6 months: 50 mg/kg every 6-8 hours to 200 mg/kg/day to maximum of 12 g/24 hours

Adults: 1-2 g every 8-12 hours, up to 2 g every 4 hours or 4 g every 8 hours for life-threatening infections

Nursing/Pharmacy Information

Administer around-the-clock to promote less variation in peak and trough serum levels; administer I.M. injections in a large muscle mass (ie, gluteus maximus)

Stability: Reconstituted solution is stable for 24 hours at room temperature and 96 hours when refrigerated; for I.V. infusion in normal saline or D_5W solution is stable for 24 hours at room temperature, 96 hours when refrigerated or 12 weeks when frozen; after freezing, thawed solution is stable for 24 hours at room temperature or 10 days when refrigerated

Dosage Forms Ceftizoxime sodium:

Injection in D_5W (frozen): 1 g (50 mL); 2 g (50 mL)

Powder for injection: 500 mg, 1 g, 2 g, 10 g

ceftriaxone (sef trye AKS one)
U.S. Brand Names Rocephin®
Mexican Brand Names Benaxona; Cefaxona; Tacex; Triaken
Generic Available No
Therapeutic Category Cephalosporin (Third Generation)
Use Treatment of sepsis, meningitis, infections of the lower respiratory tract, skin and skin structure, bone and joint, intra-abdominal and urinary tract due to susceptible organisms as a third generation cephalosporin, ceftriaxone has activity against gram-negative aerobic bacteria (ie, *H. influenzae*, Enterobacteriaceae, *Neisseria*) and variable activity against gram-positive cocci; documented or suspected infection due to susceptible organisms in home care patients and patients without I.V. line access; treatment of documented or suspected gonococcal infection or chancroid; emergency room management of patients at high risk for bacteremia, periorbital or buccal cellulitis, salmonellosis or shigellosis and pneumonia of unestablished etiology (<5 years of age)

Usual Dosage
Gonococcal ophthalmia: 25-50 mg/kg/day administered every 24 hours
Infants and Children: 50-100 mg/kg/day in 1-2 divided doses
Meningitis: 100 mg/kg/day divided every 12 hours; loading dose of 75 mg/kg may be administered at the start of therapy
Chancroid, uncomplicated gonorrhea: I.M.:
<45 kg: 125 mg as a single dose
>45 kg: 250 mg as a single dose
Adults: 1-2 g every 12-24 hours depending on the type and severity of the infection; maximum dose: 4 g/day

Nursing/Pharmacy Information
Administer around-the-clock to promote less variation in peak and trough serum levels; can be administered by I.V. intermittent infusion over 10-30 minutes; final concentration for I.V. administration should not exceed 40 mg/mL; for I.M. injection, ceftriaxone can be diluted with sterile water or 1% lidocaine to a final concentration of 250 mg/mL
Monitor CBC with differential, PT, renal and hepatic function tests periodically
Stability: Reconstituted solution (100 mg/mL) is stable for 3 days at room temperature and 3 days when refrigerated; for I.V. infusion in normal saline or D_5W solution is stable for 3 days at room temperature, 10 days when refrigerated, or 26 weeks when frozen; after freezing, thawed solution is stable for 3 days at room temperature or 10 days when refrigerated

Dosage Forms Ceftriaxone sodium:
Infusion, premixed (frozen): 1 g in $D_{3.8}W$ (50 mL); 2 g in $D_{2.4}W$ (50 mL)
Powder for injection: 250 mg, 500 mg, 1 g, 2 g, 10 g

cefuroxime (se fyoor OKS eem)
U.S. Brand Names Ceftin® Oral; Kefurox® Injection; Zinacef® Injection
Mexican Brand Names Froxal; Zinnat
Generic Available Yes
Therapeutic Category Cephalosporin (Second Generation)
Use Second generation cephalosporin useful in infections caused by susceptible staphylococci, group B streptococci, pneumococci, *H. influenzae* (type A and B), *E. coli*, *Enterobacter*, and *Klebsiella*; treatment of susceptible infections of the upper and lower respiratory tract, otitis media, urinary tract, skin and soft tissue, bone and joint, and sepsis

Usual Dosage
Children:
Oral:
<12 years: 125 mg twice daily
>12 years: 250 mg twice daily
I.M., I.V.: 75-150 mg/kg/day divided every 8 hours; maximum dose: 9 g/day
Adults:
Oral: 125-500 mg twice daily, depending on severity of infection
I.M., I.V.: 100-150 mg/kg/day in divided doses every 6-8 hours; maximum: 6 g/24 hours

Dietary Considerations May be administered with food, however, bioavailability is increased with food

Nursing/Pharmacy Information
Avoid crushing the tablet due to its bitter taste; can be administered IVP over 3-5 minutes at a maximum concentration of 100 mg/mL, or I.V. intermittent infusion over 15-30 minutes at a final concentration for administration of ≤30 mg/mL; in fluid restricted patients, a concentration of 137 mg/mL can be administered

With prolonged therapy, monitor renal, hepatic, and hematologic function periodically

Stability: Reconstituted solution is stable for 24 hours at room temperature and 48 hours when refrigerated; I.V. infusion in normal saline or D_5W solution is stable for 24 hours at room temperature, 7 days when refrigerated, or 26 weeks when frozen; after freezing, thawed solution is stable for 24 hours at room temperature or 21 days when refrigerated

Dosage Forms

Infusion, as sodium, premixed (frozen) (Zinacef®): 750 mg (50 mL); 1.5 g (50 mL)

Powder for injection, as sodium: 750 mg, 1.5 g, 7.5 g

Powder for injection, as sodium (Kefurox®, Zinacef®): 750 mg, 1.5 g, 7.5 g

Powder for oral suspension, as axetil (tutti-frutti flavor) (Ceftin®): 125 mg/5 mL (50 mL, 100 mL, 200 mL) 250 mg/5 mL (50 mL, 100 mL)

Tablet, as axetil (Ceftin®): 125 mg, 250 mg, 500 mg

♦ **Cefzil®** see cefprozil on page 124

♦ **Celebrex™** see celecoxib on page 127

celecoxib (ce le COX ib)

U.S. Brand Names Celebrex™

Generic Available No

Therapeutic Category Nonsteroidal Anti-inflammatory Drug (NSAID), COX-2 Selective

Use Short-term efficacy in rheumatoid arthritis and osteoarthritis; oral adjunct to usual care for patients with familial adenomatous polyposis

Usual Dosage Adults: Oral:

Osteoarthritis: 200 mg once/day or 100 mg twice daily

Rheumatoid arthritis: 100-200 mg twice daily

Dosage Forms Capsule: 100 mg, 200 mg

♦ **Celestoderm®-V, -EV/2** see betamethasone (topical) on page 85

♦ **Celestone® Oral** see betamethasone (systemic) on page 84

♦ **Celestone® Phosphate Injection** see betamethasone (systemic) on page 84

♦ **Celestone® Soluspan®** see betamethasone (systemic) on page 84

♦ **Celexa®** see citalopram on page 153

♦ **CellCept®** see mycophenolate on page 426

♦ **Cellufresh® [OTC]** see carboxymethylcellulose on page 115

cellulose, oxidized (SEL yoo lose, OKS i dyzed)

Synonyms absorbable cotton

U.S. Brand Names Oxycel®; Surgicel®

Generic Available No

Therapeutic Category Hemostatic Agent

Use Temporary packing for the control of capillary, venous, or small arterial hemorrhage

Usual Dosage Minimal amounts of an appropriate size are laid on the bleeding site

Nursing/Pharmacy Information Discard opened unused gauze

Dosage Forms

Pad (Oxycel®): 3" x 3", 8 ply

Pledget (Oxycel®): 2" x 1" x 1"

Strip:

Oxycel®:

18" x 2", 4 ply

5" x 1/2", 4 ply

36" x 1/2", 4 ply

Surgicel®:

2" x 14"

4" x 8"

2" x 3"

1/2" x 2"

cellulose sodium phosphate

(sel yoo lose SOW dee um FOS fate)

Synonyms CSP; sodium cellulose phosphate

U.S. Brand Names Calcibind®

Generic Available No

Therapeutic Category Urinary Tract Product

(Continued)

cellulose sodium phosphate *(Continued)*

Use Adjunct to dietary restriction to reduce renal calculi formation in absorptive hypercalciuria type I

Usual Dosage Adults: Oral: 5 g 3 times/day with meals; decrease dose to 5 g with main meal and 2.5 g with each of two other meals when urinary calcium declines to <150 mg/day

Dietary Considerations May be administered with meals

Dosage Forms Powder: 2.5 g packets (90s), 300 g bulk pack

- ♦ **Celluvisc® [OTC]** *see* carboxymethylcellulose *on page 115*
- ♦ **Celontin®** *see* methsuximide *on page 404*
- ♦ **Cel-U-Jec® Injection** *see* betamethasone (systemic) *on page 84*
- ♦ **Cenafed® [OTC]** *see* pseudoephedrine *on page 530*
- ♦ **Cenafed® Plus Tablet [OTC]** *see* triprolidine and pseudoephedrine *on page 632*
- ♦ **Cena-K®** *see* potassium chloride *on page 506*
- ♦ **Cenestin™** *see* estrogens, conjugated, a (synthetic) *New Drug on page 245*
- ♦ **Cenocort® A-40 *(Discontinued)*** *see page 743*
- ♦ **Cenocort® Forte *(Discontinued)*** *see page 743*
- ♦ **Cenolate®** *see* sodium ascorbate *on page 569*
- ♦ **Centrax Capsule & Tablet *(Discontinued)*** *see page 743*
- ♦ **Cēpacol® Anesthetic Troches [OTC]** *see* cetylpyridinium and benzocaine *on page 130*
- ♦ **Cēpacol® Troches [OTC]** *see* cetylpyridinium *on page 130*
- ♦ **Cēpastat® [OTC]** *see* phenol *on page 486*

cephalexin (sef a LEKS in)

U.S. Brand Names Biocef®; Cefanex®; Keflex®; Keftab®; Zartan®

Canadian Brand Names Apo®-Cephalex; Novo-Lexin®; Nu-Cephalex®

Mexican Brand Names Ceporex; Naxifelar

Generic Available Yes

Therapeutic Category Cephalosporin (First Generation)

Use Treatment of susceptible bacterial infections, including those caused by group A beta-hemolytic *Streptococcus*, *Staphylococcus*, *Klebsiella pneumoniae*, *E. coli*, and *Proteus mirabilis*; not active against enterococci; used to treat susceptible infections of the respiratory tract, skin and skin structure, bone, genitourinary tract, and otitis media

Usual Dosage Oral:

Children: 25-50 mg/kg/day every 6 hours; severe infections: 50-100 mg/kg/day in divided doses every 6 hours; maximum: 3 g/24 hours

Adults: 250-1000 mg every 6 hours

Dietary Considerations Should be administered on an empty stomach (ie, 1 hour prior to, or 2 hours after meals) to increase total absorption; peak antibiotic serum concentration is lowered and delayed, but total drug absorbed not affected; if GI distress, administer with food

Nursing/Pharmacy Information

Administer around-the-clock rather than 4 times/day to promote less variation in peak and trough serum levels

With prolonged therapy monitor renal, hepatic, and hematologic function periodically

Stability: Refrigerate suspension after reconstitution; discard after 14 days

Dosage Forms

Cephalexin monohydrate:

Capsule: 250 mg, 500 mg

Powder for oral suspension: 125 mg/5 mL (5 mL unit dose, 60 mL, 100 mL, 200 mL); 250 mg/5 mL (5 mL unit dose, 100 mL, 200 mL)

Suspension, oral, pediatric: 100 mg/mL [5 mg/drop] (10 mL)

Tablet: 250 mg, 500 mg, 1 g

Cephalexin hydrochloride: Tablet: 500 mg

cephalothin (sef A loe thin)

Canadian Brand Names Ceporacin®

Generic Available Yes

Therapeutic Category Cephalosporin (First Generation)

Use Treatment of respiratory tract, skin and skin structure, urinary tract, bone and joint infections, endocarditis, and septicemia due to susceptible gram-positive cocci (except enterococcus); some gram-negative bacilli including *E. coli*, *Proteus*, and *Klebsiella* may be susceptible; perioperative prophylaxis

Usual Dosage I.M., I.V.:
Children: 75-125 mg/kg/day divided every 4-6 hours; maximum dose: 10 g in a 24-hour period
Adults: 500 mg to 2 g every 4-6 hours

Nursing/Pharmacy Information
Administer around-the-clock to promote less variation in peak and trough serum levels
Stability: Reconstituted solution is stable for 12-24 hours at room temperature and 96 hours when refrigerated; for I.V. infusion in normal saline or D_5W solution is stable for 24 hours at room temperature, 96 hours when refrigerated or 12 weeks when frozen; after freezing, thawed solution is stable for 24 hours at room temperature or 96 hours when refrigerated

Dosage Forms Cephalothin sodium:
Infusion, in D_5W (frozen): 1 g (50 mL); 2 g (50 mL)
Powder for injection: 1 g, 2 g, 20 g

cephapirin (sef a PYE rin)
U.S. Brand Names Cefadyl®
Generic Available No
Therapeutic Category Cephalosporin (First Generation)
Use Treatment of respiratory tract, skin and skin structure, urinary tract, bone and joint infections, endocarditis and septicemia due to susceptible gram-positive cocci (except enterococcus); some gram-negative bacilli including *E. coli*, *Proteus*, and *Klebsiella*, may be susceptible; perioperative prophylaxis
Usual Dosage I.M., I.V.:
Children: 10-20 mg/kg every 6 hours up to 4 g/24 hours
Adults: 1 g every 6 hours up to 12 g/day

Nursing/Pharmacy Information
Administer around-the-clock rather than 4 times/day to promote less variation in peak and trough serum levels; administer I.M. doses deep into a large muscle mass (ie, gluteus maximus)
Stability: Reconstituted solution is stable for 24 hours at room temperature and 10 days when refrigerated; for I.V. infusion in normal saline or D_5W solution is stable for 24 hours at room temperature, 10 days when refrigerated or 14 days when frozen; after freezing, thawed solution is stable for 12 hours at room temperature or 10 days when refrigerated

Dosage Forms Powder for injection, as sodium: 500 mg, 1 g, 2 g, 4 g, 20 g

cephradine (SEF ra deen)
U.S. Brand Names Velosef®
Mexican Brand Names Veracef
Generic Available Yes
Therapeutic Category Cephalosporin (First Generation)
Use Treatment of susceptible bacterial infections, including those caused by group A beta-hemolytic *Streptococcus*
Usual Dosage Oral:
Children ≥9 months: 25-100 mg/kg/day in equally divided doses every 6-12 hours up to 4 g/day
Adults: 2-4 g/day in 4 equally divided doses up to 8 g/day

Dietary Considerations May administer with food to decrease GI distress; however there is delayed absorption

Nursing/Pharmacy Information
Administer around-the-clock to promote less variation in peak and trough serum levels; I.M. doses should be administered deep into a large muscle mass (ie, gluteus maximus)
Stability: Reconstituted solution is stable for 2 hours at room temperature and 24 hours when refrigerated; for I.V. infusion in normal saline or D_5W solution is stable for 10 hours at room temperature, 48 hours when refrigerated or 6 weeks when frozen; after freezing, thawed solution is stable for 10 hours at room temperature or 48 hours when refrigerated

Dosage Forms
Capsule: 250 mg, 500 mg
Powder for injection: 250 mg, 500 mg, 1 g, 2 g (in ready to use infusion bottles)
Powder for oral suspension: 125 mg/5 mL (5 mL, 100 mL, 200 mL); 250 mg/5 mL (5 mL, 100 mL, 200 mL)

♦ **Cephulac®** *see* lactulose *on page 359*
♦ **Ceporacin®** *see* cephalothin *on page 128*
♦ **Ceporex** *see* cephalexin *on page 128*
♦ **Ceptaz™** *see* ceftazidime *on page 124*
♦ **Cerebyx®** *see* fosphenytoin *on page 283*

♦ **Ceredase®** *see* alglucerase *on page 28*
♦ **Cerespan®** *(Discontinued) see page 743*
♦ **Cerezyme®** *see* imiglucerase *on page 334*

cerivastatin (se ree va STAT in)
U.S. Brand Names Baycol™
Generic Available No
Therapeutic Category HMG-CoA Reductase Inhibitor
Use Adjunct to dietary therapy to for the reduction of elevated total and LDL cholesterol levels in patients with primary hypercholesterolemia and mixed dyslipidemia when the response to dietary restriction of saturated fat and cholesterol and other nonpharmacological measures alone has been inadequate
Usual Dosage Adults: Oral: 0.3 mg once daily in the evening; may be taken with or without food
Dosage Forms Tablet, as sodium: 0.2 mg, 0.3 mg

♦ **Cerose-DM® [OTC]** *see* chlorpheniramine, phenylephrine, and dextromethorphan *on page 141*
♦ **Certiva®** *see* diphtheria, tetanus toxoids, and acellular pertussis vaccine *on page 210*
♦ **Cerubidine®** *see* daunorubicin hydrochloride *on page 183*
♦ **Cerumenex® Otic** *see* triethanolamine polypeptide oleate-condensate *on page 627*
♦ **Cervidil® Vaginal Insert** *see* dinoprostone *on page 207*
♦ **C.E.S.™** *see* estrogens, conjugated (equine) *on page 245*
♦ **Cesamet®** *see* nabilone *on page 426*
♦ **Cetacaine®** *see* benzocaine, butyl aminobenzoate, tetracaine, and benzalkonium chloride *on page 79*
♦ **Cetacort® Topical** *see* hydrocortisone (topical) *on page 324*
♦ **Cetamide®** *see* sulfacetamide *on page 584*
♦ **Cetane® *(Discontinued)*** *see page 743*
♦ **Cetapred® Ophthalmic** *see* sulfacetamide and prednisolone *on page 585*
♦ **Cetina** *see* chloramphenicol *on page 133*

cetirizine (se TI ra zeen)
Synonyms P-071; UCB-P071
U.S. Brand Names Zyrtec®
Canadian Brand Names Reactine™
Generic Available No
Therapeutic Category Antihistamine
Use Perennial and seasonal allergic rhinitis and other allergic symptoms including urticaria
Usual Dosage Children ≥6 years and Adults: Oral: 5-10 mg once daily, depending upon symptom severity
Dosage Forms Cetirizine hydrochloride:
Syrup: 5 mg/5 mL (120 mL)
Tablet: 5 mg, 10 mg

cetylpyridinium (SEE til peer i DI nee um)
U.S. Brand Names Ceepryn® [OTC]; Cēpacol® Troches [OTC]
Generic Available Yes
Therapeutic Category Local Anesthetic
Use Temporary relief of sore throat
Usual Dosage Children >6 years and Adults: Oral: Dissolve 1 lozenge in the mouth every 2 hours as needed
Nursing/Pharmacy Information Mouthwash contains 14% alcohol
Dosage Forms Cetylpyridinium chloride:
Mouthwash: 0.05% and alcohol 14% (180 mL)
Troche: 1:1500 (24s)

cetylpyridinium and benzocaine
(SEE til peer i DI nee um & BEN zoe kane)
Synonyms benzocaine and cetylpyridinium chloride; cetylpyridinium chloride and benzocaine
U.S. Brand Names Cēpacol® Anesthetic Troches [OTC]
Generic Available Yes
Therapeutic Category Local Anesthetic
Use Symptomatic relief of sore throat
Usual Dosage Oral: Use as needed for sore throat

Dosage Forms Troche: Cetylpyridinium chloride 1:1500 and benzocaine 10 mg per troche (18s)

♦ **cetylpyridinium chloride and benzocaine** *see* cetylpyridinium and benzocaine *on page 130*

♦ **Cevalin® [OTC]** *see* ascorbic acid *on page 60*

♦ **Cevi-bid® [OTC]** *see* ascorbic acid *on page 60*

♦ **Ce-Vi-Sol® [OTC]** *see* ascorbic acid *on page 60*

♦ **CFDN** *see* cefdinir *on page 120*

♦ **CG** *see* chorionic gonadotropin *on page 149*

♦ **Charcadole®, -Aqueous, -TFS** *see* charcoal *on page 131*

♦ **Charcoaid® [OTC]** *see* charcoal *on page 131*

charcoal (CHAR kole)

Synonyms activated carbon; liquid antidote; medicinal carbon

U.S. Brand Names Actidose-Aqua® [OTC]; Actidose® With Sorbitol [OTC]; Charcoaid® [OTC]; Charcocaps® [OTC]; Liqui-Char® [OTC]

Canadian Brand Names Charcadole®, -Aqueous, -TFS

Generic Available Yes

Therapeutic Category Antidote

Use Emergency treatment in poisoning by drugs and chemicals; repetitive doses for gastrointestinal dialysis in drug overdose to enhance the elimination of certain drugs (eg, theophylline, phenobarbital, and aspirin) and in uremia to adsorb various waste products

Usual Dosage Oral:

Acute poisoning: Single dose: Charcoal with sorbitol:

Children 1-12 years: 1-2 g/kg/dose or 15-30 g or approximately 5-10 times the weight of the ingested poison; 1 g adsorbs 100-1000 mg of poison; the use of repeat oral charcoal with sorbitol doses is not recommended. In young children sorbitol should be repeated no more than 1-2 times/day.

Adults: 30-100 g

Charcoal in water:

Single dose:

Infants <1 year: 1 g/kg

Children 1-12 years: 15-30 g or 1-2 g/kg

Adults: 30-100 g or 1-2 g/kg

Multiple dose:

Infants <1 year: 1 g/kg every 4-6 hours

Children 1-12 years: 20-60 g or 1-2 g/kg every 2-6 hours until clinical observations and serum drug concentration have returned to a subtherapeutic range

Adults: 20-60 g or 1-2 g/kg every 2-6 hours

Gastric dialysis: Adults: 20-50 g every 6 hours for 1-2 days

Dietary Considerations Milk, ice cream, sherbet, or marmalade may reduce charcoal's effectiveness

Nursing/Pharmacy Information

5-6 tablespoonfuls is approximately equal to 30 g of activated charcoal; minimum dilution of 240 mL water per 20-30 g activated charcoal should be mixed as an aqueous slurry

Stability: Adsorbs gases from air, store in closed container

Dosage Forms

Capsule (Charcocaps®): 260 mg

Liquid, activated:

Actidose-Aqua®: 12.5 g (60 mL); 25 g (120 mL)

Liqui-Char®: 12.5 g (60 mL); 15 g (75 mL); 25 g (120 mL); 30 g (120 mL); 50 g (240 mL)

Liquid, activated, with propylene glycol: 12.5 g (60 mL); 25 g (120 mL)

Liquid, activated, with sorbitol:

Actidose® With Sorbitol: 25 g (120 mL); 50 g (240 mL)

Charcoaid®: 30 g (150 mL)

Powder for suspension, activated: 15 g, 30 g, 40 g, 120 g, 240 g

♦ **Charcocaps® [OTC]** *see* charcoal *on page 131*

♦ **Chealamide®** *see* edetate disodium *on page 228*

♦ **Chemet®** *see* succimer *on page 582*

♦ **Chenix® Tablet (Discontinued)** *see page 743*

♦ **Cheracol®** *see* guaifenesin and codeine *on page 300*

♦ **Cheracol® D [OTC]** *see* guaifenesin and dextromethorphan *on page 300*

♦ **Chibroxin™ Ophthalmic** *see* norfloxacin *on page 448*

♦ **chicken pox vaccine** *see* varicella virus vaccine *on page 643*

- **Chiggertox®** [OTC] *see* benzocaine *on page 79*
- **Children's Advil® Suspension** *see* ibuprofen *on page 332*
- **Children's Hold®** [OTC] *see* dextromethorphan *on page 194*
- **Children's Kaopectate®** [OTC] *see* attapulgite *on page 66*
- **Children's Motrin® Suspension** [OTC] *see* ibuprofen *on page 332*
- **Children's Silfedrine®** [OTC] *see* pseudoephedrine *on page 530*
- **children's vitamins** *see* vitamin, multiple (pediatric) *on page 654*
- **Chirocaine®** *see* levobupivacaine *New Drug on page 364*
- **Chlo-Amine® Oral** [OTC] *see* chlorpheniramine *on page 138*
- **Chlorafed® Liquid** [OTC] *see* chlorpheniramine and pseudoephedrine *on page 140*
- **chloral** *see* chloral hydrate *on page 132*

chloral hydrate (KLOR al HYE drate)

Synonyms chloral; trichloroacetaldehyde monohydrate
U.S. Brand Names Aquachloral® Supprettes®
Canadian Brand Names Novo-Chlorhydrate®; PMS-Chloral Hydrate
Generic Available Yes
Therapeutic Category Hypnotic, Nonbarbiturate
Controlled Substance C-IV
Use Short-term sedative and hypnotic (<2 weeks), sedative/hypnotic prior to nonpainful therapeutic or diagnostic procedures (eg, EEG, CT scan, MRI, ophthalmic exam, dental procedure)
Usual Dosage
　Children:
　　Sedation, anxiety: Oral, rectal: 5-15 mg/kg/dose every 8 hours, maximum: 500 mg/dose
　　Prior to EEG: Oral, rectal: 20-25 mg/kg/dose, 30-60 minutes prior to EEG; may repeat in 30 minutes to maximum of 100 mg/kg or 2 g total
　　Hypnotic: Oral, rectal: 20-40 mg/kg/dose up to a maximum of 50 mg/kg/24 hours or 1 g/dose or 2 g/24 hours
　　Sedation, nonpainful procedure: Oral: 50-75 mg/kg/dose 30-60 minutes prior to procedure; may repeat 30 minutes after initial dose if needed, to a total maximum dose of 120 mg/kg or 1 g total
　Adults: Oral, rectal:
　　Sedation, anxiety: 250 mg 3 times/day
　　Hypnotic: 500-1000 mg at bedtime or 30 minutes prior to procedure, not to exceed 2 g/24 hours
Dietary Considerations May be administered with chilled liquid to mask taste
Nursing/Pharmacy Information
　May cause irritation of skin and mucous membranes; minimize unpleasant taste and gastric irritation by administering with water or other liquid; do not crush capsule; contains drug in liquid form
　Monitor vital signs, O_2 saturation and blood pressure with doses used for conscious sedation
　Stability: Sensitive to light; exposure to air causes volatilization; store in light-resistant, airtight container
Dosage Forms
　Capsule: 250 mg, 500 mg
　Suppository, rectal: 324 mg, 500 mg, 648 mg
　Syrup: 250 mg/5 mL (10 mL); 500 mg/5 mL (5 mL, 10 mL, 480 mL)

chlorambucil (klor AM byoo sil)

U.S. Brand Names Leukeran®
Generic Available No
Therapeutic Category Antineoplastic Agent
Use Management of chronic lymphocytic leukemia (CLL), Hodgkin's and non-Hodgkin's lymphoma; breast and ovarian carcinoma, testicular carcinoma, choriocarcinoma; Waldenström's macroglobulinemia, and nephrotic syndrome unresponsive to conventional therapy
Usual Dosage Children and Adults: Oral (refer to individual protocols):
　General short courses: 0.1-0.2 mg/kg/day or 4-8 mg/m^2/day for 2-3 weeks for remission induction, then adjust dose on basis of blood counts; maintenance therapy: 0.03-0.1 mg/kg/day
　Nephrotic syndrome: 0.1-0.2 mg/kg/day every day for 5-15 weeks with low-dose prednisone
　Chronic lymphocytic leukemia:
　　Biweekly regimen: Initial: 0.4 mg/kg dose is increased by 0.1 mg/kg every 2 weeks until a response occurs and/or myelosuppression occurs

Monthly regimen: Initial: 0.4 mg/kg, increase dose by 0.2 mg/kg every 4 weeks until a response occurs and/or myelosuppression occurs

Malignant lymphomas:

Non-Hodgkins: 0.1 mg/kg/day

Hodgkins: 0.2 mg/kg/day

Dietary Considerations Avoid acidic foods, hot foods, and spices; may be administered with chilled liquids

Nursing/Pharmacy Information

Monitor liver function tests, CBC, leukocyte counts, platelets, serum uric acid

Stability: Protect from light

Dosage Forms Tablet, sugar coated: 2 mg

chloramphenicol (klor am FEN i kole)

U.S. Brand Names AK-Chlor® Ophthalmic; Chloromycetin® Injection; Chloroptic® Ophthalmic; Ophthochlor® Ophthalmic

Canadian Brand Names Diochloram; Ortho-Chloram®; Pentamycetin®; Sopamycetin®

Mexican Brand Names Cetina; Clorafen; Paraxin; Quemicetina

Generic Available Yes

Therapeutic Category Antibiotic, Ophthalmic; Antibiotic, Otic; Antibiotic, Miscellaneous

Use Treatment of serious infections due to organisms resistant to other less toxic antibiotics or when its penetrability into the site of infection is clinically superior to other antibiotics to which the organism is sensitive; useful in infections caused by *Bacteroides*, *H. influenzae*, *Neisseria meningitidis*, *S. pneumoniae*, *Salmonella*, and *Rickettsia*

Usual Dosage

I.V.:

Infants and Children: 50-75 mg/kg/day divided every 6 hours; maximum daily dose: 4 g/day

Adults: 50 mg/kg/day in divided doses every 6 hours; maximum daily dose: 4 g/day

Ophthalmic: Children and Adults: Instill 1-2 drops or small amount of ointment every 3-6 hours; increase interval between applications after 48 hours

Dietary Considerations Should be administered with water on empty stomach; may decrease intestinal absorption of vitamin B_{12}; may have increased dietary need for riboflavin, pyridoxine, and vitamin B_{12}; monitor hematological status

Nursing/Pharmacy Information

Draw peak level 2 hours post oral dose or draw peak levels 90 minutes after the end of a 30-minute infusion; trough levels should be drawn just prior to the next dose; can be administered IVP over 5 minutes at a maximum concentration of 100 mg/mL, or I.V. intermittent infusion over 15-30 minutes at a final concentration for administration of ≤20 mg/mL

Monitor CBC with reticulocyte and platelet counts, periodic liver and renal function tests, serum drug concentration

Stability: Refrigerate ophthalmic solution; constituted solutions remain stable for 30 days; use only clear solutions; frozen solutions remain stable for 6 months

Dosage Forms

Capsule: 250 mg

Ointment, ophthalmic: 1% [10 mg/g] (3.5 g)

AK-Chlor®, Chloroptic® S.O.P.®: 1% [10 mg/g] (3.5 g)

Powder for injection, as sodium succinate: 1 g

Solution: 0.5% [5 mg/mL] (7.5 mL, 15 mL)

Ophthalmic (AK-Chlor®, Chloroptic®): 0.5% [5 mg/mL] (2.5 mL, 7.5 mL, 15 mL)

Otic: 0.5% (15 mL)

chloramphenicol and prednisolone

(klor am FEN i kole & pred NIS oh lone)

Synonyms prednisolone and chloramphenicol

U.S. Brand Names Chloroptic-P® Ophthalmic

Generic Available No

Therapeutic Category Antibiotic/Corticosteroid, Ophthalmic

Use Topical anti-infective and corticosteroid for treatment of ocular infections

Usual Dosage Ophthalmic: Instill 1-2 drops in eye(s) 2-4 times/day

Dosage Forms Ointment, ophthalmic: Chloramphenicol 1% and prednisolone 0.5% (3.5 g)

chloramphenicol, polymyxin B, and hydrocortisone
(klor am FEN i kole, pol i MIKS in bee, & hye droe KOR ti sone)
Generic Available No
Therapeutic Category Antibiotic/Corticosteroid, Ophthalmic
Use Topical anti-infective and corticosteroid for treatment of ocular infections
Usual Dosage Ophthalmic: Apply ½" ribbon every 3-4 hours until improvement occurs
Dosage Forms Solution, ophthalmic: Chloramphenicol 1%, polymyxin B sulfate 10,000 units, and hydrocortisone acetate 0.5% per g (3.75 g)

♦ **Chloraseptic® Oral [OTC]** *see* phenol *on page 486*
♦ **Chlorate® Oral [OTC]** *see* chlorpheniramine *on page 138*

chlordiazepoxide (klor dye az e POKS ide)
Synonyms methaminodiazepoxide
U.S. Brand Names Libritabs®; Librium®; Mitran® Oral; Reposans-10® Oral
Canadian Brand Names Apo-Chlordiazepoxide®; Corax®; Medilium®; Novo-Poxide®; Solium®
Generic Available Yes
Therapeutic Category Benzodiazepine
Controlled Substance C-IV
Use Management of anxiety and as a preoperative sedative, symptoms of alcohol withdrawal
Usual Dosage
Children >6 years: Anxiety: Oral, I.M.: 0.5 mg/kg/24 hours divided every 6-8 hours
Adults:
Anxiety: Oral: 15-100 mg divided 3-4 times/day
Severe anxiety: 20-25 mg 3-4 times/day
Preoperative sedation:
Oral: 5-10 mg 3-4 times/day, 1-day preop
I.M.: 50-100 mg 1-hour preop
Alcohol withdrawal symptoms: Oral, I.V.: 50-100 mg to start, dose may be repeated in 2-4 hours as necessary to a maximum of 300 mg/24 hours
Nursing/Pharmacy Information
Up to 300 mg may be administered I.M. or I.V. during a 6-hour period, but not more than this in any 24-hour period; assist patient with ambulation during initiation of therapy; I.V. form is a powder and should be reconstituted with 5 mL of sterile water or saline prior to administration; do not use diluent provided with ampul for I.V. administration
Monitor respiratory and cardiovascular status
Stability: Refrigerate injection; protect from light; **incompatible** when mixed with Ringer's solution, normal saline, ascorbic acid, benzquinamide, heparin, phenytoin, promethazine, secobarbital
Dosage Forms Chlordiazepoxide hydrochloride:
Capsule: 5 mg, 10 mg, 25 mg
Powder for injection: 100 mg
Tablet: 10 mg, 25 mg

♦ **chlordiazepoxide and amitriptyline** *see* amitriptyline and chlordiazepoxide *on page 40*
♦ **chlordiazepoxide and clidinium** *see* clidinium and chlordiazepoxide *on page 156*
♦ **Chloresium® [OTC]** *see* chlorophyll *on page 135*
♦ **Chlorgest-HD® Elixir** *(Discontinued)* *see page 743*

chlorhexidine gluconate (klor HEKS i deen GLOO koe nate)
U.S. Brand Names BactoShield® [OTC]; Betasept® [OTC]; Dyna-Hex® [OTC]; Exidine® Scrub [OTC]; Hibiclens® [OTC]; Hibistat® [OTC]; Peridex®; Periochip®; PerioGard®
Canadian Brand Names Bactigras®; Hibidil® 1:2000; Hibitane® Skin Cleanser; Oro-Clense
Generic Available Yes
Therapeutic Category Antibiotic, Oral Rinse; Antibiotic, Topical
Use
Dental:
Antibacterial dental rinse; chlorhexidine is active against gram-positive and gram-negative organisms, facultative anaerobes, aerobes, and yeast
Chip, for periodontal pocket insertion; indicated as an adjunct to scaling and root planing procedures for reduction of pocket depth in patients with adult periodontitis; may be used as part of a periodontal maintenance program

Medical: Skin cleanser for surgical scrub, cleanser for skin wounds, germicidal hand rinse

Usual Dosage Oral rinse (Peridex®)

Precede use of solution by flossing and brushing teeth, completely rinse toothpaste from mouth; swish 15 mL undiluted oral rinse around in mouth for 30 seconds, then expectorate. Caution patient not to swallow the medicine; avoid eating for 2-3 hours after treatment. (The cap on bottle of oral rinse is a measure for 15 mL.)

When used as a treatment of gingivitis, the regimen begins with oral prophylaxis. Patient treats mouth with 15 mL chlorhexidine; swish for 30 seconds, then expectorate; this is repeated twice daily (morning and evening). Patient should have a re-evaluation followed by a dental prophylaxis every 6 months.

Nursing/Pharmacy Information Inform patient that reduced taste perception during treatment is reversible with discontinuation of chlorhexidine

Dosage Forms

Chip, for periodontal pocket insertion (PerioChip®): 2.5 mg

Foam, topical, with isopropyl alcohol 4% (BactoShield®): 4% (180 mL)

Liquid, topical, with isopropyl alcohol 4%:

Dyna-Hex® Skin Cleanser: 2% (120 mL, 240 mL, 480 mL, 960 mL, 4000 mL); 4% (120 mL, 240 mL, 480 mL, 4000 mL)

BactoShield® 2: 2% (960 mL)

BactoShield®, Betasept®, Exidine® Skin Cleanser, Hibiclens® Skin Cleanser: 4% (15 mL, 120 mL, 240 mL, 480 mL, 960 mL, 4000 mL)

Rinse:

Oral (mint flavor) (Peridex®, PerioGard®): 0.12% with alcohol 11.6% (480 mL)

Topical (Hibistat® Hand Rinse): 0.5% with isopropyl alcohol 70% (120 mL, 240 mL)

Sponge/Brush (Hibiclens®): 4% with isopropyl alcohol 4% (22 mL)

Wipes (Hibistat®): 0.5% (50s)

♦ **2-chlorodeoxyadenosine** *see* cladribine *on page 154*

♦ **chloroethane** *see* ethyl chloride *on page 254*

♦ **Chlorofon-A® Tablet** *(Discontinued) see page 743*

♦ **Chloromycetin® Cream** *(Discontinued) see page 743*

♦ **Chloromycetin® Injection** *see* chloramphenicol *on page 133*

♦ **Chloromycetin® Kapseals** *(Discontinued) see page 743*

♦ **Chloromycetin® Ophthalmic** *(Discontinued) see page 743*

♦ **Chloromycetin® Otic** *(Discontinued) see page 743*

♦ **Chloromycetin® Palmitate Oral Suspension** *(Discontinued) see page 743*

♦ **chlorophylin** *see* chlorophyll *on page 135*

chlorophyll (KLOR oh fil)

Synonyms chlorophylin

U.S. Brand Names Chloresium® [OTC]; Derifil® [OTC]; Nullo® [OTC]; PALS® [OTC]

Generic Available No

Therapeutic Category Gastrointestinal Agent, Miscellaneous

Use Topically promotes normal healing, relieves pain and inflammation, and reduces malodors in wounds, burns, surface ulcers, abrasions and skin irritations; used orally to control fecal and urinary odors in colostomy, ileostomy, or incontinence

Usual Dosage

Oral: 1-2 tablets/day

Topical: Apply generously and cover with gauze, linen, or other appropriate dressing; do not change dressings more often than every 48-72 hours

Dosage Forms

Ointment, topical (Chloresium®): Chlorophyllin copper complex 0.5% (30 g, 120 g)

Solution, topical, in isotonic saline (Chloresium®): Chlorophyllin copper complex 0.2% (240 mL, 946 mL)

Tablet:

Chloresium®: Chlorophyllin copper complex 14 mg

Derifil®: Water soluble chlorophyll: 100 mg

Nullo®: Chlorophyllin copper complex 33.3 mg

PALS®: Chlorophyllin copper complex 100 mg

Sodium free, sugar free: 20 mg

chloroprocaine (klor oh PROE kane)

U.S. Brand Names Nesacaine®; Nesacaine®-MPF

Generic Available Yes

Therapeutic Category Local Anesthetic

Use For infiltration anesthesia and for peripheral and epidural anesthesia

Usual Dosage Dosage varies with anesthetic procedure, the area to be anesthetized, the vascularity of the tissues, depth of anesthesia required, degree of muscle relaxation required, and duration of anesthesia

Nursing/Pharmacy Information Before injecting, withdraw syringe plunger to ensure injection is not into vein or artery

Dosage Forms Chloroprocaine hydrochloride: Injection:
Preservative free (Nesacaine®-MPF): 2% (30 mL); 3% (30 mL)
With preservative (Nesacaine®): 1% (30 mL); 2% (30 mL)

♦ **Chloroptic® Ophthalmic** *see* chloramphenicol *on page 133*

♦ **Chloroptic-P® Ophthalmic** *see* chloramphenicol and prednisolone *on page 133*

chloroquine and primaquine (KLOR oh kwin & PRIM a kween)

Synonyms primaquine and chloroquine

U.S. Brand Names Aralen® Phosphate With Primaquine Phosphate

Generic Available No

Therapeutic Category Aminoquinoline (Antimalarial)

Use Prophylaxis of malaria, regardless of species, in all areas where the disease is endemic

Usual Dosage Adults: Start at least 1 day before entering the endemic area; administer 1 tablet/week on the same day each week; continue for 8 weeks after leaving the endemic area

Nursing/Pharmacy Information Monitor periodic CBC, examination for muscular weakness and ophthalmologic examination in patients receiving prolonged therapy

Dosage Forms Tablet: Chloroquine phosphate 500 mg [base 300 mg] and primaquine phosphate 79 mg [base 45 mg]

chloroquine phosphate (KLOR oh kwin FOS fate)

U.S. Brand Names Aralen® Phosphate

Generic Available Yes

Therapeutic Category Aminoquinoline (Antimalarial)

Use Suppression or chemoprophylaxis of malaria; treatment of uncomplicated or mild-moderate malaria; extraintestinal amebiasis; rheumatoid arthritis; discoid lupus erythematosus, scleroderma, pemphigus

Usual Dosage Oral:
Malaria (excluding resistant *P. falciparum*):
Suppression or prophylaxis in endemic areas (begin 1-2 weeks prior to, and continue for 6-8 weeks after the period of potential exposure):
Children: 5 mg base/kg/dose weekly, up to a maximum of 300 mg/dose
Adults: 300 mg/dose weekly
Treatment:
Children: 10 mg base/kg/dose, up to a maximum of 600 mg base/dose one time, followed by 5 mg base/kg/dose one time after 6 hours, and then daily for 2 days (total dose of 25 mg base/kg)
Adults: 600 mg base/dose one time, followed by 300 mg base/dose one time after 6 hours, and then daily for 2 days
Extraintestinal amebiasis: Dosage expressed in mg base:
Children: 10 mg/kg once daily for 2-3 weeks (up to 300 mg base/day)
Adults: 600 mg base/day for 2 days followed by 300 mg base/day for at least 2-3 weeks
Rheumatoid arthritis: Adults: 150 mg base once daily
Melanoma treatment: Children: 10 mg/kg base/dose (maximum: 600 mg) as a single dose followed by 5 mg/kg base one time after 6 hours, then daily for 2 days

Dietary Considerations May be administered with meals to decrease GI upset

Nursing/Pharmacy Information
Chloroquine phosphate tablets have also been mixed with chocolate syrup or enclosed in gelatin capsules to mask the bitter taste
Monitor periodic CBC, examination for muscular weakness and ophthalmologic examination in patients receiving prolonged therapy

Dosage Forms Tablet: 250 mg [150 mg base]; 500 mg [300 mg base]

♦ **Chloroserpine®** *(Discontinued) see page 743*

chlorothiazide (klor oh THYE a zide)

U.S. Brand Names Diurigen®; Diuril®
Generic Available Yes: Tablet
Therapeutic Category Diuretic, Thiazide
Use Management of mild to moderate hypertension; edema associated with congestive heart failure, pregnancy, or nephrotic syndrome
Usual Dosage I.V. has been limited in infants and children and is generally not recommended

Infants <6 months and patients with pulmonary interstitial edema:
Oral: 20-40 mg/kg/day in 2 divided doses
I.V.: 2-8 mg/kg/day in 2 divided doses
Infants >6 months and Children:
Oral: 20 mg/kg/day in 2 divided doses
I.V.: 4 mg/kg/day
Adults:
Oral: 500 mg to 2 g/day divided in 1-2 doses
I.V.: 100-500 mg/day

Dietary Considerations Avoid natural licorice; may need to decrease sodium and calcium, may need to increase potassium, zinc, magnesium, and riboflavin in diet; do not change your diet on your own while taking this medication, especially if you are taking potassium supplements or medications to reduce potassium loss; too much potassium can be as harmful as too little
Nursing/Pharmacy Information
Avoid extravasation of parenteral solution since it is extremely irritating to tissues; dilute 500 mg vial with 18 mL sterile water; administer by direct I.V. infusion over 3-5 minutes or infusion over 30 minutes in dextrose or normal saline
Monitor serum potassium, sodium, chloride, and bicarbonate
Stability: Reconstituted solution is stable for 24 hours at room temperature; precipitation will occur in <24 hours in pH <7.4
Dosage Forms
Powder for injection, lyophilized, as sodium: 500 mg
Suspension, oral: 250 mg/5 mL (237 mL)
Tablet: 250 mg, 500 mg

chlorothiazide and methyldopa
(klor oh THYE a zide & meth il DOE pa)
Synonyms methyldopa and chlorothiazide
U.S. Brand Names Aldoclor®
Generic Available No
Therapeutic Category Antihypertensive Agent, Combination
Use Treatment of hypertension
Usual Dosage Oral: 1 tablet 2-3 times/day for first 48 hours, then adjust
Dosage Forms Tablet:
150: Chlorothiazide 150 mg and methyldopa 250 mg
250: Chlorothiazide 250 mg and methyldopa 250 mg

chlorothiazide and reserpine
(klor oh THYE a zide & re SER peen)
Synonyms reserpine and chlorothiazide
Generic Available Yes
Therapeutic Category Antihypertensive Agent, Combination
Use Management of hypertension
Usual Dosage Oral: 1-2 tablets 1-2 times/day
Dosage Forms Tablet:
250: Chlorothiazide 250 mg and reserpine 0.125 mg
500: Chlorothiazide 500 mg and reserpine 0.125 mg

chlorotrianisene (klor oh trye AN i seen)

U.S. Brand Names TACE®
Generic Available No
Therapeutic Category Estrogen Derivative
Use Treat inoperable prostatic cancer; management of atrophic vaginitis, female hypogonadism, vasomotor symptoms of menopause; prevention of postpartum breast engorgement (no longer recommended because increased risk of thrombophlebitis)
Usual Dosage Adults: Oral:
Prostatic cancer: 12-25 mg/day
Atrophic vaginitis: 12-25 mg/day in 28-day cycles (21 days on and 7 days off)
(Continued)

chlorotrianisene *(Continued)*

Female hypogonadism: 12-25 mg for 21 days followed by I.M. progesterone 100 mg or 5 days of oral progestin; next course may begin on days of induced uterine bleeding

Menopause: 12-25 mg for 30 days

Postpartum breast engorgement: 12 mg 4 times/day for 7 days or 72 mg twice daily for 2 days

Nursing/Pharmacy Information Patients should inform their physicians if signs or symptoms of thromboembolic or thrombotic disorders including sudden severe headache or vomiting, disturbance of vision or speech, loss of vision, numbness or weakness in an extremity, sharp or crushing chest pain, calf pain, shortness of breath, severe abdominal pain or mass, mental depression or unusual bleeding.

Dosage Forms Capsule: 12 mg, 25 mg

chloroxine *(klor OKS een)*

U.S. Brand Names Capitrol®

Generic Available No

Therapeutic Category Antiseborrheic Agent, Topical

Use Treatment of dandruff or seborrheic dermatitis of the scalp

Usual Dosage Topical: Use twice weekly, massage into wet scalp, lather should remain on the scalp for approximately 3 minutes, then rinsed; application should be repeated and scalp rinsed thoroughly

Nursing/Pharmacy Information For external use only; avoid contact with eyes; if irritation, burning, or rash occurs, discontinue use; may discolor blonde, gray, or bleached hair

Dosage Forms Shampoo: 2% (120 mL)

♦ Chlorphed® [OTC] *see* brompheniramine *on page 94*

♦ Chlorphed®-LA Nasal Solution [OTC] *see* oxymetazoline *on page 463*

chlorphenesin *(klor FEN e sin)*

U.S. Brand Names Maolate®

Generic Available No

Therapeutic Category Skeletal Muscle Relaxant

Use Adjunctive treatment of discomfort in short-term, acute, painful musculoskeletal conditions

Usual Dosage Adults: Oral: 800 mg 3 times/day, then adjusted to lowest effective dosage, usually 400 mg 4 times/day for up to a maximum of 2 months

Nursing/Pharmacy Information May cause drowsiness, may impair judgment and coordination; avoid alcohol and other CNS depressants

Dosage Forms Tablet, as carbamate: 400 mg

chlorpheniramine *(klor fen IR a meen)*

U.S. Brand Names Aller-Chlor® Oral [OTC]; AL-Rr® Oral [OTC]; Chlo-Amine® Oral [OTC]; Chlorate® Oral [OTC]; Chlor-Pro® Injection; Chlor-Trimeton® Injection; Chlor-Trimeton® Oral [OTC]; Klorominr® Oral [OTC]; Telachlor® Oral; Teldrin® Oral [OTC]

Canadian Brand Names Chlor-Tripolon®

Generic Available Yes

Therapeutic Category Antihistamine

Use Perennial and seasonal allergic rhinitis and other allergic symptoms including urticaria

Usual Dosage

Children: Oral: 0.35 mg/kg/day in divided doses every 4-6 hours

2-6 years: 1 mg every 4-6 hours, not to exceed 6 mg in 24 hours

6-12 years: 2 mg every 4-6 hours, not to exceed 12 mg/day or sustained release 8 mg at bedtime

Children >12 years and Adults: Oral: 4 mg every 4-6 hours, not to exceed 24 mg/day or sustained release 8-12 mg every 8-12 hours, not to exceed 24 mg/day

Adults: Allergic reactions: I.M., I.V., S.C.: 10-20 mg as a single dose; maximum recommended dose: 40 mg/24 hours

Elderly: 4 mg once or twice daily. **Note:** Duration of action may be 36 hours or more when serum concentrations are low.

Dietary Considerations May be administered with food or water

Nursing/Pharmacy Information

Raise bed rails, institute safety measures, assist with ambulation; dilute in NS or dextrose; infuse I.V. slowly; the 100 mg/mL injection **is not for I.V. use**

Stability: The injectable form should be protected from light; **incompatible** when mixed in same syringe with calcium chloride, kanamycin, norepinephrine, pentobarbital

Dosage Forms Chlorpheniramine maleate:
Capsule: 12 mg
Timed release: 8 mg, 12 mg
Injection: 10 mg/mL (1 mL, 30 mL); 100 mg/mL (2 mL)
Syrup: 2 mg/5 mL (120 mL, 473 mL)
Tablet: 4 mg, 8 mg, 12 mg
Chewable: 2 mg
Timed release: 8 mg, 12 mg

chlorpheniramine and acetaminophen
(klor fen IR a meen & a seet a MIN oh fen)

U.S. Brand Names Coricidin® [OTC]

Generic Available Yes

Therapeutic Category Antihistamine/Analgesic

Use Symptomatic relief of congestion, headache, aches, and pains of colds and flu

Usual Dosage Adults: Oral: 2 tablets every 4 hours, up to 20 tablets/day

Dosage Forms Tablet: Chlorpheniramine maleate 2 mg and acetaminophen 325 mg

♦ **chlorpheniramine and hydrocodone** *see* hydrocodone and chlorpheniramine on page 320

chlorpheniramine and phenylephrine
(klor fen IR a meen & fen il EF rin)

Synonyms phenylephrine and chlorpheniramine

U.S. Brand Names Dallergy-D® Syrup; Ed A-Hist® Liquid; Histatab® Plus Tablet [OTC]; Histor-D® Syrup; Rolatuss® Plain Liquid; Ru-Tuss® Liquid

Generic Available Yes

Therapeutic Category Antihistamine/Decongestant Combination

Use Temporary relief of nasal congestion and eustachian tube congestion as well as runny nose, sneezing, itching of nose or throat, itchy and watery eyes

Usual Dosage Oral:
Children:
2-5 years: 2.5 mL every 4 hours
6-12 years: 5 mL every 4 hours
Adults: 10 mL every 4 hours or 1-2 regular tablets 3-4 times daily or 1 sustained release capsule every 12 hours

Dosage Forms
Capsule, sustained release: Chlorpheniramine maleate 8 mg and phenylephrine hydrochloride 20 mg
Liquid:
Dallergy-D®, Histor-D®, Rolatuss® Plain, Ru-Tuss®: Chlorpheniramine maleate 2 mg and phenylephrine hydrochloride 5 mg per 5 mL
Ed A-Hist® Liquid: Chlorpheniramine maleate 4 mg and phenylephrine hydrochloride 10 mg per 5 mL
Tablet (Histatab® Plus): Chlorpheniramine maleate 2 mg and phenylephrine hydrochloride 5 mg

chlorpheniramine and phenylpropanolamine
(klor fen IR a meen & fen il proe pa NOLE a meen)

Synonyms phenylpropanolamine and chlorpheniramine

U.S. Brand Names Allerest® 12 Hour Capsule [OTC]; A.R.M.® Caplet [OTC]; Chlor-Rest® Tablet [OTC]; Demazin® Syrup [OTC]; Genamin® Cold Syrup [OTC]; Ornade® Spansule®; Resaid®; Rescon Liquid [OTC]; Silaminic® Cold Syrup [OTC]; Temazin® Cold Syrup [OTC]; Thera-Hist® Syrup [OTC]; Triaminic® Allergy Tablet [OTC]; Triaminic® Cold Tablet [OTC]; Triaminic® Syrup [OTC]; Tri-Nefrin® Extra Strength Tablet [OTC]; Triphenyl® Syrup [OTC]

Generic Available Yes

Therapeutic Category Antihistamine/Decongestant Combination

Use Symptomatic relief of nasal congestion, runny nose, sneezing, itchy nose or throat, and itchy or watery eyes due to the common cold or allergic rhinitis

Usual Dosage Oral:
Children <12 years: 5 mL every 3-4 hours
Children >12 years and Adults: 1 sustained release capsule or tablet every 12 hours or 5-10 mL every 3-4 hours or 1-2 regular tablets 3-4 times/day

Dietary Considerations May be administered with food or water

(Continued)

chlorpheniramine and phenylpropanolamine
(Continued)

Nursing/Pharmacy Information Swallow capsule whole, do not crush or chew

Dosage Forms

Capsule, sustained release: Chlorpheniramine maleate 12 mg and phenylpropanolamine hydrochloride 75 mg

Liquid:

Triphenyl®, Genamin®: Chlorpheniramine maleate 1 mg and phenylpropanolamine hydrochloride 6.25 mg per 5 mL

Demazin®, Rescon®, Silaminic®, Temazin®, Thera-Hist®: Chlorpheniramine maleate 2 mg and phenylpropanolamine hydrochloride 12.5 mg per 5 mL

Syrup: Chlorpheniramine maleate 2 mg and phenylpropanolamine hydrochloride 12.5 mg per 5 mL

Tablet:

Triaminic® Cold: Chlorpheniramine maleate 2 mg and phenylpropanolamine hydrochloride 12.5 mg

Chlor-Rest®: Chlorpheniramine maleate 2 mg and phenylpropanolamine hydrochloride 18.7 mg

A.R.M.®, Triaminic® Allergy, Tri-Nefrin® Extra Strength: Chlorpheniramine maleate 4 mg and phenylpropanolamine hydrochloride 25 mg

Tablet, sustained release: Chlorpheniramine maleate 12 mg and phenylpropanolamine hydrochloride 75 mg

chlorpheniramine and pseudoephedrine
(klor fen IR a meen & soo doe e FED rin)

Synonyms pseudoephedrine and chlorpheniramine

U.S. Brand Names Allerest® Maximum Strength [OTC]; Anamine® Syrup [OTC]; Anaplex® Liquid [OTC]; Chlorafed® Liquid [OTC]; Chlor-Trimeton® 4 Hour Relief Tablet [OTC]; Co-Pyronil® 2 Pulvules® [OTC]; Deconamine® SR; Deconamine® Syrup [OTC]; Deconamine® Tablet [OTC]; Fedahist® Tablet [OTC]; Hayfebrol® Liquid [OTC]; Histalet® Syrup [OTC]; Klerist-D® Tablet [OTC]; Pseudo-Gest Plus® Tablet [OTC]; Rhinosyn® Liquid [OTC]; Rhinosyn-PD® Liquid [OTC]; Ryna® Liquid [OTC]; Sudafed® Plus Tablet [OTC]

Generic Available Yes

Therapeutic Category Antihistamine/Decongestant Combination

Use Relief of nasal congestion associated with the common cold, hay fever, and other allergies, sinusitis, eustachian tube blockage, and vasomotor and allergic rhinitis

Usual Dosage Oral:

Capsule: 1 capsule every 12 hours

Liquid: 5 mL 3-4 times/day

Tablet: 1 tablet 3-4 times/day

Nursing/Pharmacy Information Timesules® should not be chewed

Dosage Forms

Capsule:

Co-Pyronil® 2 Pulvules®: Chlorpheniramine maleate 4 mg and pseudoephedrine hydrochloride 60 mg

Capsule, sustained release: Chlorpheniramine maleate 4 mg and pseudoephedrine hydrochloride 60 mg; chlorpheniramine maleate 8 mg and pseudoephedrine hydrochloride 120 mg

Liquid:

Anamine®, Anaplex®, Chlorafed®, Deconamine®, Hayfebrol®, Rhinosyn-PD®, Ryna®: Chlorpheniramine maleate 2 mg and pseudoephedrine sulfate 30 mg per 5 mL

Rhinosyn®: Chlorpheniramine maleate 2 mg and pseudoephedrine sulfate 60 mg per 5 mL

Histalet®: Chlorpheniramine maleate 3 mg and pseudoephedrine sulfate 45 mg per 5 mL

Tablet:

Allerest® Maximum Strength: Chlorpheniramine maleate 2 mg and pseudoephedrine hydrochloride 30 mg

Deconamine®, Fedahist®, Klerist-D®, Pseudo-Gest Plus®, Sudafed® Plus: Chlorpheniramine maleate 4 mg and pseudoephedrine hydrochloride 60 mg

Chlor-Trimeton® 4 Hour Relief: Chlorpheniramine maleate 4 mg and pseudoephedrine sulfate 60 mg

chlorpheniramine, ephedrine, phenylephrine, and carbetapentane

(klor fen IR a meen, e FED rin, fen il EF rin, & kar bay ta PEN tane)

U.S. Brand Names Rentamine®; Rynatuss® Pediatric Suspension; Tri-Tannate Plus®

Generic Available Yes

Therapeutic Category Antihistamine/Decongestant/Antitussive

Use Symptomatic relief of cough

Usual Dosage Children: Oral:

<2 years: Titrate dose individually

2-6 years: 2.5-5 mL every 12 hours

>6 years: 5-10 mL every 12 hours

Dosage Forms Liquid: Carbetapentane tannate 30 mg, ephedrine tannate 5 mg, phenylephrine tannate 5 mg, and chlorpheniramine tannate 4 mg per 5 mL

♦ **chlorpheniramine, hydrocodone, phenylephrine, acetaminophen, and caffeine** see hydrocodone, chlorpheniramine, phenylephrine, acetaminophen, and caffeine on page 321

chlorpheniramine, phenindamine, and phenylpropanolamine

(klor fen IR a meen, fen IN dah meen, & fen il proe pa NOLE a meen)

U.S. Brand Names Nolamine®

Generic Available No

Therapeutic Category Antihistamine/Decongestant Combination

Use Relief of upper respiratory and nasal congestion

Usual Dosage Adults: Oral: 1 tablet every 8-12 hours

Dosage Forms Tablet, timed release: Chlorpheniramine maleate 4 mg, phenindamine tartrate 24 mg, and phenylpropanolamine hydrochloride 50 mg

chlorpheniramine, phenylephrine, and codeine

(klor fen IR a meen, fen il EF rin, & KOE deen)

U.S. Brand Names Pediacof®; Pedituss®

Generic Available No

Controlled Substance C-IV

Use Symptomatic relief of rhinitis, nasal congestion, and cough due to colds or allergy

Usual Dosage Children 6 months to 12 years: Oral: 1.25-10 mL every 4-6 hours

Dosage Forms Liquid: Chlorpheniramine maleate 0.75 mg, phenylephrine hydrochloride 2.5 mg, and codeine phosphate 5 mg with potassium iodide 75 mg per 5 mL

chlorpheniramine, phenylephrine, and dextromethorphan

(klor fen IR a meen, fen il EF rin, & deks troe meth OR fan)

U.S. Brand Names Cerose-DM® [OTC]

Generic Available No

Therapeutic Category Antihistamine/Decongestant/Antitussive

Use Temporary relief of cough due to minor throat and bronchial irritation; relief of nasal congestion, runny nose, and sneezing

Usual Dosage Adults: Oral: 5-10 mL 4 times/day

Dosage Forms Liquid: Chlorpheniramine maleate 4 mg, phenylephrine hydrochloride 10 mg, and dextromethorphan hydrobromide 15 mg per 5 mL

chlorpheniramine, phenylephrine, and methscopolamine

(klor fen IR a meen, fen il EF rin, & meth skoe POL a meen)

U.S. Brand Names D.A.II® Tablet; Dallergy®; Dura-Vent/DA®; Extendryl® SR; Histor-D® Timecelles®

Generic Available Yes

Therapeutic Category Antihistamine/Decongestant/Anticholinergic

Use Relief of nasal congestion, runny nose, and sneezing

Usual Dosage Adults: Oral: 1 capsule or caplet every 12 hours or 5 mL every 4-6 hours

Dosage Forms

Caplet, sustained release: Chlorpheniramine maleate 8 mg, phenylephrine hydrochloride 20 mg, and methscopolamine nitrate 2.5 mg

(Continued)

chlorpheniramine, phenylephrine, and methscopolamine *(Continued)*

Capsule, sustained release: Chlorpheniramine maleate 8 mg, phenylephrine hydrochloride 10 mg, and methscopolamine nitrate 2.5 mg

Syrup: Chlorpheniramine maleate 2 mg, phenylephrine hydrochloride 10 mg, and methscopolamine nitrate 0.625 mg per 5 mL

Tablet: Chlorpheniramine maleate 4 mg, phenylephrine hydrochloride 10 mg, and methscopolamine nitrate 1.25 mg

chlorpheniramine, phenylephrine, and phenylpropanolamine

(klor fen IR a meen, fen il EF rin, & fen il proe pa NOLE a meen)

U.S. Brand Names Hista-Vadrin® Tablet

Generic Available Yes

Therapeutic Category Antihistamine/Decongestant Combination

Use Symptomatic relief of rhinitis and nasal congestion due to colds or allergy

Usual Dosage Adults: Oral: 1 tablet every 6 hours

Dosage Forms Tablet: Chlorpheniramine maleate 6 mg, phenylephrine hydrochloride 5 mg, and phenylpropanolamine hydrochloride 40 mg

chlorpheniramine, phenylephrine, and phenyltoloxamine

(klor fen IR a meen, fen il EF rin, & fen il tole LOKS a meen)

U.S. Brand Names Comhist®; Comhist® LA

Generic Available No

Therapeutic Category Antihistamine/Decongestant Combination

Use Symptomatic relief of rhinitis and nasal congestion due to colds or allergy

Usual Dosage Oral: 1 capsule every 8-12 hours or 1-2 tablets 3 times/day

Dosage Forms

Capsule, sustained release (Comhist® LA): Chlorpheniramine maleate 4 mg, phenylephrine hydrochloride 20 mg, and phenyltoloxamine citrate 50 mg

Tablet (Comhist®): Chlorpheniramine maleate 2 mg, phenylephrine hydrochloride 10 mg, and phenyltoloxamine citrate 25 mg

chlorpheniramine, phenylephrine, phenylpropanolamine, and belladonna alkaloids

(klor fen IR a meen, fen il EF rin, fen il proe pa NOLE a meen, & bel a DON a AL ka loydz)

Synonyms phenylephrine, chlorpheniramine, phenylpropanolamine, and belladonna alkaloids; phenylpropanolamine, chlorpheniramine, phenylephrine, and belladonna alkaloids

U.S. Brand Names Atrohist® Plus; Phenahist-TR®; Phenchlor® S.H.A.; Ru-Tuss®; Stahist®

Generic Available Yes

Therapeutic Category Cold Preparation

Use Relief of symptoms resulting from irritation of sinus, nasal, and upper respiratory tract tissues, including nasal congestion, watering eyes, and postnasal drip; this product contains anticholinergic agents and should be reserved for patients who do not respond to other antihistamine/decongestants

Usual Dosage Children ≥12 years and Adults: Oral: 1 tablet morning and evening, swallowed whole

Dosage Forms Tablet, sustained release: Chlorpheniramine 8 mg, phenylephrine 25 mg, phenylpropanolamine 50 mg, hyoscyamine 0.19 mg, atropine 0.04 mg, and scopolamine 0.01 mg

chlorpheniramine, phenylpropanolamine, and acetaminophen

(klor fen IR a meen, fen il proe pa NOLE a meen, & a seet a MIN oh fen)

U.S. Brand Names Congestant D® [OTC]; Coricidin D® [OTC]; Dapacin® Cold Capsule [OTC]; Duadacin® Capsule [OTC]; Tylenol® Cold Effervescent Medication Tablet [OTC]

Generic Available Yes

Therapeutic Category Antihistamine/Decongestant/Analgesic

Use Symptomatic relief of nasal congestion and headache from colds/sinus congestion

Usual Dosage Adults: Oral: 2 capsules/tablets every 4 hours, up to 12/day

Dosage Forms
Capsule: Chlorpheniramine maleate 2 mg, phenylpropanolamine hydrochloride 12.5 mg, and acetaminophen 325 mg
Tablet: Chlorpheniramine maleate 2 mg, phenylpropanolamine hydrochloride 12.5 mg, and acetaminophen 325 mg

chlorpheniramine, phenylpropanolamine, and dextromethorphan
(klor fen IR a meen, fen il proe pa NOLE a meen, & deks troe meth OR fan)
U.S. Brand Names Triaminicol® Multi-Symptom Cold Syrup [OTC]
Generic Available Yes
Therapeutic Category Antihistamine/Decongestant/Antitussive
Use Relief of runny nose, sneezing; cough suppressant; promote nasal and sinus drainage
Usual Dosage
Children 6-12 years: 5 mL every 4 hours
Adults: 10 mL every 4 hours
Dosage Forms Liquid: Chlorpheniramine maleate 2 mg, phenylpropanolamine hydrochloride 12.5 mg, and dextromethorphan hydrobromide 10 mg per 5 mL

chlorpheniramine, phenyltoloxamine, phenylpropanolamine, and phenylephrine
(klor fen IR a meen, fen il tole LOKS a meen, fen il proe pa NOLE a meen & fen il EF rin)
U.S. Brand Names Naldecon®; Naldelate®; Nalgest®; Nalspan®; New Decongestant®; Par Decon®; Tri-Phen-Chlor®; Uni-Decon®
Generic Available Yes
Therapeutic Category Antihistamine/Decongestant Combination
Use Symptomatic treatment of nasal and eustachian tube congestion associated with sinusitis and acute upper respiratory infection; symptomatic relief of perennial and allergic rhinitis
Usual Dosage Oral:
Children:
3-6 months: 0.25 mL (pediatric drops) every 3-4 hours
6-12 months: 2.5 mL (pediatric syrup) or 0.5 mL (pediatric drops) every 3-4 hours
1-6 years: 5 mL (pediatric syrup) or 1 mL (pediatric drops) every 3-4 hours
6-12 years: 2.5 mL (syrup) or 10 mL (pediatric syrup) or ½ tablet every 3-4 hours
Children >12 years and 5 mL (syrup) or 1 tablet every 3-4 hours
Dietary Considerations May be administered with food or water
Dosage Forms
Drops, pediatric: Chlorpheniramine maleate 0.5 mg, phenyltoloxamine citrate 2 mg, phenylpropanolamine hydrochloride 5 mg, and phenylephrine hydrochloride 1.25 mg per mL
Syrup: Chlorpheniramine maleate 2.5 mg, phenyltoloxamine citrate 7.5 mg, phenylpropanolamine hydrochloride 20 mg, and phenylephrine hydrochloride 5 mg per 5 mL
Syrup, pediatric: Chlorpheniramine maleate 0.5 mg, phenyltoloxamine citrate 2 mg, phenylpropanolamine hydrochloride 5 mg, and phenylephrine hydrochloride 1.25 mg per 5 mL
Tablet, sustained release: Chlorpheniramine maleate 5 mg, phenyltoloxamine citrate 15 mg, phenylpropanolamine hydrochloride 40 mg, and phenylephrine hydrochloride 10 mg

chlorpheniramine, pseudoephedrine, and codeine
(klor fen IR a meen, soo doe e FED rin, & KOE deen)
U.S. Brand Names Codehist® DH; Decohistine® DH; Dihistine® DH; Ryna-C® Liquid
Generic Available Yes
Therapeutic Category Antihistamine/Decongestant/Antitussive
Controlled Substance C-V
Use Temporary relief of cough associated with minor throat or bronchial irritation; relief of nasal congestion due to common cold, allergic rhinitis, or sinusitis
Usual Dosage Oral:
Children:
25-50 lb: 1.25-2.50 mL every 4-6 hours, up to 4 doses in a 24-hour period
50-90 lb: 2.5-5 mL every 4-6 hours, up to 4 doses in a 24-hour period
Adults: 10 mL every 4-6 hours, up to 4 doses in a 24-hour period
(Continued)

chlorpheniramine, pseudoephedrine, and codeine
(Continued)

Dosage Forms Liquid: Chlorpheniramine maleate 2 mg, pseudoephedrine hydrochloride 30 mg, and codeine phosphate 10 mg (120 mL, 480 mL)

chlorpheniramine, pyrilamine, and phenylephrine
(klor fen IR a meen, pye RIL a meen, & fen il EF rin)

U.S. Brand Names Rhinatate® Tablet; R-Tannamine® Tablet; R-Tannate® Tablet; Rynatan® Pediatric Suspension; Rynatan® Tablet; Tanoral® Tablet; Triotann® Tablet; Tri-Tannate® Tablet

Generic Available Yes

Therapeutic Category Antihistamine/Decongestant Combination

Use Symptomatic relief of nasal congestion associated with upper respiratory tract condition

Usual Dosage Oral:
Children:
<2 years: Titrate dose individually
2-6 years: 2.5-5 mL every 12 hours
Children >6 years and Adults: 5-10 mL every 12 hours

Dosage Forms
Liquid: Chlorpheniramine tannate 2 mg, pyrilamine tannate 12.5 mg, and phenylephrine tannate 5 mg per 5 mL
Tablet: Chlorpheniramine tannate 8 mg, pyrilamine maleate 12.5 mg, and phenylephrine tannate 25 mg

chlorpheniramine, pyrilamine, phenylephrine, and phenylpropanolamine
(klor fen IR a meen, pye RIL a meen, fen il EF rin, & fen il proe pa NOLE a meen)

U.S. Brand Names Histalet Forte® Tablet

Generic Available Yes

Therapeutic Category Antihistamine/Decongestant Combination

Use Symptomatic relief of rhinitis and nasal congestion due to colds or allergy

Usual Dosage Adults: Oral: 1 tablet 2-3 times/day

Dosage Forms Tablet: Chlorpheniramine maleate 4 mg, pyrilamine maleate 25 mg, phenylephrine hydrochloride 10 mg, and phenylpropanolamine hydrochloride 50 mg

♦ Chlor-Pro® Injection *see* chlorpheniramine *on page 138*
♦ Chlorprom® *see* chlorpromazine *on page 144*
♦ Chlorpromanyl® *see* chlorpromazine *on page 144*

chlorpromazine (klor PROE ma zeen)

U.S. Brand Names Ormazine®; Thorazine®

Canadian Brand Names Apo®-Chlorpromazine; Chlorprom®; Chlorpromanyl®; Largactil®; Novo-Chlorpromazine®

Generic Available Yes

Therapeutic Category Phenothiazine Derivative

Use Treatment of nausea and vomiting; psychoses; Tourette's syndrome; mania; intractable hiccups (adults); behavioral problems (children)

Usual Dosage
Children >6 months:
Psychosis:
Oral: 0.5-1 mg/kg/dose every 4-6 hours; older children may require 200 mg/day or higher
I.M., I.V.: 0.5-1 mg/kg/dose every 6-8 hours; maximum I.M./I.V. dose for <5 years (22.7 kg): 40 mg/day; maximum I.M./I.V. for 5-12 years (22.7-45.5 kg): 75 mg/day
Nausea and vomiting:
Oral: 0.5-1 mg/kg/dose every 4-6 hours as needed
I.M., I.V.: 0.5-1 mg/kg/dose every 6-8 hours; maximum dose: Same as psychoses
Rectal: 1 mg/kg/dose every 6-8 hours as needed
Adults:
Psychosis:
Oral: Range: 30-800 mg/day in 1-4 divided doses, initiate at lower doses and titrate as needed; usual dose is 200 mg/day; some patients may require 1-2 g/day

I.M., I.V.: Initial: 25 mg, may repeat (25-50 mg) in 1-4 hours, gradually increase to a maximum of 400 mg/dose every 4-6 hours until patient controlled; usual dose: 300-800 mg/day

Nausea and vomiting:
Oral: 10-25 mg every 4-6 hours
I.M., I.V.: 25-50 mg every 4-6 hours
Rectal: 50-100 mg every 6-8 hours
Intractable hiccups: Oral, I.M.: 25-50 mg 3-4 times/day

Dietary Considerations Interferes with riboflavin metabolism and may induce depletion; some may recommend increasing riboflavin in diet; may also decrease absorption of vitamin B_{12}; undiluted oral concentrate may precipitate tube feeding

Nursing/Pharmacy Information

Dilute oral concentrate solution in juice before administration; avoid contact of oral solution or injection with skin (contact dermatitis); do not administer S.C. (tissue damage and irritation); for direct I.V. injection, must dilute with 0.9% sodium chloride, maximum concentration 1 mg/mL, administer slow I.V. at a rate not to exceed 1 mg/minute in adults and 0.5 mg/minute in children

Monitor periodic ophthalmologic exams

Stability: Protect oral dosage forms from light; a slightly yellowed solution does not indicate potency loss, but a markedly discolored solution should be discarded; diluted injection (1 mg/mL) with normal saline and stored in 5 mL vials remains stable for 30 days

Dosage Forms

Chlorpromazine hydrochloride:
Capsule, sustained action: 30 mg, 75 mg, 150 mg, 200 mg, 300 mg
Concentrate, oral: 30 mg/mL (120 mL); 100 mg/mL (60 mL, 240 mL)
Injection: 25 mg/mL (1 mL, 2 mL, 10 mL)
Syrup: 10 mg/5 mL (120 mL)
Tablet: 10 mg, 25 mg, 50 mg, 100 mg, 200 mg
Suppository, rectal, as base: 25 mg, 100 mg

chlorpropamide (klor PROE pa mide)

U.S. Brand Names Diabinese®
Canadian Brand Names Apo-Chlorpropamide®; Novo-Propamide®
Mexican Brand Names Deavynfar; Insogen®
Generic Available Yes
Therapeutic Category Antidiabetic Agent, Oral
Use Control blood sugar in adult onset, noninsulin-dependent diabetes (type II)
Usual Dosage The dosage of chlorpropamide is variable and should be individualized based upon the patient's response

Adults: Oral: 250 mg once daily; initial dose in elderly patients: 100 mg once daily; subsequent dosages may be increased or decreased by 50-125 mg/day at 3- to 5-day intervals; maximum daily dose: 750 mg

Dietary Considerations

Alcohol: A disulfiram-like reaction characterized by flushing, headache, nausea, vomiting, sweating or tachycardia; avoid alcohol; inform patient of chlorpropamide-alcohol flush (facial reddening and an increase in facial temperature)

Food: Chlorpropamide may cause GI upset; administer with food and at the same time each day; eat regularly and do not skip meals

Glucose: Decreases blood glucose concentration; hypoglycemia may occur; educate patients how to detect and treat hypoglycemia; monitor for signs and symptoms of hypoglycemia; administer glucose if necessary; evaluate patient's diet and exercise regimen; may need to decrease or discontinue dose of sulfonylurea

Sodium: Reports of hyponatremia and SIADH; those at increased risk include patients on medications or who have medical conditions that predispose them to hyponatremia; monitor sodium serum concentration and fluid status; may need to restrict water intake

Nursing/Pharmacy Information

Patients who are anorexic or NPO may need to hold the dose to avoid hypoglycemia

Monitor fasting blood glucose, normal Hgb A, C, or fructosamine levels; monitor for signs and symptoms of hypoglycemia, (fatigue, sweating, numbness of extremities); monitor urine for glucose and ketones

Dosage Forms Tablet: 100 mg, 250 mg

♦ **Chlor-Rest® Tablet [OTC]** see chlorpheniramine and phenylpropanolamine on page 139

♦ **Chlortab® (Discontinued)** see page 743

chlorthalidone (klor THAL i done)
U.S. Brand Names Hygroton®; Thalitone®
Canadian Brand Names Apo-Chlorthalidone®; Novo-Thalidone®; Uridon®
Mexican Brand Names Higroton 50
Generic Available Yes
Therapeutic Category Diuretic, Miscellaneous
Use Management of mild to moderate hypertension, used alone or in combination with other agents; treatment of edema associated with congestive heart failure, nephrotic syndrome, or pregnancy
Usual Dosage Oral:
   Children: 2 mg/kg 3 times/week
   Adults: 25-100 mg/day or 100 mg 3 times/week
Dietary Considerations This product may cause a potassium loss; your physician may prescribe a potassium supplement, another medication to help prevent the potassium loss, or recommend that you eat foods high in potassium, especially citrus fruits; do not change your diet on your own while taking this medication, especially if you are taking potassium supplements or medications to reduce potassium loss; too much potassium can be as harmful as too little
Nursing/Pharmacy Information
   Administer in the morning, check patient for orthostasis
   Monitor blood pressure, serum electrolytes, renal function
Dosage Forms
   Tablet: 25 mg, 50 mg, 100 mg
      Hygroton®: 25 mg, 50 mg, 100 mg
      Thalitone®: 15 mg, 25 mg

♦ **chlorthalidone and atenolol** see atenolol and chlorthalidone on page 63
♦ **chlorthalidone and clonidine** see clonidine and chlorthalidone on page 160
♦ **Chlor-Trimeton® 4 Hour Relief Tablet [OTC]** see chlorpheniramine and pseudoephedrine on page 140
♦ **Chlor-Trimeton® Injection** see chlorpheniramine on page 138
♦ **Chlor-Trimeton® Oral [OTC]** see chlorpheniramine on page 138
♦ **Chlor-Tripolon®** see chlorpheniramine on page 138

chlorzoxazone (klor ZOKS a zone)
U.S. Brand Names Flexaphen®; Paraflex®; Parafon Forte™ DSC
Generic Available Yes
Therapeutic Category Skeletal Muscle Relaxant
Use Symptomatic treatment of muscle spasm and pain associated with acute musculoskeletal conditions
Usual Dosage Oral:
   Children: 20 mg/kg/day or 600 mg/m²/day in 3-4 divided doses
   Adults: 250-500 mg 3-4 times/day up to 750 mg 3-4 times/day
Dietary Considerations May be administered with food or milk if GI complaints occur
Nursing/Pharmacy Information
   May discolor urine
   Monitor periodic liver functions tests
Dosage Forms
   Caplet (Parafon Forte™ DSC): 500 mg
   Capsule (Flexaphen®, Mus-Lax®): 250 mg with acetaminophen 300 mg
   Tablet: Paraflex®: 250 mg

♦ **Cholac®** see lactulose on page 359
♦ **Cholan-HMB®** see dehydrocholic acid on page 184
♦ **Cholebrine®** see radiological/contrast media (ionic) on page 539

cholecalciferol (kole e kal SI fer ole)
Synonyms D_3
U.S. Brand Names Delta-D®
Generic Available No
Therapeutic Category Vitamin D Analog
Use Dietary supplement, treatment of vitamin D deficiency or prophylaxis of deficiency
Usual Dosage Adults: Oral: 400-1000 units/day
Nursing/Pharmacy Information Do not administer more than the recommended amount. While taking this medication, your physician may want you to follow a special diet or take a calcium supplement. Follow this diet closely. Avoid taking magnesium supplements or magnesium containing antacids.

Early symptoms of hypercalcemia include weakness, fatigue, somnolence, headache, anorexia, dry mouth, metallic taste, nausea, vomiting, cramps, diarrhea, muscle pain, bone pain, and irritability.

Dosage Forms Tablet: 400 units, 1000 units

♦ **Choledyl®** *(Discontinued)* see page 743

cholera vaccine (KOL er a vak SEEN)
Generic Available No
Therapeutic Category Vaccine, Inactivated Bacteria
Use Primary immunization for cholera prophylaxis
Usual Dosage I.M., S.C.:
Children:
6 months to 4 years: 0.2 mL with same dosage schedule
5-10 years: 0.3 mL with same dosage schedule
Children >10 years and Adults: 0.5 mL in 2 doses 1 week to 1 month or more apart
Nursing/Pharmacy Information
Defer immunization in individuals with moderate or severe febrile illness; do not administer I.V.; administer I.M., S.C., or intradermally
Stability: Refrigerate, avoid freezing
Dosage Forms Injection: Suspension of killed *Vibrio cholerae* (Inaba and Ogawa types) 8 units of each serotype per mL (1.5 mL, 20 mL)

cholestyramine resin (koe LES tir a meen REZ in)
U.S. Brand Names LoCHOLEST®; LoCHOLEST® Light; Prevalite®; Questran®; Questran® Light
Canadian Brand Names PMS-Cholestyramine
Generic Available Yes
Therapeutic Category Bile Acid Sequestrant
Use Adjunct in the management of primary hypercholesterolemia; pruritus associated with elevated levels of bile acids; diarrhea associated with excess fecal bile acids; pseudomembraneous colitis
Usual Dosage Dosages are expressed in terms of anhydrous resin. Oral:
Children: 240 mg/kg/day in 3 divided doses; need to titrate dose depending on indication
Adults: 3-4 g 3-4 times/day to a maximum of 16-32 g/day in 2-4 divided doses
Dietary Considerations Cholestyramine (especially high doses or long-term therapy) may decrease the absorption of fat-soluble vitamins (vitamins A, D, E and K), folic acid, calcium, and iron; deficiencies may occur including hypoprothrombinemia and increased bleeding from vitamin K deficiency; supplementation of vitamins A, D, E, and K, folic acid, and iron may be required with high-dose, long-term therapy
Nursing/Pharmacy Information Do not administer the powder in its dry form; just prior to administration, mix with fluid or with applesauce; to minimize binding of concomitant medications, administer other drugs at least 1 hour before or at least 4-6 hours after cholestyramine
Dosage Forms
Powder: 4 g of resin/9 g of powder (9 g, 378 g)
For oral suspension:
With aspartame: 4 g of resin/5 g of powder (5 g, 210 g)
With phenylalanine: 4 g of resin/5.5 g of powder (60s)

choline magnesium trisalicylate
(KOE leen mag NEE zhum trye sa LIS i late)
U.S. Brand Names Trilisate®
Generic Available Yes
Therapeutic Category Analgesic, Non-narcotic; Nonsteroidal Anti-inflammatory Drug (NSAID)
Use Management of osteoarthritis, rheumatoid arthritis, and other arthritides
Usual Dosage Oral (based on total salicylate content):
Children: 30-60 mg/kg/day administered in 3-4 divided doses
Adults: 500 mg to 1.5 g 1-3 times/day
Dietary Considerations
Alcohol: Combination causes GI irritation, possible bleeding; avoid or limit alcohol; patients at increased risk include those prone to hypoprothrombinemia, vitamin K deficiency, thrombocytopenia, thrombotic thrombocytopenia purpura, severe hepatic impairment, and those receiving anticoagulants
(Continued)

choline magnesium trisalicylate *(Continued)*

Food:
> Food may decrease the rate but not the extent of oral absorption; may cause GI upset, bleeding, ulceration, perforation; administer with food or or large volume of water or milk to minimize GI upset
>
> Folic acid: Hyperexcretion of folate; folic acid deficiency may result, leading to macrocytic anemia; supplement with folic acid if necessary
>
> Iron: With chronic use and at doses of 3-4 g/day, iron deficiency anemia may result; supplement with iron if necessary
>
> Magnesium: Hypermagnesemia resulting from magnesium salicylate; avoid or use with caution in renal insufficiency
>
> Sodium: Hypernatremia resulting from buffered aspirin solutions or sodium salicylate containing high sodium content; avoid or use with caution in CHF or any condition where hypernatremia would be detrimental
>
> Curry powder, paprika, licorice, Benedictine liqueur, prunes, raisins, tea and gherkins: Potential salicylate salicylate accumulation; these foods contain 6 mg salicylate/100 g; an ordinary American diet contains 10-200 mg/day of salicylate; foods containing salicylates may contribute to aspirin hypersensitivity. Patients at greatest risk for aspirin hypersensitivity include those with asthma, nasal polyposis, or chronic urticaria.

Nursing/Pharmacy Information
> Liquid may be mixed with fruit juice just before drinking; do not administer with antacids
>
> Monitor serum magnesium with high dose therapy or in patients with impaired renal function; serum salicylate levels

Dosage Forms
> Liquid: 500 mg/5 mL [choline salicylate 293 mg and magnesium salicylate 362 mg per 5 mL] (237 mL)
>
> Tablet:
>> 500 mg: Choline salicylate 293 mg and magnesium salicylate 362 mg
>> 750 mg: Choline salicylate 440 mg and magnesium salicylate 544 mg
>> 1000 mg: Choline salicylate 587 mg and magnesium salicylate 725 mg

choline salicylate *(KOE leen sa LIS i late)*
U.S. Brand Names Arthropan® [OTC]
Canadian Brand Names Teejel®
Generic Available No
Therapeutic Category Analgesic, Non-narcotic; Nonsteroidal Anti-inflammatory Drug (NSAID)
Use Temporary relief of pain of rheumatoid arthritis, rheumatic fever, osteoarthritis, and other conditions for which oral salicylates are recommended; useful in patients in which there is difficulty in administering doses in a tablet or capsule dosage form, because of the liquid dosage form
Usual Dosage Adults: Oral: 5 mL every 3-4 hours, if necessary, but not more than 6 doses in 24 hours
Dietary Considerations May be administered with food
Nursing/Pharmacy Information Do not administer with antacids; watch for bleeding gums or any signs of GI bleeding; notify physician if ringing in ears or persistent GI pain occurs
Dosage Forms Liquid (mint flavor): 870 mg/5 mL (240 mL, 480 mL)

♦ **choline theophyllinate** *see* oxtriphylline *on page 461*
♦ **Cholografin® Meglumine** *see* radiological/contrast media (ionic) *on page 539*
♦ **Choloxin®** *see* dextrothyroxine *on page 195*

chondroitin sulfate-sodium hyaluronate
(kon DROY tin SUL fate-SOW de um hye a loo ROE nate)
Synonyms sodium hyaluronate-chrondroitin sulfate
U.S. Brand Names Viscoat®
Generic Available No
Therapeutic Category Ophthalmic Agent, Viscoelastic
Use Surgical aid in anterior segment procedures, protects corneal endothelium and coats intraocular lens thus protecting it
Usual Dosage Ophthalmic: Carefully introduce into anterior chamber after thoroughly cleaning the chamber with a balanced salt solution
Dosage Forms Solution: Sodium chondroitin 40 mg and sodium hyaluronate 30 mg (0.25 mL, 0.5 mL)

♦ **Chooz® [OTC]** *see* calcium carbonate *on page 103*
♦ **Chorex®** *see* chorionic gonadotropin *on page 149*

chorionic gonadotropin (kor ee ON ik goe NAD oh troe pin)
Synonyms CG; HCG
U.S. Brand Names A.P.L.®; Chorex®; Choron®; Corgonject®; Follutein®; Glukor®; Gonic®; Pregnyl®; Profasi® HP
Generic Available Yes
Therapeutic Category Gonadotropin
Use Treatment of hypogonadotropic hypogonadism, prepubertal cryptorchidism; induce ovulation
Usual Dosage Children: I.M.:
Prepubertal cryptorchidism: 1000-2000 units/m²/dose 3 times/week for 3 weeks
Hypogonadotropic hypogonadism: 500-1000 USP units 3 times/week for 3 weeks, followed by the same dose twice weekly for 3 weeks
Nursing/Pharmacy Information
I.M. administration only
Stability: Following reconstitution with the provided diluent, solutions are stable for 30-90 days, depending on the specific preparation, when stored at 2°C to 15°C
Dosage Forms Powder for injection: 200 units/mL (10 mL, 25 mL); 500 units/mL (10 mL); 1000 units/mL (10 mL); 2000 units/mL (10 mL)

- **Choron®** see chorionic gonadotropin on page 149
- **Chromagen® OB [OTC]** see vitamin, multiple (prenatal) on page 654
- **Chroma-Pak®** see trace metals on page 620
- **chromium injection** see trace metals on page 620
- **Chronulac®** see lactulose on page 359
- **Chymex® (Discontinued)** see page 743
- **Chymodiactin®** see chymopapain on page 149

chymopapain (KYE moe pa pane)
U.S. Brand Names Chymodiactin®
Generic Available No
Therapeutic Category Enzyme
Use Alternative to surgery in patients with herniated lumbar intervertebral disks
Usual Dosage 2000-4000 units/disk with a maximum cumulative dose not to exceed 8000 units for patients with multiple disk herniations
Nursing/Pharmacy Information
Patients should be well hydrated prior to chymopapain administration; anaphylactic reactions may occur up to 1 hour after injection; observe the patient closely
Stability: Store at 2°C to 8°C (36°F to 46°F); use within 2 hours of reconstitution
Dosage Forms Injection: 4000 units [4 nKat]; 10,000 units [10 nKat]

- **Cibacalcin®** see calcitonin on page 102

ciclopirox (sye kloe PEER oks)
U.S. Brand Names Loprox®
Generic Available No
Therapeutic Category Antifungal Agent
Use Treatment of tinea pedis, tinea cruris, tinea corporis, cutaneous candidiasis, tinea versicolor
Usual Dosage Children >10 years and Adults: Topical: Apply twice daily, gently massage into affected areas; safety and efficacy in children <10 years have not been established
Nursing/Pharmacy Information Avoid contact with eyes; if sensitivity or irritation occurs, discontinue use
Dosage Forms Ciclopirox olamine:
Cream, topical: 1% (15 g, 30 g, 90 g)
Gel: 1%
Lotion: 1% (30 mL)

cidofovir (si DOF o veer)
U.S. Brand Names Vistide®
Generic Available No
Therapeutic Category Antiviral Agent
Use Treatment of CMV retinitis in patients with acquired immunodeficiency syndrome (AIDS)
Usual Dosage
Induction treatment: 5 mg/kg once weekly for 2 consecutive weeks
(Continued)

cidofovir *(Continued)*

Maintenance treatment: 5 mg/kg administered once every 2 weeks
Probenecid must be administered orally with each dose of cidofovir
Probenecid dose: 2 g 3 hours prior to cidofovir dose, 1 g 2 hours and 8 hours after completion of the infusion; patients should also receive 1 L of normal saline intravenously prior to each infusion of cidofovir; saline should be infused over 1-2 hours

Nursing/Pharmacy Information Watch for signs and symptoms of renal toxicity; probenecid may be administered with food to prevent nausea and vomiting; cidofovir is a potential carcinogen in humans; women of childbearing potential should use effective contraception during and for 1 month following treatment with cidofovir; men should practice barrier contraceptive methods during and for 3 months after treatment with cidofovir

Dosage Forms Injection: 75 mg/mL (5 mL)

♦ **Cidomycin®** *see* gentamicin *on page 290*
♦ **Cilag®** *see* acetaminophen *on page 13*
♦ **cilastatin and imipenem** *see* imipenem and cilastatin *on page 334*

cilazapril *(Canada only)* (sye LAY za pril)

Canadian Brand Names Inhibace®
Generic Available No
Therapeutic Category Angiotensin-Converting Enzyme (ACE) Inhibitor
Use Management of hypertension and treatment of congestive heart failure
Usual Dosage Adults: Oral:
Congestive heart failure: Recommended starting dose is 0.5 mg once daily, usual maintenance dose: 1-2.5 mg/day
Hypertension: 2.5-5 mg once daily
Dosage Forms Tablet: 1 mg, 2.5 mg, 5 mg

cilostazol *New Drug* (sil OH sta zol)

U.S. Brand Names Pletal®
Generic Available No
Therapeutic Category Platelet Aggregation Inhibitor
Use Symptomatic management of peripheral vascular disease, primarily intermittent claudication
Usual Dosage Adults: Oral: 100 mg twice daily taken at least 30 minutes before or 2 hours after breakfast and dinner; dosage should be reduced to 50 mg twice daily during concurrent therapy with inhibitors of CYP3A4 or CYP2C19
Dosage Forms Tablet: 50 mg, 100 mg

♦ **Ciloxan™ Ophthalmic** *see* ciprofloxacin *on page 151*
♦ **Cimetase®** *see* cimetidine *on page 150*

cimetidine (sye MET i deen)

U.S. Brand Names Tagamet®; Tagamet-HB® [OTC]
Canadian Brand Names Apo®-Cimetidine; Novo-Cimetidine®; Nu-Cimet®; Peptol®
Mexican Brand Names Blocan; Cimetase®; Cimetigal; Columina; Ulcedine; Zymerol
Generic Available Yes
Therapeutic Category Histamine H_2 Antagonist
Use Short-term treatment of active duodenal ulcers and benign gastric ulcers; long-term prophylaxis of duodenal ulcer; gastric hypersecretory states; gastro-esophageal reflux
Usual Dosage Oral, I.M., I.V.:
Infants: 10-20 mg/kg/day divided every 6-12 hours
Children: 20-30 mg/kg/day in divided doses every 6 hours

Patients with an active bleed: Administer cimetidine as a continuous infusion

Adults:
Short-term treatment of active ulcers:
Oral: 300 mg 4 times/day or 800 mg at bedtime or 400 mg twice daily for up to 8 weeks
I.M., I.V.: 300 mg every 6 hours or 37.5 mg/hour by continuous infusion; I.V. dosage should be adjusted to maintain an intragastric pH of 5 or greater
Duodenal ulcer prophylaxis: Oral: 400-800 mg at bedtime
Gastric hypersecretory conditions: Oral, I.M., I.V.: 300-600 mg every 6 hours; dosage not to exceed 2.4 g/day

Dietary Considerations Limit xanthine-containing foods and beverages; may decrease iron absorption; administer with meals so that the peak effect occurs at the proper time (peak inhibition of gastric acid secretion occurs at 1 and 3 hours after dosing in fasting subjects and ~2 hours in nonfasting subjects)

Nursing/Pharmacy Information
Modify dosage in patients with renal impairment; can be administered as a slow I.V. push over a minimum of 15 minutes at a concentration not to exceed 15 mg/mL; or preferably as an I.V. intermittent or I.V. continuous infusion. Intermittent infusions are administered over 15-30 minutes at a final concentration not to exceed 6 mg/mL; for patients with an active bleed, preferred method of administration is continuous infusion

Monitor blood pressure with I.V. push administration; CBC

Stability: I.V. infusion solution with normal saline or D_5W solution is stable for 48 hours at room temperature; do not refrigerate the undiluted injection since precipitation may occur; drugs **incompatible** with cimetidine include amobarbital, amphotericin B, atropine, cefamandole, cefazolin, chlorproma-zine, methohexital, metoclopramide, pentobarbital, phenobarbital, phenytoin, secobarbital, theophylline, thiopental

Dosage Forms
Infusion, as hydrochloride, in NS: 300 mg (50 mL)
Injection, as hydrochloride: 150 mg/mL (2 mL, 8 mL)
Liquid, oral, as hydrochloride (mint-peach flavor): 300 mg/5 mL with alcohol 2.8% (5 mL, 240 mL)
Tablet: 200 mg, 300 mg, 400 mg, 800 mg

♦ **Cimetigal** see cimetidine on page 150
♦ **Cimogal** see ciprofloxacin on page 151
♦ **Cinobac® Pulvules®** see cinoxacin on page 151

cinoxacin (sin OKS a sin)

U.S. Brand Names Cinobac® Pulvules®
Mexican Brand Names Gugecin
Generic Available Yes
Therapeutic Category Quinolone
Use Urinary tract infections
Usual Dosage Children >12 years and Adults: Oral: 1 g/day in 2-4 doses
Nursing/Pharmacy Information Hold antacids for 3-4 hours after adminis-tering
Dosage Forms Capsule: 250 mg, 500 mg

♦ **Cipralan®** *(Discontinued)* see page 743
♦ **Cipro®** see ciprofloxacin on page 151
♦ **Ciproflox** see ciprofloxacin on page 151

ciprofloxacin (sip roe FLOKS a sin)

U.S. Brand Names Ciloxan™ Ophthalmic; Cipro®
Mexican Brand Names Cimogal; Ciproflox; Ciprofur; Ciproxina; Eni; Italnik®; Kenzoflex; Microrgan®; Mitroken; Nivoflox; Opthaflox; Sophixin Ofteno
Generic Available No
Therapeutic Category Antibiotic, Ophthalmic; Quinolone
Use Treatment of documented or suspected pseudomonal infection of the respi-ratory or urinary tract, acute sinusitis, skin and soft tissue, bone and joint, eye and ear; documented multidrug-resistant, aerobic gram-negative bacilli and some gram-positive staphylococci; documented infectious diarrhea due to *Campylobacter jejuni*, *Shigella*, or *Salmonella*; osteomyelitis caused by susceptible organisms in which parenteral therapy is not feasible; empiric therapy for patients with febrile neutropenia; ocular infections caused by susceptible bacterial organisms in patients with corneal ulcers or conjunctivitis

Usual Dosage
Children: Oral: 20-30 mg/kg/day in 2 divided doses; maximum dose: 1.5 g/day
Adults:
Oral: 250-750 mg every 12 hours, depending on severity of infection and susceptibility
Ophthalmic: Instill 1-2 drops in eye(s) every 2 hours while awake for 2 days and 1-2 drops every 4 hours while awake for the next 5 days
I.V.: 200-400 mg every 12 hours depending on severity of infection

Dietary Considerations
Food: Decreases rate, but not extent, of absorption; may cause GI upset; administer without regard to meals; manufacturer prefers that drug is taken two hours after meals
Dairy products, oral multivitamins, and mineral supplements: Absorption decreased by divalent and trivalent cations; these cations bind to and form
(Continued)

ciprofloxacin *(Continued)*

insoluble complexes with quinolones; avoid taking these substrates with ciprofloxacin; the manufacturer states that the usual dietary intake of calcium has not been shown to interfere with ciprofloxacin absorption

Caffeine: Possible exaggerated or prolonged effects of caffeine; ciprofloxacin reduces total body clearance of caffeine; patients consuming regular large quantities of caffeinated beverages may need to restrict caffeine intake if excessive cardiac or CNS stimulation occurs

Nursing/Pharmacy Information

Do not administer antacids with or within 4 hours of a ciprofloxacin dose; administer by slow I.V. infusion over 60 minutes to reduce the risk of venous irritation (burning, pain, erythema, and swelling); final concentration for administration should not exceed 2 mg/mL

Patients receiving concurrent ciprofloxacin, theophylline, or cyclosporine should have serum levels monitored

Stability:
Room temperature:
Prepared bags: 14 days
Premixed bags: Manufacturer expiration dating
Out of overwrap stability: 14 days
Refrigeration: Prepared bags: 14 days

Dosage Forms Ciprofloxacin hydrochloride:
Infusion in D_5W: 400 mg (200 mL)
Infusion in NS or D_5W: 200 mg (100 mL)
Injection: 200 mg (20 mL); 400 mg (40 mL)
Solution, ophthalmic: 3.5 mg/mL (2.5 mL, 5 mL)
Suspension, oral: 250 mg/5 mL (100 mL); 500 mg/5 mL (100 mL)
Tablet: 100 mg, 250 mg, 500 mg, 750 mg

ciprofloxacin and hydrocortisone

(sip roe FLOKS a sin & hye droe KOR ti sone)

U.S. Brand Names Cipro® HC Otic

Generic Available No

Therapeutic Category Antibiotic/Corticosteroid, Otic

Use Treatment of acute otitis externa, sometimes known as "swimmer's ear"

Usual Dosage Children >1 year of age and Adults: Otic: The recommended dosage for all patients is three drops of the suspension in the affected ear twice daily for seven day; twice-daily dosing schedule is more convenient for patients than that of existing treatments with hydrocortisone, which are typically administered three or four times a day; a twice-daily dosage schedule may be especially helpful for parents and caregivers of young children

Dosage Forms Suspension, otic: Ciprofloxacin hydrochloride 0.2% and hydrocortisone 1%

♦ **Ciprofur** *see ciprofloxacin on page 151*
♦ **Cipro® HC Otic** *see ciprofloxacin and hydrocortisone on page 152*
♦ **Ciproxina** *see ciprofloxacin on page 151*

cisapride (SIS a pride)

U.S. Brand Names Propulsid®

Canadian Brand Names Prepulsid®

Mexican Brand Names Enteropride; Kinestase®; Unamol

Generic Available No

Therapeutic Category Gastrointestinal Agent, Prokinetic

Use Treatment of nocturnal symptoms of gastroesophageal reflux disease (GERD), also demonstrated effectiveness for gastroparesis, refractory constipation, and nonulcer dyspepsia

Usual Dosage Adults: Oral: 10 mg 4 times/day at least 15 minutes before meals and at bedtime; in some patients the dosage will need to be increased to 20 mg to obtain a satisfactory result

Dietary Considerations May be administered before meals

Nursing/Pharmacy Information Safety and effectiveness in children have not been established. Although cisapride does not affect psychomotor function nor induce sedation or drowsiness when used alone, advise patients that the sedative effects of benzodiazepines and of alcohol may be accelerated.

Dosage Forms
Suspension, oral (cherry cream flavor): 1 mg/mL (450 mL)
Tablet, scored: 10 mg, 20 mg

cisatracurium (sis a tra KYOO ree um)

U.S. Brand Names Nimbex®
Generic Available No
Therapeutic Category Skeletal Muscle Relaxant
Use As an adjunct to general anesthesia to facilitate endotracheal intubation and to relax skeletal muscles during surgery; to facilitate mechanical ventilation in ICU patients; does not relieve pain or produce sedation
Usual Dosage I.V.: Dose to effect; doses will vary due to interpatient variability; use ideal body weight for obese patients

Surgery:
Children 2-12 years: 0.1 mg/kg, produces clinically effective block for 28 minutes
Adults: 0.15-0.2 mg/kg, then 0.03 mg/kg 40-60 minutes after initial dose to maintain neuromuscular block, followed by repeat doses of 0.03 mg/kg at 20-minute intervals; initial dose after succinylcholine for intubation: 0.1 mg/kg
Continuous infusion: At initial signs of recovery from bolus dose, begin at 3 mcg/kg/minute, block usually maintained by a rate of 1-2 mcg/kg/minute
Pretreatment/priming: 10% of intubating dose given 3-5 minutes before initial dose
ICU: Adults: 0.1 mg/kg bolus; at initial signs of recovery begin at rate of 3 mcg/kg/minute and adjust accordingly (rates of 0.5-10 mcg/kg/minute reported)
Nursing/Pharmacy Information
Neuromuscular blocking potency is 3 times that of atracurium; maximum block is up to 2 minutes longer than for equipotent doses of atracurium
Stability: Refrigerate (do not freeze); unstable in alkaline solutions; **compatible** with D_5W, D_5NS, and NS; do not dilute in lactated Ringers
Dosage Forms Injection, as besylate: 2 mg/mL (5 mL, 10 mL); 10 mg/mL (20 mL)

cisplatin (SIS pla tin)

Synonyms CDDP
U.S. Brand Names Platinol®; Platinol®-AQ
Mexican Brand Names Blastolem; Medsaplatin; Niyaplat
Generic Available No
Therapeutic Category Antineoplastic Agent
Use Management of metastatic testicular or ovarian carcinoma, advanced bladder cancer, osteosarcoma, Hodgkin's and non-Hodgkin's lymphoma, head or neck cancer, cervical cancer, lung cancer, brain tumors, neuroblastoma; used alone or in combination with other agents
Usual Dosage Children and Adults (refer to individual protocols): I.V.:
Intermittent dosing schedule: 37-75 mg/m² once every 2-3 weeks or 50-120 mg/m² once every 3-4 weeks
Daily dosing schedule: 15-20 mg/m²/day for 5 days every 3-4 weeks
Nursing/Pharmacy Information
Needles, syringes, catheters, or I.V. administration sets that contain aluminum parts should not be used for administration of drug; I.V. prehydration required to reduce toxicity of drug; I.V.: Rate of administration has varied from a 15- to 20-minute infusion, 1 mg/minute infusion, 6- to 8-hour infusion, 24-hour infusion, or per protocol
Monitor renal function tests (serum creatinine, BUN, Cl_{cr}), electrolytes (particularly magnesium, calcium, potassium); hearing test, neurologic exam (with high dose), liver function tests periodically, CBC with differential and platelet count; urine output, urinalysis
Stability: **Incompatible** with sodium bicarbonate; do not infuse in solutions containing <0.2% sodium chloride; do not refrigerate reconstituted solutions since precipitation may occur; protect from light; aluminum needles should not be used to administer the drug due to binding with the platinum
Dosage Forms
Injection, aqueous: 1 mg/mL (50 mL, 100 mL)
Powder for injection: 10 mg, 50 mg

♦ **13-*cis*-retinoic acid** *see* isotretinoin *on page 350*
♦ **Cisticid** *see* praziquantel *on page 512*

citalopram (sye TAL oh pram)

Synonyms Citalopram Hydrobromide; Nitalapram
U.S. Brand Names Celexa®
Generic Available No
Therapeutic Category Antidepressant
(Continued)

citalopram *(Continued)*

Use Depression

Usual Dosage Oral: 20-60 mg/day; reduce dosage in elderly or those with hepatic impairment

Dosage Forms Tablet, as hydrobromide: 20 mg, 40 mg, 60 mg

♦ **Citalopram Hydrobromide** *see* citalopram *on page 153*

♦ **Citanest® Forte** *see* prilocaine *on page 516*

♦ **Citanest® Plain** *see* prilocaine *on page 516*

♦ **Citax** *see* immune globulin, intravenous *on page 336*

♦ **Cithalith-S® Syrup *(Discontinued)*** *see page 743*

♦ **Citoken** *see* piroxicam *on page 497*

♦ **Citomid** *see* vincristine *on page 648*

♦ **Citracal® [OTC]** *see* calcium citrate *on page 105*

♦ **citrate of magnesia** *see* magnesium citrate *on page 380*

♦ **citric acid and d-gluconic acid irrigant** *see* citric acid bladder mixture *on page 154*

♦ **citric acid and potassium citrate** *see* potassium citrate and citric acid *on page 508*

citric acid bladder mixture (SI trik AS id BLAD dur MIKS chur)

Synonyms citric acid and d-gluconic acid irrigant; hemiacidrin

U.S. Brand Names Renacidin®

Generic Available Yes

Therapeutic Category Irrigating Solution

Use Preparing solutions for irrigating indwelling urethral catheters; to dissolve or prevent formation of calcifications

Usual Dosage 30-60 mL of 10% (sterile) solution 2-3 times/day by means of a rubber syringe

Dosage Forms

Powder for solution: Citric acid 156-171 g, magnesium hydroxycarbonate 75-87 g, D-gluconic acid 21-30 g, magnesium acid citrate 9-15 g, calcium carbonate 2-6 g (150 g, 300 g)

Solution, irrigation: Citric acid 6.602 g, magnesium hydroxycarbonate 3.177 g, glucono-delta-lactone 0.198 g and benzoic acid 0.023 g per 100 mL (500 mL)

♦ **Citrisource®** *see* enteral nutritional products *on page 233*

♦ **Citro-Nesia® Solution *(Discontinued)*** *see page 743*

♦ **Citrotein® [OTC]** *see* enteral nutritional products *on page 233*

♦ **citrovorum factor** *see* leucovorin *on page 362*

♦ **Citrucel® [OTC]** *see* methylcellulose *on page 405*

♦ **Cl-719** *see* gemfibrozil *on page 289*

♦ **CLA** *see* clarithromycin *on page 155*

cladribine (KLA dri been)

Synonyms 2-CdA; 2-chlorodeoxyadenosine

U.S. Brand Names Leustatin™

Generic Available No

Therapeutic Category Antineoplastic Agent

Use Hairy cell and chronic lymphocytic leukemias

Usual Dosage Adults: I.V. continuous infusion: 0.09 mg/kg/day

Nursing/Pharmacy Information

Monitor periodic assessment of peripheral blood counts, particularly during the first 4-8 weeks post-treatment, is recommended to detect the development of anemia, neutropenia, and thrombocytopenia and for early detection of any potential sequelae (ie, infection or bleeding)

Stability: Solutions should be administered immediately after the initial dilution or stored in the refrigerator (2°C to 8°C) for ≤8 hours. The use of dextrose 5% in water as a diluent is not recommended due to increased degradation of cladribine; should not be mixed with other intravenous drugs or additive or infused simultaneously via a common intravenous line. Admixtures for single daily infusion are stable for at least 24 hours at room temperature under normal room light in polyvinyl chloride infusion containers. Admixtures for 7-day infusion are stable (chemically and physically) for at least 7 days in the Pharmacia Deltec™ medication cassettes.

Dosage Forms Injection, preservative free: 1 mg/mL (10 mL)

♦ **Claforan®** *see* cefotaxime *on page 122*

♦ **Clamurid®** *see* carbamide peroxide *on page 112*

♦ **Clanda®** *see* vitamin, multiple (oral) *on page 654*
♦ **Claripex®** *see* clofibrate *on page 158*

clarithromycin (kla RITH roe mye sin)

Synonyms CLA
U.S. Brand Names Biaxin™
Mexican Brand Names Klaricid
Generic Available No
Therapeutic Category Macrolide (Antibiotic)
Use Treatment of upper and lower respiratory tract infections, acute otitis media, and infections of the skin and skin structure due to susceptible strains of *S. aureus*, *S. pyogenes*, *S. pneumoniae*, *H. influenzae*, *M. catarrhalis*, *Mycoplasma pneumoniae*, *C. trachomatis*, *Legionella* sp, and *M. avium*; prophylaxis of disseminated *M. avium* Complex (MAC) infections in HIV-infected patients
Usual Dosage Oral: 250-500 mg every 12 hours for 7-14 days
  Upper respiratory tract: 250-500 mg every 12 hours for 10-14 days
   Pharyngitis/tonsillitis: 250 mg every 12 hours for 10 days
   Acute maxillary sinusitis: 500 mg every 12 hours for 14 days
  Lower respiratory tract: 250-500 mg every 12 hours for 7-14 days
   Acute exacerbation of chronic bronchitis due to:
    S. pneumoniae: 250 mg every 12 hours for 7-14 days
    M. catarrhalis: 250 mg every 12 hours for 7-14 days
    H. influenzae: 500 mg every 12 hours for 7-14 days
   Pneumonia due to:
    S. pneumoniae: 250 mg every 12 hours for 7-14 days
    M. pneumoniae: 250 mg every 12 hours for 7-14 days
  Uncomplicated skin and skin structure: 250 mg every 12 hours for 7-14 days
Dietary Considerations May be administered with or without meals; slight decrease in onset of absorption; extent of absorption is increased or unaffected; may be administered with milk
Nursing/Pharmacy Information
  Administer every 12 hours rather than twice daily to avoid peak and trough variation
  Monitor patients receiving clarithromycin and drugs known to interact with erythromycin (ie, theophylline, digoxin, anticoagulants, triazolam) since there are still very few studies examining drug-drug interactions with clarithromycin; liver function tests
Dosage Forms
  Granules for oral suspension: 125 mg/5 mL (50 mL, 100 mL); 250 mg/5 mL (50 mL, 100 mL)
  Tablet, film coated: 250 mg, 500 mg

♦ **Claritin®** *see* loratadine *on page 375*
♦ **Claritin-D®** *see* loratadine and pseudoephedrine *on page 375*
♦ **Claritin-D® 24-Hour** *see* loratadine and pseudoephedrine *on page 375*
♦ **Claritin® RediTab®** *see* loratadine *on page 375*
♦ **Clarityne®** *see* loratadine *on page 375*
♦ **clavulanate potassium and amoxicillin** *see* amoxicillin and clavulanate potassium *on page 43*
♦ **clavulanic acid and ticarcillin** *see* ticarcillin and clavulanate potassium *on page 612*
♦ **Clavulin®** *see* amoxicillin and clavulanate potassium *on page 43*
♦ **Clear Away® Disc [OTC]** *see* salicylic acid *on page 557*
♦ **Clear By Design® Gel [OTC]** *see* benzoyl peroxide *on page 81*
♦ **Clear Eyes® [OTC]** *see* naphazoline *on page 431*
♦ **Clearsil® Maximum Strength [OTC]** *see* benzoyl peroxide *on page 81*
♦ **Clear Tussin® 30** *see* guaifenesin and dextromethorphan *on page 300*

clemastine (KLEM as teen)

U.S. Brand Names Antihist-1® [OTC]; Tavist®; Tavist®-1 [OTC]
Generic Available Yes
Therapeutic Category Antihistamine
Use Perennial and seasonal allergic rhinitis and other allergic symptoms including urticaria
Usual Dosage Oral:
  Children:
   <12 years: 0.67-1.34 mg every 8-12 hours as needed
   >12 years: 1.34 mg twice daily to 2.68 mg 3 times/day; do not exceed 8.04 mg/day
  Adults: 1.34 mg twice daily to 2.68 mg 3 times/day; do not exceed 8.04 mg/day
(Continued)

clemastine *(Continued)*

Nursing/Pharmacy Information
Raise bed rails, institute safety measures, assist with ambulation
Monitor for a reduction of rhinitis, urticaria, eczema, pruritus, or other allergic symptoms
Dosage Forms Clemastine fumarate:
Syrup (citrus flavor): 0.67 mg/5 mL with alcohol 5.5% (120 mL)
Tablet: 1.34 mg, 2.68 mg

clemastine and phenylpropanolamine

KLEM as teen & fen il proe pa NOLE a meen)
U.S. Brand Names Antihist-D®; Tavist-D®
Generic Available No
Therapeutic Category Antihistamine/Decongestant Combination
Use Symptomatic relief of allergic rhinitis; pruritus of the eyes, nose or throat, lacrimation and nasal congestion
Usual Dosage Children >12 years and Adults: Oral: 1 tablet every 12 hours
Dosage Forms Tablet: Clemastine fumarate 1.34 mg and phenylpropanolamine hydrochloride 75 mg

- ◆ **Cleocin HCl® Oral** *see* clindamycin *on page 156*
- ◆ **Cleocin Pediatric® Oral** *see* clindamycin *on page 156*
- ◆ **Cleocin Phosphate® Injection** *see* clindamycin *on page 156*
- ◆ **Cleocin T® Topical** *see* clindamycin *on page 156*
- ◆ **Cleocin® Vaginal** *see* clindamycin *on page 156*

clidinium and chlordiazepoxide

(kli DI nee um & klor dye az e POKS ide)
Synonyms chlordiazepoxide and clidinium
U.S. Brand Names Clindex®; Librax®
Generic Available Yes
Therapeutic Category Anticholinergic Agent
Use Adjunct treatment of peptic ulcer, treatment of irritable bowel syndrome
Usual Dosage Oral: 1-2 capsules 3-4 times/day, before meals or food and at bedtime
Dietary Considerations Should be administered before meals
Nursing/Pharmacy Information After extended therapy, abrupt discontinuation should be avoided and a gradual dose tapering schedule followed
Dosage Forms Capsule: Clidinium bromide 2.5 mg and chlordiazepoxide hydrochloride 5 mg

- ◆ **Climaderm** *see* estradiol *on page 242*
- ◆ **Climara® Transdermal** *see* estradiol *on page 242*
- ◆ **Clinda-Derm® Topical** *see* clindamycin *on page 156*

clindamycin (klin da MYE sin)

U.S. Brand Names Cleocin HCl® Oral; Cleocin Pediatric® Oral; Cleocin Phosphate® Injection; Cleocin T® Topical; Cleocin® Vaginal; Clinda-Derm® Topical
Canadian Brand Names Dalacin® C Topical; Dalacin® C Vaginal Cream
Mexican Brand Names Dalacin® C; Galecin; Klyndaken
Generic Available Yes
Therapeutic Category Acne Products; Antibiotic, Miscellaneous
Use Useful agent against most aerobic gram-positive staphylococci and streptococci (except enterococci); also useful against *Fusobacterium, Bacteroides* sp. and *Actinomyces* for treatment of respiratory tract infections, skin and soft tissue infections, sepsis, intra-abdominal infections, and infections of the female pelvis and genital tract; used topically in treatment of severe acne
Usual Dosage Avoid in neonates (contains benzyl alcohol)
Infants and Children:
Oral: 10-30 mg/kg/day in 3-4 divided doses
I.M., I.V.: 25-40 mg/kg/day in 3-4 divided doses
Children and Adults: Topical: Apply twice daily
Adults:
Oral: 150-450 mg/dose every 6-8 hours; maximum dose: 1.8 g/day
I.M., I.V.: 1.2-1.8 g/day in 2-4 divided doses; maximum dose: 4.8 g/day
Vaginal: 1 full applicator (100 mg) inserted intravaginally once daily before bedtime for 7 consecutive days
Dietary Considerations Peak concentrations may be delayed with food; may be administered with food food or a full glass of water to avoid esophageal irritation

Nursing/Pharmacy Information
Administer by I.V. intermittent infusion over at least 10-60 minutes, at a rate **not** to exceed 30 mg/minute; final concentration for administration should not exceed 12 mg/mL
Observe for changes in bowel frequency; during prolonged therapy monitor CBC, liver and renal function tests periodically
Stability: Do **not** refrigerate reconstituted oral solution because it will thicken; oral solution is stable for 2 weeks at room temperature following reconstitution; I.V. infusion solution in normal saline or D_5W solution is stable for 16 days at room temperature

Dosage Forms
Clindamycin hydrochloride:
Capsule: 75 mg, 150 mg, 300 mg
Clindamycin palmitate:
Granules for oral solution: 75 mg/5 mL (100 mL)
Clindamycin phosphate:
Cream, vaginal: 2% (40 g)
Gel, topical: 1% [10 mg/g] (7.5 g, 30 g)
Infusion in D_5W: 300 mg (50 mL); 600 mg (50 mL)
Injection: 150 mg/mL (2 mL, 4 mL, 6 mL, 50 mL, 60 mL)
Solution, topical: 1% [10 mg/mL] (30 mL, 60 mL, 480 mL)
Lotion, topical: 1% [10 mg/mL] (60 mL)

♦ **Clindex®** see clidinium and chlordiazepoxide on page 156
♦ **Clinoril®** see sulindac on page 589
♦ **Clioquinol®** see clioquinol on page 157

clioquinol (klye oh KWIN ole)
U.S. Brand Names Vioform® [OTC]
Canadian Brand Names Clioquinol®
Generic Available Yes: Cream
Therapeutic Category Antifungal Agent
Use Treatment of tinea pedis, tinea cruris, and skin infections caused by dermatophytic fungi (ring worm)
Usual Dosage Children and Adults: Topical: Apply 2-4 times/day; do not use for >7 days
Nursing/Pharmacy Information Watch affected area for increased irritation; may stain skin and clothing
Dosage Forms
Cream: 3% (30 g)
Ointment, topical: 3% (30 g)

clioquinol and hydrocortisone
(klye oh KWIN ole & hye droe KOR ti sone)
Synonyms hydrocortisone and clioquinol; iodochlorhydroxyquin and hydrocortisone
U.S. Brand Names Corque® Topical; Pedi-Cort V® Creme
Generic Available Yes
Therapeutic Category Antifungal/Corticosteroid
Use Contact or atopic dermatitis; eczema; neurodermatitis; anogenital pruritus; mycotic dermatoses; moniliasis
Usual Dosage Topical: Apply in a thin film 3-4 times/day
Dosage Forms Cream: Clioquinol 3% and hydrocortisone 1% (20 g)

♦ **Clistin®** Tablet *(Discontinued)* see page 743

clobetasol (kloe BAY ta sol)
U.S. Brand Names Cormax® Ointment; Temovate®
Canadian Brand Names Dermasone; Dermovate®; Gen-Clobetasol; Novo-Clobetasol
Generic Available Yes
Therapeutic Category Corticosteroid, Topical
Use Short-term relief of inflammation of moderate to severe corticosteroid-responsive dermatosis
Usual Dosage Topical: Apply twice daily for up to 2 weeks with no more than 50 g/week
Nursing/Pharmacy Information For external use only; do not use on open wounds; apply sparingly to occlusive dressings; should not be used in the presence of open or weeping lesions
Dosage Forms Clobetasol propionate:
Cream: 0.05% (15 g, 30 g, 45 g)
(Continued)

clobetasol *(Continued)*

Cream in emollient base: 0.05% (15 g, 30 g, 60 g)
Gel: 0.05% (15 g, 30 g, 45 g)
Ointment, topical: 0.05% (15 g, 30 g, 45 g)
Scalp application: 0.05% (25 mL, 50 mL)
Solution, topical: 0.05%

♦ **Clocort® Maximum Strength [OTC]** *see* hydrocortisone (topical) *on page 324*

clocortolone (kloe KOR toe lone)

U.S. Brand Names Cloderm® Topical
Generic Available No
Therapeutic Category Corticosteroid, Topical
Use Inflammation of corticosteroid-responsive dermatoses
Usual Dosage Topical: Apply sparingly and gently rub into affected area 1-4 times/day
Nursing/Pharmacy Information A thin film of cream or ointment is effective; do not overuse; do not use tight-fitting diapers or plastic pants on children being treated in the diaper area; use only as prescribed, and for no longer than the period prescribed; apply sparingly in light film; rub in lightly; avoid contact with eyes; notify physician if condition being treated persists or worsens
Dosage Forms Cream, as pivalate: 0.1% (15 g, 45 g)

♦ **Cloderm® Topical** *see* clocortolone *on page 158*

clofazimine (kloe FA zi meen)

U.S. Brand Names Lamprene®
Generic Available No
Therapeutic Category Leprostatic Agent
Use Treatment of dapsone-resistant lepromatous leprosy (*Mycobacterium leprae*); multibacillary dapsone-sensitive leprosy; erythema nodosum leprosum; *Mycobacterium avium-intracellulare* (MAI) infections
Usual Dosage Oral:
Children: Leprosy: 1 mg/kg/day every 24 hours in combination with dapsone and rifampin
Adults:
Dapsone-resistant leprosy: 50-100 mg/day in combination with one or more antileprosy drugs for 2 years; then alone 50-100 mg/day
Dapsone-sensitive multibacillary leprosy: 50-100 mg/day in combination with two or more antileprosy drugs for at least 2 years and continue until negative skin smears are obtained, then institute single drug therapy with appropriate agent
Erythema nodosum leprosum: 100-200 mg/day for up to 3 months or longer then taper dose to 100 mg/day when possible
MAI: Combination therapy using clofazimine 100 mg 1 or 3 times/day in combination with other antimycobacterial agents
Dietary Considerations May be administered with meals; presence of food increases the extent of absorption
Nursing/Pharmacy Information Monitor for GI complaints
Dosage Forms Capsule, as palmitate: 50 mg

clofibrate (kloe FYE brate)

U.S. Brand Names Atromid-S®
Canadian Brand Names Abitrate®; Claripex®; Novo-Fibrate®
Generic Available Yes
Therapeutic Category Antihyperlipidemic Agent, Miscellaneous
Use Adjunct to dietary therapy in the management of hyperlipidemias associated with high triglyceride levels
Usual Dosage Adults: Oral: 500 mg 4 times/day
Nursing/Pharmacy Information Monitor serum lipids, LFTs, CBC
Dosage Forms Capsule: 500 mg

♦ **Clomid®** *see* clomiphene *on page 158*

clomiphene (KLOE mi feen)

U.S. Brand Names Clomid®; Milophene®; Serophene®
Mexican Brand Names Omifin
Generic Available No
Therapeutic Category Ovulation Stimulator
Use Treatment of ovulatory failure in patients desiring pregnancy

Usual Dosage Oral: 50 mg/day for 5 days (first course); start the regimen on or about the fifth day of cycle; if ovulation occurs do not increase dosage; if not, increase next course to 100 mg/day for 5 days

Nursing/Pharmacy Information
May cause visual disturbances, dizziness, lightheadedness; if possibility of pregnancy, stop the drug and consult your physician
Stability: Protect from light

Dosage Forms Tablet, as citrate: 50 mg

clomipramine (kloe MI pra meen)
U.S. Brand Names Anafranil®
Canadian Brand Names Apo-Clomipramine®
Generic Available Yes
Therapeutic Category Antidepressant, Tricyclic (Tertiary Amine)
Use Treatment of obsessive-compulsive disorder (OCD)
Usual Dosage Oral:
Children: Initial: 25 mg/day and gradually increase, as tolerated to a maximum of 3 mg/kg or 100 mg, whichever is smaller
Adults: Initial: 25 mg/day and gradually increase, as tolerated to 100 mg/day the first 2 weeks, may then be increased to a total of 250 mg/day

Nursing/Pharmacy Information Monitor pulse rate and blood pressure prior to and during therapy, evaluate mental status

Dosage Forms Capsule, as hydrochloride: 25 mg, 50 mg, 75 mg

♦ **Clomycin®** [OTC] *see* bacitracin, neomycin, polymyxin B, and lidocaine *on page 72*

clonazepam (kloe NA ze pam)
U.S. Brand Names Klonopin™
Canadian Brand Names PMS-Clonazepam; Rivotril®
Mexican Brand Names Kenoket; Rivotril®
Generic Available Yes
Therapeutic Category Benzodiazepine
Controlled Substance C-IV
Use Prophylaxis of absence (petit mal), petit mal variant (Lennox-Gastaut), akinetic, and myoclonic seizures
Usual Dosage Oral:
Children <10 years or 30 kg:
Initial daily dose: 0.01-0.03 mg/kg/day (maximum: 0.05 mg/kg/day) administered in 2-3 divided doses; increase by no more than 0.5 mg every third day until seizures are controlled or adverse effects are seen
Maintenance dose: 0.1-0.2 mg/kg/day divided 3 times/day; not to exceed 0.2 mg/kg/day
Adults:
Initial daily dose not to exceed 1.5 mg administered in 3 divided doses; may increase by 0.5-1 mg every third day until seizures are controlled or adverse effects seen
Maintenance dose: 0.05-0.2 mg/kg; do not exceed 20 mg/day

Dietary Considerations Alcohol: Additive CNS depression; has been reported with benzodiazepines; avoid or limit alcohol

Nursing/Pharmacy Information Observe patient for excess sedation, respiratory depression, orthostasis

Dosage Forms Tablet: 0.5 mg, 1 mg, 2 mg

clonidine (KLOE ni deen)
U.S. Brand Names Catapres® Oral; Catapres-TTS® Transdermal; Duraclon™ Injection
Canadian Brand Names Apo®-Clonidine; Dixarit®; Novo-Clonidine®; Nu-Clonidine®
Mexican Brand Names Catapresan-100®
Generic Available Yes: Tablet
Therapeutic Category Alpha-Adrenergic Agonist
Use Management of hypertension; aid in the diagnosis of pheochromocytoma and growth hormone deficiency; has orphan drug status for epidural use for pain control; used for heroin withdrawal and smoking cessation therapy in adults

Investigational use: Alternate agent for the treatment of attention-deficit/hyperactivity disorder (ADHD)

Usual Dosage
Epidural infusion (continuous): 30 mcg/hour, titrated up or down depending on pain relief
(Continued)

clonidine *(Continued)*

Oral:

Children: Initial: 5-10 mcg/kg/day in divided doses every 8-12 hours; increase gradually at 5- to 7-day intervals to 25 mcg/kg/day in divided doses every 6 hours; maximum: 0.9 mg/day

Clonidine tolerance test (test of growth hormone release from pituitary): 0.15 mg/m^2 or 4 mcg/kg as single dose

Adults: Initial dose: 0.1 mg twice daily, usual maintenance dose: 0.2-1.2 mg/day in 2-4 divided doses; maximum recommended dose: 2.4 mg/day

Nicotine withdrawal symptoms: 0.1 mg twice daily to maximum of 0.4 mg/day for 3-4 weeks

Elderly: Initial: 0.1 mg once daily at bedtime, increase gradually as needed

Transdermal: Apply once every 7 days; for initial therapy start with 0.1 mg and increase by 0.1 mg at 1- to 2-week intervals; dosages >0.6 mg do not improve efficacy

Dietary Considerations Hypertensive patients may need to decrease sodium and calories in diet

Nursing/Pharmacy Information

Counsel patient/parent about compliance and danger of withdrawal reaction if doses are missed or drug is discontinued; Catapres-TTS® comes in 2 parts - the small patch containing the drug and an overlay to keep the patch in place for 1 week; both parts should be used for maximum efficacy; it may be useful to note on the patch which day it should be changed

Monitor blood pressure, standing and sitting/supine

Dosage Forms Clonidine hydrochloride:

Injection, preservative free: 100 mcg/mL (10 mL)

Patch, transdermal: 1, 2, and 3 (0.1, 0.2, 0.3 mg/day, 7-day duration)

Tablet: 0.1 mg, 0.2 mg, 0.3 mg

clonidine and chlorthalidone (KLOE ni deen & klor THAL i done)

Synonyms chlorthalidone and clonidine

U.S. Brand Names Combipres®

Generic Available No

Therapeutic Category Antihypertensive Agent, Combination

Use Management of mild to moderate hypertension

Usual Dosage Oral: 1 tablet 1-2 times/day

Dosage Forms Tablet:

0.1: Clonidine 0.1 mg and chlorthalidone 15 mg

0.2: Clonidine 0.2 mg and chlorthalidone 15 mg

0.3: Clonidine 0.3 mg and chlorthalidone 15 mg

♦ **Clonodifen®** *see* diclofenac *on page 198*

clopidogrel (kloh PID oh grel)

U.S. Brand Names Plavix®

Generic Available No

Therapeutic Category Antiplatelet Agent

Use The reduction of atherosclerotic events (myocardial infarction, stroke, vascular deaths) in patients with atherosclerosis documented by recent myocardial infarctions, recent stroke or established peripheral arterial disease

Usual Dosage Adults: Oral: 75 mg once daily

Dosage Forms Tablet, as bisulfate: 75 mg

♦ **Clopixol®** *see* zuclopenthixol *(Canada only) on page 661*
♦ **Clopixol-Acuphase®** *see* zuclopenthixol *(Canada only) on page 661*
♦ **Clopixol® Depot** *see* zuclopenthixol *(Canada only) on page 661*
♦ **Clopra®** *see* metoclopramide *on page 409*
♦ **Clorafen** *see* chloramphenicol *on page 133*

clorazepate (klor AZ e pate)

U.S. Brand Names Gen-XENE®; Tranxene®

Canadian Brand Names Apo®-Clorazepate; Novo-Clopate®

Generic Available Yes

Therapeutic Category Anticonvulsant; Benzodiazepine

Controlled Substance C-IV

Use Treatment of generalized anxiety and panic disorders; management of alcohol withdrawal; adjunct anticonvulsant in management of partial seizures

Usual Dosage Oral:

Anticonvulsant:

Children:

<9 years: Dose not established

9-12 years: Initial: 3.75-7.5 mg/dose twice daily; increase dose by 3.75 mg at weekly intervals, not to exceed 60 mg/day in 2-3 divided doses

Children >12 years and Adults: Initial: Up to 7.5 mg/dose 2-3 times/day; increase dose by 7.5 mg at weekly intervals; usual dose: 0.5-1 mg/kg/day; not to exceed 90 mg/day (up to 3 mg/kg/day has been used)

Anxiety: Adults: 7.5-15 mg 2-4 times/day, or administered as single dose of 15-22.5 mg at bedtime

Alcohol withdrawal: Adults: Initial: 30 mg, then 15 mg 2-4 times/day on first day; maximum daily dose: 90 mg; gradually decrease dose over subsequent days

Nursing/Pharmacy Information
Assist patient with ambulation during initiation of therapy; monitor for alertness
Monitor respiratory and cardiovascular status, excess CNS depression
Stability: Unstable in water

Dosage Forms Clorazepate dipotassium:
Capsule: 3.75 mg, 7.5 mg, 15 mg
Tablet: 3.75 mg, 7.5 mg, 15 mg
Tablet, single dose: 11.25 mg, 22.5 mg

♦ **Clorpactin® WCS-90** *see* oxychlorosene *on page 462*
♦ **Clorpactin® XCB Powder** *(Discontinued) see page 743*
♦ **Clotrimaderm** *see* clotrimazole *on page 161*

clotrimazole (kloe TRIM a zole)

U.S. Brand Names Gyne-Lotrimin® Vaginal [OTC]; Lotrimin AF® Topical [OTC]; Lotrimin® Topical; Mycelex®-G Topical; Mycelex®-G Vaginal [OTC]; Mycelex® Troche

Canadian Brand Names Canesten® Topical; Canesten® Vaginal; Clotrimaderm; Myclo-Derm®; Myclo-Gyne®

Generic Available Yes

Therapeutic Category Antifungal Agent

Use Treatment of susceptible fungal infections, including oropharyngeal candidiasis, dermatophytoses, superficial mycoses, cutaneous candidiasis, as well as vulvovaginal candidiasis; limited data suggests that the use of clotrimazole troches may be effective for prophylaxis against oropharyngeal candidiasis in neutropenic patients

Usual Dosage
Children >3 years and Adults:
Oral: 10 mg troche dissolved slowly 5 times/day
Topical: Apply twice daily
Adults: Vaginal: 100 mg/day for 7 days or 200 mg/day for 3 days or 500 mg single dose or 5 g (1 applicatorful) of 1% vaginal cream daily for 7-14 days

Nursing/Pharmacy Information
Administer around-the-clock rather than 4 times/day, 3 times/day, etc, (ie, 12-6-12-6, not 9-1-5-9) to promote less variation in peak and trough serum levels
Monitor periodic liver function tests during oral therapy with clotrimazole lozenges

Dosage Forms
Combination pack (Mycelex-7®): Vaginal tablet 100 mg (7's) and vaginal cream 1% (7 g)
Cream:
Topical (Lotrimin®, Lotrimin® AF, Mycelex®, Mycelex® OTC) : 1% (15 g, 30 g, 45 g, 90 g)
Vaginal (Femizole-7®, Gyne-Lotrimin®, Mycelex®-G): 1% (45 g, 90 g)
Lotion (Lotrimin®): 1% (30 mL)
Solution, topical (Fungoid®, Lotrimin®, Lotrimin® AF, Mycelex®, Mycelex® OTC): 1% (10 mL, 30 mL)
Tablet, vaginal (Gyne-Lotrimin®, Mycelex®-G): 100 mg (7s); 500 mg (1s)
Troche (Mycelex®): 10 mg
Twin pack (Mycelex®): Vaginal tablet 500 mg (1's) and vaginal cream 1% (7 g)

♦ **clotrimazole and betamethasone** *see* betamethasone and clotrimazole *on page 84*

cloxacillin (kloks a SIL in)

U.S. Brand Names Cloxapen®
Canadian Brand Names Apo®-Cloxi; Novo-Cloxin®; Nu-Cloxi®; Orbenin®; Taro-Cloxacillin®
Generic Available Yes
Therapeutic Category Penicillin
(Continued)

cloxacillin *(Continued)*

Use Treatment of susceptible bacterial infections of the respiratory tract, skin and skin structure, bone and joint caused by penicillinase-producing staphylococci

Usual Dosage Oral:
Children >1 month: 50-100 mg/kg/day in divided doses every 6 hours; up to a maximum of 4 g/day
Adults: 250-500 mg every 6 hours

Dietary Considerations Should be administered 1 hour before or 2 hours after meals with water

Nursing/Pharmacy Information
Monitor CBC with differential, urinalysis, BUN, serum creatinine, and liver enzymes
Stability: Refrigerate oral solution after reconstitution; discard after 14 days; stable for 3 days at room temperature

Dosage Forms Cloxacillin sodium:
Capsule: 250 mg, 500 mg
Powder for oral suspension: 125 mg/5 mL (100 mL, 200 mL)

♦ **Cloxapen®** *see* cloxacillin *on page 161*

clozapine *(KLOE za peen)*

U.S. Brand Names Clozaril®
Mexican Brand Names Leponex®
Generic Available No
Therapeutic Category Antipsychotic Agent, Dibenzodiazepine
Use Management of schizophrenic patients
Usual Dosage Adults: Oral: Initial: 25 mg once or twice daily, increase as tolerated to a target dose of 300-450 mg/day, may require doses as high as 600-900 mg/day
Nursing/Pharmacy Information
Benign, self-limiting temperature elevations sometimes occur during the first 3 weeks of treatment
Monitor orthostatic blood pressures; observe for signs of infection; observe for motor abnormalities
Dosage Forms Tablet: 25 mg, 100 mg

♦ **Clozaril®** *see* clozapine *on page 162*

♦ **Clysodrast®** *see* bisacodyl *on page 88*

♦ **CMV-IGIV** *see* cytomegalovirus immune globulin (intravenous-human) *on page 179*

♦ **coagulant complex inhibitor** *see* anti-inhibitor coagulant complex *on page 52*

♦ **coagulation factor VIIa** *see* factor VIIa, recombinant *New Drug on page 258*

coal tar *(KOLE tar)*

Synonyms crude coal tar; LCD; pix carbonis
U.S. Brand Names AquaTar® [OTC]; Denorex® [OTC]; DHS® Tar [OTC]; Duplex® T [OTC]; Estar® [OTC]; Fototar® [OTC]; Neutrogena® T/Derm; Pentrax® [OTC]; Polytar® [OTC]; psoriGel® [OTC]; T/Gel® [OTC]; Zetar® [OTC]
Canadian Brand Names Balnetar®; Ionil-T® Plus
Generic Available Yes
Therapeutic Category Antipsoriatic Agent; Antiseborrheic Agent, Topical
Use Topically for controlling dandruff, seborrheic dermatitis, or psoriasis
Usual Dosage
Bath: Add appropriate amount to bath water, for adults usually 60-90 mL of a 5% to 20% solution or 15-25 mL of 30% lotion; soak 5-20 minutes, then pat dry; use once daily for 3 days
Shampoo: Rub shampoo onto wet hair and scalp, rinse thoroughly; repeat; leave on 5 minutes; rinse thoroughly; apply twice weekly for the first 2 weeks then once weekly or more often if needed
Skin: Apply to the affected area 1-4 times/day; decrease frequency to 2-3 times/week once condition has been controlled
Scalp psoriasis: Tar oil bath or coal tar solution may be painted sparingly to the lesions 3-12 hours before each shampoo
Psoriasis of the body, arms, legs: Apply at bedtime; if thick scales are present, use product with salicylic acid and apply several times during the day
Nursing/Pharmacy Information For external use only
Dosage Forms
Cream: 1% to 5%
Gel: Coal tar 5%

Lotion: 2.5% to 30%
Lotion: 2%; 5%; 25%
Shampoo:
   Coal tar: 0.5% to 5%
   Coal tar extract 2% with salicylic acid 2% (60 mL)
Solution:
   Coal tar: 2.5%, 5%, 20%
   Coal tar extract: 5%
Suspension, coal tar: 30% to 33.3%

coal tar and salicylic acid (KOLE tar & sal i SIL ik AS id)

U.S. Brand Names X-seb® T [OTC]
Generic Available Yes
Therapeutic Category Antipsoriatic Agent; Antiseborrheic Agent, Topical
Use Treatment of seborrheal dermatitis, dandruff
Usual Dosage Topical: Shampoo twice weekly
Nursing/Pharmacy Information Avoid contact with eyes; for external use only
Dosage Forms Shampoo: Coal tar solution 10% and salicylic acid 4% (120 mL)

coal tar, lanolin, and mineral oil

(KOLE tar, LAN oh lin, & MIN er al oyl)
U.S. Brand Names Balnetar® [OTC]
Generic Available Yes
Therapeutic Category Antipsoriatic Agent; Antiseborrheic Agent, Topical
Use Treatment of psoriasis, seborrheal dermatitis, atopic dermatitis, eczematoid dermatitis
Usual Dosage Add to bath water, soak for 5-20 minutes then pat dry
Dosage Forms Oil, bath: Water-dispersible emollient tar 2.5%, lanolin fraction, and mineral oil (240 mL)

♦ Cobalasine® Injection *(Discontinued)* see page 743
♦ Cobex® see cyanocobalamin on page 173

cocaine (koe KANE)

Generic Available Yes
Therapeutic Category Local Anesthetic
Controlled Substance C-II
Use Topical anesthesia for mucous membranes
Usual Dosage Topical: Use lowest effective dose; do not exceed 1 mg/kg; patient tolerance, anesthetic technique, vascularity of tissue and area to be anesthetized will determine dose needed
Nursing/Pharmacy Information
   Use only on mucous membranes of the oral, laryngeal, and nasal cavities; do not use on extensive areas of broken skin
   Monitor vital signs
   Stability: Store in well closed, light-resistant containers
Dosage Forms Cocaine hydrochloride:
   Powder: 5 g, 25 g
   Solution, topical: 4% [40 mg/mL] (2 mL, 4 mL, 10 mL); 10% [100 mg/mL] (4 mL, 10 mL)
   Solution, topical, viscous: 4% [40 mg/mL] (4 mL, 10 mL); 10% [100 mg/mL] (4 mL, 10 mL)
   Tablet, soluble, for topical solution: 135 mg

coccidioidin skin test (koks i dee OH i din skin test)

U.S. Brand Names Spherulin®
Generic Available No
Therapeutic Category Diagnostic Agent
Use Intradermal skin test in diagnosis of coccidioidomycosis; differential diagnosis of this disease from histoplasmosis, sarcoidosis and other mycotic and bacterial infections. The skin test may be negative in severe forms of disease (anergy) or when prolonged periods of time have passed since infection.
Usual Dosage Children and Adults: Intradermally: 0.1 mL of 1:100 or flexor surface of forearm
   Positive reaction: Induration of 5 mm or more; erythema without induration is considered negative; read the test at 24 and 48 hours, since some reactions may not be noticeable after 36 hours. A positive reaction indicates present or past infection with *Coccidioides immitis*.
(Continued)

coccidioidin skin test *(Continued)*

Negative reaction: A negative test means the individual has not been sensitized to coccidioidin or has lost sensitivity

Nursing/Pharmacy Information
Patient should be matched for at least 15 minutes after injection for immediate hypersensitivity response
Stability: Refrigerate

Dosage Forms Injection: 1:10 (0.5 mL); 1:100 (1 mL)

♦ **Codafed® Expectorant** *see* guaifenesin, pseudoephedrine, and codeine *on page 304*

♦ **Codamine®** *see* hydrocodone and phenylpropanolamine *on page 321*

♦ **Codamine® Pediatric** *see* hydrocodone and phenylpropanolamine *on page 321*

♦ **Codehist® DH** *see* chlorpheniramine, pseudoephedrine, and codeine *on page 143*

codeine (KOE deen)

Synonyms methylmorphine

Canadian Brand Names Codeine Conhn®; Linctus Codeine Blac; Linctus With Codeine Phosphate; Paveral Stanley Syrup With Codeine Phosphate

Generic Available Yes

Therapeutic Category Analgesic, Narcotic; Antitussive

Controlled Substance C-II

Use Treatment of mild to moderate pain; antitussive in lower doses

Usual Dosage Doses should be titrated to appropriate analgesic effect; when changing routes of administration, note that oral dose is $2/3$ as effective as parenteral dose

Analgesic: Oral, I.M., S.C.:
Children: 0.5-1 mg/kg/dose every 4-6 hours as needed; maximum: 60 mg/dose
Adults: 30 mg/dose; range: 15-60 mg every 4-6 hours as needed
Antitussive: Oral (for nonproductive cough):
Children: 1-1.5 mg/kg/day in divided doses every 4-6 hours as needed; Alternatively dose according to age:
2-6 years: 2.5-5 mg every 4-6 hours as needed; maximum: 30 mg/day
6-12 years: 5-10 mg every 4-6 hours as needed; maximum: 60 mg/day
Adults: 10-20 mg/dose every 4-6 hours as needed; maximum: 120 mg/day

Dietary Considerations
Alcohol: Additive CNS effects; avoid or limit alcohol; watch for sedation
Food: Glucose may cause hyperglycemia; monitor blood glucose concentrations

Nursing/Pharmacy Information
Not intended for I.V. use due to large histamine release and cardiovascular effects
Monitor for pain relief, constipation, respiratory and mental status, blood pressure
Stability: Store injection between 15°C to 30°C, avoid freezing; do not use if injection is discolored or contains a precipitate; protect injection from light

Dosage Forms
Codeine phosphate:
Injection: 30 mg (1 mL, 2 mL); 60 mg (1 mL, 2 mL)
Tablet, soluble: 30 mg, 60 mg
Codeine sulfate:
Tablet: 15 mg, 30 mg, 60 mg
Tablet, soluble: 15 mg, 30 mg, 60 mg

♦ **codeine and acetaminophen** *see* acetaminophen and codeine *on page 14*

♦ **codeine and aspirin** *see* aspirin and codeine *on page 62*

♦ **codeine and bromodiphenhydramine** *see* bromodiphenhydramine and codeine *on page 93*

♦ **codeine and butalbital compound** *see* butalbital compound and codeine *on page 99*

♦ **codeine and guaifenesin** *see* guaifenesin and codeine *on page 300*

♦ **codeine and promethazine** *see* promethazine and codeine *on page 522*

♦ **codeine, brompheniramine, and phenylpropanolamine** *see* brompheniramine, phenylpropanolamine, and codeine *on page 95*

♦ **Codeine Conhn®** *see* codeine *on page 164*

♦ **codeine, guaifenesin, and pseudoephedrine** *see* guaifenesin, pseudoephedrine, and codeine *on page 304*

- **codeine, promethazine, and phenylephrine** *see* promethazine, phenylephrine, and codeine *on page 523*
- **Codiclear® DH** *see* hydrocodone and guaifenesin *on page 320*
- **Codimal-A® Injection** *(Discontinued) see page 743*
- **Codimal® Expectorant** *(Discontinued) see page 743*
- **cod liver oil** *see* vitamin A and vitamin D *on page 651*
- **Codoxy®** *see* oxycodone and aspirin *on page 463*
- **Cogentin®** *see* benztropine *on page 82*
- **Co-Gesic®** *see* hydrocodone and acetaminophen *on page 319*
- **Cognex®** *see* tacrine *on page 592*
- **Co-Hist® [OTC]** *see* acetaminophen, chlorpheniramine, and pseudoephedrine *on page 16*
- **Colace® [OTC]** *see* docusate *on page 214*
- **colaspase** *see* asparaginase *on page 60*
- **Co-Lav®** *see* polyethylene glycol-electrolyte solution *on page 502*
- **Colax-C®** *see* docusate *on page 214*

colchicine (KOL chi seen)
Mexican Brand Names Colchiquim; Colchiquim-30
Generic Available Yes
Therapeutic Category Antigout Agent
Use Treat acute gouty arthritis attacks and to prevent recurrences of such attacks; management of familial Mediterranean fever
Usual Dosage
  Acute gouty arthritis:
    Oral: Initial: 0.5-1.2 mg, then 0.5-0.6 mg every 1-2 hours or 1-1.2 mg every 2 hours until relief or GI side effects occur to a maximum total dose of 8 mg, wait 3 days before initiating a second course
    I.V.: Initial: 1-3 mg, then 0.5 mg every 6 hours until response, not to exceed 4 mg/day; following a full course of colchicine (4 mg), wait 7 days before initiating another course of colchicine (by any route)
  Prophylaxis of recurrent attacks: Oral:
    <1 attack/year: 0.5 or 0.6 mg/day/dose for 3-4 days/week
    >1 attack/year: 0.5 or 0.6 mg/day/dose
    Severe cases: 1-1.8 mg/day
Dietary Considerations May need low purine diet during acute gouty attack; avoid alcohol; should be administered with water (10-12 glasses fluid/day)
Nursing/Pharmacy Information
  Severe local irritation can occur following S.C. or I.M. administration; extravasation can cause tissue irritation; administer I.V. over 2-5 minutes into tubing of free-flowing I.V. with compatible fluid; administer orally with water and maintain adequate fluid intake
  Monitor CBC and renal function test
  Stability: Protect tablets from light; I.V. colchicine is **incompatible** with dextrose or I.V. solutions with preservatives
Dosage Forms
  Injection: 0.5 mg/mL (2 mL)
  Tablet: 0.5 mg, 0.6 mg

colchicine and probenecid (KOL chi seen & proe BEN e sid)
Synonyms probenecid and colchicine
Generic Available Yes
Therapeutic Category Antigout Agent
Use Treatment of chronic gouty arthritis when complicated by frequent, recurrent acute attacks of gout
Usual Dosage Adults: Oral: 1 tablet daily for 1 week, then 1 tablet twice daily thereafter
Nursing/Pharmacy Information Do not initiate therapy until an acute gouty attack has subsided
Dosage Forms Tablet: Colchicine 0.5 mg and probenecid 0.5 g

- **Colchiquim** *see* colchicine *on page 165*
- **Colchiquim-30** *see* colchicine *on page 165*
- **Cold & Allergy® Elixir [OTC]** *see* brompheniramine and phenylpropanolamine *on page 94*
- **Coldlac-LA®** *see* guaifenesin and phenylpropanolamine *on page 301*
- **Coldloc®** *see* guaifenesin, phenylpropanolamine, and phenylephrine *on page 304*
- **Coldrine® [OTC]** *see* acetaminophen and pseudoephedrine *on page 15*
- **Colestid®** *see* colestipol *on page 166*

colestipol (koe LES ti pole)
U.S. Brand Names Colestid®
Generic Available No
Therapeutic Category Antihyperlipidemic Agent, Miscellaneous
Use Adjunct in the management of primary hypercholesterolemia; to relieve pruritus associated with elevated levels of bile acids, possibly used to decrease plasma half-life of digoxin as an adjunct in the treatment of toxicity
Usual Dosage Oral: 15-30 g/day in divided doses 2-4 times/day
Nursing/Pharmacy Information Dry powder should be added to at least 90 mL of liquid and stirred until completely mixed; other drugs should be administered at least 1 hour before or 4 hours after colestipol
Dosage Forms Colestipol hydrochloride:
Granules: 5 g packet, 300 g, 500 g
Tablet: 1 g

colfosceril palmitate (kole FOS er il PALM i tate)
Synonyms dipalmitoylphosphatidylcholine; DPPC; synthetic lung surfactant
U.S. Brand Names Exosurf® Neonatal™
Generic Available No
Therapeutic Category Lung Surfactant
Use Neonatal respiratory distress syndrome (RDS):
Prophylactic therapy: Infants at risk for developing RDS with body weight <1350 g; infants with evidence of pulmonary immaturity with body weight >1350 g
Rescue therapy: Treatment of infants with RDS based on respiratory distress not attributable to any other causes and chest radiographic findings consistent with RDS
Usual Dosage
Prophylactic treatment: Administer 5 mL/kg as soon as possible; the second and third doses should be administered at 12 and 24 hours later to those infants remaining on ventilators
Rescue treatment: Administer 5 mL/kg as soon as the diagnosis of RDS is made; the second 5 mL/kg dose should be administered 12 hours later
Nursing/Pharmacy Information
For intratracheal administration only. Suction infant prior to administration; inspect solution to verify complete mixing of the suspension. Administer via sideport on the special ETT adapter without interrupting mechanical ventilation. Administer the dose in two 2.5 mL/kg aliquots. Each half-dose is instilled slowly over 1-2 minutes in small bursts with each inspiration. After the first 2.5 mL/kg dose turn the infants head and torso 45° right for 30 seconds, then return to the midline position and administer the second dose as above. Following the second dose, turn the infant's head and torso 45° to the left for 30 seconds and return the infant to the midline position. Use only the preservative-free sterile water for injection to reconstitute the drug (provided with the drug).
Continuous EKG and transcutaneous O_2 saturation should be monitored during administration; frequent ABG sampling is necessary to prevent postdosing hyperoxia and hypocarbia
Stability: Reconstituted suspension should be used immediately and unused portion discarded; store at room temperature; do not refrigerate
Dosage Forms Powder for injection, lyophilized: 108 mg (10 mL)

colistimethate (koe lis ti METH ate)
U.S. Brand Names Coly-Mycin® M Parenteral
Generic Available No
Therapeutic Category Antibiotic, Miscellaneous
Use Treatment of infections due to sensitive strains of certain gram-negative bacilli
Usual Dosage Children and Adults: I.M., I.V.: 2.5-5 mg/kg/day in 2-4 divided doses
Nursing/Pharmacy Information Freshly prepare and use within 24 hours
Dosage Forms Powder for injection, as sodium, lyophilized: 150 mg

colistin, neomycin, and hydrocortisone
(koe LIS tin, nee oh MYE sin & hye droe KOR ti sone)
Synonyms hydrocortisone, colistin, and neomycin; neomycin, colistin, and hydrocortisone
U.S. Brand Names Coly-Mycin® S Otic Drops; Cortisporin-TC® Otic
Generic Available No
Therapeutic Category Antibiotic/Corticosteroid, Otic

Use Treatment of superficial and susceptible bacterial infections of the external auditory canal; for treatment of susceptible bacterial infections of mastoidectomy and fenestration cavities

Usual Dosage Otic:
Children: 3 drops in affected ear 3-4 times/day
Adults: 4 drops in affected ear 3-4 times/day

Nursing/Pharmacy Information Shake well for 10 seconds before administering

Dosage Forms Suspension, otic:
Coly-Mycin® S Otic Drops: Colistin sulfate 0.3%, neomycin sulfate 0.47%, and hydrocortisone acetate 1% (5 mL, 10 mL)
Cortisprorin-TC®: Colistin sulfate 0.3%, neomycin sulfate 0.33%, and hydrocortisone acetate 1% (5 mL, 10 mL)

collagenase (KOL la je nase)

U.S. Brand Names Biozyme-C®; Santyl®
Generic Available No
Therapeutic Category Enzyme
Use Promote debridement of necrotic tissue in dermal ulcers and severe burns
Usual Dosage Topical: Apply daily or every other day
Nursing/Pharmacy Information Do not introduce into major body cavities; monitor debilitated patients for systemic bacterial infections; prior to application, cleanse lesion of debris and digested material; when infection is present, neomycin-bacitracin-polymyxin B may be used with collagenase; excess ointment should be removed each time the dressing is changed; treatment should be discontinued when debridement is complete and granulation tissue is well established

Dosage Forms Ointment, topical: 250 units/g (15 g, 30 g)

collagen implants (KOL a jen im PLANTS)

Generic Available No
Therapeutic Category Ophthalmic Agent, Miscellaneous
Use Relief of dry eyes; enhance the effect of ocular medications
Usual Dosage Implants inserted by physician
Dosage Forms Implant: 0.2 mm, 0.3 mm, 0.4 mm, 0.5 mm, 0.6 mm

- ♦ **Collyrium Fresh® Ophthalmic [OTC]** *see* tetrahydrozoline *on page 602*
- ♦ **Colovage®** *see* polyethylene glycol-electrolyte solution *on page 502*
- ♦ **Columina** *see* cimetidine *on page 150*
- ♦ **Coly-Mycin® M Parenteral** *see* colistimethate *on page 166*
- ♦ **Coly-Mycin® S Oral (Discontinued)** *see page 743*
- ♦ **Coly-Mycin® S Otic Drops** *see* colistin, neomycin, and hydrocortisone *on page 166*
- ♦ **CoLyte®** *see* polyethylene glycol-electrolyte solution *on page 502*
- ♦ **CoLyte®-Flavored** *see* polyethylene glycol-electrolyte solution *on page 502*
- ♦ **Comalose-R** *see* lactulose *on page 359*
- ♦ **Combantrin®** *see* protirelin *on page 529*
- ♦ **Combipres®** *see* clonidine and chlorthalidone *on page 160*
- ♦ **Combivent®** *see* ipratropium and albuterol *on page 345*
- ♦ **Combivir®** *see* zidovudine and lamivudine *on page 659*
- ♦ **Comfort® Ophthalmic [OTC]** *see* naphazoline *on page 431*
- ♦ **Comfort® Tears Solution [OTC]** *see* artificial tears *on page 59*
- ♦ **Comhist®** *see* chlorpheniramine, phenylephrine, and phenyltoloxamine *on page 142*
- ♦ **Comhist® LA** *see* chlorpheniramine, phenylephrine, and phenyltoloxamine *on page 142*
- ♦ **Compazine®** *see* prochlorperazine *on page 519*
- ♦ **Complan** *see* vitamin, multiple (oral) *on page 654*
- ♦ **compound E** *see* cortisone acetate *on page 169*
- ♦ **compound F** *see* hydrocortisone (systemic) *on page 323*
- ♦ **compound S** *see* zidovudine *on page 658*
- ♦ **Compoz® Gel Caps [OTC]** *see* diphenhydramine *on page 208*
- ♦ **Compoz® Nighttime Sleep Aid [OTC]** *see* diphenhydramine *on page 208*
- ♦ **Comprecin** *see* enoxacin *on page 232*
- ♦ **Comtan®** *see* entacapone *New Drug on page 233*
- ♦ **Comtrex® Maximum Strength Non-Drowsy [OTC]** *see* acetaminophen, dextromethorphan, and pseudoephedrine *on page 16*
- ♦ **Comvax®** *see* Haemophilus B conjugate and hepatitis B vaccine *New Drug on page 306*

- **Conazol** *see* ketoconazole *on page 354*
- **Condylox®** *see* podofilox *on page 500*
- **Conex® [OTC]** *see* guaifenesin and phenylpropanolamine *on page 301*
- **Congess® Jr** *see* guaifenesin and pseudoephedrine *on page 302*
- **Congess® Sr** *see* guaifenesin and pseudoephedrine *on page 302*
- **Congest** *see* estrogens, conjugated (equine) *on page 245*
- **Congestac®** *see* guaifenesin and pseudoephedrine *on page 302*
- **Congestant D® [OTC]** *see* chlorpheniramine, phenylpropanolamine, and acetaminophen *on page 142*
- **conjugated estrogen and methyltestosterone** *see* estrogens and methyltestosterone *on page 244*
- **conjugated estrogens** *see* estrogens, conjugated (equine) *on page 245*
- **Conray®** *see* radiological/contrast media (ionic) *on page 539*
- **Constant-T® Tablet** *(Discontinued) see page 743*
- **Constilac®** *see* lactulose *on page 359*
- **Constulose®** *see* lactulose *on page 359*
- **Consupren** *see* cyclosporine *on page 176*
- **Contac® Cough Formula Liquid [OTC]** *see* guaifenesin and dextromethorphan *on page 300*
- **Contergan®** *see* thalidomide *on page 602*
- **Control® [OTC]** *see* phenylpropanolamine *on page 489*
- **Control-L®** *(Discontinued) see page 743*
- **Contuss®** *see* guaifenesin, phenylpropanolamine, and phenylephrine *on page 304*
- **Contuss® XT** *see* guaifenesin and phenylpropanolamine *on page 301*
- **Copaxone®** *see* glatiramer acetate *on page 291*
- **Cophene-B®** *see* brompheniramine *on page 94*
- **Cophene XP®** *see* hydrocodone, pseudoephedrine, and guaifenesin *on page 322*
- **copolymer-1** *see* glatiramer acetate *on page 291*
- **copper injection** *see* trace metals *on page 620*
- **Coptin®** *see* sulfadiazine *on page 586*
- **Co-Pyronil® 2 Pulvules® [OTC]** *see* chlorpheniramine and pseudoephedrine *on page 140*
- **Coradur®** *see* isosorbide dinitrate *on page 349*
- **Corax®** *see* chlordiazepoxide *on page 134*
- **Cordarone®** *see* amiodarone *on page 39*
- **Cordran®** *see* flurandrenolide *on page 277*
- **Cordran® SP** *see* flurandrenolide *on page 277*
- **Coreg®** *see* carvedilol *on page 117*
- **Corgard®** *see* nadolol *on page 427*
- **Corgonject®** *see* chorionic gonadotropin *on page 149*
- **Coricidin® [OTC]** *see* chlorpheniramine and acetaminophen *on page 139*
- **Coricidin D® [OTC]** *see* chlorpheniramine, phenylpropanolamine, and acetaminophen *on page 142*
- **Corlopam®** *see* fenoldopam *on page 261*
- **Cormax® Ointment** *see* clobetasol *on page 157*
- **Corogal** *see* nifedipine *on page 442*
- **Corotrend** *see* nifedipine *on page 442*
- **Corotrend Retard** *see* nifedipine *on page 442*
- **Corque® Topical** *see* clioquinol and hydrocortisone *on page 157*
- **CortaGel® Topical [OTC]** *see* hydrocortisone (topical) *on page 324*
- **Cortaid® Maximum Strength Topical [OTC]** *see* hydrocortisone (topical) *on page 324*
- **Cortaid® Ointment** *(Discontinued) see page 743*
- **Cortaid® with Aloe Topical [OTC]** *see* hydrocortisone (topical) *on page 324*
- **Cortamed®** *see* hydrocortisone (topical) *on page 324*
- **Cortate®** *see* hydrocortisone (topical) *on page 324*
- **Cortatrigen® Otic** *see* neomycin, polymyxin B, and hydrocortisone *on page 437*
- **Cort-Dome® Topical** *see* hydrocortisone (topical) *on page 324*
- **Cortef® Feminine Itch Topical** *see* hydrocortisone (topical) *on page 324*
- **Cortenema® Rectal** *see* hydrocortisone (rectal) *on page 322*
- **Corticaine® Topical** *see* dibucaine and hydrocortisone *on page 197*

corticotropin (kor ti koe TROE pin)
Synonyms ACTH; adrenocorticotropic hormone
U.S. Brand Names Acthar®; H.P. Acthar® Gel
Generic Available Yes
Therapeutic Category Adrenal Corticosteroid
Use Infantile spasms; diagnostic aid in adrenocortical insufficiency; acute exacerbations of multiple sclerosis; severe muscle weakness in myasthenia gravis
Usual Dosage
Acute exacerbation of multiple sclerosis: I.M.: 80-120 units/day for 2-3 weeks
Diagnostic purposes:
I.M., S.C.: 20 units 4 times/day
I.V.: 10-25 units in 500 mL 5% dextrose in water over 8 hours
Dietary Considerations May increase renal loss of potassium, calcium, zinc, and vitamin C; may need to increase dietary intake or give supplements
Nursing/Pharmacy Information
Do not administer zinc hydroxide suspension S.C. or I.V.; do not abruptly discontinue the medication
Stability: Store repository injection in the refrigerator; reconstituted solution remains stable for 24 hours to 7 days when refrigerated depending on product; warm gel before administration
Dosage Forms
Injection, repository (H.P. Acthar® Gel): 40 units/mL (1 mL, 5 mL); 80 units/mL (1 mL, 5 mL)
Powder for injection (Acthar®): 25 units, 40 units

- **Corticreme®** *see* hydrocortisone (topical) *on page 324*
- **Cortifoam® Rectal** *see* hydrocortisone (rectal) *on page 322*
- **Cortiment®** *see* hydrocortisone (topical) *on page 324*

cortisone acetate (KOR ti sone AS e tate)
Synonyms compound E
U.S. Brand Names Cortone® Acetate
Generic Available Yes
Therapeutic Category Adrenal Corticosteroid
Use Management of adrenocortical insufficiency
Usual Dosage Depends upon the condition being treated and the response of the patient
Children:
Anti-inflammatory or immunosuppressive:
Oral: 2.5-10 mg/kg/day or 20-300 mg/m²/day in divided doses every 6-8 hours
I.M.: 1-5 mg/kg/day or 14-375 mg/m²/day in divided doses every 12-24 hours
Physiologic replacement:
Oral: 0.5-0.75 mg/kg/day in divided doses every 8 hours
I.M.: 0.25-0.35 mg/kg/day once daily
Stress coverage for surgery: I.M.: 1 and 2 days before preanesthesia, and 1-3 days after surgery: 50-62.5 mg/m²/day; 4 days after surgery: 31-50 mg/m²/day
Adults: Oral, I.M.: 20-300 mg/day
Dietary Considerations Limit caffeine; may need diet with increased potassium, pyridoxine, vitamin C, vitamin D, folate, calcium, and phosphorus and decreased sodium; may be administered with food to decrease GI distress
Nursing/Pharmacy Information I.M. use only, not to be administered I.V.; administer I.M. daily dose before 9 AM to minimize adrenocortical suppression; shake vial before withdrawing dose
Dosage Forms Cortisone acetate:
Injection: 50 mg/mL (10 mL)
Tablet: 5 mg, 10 mg, 25 mg

- **Cortisporin® Ophthalmic Ointment** *see* bacitracin, neomycin, polymyxin B, and hydrocortisone *on page 72*
- **Cortisporin® Ophthalmic Suspension** *see* neomycin, polymyxin B, and hydrocortisone *on page 437*
- **Cortisporin® Otic** *see* neomycin, polymyxin B, and hydrocortisone *on page 437*
- **Cortisporin-TC® Otic** *see* colistin, neomycin, and hydrocortisone *on page 166*
- **Cortisporin®-TC Otic Suspension** *see* neomycin, colistin, hydrocortisone, and thonzonium *on page 436*

- **Cortisporin® Topical Cream** *see* neomycin, polymyxin B, and hydrocortisone *on page 437*
- **Cortisporin® Topical Ointment** *see* bacitracin, neomycin, polymyxin B, and hydrocortisone *on page 72*
- **Cortizone®-5 Topical [OTC]** *see* hydrocortisone (topical) *on page 324*
- **Cortizone®-10 Topical [OTC]** *see* hydrocortisone (topical) *on page 324*
- **Cortoderm** *see* hydrocortisone (topical) *on page 324*
- **Cortone® Acetate** *see* cortisone acetate *on page 169*
- **Cortrophin-Zinc®** *(Discontinued)* *see page 743*
- **Cortrosyn®** *see* cosyntropin *on page 170*
- **Corvert®** *see* ibutilide *on page 332*
- **Coryphen® Codeine** *see* aspirin and codeine *on page 62*
- **Cosmegen®** *see* dactinomycin *on page 180*
- **Cosopt™** *see* dorzolamide and timolol *on page 218*

cosyntropin (koe sin TROE pin)

Synonyms synacthen; tetracosactide
U.S. Brand Names Cortrosyn®
Canadian Brand Names Synacthen® Depot
Generic Available No
Therapeutic Category Diagnostic Agent
Use Diagnostic test to differentiate primary adrenal from secondary (pituitary) adrenocortical insufficiency
Usual Dosage
Adrenocortical insufficiency: I.M., I.V.:
Children <2 years: 0.125 mg injected over 2 minutes
Children >2 years and Adults: 0.25 mg injected over 2 minutes
When greater cortisol stimulation is needed, an I.V. infusion may be used: I.V. infusion: 0.25 mg administered over 4-8 hours

Congenital adrenal hyperplasia evaluation: 1 mg/m^2/dose up to a maximum of 1 mg
Nursing/Pharmacy Information
Patient should not receive corticosteroids or spironolactone the day prior and the day of the test; administer I.V. doses over 2 minutes
Stability: Reconstituted solution is stable for 24 hours at room temperature and 21 days when refrigerated; for I.V. infusion in normal saline or D$_5$W solution is stable for 12 hours at room temperature
Dosage Forms Powder for injection: 0.25 mg

- **Cotazym®** *see* pancrelipase *on page 467*
- **Cotazym-S®** *see* pancrelipase *on page 467*
- **Cotrim®** *see* co-trimoxazole *on page 170*
- **Cotrim® DS** *see* co-trimoxazole *on page 170*

co-trimoxazole (koe trye MOKS a zole)

Synonyms SMX-TMP; sulfamethoxazole and trimethoprim; TMP-SMX; trimethoprim and sulfamethoxazole
U.S. Brand Names Bactrim™; Bactrim™ DS; Cotrim®; Cotrim® DS; Septra®; Septra® DS; Sulfamethoprim®; Sulfatrim®; Sulfatrim® DS; Uroplus® DS; Uroplus® SS
Canadian Brand Names Apo®-Sulfatrim; Novo-Trimel®; Nu-Cotrimox®; Pro-Trin®; Roubac®; Trisulfa®; Trisulfa-S®
Mexican Brand Names Anitrim; Bactelan; Batrizol; Ectaprim®; Ectaprim®-F; Enterobacticel; Esteprim; Isobac; Kelfiprim; Metoxiprim; Syraprim; Tribakin; Trimesuxol; Trimetoger; Trimetox; Trimzol
Generic Available Yes
Therapeutic Category Sulfonamide
Use Treatment of urinary tract infections caused by susceptible *E. coli*, *Klebsiella*, *Enterobacter*, *Proteus mirabilis*, *Proteus* (indole positive); acute otitis media due to amoxicillin-resistant *H. influenzae*, *S. pneumoniae*, and *M. catarrhalis*; acute exacerbations of chronic bronchitis; prophylaxis and treatment of *Pneumocystis carinii* pneumonitis (PCP); treatment of susceptible shigellosis, typhoid fever, *Nocardia asteroides* infection, and *Xanthomonas maltophilia* infection; the I.V. preparation is used for treatment of *Pneumocystis carinii* pneumonitis, *Shigella*, and severe urinary tract infections
Usual Dosage Oral, I.V. (dosage recommendations are based on the trimethoprim component):

Children >2 months:

Mild to moderate infections: 6-12 mg TMP/kg/day in divided doses every 12 hours

Serious infection/*Pneumocystis*: 15-20 mg TMP/kg/day in divided doses every 6 hours

Urinary tract infection prophylaxis: 2 mg TMP/kg/dose daily

Prophylaxis of *Pneumocystis*: 5-10 mg TMP/kg/day or 150 mg TMP/m^2/day in divided doses every 12 hours 3 days/week; dose should not exceed 320 mg trimethoprim and 1600 mg sulfamethoxazole 3 days/week; Mon, Tue, Wed

Adults: Urinary tract infection/chronic bronchitis: 1 double strength tablet every 12 hours for 10-14 days

Dietary Considerations Should be administered with a glass of water on empty stomach

Nursing/Pharmacy Information

Maintain adequate fluid intake to prevent crystalluria; infuse I.V. co-trimoxazole over 60-90 minutes; must be further diluted 1:25 (5 mL drug to 125 mL diluent, ie, D$_5$W); in patients who require fluid restriction, a 1:15 dilution (5 mL drug to 75 mL diluent, ie, D$_5$W) or a 1:10 dilution (5 mL drug to 50 mL diluent, ie, D$_5$W) can be administered

Monitor CBC, renal function test, liver function test, urinalysis

Stability: Do not refrigerate injection; less soluble in more alkaline pH; protect from light; do not use normal saline as a diluent; injection vehicle contains benzyl alcohol and sodium metabisulfite

Stability of parenteral admixture at room temperature (25°C):

5 mL/125 mL D$_5$W: 6 hours
5 mL/100 mL D$_5$W: 4 hours
5 mL/75 mL D$_5$W: 2 hours

Dosage Forms The 5:1 ratio (SMX to TMP) remains constant in all dosage forms:

Injection: Sulfamethoxazole 80 mg and trimethoprim 16 mg per mL (5 mL, 10 mL, 20 mL, 30 mL, 50 mL)

Suspension, oral: Sulfamethoxazole 200 mg and trimethoprim 40 mg per 5 mL (20 mL, 100 mL, 150 mL, 200 mL, 480 mL)

Tablet: Sulfamethoxazole 400 mg and trimethoprim 80 mg

Double strength: Sulfamethoxazole 800 mg and trimethoprim 160 mg

- ◆ **Coumadin**® *see* warfarin *on page 655*
- ◆ **Covera-HS**® *see* verapamil *on page 646*
- ◆ **Coversyl**® *see* perindopril erbumine *on page 481*
- ◆ **Cozaar**® *see* losartan *on page 376*
- ◆ **CP-99,219-27** *see* trovafloxacin *on page 634*
- ◆ **CPM** *see* cyclophosphamide *on page 175*
- ◆ **Credaxol** *see* ranitidine hydrochloride *on page 541*
- ◆ **Crema Blanca Bustillos** *see* hydroquinone *on page 325*
- ◆ **Creon**® *see* pancreatin *on page 467*
- ◆ **Creon**® **10** *see* pancrelipase *on page 467*
- ◆ **Creon**® **20** *see* pancrelipase *on page 467*
- ◆ **Creo-Terpin**® **[OTC]** *see* dextromethorphan *on page 194*
- ◆ **Cresylate**® *see* m-cresyl acetate *on page 386*
- ◆ **Crinone**™ *see* progesterone *on page 520*
- ◆ **Crinone**® **V** *see* progesterone *on page 520*
- ◆ **Criticare HN**® **[OTC]** *see* enteral nutritional products *on page 233*
- ◆ **Crixivan**® *see* indinavir *on page 337*
- ◆ **Crolom**® *see* cromolyn sodium *on page 171*
- ◆ **cromoglicic acid** *see* cromolyn sodium *on page 171*

cromolyn sodium (KROE moe lin SOW dee um)

Synonyms cromoglicic acid; disodium cromoglycate; DSCG

U.S. Brand Names Crolom®; Gastrocrom®; Intal®; Nasalcrom® [OTC]; Opticrom®

Canadian Brand Names Novo-Cromolyn®; PMS-Sodium Cromoglycate; Rynacrom®

Generic Available Yes

Therapeutic Category Mast Cell Stabilizer

Use Adjunct in the prophylaxis of allergic disorders, including rhinitis, conjunctivitis, and asthma; inhalation product may be used for prevention of exercise-induced bronchospasm

(Continued)

cromolyn sodium *(Continued)*

Ophthalmologic: Vernal conjunctivitis, vernal keratoconjunctivitis, and vernal keratitis

Systemic: Mastocytosis, food allergy, and treatment of inflammatory bowel disease

Usual Dosage

Children:

Inhalation: >2 years: 20 mg 4 times/day

Nebulization solution: >5 years: 2 inhalations 4 times/day by metered spray, or 20 mg 4 times/day (Spinhaler®); taper frequency to the lowest effective level

For prevention of exercise-induced bronchospasm: Single dose of 2 inhalations (aerosol) just prior to exercise

Nasal: >6 years: 1 spray in each nostril 3-4 times/day

Adults: Nasal: 1 spray in each nostril 3-4 times/day

Systemic mastocytosis: Oral:

Infants ≤2 years: 20 mg/kg/day in 4 divided doses, not to exceed 30 mg/kg/day

Children 2-12 years: 100 mg 4 times/day; not to exceed 40 mg/kg/day

Adults: 200 mg 4 times/day

Food allergy and inflammatory bowel disease: Oral:

Children: 100 mg 4 times/day 15-20 minutes before meals, not to exceed 40 mg/kg/day

Adults: 200 mg 4 times/day 15-20 minutes before meal, up to 400 mg 4 times/day

Dietary Considerations Do not mix with food, fruit juice, or milk; should be administered at least 30 minutes before meals

Nursing/Pharmacy Information

Advise patient to clear as much mucus as possible before inhalation treatments; for oral use, cromolyn powder is dissolved in water

Monitor periodic pulmonary function tests

Stability: Nebulizer solution is **compatible** with metaproterenol sulfate, isoproterenol hydrochloride, 0.25% isoetharine hydrochloride, epinephrine hydrochloride, terbutaline sulfate, and 20% acetylcysteine solution for at least 1 hour after their admixture; store nebulizer solution protected from direct light

Dosage Forms

Capsule: Oral (Gastrocrom®): 100 mg

Solution:

For nebulization: 10 mg/mL (2 mL)

Intal®: 10 mg/mL (2 mL)

Nasal (Nasalcrom®): 40 mg/mL (13 mL)

Ophthalmic (Crolom®): 4% (2.5 mL, 10 mL)

♦ **crotaline antivenin, polyvalent** *see* antivenin (*Crotalidae*) polyvalent *on page 54*

crotamiton *(kroe TAM i tonn)*

U.S. Brand Names Eurax® Topical

Generic Available No

Therapeutic Category Scabicides/Pediculicides

Use Treatment of scabies (*Sarcoptes scabiei*) in infants and children

Usual Dosage Scabicide: Children and Adults: Topical: Wash thoroughly and scrub away loose scales, then towel dry; apply a thin layer and massage drug onto skin of the entire body from the neck to the toes (with special attention to skin folds, creases, and interdigital spaces). Repeat application in 24 hours; patient should take a cleansing bath 48 hours after the final application.

Nursing/Pharmacy Information Lotion: Shake well before using; avoid contact with face, eyes, mucous membranes, and urethral meatus

Dosage Forms

Cream: 10% (60 g)

Lotion: 10% (60 mL, 454 mL)

♦ **crude coal tar** *see* coal tar *on page 162*

♦ **Cryocriptina** *see* bromocriptine *on page 93*

♦ **Cryopril** *see* captopril *on page 110*

♦ **Cryosolona** *see* methylprednisolone *on page 407*

♦ **Cryoval** *see* valproic acid and derivatives *on page 641*

♦ **Cryoxifeno** *see* tamoxifen *on page 592*

♦ **crystalline penicillin** *see* penicillin G, parenteral, aqueous *on page 475*

♦ **Crystamine®** *see* cyanocobalamin *on page 173*

♦ **Crysticillin® 300 A.S.** *(Discontinued)* *see page 743*
♦ **Crysticillin® 600 A.S.** *(Discontinued)* *see page 743*
♦ **Crysticillin® A.S.** *see* penicillin G procaine *on page 476*
♦ **Crystodigin®** *see* digitoxin *on page 202*
♦ **Crystodigin® 0.05 mg & 0.15 mg Tablet** *(Discontinued)* *see page 743*
♦ **CSP** *see* cellulose sodium phosphate *on page 127*
♦ **CTX** *see* cyclophosphamide *on page 175*
♦ **Cuprimine®** *see* penicillamine *on page 473*
♦ **Curretab® Oral** *see* medroxyprogesterone acetate *on page 389*
♦ **Cutivate™** *see* fluticasone (topical) *on page 280*
♦ **CYA** *see* cyclosporine *on page 176*

cyanide antidote kit (SYE a nide AN tee dote kit)

Generic Available Yes

Therapeutic Category Antidote

Use Treatment of cyanide poisoning

Usual Dosage Cyanide poisoning: 0.3 mL ampul of amyl nitrite is crushed every minute and vapor is inhaled for 15-30 seconds until an I.V. sodium nitrite infusion is available. Following administration of 300 mg I.V. sodium nitrite, inject 12.5 g sodium thiosulfate I.V. (over ~10 minutes), if needed; injection of both may be repeated at ½ the original dose.

Nursing/Pharmacy Information Sodium nitrate infusion is limited by hypotension; sodium thiosulfate infusion rate is 2.5-5 mL/minute

Dosage Forms Kit: Sodium nitrite 300 mg/10 mL (#2); sodium thiosulfate 12.5 g/50 mL (#2); amyl nitrite 0.3 mL (#12); also disposable syringes, stomach tube, tourniquet and instructions

cyanocobalamin (sye an oh koe BAL a min)

Synonyms vitamin B_{12}

U.S. Brand Names Berubigen®; Cobex®; Crystamine®; Cyanoject®; Cyomin®; Ener-B® [OTC]; Kaybovite-1000®; Redisol®; Rubramin-PC®; Sytobex®

Canadian Brand Names Rubramin®

Generic Available Yes

Therapeutic Category Vitamin, Water Soluble

Use Pernicious anemia; vitamin B_{12} deficiency; increased B_{12} requirements due to pregnancy, thyrotoxicosis, hemorrhage, malignancy, liver or kidney disease

Usual Dosage

Congenital pernicious anemia (if evidence of neurologic involvement): I.M.: 1000 mcg/day for at least 2 weeks; maintenance: 50 mcg/month

Vitamin B_{12} deficiency: I.M., S.C. (oral is not recommended due to poor absorption):

Children: 100 mcg/day for 10-15 days (total dose of 1-1.5 mg), then once or twice weekly for several months; may taper to 250-1000 mcg every month

Adults: 100 mcg/day for 6-7 days

Hematologic signs only:

Children: 10-50 mcg/day for 5-10 days, then maintenance: 100-250 mcg/ dose every 2-4 weeks

Adults: 30 mcg/day for 5-10 days, followed by 100-200 mcg/month

Methylmalonic aciduria: I.M.: 1 mg/day

Nursing/Pharmacy Information

I.M. or deep S.C. are preferred routes of administration; oral therapy is markedly inferior to parenteral therapy; folate therapy may be necessary in first month B_{12} replacement

Monitor serum potassium, erythrocyte and reticulocyte count, hemoglobin, hematocrit

Stability: Clear pink to red solutions are stable at room temperature; protect from light; **incompatible** with chlorpromazine, phytonadione, prochlorperazine, warfarin, ascorbic acid, dextrose, heavy metals, oxidizing or reducing agents

Dosage Forms

Gel, nasal:

Ener-B®: 400 mcg/0.1 mL

Nascobal®: 500 mcg/0.1 mL (5 mL)

Injection: 30 mcg/mL (30 mL); 100 mcg/mL (1 mL, 10 mL, 30 mL); 1000 mcg/ mL (1 mL, 10 mL, 30 mL)

Tablet [OTC]: 25 mcg, 50 mcg, 100 mcg, 250 mcg, 500 mcg, 1000 mcg

♦ **Cyanoject®** *see* cyanocobalamin *on page 173*

cyclandelate (sye KLAN de late)
Generic Available Yes

Therapeutic Category Vasodilator, Peripheral

Use Considered as "possibly effective" for adjunctive therapy in peripheral vascular disease and possibly senility due to cerebrovascular disease or multi-infarct dementia; migraine prophylaxis, vertigo, tinnitus, and visual disturbances secondary to cerebrovascular insufficiency and diabetic peripheral polyneuropathy

Usual Dosage Adults: Oral: Initial: 1.2-1.6 g/day in divided doses before meals and at bedtime until response; maintenance therapy: 400-800 mg/day in 2-4 divided doses; start with lowest dose in elderly due to hypotensive potential; decrease dose by 200 mg decrements to achieve minimal maintenance dose; improvement can usually be seen over weeks of therapy and prolonged use; short courses of therapy are usually ineffective and not recommended

Dosage Forms Tablet: 200 mg

cyclizine (SYE kli zeen)
U.S. Brand Names Marezine® Oral [OTC]

Generic Available No

Therapeutic Category Antihistamine

Use Prevention and treatment of nausea, vomiting and vertigo associated with motion sickness; control of postoperative nausea and vomiting

Usual Dosage Oral:
Children 6-12 years: 25 mg up to 3 times/day
Adults: 50 mg taken 30 minutes before departure, may repeat in 4-6 hours if needed, up to 200 mg/day

Nursing/Pharmacy Information Monitor CNS effects or unusual movements

Dosage Forms Tablet, as hydrochloride: 50 mg

cyclobenzaprine (sye kloe BEN za preen)
U.S. Brand Names Flexeril®

Canadian Brand Names Novo-Cycloprine®

Generic Available Yes

Therapeutic Category Skeletal Muscle Relaxant

Use Treatment of muscle spasm associated with acute painful musculoskeletal conditions; supportive therapy in tetanus

Usual Dosage Oral:
Children: Dosage has not been established
Adults: 20-40 mg/day in 2-4 divided doses; maximum dose: 60 mg/day

Nursing/Pharmacy Information Raise bed rails, institute safety measures, assist with ambulation

Dosage Forms Tablet, as hydrochloride: 10 mg

- ♦ **Cyclocort® Topical** *see* amcinonide *on page 36*
- ♦ **Cyclogyl®** *see* cyclopentolate *on page 174*
- ♦ **Cyclomen®** *see* danazol *on page 181*
- ♦ **Cyclomydril® Ophthalmic** *see* cyclopentolate and phenylephrine *on page 175*

cyclopentolate (sye kloe PEN toe late)
U.S. Brand Names AK-Pentolate®; Cyclogyl®; I-Pentolate®

Generic Available Yes

Therapeutic Category Anticholinergic Agent

Use Diagnostic procedures requiring mydriasis and cycloplegia

Usual Dosage Ophthalmic:
Infants: Instill 1 drop of 0.5% into each eye 5-10 minutes before examination
Children: Instill 1 drop of 0.5%, 1%, or 2% in eye followed by 1 drop of 0.5% or 1% in 5 minutes, if necessary
Adults: Instill 1 drop of 1% followed by another drop in 5 minutes; 2% solution in heavily pigmented iris

Nursing/Pharmacy Information
Ophthalmic: To avoid excessive systemic absorption, finger pressure should be applied on the lacrimal sac during and for 1-2 minutes following application

Stability: Store in tight containers

Dosage Forms Solution, ophthalmic, as hydrochloride: 0.5% (2 mL, 5 mL, 15 mL); 1% (2 mL, 5 mL, 15 mL); 2% (2 mL, 5 mL, 15 mL)

cyclopentolate and phenylephrine
(sye kloe PEN toe late & fen il EF rin)

Synonyms phenylephrine and cyclopentolate

U.S. Brand Names Cyclomydril® Ophthalmic

Generic Available No

Therapeutic Category Anticholinergic/Adrenergic Agonist

Use Induce mydriasis greater than that produced with cyclopentolate HCl alone

Usual Dosage Ophthalmic: Instill 1 drop every 5-10 minutes, not to exceed 3 instillations

Nursing/Pharmacy Information

Finger pressure should be applied to lacrimal sac for 1-2 minutes after instillation to decrease risk of absorption and systemic reactions

Stability: Store in tight containers and protect from light

Dosage Forms Solution, ophthalmic: Cyclopentolate hydrochloride 0.2% and phenylephrine hydrochloride 1% (2 mL, 5 mL)

cyclophosphamide (sye kloe FOS fa mide)

Synonyms CPM; CTX; CYT

U.S. Brand Names Cytoxan®; Neosar®

Canadian Brand Names Procytox®

Mexican Brand Names Genoxal; Ledoxina

Generic Available No

Therapeutic Category Antineoplastic Agent

Use Management of Hodgkin's disease, malignant lymphomas, multiple myeloma, leukemias, sarcomas, mycosis fungoides, neuroblastoma, ovarian carcinoma, breast carcinoma, a variety of other tumors; nephrotic syndrome, lupus erythematosus, severe rheumatoid arthritis, and rheumatoid vasculitis

Usual Dosage

Children (with no hematologic problems):

Induction:

Oral: 2-8 mg/kg/day

I.V.: 10-20 mg/kg/day divided once daily

Maintenance: Oral: 2-5 mg/kg (50-150 mg/m^2) twice weekly

Pediatric solid tumors: I.V.: 250-1800 mg/m^2 once daily for 1-5 days every 21-28 days

Adults with no hematologic problems:

Induction:

Oral: 1-5 mg/kg/day

I.V.: 40-50 mg/kg (1.5-1.8 g/m^2) in divided doses over 2-5 days

Maintenance:

Oral: 1-5 mg/kg/day

I.V.: 10-15 mg/kg (350-550 mg/m^2) every 7-10 days or 3-5 mg/kg (110-185 mg/m^2) twice weekly

Children and Adults: I.V.:

SLE: 500-750 mg/m^2 every month; maximum: 1 g/m^2

JRA/vasculitis: 10 mg/kg every 2 weeks

BMT conditioning regimen: I.V.: 50 mg/kg/day once daily for 3-4 days

Nephrotic syndrome: Oral: 2-3 mg/kg/day every day for up to 12 weeks when corticosteroids are unsuccessful

Dietary Considerations Tablets should be administered during or after meals

Nursing/Pharmacy Information

Encourage adequate hydration and frequent voiding to help prevent hemorrhagic cystitis; can be administered IVP, I.V. intermittent, or continuous infusion at a final concentration for administration of 20-25 mg/mL

Monitor CBC with differential and platelet count, ESR, BUN, urinalysis, serum electrolytes, serum creatinine

Stability: I.V. solution is usually reconstituted in 20 mg/mL concentrations; solutions may be administered I.V., I.M., intraperitoneally, or intrapleurally; they may be infused I.V. in D$_5$W, 0.9% sodium chloride, D$_5$LR, lactated Ringer's, or 0.45% sodium chloride; prepared solutions should be used within 24 hours or may be stored up to 6 days under refrigeration; oral elixir may be prepared from the injectable preparation and is stable for 14 days if refrigerated

Dosage Forms

Powder for injection: 100 mg, 200 mg, 500 mg, 1 g, 2 g

Powder for injection, lyophilized: 100 mg, 200 mg, 500 mg, 1 g, 2 g

Tablet: 25 mg, 50 mg

cycloserine (sye kloe SER een)

U.S. Brand Names Seromycin® Pulvules®

Generic Available No

Therapeutic Category Antibiotic, Miscellaneous

Use Adjunctive treatment in pulmonary or extrapulmonary tuberculosis; treatment of acute urinary tract infections caused by *E. coli* or *Enterobacter* sp when less toxic conventional therapy has failed or is contraindicated

Usual Dosage Oral:

Tuberculosis:

Children: 10-20 mg/kg/day in 2 divided doses up to 1000 mg/day

Adults: Initial: 250 mg every 12 hours for 14 days, then administer 500 mg to 1 g/day in 2 divided doses

Urinary tract infection: Adults: 250 mg every 12 hours for 14 days

Dietary Considerations May be administered with food; may increase vitamin B_{12} and folic acid dietary requirements

Nursing/Pharmacy Information

Some of the neurotoxic effects may be relieved or prevented by the concomitant administration of pyridoxine

Monitor periodic renal, hepatic, hematological tests, and plasma cycloserine concentrations

Dosage Forms Capsule: 250 mg

♦ **Cyclospasmol®** *(Discontinued) see page 743*

♦ **cyclosporin A** *see* cyclosporine *on page 176*

cyclosporine (SYE kloe spor een)

Synonyms CYA; cyclosporin A

U.S. Brand Names Neoral®; Sandimmune®; SangCya™

Mexican Brand Names Consupren; Sandimmun Neoral®

Generic Available No

Therapeutic Category Immunosuppressant Agent

Use Immunosuppressant used with corticosteroids to prevent graft vs host disease in patients with kidney, liver, heart, and bone marrow transplants; has been used in the treatment of nephrotic syndrome in patients with documented focal glomerulosclerosis when corticosteroids and cyclophosphamide were unsuccessful; monotherapy or in combination with methotrexate for treatment of severe active rheumatoid arthritis where the disease has not adequately responded to methotrexate

Usual Dosage Children and Adults:

Oral: Initial: 14-18 mg/kg/dose daily, beginning 4-12 hours prior to organ transplantation; maintenance: 5-10 mg/kg/day

I.V.: Initial: 5-6 mg/kg/day in divided doses every 12-24 hours; patients should be switched to oral cyclosporine as soon as possible

Dietary Considerations Grapefruit juice will increase absorption; mix at room temperature, may use milk, chocolate milk, or orange juice

Nursing/Pharmacy Information

Use glass dropper or container (not plastic or styrofoam) when administering this medication orally; do not allow to stand before drinking; rinse with more diluent to ensure that the total dose is taken; after use, dry outside of pipette, do not rinse with water or other cleaning agents; adequate airway and other supportive measures and agents for treating anaphylaxis should be present when I.V. cyclosporine is administered I.V.; cyclosporine can be administered by I.V. intermittent infusion or continuous infusion; for intermittent infusion, administer over 2-6 hours at a final concentration not to exceed 2.5 mg/mL

Monitor cyclosporine levels, serum electrolytes, renal function, hepatic function, blood pressure, pulse

Stability: Do **not** store oral solution in the refrigerator; use contents of oral solution within 2 months after opening; I.V. cyclosporine prepared in normal saline or D_5W is stable 6 hours in PVC or 24 hours in a glass container or PAB container or Excell® container; do not freeze

Dosage Forms

Capsule (Sandimmune®): 25 mg, 100 mg

Soft gel (Sandimmune®): 50 mg

Soft gel for microemulsion (Neoral®): 25 mg, 100 mg

Injection (Sandimmune®): 50 mg/mL (5 mL)

Solution:

Oral (Sandimmune®): 100 mg/mL (50 mL)

Oral for microemulsion (Neoral®): 100 mg/mL (50 mL)

- **Cycofed® Pediatric** *see guaifenesin, pseudoephedrine, and codeine on page 304*
- **Cycrin® 10 mg Tablet *(Discontinued)*** *see page 743*
- **Cycrin® Oral** *see medroxyprogesterone acetate on page 389*
- **Cyklokapron®** *see tranexamic acid on page 621*
- **Cylert®** *see pemoline on page 473*
- **Cylex® [OTC]** *see benzocaine on page 79*
- **Cymevene** *see ganciclovir on page 287*
- **Cyomin®** *see cyanocobalamin on page 173*

cyproheptadine (si proe HEP ta deen)
U.S. Brand Names Periactin®
Canadian Brand Names PMS-Cyproheptadine
Generic Available Yes
Therapeutic Category Antihistamine
Use Perennial and seasonal allergic rhinitis and other allergic symptoms including urticaria
Usual Dosage Oral:
  Children: 0.25 mg/kg/day in 2-3 divided doses **or**
    2-6 years: 2 mg every 8-12 hours (not to exceed 12 mg/day)
    7-14 years: 4 mg every 8-12 hours (not to exceed 16 mg/day)
  Adults: 12-16 mg/day every 8 hours (not to exceed 0.5 mg/kg/day)
Dietary Considerations May be administered with food, water, or milk
Nursing/Pharmacy Information Monitor for relief of symptoms, weight, eating habits
Dosage Forms Cyproheptadine hydrochloride:
  Syrup: 2 mg/5 mL with alcohol 5% (473 mL)
  Tablet: 4 mg

cyproterone *(Canada only)* (sye PROE ter one)
Canadian Brand Names Androcur®; Androcur® Depot
Generic Available No
Therapeutic Category Antiandrogen; Progestin
Use Palliative treatment of patients with advanced prostatic carcinoma
Usual Dosage Adults:
  I.M.: 300 mg (3 mL) once a week
  Oral: 200-300 mg divided into 2-3 doses and taken after meals
Dosage Forms
  Injection, as acetate: 100 mg/mL (3 mL)
  Tablet, as acetate: 50 mg

- **Cystadane®** *see betaine anhydrous on page 84*
- **Cystagon®** *see cysteamine on page 177*

cysteamine (sis TEE a meen)
U.S. Brand Names Cystagon®
Generic Available No
Therapeutic Category Urinary Tract Product
Use Nephropathic cystinosis in children and adults
Usual Dosage Initiate therapy with 1/4 to 1/8 of maintenance dose; titrate slowly upward over 4-6 weeks
  Children <12 years: Oral: Maintenance: 1.3 g/m²/day divided into 4 doses
  Children >12 years and Adults (>110 lbs): Oral: 2 g/day in 4 divided doses; dosage may in increased to 1.95 g/m²/day if cystine levels are <1 nmol/¹/₂ cystine/mg protein, although intolerance and incidence of adverse events may be increased
Dosage Forms Capsule, as bitartrate: 50 mg, 150 mg

cysteine (SIS teen)
Generic Available Yes
Therapeutic Category Nutritional Supplement
Use Total parenteral nutrition of infants as an additive to meet the I.V. amino acid requirements
Usual Dosage Combine 500 mg of cysteine with 12.5 g of amino acid, then dilute with 50% dextrose
Nursing/Pharmacy Information Avoid excessive heat, do not freeze
Dosage Forms Injection, as hydrochloride: 50 mg/mL (10 mL)

- **Cystografin®** *see radiological/contrast media (ionic) on page 539*
- **Cystospaz®** *see hyoscyamine on page 329*

- **Cystospaz-M®** *see* hyoscyamine *on page 329*
- **CYT** *see* cyclophosphamide *on page 175*
- **Cytadren®** *see* aminoglutethimide *on page 38*

cytarabine (sye TARE a been)

Synonyms arabinosylcytosine; ARA-C; cytosine arabinosine

U.S. Brand Names Cytosar-U®; Tarabine® PFS

Generic Available Yes

Therapeutic Category Antineoplastic Agent

Use In combination regimens for the treatment of leukemias and non-Hodgkin's lymphomas

Usual Dosage Children and Adults (refer to individual protocols):

Induction remission:

I.T.: 5-75 mg/m² once daily for 4 days or 1 every 4 days until CNS

I.V.: 200 mg/m²/day for 5 days at 2-week intervals; 100-200 mg/m²/day for 5- to 10-day therapy course or every day until remission administered I.V. continuous drip, or in 2-3 divided doses findings normalize

Maintenance remission:

I.M., S.C.: 1-1.5 mg/kg single dose for maintenance at 1- to 4-week intervals

I.V.: 70-200 mg/m²/day for 2-5 days at monthly intervals

High-dose therapies: Doses as high as 1-3 g/m² have been used for refractory or secondary leukemias or refractory non-Hodgkins lymphoma; dosages of 3 g/m² every 12 hours for up to 12 doses have been used

Nursing/Pharmacy Information

Administer corticosteroid eye drops around the clock prior to, during, and after high-dose Ara-C for prophylaxis of conjunctivitis; pyridoxine has been administered on days of high-dose Ara-C therapy for prophylaxis of CNS toxicity. Can be administered I.M., IVP, I.V. infusion, or S.C. at a concentration not to exceed 100 mg/mL; high-dose regimens are usually administered by I.V. infusion over 1-3 hours or as I.V. continuous infusion; for I.T. use, reconstitute with preservative free saline or preservative free lactated Ringer's solution.

Monitor liver function tests, CBC with differential and platelet count, serum creatinine, BUN, serum uric acid

Stability: Keep in refrigerator until reconstituted; after reconstitution, solutions remain stable for 48 hours at room temperature; discard hazy solutions; I.V. infusion solution in normal saline or D_5W solution is stable for 192 hours at room temperature; I.T. Ara-C is **compatible** with methotrexate and hydrocortisone mixed in the same syringe. **Compatible** with vincristine, potassium chloride, calcium, magnesium, and idarubicin. **Incompatible** with 5-FU, gentamicin, heparin, insulin, methylprednisolone, nafcillin, oxacillin, penicillin G sodium. For intrathecal administration, use Elliott's B solution, 0.9% sodium chloride, or patient's CSF as diluent.

Dosage Forms Cytarabine hydrochloride:

Powder for injection: 100 mg, 500 mg, 1 g, 2 g

Powder for injection (Cytosar-U®): 100 mg, 500 mg, 1 g, 2 g

cytarabine (liposomal) *New Drug*

(sye TARE a been lip po SOE mal)

U.S. Brand Names DepoCyt™

Generic Available No

Therapeutic Category Antineoplastic Agent, Antimetabolite (Purine)

Use Intrathecal treatment of lymphomatous meningitis

Usual Dosage Adults:

Induction: 50 mg intrathecally every 14 days for a total of 2 doses (weeks 1 and 3)

Consolidation: 50 mg intrathecally every 14 days for 3 doses (weeks 5, 7, and 9), followed by an additional dose at week 13

Maintenance: 50 mg intrathecally every 28 days for 4 doses (weeks 17, 21, 25, and 29)

If drug-related neurotoxicity develops, the dose should be reduced to 25 mg; if toxicity persists, treatment with liposomal cytarabine should be discontinued

Note: Patients should be started on dexamethasone 4 mg twice daily (oral or I.V.) for 5 days, beginning on the day of liposomal cytarabine injection

Dosage Forms Injection: 10 mg/mL (5 mL)

- **CytoGam™** *see* cytomegalovirus immune globulin (intravenous-human) *on page 179*

cytomegalovirus immune globulin (intravenous-human)

(sye toe meg a low VYE rus i MYUN GLOB yoo lin in tra VEE nus, HYU man)

Synonyms CMV-IGIV

U.S. Brand Names CytoGam™

Generic Available No

Therapeutic Category Immune Globulin

Use Attenuation of primary CMV disease associated with kidney transplantation

Usual Dosage I.V.: Initial: Administer at 15 mg/kg/hour, then increase to 30 mg/kg/hour after 30 minutes if no untoward reactions, then increase to 60 mg/kg/hour after another 30 minutes, volume not to exceed 75 mL/hour

Nursing/Pharmacy Information

I.V. use only; administer as separate infusion if pre-existing line; must be used diluted no more than 1:2

Stability: Use reconstituted product within 6 hours

Dosage Forms Powder for injection, lyophilized, detergent treated: 2500 mg ±250 mg (50 mL)

- ◆ **Cytomel® Oral** *see* liothyronine *on page 371*
- ◆ **Cytosar-U®** *see* cytarabine *on page 178*
- ◆ **cytosine arabinosine** *see* cytarabine *on page 178*
- ◆ **Cytotec®** *see* misoprostol *on page 417*
- ◆ **Cytovene®** *see* ganciclovir *on page 287*
- ◆ **Cytoxan®** *see* cyclophosphamide *on page 175*
- ◆ **D₃** *see* cholecalciferol *on page 146*
- ◆ **25-D₃** *see* calcifediol *on page 101*
- ◆ **d-3-mercaptovaline** *see* penicillamine *on page 473*
- ◆ **d4T** *see* stavudine *on page 579*
- ◆ **Dabex** *see* metformin *on page 398*

dacarbazine (da KAR ba zeen)

Synonyms DIC; imidazole carboxamide

U.S. Brand Names DTIC-Dome®

Generic Available Yes

Therapeutic Category Antineoplastic Agent

Use Singly or in various combination therapy to treat malignant melanoma, Hodgkin's disease, soft-tissue sarcomas (fibrosarcomas, rhabdomyosarcoma), islet cell carcinoma, medullary carcinoma of the thyroid, and neuroblastoma

Usual Dosage Refer to individual protocols. I.V.:

Children:

Solid tumors: 200-470 mg/m²/day over 5 days every 21-28 days

Neuroblastoma: 800-900 mg/m² as a single dose every 3-4 weeks in combination therapy

Adults:

Malignant melanoma: 2-4.5 mg/kg/day for 10 days, repeat in 4 weeks or may use 250 mg/m²/day for 5 days, repeat in 3 weeks

Hodgkin's disease: 150 mg/m²/day for 5 days, repeat every 4 weeks or 375 mg/m² on day 1, repeat in 15 days of each 28-day cycle in combination with other agents

Nursing/Pharmacy Information

Local pain, burning sensation, and irritation at the injection site may be relieved by local application of hot packs, slowing the I.V. rate, or further dilution in I.V. fluid; administer by slow IVP over 2-3 minutes at a concentration not to exceed 10 mg/mL or by I.V. infusion over 15-30 minutes

Monitor CBC with differential, erythrocyte, and platelet count, liver function tests

Stability: Vials require refrigeration and are stable for up to 72 hours under refrigeration and up to 8 hours at room temperature once reconstituted. DTIC® should be protected from light. Solutions further diluted in D₅W or normal saline are stable under refrigeration for up to 24 hours

Dosage Forms Injection: 100 mg (10 mL, 20 mL); 200 mg (20 mL, 30 mL); 500 mg (50 mL)

daclizumab (da KLIK si mab)

U.S. Brand Names Zenapax®

Generic Available No

Therapeutic Category Immunosuppressant Agent

(Continued)

daclizumab (Continued)

Use In combination with an immunosuppressive regimen, including cyclosporine and corticosteroids, for prophylaxis of acute organ rejection in patients receiving renal transplants

Usual Dosage Children and Adults: IVPB: 1 mg/kg, used as part of an immunosuppressive regimen that includes cyclosporine and corticosteroids for a total of 5 doses; give the first dose ≤24 hours before transplantation. The 4 remaining doses should be administered at intervals of 14 days.

Dosage Forms Injection: 5 mg/mL (5 mL)

◆ **Dacodyl® [OTC]** see bisacodyl on page 88

dactinomycin (dak ti noe MYE sin)

Synonyms ACT; actinomycin D

U.S. Brand Names Cosmegen®

Generic Available No

Therapeutic Category Antineoplastic Agent

Use Management, either alone or in combination with other treatment modalities of Wilms' tumor, rhabdomyosarcoma, neuroblastoma, retinoblastoma, Ewing's sarcoma, trophoblastic neoplasms, testicular carcinoma, and other malignancies

Usual Dosage Refer to individual protocols; dosage should be based on body surface area in obese or edematous patients

Children >6 months and Adults: I.V.: 15 mcg/kg/day or 400-600 mcg/m^2/day for 5 days, may repeat every 3-6 weeks; or 2.5 mg/m^2 administered in divided doses over 1 week; 0.75-2 mg/m^2 as a single dose administered at intervals of 1-4 weeks have been used

Nursing/Pharmacy Information

For I.V. administration only; since drug is extremely irritating to tissues, **do not administer I.M. or S.C.**; administer IVP over a few minutes at a concentration not to exceed 500 mcg/mL through a freely flowing I.V.

Monitor CBC with differential and platelet count, liver function tests, and renal function tests

Stability: Although chemically stable after reconstitution, there is no preservative present, discard any used portion; use of a diluent containing preservatives to reconstitute will result in a precipitate. Reconstituted solutions should be discarded within a few hours; may exhibit considerable binding to Millex or Millex GV filters; binds to cellulose filters, so avoid in-line filtration; adsorbs to glass and plastic so dactinomycin should not be administered by continuous or intermittent infusion; use of a diluent containing preservatives for reconstitution may result in a precipitate

Dosage Forms Powder for injection, lyophilized: 0.5 mg

◆ **Dafloxen®** see naproxen on page 432
◆ **D.A.II® Tablet** see chlorpheniramine, phenylephrine, and methscopolamine on page 141
◆ **Dairy Ease® [OTC]** see lactase on page 357
◆ **Dakin's solution** see sodium hypochlorite solution on page 572
◆ **Dakrina® Ophthalmic Solution [OTC]** see artificial tears on page 59
◆ **Daktarin** see miconazole on page 413
◆ **Dalacin® C** see clindamycin on page 156
◆ **Dalacin® C Topical** see clindamycin on page 156
◆ **Dalacin® C Vaginal Cream** see clindamycin on page 156
◆ **Dalgan®** see dezocine on page 195
◆ **Dalisol** see leucovorin on page 362
◆ **Dallergy®** see chlorpheniramine, phenylephrine, and methscopolamine on page 141
◆ **Dallergy-D® Syrup** see chlorpheniramine and phenylephrine on page 139
◆ **Dalmane®** see flurazepam on page 278
◆ **d-alpha tocopherol** see vitamin E on page 652

dalteparin (dal TE pa rin)

U.S. Brand Names Fragmin®

Generic Available No

Therapeutic Category Anticoagulant

Use Prevent deep vein thrombosis following abdominal surgery

Usual Dosage Adults: S.C.: 2500 units 1-2 hours prior to surgery, then once daily for 5-10 days postoperatively

Dosage Forms Injection: Prefilled syringe: 2500 units (16 mg) in 0.2 mL

♦ **Damason-P®** *see* hydrocodone and aspirin *on page 319*
♦ **D-Amp®** *(Discontinued) see page 743*

danaparoid (da NAP a roid)
U.S. Brand Names Orgaran®
Generic Available No
Therapeutic Category Anticoagulant
Use Prophylaxis of postoperative deep vein thrombosis (DVT)
Usual Dosage Adults: S.C.: 750 anti-Xa units twice daily beginning 1-4 hours preoperatively, and then not sooner than 2 hours hours after surgery
Dosage Forms Injection, as sodium: 750 anti-Xa units/0.6 mL

danazol (DA na zole)
U.S. Brand Names Danocrine®
Canadian Brand Names Cyclomen®
Mexican Brand Names Ladogal; Norciden; Zoldan-A
Generic Available Yes
Therapeutic Category Androgen
Use Treatment of endometriosis, fibrocystic breast disease, and hereditary angi-oedema
Usual Dosage Adults: Oral:
  Endometriosis: 100-400 mg twice daily
  Fibrocystic breast disease: 50-200 mg twice daily for 2-6 months
  Hereditary angioedema: 400-600 mg/day in 2-3 divided doses
Nursing/Pharmacy Information Notify physician if masculinity effects occur
Dosage Forms Capsule: 50 mg, 100 mg, 200 mg

♦ **Danex® Shampoo** *(Discontinued) see page 743*
♦ **Danocrine®** *see* danazol *on page 181*
♦ **Dantrium®** *see* dantrolene *on page 181*

dantrolene (DAN troe leen)
U.S. Brand Names Dantrium®
Generic Available No
Therapeutic Category Skeletal Muscle Relaxant
Use Treatment of spasticity associated with upper motor neuron disorders such as spinal cord injury, stroke, cerebral palsy, or multiple sclerosis; also used as treatment of malignant hyperthermia
Usual Dosage
  Spasticity: Oral:
    Children: Initial: 0.5 mg/kg/dose twice daily, increase frequency to 3-4 times/day at 4- to 7-day intervals, then increase dose by 0.5 mg/kg to a maximum of 3 mg/kg/dose 2-4 times/day up to 400 mg/day
    Adults: 25 mg/day to start, increase frequency to 3-4 times/day, then increase dose by 25 mg every 4-7 days to a maximum of 100 mg 2-4 times/day or 400 mg/day
  Hyperthermia: Children and Adults:
    Oral: 4-8 mg/kg/day in 4 divided doses
    I.V.: 1 mg/kg; may repeat dose up to cumulative dose of 10 mg/kg (mean effective dose: 2.5 mg/kg), then switch to oral dosage
Nursing/Pharmacy Information
  Avoid extravasation as is a tissue irritant; reconstitute by adding 60 mL sterile water (**not bacteriostatic water for injection**); administer by rapid I.V. injection; for infusion, **do not** further dilute with normal saline or dextrose; place solution in plastic container for continuous infusion
  Motor performance should be monitored for therapeutic outcomes; nausea, vomiting, and liver function tests should be monitored for potential hepatotoxicity
  Stability: Reconstitute vial by adding 60 mL of sterile water for injection USP (**not bacteriostatic water for injection**); protect from light; use within 6 hours; avoid glass bottles for I.V. infusion
Dosage Forms Dantrolene sodium:
  Capsule: 25 mg, 50 mg, 100 mg
  Powder for injection: 20 mg

♦ **Daonil** *see* glyburide *on page 294*
♦ **Dapa® [OTC]** *see* acetaminophen *on page 13*
♦ **Dapacin® [OTC]** *see* acetaminophen *on page 13*
♦ **Dapacin® Cold Capsule [OTC]** *see* chlorpheniramine, phenylpropanolamine, and acetaminophen *on page 142*
♦ **Dapex-37.5®** *(Discontinued) see page 743*

dapiprazole (DA pi pray zole)
U.S. Brand Names Rēv-Eyes™
Generic Available No
Therapeutic Category Alpha-Adrenergic Blocking Agent
Use Treatment of iatrogenically induced mydriasis produced by adrenergic or parasympatholytic agents
Usual Dosage Ophthalmic: Instill 2 drops followed 5 minutes later by an additional 2 drops applied to the conjunctiva
Nursing/Pharmacy Information
  Finger pressure should be applied to lacrimal sac for 1-2 minutes after instillation to decrease risk of absorption and systemic reactions; do not touch eye with dropper
  Stability: After reconstitution, drops are stable at room temperature for 21 days
Dosage Forms Powder, lyophilized, as hydrochloride: 25 mg [0.5% solution when mixed with supplied diluent]

dapsone (DAP sone)
Synonyms DDS; diaminodiphenylsulfone
U.S. Brand Names Avlosulfon®
Generic Available Yes
Therapeutic Category Sulfone
Use Treatment of leprosy due to susceptible strains of *M. leprae*; treatment of dermatitis herpetiformis; prophylaxis against *Pneumocystis carinii* in children who cannot tolerate sulfamethoxazole/trimethoprim or aerosolized pentamidine
Usual Dosage Oral:
  Children: Leprosy: 1-2 mg/kg/24 hours; maximum: 100 mg/day
  Adults:
    Leprosy: 50-100 mg/day
    Dermatitis herpetiformis: Start at 50 mg/day, increase to 300 mg/day, or higher to achieve full control, reduce dosage to minimum level as soon as possible
Dietary Considerations Do not administer with antacids, alkaline foods or drugs (may decrease dapsone absorption)
Nursing/Pharmacy Information
  Monitor for signs of jaundice and hemolysis
  Stability: Protect from light
Dosage Forms Tablet: 25 mg, 100 mg

- **Daranide®** *see* dichlorphenamide *on page 198*
- **Daraprim®** *see* pyrimethamine *on page 534*
- **Darbid® Tablet *(Discontinued)*** *see page 743*
- **Daricon® *(Discontinued)*** *see page 743*
- **Darvocet-N®** *see* propoxyphene and acetaminophen *on page 526*
- **Darvocet-N® 100** *see* propoxyphene and acetaminophen *on page 526*
- **Darvon®** *see* propoxyphene *on page 526*
- **Darvon® 32 mg Capsule *(Discontinued)*** *see page 743*
- **Darvon® Compound-65 Pulvules®** *see* propoxyphene and aspirin *on page 526*
- **Darvon-N®** *see* propoxyphene *on page 526*
- **Darvon-N® Oral Suspension *(Discontinued)*** *see page 743*
- **Datril® Extra Strength *(Discontinued)*** *see page 743*
- **daunomycin** *see* daunorubicin hydrochloride *on page 183*

daunorubicin citrate (liposomal)
(daw noe ROO bi sin SI trate lip po SOE mal)
U.S. Brand Names DaunoXome®
Generic Available No
Therapeutic Category Antineoplastic Agent
Use Advanced HIV-associated Kaposi's sarcoma
Usual Dosage I.V. (refer to individual protocols):
  Children:
    ALL combination therapy: Remission induction: 25-45 mg/m^2 on day 1 every week for 4 cycles **or** 30-45 mg/m^2/day for 3 days
    In children <2 years or <0.5 m^2, daunorubicin should be based on weight (mg/kg): 1 mg/kg per protocol with frequency dependent on regimen employed
    Cumulative dose should not exceed 300 mg/m^2 in children >2 years or 10 mg/kg in children <2 years

Adults: 30-60 mg/m²/day for 3-5 days, repeat dose in 3-4 weeks
Single agent induction for AML: 60 mg/m²/day for 3 days; repeat every 3-4 weeks
Combination therapy induction for AML: 45 mg/m²/day for 3 days of the first course of induction therapy; subsequent courses: Every day for 2 days
ALL combination therapy: 45 mg/m²/day for 3 days
Cumulative dose should not exceed 400-600 mg/m²

Dosage Forms Injection: 2 mg/mL equivalent to 50 mg daunorubicin base

daunorubicin hydrochloride
(daw noe ROO bi sin hye droe KLOR ide)
Synonyms daunomycin; DNR; rubidomycin
U.S. Brand Names Cerubidine®
Mexican Brand Names Rubilem; Trixilem
Generic Available No
Therapeutic Category Antineoplastic Agent
Use In combination with other agents in the treatment of leukemias (ALL, AML)
Usual Dosage I.V.:
Children:
Combination therapy: Remission induction for ALL: 25-45 mg/m² on day 1 every week for 4 cycles
<2 years or <0.5 m²: Manufacturer recommends that the dose is based on body weight rather than body surface area
Adults: 30-60 mg/m²/day for 3-5 days, repeat dose in 3-4 weeks; total cumulative dose should not exceed 400-600 mg/m²
Single agent induction for AML: 60 mg/m²/day for 3 days; repeat every 3-4 weeks
Combination therapy induction for AML: 45 mg/m²/day for 3 days; Subsequent courses: Every day for 2 days
Combination therapy: Remission induction for ALL: 45 mg/m² on days 1, 2, and 3
Nursing/Pharmacy Information
Drug is very irritating, do not inject I.M. or S.C.; avoid extravasation; for extravasation, infiltrate area with hydrocortisone and/or sodium bicarbonate and apply cold packs for 15 minutes 4 times/day
Monitor CBC with differential and platelet count, liver function test, EKG, ventricular ejection fraction, renal function test
Stability: Reconstituted solution is stable for 24 hours at room temperature and 48 hours when refrigerated; unstable in solutions with a pH >8; reconstituted solution should be protected from sunlight; **incompatible** with sodium bicarbonate and 5-FU, heparin, dexamethasone
Dosage Forms Powder for injection, lyophilized: 20 mg

- **Decholin®** *see* dehydrocholic acid *on page 184*
- **Declomycin®** *see* demeclocycline *on page 185*
- **Decofed® Syrup [OTC]** *see* pseudoephedrine *on page 530*
- **Decohistine® DH** *see* chlorpheniramine, pseudoephedrine, and codeine *on page 143*
- **Decohistine® Expectorant** *see* guaifenesin, pseudoephedrine, and codeine *on page 304*
- **Deconamine® SR** *see* chlorpheniramine and pseudoephedrine *on page 140*
- **Deconamine® Syrup [OTC]** *see* chlorpheniramine and pseudoephedrine *on page 140*
- **Deconamine® Tablet [OTC]** *see* chlorpheniramine and pseudoephedrine *on page 140*
- **Deconsal® II** *see* guaifenesin and pseudoephedrine *on page 302*
- **Deconsal® Sprinkle®** *see* guaifenesin and phenylephrine *on page 301*
- **Decorex** *see* dexamethasone (systemic) *on page 190*
- **Defen-LA®** *see* guaifenesin and pseudoephedrine *on page 302*

deferoxamine (de fer OKS a meen)

U.S. Brand Names Desferal® Mesylate
Generic Available No
Therapeutic Category Antidote
Use Acute iron intoxication; chronic iron overload secondary to multiple transfusions; diagnostic test for iron overload

> **Investigational use:** Treatment of aluminum accumulation in renal failure

Usual Dosage

Children and Adults: Acute iron toxicity: I.V. route is used when severe toxicity is evidenced by systemic symptoms (coma, shock, metabolic acidosis, or severe gastrointestinal bleeding) or potentially severe intoxications (serum iron level >500 µg/dL). When severe symptoms are not present, the I.M. route may be preferred; however, the use of deferoxamine in situations where the serum iron concentration is <500 µg/dL or when severe toxicity is not evident is a subject of some clinical debate.

Dose: 15 mg/kg/hour (although rates up to 40-50 mg/kg/hour have been given in patients with massive iron intoxication); maximum recommended dose: 6 g/day (however, doses as high as 16-37 g have been administered)

Children:
Chronic iron overload:
I.V.: 15 mg/kg/hour
S.C.: 20-40 mg/kg/day over 8-12 hours
Aluminum-induced bone disease: 20-40 mg/kg every hemodialysis treatment, frequency dependent on clinical status of the patient

Adults:
Chronic iron overload:
I.M.: 0.5-1 g every day
S.C.: 1-2 g every day over 8-24 hours

Nursing/Pharmacy Information

May cause the urine to turn a reddish color; add 2 mL sterile water to 500 mg vial; for I.M. or S.C. administration, no further dilution is required; for I.V. infusion, dilute in dextrose, normal saline, or lactated Ringer's; 10 mg/mL (maximum: 25 mg/mL); maximum rate of infusion: 15 mg/kg/hour

Monitor serum iron, total iron binding capacity; ophthalmologic exam and audiometry with chronic therapy

Stability: Protect from light; reconstituted solutions (sterile water) may be stored at room temperature for 7 days

Dosage Forms Powder for injection, as mesylate: 500 mg

- **Deficol® [OTC]** *see* bisacodyl *on page 88*
- **Degas® [OTC]** *see* simethicone *on page 566*
- **Degest® 2 Ophthalmic [OTC]** *see* naphazoline *on page 431*
- **Dehist® *(Discontinued)*** *see page 743*
- **Dehydral™** *see* methenamine *on page 400*
- **Dehydrobenzperidol** *see* droperidol *on page 223*

dehydrocholic acid (dee hye droe KOE lik AS id)

U.S. Brand Names Cholan-HMB®; Decholin®
Generic Available Yes
Therapeutic Category Laxative
Use Relief of constipation; adjunct to various biliary tract conditions

Usual Dosage Children >12 years and Adults: Oral: 250-500 mg 2-3 times/day after meals up to 1.5 g/day
Dietary Considerations Administer on empty stomach for rapid effect
Dosage Forms Tablet: 250 mg

- ◆ **Deladumone®** see estradiol and testosterone on page 243
- ◆ **Del Aqua-5® Gel** see benzoyl peroxide on page 81
- ◆ **Del Aqua-10® Gel** see benzoyl peroxide on page 81
- ◆ **Delatest® Injection** see testosterone on page 598
- ◆ **Delatestryl® Injection** see testosterone on page 598

delavirdine (de la VIR deen)
Synonyms U-90152S
U.S. Brand Names Rescriptor®
Generic Available No
Therapeutic Category Antiviral Agent
Use Treatment of HIV-1 infection in combination with appropriate antiretrovirals
Usual Dosage Adults: Oral: 400 mg 3 times/day
Dosage Forms Tablet: 100 mg

- ◆ **Delcort® Topical** see hydrocortisone (topical) on page 324
- ◆ **Delfen® [OTC]** see nonoxynol 9 on page 446
- ◆ **Del-Mycin® Topical** see erythromycin (ophthalmic/topical) on page 239
- ◆ **Delsym® [OTC]** see dextromethorphan on page 194
- ◆ **Delta-Cortef® Oral** see prednisolone (systemic) on page 514
- ◆ **deltacortisone** see prednisone on page 515
- ◆ **Delta-D®** see cholecalciferol on page 146
- ◆ **deltadehydrocortisone** see prednisone on page 515
- ◆ **deltahydrocortisone** see prednisolone (systemic) on page 514
- ◆ **Deltalin® Capsule (Discontinued)** see page 743
- ◆ **Deltasone®** see prednisone on page 515
- ◆ **Delta-Tritex® Topical** see triamcinolone (topical) on page 624
- ◆ **Del-Vi-A®** see vitamin A on page 650
- ◆ **Demadex®** see torsemide on page 619
- ◆ **Demazin® Syrup [OTC]** see chlorpheniramine and phenylpropanolamine on page 139

demecarium (dem e KARE ee um)
U.S. Brand Names Humorsol® Ophthalmic
Generic Available No
Therapeutic Category Cholinesterase Inhibitor
Use Management of chronic simple glaucoma, chronic and acute angle-closure glaucoma; counter effects of cycloplegics
Usual Dosage Ophthalmic:
Children: Instill 1 drop into eyes twice weekly to a maximum dosage of 1 or 2 drops twice daily for up to 4 months
Adults: Instill 1-2 drops into eyes twice weekly to a maximum dosage of 1 or 2 drops twice daily for up to 4 months
Nursing/Pharmacy Information
Do not touch dropper to eye; transient burning or stinging may occur; do not use more often than directed
Stability: Protect from heat
Dosage Forms Solution, ophthalmic, as bromide: 0.125% (5 mL); 0.25% (5 mL)

demeclocycline (dem e kloe SYE kleen)
Synonyms demethylchlortetracycline
U.S. Brand Names Declomycin®
Mexican Brand Names Ledermicina
Generic Available No
Therapeutic Category Tetracycline Derivative
Use Treatment of susceptible bacterial infections (acne, gonorrhea, pertussis, chronic bronchitis, and urinary tract infections) caused by both gram-negative and gram-positive organisms; treatment of chronic syndrome of inappropriate antidiuretic hormone (SIADH) secretion
Usual Dosage Oral:
Children ≥8 years: 8-12 mg/kg/day divided every 6-12 hours
Adults: 150 mg 4 times/day or 300 mg twice daily
Uncomplicated gonorrhea: 600 mg stat, 300 mg every 12 hours for 4 days (3 g total)
(Continued)

demeclocycline *(Continued)*

SIADH: Initial: 900-1200 mg/day or 13-15 mg/kg/day divided every 6-8 hours, then decrease to 0.6-0.9 g/day

Dietary Considerations Should be administered 2 hours before or after milk, milk formulas, or dairy products, with plenty of fluid

Nursing/Pharmacy Information
Monitor CBC, renal and hepatic function
Stability: Tetracyclines form toxic products when outdated or when exposed to light, heat, or humidity (Fanconi-like syndrome)

Dosage Forms Demeclocycline hydrochloride:
Capsule: 150 mg
Tablet: 150 mg, 300 mg

- **Demerol®** *see* meperidine *on page 392*
- **4-demethoxydaunorubicin** *see* idarubicin *on page 333*
- **demethylchlortetracycline** *see* demeclocycline *on page 185*
- **Demolox** *see* amoxapine *on page 42*
- **Demser®** *see* metyrosine *on page 412*
- **Demulen®** *see* ethinyl estradiol and ethynodiol diacetate *on page 249*
- **Denavir™** *see* penciclovir *on page 473*

denileukin deftitox *New Drug* (de ne LU kin DEFT e tox)

U.S. Brand Names Ontak®
Generic Available No
Therapeutic Category Antineoplastic Agent, Miscellaneous
Use Treatment of patients with persistent or recurrent cutaneous T-cell lymphoma whose malignant cells express the CD25 component of the IL-2 receptor
Usual Dosage Adults: I.V.: A treatment cycle consists of 9 or 18 mcg/kg/day for 5 consecutive days administered every 21 days. The optimal duration of therapy has not been determined. Only 2% of patients who failed to demonstrate a response (at least a 25% decrease in tumor burden) prior to the fourth cycle responded to subsequent treatment.
Dosage Forms Injection: 150 mcg/mL (2 mL)

- **Denorex® [OTC]** *see* coal tar *on page 162*
- **Denvar** *see* cefixime *on page 121*
- **deodorized opium tincture** *see* opium tincture *on page 456*
- **2'-deoxycoformycin** *see* pentostatin *on page 480*
- **Depacon®** *see* valproic acid and derivatives *on page 641*
- **Depade®** *see* naltrexone *on page 430*
- **Depakene®** *see* valproic acid and derivatives *on page 641*
- **Depakote®** *see* valproic acid and derivatives *on page 641*
- **depAndrogyn®** *see* estradiol and testosterone *on page 243*
- **depAndro® Injection** *see* testosterone *on page 598*
- **Depen®** *see* penicillamine *on page 473*
- **depGynogen® Injection** *see* estradiol *on page 242*
- **depMedalone® Injection** *see* methylprednisolone *on page 407*
- **DepoCyt™** *see* cytarabine (liposomal) *New Drug on page 178*
- **Depo®-Estradiol Injection** *see* estradiol *on page 242*
- **Depogen® Injection** *see* estradiol *on page 242*
- **Depoject® Injection** *see* methylprednisolone *on page 407*
- **Depo-Medrol® Injection** *see* methylprednisolone *on page 407*
- **Deponit® Patch** *see* nitroglycerin *on page 444*
- **Depopred® Injection** *see* methylprednisolone *on page 407*
- **Depo-Provera® 100 mg/mL *(Discontinued)*** *see page 743*
- **Depo-Provera® Injection** *see* medroxyprogesterone acetate *on page 389*
- **Depo-Testadiol®** *see* estradiol and testosterone *on page 243*
- **Depotest® Injection** *see* testosterone *on page 598*
- **Depotestogen®** *see* estradiol and testosterone *on page 243*
- **Depo®-Testosterone Injection** *see* testosterone *on page 598*
- **deprenyl** *see* selegiline *on page 562*
- **Deproist® Expectorant With Codeine** *see* guaifenesin, pseudoephedrine, and codeine *on page 304*
- **Deprol® *(Discontinued)*** *see page 743*
- **Dequadin®** *see* dequalínium (Canada only) *on page 187*

dequalinium *(Canada only)* (de kwal LI ne um)
Canadian Brand Names Dequadin®
Generic Available No
Therapeutic Category Antibacterial, Topical; Antifungal Agent, Topical
Use Treatment of mouth and throat infections
Usual Dosage Adults:
Lozenge: One lozenge sucked slowly every 2-3 hours
Oral paint: Apply freely to infected area, every 2-3 hours, or as directed by physician
Dosage Forms
Lozenge, as chloride: 0.25 mg (20s)
Oral paint, as chloride: 0.5% (25 mL)

♦ **Derifil® [OTC]** *see* chlorophyll *on page 135*

♦ **Dermacort® Topical** *see* hydrocortisone (topical) *on page 324*

♦ **Dermarest Dricort® Topical** *see* hydrocortisone (topical) *on page 324*

♦ **Derma-Smoothe/FS® Topical** *see* fluocinolone *on page 273*

♦ **Dermasone** *see* clobetasol *on page 157*

♦ **Dermatop®** *see* prednicarbate *on page 513*

♦ **Dermatophytin®** *see* Trichophyton skin test *on page 626*

♦ **Dermatophytin-O** *see* Candida albicans (Monilia) *on page 109*

♦ **Dermazin™** *see* silver sulfadiazine *on page 566*

♦ **Dermifun** *see* miconazole *on page 413*

♦ **Dermolate® Topical [OTC]** *see* hydrocortisone (topical) *on page 324*

♦ **Dermoplast® [OTC]** *see* benzocaine *on page 79*

♦ **Dermovate®** *see* clobetasol *on page 157*

♦ **Dermoxyl® Gel *(Discontinued)*** *see page 743*

♦ **Dermtex® HC with Aloe Topical [OTC]** *see* hydrocortisone (topical) *on page 324*

♦ **DES** *see* diethylstilbestrol *on page 201*

♦ **Desenex® [OTC]** *see* tolnaftate *on page 618*

♦ **deserpidine and methyclothiazide** *see* methyclothiazide and deserpidine *on page 405*

♦ **Desferal® Mesylate** *see* deferoxamine *on page 184*

desflurane (des FLOO rane)
U.S. Brand Names Suprane®
Generic Available No
Therapeutic Category General Anesthetic
Use Induction or maintenance of anesthesia for adults in outpatient and inpatient surgery
Usual Dosage
Children: Maintenance: Surgical levels of anesthesia may be maintained with concentrations of 5.2% to 10% desflurane, with or without nitrous oxide
Adults: Titrate dose based on individual response; see table in the product packaging for specific details; minimum alveolar concentration (MAC) should be reduced in elderly patients
Induction: Frequent starting concentration 3%; increased in 0.5% to 1% increments every 2-3 breaths; end tidal concentrations of 4% to 11% desflurane with and without nitrous oxide produce anesthesia within 2-4 minutes
Maintenance: Surgical levels of anesthesia in adults may be maintained with concentrations of 2.5% to 8.5% desflurane, with or without nitrous oxide
Note: Because of the higher vapor pressure and higher MAC of desflurane, special vaporizer canisters must be used. Equipment is **not** interchangeable with that for isoflurane.
Dosage Forms Liquid: 240 mL

♦ **desiccated thyroid** *see* thyroid *on page 610*

desipramine (des IP ra meen)
Synonyms desmethylimipramine
U.S. Brand Names Norpramin®
Canadian Brand Names PMS-Desipramine
Generic Available Yes: Tablet
Therapeutic Category Antidepressant, Tricyclic (Secondary Amine)
Use Treatment of various forms of depression, often in conjunction with psychotherapy; analgesic in chronic pain, peripheral neuropathies
(Continued)

desipramine *(Continued)*

Usual Dosage Oral (not recommended for use in children <12 years):

Adolescents: Initial: 25-50 mg/day; gradually increase to 100 mg/day in single or divided doses; maximum: 150 mg/day

Adults: Initial: 75 mg/day in divided doses; increase gradually to 150-200 mg/day in divided or single dose; maximum: 300 mg/day

Dietary Considerations Limit caffeine; may need diet with increased riboflavin; may be administered with food to decrease GI distress

Nursing/Pharmacy Information

May increase appetite

Monitor blood pressure and pulse rate prior to and during initial therapy; evaluate mental status; monitor weight

Dosage Forms Tablet, as hydrochloride: 10 mg, 25 mg, 50 mg, 75 mg, 100 mg, 150 mg

♦ **Desitin® [OTC]** *see* zinc oxide, cod liver oil, and talc *on page 660*

♦ **desmethylimipramine** *see* desipramine *on page 187*

desmopressin acetate *(des moe PRES in AS e tate)*

Synonyms 1-deamino-8-d-arginine vasopressin

U.S. Brand Names DDAVP®; Stimate®

Canadian Brand Names Octostim®

Mexican Brand Names Minirin

Generic Available No

Therapeutic Category Vasopressin Analog, Synthetic

Use Treatment of diabetes insipidus and controlling bleeding in certain types of hemophilia

Usual Dosage

Children:

Diabetes insipidus: 3 months to 12 years: Intranasal: Initial: 5 mcg/day divided 1-2 times/day; range: 5-30 mcg/day divided 1-2 times/day

Hemophilia: >3 months: I.V.: 0.3 mcg/kg by slow infusion; may repeat dose if needed

Nocturnal enuresis: ≥6 years: Intranasal: Initial: 20 mcg at bedtime; range: 10-40 mcg

Adults:

Diabetes insipidus: I.V., S.C.: 2-4 mcg/day in 2 divided doses or $1/10$ of the maintenance intranasal dose; intranasal: 5-40 mcg/day 1-3 times/day

Hemophilia: I.V.: 0.3 mcg/kg by slow infusion

Nursing/Pharmacy Information

Parenteral: Dilute to a maximum concentration of 0.5 mcg/mL in normal saline and infuse over 15-30 minutes

Monitor blood pressure and pulse should be monitored during I.V. infusion

Diabetes insipidus: Fluid intake, urine volume, specific gravity, plasma and urine osmolality, serum electrolytes

Hemophilia: Factor VIII antigen levels, APTT

Stability: Store in refrigerator, avoid freezing; discard discolored solutions; nasal solution stable for 3 weeks at room temperature

Dosage Forms Desmopressin acetate:

Injection (DDAVP®): 4 mcg/mL (1 mL)

Solution, nasal:

DDAVP®: 100 mcg/mL (2.5 mL, 5 mL)

Stimate®: 1.5 mg/mL (2.5 mL)

Tablet (DDAVP®): 0.1 mg, 0.2 mg

♦ **Desocort®** *see* desonide *on page 188*

♦ **Desogen®** *see* ethinyl estradiol and desogestrel *on page 248*

♦ **desogestrel and ethinyl estradiol** *see* ethinyl estradiol and desogestrel *on page 248*

desonide *(DES oh nide)*

U.S. Brand Names DesOwen® Topical; Tridesilon® Topical

Canadian Brand Names Desocort®

Generic Available Yes

Therapeutic Category Corticosteroid, Topical

Use Adjunctive therapy for inflammation in acute and chronic corticosteroid responsive dermatosis

Usual Dosage Topical: Apply 2-4 times/day

Nursing/Pharmacy Information For external use only; do not use on open wounds; apply sparingly to occlusive dressings; should not be used in the presence of open or weeping lesions

Dosage Forms
Cream, topical: 0.05% (15 g, 60 g)
Lotion: 0.05% (60 mL, 120 mL)
Ointment, topical: 0.05% (15 g, 60 g)

♦ **DesOwen® Topical** *see* desonide *on page 188*

desoximetasone (des oks i MET a sone)
U.S. Brand Names Topicort®; Topicort®-LP
Generic Available Yes
Therapeutic Category Corticosteroid, Topical
Use Relief of inflammation and pruritic symptoms of corticosteroid-responsive dermatosis
Usual Dosage Topical:
Children: Apply sparingly in a very thin film to affected area 1-2 times/day
Adults: Apply sparingly in a thin film twice daily
Nursing/Pharmacy Information For external use only; apply sparingly with occlusive dressings; should not be used in the presence of open or weeping lesions
Dosage Forms
Cream, topical:
Topicort®: 0.25% (15 g, 60 g, 120 g)
Topicort®-LP: 0.05% (15 g, 60 g)
Gel, topical: 0.05% (15 g, 60 g)
Ointment, topical (Topicort®): 0.25% (15 g, 60 g)

♦ **desoxyephedrine** *see* methamphetamine *on page 400*
♦ **Desoxyn®** *see* methamphetamine *on page 400*
♦ **desoxyphenobarbital** *see* primidone *on page 517*
♦ **Despec® Liquid (Discontinued)** *see page 743*
♦ **Desquam-E™ Gel** *see* benzoyl peroxide *on page 81*
♦ **Desquam-X® Gel** *see* benzoyl peroxide *on page 81*
♦ **Desquam-X® Wash** *see* benzoyl peroxide *on page 81*
♦ **Desyrel®** *see* trazodone *on page 622*
♦ **Detensol®** *see* propranolol *on page 527*
♦ **Detrol™** *see* tolterodine *on page 618*
♦ **Detussin® Expectorant** *see* hydrocodone, pseudoephedrine, and guaifenesin *on page 322*
♦ **Detussin® Liquid** *see* hydrocodone and pseudoephedrine *on page 321*
♦ **Devrom® [OTC]** *see* bismuth subgallate *on page 88*
♦ **Dexacen-4® (Discontinued)** *see page 743*
♦ **Dexacen® LA-8 (Discontinued)** *see page 743*
♦ **Dexacidin®** *see* neomycin, polymyxin B, and dexamethasone *on page 436*
♦ **Dexacort® Phosphate in Respihaler®** *see* dexamethasone (oral inhalation) *on page 190*
♦ **Dexacort® Phosphate Turbinaire®** *see* dexamethasone (nasal) *on page 189*
♦ **dexamethasone and neomycin** *see* neomycin and dexamethasone *on page 435*
♦ **dexamethasone and tobramycin** *see* tobramycin and dexamethasone *on page 616*

dexamethasone (nasal) (deks a METH a sone)
U.S. Brand Names Dexacort® Phosphate Turbinaire®
Generic Available Yes
Therapeutic Category Adrenal Corticosteroid
Use Chronic inflammation and/or allergic conditions
Dietary Considerations May be administered with meals to decrease GI upset; limit caffeine; may need diet with increased potassium, pyridoxine, vitamin C, vitamin D, folate, calcium, and phosphorus
Dosage Forms Dexamethasone sodium phosphate: Aerosol, nasal 84 mcg/ activation [170 metered doses] (12.6 g)

♦ **dexamethasone, neomycin, and polymyxin B** *see* neomycin, polymyxin B, and dexamethasone *on page 436*

dexamethasone (ophthalmic) (deks a METH a sone)
U.S. Brand Names AK-Dex® Ophthalmic; Baldex®; Decadron® Ophthalmic; Maxidex®
Generic Available Yes
Therapeutic Category Adrenal Corticosteroid
(Continued)

dexamethasone (ophthalmic) *(Continued)*

Use Inflammatory or allergic conjunctivitis
Usual Dosage Ophthalmic: Instill 3-4 times/day
Dosage Forms Dexamethasone base:
Suspension, ophthalmic: 0.1% (5 mL)
Ointment, ophthalmic: 0.05% (3.5 g)
Solution, ophthalmic: 0.1% (5 mL)

dexamethasone (oral inhalation) (deks a METH a sone)

U.S. Brand Names Dexacort® Phosphate in Respihaler®
Generic Available Yes
Therapeutic Category Adrenal Corticosteroid
Use Chronic inflammation or allergic conditions
Dosage Forms Aerosol, oral: 84 mcg/activation [170 metered doses] (12.6 g)

dexamethasone (systemic) (deks a METH a sone)

U.S. Brand Names Decadron® Injection; Decadron®-LA; Decadron® Oral; Decaject®; Decaject-LA®; Dexasone®; Dexasone® L.A.; Dexone®; Dexone® LA; Hexadrol®; Solurex L.A.®
Mexican Brand Names Alin; Alin Depot; Decadronal®; Decorex; Dibasona
Generic Available Yes
Therapeutic Category Adrenal Corticosteroid
Use Systemically for chronic inflammation, allergic, hematologic, neoplastic, and autoimmune diseases; may be used in management of cerebral edema, septic shock, and as a diagnostic agent
Usual Dosage
Children:
Antiemetic (prior to chemotherapy): 10 mg/m^2/dose for first dose then 5 mg/m^2/dose every 6 hours as needed
Physiologic replacement: Oral, I.M., I.V.: 0.03-0.15 mg/kg/day or 0.6-0.75 mg/m^2/day in divided doses every 6-12 hours
Extubation or airway edema: Oral, I.M., I.V.: 0.5-1 mg/kg/day in divided doses every 6 hours beginning 24 hours prior to extubation and continuing for 4-6 doses afterwards
Anti-inflammatory: Oral, I.M., I.V.: 0.75-9 mg/day in divided doses every 6-12 hours
Cerebral edema: I.V. 10 mg stat, 4 mg I.M./I.V. every 6 hours until response is maximized, then switch to oral regimen, then taper off if appropriate
Diagnosis for Cushing's syndrome: Oral: 1 mg at 11 PM, draw blood at 8 AM
ANLL protocol: I.V.: 2 mg/m^2/dose every 8 hours for 12 doses
Dietary Considerations May be administered with meals to decrease GI upset; limit caffeine; may need diet with increased potassium, pyridoxine, vitamin C, vitamin D, folate, calcium, and phosphorus
Nursing/Pharmacy Information
Parenteral: Administer undiluted solution IVP over 1-4 minutes if dose is <10 mg; high dose therapy must be administered by I.V. intermittent infusion over 15-30 minutes; acetate injection is not for I.V. use
Monitor hemoglobin, occult blood loss, serum potassium, and glucose
Stability: Injection of parenteral admixture:
Room temperature (25°C): 24 hours
Refrigeration (4°C): 2 days
Protect from light and freezing
Dosage Forms
Dexamethasone acetate:
Injection:
Dalalone L.A.®, Decadron®-LA, Decaject-LA®, Dexasone® L.A., Dexone® LA, Solurex L.A.®: 8 mg/mL (1 mL, 5 mL)
Dalalone D.P.®: 16 mg/mL (1 mL, 5 mL)
Dexamethasone base:
Elixir (Decadron®, Hexadrol®): 0.5 mg/5 mL (5 mL, 20 mL, 100 mL, 120 mL, 240 mL, 500 mL)
Solution, oral: 0.5 mg/5 mL (5 mL, 20 mL, 500 mL)
Solution, oral concentrate: 0.5 mg/0.5 mL (30 mL)
Tablet (Decadron®, Dexone®, Hexadrol®): 0.25 mg, 0.5 mg, 0.75 mg, 1 mg, 1.5 mg, 2 mg, 4 mg, 6 mg
Therapeutic pack: Six 1.5 mg tablets and eight 0.75 mg tablets
Injection:
Dalalone®, Decadron® Phosphate, Decaject®, Dexasone®, Hexadrol® Phosphate, Solurex®: 4 mg/mL (1 mL, 2 mL, 2.5 mL, 5 mL, 10 mL, 30 mL)

Hexadrol® Phosphate: 10 mg/mL (1 mL, 10 mL); 20 mg/mL (5 mL)
Decadron® Phosphate: 24 mg/mL (5 mL, 10 mL)

dexamethasone (topical) (deks a METH a sone)

U.S. Brand Names Aeroseb-Dex®; Decadron® Phosphate
Generic Available Yes
Therapeutic Category Adrenal Corticosteroid
Use For chronic inflammation and/or allergic conditions
Usual Dosage Topical: Apply 2-4 times daily
Nursing/Pharmacy Information Do not use topical products on open wounds
Dosage Forms Dexamethasone base:
Aerosol, topical: 0.01% (58 g)
Cream: 0.1% (15 g, 30 g)

• **Dexasone®** see dexamethasone (systemic) *on page 190*
• **Dexasone® L.A.** *see* dexamethasone (systemic) *on page 190*
• **Dexasporin®** *see* neomycin, polymyxin B, and dexamethasone *on page 436*
• **Dexatrim® Pre-Meal [OTC]** *see* phenylpropanolamine *on page 489*

dexbrompheniramine and pseudoephedrine

(deks brom fen EER a meen & soo doe e FED rin)
Synonyms pseudoephedrine and dexbrompheniramine
U.S. Brand Names Disobrom® [OTC]; Disophrol® Chronotabs® [OTC]; Disophrol® Tablet [OTC]; Drixomed®; Drixoral® [OTC]
Generic Available Yes
Therapeutic Category Antihistamine/Decongestant Combination
Use Relief of symptoms of upper respiratory mucosal congestion in seasonal and perennial nasal allergies, acute rhinitis, rhinosinusitis and eustachian tube blockage
Usual Dosage Children >12 years and Adults: Oral: 1 tablet every 12 hours, may require 1 tablet every 8 hours
Dietary Considerations May be administered with food or water
Nursing/Pharmacy Information Swallow whole, do not crush or chew
Dosage Forms
Tablet (Disophrol®): Dexbrompheniramine maleate 2 mg and pseudoephedrine sulfate 60 mg
Timed release (Disobrom®, Disophrol® Chrontabs®, Drixomed®, Drixoral®, Histrodrix®, Resporal®): Dexbrompheniramine maleate 6 mg and pseudoephedrine sulfate 120 mg

• **Dexchlor®** see dexchlorpheniramine *on page 191*

dexchlorpheniramine (deks klor fen EER a meen)

U.S. Brand Names Dexchlor®; Poladex®; Polaramine®
Generic Available Yes
Therapeutic Category Antihistamine
Use Perennial and seasonal allergic rhinitis and other allergic symptoms including urticaria
Usual Dosage Oral:
Children:
2-5 years: 0.5 mg every 4-6 hours
6-11 years: 1 mg every 4-6 hours or 4 mg timed release at bedtime
Adults: 2 mg every 4-6 hours or 4-6 mg timed release at bedtime or 8-10 hours
Dietary Considerations May be administered with food or water
Nursing/Pharmacy Information May cause drowsiness; swallow whole, do not crush or chew sustained release product; avoid alcohol, may impair coordination and judgment
Dosage Forms Dexchlorpheniramine maleate:
Syrup (orange flavor): 2 mg/5 mL with alcohol 6% (480 mL)
Tablet: 2 mg
Tablet, sustained action: 4 mg, 6 mg

• **Dexedrine®** *see* dextroamphetamine *on page 193*
• **Dexedrine® Elixir *(Discontinued)* see page 743*
• **Dexferrum®** *see* iron dextran complex *on page 346*
• **Dexone®** *see* dexamethasone (systemic) *on page 190*
• **Dexone® LA** *see* dexamethasone (systemic) *on page 190*

dexpanthenol (deks PAN the nole)
Synonyms pantothenyl alcohol
U.S. Brand Names Ilopan-Choline® Oral; Ilopan® Injection; Panthoderm® Cream [OTC]
Generic Available Yes
Therapeutic Category Gastrointestinal Agent, Stimulant
Use Prophylactic use to minimize paralytic ileus, treatment of postoperative distention
Usual Dosage
Children and Adults: Relief of itching and aid in skin healing: Topical: Apply to affected area 1-2 times/day
Adults:
Relief of gas retention: Oral: 2-3 tablets 3 times/day
Prevention of postoperative ileus: I.M.: 250-500 mg stat, repeat in 2 hours, followed by doses every 6 hours until danger passes
Paralyzed ileus: I.M.: 500 mg stat, repeat in 2 hours, followed by doses every 6 hours, if needed
Nursing/Pharmacy Information Not for direct I.V. administration
Dosage Forms
Cream: 2% (30 g, 60 g)
Injection (Ilopan®): 250 mg/mL (2 mL, 10 mL, 30 mL)
Tablet (Ilopan-Choline®): 50 mg with choline bitartrate 25 mg

dexrazoxane (deks ray ZOKS ane)
Synonyms ICRF-187
U.S. Brand Names Zinecard®
Generic Available No
Therapeutic Category Cardiovascular Agent, Other
Use Prevention of cardiomyopathy associated with doxorubicin administration
Usual Dosage I.V.: 1000 mg/m^2 30 minutes before administration of doxorubicin; maximal doses in patients with and without prior treatment with nitrosoureas, respectively = 750 mg/m^2 and 120 mg/m^2; 3500 mg/m^2/day for 3 days has been maximally used in pediatric patients. The recommended dosage ratio of dexrazoxane:doxorubicin is 10:1.
Dosage Forms Powder for injection, lyophilized: 250 mg, 500 mg (10 mg/mL when reconstituted)

dextran (DEKS tran)
Synonyms dextran, high molecular weight; dextran, low molecular weight
U.S. Brand Names Gentran®; LMD®; Macrodex®; Rheomacrodex®
Mexican Brand Names Alpha-Dextrano"40"
Generic Available Yes
Therapeutic Category Plasma Volume Expander
Use Fluid replacement and blood volume expander used in the treatment of hypovolemia, shock, or near shock states
Usual Dosage I.V.:
Children: Total dose should not be >20 mL/kg during first 24 hours
Adults: 500-1000 mL at rate of 20-40 mL/minute
Nursing/Pharmacy Information
I.V. infusion only; observe patient for signs of circulatory overload and/or monitor central venous pressure; observe patients closely during the first minute of infusion and have other means of maintaining circulation should dextran therapy result in an anaphylactoid reaction; patients should be well hydrated at the start of therapy; discontinue dextran if urine specific gravity is low, and/or if oliguria or anuria occurs, or if there is a precipitous rise in central venous pressure or sign of circulatory overloading
Stability: Store at room temperature; discard partially used containers
Dosage Forms Injection:
High molecular weight:
6% dextran 75 in dextrose 5% (500 mL)
Gentran®: 6% dextran 75 in sodium chloride 0.9% (500 mL)
Gentran®, Macrodex®: 6% dextran 70 in sodium chloride 0.9% (500 mL)
Macrodex®: 6% dextran 70 in dextrose 5% (500 mL)
Low molecular weight: Gentran®, LMD®, Rheomacrodex®:
10% dextran 40 in dextrose 5% (500 mL)
10% dextran 40 in sodium chloride 0.9% (500 mL)

dextran 1 (DEKS tran won)
U.S. Brand Names Promit®
Generic Available No

Therapeutic Category Plasma Volume Expander

Use Prophylaxis of serious anaphylactic reactions to I.V. infusion of dextran

Usual Dosage I.V. (time between dextran 1 and dextran solution should not exceed 15 minutes):

Children: 0.3 mL/kg 1-2 minutes before I.V. infusion of dextran

Adults: 20 mL 1-2 minutes before I.V. infusion of dextran

Nursing/Pharmacy Information

Do not dilute or admix with dextrans

Stability: Protect from freezing

Dosage Forms Injection: 150 mg/mL (20 mL)

◆ **dextran, high molecular weight** *see* dextran *on page 192*

◆ **dextran, low molecular weight** *see* dextran *on page 192*

dextranomer (deks TRAN oh mer)

U.S. Brand Names Debrisan® [OTC]

Generic Available No

Therapeutic Category Topical Skin Product

Use Clean exudative wounds; no controlled studies have found dextranomer to be more effective than conventional therapy

Usual Dosage Topical: Apply to affected area once or twice daily

Nursing/Pharmacy Information Sprinkle beads into ulcer (or apply paste) to ¼" thickness; change dressings 1-4 times/day depending on drainage; change dressing before it is completely dry to facilitate removal. Remove beads or paste when they become saturated. Occasionally vigorous irrigation, soaking, or whirlpool may be needed to remove the product. Discontinue treatment when the area is free of exudate and edema or when healthy granulation tissue is present. Each container should only be used for one patient to avoid cross-contamination.

Dosage Forms

Beads: 4 g, 25 g, 60 g, 120 g

Paste: 10 g foil packets

dextroamphetamine (deks troe am FET a meen)

U.S. Brand Names Dexedrine®

Generic Available Yes

Therapeutic Category Amphetamine

Controlled Substance C-II

Use Adjunct in treatment of attention-deficit/hyperactivity disorder (ADHD) in children, narcolepsy, exogenous obesity

Usual Dosage Oral:

Children:

Narcolepsy: 6-12 years: Initial: 5 mg/day, may increase at 5 mg increments in weekly intervals until side effects appear; maximum dose: 60 mg/day

Attention deficit disorder:

3-5 years: Initial: 2.5 mg/day administered every morning; increase by 2.5 mg/day in weekly intervals until optimal response is obtained, usual range is 0.1-0.5 mg/kg/dose every morning with maximum of 40 mg/day

≥6 years: 5 mg once or twice daily; increase in increments of 5 mg/day at weekly intervals until optimal response is reached, usual range is 0.1-0.5 mg/kg/dose every morning (5-20 mg/day) with maximum of 40 mg/day

Adults:

Narcolepsy: Initial: 10 mg/day, may increase at 10 mg increments in weekly intervals until side effects appear; maximum: 60 mg/day

Exogenous obesity: 5-30 mg/day in divided doses of 5-10 mg 30-60 minutes before meals

Dietary Considerations Should be administered 30 minutes before meals and at least 6 hours before bedtime; acidic foods, juices, or vitamin C may decrease GI absorption

Nursing/Pharmacy Information

Daily dose may be administered in 1-3 divided doses/day; sustained release preparations should be used for once daily dosing; last daily dose should be administered 6 hours before retiring; do not crush or allow patient to chew sustained release preparations

Monitor CNS activity

Stability: Protect from light

Dosage Forms Dextroamphetamine sulfate:

Capsule, sustained release: 5 mg, 10 mg, 15 mg

Tablet: 5 mg, 10 mg (5 mg tablets contain tartrazine)

dextroamphetamine and amphetamine
(deks troe am FET a meen & am FET a meen)

U.S. Brand Names Adderall®

Generic Available No

Therapeutic Category Amphetamine

Use Treatment of narcolepsy; exogenous obesity; abnormal behavioral syndrome in children (minimal brain dysfunction); attention-deficit/hyperactivity disorder (ADHD)

Usual Dosage Oral:

Narcolepsy:

Children:

6-12 years: 5 mg/day, increase by 5 mg at weekly intervals

>12 years: 10 mg/day, increase by 10 mg at weekly intervals

Adults: 5-60 mg/day in 2-3 divided doses

Attention deficit disorder: Children:

3-5 years: 2.5 mg/day, increase by 2.5 mg at weekly intervals

>6 years: 5 mg/day, increase by 5 mg at weekly intervals not to exceed 40 mg/day

Short-term adjunct to exogenous obesity: Children >12 years and Adults: 5-30 mg/day in divided doses

Dosage Forms Tablet:

10 mg [dextroamphetamine sulfate 2.5 mg, dextroamphetamine saccharate 2.5 mg and amphetamine aspartate 2.5 mg, amphetamine sulfate 2.5 mg]

30 mg [dextroamphetamine sulfate 7.5 mg, dextroamphetamine saccharate 7.5 mg and amphetamine aspartate 7.55 mg, amphetamine sulfate 7.5 mg]

dextromethorphan (deks troe meth OR fan)

U.S. Brand Names Benylin DM® [OTC]; Benylin® Pediatric [OTC]; Children's Hold® [OTC]; Creo-Terpin® [OTC]; Delsym® [OTC]; Drixoral® Cough Liquid Caps [OTC]; Hold® DM [OTC]; Pertussin® CS [OTC]; Pertussin® ES [OTC]; Robitussin® Cough Calmers [OTC]; Robitussin® Pediatric [OTC]; Scot-Tussin DM® Cough Chasers [OTC]; Silphen DM® [OTC]; St. Joseph® Cough Suppressant [OTC]; Sucrets® Cough Calmers [OTC]; Suppress® [OTC]; Trocal® [OTC]; Vicks Formula 44® [OTC]; Vicks Formula 44® Pediatric Formula [OTC]

Canadian Brand Names Balminil®-DM, -DM Children; Koffex® DM, -DM Children; Triaminic DM

Generic Available Yes

Therapeutic Category Antitussive

Use Symptomatic relief of coughs caused by minor viral upper respiratory tract infections or inhaled irritants; most effective for a chronic nonproductive cough

Usual Dosage Oral:

Children:

2-5 years: 2.5-5 mg every 4 hours or 7.5 mg every 6-8 hours; extended release is 50 mg twice daily

6-11 years: 5-10 mg every 4 hours or 15 mg every 6-8 hours; extended release is 30 mg twice daily

Adults: 10-20 mg every 4 hours or 30 mg every 6-8 hours; extended release is 60 mg twice daily

Nursing/Pharmacy Information Raise side rails, institute safety measures

Dosage Forms

Capsule (Drixoral® Cough Liquid Caps): 30 mg

Liquid:

Creo-Terpin®: 10 mg/15 mL (120 mL)

Pertussin® CS: 3.5 mg/5 mL (120 mL)

Robitussin® Pediatric, St. Joseph® Cough Suppressant: 7.5 mg/5 mL (60 mL, 120 mL, 240 mL)

Pertussin® ES, Vicks Formula 44®: 15 mg/5 mL (120 mL, 240 mL)

Liquid, sustained release, as polistirex (Delsym®): 30 mg/5 mL (89 mL)

Lozenges:

Scot-Tussin DM® Cough Chasers: 2.5 mg

Children's Hold®, Hold® DM, Robitussin® Cough Calmers, Sucrets® Cough Calmers: 5 mg

Suppress®, Trocal®: 7.5 mg

Syrup:

Benylin® Pediatric: 7.5 mg/mL (118 mL)

Benylin DM®, Silphen DM®: 10 mg/5 mL (120 mL, 3780 mL)

Vicks Formula 44® Pediatric Formula: 15 mg/15 mL (120 mL)

♦ **dextromethorphan, acetaminophen, and pseudoephedrine** see acetaminophen, dextromethorphan, and pseudoephedrine on page 16

- **dextromethorphan and guaifenesin** *see* guaifenesin and dextromethorphan *on page 300*
- **dextromethorphan and promethazine** *see* promethazine and dextromethorphan *on page 523*
- **dextromethorphan, guaifenesin, and phenylpropanolamine** *see* guaifenesin, phenylpropanolamine, and dextromethorphan *on page 303*
- **dextromethorphan, guaifenesin, and pseudoephedrine** *see* guaifenesin, pseudoephedrine, and dextromethorphan *on page 304*
- **dextropropoxyphene** *see* propoxyphene *on page 526*
- **dextrose, levulose and phosphoric acid** *see* phosphorated carbohydrate solution *on page 492*

dextrothyroxine (deks troe thye ROKS een)
U.S. Brand Names Choloxin®
Generic Available No
Therapeutic Category Antihyperlipidemic Agent, Miscellaneous
Use Reduction of elevated serum cholesterol
Usual Dosage Oral:
  Children: 0.1 mg/kg/day
  Adults: 1-2 mg/day, up to 8 mg/day
Dietary Considerations Low-fat, low-cholesterol may be recommended
Nursing/Pharmacy Information If chest pain, palpitations, sweating, and/or diarrhea develop during therapy, discontinue drug
Dosage Forms Tablet, as sodium: 2 mg, 4 mg, 6 mg

- **Dey-Dose® Isoproterenol** *see* isoproterenol *on page 348*
- **Dey-Dose® Metaproterenol** *see* metaproterenol *on page 397*
- **Dey-Drop® Ophthalmic Solution** *see* silver nitrate *on page 565*
- **Dey-Lute® Isoetharine** *see* isoetharine *on page 346*

dezocine (DEZ oh seen)
U.S. Brand Names Dalgan®
Generic Available No
Therapeutic Category Analgesic, Narcotic
Use Relief of moderate to severe postoperative, acute renal and ureteral colic, and cancer pain
Usual Dosage Adults:
  I.M.: Initial: 5-20 mg; may be repeated every 3-6 hours as needed; maximum: 120 mg/day
  I.V.: Initial: 2.5-10 mg; may be repeated every 2-4 hours as needed
Nursing/Pharmacy Information
  Avoid driving or operating machinery until the effect of drug wears off; may be addicting with prolonged use
  Stability: Store at room temperature; protect from light
Dosage Forms Injection, single-dose vial: 5 mg/mL (2 mL); 10 mg/mL (2 mL); 15 mg/mL (2 mL)

- **DFP** *see* isoflurophate *on page 347*
- **DHAD** *see* mitoxantrone *on page 418*
- **DHC Plus®** *see* dihydrocodeine compound *on page 204*
- **D.H.E. 45® Injection** *see* dihydroergotamine *on page 204*
- **DHPG sodium** *see* ganciclovir *on page 287*
- **DHS® Tar [OTC]** *see* coal tar *on page 162*
- **DHS Zinc® [OTC]** *see* pyrithione zinc *on page 535*
- **DHT™** *see* dihydrotachysterol *on page 204*
- **Diaβeta®** *see* glyburide *on page 294*
- **Diabetic Tussin DM® [OTC]** *see* guaifenesin and dextromethorphan *on page 300*
- **Diabetic Tussin® EX [OTC]** *see* guaifenesin *on page 299*
- **Diabinese®** *see* chlorpropamide *on page 145*
- **Dialose® Capsule** *(Discontinued) see page 743*
- **Dialose® Plus Capsule [OTC]** *see* docusate and casanthranol *on page 215*
- **Dialose® Tablet [OTC]** *see* docusate *on page 214*
- **Dialume® [OTC]** *see* aluminum hydroxide *on page 33*
- **Diamicron®** *see* gliclazide *(Canada only) on page 292*
- **Diamine T.D.® [OTC]** *see* brompheniramine *on page 94*
- **diaminodiphenylsulfone** *see* dapsone *on page 182*
- **Diamox®** *see* acetazolamide *on page 17*
- **Diamox Sequels®** *see* acetazolamide *on page 17*

- **Diaparene® [OTC]** *see* methylbenzethonium chloride *on page 405*
- **Diaparene® Cradol® (Discontinued)** *see page 743*
- **Diapid® Nasal Spray** *see* lypressin *on page 379*
- **Diar-aid® [OTC]** *see* loperamide *on page 374*
- **Diasorb® [OTC]** *see* attapulgite *on page 66*
- **Diastat® Rectal Delivery System** *see* diazepam *on page 196*
- **Diatex** *see* diazepam *on page 196*
- **Diaval** *see* tolbutamide *on page 617*
- **Diazemuls® Injection** *see* diazepam *on page 196*

diazepam (dye AZ e pam)

U.S. Brand Names Diastat® Rectal Delivery System; Diazemuls® Injection; Diazepam Intensol®; Dizac® Injectable Emulsion; Valium® Injection; Valium® Oral

Canadian Brand Names Apo®-Diazepam; E Pam®; Meval®; Novo-Dipam®; PMS-Diazepam; Vivol®

Mexican Brand Names Diatex

Generic Available Yes

Therapeutic Category Benzodiazepine

Controlled Substance C-IV

Use Management of general anxiety disorders, panic disorders; to provide preoperative sedation, light anesthesia, and amnesia; treatment of status epilepticus, alcohol withdrawal symptoms; used as a skeletal muscle relaxant

Usual Dosage

Children:

Sedation or muscle relaxation or anxiety:

Oral: 0.12-0.8 mg/kg/day in divided doses every 6-8 hours

I.M., I.V.: 0.04-0.3 mg/kg/dose every 2-4 hours to a maximum of 0.6 mg/kg within an 8-hour period if needed

Status epilepticus: I.V.:

Infants 30 days to 5 years: 0.05-0.3 mg/kg/dose administered over 2-3 minutes, every 15-30 minutes to a maximum total dose of 5 mg; repeat in 2-4 hours as needed or 0.2-0.5 mg/dose every 2-5 minutes to a maximum total dose of 5 mg

>5 years: 0.05-0.3 mg/kg/dose administered over 2-3 minutes, every 15-30 minutes to a maximum total dose of 10 mg; repeat in 2-4 hours as needed or 1 mg/dose every 2-5 minutes to a maximum of 10 mg;

Adults:

Anxiety:

Oral: 2-10 mg 2-4 times/day

I.M., I.V.: 2-10 mg, may repeat in 3-4 hours if needed

Skeletal muscle relaxation:

Oral: 2-10 mg 2-4 times/day

I.M., I.V.: 5-10 mg, may repeat in 2-4 hours

Status epilepticus: I.V.: 0.2-0.5 mg/kg/dose every 15-30 minutes for 2-3 doses; maximum dose: 30 mg

Dietary Considerations May be administered with food or water; alcohol: additive CNS depression; has been reported with benzodiazepines; avoid or limit alcohol

Nursing/Pharmacy Information

Do not exceed 5 mg/minute IVP; rapid injection may cause respiratory depression or hypotension; provide safety measures (ie, side rails, night light, and call button); remove smoking materials from area; supervise ambulation

Monitor respiratory, cardiovascular, and mental status; check for orthostasis

Stability: Protect parenteral dosage form from light; potency is retained for up to 3 months when kept at room temperature; most stable at pH 4-8, hydrolysis occurs at pH <3; do not mix I.V. product with other medications

Dosage Forms

Gel, rectal:

Adult: 10 mg, 15 mg, 20 mg

Pediatric: 2.5 mg, 5 mg, 10 mg

Injection: 5 mg/mL (1 mL, 2 mL, 5 mL, 10 mL)

Injection, emulsified (Dizac®): 5 mg/mL (3 mL)

Solution, oral (wintergreen-spice flavor): 5 mg/5 mL (5 mL, 10 mL, 500 mL)

Solution, oral concentrate: 5 mg/mL (30 mL)

Tablet: 2 mg, 5 mg, 10 mg

- **Diazepam Intensol®** *see* diazepam *on page 196*

diazoxide (dye az OKS ide)

U.S. Brand Names Hyperstat® I.V.; Proglycem® Oral

Mexican Brand Names Sefulken

Generic Available Yes: Injection

Therapeutic Category Antihypoglycemic Agent; Vasodilator

Use I.V.: Emergency lowering of blood pressure; Oral: Hypoglycemia related to hyperinsulinism secondary to islet cell adenoma, carcinoma, or hyperplasia; adenomatosis; nesidioblastosis (persistent hyperinsulinemic hypoglycemia of infancy); leucine sensitivity, or extrapancreatic malignancy

Usual Dosage

Hyperinsulinemic hypoglycemia: Oral:

Newborns and Infants: 8-15 mg/kg/day in divided doses every 8-12 hours

Children and Adults: 3-8 mg/kg/day in divided doses every 8-12 hours

Hypertension: Children and Adults: I.V.: 1-3 mg/kg (maximum: 150 mg in a single injection); repeat dose in 5-15 minutes until blood pressure adequately reduced; repeat administration every 4-24 hours; monitor blood pressure closely

Nursing/Pharmacy Information

Shake suspension well before using; do not administer I.M. or S.C.; administer I.V. (undiluted) by rapid I.V. injection over a period of 30 seconds or less

Monitor blood pressure, blood glucose, serum uric acid

Stability: Protect from light, heat, and freezing; avoid using darkened solutions

Dosage Forms

Capsule (Proglycem®): 50 mg

Injection (Hyperstat®): 15 mg/mL (1 mL, 20 mL)

Suspension, oral (chocolate-mint flavor) (Proglycem®): 50 mg/mL (30 mL)

♦ **Dibacilina** see ampicillin on page 46
♦ **Dibasona** see dexamethasone (systemic) on page 190
♦ **Dibent® Injection** see dicyclomine on page 199
♦ **Dibenzyline®** see phenoxybenzamine on page 486

dibucaine (DYE byoo kane)

U.S. Brand Names Nupercainal® [OTC]

Generic Available Yes

Therapeutic Category Local Anesthetic

Use Fast, temporary relief of pain and itching due to hemorrhoids, minor burns, other minor skin conditions

Usual Dosage Children and Adults:

Rectal: Hemorrhoids: Insert ointment into rectum using a rectal applicator; administer each morning, evening, and after each bowel movement

Topical: Apply gently to the affected areas; no more than 30 g for adults or 7.5 g for children should be used in any 24-hour period

Nursing/Pharmacy Information Do not use near the eyes or over denuded surfaces or blistered areas

Dosage Forms

Cream: 0.5% (45 g)

Ointment, topical: 1% (30 g, 60 g)

dibucaine and hydrocortisone

(DYE byoo kane & hye droe KOR ti sone)

Synonyms hydrocortisone and dibucaine

U.S. Brand Names Corticaine® Topical

Generic Available Yes

Therapeutic Category Anesthetic/Corticosteroid

Use Relief of the inflammatory and pruritic manifestations of corticosteroid-responsive dermatoses and for external anal itching

Usual Dosage Topical: Apply to affected areas 2-4 times/day

Nursing/Pharmacy Information For external use only

Dosage Forms Cream: Dibucaine 5% and hydrocortisone 5%

♦ **Dibufen** see ibuprofen on page 332
♦ **DIC** see dacarbazine on page 179
♦ **dicalcium phosphate** see calcium phosphate, dibasic on page 107
♦ **Dicarbosil® [OTC]** see calcium carbonate on page 103
♦ **Dicetel®** see pinaverium (Canada only) on page 495

dichlorodifluoromethane and trichloromonofluoromethane
(dye klor oh dye flor oh METH ane & tri klor oh mon oh flor oh METH ane)

U.S. Brand Names Fluori-Methane® Topical Spray

Generic Available No

Therapeutic Category Analgesic, Topical

Use Management of myofascial pain, restricted motion, muscle pain; control of pain associated with injections

Usual Dosage Topical: Apply to area from approximately 12" away

Nursing/Pharmacy Information Do not spray on abraded skin, wounds, or burns

Dosage Forms Spray, topical: Dichlorodifluoromethane 15% and trichloromonofluoromethane 85%

♦ **dichlorotetrafluoroethane and ethyl chloride** *see* ethyl chloride and dichlorotetrafluoroethane *on page 254*

dichlorphenamide (dye klor FEN a mide)
Synonyms diclofenamide

U.S. Brand Names Daranide®

Generic Available No

Therapeutic Category Carbonic Anhydrase Inhibitor

Use Adjunct in treatment of open-angle glaucoma and perioperative treatment for angle-closure glaucoma

Usual Dosage Adults: Oral: 100-200 mg to start followed by 100 mg every 12 hours until desired response is obtained; maintenance dose: 25-50 mg 1-3 times/day

Nursing/Pharmacy Information Monitor electrolytes

Dosage Forms Tablet: 50 mg

♦ **dichysterol** *see* dihydrotachysterol *on page 204*

diclofenac (dye KLOE fen ak)
U.S. Brand Names Cataflam® Oral; Voltaren® Ophthalmic; Voltaren® Oral; Voltaren®-XR Oral

Canadian Brand Names Apo®-Diclo; Novo-Difenac®; Novo-Difenac-SR®; Nu-Diclo®

Mexican Brand Names Artrenac; Clonodifen®; Dolo Pangavit-D; Fustaren Retard; Galedol; Lifenal; Liroken; Logesic

Generic Available Yes

Therapeutic Category Analgesic, Non-narcotic; Nonsteroidal Anti-inflammatory Drug (NSAID)

Use Acute treatment of mild to moderate pain; acute and chronic treatment of rheumatoid arthritis, ankylosing spondylitis, and osteoarthritis; used for juvenile rheumatoid arthritis, gout, dysmenorrhea; ophthalmic solution for postoperative inflammation after cataract extraction; temporary relief of pain and photophobia in patients undergoing corneal refractive surgery

Usual Dosage Adults:
Oral:
Rheumatoid arthritis: 150-200 mg/day in 2-4 divided doses
Osteoarthritis: 100-150 mg/day in 2-3 divided doses
Ankylosing spondylitis: 100-125 mg/day in 4-5 divided doses
Ophthalmic: Instill 1 drop into affected eye 4 times/day beginning 24 hours after cataract surgery and continuing for 2 weeks

Dietary Considerations May be administered with food to decrease GI distress; delayed oral absorption has been reported with food for single doses but not with chronic multiple-dose administration

Nursing/Pharmacy Information
Do not crush tablets
Monitor CBC, liver enzymes; urine output, BUN/serum creatinine; occult blood loss

Dosage Forms
Diclofenac sodium:
Solution, ophthalmic (Voltaren®): 0.1% (2.5 mL, 5 mL)
Tablet, delayed release (Voltaren®): 25 mg, 50 mg, 75 mg
Tablet, extended release, as sodium (Voltaren® XR): 100 mg
Diclofenac potassium:
Tablet (Cataflam®): 50 mg

diclofenac and misoprostol (dye KLOE fen ak & mye soe PROST ole)

Synonyms misoprostol and diclofenac

U.S. Brand Names Arthrotec®

Generic Available No

Therapeutic Category Analgesic, Non-narcotic; Prostaglandin

Use The diclofenac component is indicated for the treatment of osteoarthritis and rheumatoid arthritis; the misoprostol component is indicated for the prophylaxis of NSAID-induced gastric and duodenal ulceration

Usual Dosage Adults: Oral: 1 tablet 2-3 times/day with food; tablets should be swallowed whole, not chewed

Dosage Forms Tablet: Diclofenac 50 mg and misoprostol 200 mcg; diclofenac 75 mg and misoprostol 200 mcg

♦ **diclofenamide** see dichlorphenamide on page 198

♦ **Diclotride®** see hydrochlorothiazide on page 317

dicloxacillin (dye kloks a SIL in)

U.S. Brand Names Dycill®; Dynapen®; Pathocil®

Mexican Brand Names Brispen; Posipen

Generic Available Yes

Therapeutic Category Penicillin

Use Treatment of skin and soft tissue infections, pneumonia and follow-up therapy of osteomyelitis caused by susceptible penicillinase-producing staphylococci

Usual Dosage Oral:

Children <40 kg: 12.5-50 mg/kg/day divided every 6 hours; doses of 50-100 mg/kg/day in divided doses every 6 hours have been used for follow-up therapy of osteomyelitis

Children >40 kg and Adults: 125-500 mg every 6 hours

Dietary Considerations Should be administered with a full glass of water 1 hour before or 2 hours after meals on an empty stomach unless otherwise directed, decreases drug absorption rate; decreases drug serum concentration

Nursing/Pharmacy Information

Administer around-the-clock rather than 4 times/day, 3 times/day, etc, (ie, 12-6-12-6, not 9-1-5-9) to promote less variation in peak and trough serum levels

Monitor periodic monitoring of CBC, urinalysis, BUN, serum creatinine, and liver enzymes during prolonged therapy

Stability: Refrigerate suspension after reconstitution; discard after 14 days if refrigerated or 7 days if kept at room temperature

Dosage Forms Dicloxacillin sodium:

Capsule: 125 mg, 250 mg, 500 mg

Powder for oral suspension: 62.5 mg/5 mL (80 mL, 100 mL, 200 mL)

dicumarol (dye KOO ma role)

Synonyms bishydroxycoumarin

Generic Available Yes

Therapeutic Category Anticoagulant

Use Prophylaxis and treatment of thromboembolic disorders

Usual Dosage Adults: Oral: 25-200 mg/day based on prothrombin time (PT) determinations

Dietary Considerations Avoid proteolytic enzymes (papain), fried/boiled onions & soybean oil

Dosage Forms Tablet: 25 mg, 50 mg, 100 mg

dicyclomine (dye SYE kloe meen)

Synonyms dicycloverine

U.S. Brand Names Antispas® Injection; Bentyl® Hydrochloride Injection; Bentyl® Hydrochloride Oral; Byclomine® Injection; Dibent® Injection; Dilomine® Injection; Di-Spaz® Injection; Di-Spaz® Oral; Or-Tyl® Injection

Canadian Brand Names Bentylol®

Generic Available Yes

Therapeutic Category Anticholinergic Agent

Use Treatment of functional disturbances of GI motility such as irritable bowel syndrome

Usual Dosage

Oral:

Infants >6 months: 5 mg/dose 3-4 times/day

Children: 10 mg/dose 3-4 times/day

(Continued)

dicyclomine *(Continued)*

Adults: Begin with 80 mg/day in 4 equally divided doses, then increase up to 160 mg/day

I.M. **(should not be used I.V.):** 80 mg/day in 4 divided doses (20 mg/dose)

Dietary Considerations Should be administered 30 minutes before food

Nursing/Pharmacy Information

Do not administer I.V.

Stability: Protect from light

Dosage Forms Dicyclomine hydrochloride:

Capsule: 10 mg, 20 mg

Injection: 10 mg/mL (2 mL, 10 mL)

Syrup: 10 mg/5 mL (118 mL, 473 mL, 946 mL)

Tablet: 20 mg

♦ **dicycloverine** *see dicyclomine on page 199*

didanosine *(dye DAN oh seen)*

Synonyms ddI

U.S. Brand Names Videx®

Generic Available No

Therapeutic Category Antiviral Agent

Use Treatment of patients with advanced HIV infection which is resistant to zidovudine therapy or in those patients with zidovudine intolerance; has been used in asymptomatic patients with very low CD4+ lymphocyte counts (<200 cells/mm³) with or without AIDS-related complex

Usual Dosage Administer on an empty stomach: Oral:

Children (dosing is based on body surface area (m²)):

<0.4: 25 mg tablets twice daily or 31 mg powder twice daily

0.5-0.7: 50 mg tablets twice daily or 62 mg powder twice daily

0.8-1: 75 mg tablets twice daily or 94 mg powder twice daily

1.1-1.4: 100 mg tablets twice daily or 125 mg powder twice daily

Adults: Dosing is based on patient weight:

35-49 kg: 125 mg tablets twice daily or 167 mg buffered powder twice daily

50-74 kg: 200 mg tablets twice daily or 250 mg buffered powder twice daily

≥75 mg: 300 mg tablets twice daily or 375 mg buffered powder twice daily

Note: Children >1 year and Adults should receive 2 tablets per dose and children <1 year should receive 1 tablet per dose for adequate buffering and absorption; tablets should be chewed

Dietary Considerations Do not mix with fruit juice or other acid containing liquid; administer at least 1 hour before or 2 hours after eating

Nursing/Pharmacy Information

Avoid creating dust if powder spilled, use wet mop or damp sponge; tablets should be chewed, crushed, or dispersed in water for oral administration

Monitor serum potassium, uric acid, creatinine; hemoglobin, CBC with neutrophil, and platelet count, CD4 cells; liver function tests, amylase; weight gain; perform dilated retinal exam every 6 months

Stability: Pediatric oral solution is stable 30 days under refrigeration

Dosage Forms

Powder for oral solution:

Buffered (single dose packet): 100 mg, 167 mg, 250 mg, 375 mg

Pediatric: 2 g, 4 g

Tablet, buffered, chewable (mint flavor): 25 mg, 50 mg, 100 mg, 150 mg

♦ **dideoxycytidine** *see zalcitabine on page 657*

♦ **Didrex®** *see benzphetamine on page 81*

♦ **Didronel®** *see etidronate disodium on page 254*

dienestrol *(dye en ES trole)*

U.S. Brand Names DV® Vaginal Cream; Ortho®-Dienestrol Vaginal

Generic Available No

Therapeutic Category Estrogen Derivative

Use Symptomatic management of atrophic vaginitis in postmenopausal women

Usual Dosage Adults: Vaginal: 1-2 applicatorfuls/day for 2 weeks and then ½ of that dose for 2 weeks; maintenance dose: 1 applicatorful 1-3 times/week for 3 weeks each month

Nursing/Pharmacy Information Insert applicator high into vagina. Patients should inform their physician if signs or symptoms of any of the following occur: Thromboembolic or thrombotic disorders including sudden severe headache or vomiting, disturbance of vision or speech, loss of vision, numbness or weakness in an extremity, sharp or crushing chest pain, calf pain, shortness of breath, severe abdominal pain or mass, mental depression, or unusual bleeding. Patients should discontinue taking the medication if they suspect they are pregnant or become pregnant.

Dosage Forms Cream, vaginal: 0.01% (30 g, 78 g)

♦ **dietary supplements** *see* enteral nutritional products *on page 233*

diethylpropion (dye eth il PROE pee on)

Synonyms amfepramone
U.S. Brand Names Tenuate®; Tenuate® Dospan®
Canadian Brand Names Nobesine®
Generic Available Yes
Therapeutic Category Anorexiant
Controlled Substance C-IV
Use Short-term adjunct in exogenous obesity
Usual Dosage Adults: Oral: 25 mg 3 times/day before meals or food or 75 mg controlled release tablet at midmorning
Dietary Considerations Should be administered before meals
Nursing/Pharmacy Information Monitor CNS
Dosage Forms Diethylpropion hydrochloride:
Tablet: 25 mg
Tablet, controlled release: 75 mg

diethylstilbestrol (dye eth il stil BES trole)

Synonyms DES; stilbestrol
U.S. Brand Names Stilphostrol®
Canadian Brand Names Honvol®
Generic Available Yes
Therapeutic Category Estrogen Derivative
Use Management of severe vasomotor symptoms of menopause, for estrogen replacement, and for palliative treatment of inoperable metastatic prostatic carcinoma
Usual Dosage Adults:
Hypogonadism and ovarian failure: Oral: 0.2-0.5 mg/day
Menopausal symptoms: Oral: 0.1-2 mg/day for 3 weeks and then off 1 week
Postmenopausal breast carcinoma: Oral: 15 mg/day
Prostate carcinoma: Oral: 1-3 mg/day
Prostatic cancer: I.V.: 0.5 g to start, then 1 g every 2-5 days followed by 0.25-0.5 g 1-2 times/week as maintenance
Diphosphate:
Oral: 50 mg 3 times/day; increase up to 200 mg or more 3 times/day
I.V.: Administer 0.5 g, dissolved in 250 mL of saline or D_5W, administer slowly the first 10-15 minutes then adjust rate so that the entire amount is administered in 1 hour
Dietary Considerations Should be administered with food to decrease GI distress
Nursing/Pharmacy Information
Administer 0.5 g I.V., dissolved in 250 mL of saline or D_5W, administer slowly the first 10-15 minutes then adjust rate so that the entire amount is administered in 1 hour
Stability: Intravenous solution should be stored at room temperature and away from direct light; solution is stable for 3 days as long as cloudiness or precipitation has not occurred
Dosage Forms
Diethylstilbestrol base:
Tablet: 1 mg, 2.5 mg, 5 mg
Diethylstilbestrol diphosphate sodium:
Injection (Stilphostrol®): 0.25 g (5 mL)
Tablet (Stilphostrol®): 50 mg

difenoxin and atropine (dye fen OKS in & A troe peen)

Synonyms atropine and difenoxin
U.S. Brand Names Motofen®
Generic Available No
Therapeutic Category Antidiarrheal
Controlled Substance C-IV
Use Treatment of diarrhea
Usual Dosage Adults: Oral: Initial: 2 tablets, then 1 tablet after each loose stool; 1 tablet every 3-4 hours, up to 8 tablets in a 24-hour period; if no improvement after 48 hours, continued administration is not indicated
Dosage Forms Tablet: Difenoxin hydrochloride 1 mg and atropine sulfate 0.025 mg

♦ **Differin®** *see* adapalene *on page 22*

diflorasone (dye FLOR a sone)
U.S. Brand Names Florone®; Florone E®; Maxiflor®; Psorcon™
Generic Available No
Therapeutic Category Corticosteroid, Topical
Use Relief of inflammation and pruritic symptoms of corticosteroid-responsive dermatosis
Usual Dosage Topical:
Cream: Apply 2-4 times/day
Ointment: Apply sparingly 1-3 times/day
Nursing/Pharmacy Information For external use only; do not use on open wounds; apply sparingly to occlusive dressings; should not be used in the presence of open or weeping lesions
Dosage Forms Diflorasone diacetate:
Cream: 0.05% (15 g, 30 g, 60 g)
Ointment, topical: 0.05% (15 g, 30 g, 60 g)

♦ **Diflucan®** *see* fluconazole *on page 270*

diflunisal (dye FLOO ni sal)
U.S. Brand Names Dolobid®
Canadian Brand Names Apo-Diflunisal®; Novo-Diflunisal; Nu-Diflunisal
Generic Available Yes
Therapeutic Category Analgesic, Non-narcotic; Nonsteroidal Anti-inflammatory Drug (NSAID)
Use Management of inflammatory disorders usually including rheumatoid arthritis and osteoarthritis; can be used as an analgesic for treatment of mild to moderate pain
Usual Dosage Adults: Oral:
Pain: Initial: 500-1000 mg followed by 250-500 mg every 8-12 hours
Inflammatory condition: 500-1000 mg/day in 2 divided doses
Dietary Considerations Should be administered with food to decrease GI distress
Nursing/Pharmacy Information Do not crush tablet
Dosage Forms Tablet: 250 mg, 500 mg

♦ **Di-Gel® [OTC]** *see* aluminum hydroxide, magnesium hydroxide, and simethicone *on page 34*
♦ **Digepepsin®** *see* pancreatin *on page 467*
♦ **Digess®8000** *see* pancrelipase *on page 467*
♦ **Digibind®** *see* digoxin immune Fab *on page 203*
♦ **Digitaline®** *see* digitoxin *on page 202*

digitoxin (di ji TOKS in)
U.S. Brand Names Crystodigin®
Canadian Brand Names Digitaline®
Generic Available Yes
Therapeutic Category Antiarrhythmic Agent, Miscellaneous; Cardiac Glycoside
Use Congestive heart failure; atrial fibrillation; atrial flutter; paroxysmal atrial tachycardia; and cardiogenic shock
Usual Dosage Oral:
Children: Doses are very individualized; the maintenance range after neonatal period, the recommended digitalizing dose is as follows:
<1 year: 0.045 mg/kg
1-2 years: 0.04 mg/kg
2 years: 0.03 mg/kg which is equivalent to 0.75 mg/m²
Maintenance: Approximately $\frac{1}{10}$ of the digitalizing dose
Adults:
Rapid loading dose: Initial: 0.6 mg followed by 0.4 mg and then 0.2 mg at intervals of 4-6 hours
Slow loading dose: 0.2 mg twice daily for a period of 4 days followed by a maintenance dose
Maintenance: 0.05-0.3 mg/day
Most common dose: 0.15 mg/day
Dietary Considerations Should be administered with water 30 minutes before or 2 hours after meals, with high-fiber foods and foods high in calcium; avoid natural licorice
Nursing/Pharmacy Information
Check apical pulse before administering

Monitor blood pressure, EKG
Dosage Forms Tablet: 0.1 mg, 0.2 mg

digoxin (di JOKS in)

U.S. Brand Names Lanoxicaps®; Lanoxin®
Canadian Brand Names Novo-Digoxin®
Mexican Brand Names Mapluxin®
Generic Available Yes
Therapeutic Category Antiarrhythmic Agent, Miscellaneous; Cardiac Glycoside
Use Treatment of congestive heart failure; slows the ventricular rate in tachyarrhythmias such as atrial fibrillation, atrial flutter, supraventricular tachycardia
Usual Dosage Adults (based on lean body weight and normal renal function for age. Decrease dose in patients with decreased renal function)

Total digitalizing dose: Administer $\frac{1}{2}$ as initial dose, then administer $\frac{1}{4}$ of the total digitalizing dose (TDD) in each of 2 subsequent doses at 8- to 12-hour intervals; obtain EKG 6 hours after each dose to assess potential toxicity
Oral: 0.75-1.5 mg
I.M., I.V.: 0.5-1 mg
Daily maintenance dose:
Oral: 0.125-0.5 mg
I.M., I.V.: 0.1-0.4 mg

Dietary Considerations Meals containing increased fiber (bran) or foods high in pectin, may decrease oral absorption of digoxin; avoid natural licorice (causes sodium and water retention and increases potassium loss); maintain adequate amounts of potassium in diet to decrease risk of hypokalemia (hypokalemia may increase risk of digoxin toxicity)

Nursing/Pharmacy Information

Check apical pulse before administering; administer I.V. doses slowly over 5 minutes; I.M. route not usually recommended due to local irritation, pain, and tissue damage
Monitor blood pressure and EKG closely; routine serum level monitoring not recommended but is indicated to rule out toxicity, serum electrolytes (potassium, magnesium, calcium), heart rate
Stability: Protect elixir and injection from light; solution **compatibility**: D_5W, $D_{10}W$, normal saline, sterile water for injection (when diluted fourfold or greater)

Dosage Forms
Capsule: 50 mcg, 100 mcg, 200 mcg
Elixir: 50 mcg/mL with alcohol 10% (60 mL)
Injection: 250 mcg/mL (1 mL, 2 mL)
Injection, pediatric: 100 mcg/mL (1 mL)
Tablet: 125 mcg, 250 mcg, 500 mcg

digoxin immune Fab (di JOKS in i MYUN fab)

Synonyms antidigoxin Fab fragments
U.S. Brand Names Digibind®
Generic Available No
Therapeutic Category Antidote
Use Treatment of potentially life-threatening digoxin or digitoxin intoxication in carefully selected patients
Usual Dosage Each vial of Digibind® will bind approximately 0.5 mg of digoxin or digitoxin

I.V.: To determine the dose of digoxin immune Fab, first determine the total body load of digoxin (TBL using either an approximation of the amount ingested or a postdistribution serum digoxin concentration). If neither ingestion amount or serum level is known: Adult dosage is 20 vials (760 mg) I.V. infusion.

Nursing/Pharmacy Information

Parenteral: Digoxin immune Fab is reconstituted by adding 4 mL sterile water, resulting in 10 mg/mL for I.V. infusion, the reconstituted solution may be further diluted with NS to a convenient volume (eg, 1 mg/mL); infuse over 15-30 minutes; to remove protein aggregates, 0.22 micron in-line filter is needed
Monitor serum potassium, serum digoxin concentration prior to first dose of digoxin immune Fab; digoxin levels will greatly increase with Digibind® use
Stability: Use reconstituted product promptly; if not used immediately, may be kept in refrigerator for up to 4 hours only

Dosage Forms Powder for injection, lyophilized: 38 mg

♦ **Dihistine® DH** see chlorpheniramine, pseudoephedrine, and codeine on page 143

♦ **Dihistine® Expectorant** *see* guaifenesin, pseudoephedrine, and codeine *on page 304*

dihydrocodeine compound (dye hye droe KOE deen KOM pound)
U.S. Brand Names DHC Plus®; Synalgos®-DC
Generic Available Yes
Therapeutic Category Analgesic, Narcotic
Controlled Substance C-III
Use Management of mild to moderate pain that requires relaxation
Usual Dosage Adults: Oral: 1-2 capsules every 4-6 hours as needed for pain
Dietary Considerations Should be administered with food or full glass of water
Nursing/Pharmacy Information Observe patient for excessive sedation, respiratory depression; implement safety measures, assist with ambulation
Dosage Forms Capsule:
DHC Plus®: Dihydrocodeine bitartrate 16 mg, acetaminophen 356.4 mg, and caffeine 30 mg
Synalgos®-DC: Dihydrocodeine bitartrate 16 mg, aspirin 356.4 mg, and caffeine 30 mg

dihydroergotamine (dye hye droe er GOT a meen)
U.S. Brand Names D.H.E. 45® Injection; Migranal® Nasal Spray
Generic Available Yes
Therapeutic Category Ergot Alkaloid and Derivative
Use Abort or prevent vascular headaches
Usual Dosage Adults:
I.M.: 1 mg at first sign of headache; repeat hourly to a maximum dose of 3 mg total
I.V.: Up to 2 mg maximum dose for faster effects; maximum dose: 6 mg/week
Intranasal: One spray (0.5 mg) of nasal spray should be administered into each nostril; if the condition has not sufficiently improved approximately fifteen minutes later, an additional spray should be administered to each nostril. The usual dosage required to obtain optimal efficacy is a total dosage of 4 sprays (2 mg); nasal spray is exclusively indicated for the symptomatic treatment of migraine attacks; no more than 4 sprays (2 mg) should be administered for any single migraine attack; an interval of at least 6-8 hours should be observed before treating another migraine attack with the nasal spray or any drug containing dihydroergotamine or ergotamine; no more than 8 sprays (4 mg) (corresponding to the use of 2 ampuls) should be administered during any 24-hour period; the maximum weekly dosage is 24 sprays (12 mg)
Nursing/Pharmacy Information Stability: Store in refrigerator
Dosage Forms Dihydroergotamine mesylate:
Injection: 1 mg/mL (1 mL)
Spray, nasal: 4 mg/mL [0.5 mg/spray] (1 mL)

♦ **dihydroergotoxine** *see* ergoloid mesylates *on page 238*
♦ **dihydrohydroxycodeinone** *see* oxycodone *on page 462*
♦ **dihydromorphinone** *see* hydromorphone *on page 325*

dihydrotachysterol (dye hye droe tak IS ter ole)
Synonyms dichysterol
U.S. Brand Names DHT™; Hytakerol®
Generic Available Yes
Therapeutic Category Vitamin D Analog
Use Treatment of hypocalcemia associated with hypoparathyroidism; prophylaxis of hypocalcemic tetany following thyroid surgery; suppress hyperparathyroidism and treat renal osteodystrophy in patients with chronic renal failure
Usual Dosage Oral:
Hypoparathyroidism:
Infants and young Children: 0.1-0.5 mg/day
Older Children and Adults: 0.5-1 mg/day
Nutritional rickets: 0.5 mg as a single dose or 13-50 mcg/day until healing occurs
Renal osteodystrophy: 0.6-6 mg/24 hours; maintenance: 0.25-0.6 mg/24 hours adjusted as necessary to achieve normal serum calcium levels and promote bone healing
Nursing/Pharmacy Information
Monitor calcium and phosphate levels closely; monitor symptoms of hypercalcemia
Stability: Protect from light

Dosage Forms
Capsule (Hytakerol®): 0.125 mg
Solution:
Oral Concentrate (DHT™): 0.2 mg/mL (30 mL)
Oral, in oil (Hytakerol®): 0.25 mg/mL (15 mL)
Tablet (DHT™): 0.125 mg, 0.2 mg, 0.4 mg

dihydroxyaluminum sodium carbonate
(dye hye DROKS i a LOO mi num SOW dee um KAR bun ate)
U.S. Brand Names Rolaids® [OTC]
Generic Available Yes
Therapeutic Category Antacid
Use Symptomatic relief of upset stomach associated with hyperacidity
Usual Dosage Oral: Chew 1-2 tablets as needed
Nursing/Pharmacy Information Chew tablets thoroughly and follow with water
Dosage Forms Tablet, chewable: 334 mg

- ♦ **1,25 dihydroxycholecalciferol** see calcitriol on page 103
- ♦ **dihydroxypropyl theophylline** see dyphylline on page 226
- ♦ **Dihyrex® Injection** see diphenhydramine on page 208
- ♦ **diiodohydroxyquin** see iodoquinol on page 344
- ♦ **diisopropyl fluorophosphate** see isoflurophate on page 347
- ♦ **Dilacoran** see verapamil on page 646
- ♦ **Dilacoran HTA** see verapamil on page 646
- ♦ **Dilacoran Retard** see verapamil on page 646
- ♦ **Dilacor XR®** see diltiazem on page 205
- ♦ **Dilafed** see nifedipine on page 442
- ♦ **Dilantin®** see phenytoin on page 490
- ♦ **Dilantin-30® Pediatric Suspension** *(Discontinued)* see page 743
- ♦ **Dilantin® With Phenobarbital** *(Discontinued)* see page 743
- ♦ **Dilatrate®-SR** see isosorbide dinitrate on page 349
- ♦ **Dilaudid® 1 mg & 3 mg Tablet** *(Discontinued)* see page 743
- ♦ **Dilaudid® Cough Syrup** see hydromorphone on page 325
- ♦ **Dilaudid-HP® Injection** see hydromorphone on page 325
- ♦ **Dilaudid® Injection** see hydromorphone on page 325
- ♦ **Dilaudid® Oral** see hydromorphone on page 325
- ♦ **Dilaudid® Suppository** see hydromorphone on page 325
- ♦ **Dilocaine® Injection** see lidocaine on page 368
- ♦ **Dilomine® Injection** see dicyclomine on page 199
- ♦ **Dilor®** see dyphylline on page 226

diltiazem (dil TYE a zem)
U.S. Brand Names Cardizem® CD; Cardizem® Injectable; Cardizem® SR; Cardizem® Tablet; Dilacor XR®; Tiamate®; Tiazac®
Canadian Brand Names Apo®-Diltiaz; Novo-Diltazem®; Nu-Diltiaz®; Syn-Diltiazem®
Mexican Brand Names Angiotrofin; Angiotrofin A.P.; Angiotrofin Retard; Presoken; Presoquim; Tilazem
Generic Available Yes
Therapeutic Category Calcium Channel Blocker
Use
Oral: Hypertension; chronic stable angina or angina from coronary artery spasm
Injection: Atrial fibrillation or atrial flutter; paroxysmal supraventricular tachycardias (PSVT)
Usual Dosage Adults:
Oral: 30-120 mg 3-4 times/day; dosage should be increased gradually, at 1- to 2-day intervals until optimum response is obtained; usual maintenance dose: 240-360 mg/day
Sustained-release capsules (SR): Initial dose of 60-120 mg twice daily
Sustained-release capsules (CD, XR): 180-300 mg once daily
I.V.: Initial: 0.25 mg/kg as a bolus over 2 minutes, then continuous infusion of 5-15 mg/hour for up to 24 hours
Dietary Considerations Should be administered 1 hour before or 2 hours after meals; food may increase absorption of diltiazem from sustained-release preparation
Nursing/Pharmacy Information Do not crush sustained release capsules
(Continued)

diltiazem *(Continued)*

Dosage Forms
Capsule, sustained release, as hydrochloride:
Cardizem® CD: 120 mg, 180 mg, 240 mg, 300 mg
Cardizem® SR: 60 mg, 90 mg, 120 mg
Dilacor™ XR: 180 mg, 240 mg
Tiazac™: 120 mg, 180 mg, 240 mg, 300 mg, 360 mg
Injection, as hydrochloride: 5 mg/mL (5 mL, 10 mL)
Cardizem®: 5 mg/mL (5 mL, 10 mL)
Tablet, as hydrochloride (Cardizem®): 30 mg, 60 mg, 90 mg, 120 mg
Tablet, extended release, as hydrochloride (Tiamate®): 120 mg, 180 mg, 240 mg

♦ **Dimacol® Caplets [OTC]** *see* guaifenesin, pseudoephedrine, and dextromethorphan *on page 304*

♦ **Dimantil** *see* warfarin *on page 655*

♦ **Dimaphen® Elixir [OTC]** *see* brompheniramine and phenylpropanolamine *on page 94*

♦ **Dimaphen® Tablets [OTC]** *see* brompheniramine and phenylpropanolamine *on page 94*

dimenhydrinate *(dye men HYE dri nate)*

U.S. Brand Names Calm-X® Oral [OTC]; Dimetabs® Oral; Dinate® Injection; Dramamine® Oral [OTC]; Dramilin® Injection; Dymenate® Injection; Hydrate® Injection; Marmine® Injection; Marmine® Oral [OTC]; Tega-Vert® Oral; TripTone® Caplets® [OTC]

Canadian Brand Names Apo®-Dimenhydrinate; Gravol®; PMS-Dimenhydrinate; Travel Aid®; Travel Tabs

Generic Available Yes

Therapeutic Category Antihistamine

Use Treatment and prevention of nausea, vertigo, and vomiting associated with motion sickness

Usual Dosage Oral:
Children:
2-5 years: 12.5-25 mg every 6-8 hours, maximum: 75 mg/day
6-12 years: 25-50 mg every 6-8 hours, maximum: 75 mg/day
or
Alternately: 5 mg/kg/day in 4 divided doses, not to exceed 300 mg/day
Adults: 50-100 mg every 4-6 hours, not to exceed 400 mg/day

Dietary Considerations May be administered with food or water

Nursing/Pharmacy Information
I.V. injection must be diluted to 10 mL with NS and administered at 25 mg/minute over at least 2 minutes
Stability: When mixed in the same syringe, drugs reported to be **incompatible** include aminophylline, barbiturates, butorphanol, chlorpromazine, glycopyrrolate, heparin, hydrocortisone, hydroxyzine, midazolam, phenytoin, prednisolone, prochlorperazine, promethazine, tetracycline, trifluoperazine

Dosage Forms
Capsule: 50 mg
Injection: 50 mg/mL (1 mL, 5 mL, 10 mL)
Liquid: 12.5 mg/4 mL (90 mL, 473 mL); 16.62 mg/5 mL (480 mL)
Tablet: 50 mg
Chewable: 50 mg

dimercaprol *(dye mer KAP role)*

Synonyms BAL; British anti-lewisite; dithioglycerol

U.S. Brand Names BAL in Oil®

Generic Available No

Therapeutic Category Chelating Agent

Use Antidote to gold, arsenic, and mercury poisoning; adjunct to edetate calcium disodium in lead poisoning

Usual Dosage Children and Adults: I.M.:
Mild arsenic and gold poisoning: 2.5 mg/kg/dose every 6 hours for 2 days, then every 12 hours on the third day, and once daily thereafter for 10 days
Severe arsenic and gold poisoning: 3 mg/kg/dose every 4 hours for 2 days then every 6 hours on the third day, then every 12 hours thereafter for 10 days
Mercury poisoning: Initial: 5 mg/kg followed by 2.5 mg/kg/dose 1-2 times/day for 10 days
Lead poisoning (use with edetate calcium disodium):
Mild: 3 mg/kg/dose every 4 hours for 5-7 days

Severe: 4 mg/kg/dose every 4 hours for 5-7 days
Acute encephalopathy: Initial: 4 mg/kg/dose, then every 4 hours
Nursing/Pharmacy Information
Urine should be kept alkaline; administer undiluted, deep I.M.
Monitor specific heavy metal levels, urine pH
Dosage Forms Injection: 100 mg/mL (3 mL)

♦ **Dimetabs® Oral** see dimenhydrinate on page 206
♦ **Dimetane®-DC** see brompheniramine, phenylpropanolamine, and codeine on page 95
♦ **Dimetane® Decongestant Elixir [OTC]** see brompheniramine and phenylephrine on page 94
♦ **Dimetane® (Discontinued)** see page 743
♦ **Dimetane® Extentabs® [OTC]** see brompheniramine on page 94
♦ **Dimetapp® 4-Hour Liqui-Gel Capsule [OTC]** see brompheniramine and phenylpropanolamine on page 94
♦ **Dimetapp® Elixir [OTC]** see brompheniramine and phenylpropanolamine on page 94
♦ **Dimetapp® Extentabs® [OTC]** see brompheniramine and phenylpropanolamine on page 94
♦ **Dimetapp® Sinus Caplets [OTC]** see pseudoephedrine and ibuprofen on page 531
♦ **Dimetapp® Tablet [OTC]** see brompheniramine and phenylpropanolamine on page 94
♦ **β,β-dimethylcysteine** see penicillamine on page 473

dimethyl sulfoxide (dye meth il sul FOKS ide)
Synonyms DMSO
U.S. Brand Names Rimso®-50
Generic Available No
Therapeutic Category Urinary Tract Product
Use Symptomatic relief of interstitial cystitis
Usual Dosage Instill 50 mL directly into bladder and allow to remain for 15 minutes; repeat every 2 weeks until maximum symptomatic relief is obtained
Dosage Forms Solution: 50% [500 mg/mL] (50 mL)

♦ **dimethyl tubocurarine iodide** see metocurine iodide on page 410
♦ **Dimodan** see disopyramide on page 213
♦ **Dinate® Injection** see dimenhydrinate on page 206

dinoprostone (dye noe PROST one)
Synonyms PGE_2; prostaglandin E_2
U.S. Brand Names Cervidil® Vaginal Insert; Prepidil® Vaginal Gel; Prostin E_2® Vaginal Suppository
Mexican Brand Names Propress
Generic Available No
Therapeutic Category Prostaglandin
Use Terminate pregnancy from 12th through 28th week of gestation; evacuate uterus in cases of missed abortion or intrauterine fetal death; manage benign hydatidiform mole
Usual Dosage Vaginal: Insert 1 suppository high in vagina, repeat at 3- to 5-hour intervals until abortion occurs up to 240 mg (maximum dose)
Nursing/Pharmacy Information
Bring suppository to room temperature just prior to use; patient should remain supine for 10 minutes following insertion; commercially available suppositories should not be used for extemporaneous preparation of any other dosage form of drug
Stability: Suppositories must be kept frozen, store in freezer not above -20°F (-4°C)
Dosage Forms
Insert, vaginal (Cervidil®): 10 mg
Gel, vaginal: 0.5 mg in 3 g syringes [each package contains a 10-mm and 20-mm shielded catheter]
Suppository, vaginal: 20 mg

dinoprost tromethamine (DYE noe prost tro METH a meen)
Synonyms $PGF_{2\alpha}$; prostaglandin F_2 alpha
U.S. Brand Names Prostin F_2 Alpha®
Generic Available No
Therapeutic Category Prostaglandin
Use Abort 2nd trimester pregnancy
(Continued)

dinoprost tromethamine *(Continued)*

Usual Dosage 40 mg (8 mL) via transabdominal tap; if abortion not completed in 24 hours, another 10-40 mg may be administered

Dosage Forms Injection: 5 mg/mL (4 mL, 8 mL)

- ♦ **Diocaine** *see* proparacaine *on page 524*
- ♦ **Diocarpine** *see* pilocarpine *on page 493*
- ♦ **Diochloram** *see* chloramphenicol *on page 133*
- ♦ **Diocto®** [OTC] *see* docusate *on page 214*
- ♦ **Diocto C®** [OTC] *see* docusate and casanthranol *on page 215*
- ♦ **Diocto-K®** [OTC] *see* docusate *on page 214*
- ♦ **Diocto-K Plus®** [OTC] *see* docusate and casanthranol *on page 215*
- ♦ **Dioctolose Plus®** [OTC] *see* docusate and casanthranol *on page 215*
- ♦ **dioctyl calcium sulfosuccinate** *see* docusate *on page 214*
- ♦ **dioctyl potassium sulfosuccinate** *see* docusate *on page 214*
- ♦ **dioctyl sodium sulfosuccinate** *see* docusate *on page 214*
- ♦ **Diodoquin®** *see* iodoquinol *on page 344*
- ♦ **Dioeze®** [OTC] *see* docusate *on page 214*
- ♦ **Diomycin** *see* erythromycin (systemic) *on page 240*
- ♦ **Dionephrine** *see* phenylephrine *on page 487*
- ♦ **Dionosil Oily®** *see* radiological/contrast media (ionic) *on page 539*
- ♦ **Diotrope** *see* tropicamide *on page 634*
- ♦ **Dioval® Injection** *see* estradiol *on page 242*
- ♦ **Diovan™** *see* valsartan *on page 642*
- ♦ **Diovan HCT™** *see* valsartan and hydrochlorothiazide *on page 642*
- ♦ **dipalmitoylphosphatidylcholine** *see* colfosceril palmitate *on page 166*
- ♦ **Dipedyne** *see* zidovudine *on page 658*
- ♦ **Dipentum®** *see* olsalazine *on page 454*
- ♦ **Diphenacen-50® Injection** [OTC] *see* diphenhydramine *on page 208*
- ♦ **Diphen® Cough** [OTC] *see* diphenhydramine *on page 208*
- ♦ **Diphenhist** [OTC] *see* diphenhydramine *on page 208*

diphenhydramine *(dye fen HYE dra meen)*

U.S. Brand Names AllerMax® Oral [OTC]; Banophen® Oral [OTC]; Belix® Oral [OTC]; Benadryl® Injection; Benadryl® Oral [OTC]; Benadryl® Topical; Ben-Allergin-50® Injection; Benylin® Cough Syrup [OTC]; Bydramine® Cough Syrup [OTC]; Compoz® Gel Caps [OTC]; Compoz® Nighttime Sleep Aid [OTC]; Dihyrex® Injection; Diphenacen-50® Injection [OTC]; Diphen® Cough [OTC]; Diphenhist [OTC]; Dormarex® 2 Oral [OTC]; Dormin® Oral [OTC]; Genahist® Oral; Hydramyn® Syrup [OTC]; Hyrexin-50® Injection; Maximum Strength Nytol® [OTC]; Miles Nervine® Caplets [OTC]; Nordryl® Injection; Nordryl® Oral; Nytol® Oral [OTC]; Phendry® Oral [OTC]; Siladryl® Oral [OTC]; Silphen® Cough [OTC]; Sleep-eze 3® Oral [OTC]; Sleepinal® [OTC]; Sleepwell 2-nite® [OTC]; Sominex® Oral [OTC]; Tusstat® Syrup; Twilite® Oral [OTC]; Uni-Bent® Cough Syrup; Winks® [OTC]

Canadian Brand Names Allerdryl®; Allernix®

Generic Available Yes

Therapeutic Category Antihistamine

Use Symptomatic relief of allergic symptoms caused by histamine release which include nasal allergies and allergic dermatosis; mild nighttime sedation, prevention of motion sickness, as an antitussive; treatment of phenothiazine-induced dystonic reactions

Usual Dosage

Children: Oral, I.M., I.V.: 5 mg/kg/day or 150 mg/m²/day in divided doses every 6-8 hours, not to exceed 300 mg/day

Adults:

Oral: 25-50 mg every 4-6 hours

I.M., I.V.: 10-50 mg in a single dose every 2-4 hours, not to exceed 400 mg/day

Topical: For external application, not longer than 7 days

Dietary Considerations May be administered with food or water

Nursing/Pharmacy Information

I.V. must be administered slowly; dilute to a maximum concentration of 25 mg/mL and infuse over 10-15 minutes (maximum rate of infusion: 25 mg/minute); monitor patient for sedation

Stability: Protect from light; the following drugs are **incompatible** with diphenhydramine when mixed in the same syringe: Amobarbital, amphotericin B, cephalothin, diatrizoate, foscarnet, heparin, hydrocortisone, hydroxyzine, pentobarbital, phenobarbital, phenytoin, prochlorperazine, promazine, promethazine, tetracycline, thiopental

Dosage Forms Diphenhydramine hydrochloride:

Capsule: 25 mg, 50 mg

Cream: 1%, 2%

Elixir: 12.5 mg/5 mL (5 mL, 10 mL, 20 mL, 120 mL, 480 mL, 3780 mL)

Injection: 10 mg/mL (10 mL, 30 mL); 50 mg/mL (1 mL, 10 mL)

Lotion: 1% (75 mL)

Solution, topical spray: 1% (60 mL)

Syrup: 12.5 mg/5 mL (5 mL, 120 mL, 240 mL, 480 mL, 3780 mL)

Tablet: 25 mg, 50 mg

diphenhydramine and pseudoephedrine
(dye fen HYE dra meen & soo doe e FED rin)

U.S. Brand Names Actifed® Allergy Tablet (Night) [OTC]; Banophen® Decongestant Capsule [OTC]; Benadryl® Decongestant Allergy Tablet [OTC]

Generic Available Yes

Therapeutic Category Antihistamine/Decongestant Combination

Use Relief of symptoms of upper respiratory mucosal congestion in seasonal and perennial nasal allergies, acute rhinitis, rhinosinusitis, and eustachian tube blockage

Usual Dosage Adults: Oral: 1 capsule or tablet every 4-6 hours, up to 4/day

Dosage Forms

Capsule: Diphenhydramine hydrochloride 25 mg and pseudoephedrine hydrochloride 60 mg

Tablet:

Actifed® Allergy (Night): Diphenhydramine hydrochloride 25 mg and pseudoephedrine hydrochloride 30 mg

Benadryl® Decongestant Allergy: Diphenhydramine hydrochloride 25 mg and pseudoephedrine hydrochloride 60 mg

diphenoxylate and atropine (dye fen OKS i late & A troe peen)

Synonyms atropine and diphenoxylate

U.S. Brand Names Logen®; Lomanate®; Lomotil®; Lonox®

Generic Available Yes

Therapeutic Category Antidiarrheal

Controlled Substance C-V

Use Treatment of diarrhea

Usual Dosage Oral (as diphenoxylate): Initial dose:

Children: 0.3-0.4 mg/kg/day in 2-4 divided doses

<2 years: Not recommended

2-5 years: 2 mg 3 times/day

5-8 years: 2 mg 4 times/day

8-12 years: 2 mg 5 times/day

Adults: 15-20 mg/day in 3-4 divided doses

Reduce dosage as soon as initial control of symptoms is achieved

Dietary Considerations May be administered with food

Nursing/Pharmacy Information

Watch for signs of atropinism (dryness of skin and mucous membranes, tachycardia, thirst, flushing), hypotension, respiratory depression, confusion

Stability: Protect from light

Dosage Forms

Solution, oral: Diphenoxylate hydrochloride 2.5 mg and atropine sulfate 0.025 mg per 5 mL (4 mL, 10 mL, 60 mL)

Tablet: Diphenoxylate hydrochloride 2.5 mg and atropine sulfate 0.025 mg

♦ **Diphenylan Sodium®** see phenytoin on page 490

♦ **diphenylhydantoin** see phenytoin on page 490

diphtheria and tetanus toxoid
(dif THEER ee a a & TET a nus TOKS oyd)

Synonyms DT; Td; tetanus and diphtheria toxoid

Generic Available Yes

Therapeutic Category Toxoid

Use Active immunity against diphtheria and tetanus

Usual Dosage I.M.:

Infants and Children:

6 weeks to 1 year: Three 0.5 mL doses at least 4 weeks apart; administer a reinforcing dose 6-12 months after the third injection

(Continued)

diphtheria and tetanus toxoid *(Continued)*

1-6 years: Administer two 0.5 mL doses at least 4 weeks apart; reinforcing dose 6-12 months after second injection; if final dose is administered after seventh birthday, use adult preparation

4-6 years (booster immunization): 0.5 mL; not necessary if all 4 doses were administered after fourth birthday - routinely administer booster doses at 10-year intervals with the adult preparation

Children >7 years and Adults: 2 primary doses of 0.5 mL each, administered at an interval of 4-6 weeks; third (reinforcing) dose of 0.5 mL 6-12 months later; boosters every 10 years

Nursing/Pharmacy Information

Shake well before administering; advise patient of adverse reactions; must be administered I.M.; do not inject the same site more than once; federal law requires that the date of administration, the vaccine manufacturer, lot number of vaccine, and the administering person's name, title, and address be entered into the patient's permanent medical record

Stability: Refrigerate

Dosage Forms Injection:

Pediatric use:

Diphtheria 6.6 Lf units and tetanus 5 Lf units per 0.5 mL (5 mL)

Diphtheria 10 Lf units and tetanus 5 Lf units per 0.5 mL (0.5 mL, 5 mL)

Diphtheria 12.5 Lf units and tetanus 5 Lf units per 0.5 mL (5 mL)

Diphtheria 15 Lf units and tetanus 10 Lf units per 0.5 mL (5 mL)

Adult use:

Diphtheria 1.5 Lf units and tetanus 5 Lf units per 0.5 mL (0.5 mL, 5 mL)

Diphtheria 2 Lf units and tetanus 5 Lf units per 0.5 mL (5 mL)

Diphtheria 2 Lf units and tetanus 10 Lf units per 0.5 mL (5 mL)

diphtheria antitoxin (dif THEER ee a an tee TOKS in)

Generic Available Yes

Therapeutic Category Antitoxin

Use Passive prevention and treatment of diphtheria

Usual Dosage I.M. or slow I.V. infusion: Dosage varies; range: 20,000-120,000 units

Dosage Forms Injection: 500 units/mL (20 mL, 40 mL)

diphtheria, tetanus toxoids, and acellular pertussis vaccine

(dif THEER ee a, TET a nus TOKS oyds & ay CEL yoo lar per TUS sis vak SEEN)

Synonyms DTAP

U.S. Brand Names Acel-Imune®; Certiva®; Infanrix™; Tripedia®

Generic Available No

Therapeutic Category Toxoid

Use Fourth or fifth immunization of children 15 months to 7 years of age (prior to seventh birthday) who have been previously immunized with 3 or 4 doses of whole-cell pertussis DTP vaccine

Usual Dosage I.M.: After at least 3 doses of whole-cell DTP, administer 0.5 mL at ~18 months (at least 6 months after third DTWP dose), then another dose at 4-5 years of age

Nursing/Pharmacy Information

This preparation contains less endotoxin relative to DTP and, although immunogenic, it apparently is less reactogenic than DTP. Federal law requires that the date of administration, the vaccine manufacturer, lot number of vaccine, and the administering person's name, title, and address be entered into the patient's permanent medical record.

Stability: Refrigerate

Dosage Forms Injection:

Acel-Imune®: Diphtheria 7.5 Lf units, tetanus 5 Lf units, and acellular pertussis vaccine 40 mcg per 0.5 mL (7.5 mL)

Certiva®: Diphtheria 15 Lf units, tetanus 6 Lf units, and acellular pertussis vaccine 40 mcg per 0.5 mL (7.5 mL)

Infanrix™: Diphtheria 25 Lf units, tetanus 10 Lf units, and acellular pertussis vaccine 25 mcg per 0.5 mL (7.5 mL)

Tripedia®: Diphtheria 6.7 Lf units, tetanus 5 Lf units, and acellular pertussis vaccine 46.8 mcg per 0.5 mL (7.5 mL)

diphtheria, tetanus toxoids, and whole-cell pertussis vaccine

(dif THEER ee a & TET a nus TOKS oyds & hole-sel per TUS sis vak SEEN)

Synonyms DPT

U.S. Brand Names Tri-Immunol®

Generic Available Yes

Therapeutic Category Toxoid

Use Active immunization of infants and children through 6 years of age (between 2 months and the seventh birthday) against diphtheria, tetanus, and pertussis; recommended for both primary immunization and routine recall; start immunization at once if whooping cough or diphtheria is present in the community

Usual Dosage The primary immunization for children 2 months to 6 years of age, ideally beginning at the age of 2-3 months or at 6-week check-up. Administer 0.5 mL I.M. on 3 occasions at 4- to 8-week intervals with a re-enforcing dose administered 1 year after the third injection. The booster doses (0.5 mL I.M.) are administered when the child is 4-6 years of age.

Nursing/Pharmacy Information

Acellular pertussis vaccine indicated for fourth or fifth booster dose of the five-part DTP series for children, indicated specifically for children 15 months of age

Stability: Refrigerate

Dosage Forms Injection:

Diphtheria 6.7 Lf units, tetanus 5 Lf units, and pertussis 4 protective units per 0.5 mL (7.5 mL)

Tri-Immunol®: Diphtheria 12.5 Lf units, tetanus 5 Lf units, and pertussis 4 protective units per 0.5 mL (7.5 mL)

diphtheria, tetanus toxoids, whole-cell pertussis, and *Haemophilus* B conjugate vaccine

(dif THEER ee a, TET a nus TOKS oyds, hole-sel per TUS sis, & hem OF fil us bee KON joo gate vak SEEN)

Synonyms DTwP-HIB

U.S. Brand Names Tetramune®

Generic Available No

Therapeutic Category Toxoid

Use Active immunization of infants and children through 5 years of age (between 2 months and the sixth birthday) against diphtheria, tetanus, and pertussis and *Haemophilus* B disease when indications for immunization with DTP vaccine and HIB vaccine coincide

Usual Dosage The primary immunization for children 2 months to 5 years of age, ideally beginning at the age of 2-3 months or at 6-week check-up; administer 0.5 mL I.M. on 3 occasions at ~2 month intervals, followed by a fourth 0.5 mL dose at ~15 months of age

Nursing/Pharmacy Information Refrigerate

Dosage Forms Injection: Diphtheria toxoid 12.5 Lf units, tetanus toxoid 5 Lf units, and whole-cell pertussis vaccine 4 units, and *Haemophilus influenzae* type B oligosaccharide 10 mcg per 0.5 mL (5 mL)

♦ **dipivalyl epinephrine** *see* dipivefrin *on page 211*

dipivefrin (dye PI ve frin)

Synonyms dipivalyl epinephrine; DPE

U.S. Brand Names Propine®

Canadian Brand Names DPE™; Optho-Dipivefrin™

Generic Available Yes

Therapeutic Category Adrenergic Agonist Agent

Use Reduces elevated intraocular pressure in chronic open-angle glaucoma; treatment of ocular hypertension

Usual Dosage Adults: Ophthalmic: Initial: 1 drop every 12 hours

Nursing/Pharmacy Information

Instruct on how to administer eye drops

Monitor intraocular pressure

Stability: Avoid exposure to light and air; discolored or darkened solutions indicate loss of potency

Dosage Forms Solution, ophthalmic, as hydrochloride: 0.1% (5 mL, 10 mL, 15 mL)

♦ **Diprivan®** *see* propofol *on page 525*

- ♦ **Diprolene® AF Topical** *see* betamethasone (topical) *on page 85*
- ♦ **Diprolene® Glycol** *see* betamethasone (topical) *on page 85*
- ♦ **Diprolene® Topical** *see* betamethasone (topical) *on page 85*
- ♦ **dipropylacetic acid** *see* valproic acid and derivatives *on page 641*
- ♦ **Diprosone® Topical** *see* betamethasone (topical) *on page 85*

dipyridamole (dye peer ID a mole)
U.S. Brand Names Persantine®
Canadian Brand Names Apo®-Dipyridamole FC; Apo®-Dipyridamole SC; Asasantine® [with Aspirin also]; Novo-Dipiradol®
Mexican Brand Names Dirinol; Lodimil; Trompersantin
Generic Available Yes
Therapeutic Category Antiplatelet Agent; Vasodilator
Use Maintain patency after surgical grafting procedures including coronary artery bypass; with warfarin to decrease thrombosis in patients after artificial heart valve replacement; for chronic management of angina pectoris; with aspirin to prevent coronary artery thrombosis; in combination with aspirin or warfarin to prevent other thromboembolic disorders; dipyridamole may also be administered 2 days prior to open heart surgery to prevent platelet activation by extracorporeal bypass pump; diagnostic agent I.V. (dipyridamole stress test) for coronary artery disease
Usual Dosage
Children: Oral: 3-6 mg/kg/day in 3 divided doses
Dipyridamole stress test (for evaluation of myocardial perfusion): I.V.: 0.14 mg/kg/minute for a total of 4 minutes
Adults: Oral: 75-400 mg/day in 3-4 divided doses
Dietary Considerations Should be administered with water 1 hour before meals
Nursing/Pharmacy Information
Parenteral: I.V.: Dilute in at least a 1:2 ratio with NS, $\frac{1}{2}$NS, or D_5W; infusion of undiluted dipyridamole may cause local irritation
Monitor blood pressure, heart rate
Stability: Do not freeze, protect I.V. preparation from light
Dosage Forms
Injection: 10 mg/2 mL
Tablet: 25 mg, 50 mg, 75 mg

dipyridamole and aspirin *New Drug*
(dye peer ID a mole & AS pir in)
U.S. Brand Names Aggrenox®
Canadian Brand Names Asasantine®
Generic Available No
Therapeutic Category Antiplatelet Agent
Use Combined therapy with dipyridamole and aspirin is indicated in patients who are recovering from a myocardial infarction; the rate of reinfarction is significantly reduced by such therapy; combined treatment is also indicated for the prevention of occlusion of saphenous vein coronary artery bypass grafts
Usual Dosage Adults: Oral:
Prevention of recurrent myocardial infarction: The recommended oral dose is one capsule 3 times/day, in patients who have suffered a previous myocardial infarction
Prevention of occlusion of saphenous vein coronary artery bypass grafts:
For 2 days preoperatively: Dipyridamole 100 mg four times/day;
Day of surgery: Morning of operation: Dipyridamole 100 mg; 1 hour post-op: Dipyridamole 100 mg (via nasogastric tube); 7 hours post-op: Asasantine® capsule; daily maintenance dosage: (for the next 12 months): One Asasantine® capsule three times/daily
Dosage Forms Capsule: Dipyridamole 75 mg and aspirin 330 mg

- ♦ **Dirinol** *see* dipyridamole *on page 212*

dirithromycin (dye RITH roe mye sin)
U.S. Brand Names Dynabac®
Generic Available No
Therapeutic Category Macrolide (Antibiotic)
Use Treatment of mild to moderate upper and lower respiratory tract infections, infections of the skin and skin structure, and sexually transmitted diseases due to susceptible strains
Usual Dosage Adults: Oral: 500 mg once daily for 7-14 days
Dietary Considerations Administer with food or within 1 hour of eating
Dosage Forms Tablet, enteric coated: 250 mg

♦ **Disalcid®** *see* salsalate *on page 559*
♦ **disalicylic acid** *see* salsalate *on page 559*
♦ **Disanthrol® [OTC]** *see* docusate and casanthranol *on page 215*
♦ **Disobrom® [OTC]** *see* dexbrompheniramine and pseudoephedrine *on page 191*
♦ **disodium cromoglycate** *see* cromolyn sodium *on page 171*
♦ **d-isoephedrine** *see* pseudoephedrine *on page 530*
♦ **Disonate® [OTC]** *see* docusate *on page 214*
♦ **Disophrol® Chronotabs® [OTC]** *see* dexbrompheniramine and pseudoephedrine *on page 191*
♦ **Disophrol® Tablet [OTC]** *see* dexbrompheniramine and pseudoephedrine *on page 191*

disopyramide (dye soe PEER a mide)

U.S. Brand Names Norpace®; Norpace® CR
Canadian Brand Names Rythmodan®, -LA
Mexican Brand Names Dimodan
Generic Available Yes
Therapeutic Category Antiarrhythmic Agent, Class I-A
Use Suppression and prevention of unifocal and multifocal ventricular premature complexes, coupled ventricular premature complexes, and/or paroxysmal ventricular tachycardia; also effective in the conversion and prevention of recurrence of atrial fibrillation, atrial flutter, and paroxysmal atrial tachycardia
Usual Dosage Oral:
  Children:
    <1 year: 10-30 mg/kg/24 hours in 4 divided doses
    1-4 years: 10-20 mg/kg/24 hours in 4 divided doses
    4-12 years: 10-15 mg/kg/24 hours in 4 divided doses
    12-18 years: 6-15 mg/kg/24 hours in 4 divided doses
  Adults:
    <50 kg: 100 mg every 6 hours or 200 mg every 12 hours (controlled release)
    >50 kg: 150 mg every 6 hours or 300 mg every 12 hours (controlled release); if no response, may increase to 200 mg every 6 hours; maximum dose required for patients with severe refractory ventricular tachycardia is 400 mg every 6 hours
Dietary Considerations Should be administered on an empty stomach
Nursing/Pharmacy Information
  Do not crush, break, or chew controlled release capsules
  Monitor EKG, blood pressure, disopyramide drug level
Dosage Forms Disopyramide phosphate:
  Capsule: 100 mg, 150 mg
  Capsule, sustained action: 100 mg, 150 mg

♦ **Disotate®** *see* edetate disodium *on page 228*
♦ **Di-Spaz® Injection** *see* dicyclomine *on page 199*
♦ **Di-Spaz® Oral** *see* dicyclomine *on page 199*
♦ **Dispos-a-Med® Isoproterenol** *(Discontinued) see page 743*
♦ **Distaval®** *see* thalidomide *on page 602*

disulfiram (dye SUL fi ram)

U.S. Brand Names Antabuse®
Generic Available Yes
Therapeutic Category Aldehyde Dehydrogenase Inhibitor Agent
Use Management of chronic alcoholics
Usual Dosage Oral:
  Maximum daily dose: 500 mg/day in a single dose for 1-2 weeks
  Average maintenance dose: 250 mg/day; range: 125-500 mg; duration of therapy is to continue until the patient is fully recovered socially and a basis for permanent self control has been established; maintenance therapy may be required for months or even years
Nursing/Pharmacy Information Monitor hypokalemia
Dosage Forms Tablet: 250 mg, 500 mg

♦ **Dital®** *see* phendimetrazine *on page 484*
♦ **dithioglycerol** *see* dimercaprol *on page 206*
♦ **dithranol** *see* anthralin *on page 50*
♦ **Ditropan®** *see* oxybutynin *on page 461*
♦ **Ditropan® XL** *see* oxybutynin *on page 461*
♦ **Diucardin®** *see* hydroflumethiazide *on page 324*
♦ **Diuchlor®** *see* hydrochlorothiazide *on page 317*

- **Diupress®** *(Discontinued)* see page 743
- **Diurigen®** see chlorothiazide *on page 137*
- **Diuril®** see chlorothiazide *on page 137*
- **Dixaparine** see heparin *on page 310*
- **Dixarit®** see clonidine *on page 159*
- **Dixonal** see piroxicam *on page 497*
- **Dizac® Injectable Emulsion** see diazepam *on page 196*
- **Dizmiss® [OTC]** see meclizine *on page 387*
- **Dizymes® Tablet** *(Discontinued)* see page 743
- ***dl*-alpha tocopherol** see vitamin E *on page 652*
- ***dl*-norephedrine** see phenylpropanolamine *on page 489*
- ***d*-mannitol** see mannitol *on page 383*
- **4-dmdr** see idarubicin *on page 333*
- **D-Med® Injection** see methylprednisolone *on page 407*
- **DMSO** see dimethyl sulfoxide *on page 207*
- **DNASE** see dornase alfa *on page 218*
- **DNR** see daunorubicin hydrochloride *on page 183*
- **Doan's®, Original [OTC]** see magnesium salicylate *on page 382*
- **Dobuject** see dobutamine *on page 214*

dobutamine (doe BYOO ta meen)
U.S. Brand Names Dobutrex®
Mexican Brand Names Dobuject; Oxiken
Generic Available Yes
Therapeutic Category Adrenergic Agonist Agent
Use Short-term management of patients with cardiac decompensation
Usual Dosage I.V. infusion:
  Children: 2.5-15 mcg/kg/minute, titrate to desired response
  Adults: 2.5-15 mcg/kg/minute; maximum: 40 mcg/kg/minute, titrate to desired response
Nursing/Pharmacy Information
  Administer into large vein; use infusion device to control rate of flow; dilute in dextrose or normal saline; maximum recommended concentration: 6000 mcg/mL (6 mg/mL); rate of infusion (mL/hour) = dose (mcg/kg/minute) x weight (kg) x 60 minutes/hour divided by the concentration (mcg/mL)
  Monitor blood pressure, EKG, heart rate, CVP, RAP, MAP, urine output; if pulmonary artery catheter is in place, monitor CI, PCWP, and SVR; also monitor serum glucose
  Stability: Remix solution every 24 hours; **incompatible** with sodium bicarbonate solutions; store reconstituted solution under refrigeration for 48 hours or 6 hours at room temperature; pink discoloration of solution indicates slight oxidation but **no** significant loss of potency.
Dosage Forms Infusion, as hydrochloride: 12.5 mg/mL (20 mL)

- **Dobutrex®** see dobutamine *on page 214*

docetaxel (doe se TAKS el)
U.S. Brand Names Taxotere®
Generic Available No
Therapeutic Category Antineoplastic Agent
Use Treatment of breast cancer; advanced or metastatic nonsmall-cell lung cancer in patients whose disease has progressed after platinum-based chemotherapy
Usual Dosage Adults: I.V.: 60-100 mg/m^2 administered over 1 hour every 3 weeks
Dosage Forms Injection: 40 mg/mL (0.5 mL, 2 mL)

docusate (DOK yoo sate)
Synonyms dioctyl calcium sulfosuccinate; dioctyl potassium sulfosuccinate; dioctyl sodium sulfosuccinate; DOSS; DSS
U.S. Brand Names Colace® [OTC]; DC 240® Softgel [OTC]; Dialose® Tablet [OTC]; Diocto® [OTC]; Diocto-K® [OTC]; Dioeze® [OTC]; Disonate® [OTC]; DOK® [OTC]; DOS® Softgel® [OTC]; D-S-S® [OTC]; Kasof® [OTC]; Modane® Soft [OTC]; Pro-Cal-Sof® [OTC]; Regulax SS® [OTC]; Sulfalax® [OTC]; Surfak® [OTC]
Canadian Brand Names Albert® Docusate; Colax-C®; PMS-Docusate Calcium; Regulex®; Selax®; Soflax™
Generic Available Yes
Therapeutic Category Stool Softener

Use Stool softener in patients who should avoid straining during defecation and constipation associated with hard, dry stools

Usual Dosage Docusate salts are interchangeable; the amount of sodium, calcium, or potassium per dosage unit is clinically insignificant

Infants and Children <3 years: Oral: 10-40 mg/day in 1-4 divided doses
Children: Oral:
3-6 years: 20-60 mg/day in 1-4 divided doses
6-12 years: 40-150 mg/day in 1-4 divided doses
Adolescents and Adults: Oral: 50-500 mg/day in 1-4 divided doses
Older Children and Adults: Rectal: Add 50-100 mg of docusate liquid to enema fluid (saline or water); administer as retention or flushing enema

Dietary Considerations Should be administered with a full glass of water, milk, or fruit juice

Nursing/Pharmacy Information Docusate liquid should be administered with milk, fruit juice, or infant formula to mask the bitter taste

Dosage Forms
Capsule:
As calcium:
DC 240® Softgels®, Pro-Cal-Sof®, Sulfalax®: 240 mg
Surfak®: 50 mg, 240 mg
As potassium:
Diocto-K®: 100 mg
Kasof®: 240 mg
As sodium:
Colace®: 50 mg, 100 mg
Dioeze®: 250 mg
Disonate®: 100 mg, 240 mg
DOK®: 100 mg, 250 mg
DOS® Softgel®: 100 mg, 250 mg
D-S-S®: 100 mg
Modane® Soft: 100 mg
Regulax SS®: 100 mg, 250 mg
Liquid, as sodium (Diocto®, Colace®, Disonate®, DOK®): 150 mg/15 mL (30 mL, 60 mL, 480 mL)
Solution, oral, as sodium (Doxinate®): 50 mg/mL with alcohol 5% (60 mL, 3780 mL)
Syrup, as sodium:
50 mg/15 mL (15 mL, 30 mL)
Colace®, Diocto®, Disonate®, DOK®: 60 mg/15 mL (240 mL, 480 mL, 3780 mL)
Tablet, as sodium: 100 mg

docusate and casanthranol (DOK yoo sate & ka SAN thra nole)

Synonyms casanthranol and docusate; dss with casanthranol

U.S. Brand Names Dialose® Plus Capsule [OTC]; Diocto C® [OTC]; Diocto-K Plus® [OTC]; Dioctolose Plus® [OTC]; Disanthrol® [OTC]; DSMC Plus® [OTC]; Genasoft® Plus [OTC]; Peri-Colace® [OTC]; Pro-Sof® Plus [OTC]; Regulace® [OTC]; Silace-C® [OTC]

Generic Available Yes

Therapeutic Category Laxative/Stool Softener

Use Treatment of constipation generally associated with dry, hard stools and decreased intestinal motility

Usual Dosage Oral:
Children: 5-15 mL of syrup at bedtime or 1 capsule at bedtime
Adults: 1-2 capsules or 15-30 mL syrup at bedtime, may be increased to 2 capsules or 30 mL twice daily or 3 capsules at bedtime

Nursing/Pharmacy Information
Monitor bowel frequency
Stability: Store in tight, light-resistant containers

Dosage Forms
Capsule:
Dialose® Plus, Diocto-K Plus®, Dioctolose Plus®, DSMC Plus®: Docusate potassium 100 mg and casanthranol 30 mg
Disanthrol®, Genasoft® Plus, Peri-Colace®, Pro-Sof® Plus, Regulace®: Docusate sodium 100 mg and casanthranol 30 mg
Syrup (Diocto C®, Peri-Colace®, Silace-C®): Docusate sodium 60 mg and casanthranol 30 mg per 15 mL with alcohol 10% (240 mL, 480 mL, 4000 mL)

dofetilide *New Drug* (doe FET il ide)

Synonyms UK-68-798

U.S. Brand Names Tikosyn™

(Continued)

dofetilide *New Drug* *(Continued)*

Therapeutic Category Antiarrhythmic Agent, Class III

Use Prevention and treatment of fibrillation (atrial), flutter (atrial), paroxysmal tachycardia (ventricular), tachycardia (ventricular), fibrillation (ventricular); used in conjunction of implantable defibrillator

Usual Dosage

Oral: 0.25-1 mg twice daily in patients with sustained tachycardia (ventricular) (lower dose in patients with renal insufficiency)

I.V.:

Supraventricular tachycardia: 1-10 mcg/kg over 15 minutes followed by 0.12-0.5 mcg/kg maintenance infusion

Ventricular arrhythmia: 1.5-15 mcg/kg

- ◆ **DOK® [OTC]** *see* docusate *on page 214*
- ◆ **Doktors® Nasal Solution [OTC]** *see* phenylephrine *on page 487*
- ◆ **Dolacet®** *see* hydrocodone and acetaminophen *on page 319*
- ◆ **Dolac Inyectable** *see* ketorolac tromethamine *on page 355*
- ◆ **Dolac Oral** *see* ketorolac tromethamine *on page 355*
- ◆ **Dolaren (Carisoprodol With Diclofenac)** *see* carisoprodol *on page 116*

dolasetron *(dol A se tron)*

U.S. Brand Names Anzemet®

Generic Available No

Therapeutic Category Selective 5-HT$_3$ Receptor Antagonist

Use The prevention of nausea and vomiting associated with moderately emetogenic cancer chemotherapy, including initial and repeat courses; the prevention of postoperative nausea and vomiting.

Usual Dosage

Oral:

Prevention of cancer chemotherapy-induced nausea and vomiting:

Children 2-16 years: 1.8 mg/kg given within 1 hour before chemotherapy, up to a maximum of 100 mg; safety and effectiveness in pediatric patients <2 years of age have not been established

Adults: 100 mg given within 1 hour before chemotherapy

Use in the elderly, renal failure patients, or hepatically impaired patients: No dosage adjustment is recommended

Prevention of postoperative nausea and vomiting:

Children 2-16 years: 1.2 mg/kg given within 2 hours before surgery, up to a maximum of 100 mg; safety and effectiveness in pediatric patients <2 years of age have not been established

Adults: 100 mg within 2 hours before surgery

Use in the elderly, renal failure patients, or hepatically impaired patients: No dosage adjustment is recommended

Parenteral (injection):

Prevention of cancer chemotherapy-induced nausea and vomiting:

Children 2-16 years: 1.8 mg/kg given as a single dose approximately 30 minutes before chemotherapy, up to a maximum of 100 mg; safety and effectiveness in pediatric patients <2 years of age have not been established. Injection mixed in apple or apple-grape juice may be used for oral dosing of pediatric patients. When injection is administered orally, the recommended dosage in pediatric patients 2-16 years of age is 1.8 mg/kg up to a maximum 100 mg dose given within 1 hour before chemotherapy. The diluted product may be kept up to 2 hours at room temperature before use.

Adults: From clinical trials, the dose is 1.8 mg/kg given as a single dose approximately 30 minutes before chemotherapy; alternatively, for most patients, a fixed dose of 100 mg can be administered over 30 seconds

Use in the elderly, renal failure patients, or hepatically impaired patients: No dosage adjustment is recommended

Prevention of postoperative nausea and/or vomiting:

Children 2-16 years: 0.35 mg/kg, with a maximum dose of 12.5 mg, given as a single dose approximately 15 minutes before the cessation of anesthesia or as soon as nausea or vomiting presents. Safety and effectiveness in pediatric patients <2 years of age have not been established. Injection mixed in apple or apple-grape juice may be used for oral dosing of pediatric patients; dosage in pediatric patients 2-16 years is 1.2 mg/kg up to a maximum 100 mg dose given before surgery.

Adults: 12.5 mg given as a single dose approximately 15 minutes before the cessation of anesthesia (prevention) or as soon as nausea or vomiting presents (treatment)

Dosage Forms Dolasetron mesylate:
Injection: 20 mg/mL
Tablet: 50 mg, 100 mg

- ♦ **Dolene®** *see* propoxyphene *on page 526*
- ♦ **Dolobid®** *see* diflunisal *on page 202*
- ♦ **Dolo Pangavit-D** *see* diclofenac *on page 198*
- ♦ **Dolophine®** *see* methadone *on page 399*
- ♦ **Dolorac™ [OTC]** *see* capsaicin *on page 110*
- ♦ **Dolotic®** *see* antipyrine and benzocaine *on page 53*
- ♦ **Domeboro® Topical [OTC]** *see* aluminum acetate and calcium acetate *on page 32*
- ♦ **Dommanate® Injection *(Discontinued)*** *see page 743*

domperidone *(Canada only)* (dom PE ri done)
Canadian Brand Names Motilium®
Generic Available No
Therapeutic Category Dopamine Antagonist
Use Symptomatic management of upper gastrointestinal motility disorders associated with chronic and subacute gastritis and diabetic gastroparesis; may also be used to prevent gastrointestinal symptoms associated with the use of dopamine agonist antiparkinsonian agents
Usual Dosage Adults: Oral:
Upper gastrointestinal motility disorders: Usual dosage in adults: 10 mg 3-4 times/day, 15-30 minutes before meals and at bedtime if required. In severe or resistant cases the dose may be increased to a maximum of 20 mg 3-4 times/day.
Nausea and vomiting associated with dopamine agonist antiparkinsonian agents: Usual dosage in adults: 20 mg 3-4 times/day. Higher doses may be required to achieve symptom control while titration of the antiparkinsonian medication is occurring.

donepezil (don EH pa zil)
Synonyms E2020
U.S. Brand Names Aricept®
Generic Available No
Therapeutic Category Acetylcholinesterase Inhibitor
Use Treatment of mild to moderate dementia of the Alzheimer's type
Usual Dosage Adults: Oral: Initial: 5 mg at bedtime; may be increased to 10 mg at bedtime after 4-6 weeks; a 10 mg dose may provide additional benefit for some patients
Dosage Forms Tablet: 5 mg, 10 mg

- ♦ **Donnagel®-MB** *see* kaolin and pectin *on page 352*
- ♦ **Donnamar®** *see* hyoscyamine *on page 329*
- ♦ **Donnapectolin-PG®** *see* hyoscyamine, atropine, scopolamine, kaolin, pectin, and opium *on page 331*
- ♦ **Donnatal®** *see* hyoscyamine, atropine, scopolamine, and phenobarbital *on page 330*
- ♦ **Donnazyme®** *see* pancreatin *on page 467*
- ♦ **Donphen® Tablet *(Discontinued)*** *see page 743*
- ♦ **Dopamet®** *see* methyldopa *on page 406*

dopamine (DOE pa meen)
U.S. Brand Names Intropin®
Generic Available Yes
Therapeutic Category Adrenergic Agonist Agent
Use Adjunct in the treatment of shock which persists after adequate fluid volume replacement
Usual Dosage I.V. infusion:
Children: 1-20 mcg/kg/minute, maximum: 50 mcg/kg/minute continuous infusion, titrate to desired response
Adults: 1 mcg/kg/minute up to 50 mcg/kg/minute, titrate to desired response
If dosages >20-30 mcg/kg/minute are needed, a more direct acting pressor may be more beneficial (ie, epinephrine, norepinephrine)

Hemodynamic effects of dopamine are dose-dependent:
Low-dose: 1-5 mcg/kg/minute, increased renal blood flow and urine output
Intermediate-dose: 5-15 mcg/kg/minute, increased renal blood flow, heart rate, cardiac contractility, and cardiac output
(Continued)

dopamine *(Continued)*

High-dose: >15 mcg/kg/minute, alpha-adrenergic effects begin to predominate, vasoconstriction, increased blood pressure

Nursing/Pharmacy Information

Administer into large vein to prevent the possibility of extravasation; use infusion device to control rate of flow; administration into an umbilical arterial catheter is **not** recommended; must be diluted prior to administration; maximum concentration: 6000 mcg/mL (6 mg/mL); rate of infusion (mL/hour): dose (mcg/kg/minute) x weight (kg) x 60 minutes/hour divided by concentration (mcg/mL)

Monitor blood pressure, EKG, heart rate, CVP, RAP, MAP, urine output; if pulmonary artery catheter is in place, monitor CI, PCWP, SVR, and PVR

Stability: Protect from light; solutions that are darker than slightly yellow should not be used; **incompatible** with alkaline solutions or iron salts; **compatible** when coadministered with dobutamine, epinephrine, isoproterenol, and lidocaine

Dosage Forms Dopamine hydrochloride:

Infusion in D_5W: 0.8 mg/mL (250 mL, 500 mL); 1.6 mg/mL (250 mL, 500 mL); 3.2 mg/mL (250 mL, 500 mL)

Injection: 40 mg/mL (5 mL, 10 mL, 20 mL); 80 mg/mL (5 mL, 20 mL); 160 mg/mL (5 mL)

♦ **Dopar®** *see* levodopa *on page 365*
♦ **Dopastat® Injection** *(Discontinued) see page 743*
♦ **Dopram®** *see* doxapram *on page 219*
♦ **Doral®** *see* quazepam *on page 535*
♦ **Dorcol® [OTC]** *see* acetaminophen *on page 13*
♦ **Doriden® Tablet** *(Discontinued) see page 743*
♦ **Dormarex® 2 Oral [OTC]** *see* diphenhydramine *on page 208*
♦ **Dormicum** *see* midazolam *on page 415*
♦ **Dormin® Oral [OTC]** *see* diphenhydramine *on page 208*

dornase alfa *(DOOR nase AL fa)*

Synonyms DNASE; recombinant human deoxyribonuclease
U.S. Brand Names Pulmozyme®
Generic Available No
Therapeutic Category Enzyme
Use Management of cystic fibrosis patients to reduce the frequency of respiratory infections and to improve pulmonary function
Usual Dosage Children >5 years and Adults: Inhalation: 2.5 mg once daily through selected nebulizers in conjunction with a Pulmo-Aide® or a Pari-Proneb® compressor
Nursing/Pharmacy Information
Should not be diluted or mixed with any other drugs in the nebulizer, this may inactivate the drug
Stability: Most be stored in the refrigerator at 2°C to 8°C (36°F to 46°F) and protected from strong light; should not be exposed to room temperature for a total of 24 hours
Dosage Forms Solution, inhalation: 1 mg/mL (2.5 mL)

♦ **Doryx®** *see* doxycycline *on page 222*

dorzolamide *(dor ZOLE a mide)*

U.S. Brand Names Trusopt®
Generic Available No
Therapeutic Category Carbonic Anhydrase Inhibitor
Use Lower intraocular pressure to treat glaucoma
Usual Dosage Adults: Ophthalmic: 1 drop in eye(s) 3 times/day
Dosage Forms Solution, ophthalmic, as hydrochloride: 2%

dorzolamide and timolol *(dor ZOLE a mide & TYE moe lole)*

U.S. Brand Names Cosopt™
Generic Available No
Therapeutic Category Beta-Adrenergic Blocker; Carbonic Anhydrase Inhibitor
Use Lowers intraocular pressure to treat glaucoma in patients with ocular hypertension or open-angle glaucoma
Usual Dosage Adults: ophthalmic: One drop in eye(s) twice daily
Dosage Forms Solution, ophthalmic: Dorzolamide 2% and timolol 0.5% (5 mL, 10 mL)

- ◆ **DOSS** *see docusate on page 214*
- ◆ **DOS® Softgel® [OTC]** *see docusate on page 214*
- ◆ **Dostinex®** *see cabergoline on page 101*
- ◆ **Dovonex®** *see calcipotriene on page 102*

doxacurium (doks a KYOO ri um)

U.S. Brand Names Nuromax®

Generic Available No

Therapeutic Category Skeletal Muscle Relaxant

Use Doxacurium is indicated for use as an adjunct to general anesthesia. It provides skeletal muscle relaxation during surgery or endotracheal intubation; increases pulmonary compliance during mechanical ventilation

Usual Dosage I.V. (in obese patients, use ideal body weight to calculate dosage):

Children >2 years: Initial: 0.03-0.05 mg/kg followed by maintenance doses of 0.005-0.01 mg/kg after 30-45 minutes

Adults: Surgery: 0.05 mg/kg with thiopental/narcotic or 0.025 mg/kg with succinylcholine; maintenance dose: 0.005-0.01 mg/kg after 60-100 minutes

Nursing/Pharmacy Information

Parenteral: May be administered rapid I.V. injection undiluted

Blockade is monitored with a peripheral nerve stimulator, should also evaluate EKG, blood pressure, and heart rate

Stability: Stable for 24 hours at room temperature when diluted, up to 0.1 mg/mL in dextrose 5% or normal saline; **compatible** with sufentanil, alfentanil, and fentanyl

Dosage Forms Injection, as chloride: 1 mg/mL (5 mL)

doxapram (DOKS a pram)

U.S. Brand Names Dopram®

Generic Available No

Therapeutic Category Respiratory Stimulant

Use Respiratory and CNS stimulant; idiopathic apnea of prematurity refractory to xanthines

Usual Dosage I.V.:

Neonatal apnea (apnea of prematurity):

Initial: 0.5 mg/kg/hour

Maintenance: 0.5-2.5 mg/kg/hour, titrated to the lowest rate at which apnea is controlled

Adults: Respiratory depression following anesthesia:

Initial: 0.5-1 mg/kg; may repeat at 5-minute intervals; maximum total dose: 2 mg/kg; single doses should not exceed 1.5 mg/kg

I.V. infusion: Initial: 5 mg/minute until adequate response or adverse effects seen; decrease to 1-3 mg/minute; usual total dose: 0.5-4 mg/kg; maximum: 300 mg

Nursing/Pharmacy Information

Dilute loading dose to a maximum concentration of 2 mg/mL and infuse over 15-30 minutes; for infusion, dilute in normal saline or dextrose to 1 mg/mL (maximum: 2 mg/mL); irritating to tissues; avoid extravasation

Monitor heart rate, blood pressure, reflexes, CNS status

Stability: **Incompatible** with aminophylline, thiopental, or sodium bicarbonate (alkali drugs)

Dosage Forms Injection, as hydrochloride: 20 mg/mL (20 mL)

doxazosin (doks AYE zoe sin)

U.S. Brand Names Cardura®

Generic Available No

Therapeutic Category Alpha-Adrenergic Blocking Agent

Use Alpha-adrenergic blocking agent for treatment of hypertension

Usual Dosage Adults: Oral: 1 mg once daily, may be increased to 2 mg once daily thereafter up to 16 mg if needed

Nursing/Pharmacy Information

Syncope may occur, usually within 90 minutes of the initial dose

Monitor blood pressure, standing and sitting/supine

Dosage Forms Tablet: 1 mg, 2 mg, 4 mg, 8 mg

doxepin (DOKS e pin)

U.S. Brand Names Adapin® Oral; Sinequan® Oral; Zonalon® Topical Cream

Canadian Brand Names Apo®-Doxepin; Novo-Doxepin®; Triadapin®

Generic Available Yes

(Continued)

doxepin *(Continued)*

Therapeutic Category Antidepressant, Tricyclic (Tertiary Amine); Topical Skin Product

Use

Oral: Treatment of various forms of depression, usually in conjunction with psychotherapy; treatment of anxiety disorders; analgesic for certain chronic and neuropathic pain

Topical: Adults: Short-term (<8 days) therapy of moderate pruritus due to atopic dermatitis or lichen simplex chronicus

Usual Dosage

Oral:

Adolescents: Initial: 25-50 mg/day in single or divided doses; gradually increase to 100 mg/day

Adults: Initial: 30-150 mg/day at bedtime or in 2-3 divided doses; may increase up to 300 mg/day; single dose should not exceed 150 mg; select patients may respond to 25-50 mg/day

Topical: Apply in a thin film 4 times/day

Dietary Considerations Do not mix oral concentrate with carbonated beverages (physically incompatible); may be administered with food to decrease GI distress

Nursing/Pharmacy Information

Oral concentrate should be diluted in 120 mL of water, milk, juice (but not grape juice) prior to administration; may increase appetite

Monitor sitting and standing blood pressure and pulse rate prior to and during initial therapy; evaluate mental status; monitor weight

Stability: Protect from light

Dosage Forms Doxepin hydrochloride:

Capsule: 10 mg, 25 mg, 50 mg, 75 mg, 100 mg, 150 mg

Concentrate, oral: 10 mg/mL (120 mL)

Cream (Zonalon®): 5% (30 g)

doxercalciferol *New Drug* (dox er kal si fe FEER ole)

U.S. Brand Names Hectorol®

Generic Available No

Therapeutic Category Vitamin D Analog

Use Reduction of elevated intact parathyroid hormone (iPTH) in the management of secondary hyperparathyroidism in patients on chronic hemodialysis.

Usual Dosage

Adults: Oral: If the iPTH >400 pg/mL, then the initial dose is 10 mcg 3 times/week at dialysis. The dose is adjusted at 8-week intervals based upon the iPTH levels. If the iPTH level is decreased by 50% and above 300 pg/mL, then the dose can be increased to 12.5 mcg 3 times/week for 8 more weeks. This titration process can continue at 8-week intervals up to a maximum dose of 20 mcg 3 times/week. Each increase should be by 2.5 mcg/dose. If the iPTH is between 150-300 pg/mL, maintain the current dose. If the iPTH is <100 pg/mL, then suspend the drug for 1 week. Resume doxercalciferol at a reduced dose. Decrease each dose (not weekly dose) by at least 2.5 mcg.

Dosage Forms Capsule: 2.5 mcg

♦ **Doxil®** *see* doxorubicin (liposomal) *on page 221*

♦ **Doxinate® Capsule *(Discontinued)*** *see page 743*

♦ **Doxolem** *see* doxorubicin *on page 220*

doxorubicin (doks oh ROO bi sin)

Synonyms ADR; hydroxydaunomycin

U.S. Brand Names Adriamycin PFS™; Adriamycin RDF®; Rubex®

Mexican Brand Names Doxolem

Generic Available Yes

Therapeutic Category Antineoplastic Agent

Use Treatment of various solid tumors including ovarian, breast, and bladder tumors; various lymphomas and leukemias (ANL, ALL), soft tissue sarcomas, neuroblastoma, osteosarcoma

Usual Dosage I.V. (refer to individual protocols; patient's ideal weight should be used to calculate body surface area):

Children: 35-75 mg/m² as a single dose, repeat every 21 days; or 20 mg/m² once weekly

Adults: 60-75 mg/m² as a single dose, repeat every 21 days or other dosage regimens like 20-30 mg/m²/day for 2-3 days, repeat in 4 weeks or 20 mg/m² once weekly

The lower dose regimen should be administered to patients with decreased bone marrow reserve, prior therapy or marrow infiltration with malignant cells

Nursing/Pharmacy Information

Local erythematous streaking along the vein and/or facial flushing may indicate too rapid a rate of administration; drug is very irritating; avoid extravasation; if extravasation occurs, apply cold packs. Local infiltration with a corticosteroid and irrigating the site with normal saline may also be helpful. Administer slow IVP at a rate no faster than over 3-5 minutes or by I.V. infusion over 1-4 hours at a concentration not to exceed 2 mg/mL

Monitor CBC with differential and platelet count, echocardiogram, liver function tests

Stability: Protect from light, must be dispensed in an amber bag; store powder vials at room temperature, refrigerate liquid vials; reconstituted powder vials stable for 24 hours at room temperature and 48 hours if refrigerated; unstable in solutions with a pH <3 or >7. **Incompatible** with heparin, fluorouracil, aminophylline, cephalothin, methotrexate, dexamethasone, diazepam, hydrocortisone, furosemide. Y-site is **compatible** with doxorubicin, vincristine, cyclophosphamide, dacarbazine, bleomycin, vinblastine.

Dosage Forms Doxorubicin hydrochloride:

Aqueous injection with NS: 2 mg/mL (5 mL, 10 mL, 25 mL)

Preservative free injection: 2 mg/mL (5 mL, 10 mL, 25 mL, 100 mL)

Powder for injection, lyophilized: 10 mg, 20 mg, 50 mg, 100 mg

Powder for injection, lyophilized, rapid dissolution formula: 10 mg, 20 mg, 50 mg, 150 mg

doxorubicin (liposomal) (doks oh ROO bi sin lip pah SOW mal)

U.S. Brand Names Doxil®

Generic Available No

Therapeutic Category Antineoplastic Agent

Use Treatment of AIDS-related Kaposi's sarcoma in patients with disease that has progressed on prior combination chemotherapy or in patients who are intolerant to such therapy; treatment of metastatic carcinoma of the ovary in patients with disease that is refractory to both paclitaxel and platinum-based regimens

Usual Dosage Refer to individual protocols

I.V. (patient's ideal weight should be used to calculate body surface area): 20 mg/m^2 over 30 minutes, once every 3 weeks, for as long as patients respond satisfactorily and tolerate treatment.

AIDS-KS patients: I.V.: 20 mg/m^2/dose over 30 minutes once every 3 weeks for as long as patients respond satisfactorily and tolerate treatment

Breast cancer: I.V.: 20-80 mg/m^2/dose has been studied in a limited number of phase I/II trials

Ovarian cancer: I.V.: 50 mg/m^2/dose repeated every 4 weeks (minimum of 4 courses is recommended)

Solid tumors: I.V.: 50-60 mg/m^2/dose repeated every 3-4 weeks has been studied in a limited number of phase I/II trials

Nursing/Pharmacy Information Store intact vials of solution under refrigeration (2°C to 8°C) and avoid freezing. Prolonged freezing may adversely affect liposomal drug products, however, short-term freezing (<1 month) does not appear to have a deleterious effect.

The appropriate dose (up to a maximum of 90 mg) must be diluted in 250 mL of dextrose 5% in water prior to administration. Diluted doxorubicin hydrochloride liposome injection should be refrigerated at 2°C to 8°C and administered within 24 hours. **Do not use with in-line filters.**

Local erythematous streaking along the vein and/or facial flushing may indicate too rapid a rate of administration

Extravasation management:

Apply ice immediately for 30-60 minutes; then alternate off/on every 15 minutes for one day

Topical cooling may be achieved using ice packs or cooling pad with circulating ice water; cooling of site for 24 hours as tolerated by the patient. Elevate and rest extremity 24-48 hours, then resume normal activity as tolerated. Application of cold inhibits vesicant's cytotoxicity.

Application of heat or sodium bicarbonate can be harmful and is contraindicated

If pain, erythema, and/or swelling persist beyond 48 hours, refer patient immediately to plastic surgeon for consultation and possible debridement. Discolors urine red/orange; immediately report any change in sensation

(Continued)

doxorubicin (liposomal) *(Continued)*

(eg, stinging) at injection site during infusion (may be an early sign of infiltration).

Dosage Forms Injection, as hydrochloride: 2 mg/mL (10 mL)

♦ **Doxy-200®** *see* doxycycline *on page 222*
♦ **Doxy-Caps®** *see* doxycycline *on page 222*
♦ **Doxychel®** *see* doxycycline *on page 222*
♦ **Doxycin** *see* doxycycline *on page 222*

doxycycline (doks i SYE kleen)

U.S. Brand Names Bio-Tab®; Doryx®; Doxy-200®; Doxy-Caps®; Doxychel®; Doxy-Tabs®; Dynacin®; Monodox®; Vibramycin®; Vibra-Tabs®
Canadian Brand Names Apo®-Doxy; Apo®-Doxy Tabs; Doxycin; Doxytec; Novo-Doxylin®; Nu-Doxycycline®
Mexican Brand Names Vibramicina®
Generic Available Yes
Therapeutic Category Tetracycline Derivative
Use
Children, Adolescents, and Adults: Treatment of Rocky Mountain spotted fever caused by susceptible *Rickettsia* or brucellosis
Older Children, Adolescents, and Adults: Treatment of Lyme disease, mycoplasmal disease, or *Legionella*; management of malignant pleural effusions when intrapleural therapy is indicated
Adolescents and Adults: Treatment of nongonococcal pelvic inflammatory disease and urethritis due to *Chlamydia*; treatment for victims of sexual assault
Adults: Periostat™ (20 mg capsule) is used as an adjunct to scaling and root planing to promote attachment level gain and to reduce pocket depth in patients with adult periodontitis
Unapproved use: Treatment for syphilis in penicillin-allergic patients; sclerosing agent for pleural effusions
Usual Dosage Oral, I.V.:
Children ≥8 years (<45 kg): 2-5 mg/kg/day in 1-2 divided doses, not to exceed 200 mg/day
Children >8 years (>45 kg) and Adults: 100-200 mg/day in 1-2 divided doses
Sclerosing agent for pleural effusion injection: 500 mg as a single dose in 30-50 mL of NS or SWI
Adults: Periodontitis: 20 mg twice/day for up to 9 months; safety beyond 12 months and efficacy beyond 9 months have not been established
Dietary Considerations Administration with iron, calcium, milk or dairy products may decrease doxycycline absorption; may decrease absorption of calcium, iron, magnesium, zinc and amino acids
Nursing/Pharmacy Information
I.V. doxycycline should not be administered I.M. or S.C.; avoid extravasation; administer by slow I.V. intermittent infusion over a minimum of 1-2 hours at a concentration not to exceed 1 mg/mL (can be infused over 1-4 hours); concentrations <0.1 mg/mL are not recommended
Monitor periodic monitoring of renal, hepatic, and hematologic function tests; check for signs of phlebitis
Stability: Tetracyclines form toxic products when outdated or when exposed to light, heat, or humidity; reconstituted solution is stable for 72 hours (refrigerated); for I.V. infusion in normal saline or D_5W solution, complete infusion should be completed within 12 hours; discard remaining solution
Dosage Forms
Doxycycline calcium:
Syrup (raspberry-apple flavor) (Vibramycin®): 50 mg/5 mL (30 mL, 473 mL)
Doxycycline hyclate:
Capsule:
Periostat™: 20 mg
Doxychel®, Vibramycin®: 50 mg
Doxy®, Doxychel®, Vibramycin®: 100 mg
Capsule, coated pellets (Doryx®): 100 mg
Powder for injection (Doxy®, Doxychel®, Vibramycin® IV): 100 mg, 200 mg
Tablet:
Doxychel®: 50 mg
Bio-Tab®, Doxychel®, Vibra-Tabs®: 100 mg
Doxycycline monohydrate:
Capsule (Monodox®): 50 mg, 100 mg
Powder for oral suspension (raspberry flavor) (Vibramycin®): 25 mg/5 mL (60 mL)

- **Doxy-Tabs®** *see* doxycycline *on page 222*
- **Doxytec** *see* doxycycline *on page 222*
- **DPA** *see* valproic acid and derivatives *on page 641*
- **DPE™** *see* dipivefrin *on page 211*
- **d-penicillamine** *see* penicillamine *on page 473*
- **DPH** *see* phenytoin *on page 490*
- **DPPC** *see* colfosceril palmitate *on page 166*
- **DPT** *see* diphtheria, tetanus toxoids, and whole-cell pertussis vaccine *on page 211*
- **Dramamine® II [OTC]** *see* meclizine *on page 387*
- **Dramamine® Injection *(Discontinued)*** *see page 743*
- **Dramamine® Oral [OTC]** *see* dimenhydrinate *on page 206*
- **Dramilin® Injection** *see* dimenhydrinate *on page 206*
- **Dramocen® *(Discontinued)*** *see page 743*
- **Dramoject® *(Discontinued)*** *see page 743*
- **Drenison®** *see* flurandrenolide *on page 277*
- **Dri-Ear® Otic [OTC]** *see* boric acid *on page 90*
- **Driken** *see* iron dextran complex *on page 346*
- **Drisdol®** *see* ergocalciferol *on page 237*
- **Dristan® Cold Caplets [OTC]** *see* acetaminophen and pseudoephedrine *on page 15*
- **Dristan® Long Lasting Nasal Solution [OTC]** *see* oxymetazoline *on page 463*
- **Dristan® Saline Spray [OTC]** *see* sodium chloride *on page 571*
- **Dristan® Sinus Caplets [OTC]** *see* pseudoephedrine and ibuprofen *on page 531*
- **Drithocreme®** *see* anthralin *on page 50*
- **Drithocreme® HP 1%** *see* anthralin *on page 50*
- **Dritho-Scalp®** *see* anthralin *on page 50*
- **Drixomed®** *see* dexbrompheniramine and pseudoephedrine *on page 191*
- **Drixoral® [OTC]** *see* dexbrompheniramine and pseudoephedrine *on page 191*
- **Drixoral® Cough & Congestion Liquid Caps [OTC]** *see* pseudoephedrine and dextromethorphan *on page 531*
- **Drixoral® Cough Liquid Caps [OTC]** *see* dextromethorphan *on page 194*
- **Drixoral® Cough & Sore Throat Liquid Caps [OTC]** *see* acetaminophen and dextromethorphan *on page 15*
- **Drixoral® Nasal** *see* oxymetazoline *on page 463*
- **Drixoral® Non-Drowsy [OTC]** *see* pseudoephedrine *on page 530*
- **Drixoral® Syrup [OTC]** *see* brompheniramine and pseudoephedrine *on page 95*

dronabinol (droe NAB i nol)

Synonyms tetrahydrocannabinol; THC
U.S. Brand Names Marinol®
Generic Available No
Therapeutic Category Antiemetic
Controlled Substance C-III
Use Treatment of nausea and vomiting secondary to cancer chemotherapy in patients who have not responded to conventional antiemetics; treatment of anorexia associated with weight loss in AIDS patients
Usual Dosage Oral:
Children: NCI protocol recommends 5 mg/m² starting 6-8 hours before chemotherapy and every 4-6 hours after to be continued for 12 hours after chemotherapy is discontinued
Adults: 5 mg/m² 1-3 hours before chemotherapy, then administer 5 mg/m²/dose every 2-4 hours after chemotherapy for a total of 4-6 doses/day; dose may be increased up to a maximum of 15 mg/m²/dose if needed (dosage may be increased by 2.5 mg/m² increments)
Nursing/Pharmacy Information
Monitor CNS effects, heart rate, blood pressure
Stability: Store in a cool place
Dosage Forms Capsule: 2.5 mg, 5 mg, 10 mg

droperidol (droe PER i dole)

U.S. Brand Names Inapsine®
Mexican Brand Names Dehydrobenzperidol
Generic Available Yes
(Continued)

droperidol *(Continued)*

Therapeutic Category Antiemetic; Antipsychotic Agent, Butyrophenone

Use Tranquilizer and antiemetic in surgical and diagnostic procedures; antiemetic for cancer chemotherapy; preoperative medication

Usual Dosage Titrate carefully to desired effect

Children 2-12 years:

Premedication: I.M.: 0.088-0.165 mg/kg; smaller doses may be sufficient for control of nausea or vomiting

Adjunct to general anesthesia: I.V. induction: 0.088-0.165 mg/kg

Nausea and vomiting: I.M., I.V.: 0.05-0.06 mg/kg/dose every 4-6 hours as needed

Adults:

Premedication: I.M., I.V.: 2.5-10 mg 30 minutes to 1 hour preoperatively

Adjunct to general anesthesia: I.V. induction: 0.22-0.275 mg/kg; maintenance: 1.25-2.5 mg/dose

Alone in diagnostic procedures: I.M.: Initial: 2.5-10 mg 30 minutes to 1 hour before; then 1.25-2.5 mg if needed

Nausea and vomiting: I.M., I.V.: 2.5-5 mg/dose every 3-4 hours as needed

Nursing/Pharmacy Information

Parenteral: I.V. over 2-5 minutes

Monitor blood pressure, heart rate, respiratory rate

Stability: Parenteral admixture at room temperature (25°C): 24 hours

Dosage Forms Injection: 2.5 mg/mL (1 mL, 2 mL, 5 mL, 10 mL)

droperidol and fentanyl (droe PER i dole & FEN ta nil)

Synonyms fentanyl and droperidol

U.S. Brand Names Innovar®

Generic Available Yes

Therapeutic Category Analgesic, Narcotic

Use Produce and maintain analgesia and sedation during diagnostic or surgical procedures (neuroleptanalgesia and neuroleptanesthesia); adjunct to general anesthesia

Usual Dosage

Children:

Premedication: I.M.: 0.03 mL/kg 30-60 minutes prior to surgery

Adjunct to general anesthesia: I.V.: Total dose: 0.05 mL/kg as slow infusion (1 mL/1-2 minutes) until sleep occurs

Adults:

Premedication: I.M.: 0.5-2 mL 30-60 minutes prior to surgery

Adjunct to general anesthesia: I.V.: 0.09-0.11 mL/kg as slow infusion (1 mL/1-2 minutes) until sleep occurs

Nursing/Pharmacy Information

An opioid antagonist, resuscitative and intubation equipment, and oxygen should be available

Monitor O$_2$ saturation, blood pressure, vital signs

Dosage Forms Injection: Droperidol 2.5 mg and fentanyl 50 mcg per mL (2 mL, 5 mL)

- **Duadacin® Capsule [OTC]** *see* chlorpheniramine, phenylpropanolamine, and acetaminophen *on page 142*
- **Dulcolax® [OTC]** *see* bisacodyl *on page 88*
- **Dull-C® [OTC]** *see* ascorbic acid *on page 60*
- **DuoCet™** *see* hydrocodone and acetaminophen *on page 319*
- **Duo-CVP®** *see* ascorbic acid *on page 60*
- **Duo-Cyp®** *see* estradiol and testosterone *on page 243*
- **Duofilm® Solution** *see* salicylic acid and lactic acid *on page 557*
- **Duoforte® 27** *see* salicylic acid *on page 557*
- **Duo-Medihaler®** *(Discontinued)* *see page 743*
- **Duo-Trach® Injection** *see* lidocaine *on page 368*
- **Duotrate®** *see* pentaerythritol tetranitrate *on page 477*
- **DuP 753** *see* losartan *on page 376*
- **Duphalac®** *see* lactulose *on page 359*
- **Duplex® T [OTC]** *see* coal tar *on page 162*
- **Duracef®** *see* cefadroxil *on page 119*
- **Duracid®** *(Discontinued)* *see page 743*
- **Duraclon™ Injection** *see* clonidine *on page 159*
- **Duract®** *(Discontinued)* *see page 743*
- **Duradoce®** *see* hydroxocobalamin *on page 326*
- **Duradyne DHC®** *see* hydrocodone and acetaminophen *on page 319*
- **Duragesic® Transdermal** *See* fentanyl *on page 263*
- **Dura-Gest®** *see* guaifenesin, phenylpropanolamine, and phenylephrine *on page 304*
- **Duralith®** *see* lithium *on page 372*
- **Duralone® Injection** *see* methylprednisolone *on page 407*
- **Duramist Plus® [OTC]** *see* oxymetazoline *on page 463*
- **Duramorph® Injection** *see* morphine sulfate *on page 422*
- **Duranest®** *see* etidocaine *on page 254*
- **Durater** *see* famotidine *on page 259*
- **Duratest® Injection** *see* testosterone *on page 598*
- **Duratestrin®** *see* estradiol and testosterone *on page 243*
- **Durathate® Injection** *see* testosterone *on page 598*
- **Duration® Nasal Solution [OTC]** *see* oxymetazoline *on page 463*
- **Duratuss-G®** *see* guaifenesin *on page 299*
- **Dura-Vent®** *see* guaifenesin and phenylpropanolamine *on page 301*
- **Dura-Vent/DA®** *see* chlorpheniramine, phenylephrine, and methscopolamine *on page 141*
- **Duricef®** *see* cefadroxil *on page 119*
- **Durogesic** *see* fentanyl *on page 263*
- **Durrax® Oral** *see* hydroxyzine *on page 328*
- **Duvoid®** *see* bethanechol *on page 86*
- **DV® Vaginal Cream** *see* dienestrol *on page 200*
- **Dwelle® Ophthalmic Solution [OTC]** *see* artificial tears *on page 59*

d-xylose (dee ZYE lose)

Synonyms wood sugar

U.S. Brand Names Xylo-Pfan® [OTC]

Generic Available Yes

Therapeutic Category Diagnostic Agent

Use Evaluating intestinal absorption and diagnosing malabsorptive states

Usual Dosage Oral:

Infants and young Children: 500 mg/kg as a 5% to 10% aqueous solution

Children: 5 g is dissolved in 250 mL water; additional fluids are permitted and are encouraged for children

Adults: 25 g dissolved in 200-300 mL water followed with an additional 200-400 mL water **or** 5 g dissolved in 200-300 mL water followed by an additional 200-400 mL water

Nursing/Pharmacy Information Monitor urinary and blood xylose concentration

Dosage Forms Powder for oral solution: 25 g

- **Dyazide®** *see* hydrochlorothiazide and triamterene *on page 318*
- **Dycill®** *see* dicloxacillin *on page 199*
- **Dyclone®** *see* dyclonine *on page 226*

dyclonine (DYE kloe neen)
U.S. Brand Names Dyclone®; Sucrets® [OTC]
Generic Available No
Therapeutic Category Local Anesthetic
Use Local anesthetic prior to laryngoscopy, bronchoscopy, or endotracheal intubation; used topically for temporary relief of pain associated with oral mucosa, skin, episiotomy, or anogenital lesions; the 0.5% topical solution may be used to block the gag reflex, and to relieve the pain of oral ulcers or stomatitis
Usual Dosage
    Children and Adults: Topical solution:
        Mouth sores: 5-10 mL of 0.5% or 1% to oral mucosa (swab or swish and then spit) 3-4 times/day as needed; maximum single dose: 200 mg (40 mL of 0.5% solution or 20 mL of 1% solution)
        Bronchoscopy: Use 2 mL of the 1% solution or 4 mL of the 0.5% solution sprayed onto the larynx and trachea every 5 minutes until the reflex has been abolished
    Children >3 years and Adults: Lozenge: Dissolve 1 in mouth slowly every 2 hours
Dietary Considerations Food should not be ingested for 60 minutes following application in the mouth or throat area
Nursing/Pharmacy Information
    Use the lowest dose needed to provide effective anesthesia; not for injection; do not apply nasally or to the eye
    Stability: Store in tight, light-resistant containers
Dosage Forms Dyclonine hydrochloride:
    Lozenges: 1.2 mg, 3 mg
    Solution, topical: 0.5% (30 mL); 1% (30 mL)

♦ **Dyflex-400® Tablet** *(Discontinued)* see page 743
♦ **dyflos** see isoflurophate on page 347
♦ **Dymelor®** see acetohexamide on page 18
♦ **Dymenate® Injection** see dimenhydrinate on page 206
♦ **Dynabac®** see dirithromycin on page 212
♦ **Dynacin®** see doxycycline on page 222
♦ **Dynacin® Oral** see minocycline on page 416
♦ **DynaCirc®** see isradipine on page 350
♦ **DynaCirc SRO®** see isradipine on page 350
♦ **Dynafed®, Maximum Strength [OTC]** see acetaminophen and pseudoephedrine on page 15
♦ **Dyna-Hex® [OTC]** see chlorhexidine gluconate on page 134
♦ **Dynapen®** see dicloxacillin on page 199

dyphylline (DYE fi lin)
Synonyms dihydroxypropyl theophylline
U.S. Brand Names Dilor®; Lufyllin®
Generic Available Yes
Therapeutic Category Theophylline Derivative
Use Bronchodilator in reversible airway obstruction due to asthma or COPD
Usual Dosage
    Children: I.M.: 4.4-6.6 mg/kg/day in divided doses
    Adults:
        Oral: Up to 15 mg/kg 4 times/day, individualize dosage
        I.M.: 250-500 mg, do not exceed total dosage of 15 mg/kg every 6 hours
Dietary Considerations Should be administered with water 1 hour before or 1 hour after meals
Nursing/Pharmacy Information Not for I.V. administration, inject slowly; administer oral form around-the-clock rather than 4 times/day, 3 times/day, etc, (ie, 12-6-12-6, not 9-1-5-9) to promote less variation in peak and trough serum levels; monitor vital signs, serum concentrations, and CNS effects (insomnia, irritability); encourage patient to drink adequate fluids (2 L/day) to decrease mucous viscosity in airways
Dosage Forms
    Elixir:
        Lufyllin®: 100 mg/15 mL with alcohol 20% (473 mL, 3780 mL)
        Dilor®: 160 mg/15 mL with alcohol 18% (473 mL)
    Injection (Dilor®, Lufyllin®): 250 mg/mL (2 mL)
    Tablet: 200 mg, 400 mg
        Dilor®, Lufyllin®: 200 mg, 400 mg

♦ **Dyrenium®** *see* triamterene *on page 625*
♦ **Dyrexan-OD®** *see* phendimetrazine *on page 484*
♦ **E2020** *see* donepezil *on page 217*
♦ **Easprin®** *see* aspirin *on page 61*
♦ **Ecapresan** *see* captopril *on page 110*
♦ **Ecaten** *see* captopril *on page 110*

echothiophate iodide (ek oh THYE oh fate EYE oh dide)

Synonyms ecostigmine iodide
U.S. Brand Names Phospholine Iodide® Ophthalmic
Generic Available No
Therapeutic Category Cholinesterase Inhibitor
Use Reverse toxic CNS effects caused by anticholinergic drugs; used as miotic in treatment of glaucoma
Usual Dosage Adults: Ophthalmic: Glaucoma: Instill 1 drop twice daily into eyes with one dose just prior to bedtime; some patients have been treated with 1 dose/day or every other day. Use lowest concentration and frequency which gives satisfactory response, with a maximum dose of 0.125% once daily, although more intensive therapy may be used for short periods of time
Nursing/Pharmacy Information
Instruct patient on how to administer drops
Stability: Store at room temperature; reconstituted solutions remain stable for 30 days at room temperature or 6 months when refrigerated
Dosage Forms Powder for reconstitution, ophthalmic: 1.5 mg [0.03%] (5 mL); 3 mg [0.06%] (5 mL); 6.25 mg [0.125%] (5 mL); 12.5 mg [0.25%] (5 mL)

♦ **E-Complex-600® [OTC]** *see* vitamin E *on page 652*

econazole (e KONE a zole)

U.S. Brand Names Spectazole™
Canadian Brand Names Ecostatin®
Mexican Brand Names Micostyl
Generic Available No
Therapeutic Category Antifungal Agent
Use Topical treatment of tinea pedis, tinea cruris, tinea corporis, tinea versicolor, and cutaneous candidiasis
Usual Dosage Children and Adults: Topical: Apply a sufficient amount to cover affected areas once daily; for cutaneous candidiasis: apply twice daily; candidal infections and tinea cruris, versicolor, and corporis should be treated for 2 weeks and tinea pedis for 1 month; occasionally, longer treatment periods may be required
Nursing/Pharmacy Information Candidal infections and tinea cruris, versicolor, and corporis should be treated for 2 weeks and tinea pedis for 1 month; occasionally, longer treatment periods may be required
Dosage Forms Cream, as nitrate: 1% (15 g, 30 g, 85 g)

♦ **Econopred® Ophthalmic** *see* prednisolone (ophthalmic) *on page 514*
♦ **Econopred® Plus Ophthalmic** *see* prednisolone (ophthalmic) *on page 514*
♦ **Ecostatin®** *see* econazole *on page 227*
♦ **ecostigmine iodide** *see* echothiophate iodide *on page 227*
♦ **Ecotrin® [OTC]** *see* aspirin *on page 61*
♦ **Ectaprim®** *see* co-trimoxazole *on page 170*
♦ **Ectaprim®-F** *see* co-trimoxazole *on page 170*
♦ **Ectosone** *see* betamethasone (topical) *on page 85*
♦ **Ed A-Hist® Liquid** *see* chlorpheniramine and phenylephrine *on page 139*
♦ **edathamil disodium** *see* edetate disodium *on page 228*
♦ **Edecrin®** *see* ethacrynic acid *on page 247*
♦ **Edenol** *see* furosemide *on page 285*

edetate calcium disodium

(ED e tate KAL see um dye SOW dee um)
Synonyms calcium edta
U.S. Brand Names Calcium Disodium Versenate®
Generic Available No
Therapeutic Category Chelating Agent
Use Treatment of acute and chronic lead poisoning; also used as an aid in the diagnosis of lead poisoning
(Continued)

edetate calcium disodium *(Continued)*

Usual Dosage
Children:
Diagnosis of lead poisoning: Mobilization test: (Asymptomatic patients or lead levels <55 mcg/dL): **(Note:** Urine is collected for 24 hours after first EDTA dose and analyzed for lead content; if the ratio of mcg of lead in urine to mg calcium EDTA given is >1, then test is considered positive): Children: 500 mg/m^2 (maximum: 1 g/dose) I.M. or I.V. over 1 hour **or** 2 doses of 500 mg/m^2 at 12-hour intervals

Asymptomatic lead poisoning: (Blood lead concentration >55 mcg/dL or blood lead concentrations of 25-55 mcg/dL with blood erythrocyte protoporphyrin concentrations of ≥35 mcg/dL and positive mobilization test) or symptomatic lead poisoning without encephalopathy with lead level <100 mcg/dL: 1 g/m^2/day I.M./I.V. in divided doses every 8-12 hours for 3-5 days (usually 5 days); maximum: 1 g/24 hours or 50 mg/kg/day

Symptomatic lead poisoning with encephalopathy with lead level >100 mcg/dL (treatment with calcium EDTA and dimercaprol is preferred): 250 mg/m^2 I.M. or intermittent I.V. infusion 4 hours after dimercaprol, then at 4-hour intervals thereafter for 5 days (1.5 g/m^2/day); dose (1.5 g/m^2/day) can also be administered as a single I.V. continuous infusion over 12-24 hours/day for 5 days; maximum: 1 g/24 hours or 75 mg/kg/day

Note: Course of therapy may be repeated in 2-3 weeks until blood lead level is normal

Adults: I.M., I.V.:
Diagnosis of lead poisoning: 500 mg/m^2 (maximum: 1 g/dose) over 1 hour
Treatment: 2 g/day or 1.5 g/m^2/day in divided doses every 12-24 hours for 5 days; may repeat course one time after at least 2 days (usually after 2 weeks)

Nursing/Pharmacy Information
Parenteral: For intermittent I.V. infusion, administer the dose I.V. over at least 1 hour in asymptomatic patients, 2 hours in symptomatic patients; for single daily I.V. (continuous infusion), dilute to 2-4 mg/mL in D$_5$W or NS and infuse over at least 8 hours, usually over 12-24 hours; for I.M. injection, 1 mL of 1% lidocaine or procaine hydrochloride may be added to each mL of EDTA calcium to minimize pain at I.M. injection site
Monitor BUN, creatinine, urinalysis, I & O, and EKG during therapy
Stability: Dilute with 0.9% sodium chloride or D$_5$W; physically **incompatible** with D$_{10}$W, lactated Ringer's, Ringer's
Dosage Forms Injection: 200 mg/mL (5 mL)

edetate disodium *(ED e tate dye SOW dee um)*

Synonyms edathamil disodium; EDTA; sodium edetate
U.S. Brand Names Chealamide®; Disotate®; Endrate®
Generic Available Yes
Therapeutic Category Chelating Agent
Use Emergency treatment of hypercalcemia; control digitalis-induced cardiac dysrhythmias (ventricular arrhythmias)
Usual Dosage I.V.:
Hypercalcemia:
Children: 40-70 mg/kg slow infusion over 3-4 hours
Adults: 50 mg/kg/day over 3 or more hours
Dysrhythmias: Children and Adults: 15 mg/kg/hour up to 60 mg/kg/day
Nursing/Pharmacy Information
Avoid extravasation; patient should remain supine for a short period after infusion; must be diluted before use in 500 mL D$_5$W or NS to <30 mg/mL
Monitor serum calcium
Dosage Forms Injection: 150 mg/mL (20 mL)

♦ **Edex® Injection** *see* alprostadil *on page 30*

edrophonium *(ed roe FOE nee um)*

U.S. Brand Names Enlon®; Reversol®; Tensilon®
Generic Available No
Therapeutic Category Cholinergic Agent
Use Diagnosis of myasthenia gravis; differentiation of cholinergic crises from myasthenia crises; reversal of nondepolarizing neuromuscular blockers; treatment of paroxysmal atrial tachycardia
Usual Dosage
Infants: I.V.: Initial: 0.1 mg, followed by 0.4 mg if no response; total dose: 0.5 mg

Children:

Diagnosis: Initial: 0.04 mg/kg followed by 0.16 mg/kg if no response, to a maximum total dose of 5 mg for children ≤34 kg, or 10 mg for children >34 kg

Titration of oral anticholinesterase therapy: 0.04 mg/kg once; if strength improves, an increase in neostigmine or pyridostigmine dose is indicated

Adults:

Diagnosis: I.V.: 2 mg test dose administered over 15-30 seconds; 8 mg administered 45 seconds later if no response is seen. Test dose may be repeated after 30 minutes.

Titration of oral anticholinesterase therapy: 1-2 mg administered 1 hour after oral dose of anticholinesterase; if strength improves, an increase in neostigmine or pyridostigmine dose is indicated

Differentiation of cholinergic from myasthenic crisis: I.V.: 1 mg, may repeat after 1 minute (**Note:** Intubation and controlled ventilation may be required if patient has cholinergic crises.)

Reversal of nondepolarizing neuromuscular blocking agents (neostigmine with atropine usually preferred): I.V.: 10 mg, may repeat every 5-10 minutes up to 40 mg

Termination of paroxysmal atrial tachycardia: I.V.: 5-10 mg

Nursing/Pharmacy Information

Parenteral: Edrophonium is administered by direct I.V. injection

Monitor pre- and postinjection strength (cranial musculature is most useful); heart rate, respiratory rate, blood pressure

Dosage Forms Injection, as chloride: 10 mg/mL (1 mL, 10 mL, 15 mL)

- ♦ **ED-SPAZ®** see hyoscyamine on page 329
- ♦ **EDTA** see edetate disodium on page 228
- ♦ **E.E.S.®** see erythromycin (systemic) on page 240
- ♦ **E.E.S.® Chewable** see erythromycin (systemic) on page 240
- ♦ **E.E.S.® Granules** see erythromycin (systemic) on page 240

efavirenz (e FAV e renz)

U.S. Brand Names Sustiva™

Generic Available No

Therapeutic Category Non-nucleoside Reverse Transcriptase Inhibitor (NNRTI)

Use Treatment of HIV-1 infections in combination with at least 2 other antiretroviral agents. Also has some activity against hepatitis B virus and herpes viruses.

Usual Dosage Dosing at bedtime is recommended to limit central nervous system effects; should not be used as single-agent therapy

Oral:

Adults: 600 mg once daily

Children: Dosage is based on body weight

10 to <15 kg: 200 mg

15 to <20 kg: 250 mg

20 to <25 kg: 300 mg

25 to <32.5 kg: 350 mg

32.5 to <40 kg: 400 mg

≥40 kg: 600 mg

Dietary Considerations Avoid high-fat meals when taking this medication. May be taken with or without food

Dosage Forms Capsule: 50 mg, 100 mg, 200 mg

- ♦ **Effer-K™** see potassium bicarbonate and potassium citrate, effervescent on page 506
- ♦ **Effer-Syllium® [OTC]** see psyllium on page 531
- ♦ **Effexor®** see venlafaxine on page 646
- ♦ **Effexor-XR®** see venlafaxine on page 646
- ♦ **Efidac/24® [OTC]** see pseudoephedrine on page 530

eflornithine (ee FLOR ni theen)

U.S. Brand Names Ornidyl®

Generic Available No

Therapeutic Category Antiprotozoal

Use Treatment of meningoencephalitic stage of *Trypanosoma brucei gambiense* infection (sleeping sickness)

Usual Dosage I.V. infusion: 100 mg/kg/dose administered every 6 hours (over 45 minutes) for 14 days

(Continued)

eflornithine *(Continued)*

Nursing/Pharmacy Information
Monitor CBC with platelet counts
Stability: Must be diluted before use and used within 24 hours of preparation
Dosage Forms Injection, as hydrochloride: 200 mg/mL (100 mL)

- **Efodine®** [OTC] *see* povidone-iodine *on page 510*
- **Efudex® Topical** *see* fluorouracil *on page 275*
- **Efudix** *see* fluorouracil *on page 275*
- **EHDP** *see* etidronate disodium *on page 254*
- **Elantan** *see* isosorbide mononitrate *on page 349*
- **Elase®-Chloromycetin® Ointment** *(Discontinued) see page 743*
- **Elase® Ointment** *(Discontinued) see page 743*
- **Elavil®** *see* amitriptyline *on page 40*
- **Eldecort® Topical** *see* hydrocortisone (topical) *on page 324*
- **Eldepryl®** *see* selegiline *on page 562*
- **Eldepryl® Tablet (only)** *(Discontinued) see page 743*
- **Eldercaps®** [OTC] *see* vitamin, multiple (oral) *on page 654*
- **Eldopaque®** [OTC] *see* hydroquinone *on page 325*
- **Eldopaque Forte®** *see* hydroquinone *on page 325*
- **Eldoquin®** [OTC] *see* hydroquinone *on page 325*
- **Eldoquin® Forte®** *see* hydroquinone *on page 325*
- **Eldoquin® Lotion** *(Discontinued) see page 743*
- **electrolyte lavage solution** *see* polyethylene glycol-electrolyte solution *on page 502*
- **Elequine** *see* levofloxacin *on page 366*
- **Elimite™ Cream** *see* permethrin *on page 482*
- **Elixomin®** *see* theophylline *on page 603*
- **Elixophyllin®** *see* theophylline *on page 603*
- **Elixophyllin SR®** *(Discontinued) see page 743*
- **Ellence™** *see* epirubicin *New Drug on page 235*
- **Elmiron®** *see* pentosan polysulfate sodium *on page 480*
- **Elocom** *see* mometasone furoate *on page 420*
- **Elocon®** *see* mometasone furoate *on page 420*
- **E-Lor® Tablet** *(Discontinued) see page 743*
- **Elspar®** *see* asparaginase *on page 60*
- **Eltor®** *see* pseudoephedrine *on page 530*
- **Eltroxin®** *see* levothyroxine *on page 367*
- **Emcyt®** *see* estramustine *on page 244*
- **Emecheck®** [OTC] *see* phosphorated carbohydrate solution *on page 492*
- **Emete-Con Injection** *(Discontinued) see page 743*
- **Emetine Hydrochloride** *(Discontinued) see page 743*
- **Emetrol®** [OTC] *see* phosphorated carbohydrate solution *on page 492*
- **Emgel™ Topical** *see* erythromycin (ophthalmic/topical) *on page 239*
- **Eminase®** *see* anistreplase *on page 50*
- **Emitrip®** *see* amitriptyline *on page 40*
- **Emko®** [OTC] *see* nonoxynol 9 *on page 446*
- **EMLA®** *see* lidocaine and prilocaine *on page 369*
- **Emo-Cort™** *see* hydrocortisone (topical) *on page 324*
- **Empirin®** [OTC] *see* aspirin *on page 61*
- **Empirin® With Codeine** *see* aspirin and codeine *on page 62*
- **Empracet®-30, -60** *see* acetaminophen and codeine *on page 14*
- **Emtec-30®** *see* acetaminophen and codeine *on page 14*
- **Emulsan 20%** *see* fat emulsion *on page 259*
- **Emulsoil®** [OTC] *see* castor oil *on page 118*
- **E-Mycin®** *see* erythromycin (systemic) *on page 240*
- **E-Mycin-E®** *see* erythromycin (systemic) *on page 240*
- **Enaladil** *see* enalapril *on page 230*

enalapril *(e NAL a pril)*
U.S. Brand Names Vasotec® I.V.; Vasotec® Oral
Canadian Brand Names Apo®-Enalapril
Mexican Brand Names Enaladil; Glioten; Kenopril; Renitec
Generic Available No
Therapeutic Category Angiotensin-Converting Enzyme (ACE) Inhibitor

Use Management of mild to severe hypertension, congestive heart failure, and asymptomatic left ventricular dysfunction

Usual Dosage Use lower listed initial dose in patients with hyponatremia, hypovolemia, severe congestive heart failure, decreased renal function, or in those receiving diuretics

Children:

Investigational initial oral doses of enalapril of 0.1 mg/kg/day increasing over 2 weeks to 0.12-0.43 mg/kg/day have been used to treat severe congestive heart failure in infants (n=8)

Investigational I.V. doses of enalaprilat of 5-10 mcg/kg/dose administered every 8-24 hours (as determined by blood pressure readings) have been used for the treatment of neonatal hypertension (n=10); monitor patients carefully; select patients may require higher doses

Adults:

Oral: **Enalapril:** 2.5-5 mg/day then increase as required, usually 10-40 mg/day in 1-2 divided doses

I.V.: **Enalaprilat:** 0.625-1.25 mg/dose, administered over 5 minutes every 6 hours

Dietary Considerations Limit salt substitutes or potassium-rich diet; avoid natural licorice (causes sodium and water retention and increases potassium loss)

Nursing/Pharmacy Information

May cause depression in some patients; discontinue if angioedema of the face, extremities, lips, tongue, or glottis occurs; watch for hypotensive effect within 1-3 hours of first dose or new higher dose; administer as I.V. infusion (undiluted solution or further diluted) over 5 minutes

Monitor blood pressure, serum potassium

Stability: Solutions for I.V. infusion mixed in normal saline or D_5W are stable for 24 hours at room temperature

Dosage Forms

Enalaprilat: Injection: 1.25 mg/mL (1 mL, 2 mL)

Enalapril maleate: Tablet: 2.5 mg, 5 mg, 10 mg, 20 mg

enalapril and diltiazem (e NAL a pril & dil TYE a zem)

U.S. Brand Names Teczem®

Generic Available No

Therapeutic Category Antihypertensive Agent, Combination

Use Combination drug for treatment of hypertension

Usual Dosage Adults: Oral: One tablet daily, if further blood pressure control is required, increase dosage to two tablets daily

Dosage Forms Tablet, extended release: Enalapril maleate 5 mg and diltiazem maleate 180 mg

enalapril and felodipine (e NAL a pril & fe LOE di peen)

U.S. Brand Names Lexxel™

Generic Available No

Therapeutic Category Antihypertensive Agent, Combination

Use Treatment of hypertension

Usual Dosage Adults: Oral: The dose of this combination when given as a replacement to patients taking both components separately should be equal to the component doses previously used. Patients whose blood pressure is not sufficiently controlled on either component may be switched to one combination tablet (5 mg enalapril and 5 mg extended-release felodipine) daily. If control remains inadequate after 1 or 2 weeks, the dosage may be increased to two tablets daily, and if lack of control persists, a thiazide diuretic may be added

Dosage Forms Tablet, extended release: Enalapril maleate 5 mg and felodipine 5 mg

enalapril and hydrochlorothiazide

(e NAL a pril & hye droe klor oh THYE a zide)

Synonyms hydrochlorothiazide and enalapril

U.S. Brand Names Vaseretic® 10-25

Generic Available No

Therapeutic Category Antihypertensive Agent, Combination

Use Treatment of hypertension

Usual Dosage Oral: Dose is individualized

Dosage Forms Tablet:

Enalapril maleate 5 mg and hydrochlorothiazide 12.5 mg

Enalapril maleate 10 mg and hydrochlorothiazide 25 mg

- **Enbrel®** see etanercept on page 247
- **Encare®** [OTC] see nonoxynol 9 on page 446
- **Endal®** see guaifenesin and phenylephrine on page 301
- **Endantadine™** see amantadine on page 35
- **Endep®** *(Discontinued)* see page 743
- **End Lice® Liquid** [OTC] see pyrethrins and piperonyl butoxide on page 533
- **Endocet®** see oxycodone and acetaminophen on page 462
- **Endodan®** see oxycodone and aspirin on page 463
- **Endolor®** see butalbital compound and acetaminophen on page 99
- **Endrate®** see edetate disodium on page 228
- **Enduron®** see methyclothiazide on page 405
- **Enduron® 2.5 mg Tablet** *(Discontinued)* see page 743
- **Enduronyl®** see methyclothiazide and deserpidine on page 405
- **Enduronyl® Forte** see methyclothiazide and deserpidine on page 405
- **Enecat®** see radiological/contrast media (ionic) on page 539
- **Enemol™** see sodium phosphates on page 573
- **Ener-B®** [OTC] see cyanocobalamin on page 173

enflurane (EN floo rane)
U.S. Brand Names Ethrane®
Generic Available No
Therapeutic Category General Anesthetic
Use General induction and maintenance of anesthesia (inhalation)
Usual Dosage Inhalation: 0.5% to 3%
Dosage Forms Liquid: 125 mL, 250 mL

- **Engerix-B®** see hepatitis B vaccine on page 312
- **Eni** see ciprofloxacin on page 151
- **Enisyl®** [OTC] see l-lysine on page 373
- **Enkaid®** *(Discontinued)* see page 743
- **Enlon®** see edrophonium on page 228
- **Enomine®** see guaifenesin, phenylpropanolamine, and phenylephrine on page 304
- **Enovid®** *(Discontinued)* see page 743
- **Enovil®** see amitriptyline on page 40

enoxacin (en OKS a sin)
U.S. Brand Names Penetrex™
Mexican Brand Names Comprecin
Generic Available No
Therapeutic Category Quinolone
Use Complicated and uncomplicated urinary tract infections caused by susceptible gram-negative and gram-positive bacteria
Usual Dosage Adults: Oral: 400 mg twice daily
Nursing/Pharmacy Information
Hold antacids for 3-4 hours before or after administering; administer on an empty stomach; encourage fluids
Patients receiving concurrent enoxacin and theophylline should have serum levels of theophylline monitored
Dosage Forms Tablet: 200 mg, 400 mg

enoxaparin (ee noks a PA rin)
U.S. Brand Names Lovenox®
Generic Available No
Therapeutic Category Anticoagulant
Use Prophylaxis and treatment of thromboembolic disorders (deep vein thrombosis)
Usual Dosage Adults: S.C.: 30 mg twice daily
Nursing/Pharmacy Information
Administer S.C. only; do not administer I.M. injection
Monitor platelets, occult blood, and anti-Xa activity, if available
Stability: Do not mix with other injections or infusions; store at ≤25°C (77°F); do not freeze
Dosage Forms Injection, as sodium, preservative free: 30 mg/0.3 mL; 40 mg/0.4 mL; 60 mg/0.6 mL; 80 mg/0.8 mL; 100 mg/mL

- **Ensure®** [OTC] see enteral nutritional products on page 233
- **Ensure Plus®** [OTC] see enteral nutritional products on page 233

entacapone *New Drug* (en TA ka pone)
U.S. Brand Names Comtan®
Therapeutic Category Anti-Parkinson's Agent; Reverse COMT Inhibitor
Controlled Substance [EZ100,MG250]parkinsonism
Use Adjunct to levodopa/carbidopa therapy in patients with idiopathic Parkinson's disease who experience "wearing-off" symptoms at the end of a dosing interval
Usual Dosage
Adults: Oral: 200 mg dose, up to a maximum of 8 times/day; maximum daily dose: 1600 mg/day. Always administer with levodopa/carbidopa. To optimize therapy the levodopa/carbidopa dosage must be reduced, usually by 25%. This reduction is usually necessary when the patient is taking more than 800 mg of levodopa daily.
Dosage Forms Tablet: 200 mg

♦ **E.N.T.®** *(Discontinued) see page 743*

enteral nutritional products
(noo TRISH un al FOR myoo la, EN ter al/OR al)
Synonyms dietary supplements
U.S. Brand Names Carnation Instant Breakfast® [OTC]; Citrotein® [OTC]; Criticare HN® [OTC]; Ensure® [OTC]; Ensure Plus® [OTC]; Isocal® [OTC]; Magnacal® [OTC]; Microlipid™ [OTC]; Osmolite® HN [OTC]; Pedialyte® [OTC]; Portagen® [OTC]; Pregestimil® [OTC]; Propac™ [OTC]; Soyalac® [OTC]; Vital HN® [OTC]; Vitaneed™ [OTC]; Vivonex® [OTC]; Vivonex® T.E.N. [OTC]
Canadian Brand Names Citrisource®; Glucerna™; Isocal® with Fibre; Isosource®; Nutrisource™; Optifast® 900; Palmocare®; Pediasure™; Resource®; Sandosource™ Peptide, Sustacal®; Tolerex®; Travasol®; Vivonex® Plus
Generic Available Yes
Therapeutic Category Nutritional Supplement
Dosage Forms
Liquid: Calcium and sodium caseinate, maltodextrin, sucrose, partially hydrogenated soy oil, soy lecithin
Powder: Amino acids, predigested carbohydrates, safflower oil

♦ **Enterobacticel** *see co-trimoxazole on page 170*
♦ **Enteropride** *see cisapride on page 152*
♦ **Entertainer's Secret® Spray [OTC]** *see saliva substitute on page 558*
♦ **Entex®** *see guaifenesin, phenylpropanolamine, and phenylephrine on page 304*
♦ **Entex® LA** *see guaifenesin and phenylpropanolamine on page 301*
♦ **Entex® PSE** *see guaifenesin and pseudoephedrine on page 302*
♦ **Entocort®** *see budesonide on page 96*
♦ **Entoplus** *see albendazole on page 24*
♦ **Entozyme®** *(Discontinued) see page 743*
♦ **Entrobar®** *see radiological/contrast media (ionic) on page 539*
♦ **Entrophen®** *see aspirin on page 61*
♦ **Entuss-D® Liquid** *see hydrocodone and pseudoephedrine on page 321*
♦ **Enulose®** *see lactulose on page 359*
♦ **Enzone®** *see pramoxine and hydrocortisone on page 512*
♦ **E Pam®** *see diazepam on page 196*
♦ **EPEG** *see etoposide on page 255*

ephedrine (e FED rin)
U.S. Brand Names Kondon's Nasal® [OTC]; Pretz-D® [OTC]
Generic Available Yes
Therapeutic Category Adrenergic Agonist Agent
Use Bronchial asthma; nasal congestion; acute bronchospasm; acute hypotensive states
Usual Dosage
Children:
Oral, S.C.: 3 mg/kg/day or 25-100 mg/m^2/day in 4-6 divided doses every 4-6 hours
I.M., slow I.V. push: 0.2-0.3 mg/kg/dose every 4-6 hours
Adults:
Oral: 25-50 mg every 3-4 hours as needed
I.M., S.C.: 25-50 mg, parenteral adult dose should not exceed 150 mg in 24 hours
(Continued)

ephedrine *(Continued)*

I.V.: 5-25 mg/dose slow I.V. push repeated after 5-10 minutes as needed, then every 3-4 hours not to exceed 150 mg/24 hours

Nursing/Pharmacy Information

Protect from light; do not administer unless solution is clear

Monitor heart rate, EKG, blood pressure, urine output, mental status

Stability: Protect all dosage forms from light

Dosage Forms Ephedrine sulfate:

Injection: 25 mg/mL (1 mL); 50 mg/mL (1 mL, 10 mL)

Jelly (Kondon's Nasal®): 1% (20 g)

Spray (Pretz-D®): 0.25% (15 mL)

- ◆ **ephedrine, theophylline, and hydroxyzine** *see* theophylline, ephedrine, and hydroxyzine *on page 605*
- ◆ **ephedrine, theophylline, and phenobarbital** *see* theophylline, ephedrine, and phenobarbital *on page 605*
- ◆ **Epi-C®** *see* radiological/contrast media (ionic) *on page 539*
- ◆ **Epi E-Z Pen™, -Jr** *see* epinephrine *on page 234*
- ◆ **Epifrin®** *see* epinephrine *on page 234*
- ◆ **E-Pilo-x® Ophthalmic** *see* pilocarpine and epinephrine *on page 494*
- ◆ **Epimorph®** *see* morphine sulfate *on page 422*
- ◆ **Epinal®** *see* epinephryl borate *on page 235*

epinephrine *(ep i NEF rin)*

Synonyms adrenaline

U.S. Brand Names Adrenalin® Chloride; AsthmaHaler® Mist [OTC]; AsthmaNefrin® [OTC]; Bronitin® Mist [OTC]; Bronkaid® Mist [OTC]; Epifrin®; EpiPen®; EpiPen® Jr; Glaucon®; microNefrin® [OTC]; Primatene® Mist [OTC]; Sus-Phrine®; Vaponefrin® [OTC]

Canadian Brand Names Epi E-Z Pen™, -Jr

Generic Available Yes

Therapeutic Category Adrenergic Agonist Agent

Use Treatment of bronchospasm, anaphylactic reactions, cardiac arrest, and management of open-angle (chronic simple) glaucoma

Usual Dosage

Bronchodilator:

Children: S.C.: 10 mcg/kg (0.01 mL/kg of 1:1000) (single doses not to exceed 0.5 mg); injection suspension (1:200): 0.005 mL/kg/dose (0.025 mg/kg/dose) to a maximum of 0.15 mL (0.75 mg for single dose) every 8-12 hours

Adults:

I.M., S.C. (1:1000): 0.1-0.5 mg every 10-15 minutes to 4 hours

Suspension (1:200) S.C.: 0.1-0.3 mL (0.5-1.5 mg)

I.V.: 0.1-0.25 mg (single dose maximum: 1 mg)

Cardiac arrest:

Neonates: I.V. or intratracheal: 0.01-0.03 mg/kg (0.1-0.3 mL/kg of 1:10,000 solution) every 3-5 minutes as needed; dilute intratracheal doses in 1-2 mL of normal saline

Infants and Children: Asystole or pulseless arrest:

I.V., intraosseous: First dose: 0.01 mg/kg (0.1 mL/kg of a 1:10,000 solution); subsequent doses: 0.1 mg/kg (0.1 mL/kg of a 1:1000 solution); doses as high as 0.2 mg/kg may be effective; repeat every 3-5 minutes

Intratracheal: 0.1 mg/kg (0.1 mL/kg of a 1:1000 solution); doses as high as 0.2 mg/kg may be effective

Adults: Asystole:

I.V.: 1 mg every 3-5 minutes; if this approach fails, alternative regimens include: Intermediate: 2-5 mg every 3-5 minutes; Escalating: 1 mg, 3 mg, 5 mg at 3-minute intervals; High: 0.1 mg/kg every 3-5 minutes

Intratracheal: Although optimal dose is unknown, doses of 2-2.5 times the I.V. dose may be needed

Bradycardia: Children:

I.V.: 0.01 mg/kg (0.1 mL/kg of 1:10,000 solution) every 3-5 minutes as needed (maximum: 1 mg/10 mL)

Intratracheal: 0.1 mg/kg (0.1 mL/kg of 1:1000 solution every 3-5 minutes); doses as high as 0.2 mg/kg may be effective

Refractory hypotension (refractory to dopamine/dobutamine): I.V. infusion administration requires the use of an infusion pump:

Children: Infusion rate 0.1-4 mcg/kg/minute

Adults: I.V. infusion: 1 mg in 250 mL NS/D$_5$W at 0.1-1 mcg/kg/minute; titrate to desired effect

Hypersensitivity reaction:
   Children: S.C.: 0.01 mg/kg every 15 minutes for 2 doses then every 4 hours as needed (single doses not to exceed 0.5 mg)
   Adults: I.M., S.C.: 0.2-0.5 mg every 20 minutes to 4 hours (single dose maximum: 1 mg)

Nebulization:
   Children <2 years: 0.25 mL of 1:1000 diluted in 3 mL NS with treatments ordered individually
   Children >2 years and Adolescents: 0.5 mL of 1:1000 concentration diluted in 3 mL NS
   Children >2 years and Adults (racemic epinephrine):
      <10 kg: 2 mL of 1:8 dilution over 15 minutes every 1-4 hours
      10-15 kg: 2 mL of 1:6 dilution over 15 minutes every 1-4 hours
      15-20 kg: 2 mL of 1:4 dilution over 15 minutes every 1-4 hours
      >20 kg: 2 mL of 1:3 dilution over 15 minutes every 1-4 hours
   Adults: Instill 8-15 drops into nebulizer reservoirs; administer 1-3 inhalations 4-6 times/day
Ophthalmic: Instill 1-2 drops in eye(s) once or twice daily
Intranasal: Children ≥6 years and Adults: Apply locally as drops or spray or with sterile swab

Nursing/Pharmacy Information
Tissue irritant; extravasation may be treated by local small injections of a diluted phentolamine solution (mix 5 mg with 9 mL normal saline); for continuous infusion: rate of infusion (mL/hour) = dose (mcg/kg/minute) x weight (kg) x 60 minutes/hour divided by the concentration (mcg/mL); maximum concentration: 64 mcg/mL
Monitor heart rate, blood pressure
Stability: Protect from light, oxidation turns drug pink, then a brown color; solutions should not be used if they are discolored or contain a precipitate; stability of injection of parenteral admixture at room temperature and refrigeration: 24 hours; unstable in alkali solutions

Dosage Forms
Aerosol, oral:
   Bitartrate (AsthmaHaler®, Bronitin®): 0.3 mg/spray [epinephrine base 0.16 mg/spray] (10 mL, 15 mL, 22.5 mL)
   Bronkaid®: 0.5% (10 mL, 15 mL, 22.5 mL)
   Primatene® Mist: 0.2 mg/spray (15 mL, 22.5 mL)
Auto-injector:
   EpiPen®: Delivers 0.3 mg I.M. of epinephrine 1:1000 (2 mL)
   EpiPen® Jr.: Delivers 0.15 mg I.M. of epinephrine 1:2000 (2 mL)
Solution:
   Inhalation:
      Adrenalin®: 1% [10 mg/mL, 1:100] (7.5 mL)
   Injection:
      Adrenalin®: 0.01 mg/mL [1:100,000] (5 mL); 0.1 mg/mL [1:10,000] (3 mL, 10 mL); 1 mg/mL [1:1000] (1 mL, 2 mL, 30 mL)
      Suspension (Sus-Phrine®): 5 mg/mL [1:200] (0.3 mL, 5 mL)
   Nasal (Adrenalin®): 0.1% [1 mg/mL, 1:1000] (30 mL)
   Ophthalmic, as hydrochloride (Epifrin®, Glaucon®): 0.1% (1 mL, 30 mL); 0.5% (15 mL); 1% (1 mL, 10 mL, 15 mL); 2% (10 mL, 15 mL)
   Topical (Adrenalin®): 0.1% [1 mg/mL, 1:1000] (10 mL, 30 mL)

♦ **epinephrine and lidocaine** *see* lidocaine and epinephrine *on page 369*
♦ **epinephrine and pilocarpine** *see* pilocarpine and epinephrine *on page 494*

epinephryl borate (ep i NEF ril BOR ate)
U.S. Brand Names Epinal®
Generic Available No
Therapeutic Category Adrenergic Agonist Agent
Use Reduces elevated intraocular pressure in chronic open-angle glaucoma
Usual Dosage Adults: Ophthalmic: Instill 1 drop into the eyes once or twice daily
Dosage Forms Solution, ophthalmic: 0.5% (7.5 mL); 1% (7.5 mL)

♦ **EpiPen®** *see* epinephrine *on page 234*
♦ **EpiPen® Jr** *see* epinephrine *on page 234*

epirubicin *New Drug* (ep i ROO bi sin)
U.S. Brand Names Ellence™
Generic Available No
Therapeutic Category Antineoplastic Agent, Anthracycline; Antineoplastic Agent, Antibiotic
(Continued)

epirubicin *New Drug* (Continued)

Use As a component of adjuvant therapy following primary resection of primary breast cancer in patients with evidence of axillary node tumor involvement

Usual Dosage Adults: I.V. (refer to individual protocols): 100-120 mg/m², repeated in 3- to 4-week cycles. The total dose of epirubicin may be given on Day 1 of each cycle or the dose may be divided equally and given on Day 1 and Day 8 of each cycle.

Dosage Forms Injection: 2 mg/mL (25 mL, 100 mL)

♦ **Epitol®** *see* carbamazepine *on page 112*

♦ **Epival®** *see* valproic acid and derivatives *on page 641*

♦ **Epivir®** *see* lamivudine *on page 359*

♦ **Epivir®-HBV™** *see* lamivudine *on page 359*

♦ **E.P. Mycin® Capsule** *(Discontinued) see page 743*

♦ **EPO** *see* epoetin alfa *on page 236*

epoetin alfa (e POE e tin AL fa)

Synonyms EPO; erythropoietin; RHUEPO-α

U.S. Brand Names Epogen®; Procrit®

Canadian Brand Names Eprex®

Mexican Brand Names Eprex®

Generic Available No

Therapeutic Category Colony-Stimulating Factor

Use Anemia associated with end-stage renal disease; anemia related to therapy with AZT-treated HIV-infected patients; anemia in cancer patients receiving chemotherapy; anemia of prematurity

Usual Dosage

In patients on dialysis, epoetin alfa usually has been administered as an I.V. bolus 3 times/week; while the administration is independent of the dialysis procedure, it may be administered into the venous line at the end of the dialysis procedure to obviate the need for additional venous access. In patients with CRF not on dialysis, epoetin alfa may be administered either as an I.V. or S.C. injection.

AZT-treated HIV-infected patients: I.V., S.C.: Initial: 100 units/kg/dose 3 times/week for 8 weeks; after 8 weeks of therapy the dose can be adjusted by 50-100 units/kg increments 3 times/week to a maximum dose of 300 units/kg 3 times/week; if the hematocrit exceeds 40%, the dose should be discontinued until the hematocrit drops to 36%

Anemia of prematurity: S.C.: 25-100 units/kg/dose 3 times/week

Nursing/Pharmacy Information

Dilute with an equal volume of normal saline and infuse over 1-3 minutes; may be administered into the venous line at the end of the dialysis procedure

Careful monitoring of blood pressure is indicated; problems with hypertension have been noted in renal failure patients treated with rHuEPO-α. Other patients are less likely to develop this complication. Follow serum ferritin and serum transferrin saturation monthly. Hematocrit should be determined twice weekly until stabilization within the target range (30% to 33%), and twice weekly at least 2 to 6 weeks after a dose increase. Baseline and follow-up of blood urea nitrogen (BUN), uric acid, serum creatinine, phosphorous, and potassium.

Stability: Refrigerate; vials are stable 2 weeks at room temperature; do not shake vial

Dosage Forms

1 mL single-dose vials: Preservative-free solution
2000 units/mL
3000 units/mL
4000 units/mL
10,000 units/mL
20,000 units/mL
40,000 units/mL
2 mL multidose vials: Preserved solution: 10,000 units/mL

♦ **Epogen®** *see* epoetin alfa *on page 236*

epoprostenol (e poe PROST en ole)

U.S. Brand Names Flolan®

Generic Available No

Therapeutic Category Platelet Inhibitor

Use Long-term intravenous treatment of primary pulmonary hypertension (PPH)

Usual Dosage I.V. continuous infusion: 2 ng/kg/minute

Dosage Forms Injection, as sodium: 0.5 mg/vial and 1.5 mg/vial, each supplied with 50 mL of sterile diluent

- ◆ **Eprex®** *see* epoetin alfa *on page 236*
- ◆ **epsom salts** *see* magnesium sulfate *on page 382*
- ◆ **EPT** *see* teniposide *on page 595*

eptifibatide (ep TIF i ba tide)

U.S. Brand Names Integrilin®
Generic Available No
Therapeutic Category Antiplatelet Agent
Use Treatment of patients with acute coronary syndrome (UA/NQMI), including patients who are to be managed medically and those undergoing percutaneous coronary intervention (PCI); it has been shown to decrease the rate of a combined endpoint of death or new myocardial infarction. For the treatment of patients undergoing PCI, it has been shown to decrease the rate of a combined endpoint of death, new myocardial infarction, or need for urgent intervention.
Usual Dosage Adults: I.V.:

Acute coronary syndrome: Bolus of 180 mcg/kg as soon as possible following diagnosis, followed by a continuous infusion of 2 mcg/kg/minute until hospital discharge or initiation of CABG surgery, up to 72 hours. If a patient is to undergo a percutaneous coronary intervention (PCI) while receiving eptifibatide, consideration can be given to decreasing the infusion rate to 0.5 mcg/kg/minute (the infusion rate in IMPACT II) at the time of the procedure. Infusion should be continued for an additional 20-24 hours after the procedure, allowing for up to 96 hours of therapy.

Percutaneous coronary intervention (PCI) in patients not presenting with an acute coronary syndrome: Bolus of 135 mcg/kg administered immediately before the initiation of PCI followed by a continuous infusion of 0.5 mcg/kg/minute for 20-24 hours. In the IMPACT II Study, there was little experience in patients weighing more than 143 kg.

Dosage Forms Injection: 0.75 mg/mL (100 mL); 2 mg/mL (10 mL)

- ◆ **Equagesic®** *see* aspirin and meprobamate *on page 62*
- ◆ **Equalactin® Chewable Tablet [OTC]** *see* calcium polycarbophil *on page 107*
- ◆ **Equanil®** *see* meprobamate *on page 394*
- ◆ **Equilet® [OTC]** *see* calcium carbonate *on page 103*
- ◆ **Ercaf®** *see* ergotamine *on page 238*
- ◆ **Ergamisol®** *see* levamisole *on page 364*
- ◆ **Ergocaf** *see* ergotamine *on page 238*

ergocalciferol (er goe kal SIF e role)

Synonyms activated ergosterol; viosterol; vitamin D_2
U.S. Brand Names Calciferol™; Drisdol®
Canadian Brand Names Ostoforte®; Radiostol®
Generic Available Yes
Therapeutic Category Vitamin D Analog
Use Refractory rickets; hypophosphatemia; hypoparathyroidism
Usual Dosage

Dietary supplementation: Oral:
  Premature infants: 10-20 mcg/day (400-800 units), up to 750 mcg/day (30,000 units)
  Infants and healthy Children: 10 mcg/day (400 units)
Renal failure: Oral:
  Children: 0.1-1 mg/day (4000-40,000 units)
  Adults: 0.5 mg/day (20,000 units)
Hypoparathyroidism: Oral:
  Children: 1.25-5 mg/day (50,000-200,000 units) and calcium supplements
  Adults: 625 mcg to 5 mg/day (25,000-200,000 units) and calcium supplements
Vitamin D-dependent rickets: Oral:
  Children: 75-125 mcg/day (3000-5000 units)
  Adults: 250 mcg to 1.5 mg/day (10,000-60,000 units)
Nutritional rickets and osteomalacia:
  Oral:
    Children and Adults (with normal absorption): 25 mcg/day (1000 units)
    Children with malabsorption: 250-625 mcg/day (10,000-25,000 units)
  I.M.: Adults: 250 mcg/day
(Continued)

ergocalciferol *(Continued)*

Nursing/Pharmacy Information
Parenteral injection for I.M. use only
Measure serum calcium, BUN, and phosphorus routinely
Stability: Protect from light

Dosage Forms
Capsule (Drisdol®): 50,000 units [1.25 mg]
Injection (Calciferol™): 500,000 units/mL [12.5 mg/mL] (1 mL)
Liquid (Calciferol™, Drisdol®): 8000 units/mL [200 mcg/mL] (60 mL)
Tablet (Calciferol™): 50,000 units [1.25 mg]

ergoloid mesylates *(ER goe loid MES i lates)*

Synonyms dihydroergotoxine; hydrogenated ergot alkaloids
U.S. Brand Names Germinal®; Hydergine®; Hydergine® LC
Generic Available Yes
Therapeutic Category Ergot Alkaloid and Derivative
Use Treatment of cerebrovascular insufficiency in primary progressive dementia, Alzheimer's dementia, and senile onset
Usual Dosage Adults: Oral: 1 mg 3 times/day up to 4.5-12 mg/day; up to 6 months of therapy may be necessary
Dietary Considerations Should not eat or drink while tablet dissolves under tongue
Nursing/Pharmacy Information Monitor blood pressure, heart rate
Dosage Forms
Capsule, liquid (Hydergine® LC): 1 mg
Liquid (Hydergine®): 1 mg/mL (100 mL)
Tablet:
Oral: 0.5 mg
Gerimal®, Hydergine®: 1 mg
Sublingual: Gerimal®, Hydergine®: 0.5 mg, 1 mg

♦ **Ergomar®** *see* ergotamine *on page 238*
♦ **Ergostat** *(Discontinued) see page 743*

ergotamine *(er GOT a meen)*

Synonyms ergotamine tartrate; ergotamine tartrate and caffeine; ergotamine tartrate with belladonna alkaloids, and phenobarbital
U.S. Brand Names Cafatine-PB®; Cafergot®; Cafetrate®; Ercaf®; Ergomar®; Ergotamine Tartrate and Caffeine Cafatine®; Phenerbel-S®; Wigraine®
Canadian Brand Names Gynergen®
Mexican Brand Names Ergocaf; Sydolil
Generic Available Yes
Therapeutic Category Ergot Alkaloid and Derivative
Use Prevent or abort vascular headaches, such as migraine or cluster
Usual Dosage
Older Children and Adolescents: Oral: 1 tablet at onset of attack; then 1 tablet every 30 minutes as needed, up to a maximum of 3 tablets per attack
Adults:
Oral (Cafergot®): 2 tablets at onset of attack; then 1 tablet every 30 minutes as needed; maximum: 6 tablets per attack; do not exceed 10 tablets/week
Oral (Ergostat®): 1 tablet under tongue at first sign, then 1 tablet every 30 minutes, 3 tablets/24 hours, 5 tablets/week
Rectal (Cafergot® suppositories, Wigraine® suppositories, Cafatine-PB® suppositories): 1 at first sign of an attack; follow with second dose after 1 hour, if needed; maximum dose: 2 per attack; do not exceed 5/week
Dietary Considerations Avoid tea, cola, and coffee, caffeine may increase GI absorption of ergotamine
Nursing/Pharmacy Information Do not crush sublingual drug product
Dosage Forms
Suppository, rectal (Cafatine®, Cafergot®, Cafetrate®, Wigraine®): Ergotamine tartrate 2 mg and caffeine 100 mg (12s)
Tablet (Ercaf®, Wigraine®): Ergotamine tartrate 1 mg and caffeine 100 mg
Sublingual (Ergomar®): Ergotamine tartrate 2 mg

♦ **ergotamine tartrate** *see* ergotamine *on page 238*
♦ **ergotamine tartrate and caffeine** *see* ergotamine *on page 238*
♦ **Ergotamine Tartrate and Caffeine Cafatine®** *see* ergotamine *on page 238*
♦ **ergotamine tartrate, belladonna, and phenobarbital** *see* belladonna, phenobarbital, and ergotamine tartrate *on page 76*
♦ **ergotamine tartrate with belladonna alkaloids, and phenobarbital** *see* ergotamine *on page 238*

- **Ergotrate® Maleate** *(Discontinued)* *see page 743*
- **Eridium®** *(Discontinued)* *see page 743*
- **Eritroquim** *see erythromycin (systemic)* *on page 240*
- **E•R•O Ear [OTC]** *see carbamide peroxide* *on page 112*
- **Erybid™** *see erythromycin (systemic)* *on page 240*
- **Eryc®** *see erythromycin (systemic)* *on page 240*
- **Eryderm® Topical** *see erythromycin (ophthalmic/topical)* *on page 239*
- **Erygel® Topical** *see erythromycin (ophthalmic/topical)* *on page 239*
- **Erymax® Topical** *see erythromycin (ophthalmic/topical)* *on page 239*
- **Ery-Sol® Topical Solution** *(Discontinued)* *see page 743*
- **Ery-Tab®** *see erythromycin (systemic)* *on page 240*

erythrityl tetranitrate (e RI thri til te tra NYE trate)
U.S. Brand Names Cardilate®
Generic Available No
Therapeutic Category Vasodilator
Use Prophylaxis and long-term treatment of frequent or recurrent anginal pain and reduced exercise tolerance associated with angina pectoris
Usual Dosage Adults: Oral: 5 mg under the tongue or in the buccal pouch 3 times/day or 10 mg before meals or food, chewed 3 times/day, increasing in 2-3 days if needed
Dietary Considerations Should be administered before meals
Nursing/Pharmacy Information
Do not crush sublingual drug product
Monitor blood pressure reduction for maximal effect and orthostatic hypotension
Dosage Forms Tablet, oral or sublingual: 10 mg

- **Erythro-Base®** *see erythromycin (systemic)* *on page 240*
- **Erythrocin®** *see erythromycin (systemic)* *on page 240*

erythromycin and benzoyl peroxide
(er ith roe MYE sin & BEN zoe il per OKS ide)
Synonyms benzoyl peroxide and erythromycin
U.S. Brand Names Benzamycin®
Generic Available No
Therapeutic Category Acne Products
Use Topical control of acne vulgaris
Usual Dosage Topical: Apply twice daily (morning and evening)
Nursing/Pharmacy Information Apply after skin is washed, rinsed with warm water, and gently patted dry
Dosage Forms Gel: Erythromycin 30 mg and benzoyl peroxide 50 mg per g

erythromycin and sulfisoxazole
(er ith roe MYE sin & sul fi SOKS a zole)
Synonyms sulfisoxazole and erythromycin
U.S. Brand Names Eryzole®; Pediazole®
Generic Available Yes
Therapeutic Category Macrolide (Antibiotic); Sulfonamide
Use Treatment of susceptible bacterial infections of the upper and lower respiratory tract; otitis media in children caused by susceptible strains of *Haemophilus influenzae*; other infections in patients allergic to penicillin
Usual Dosage Dosage recommendation is based on the product's erythromycin content; Oral:
Children ≥2 months: 40-50 mg/kg/day of erythromycin in divided doses every 6-8 hours; not to exceed 2 g erythromycin or 6 g sulfisoxazole/day or approximately 1.25 mL/kg/day divided every 6-8 hours
Adults: 400 mg erythromycin and 1200 mg sulfisoxazole every 6 hours
Nursing/Pharmacy Information
Monitor CBC and periodic liver function test
Stability: Reconstituted suspension is stable for 14 days when refrigerated
Dosage Forms Suspension, oral: Erythromycin ethylsuccinate 200 mg and sulfisoxazole acetyl 600 mg per 5 mL (100 mL, 150 mL, 200 mL, 250 mL)

erythromycin (ophthalmic/topical)
(er ith roe MYE sin TOP i kal)
U.S. Brand Names Akne-Mycin® Topical; A/T/S® Topical; Del-Mycin® Topical; Emgel™ Topical; Eryderm® Topical; Erygel® Topical; Erymax® Topical; E-Solve-2® Topical; ETS-2%® Topical; Ilotycin® Ophthalmic; Staticin® Topical; T-Stat® Topical
(Continued)

erythromycin (ophthalmic/topical) *(Continued)*

Generic Available Yes

Therapeutic Category Acne Products; Antibiotic, Ophthalmic; Antibiotic, Topical

Use Topical treatment of acne vulgaris

Usual Dosage Children and Adults:

Ophthalmic: Instill one or more times daily depending on the severity of the infection

Topical: Apply 2% solution over the affected area twice daily after the skin has been thoroughly washed and patted dry

Nursing/Pharmacy Information

Contains benzoyl peroxide which may bleach or stain clothing

Stability: Must be stored in a cool place such as a refrigerator following reconstitution

Dosage Forms

Gel: 2% (30 g, 60 g)

Gel (A/T/S®, Emgel™, Erygel®): 2% (27 g, 30 g, 60 g)

Ointment:

Ophthalmic: 0.5% [5 mg/g] (3.5 g)

Ilotycin®: 0.5% [5 mg/g] (3.5 g)

Topical (Akne-Mycin®): 2% (25 g)

Solution, topical:

Staticin®: 1.5% (60 mL)

Akne-Mycin®, A/T/S®, Del-Mycin®, EryDerm®, ETS-2%®, Romycin®, Theramycin Z®, T-Stat®: 2% (60 mL, 66 mL, 120 mL)

Pad (T-Stat®): 2% (60s)

Pledgets: 2% (60s)

Swab: 2% (60s)

erythromycin (systemic) (er ith roe MYE sin)

U.S. Brand Names AK-Mycin®; E.E.S.®; E.E.S.® Chewable; E.E.S.® Granules; E-Mycin®; E-Mycin-E®; Eryc®; Ery-Tab®; Erythrocin®; Ilosone®; Ilosone® Pulvules®; Ilotycin®; PCE®; Wyamycin® S

Canadian Brand Names Apo®-Erythro E-C; Diomycin; Erybid™; Erythro-Base®; Ilotycin®; Novo-Rythro Encap; PMS-Erythromycin

Mexican Brand Names Eritroquim; Latotryd®; Lauricin; Lederpax; Luritran®; Pantomicina; Tromigal

Generic Available Yes

Therapeutic Category Macrolide (Antibiotic)

Use Treatment of mild to moderately severe infections of the upper and lower respiratory tract, pharyngitis and skin infections due to susceptible streptococci and staphylococci; other susceptible bacterial infections including *Mycoplasma* pneumonia, *Legionella* pneumonia, diphtheria, pertussis, chancroid, *Chlamydia*, and *Campylobacter* gastroenteritis; used in conjunction with neomycin for decontaminating the bowel for surgery; dental procedure prophylaxis in penicillin allergic patients

Usual Dosage

Infants and Children:

Oral: Do not exceed 2 g/day

Base and ethylsuccinate: 30-50 mg/kg/day divided every 6-8 hours

Estolate: 30-50 mg/kg/day divided every 8-12 hours

Stearate: 20-40 mg/kg/day divided every 6 hours

Pre-op bowel preparation: 20 mg/kg erythromycin base at 1, 2, and 11 PM on the day before surgery combined with mechanical cleansing of the large intestine and oral neomycin

I.V.: Lactobionate: 20-40 mg/kg/day divided every 6 hours, not to exceed 4 g/day

Adults:

Oral:

Base: 333 mg every 8 hours

Estolate, stearate or base: 250-500 mg every 6-12 hours

Ethylsuccinate: 400-800 mg every 6-12 hours

Pre-op bowel preparation: 1 g erythromycin base at 1, 2, and 11 PM on the day before surgery combined with mechanical cleansing of the large intestine and oral neomycin

I.V.: 15-20 mg/kg/day divided every 6 hours or administered as a continuous infusion over 24 hours

Dietary Considerations Decreased absorption with food; avoid milk and acidic beverages 1 hour before or 2 hours after a dose; ethylsuccinate, estolate, and enteric coated products are **not** affected by food; administer PCE® polymer coated particles tablet without food

Nursing/Pharmacy Information

Do not crush enteric coated drug product; administer by I.V. intermittent or continuous infusion at a concentration of 1-2.5 mg/mL; maximum concentration: 5 mg/mL; I.V. intermittent infusions can be administered over 20-60 minutes

Monitor liver function tests

Stability: Erythromycin lactobionate should be reconstituted with sterile water for injection without preservatives to avoid gel formation; the reconstituted solution is stable for 2 weeks when refrigerated or 24 hours at room temperature. Erythromycin I.V. infusion solution is stable at pH 6-8. Do not use D_5W as a diluent unless sodium bicarbonate is added to solution.

Dosage Forms

Erythromycin base:
Capsule:
Delayed release: 250 mg
Delayed release, enteric coated pellets (Eryc®): 250 mg
Tablet:
Delayed release: 333 mg
Enteric coated (E-Mycin®, Ery-Tab®, E-Base®): 250 mg, 333 mg, 500 mg
Film coated: 250 mg, 500 mg
Polymer coated particles (PCE®): 333 mg, 500 mg
Erythromycin estolate:
Capsule (Ilosone® Pulvules®): 250 mg
Suspension, oral (Ilosone®): 125 mg/5 mL (480 mL); 250 mg/5 mL (480 mL)
Tablet (Ilosone®): 500 mg
Erythromycin ethylsuccinate:
Granules for oral suspension (EryPed®): 400 mg/5 mL (60 mL, 100 mL, 200 mL)
Powder for oral suspension (E.E.S.®): 200 mg/5 mL (100 mL, 200 mL)
Suspension:
Oral (E.E.S.®, EryPed®): 200 mg/5 mL (5 mL, 100 mL, 200 mL, 480 mL); 400 mg/5 mL (5 mL, 60 mL, 100 mL, 200 mL, 480 mL)
Oral [drops] (EryPed®): 100 mg/2.5 mL (50 mL)
Tablet (E.E.S.®): 400 mg
Tablet, chewable (EryPed®): 200 mg
Erythromycin gluceptate: Injection: 1000 mg (30 mL)
Erythromycin lactobionate: Powder for injection: 500 mg, 1000 mg
Erythromycin stearate: Tablet, film coated (Eramycin®, Erythrocin®): 250 mg, 500 mg

♦ **erythropoietin** see epoetin alfa on page 236
♦ **Eryzole®** see erythromycin and sulfisoxazole on page 239
♦ **Esclim® Transdermal** see estradiol on page 242
♦ **Esgic®** see butalbital compound and acetaminophen on page 99
♦ **Esgic-Plus®** see butalbital compound and acetaminophen on page 99
♦ **Esidrix®** see hydrochlorothiazide on page 317
♦ **Esidrix® 100 mg Tablet (Discontinued)** see page 743
♦ **Eskalith®** see lithium on page 372
♦ **Eskazole** see albendazole on page 24

esmolol (ES moe lol)

U.S. Brand Names Brevibloc®

Generic Available No

Therapeutic Category Antiarrhythmic Agent, Class II; Beta-Adrenergic Blocker

Use Supraventricular tachycardia (primarily to control ventricular rate) and hypertension (especially perioperatively)

Usual Dosage Must be adjusted to individual response and tolerance

Children: An extremely limited amount of information regarding esmolol use in pediatric patients is currently available. Some centers have utilized doses of 100-500 mcg/kg administered over 1 minute for control of supraventricular tachycardias. Loading doses of 500 mcg/kg/minute over 1 minute with maximal doses of 50-250 mcg/kg/minute (mean 173) have been used in addition to nitroprusside in a small number of patients (7 patients; 7-19 years of age; median 13 years) to treat postoperative hypertension after coarctation of aorta repair.

(Continued)

esmolol (Continued)

Adults: I.V.: Loading dose: 500 mcg/kg over 1 minute; follow with a 50 mcg/kg/ minute infusion for 4 minutes; if response is inadequate, rebolus with another 500 mcg/kg loading dose over 1 minute, and increase the maintenance infusion to 100 mcg/kg/minute. Repeat this process until a therapeutic effect has been achieved or to a maximum recommended maintenance dose of 200 mcg/kg/minute. Usual dosage range: 50-200 mcg/kg/minute with average dose = 100 mcg/kg/minute.

Dietary Considerations Avoid xanthine-containing foods or beverages

Nursing/Pharmacy Information

Decrease infusion or discontinue if hypotension, congestive heart failure, etc occur; The 250 mg/mL ampul is **not** for direct I.V. injection, but must first be diluted to a final concentration not to exceed 10 mg/mL (ie, 2.5 g in 250 mL or 5 g in 500 mL).

Monitor blood pressure, heart rate, MAP, EKG, respiratory rate

Stability: Diluted I.V. infusion solution is stable for 24 hours at room temperature

Dosage Forms Injection, as hydrochloride: 10 mg/mL (10 mL); 250 mg/mL (10 mL)

- ♦ **E-Solve-2® Topical** see erythromycin (ophthalmic/topical) on page 239
- ♦ **Esoterica® Facial [OTC]** see hydroquinone on page 325
- ♦ **Esoterica® Regular [OTC]** see hydroquinone on page 325
- ♦ **Esoterica® Sensitive Skin Formula [OTC]** see hydroquinone on page 325
- ♦ **Esoterica® Sunscreen [OTC]** see hydroquinone on page 325
- ♦ **Estar® [OTC]** see coal tar on page 162

estazolam (es TA zoe lam)

U.S. Brand Names ProSom™

Mexican Brand Names Tasedan

Generic Available Yes

Therapeutic Category Benzodiazepine

Controlled Substance C-IV

Use Short-term management of insomnia

Usual Dosage Adults: Oral: 1 mg at bedtime, some patients may require 2 mg

Nursing/Pharmacy Information

Provide safety measures (ie, side rails, night light, and call button); remove smoking materials from area; supervise ambulation

Monitor respiratory and cardiovascular status

Dosage Forms Tablet: 1 mg, 2 mg

- ♦ **Esteprim** see co-trimoxazole on page 170
- ♦ **esterified estrogen and methyltestosterone** see estrogens and methyltestosterone on page 244
- ♦ **esterified estrogens** see estrogens, esterified on page 246
- ♦ **Estinyl®** see ethinyl estradiol on page 248
- ♦ **Estivin® II Ophthalmic [OTC]** see naphazoline on page 431
- ♦ **Estrace® Oral** see estradiol on page 242
- ♦ **Estraderm® Transdermal** see estradiol on page 242

estradiol (es tra DYE ole)

Synonyms Estradiol Hemihydrate

U.S. Brand Names Alora® Transdermal; Climara® Transdermal; depGynogen® Injection; Depo®-Estradiol Injection; Depogen® Injection; Dioval® Injection; Esclim® Transdermal; Estrace® Oral; Estraderm® Transdermal; Estra-L® Injection; Estring®; Estro-Cyp® Injection; Gynogen L.A.® Injection; Vagifem®; Vivelle™ Transdermal

Mexican Brand Names Climaderm; Ginedisc®; Oestrogel; Systen

Generic Available Yes

Therapeutic Category Estrogen Derivative

Use Atrophic vaginitis, atrophic dystrophy of vulva, menopausal symptoms, female hypogonadism

Usual Dosage Adults (all dosage needs to be adjusted based upon the patient's response):

Male: Prostate cancer: Valerate:
I.M.. ≥30 mg or more every 1-2 weeks
Oral: 1-2 mg 3 times/day

Female:

Hypogonadism:

Oral: 1-2 mg/day in a cyclic regimen for 3 weeks on drug, then 1 week off drug

I.M.: Cypionate: 1.5-2 mg/month; valerate: 10-20 mg/month

Transdermal: 0.05 mg patch initially (titrate dosage to response) applied twice weekly in a cyclic regimen, for 3 weeks on drug and 1 week off drug

Atrophic vaginitis, kraurosis vulvae: Vaginal: Insert 2-4 g/day for 2 weeks then gradually reduce to $1/2$ the initial dose for 2 weeks followed by a maintenance dose of 1 g 1-3 times/week

Moderate to severe vasomotor symptoms: I.M.:

Cypionate: 1-5 mg every 3-4 weeks

Valerate: 10-20 mg every 4 weeks

Postpartum breast engorgement: I.M.: Valerate: 10-25 mg at end of first stage of labor

Dietary Considerations Larger doses of vitamin C (eg 1 g/day in adults) may increase the serum concentrations and adverse effects of estradiol; vitamin C supplements are not recommended, but this effect may be decreased if vitamin C supplement is administered 2-3 hours after estrogen; dietary intake of folate and pyridoxine may need to be increased

Nursing/Pharmacy Information Injection for I.M. use only

Dosage Forms

Cream, vaginal (Estrace®): 0.1 mg/g (42.5 g)

Injection, as cypionate (depGynogen®, Depo®-Estradiol, Depogen®, Dura-Estrin®, Estra-D®, Estro-Cyp®): 5 mg/mL (5 mL, 10 mL):

Injection, as valerate:

Dioval®, Duragen®, Estra-L®, Gynogen L.A.®: 20 mg/mL (10 mL); 40 mg/mL (10 mL)

Tablet, micronized (Estrace®): 1 mg, 2 mg

Tablet, vaginal (Vagifem®): 25 mcg (with applicator)

Transdermal system

Alora®:

0.05 mg/24 hours [18 cm²], total estradiol 1.5 mg

0.075 mg/24 hours [27 cm²], total estradiol 2.3 mg

0.1 mg/24 hours [36 cm²], total estradiol 3 mg

Climara®:

0.05 mg/24 hours [12.5 cm²], total estradiol 3.9 mg

0.1 mg/24 hours [25 cm²], total estradiol 7.8 mg

Esclim®:

0.025 mg/day

0.0375 mg/day

0.05 mg/day

0.075 mg/day

0.1 mg/day

Estraderm®:

0.05 mg/24 hours [10 cm²], total estradiol 4 mg

0.1 mg/24 hours [20 cm²], total estradiol 8 mg

Vivelle®:

0.0375 mg/day

0.05 mg/day

0.075 mg/day

Vaginal ring (Estring®): 2 mg gradually released over 90 days

estradiol and norethindrone (es tra DYE ole & nor eth IN drone)

U.S. Brand Names Activelle™

Generic Available No

Therapeutic Category Estrogen and Progestin Combination

Use Treatment of moderate to severe vasomotor symptoms associated with menopause; treatment of vulvar and vaginal atrophy

Usual Dosage Adults: Oral: Take one tablet daily

Dosage Forms Tablet: Estradiol 1 mg and norethindrone acetate 0.5 mg (28s)

estradiol and testosterone (es tra DYE ole & tes TOS ter one)

U.S. Brand Names Andro/Fem®; Deladumone®; depAndrogyn®; Depo-Testadiol®; Depotestogen®; Duo-Cyp®; Duratestrin®; Valertest No.1®

Generic Available No

Therapeutic Category Estrogen and Androgen Combination

Use Vasomotor symptoms associated with menopause; postpartum breast engorgement

Usual Dosage Adults (all dosage needs to be adjusted based upon the patient's response)

(Continued)

estradiol and testosterone *(Continued)*

Dosage Forms Injection:
Andro/Fem®, depAndrogyn®, Depo-Testadiol®, Depotestogen®, Duo-Cyp®, Duratestrin®: Estradiol cypionate 2 mg and testosterone cypionate 50 mg per mL in cottonseed oil (1 mL, 10 mL)
Androgyn L.A.®, Deladumone®, Estra-Testrin®, Valertest No.1®: Estradiol valerate 4 mg and testosterone enanthate 90 mg per mL in sesame oil (5 mL, 10 mL)

♦ **Estradiol Hemihydrate** *see* estradiol *on page 242*
♦ **Estradurin® Injection** *(Discontinued) see page 743*
♦ **Estra-L® Injection** *see* estradiol *on page 242*

estramustine (es tra MUS teen)

U.S. Brand Names Emcyt®
Generic Available No
Therapeutic Category Antineoplastic Agent
Use Palliative treatment of prostatic carcinoma
Usual Dosage Oral: 1 capsule for each 22 lb/day, in 3-4 divided doses
Dietary Considerations Administer at least 1 hour before or 2 hours after eating
Nursing/Pharmacy Information
Administer on an empty stomach, particularly avoid taking with milk
Stability: Refrigerate at 2°C to 8°C (36°F to 46°F); capsules may be stored outside of refrigerator for up to 30 days
Dosage Forms Capsule, as phosphate sodium: 140 mg

♦ **Estratab®** *see* estrogens, esterified *on page 246*
♦ **Estratest®** *see* estrogens and methyltestosterone *on page 244*
♦ **Estratest® H.S.** *see* estrogens and methyltestosterone *on page 244*
♦ **Estring®** *see* estradiol *on page 242*
♦ **Estro-Cyp® Injection** *see* estradiol *on page 242*
♦ **estrogenic substance aqueous** *see* estrone *on page 246*

estrogens and medroxyprogesterone

(ES troe jenz & me DROKS ee proe JES te rone)
Synonyms medroxyprogesterone and estrogens
U.S. Brand Names Premphase™; Prempro™
Generic Available Yes
Therapeutic Category Estrogen and Progestin Combination
Use Women with an intact uterus for the treatment of moderate to severe vasomotor symptoms associated with the menopause; treatment of atrophic vaginitis; primary ovarian failure; osteoporosis prophylactic
Usual Dosage Adults: Oral:
Premphase™: Conjugated estrogen 0.625 mg [Premarin®] and taken orally for 28 days and medroxyprogesterone acetate [Cycrin®] 5 mg (14s) which are taken orally with a Premarin® tablet on days 15 through 28
Prempro™: Conjugated estrogen 0.625 mg [Premarin®] and medroxyprogesterone acetate [Cycrin®] 2.5 mg are taken continuously one each day
Dietary Considerations Administration with food decreases nausea, administer with food
Nursing/Pharmacy Information Prempro™ is now a single-tablet product which replaces the two-tablet product
Dosage Forms
Premphase™: Two separate tablets in therapy pack: Conjugated estrogens 0.625 mg [Premarin®] (28s) taken orally for 28 days and medroxyprogesterone acetate [Cycrin®] 5 mg (14s) which are taken orally with a Premarin® tablet on days 15 through 28
Prempro™: Conjugated estrogens 0.625 mg and medroxyprogesterone acetate 2.5 mg (14s)

estrogens and methyltestosterone

(ES troe jenz & meth il tes TOS te rone)
Synonyms conjugated estrogen and methyltestosterone; esterified estrogen and methyltestosterone
U.S. Brand Names Estratest®; Estratest® H.S.; Premarin® With Methyltestosterone
Generic Available No
Therapeutic Category Estrogen and Androgen Combination

Use Atrophic vaginitis; hypogonadism; primary ovarian failure; vasomotor symptoms of menopause; prostatic carcinoma; osteoporosis prophylactic

Usual Dosage Oral: Lowest dose that will control symptoms should be chosen, normally administered 3 weeks on and 1 week off

Dietary Considerations Should be administered with food at same time each day

Nursing/Pharmacy Information Women should inform their physicians if signs or symptoms of any of the following occur: thromboembolic or thrombotic disorders including sudden severe headache or vomiting, disturbance of vision or speech, loss of vision, numbness or weakness in an extremity, sharp or crushing chest pain, calf pain, shortness of breath, severe abdominal pain or mass, mental depression or unusual bleeding; women should discontinue taking the medication if they suspect they are pregnant or become pregnant.

Dosage Forms Tablet:

Estratest®, Menogen®: Esterified estrogen 1.25 mg and methyltestosterone 2.5 mg

Estratest® H.S., Menogen H.S.®: Esterified estrogen 0.625 mg and methyltestosterone 1.25 mg

Premarin® With Methyltestosterone: Conjugated estrogen 0.625 mg and methyltestosterone 5 mg; conjugated estrogen 1.25 mg and methyltestosterone 10 mg

estrogens, conjugated, a (synthetic) *New Drug*
(ES troe jenz, KON joo gate ed, aye, sin THET ik)

U.S. Brand Names Cenestin™

Generic Available No

Therapeutic Category Estrogen Derivative

Use Treatment of moderate to severe vasomotor symptoms of menopause

Usual Dosage Moderate to severe vasomotor symptoms: Oral: 0.625 mg/day; may be titrated up to 1.25 mg daily. Attempts to discontinue medication should be made at 3-6 month intervals.

Dosage Forms Tablet: 0.625 mg, 1.25 mg

estrogens, conjugated (equine) (ES troe jenz KON joo gate ed)

Synonyms CES; conjugated estrogens

U.S. Brand Names Premarin®

Canadian Brand Names C.E.S.™; Congest

Generic Available No

Therapeutic Category Estrogen Derivative

Use Dysfunctional uterine bleeding, atrophic vaginitis, hypogonadism, vasomotor symptoms of menopause

Usual Dosage Adults:

Male: Prostate cancer: Oral: 1.25-2.5 mg 3 times/day

Female:

Hypogonadism: Oral: 2.5-7.5 mg/day for 20 days, off 10 days and repeat until menses occur

Abnormal uterine bleeding:

Oral: 2.5-5 mg/day for 7-10 days; then decrease to 1.25 mg/day for 2 weeks

I.V.: 25 mg every 6-12 hours until bleeding stops

Moderate to severe vasomotor symptoms: Oral: 0.625-1.25 mg/day

Postpartum breast engorgement: Oral: 3.75 mg every 4 hours for 5 doses, then 1.25 mg every 4 hours for 5 days

Dietary Considerations Larger doses of vitamin C (eg, 1 g/day in adults) may increase the serum concentrations and adverse effects of estrogens; vitamin C supplements are not recommended, but this effect may be decreased if vitamin C supplement is administered 2-3 hours after estrogen; dietary intake of folate and pyridoxine may need to be increased

Nursing/Pharmacy Information

May also be administered intramuscularly; administer at bedtime to minimize occurrence of adverse effects; when administered I.V., drug should be administered slowly to avoid the occurrence of a flushing reaction may also be administered intramuscularly

Stability: Refrigerate injection; reconstituted solution is stable for 60 days; injection is **compatible** with normal saline, dextrose, and invert sugar solutions; **incompatible** with proteins, ascorbic acid, or solutions with acidic pH

Dosage Forms

Cream, vaginal: 0.625 mg/g (42.5 g)

Injection: 25 mg (5 mL)

Tablet: 0.3 mg, 0.625 mg, 0.9 mg, 1.25 mg, 2.5 mg

estrogens, esterified (ES troe jenz, es TER i fied)
Synonyms esterified estrogens
U.S. Brand Names Estratab®; Menest®
Generic Available No
Therapeutic Category Estrogen Derivative
Use Atrophic vaginitis; hypogonadism; primary ovarian failure; vasomotor symptoms of menopause; prostatic carcinoma; osteoporosis prophylactic
Usual Dosage Adults: Oral:
Male: Prostate cancer: 1.25-2.5 mg 3 times/day
Female:
Hypogonadism: 2.5-7.5 mg/day for 20 days, off 10 days and repeat until menses occur
Moderate to severe vasomotor symptoms: 0.3-1.25 mg/day
Dietary Considerations Should be administered with food at same time each day
Nursing/Pharmacy Information Esterified estrogens are a combination of the sodium salts of the sulfate esters of estrogenic substances; the principal component is estrone, with preparations containing 75% to 85% sodium estrone sulfate and 6% to 15% sodium equilin sulfate such that the total is not <90%
Dosage Forms Tablet: 0.3 mg, 0.625 mg, 1.25 mg, 2.5 mg

♦ **Estroject-2® Injection** *(Discontinued)* *see page 743*
♦ **Estroject-L.A.® Injection** *(Discontinued)* *see page 743*

estrone (ES trone)
Synonyms estrogenic substance aqueous
U.S. Brand Names Aquest®; Kestrone®
Canadian Brand Names Femogen®; Neo-Estrone®; Oestrillin®
Generic Available Yes
Therapeutic Category Estrogen Derivative
Use Atrophic vaginitis; hypogonadism; primary ovarian failure; vasomotor symptoms of menopause; prostatic carcinoma; osteoporosis prophylactic
Usual Dosage Adults: I.M.:
Vasomotor symptoms, atrophic vaginitis: 0.1-0.5 mg 2-3 times/week
Primary ovarian failure, hypogonadism: 0.1-1 mg/week, up to 2 mg/week
Prostatic carcinoma: 2-4 mg 2-3 times/week
Nursing/Pharmacy Information May also be administered intramuscularly; administer at bedtime to minimize occurrence of adverse effects; when administered I.V., drug should be administered slowly to avoid the occurrence of a flushing reaction
Dosage Forms Injection: 2 mg/mL (10 mL, 30 mL); 5 mg/mL (10 mL)

♦ **Estronol® Injection** *(Discontinued)* *see page 743*

estropipate (ES troe pih pate)
Synonyms piperazine estrone sulfate
U.S. Brand Names Ogen® Oral; Ogen® Vaginal; Ortho-Est® Oral
Generic Available Yes
Therapeutic Category Estrogen Derivative
Use Atrophic vaginitis; hypogonadism; primary ovarian failure; vasomotor symptoms of menopause; prostatic carcinoma; osteoporosis prophylactic
Usual Dosage Adults: Female:
Moderate to severe vasomotor symptoms: Oral: 0.625-5 mg/day
Hypogonadism: Oral: 1.25-7.5 mg/day for 3 weeks followed by an 8- to 10-day rest period
Atrophic vaginitis or kraurosis vulvae: Vaginal: Instill 2-4 g/day 3 weeks on and 1 week off
Nursing/Pharmacy Information Patients should inform their physicians if signs or symptoms of any of the following occur: Thromboembolic or thrombotic disorders including sudden severe headache or vomiting, disturbance of vision or speech, loss of vision, numbness or weakness in an extremity, sharp or crushing chest pain, calf pain, shortness of breath, severe abdominal pain or mass, mental depression or unusual bleeding; patients should discontinue taking the medication if they suspect they are pregnant or become pregnant. Patient package insert is available; insert product high into the vagina.
Dosage Forms Piperazine estrone sulfate:
Cream, vaginal: 0.15% [estropipate 1.5 mg/g] (42.5 g tube)
Tablet: 0.625 mg [estropipate 0.75 mg]; 1.25 mg [estropipate 1.5 mg]; 2.5 mg [estropipate 3 mg]; 5 mg [estropipate 6 mg]

♦ **Estrostep® 21** *see ethinyl estradiol and norethindrone on page 250*

♦ **Estrostep® Fe** *see* ethinyl estradiol and norethindrone *on page 250*
♦ **Estrovis®** *(Discontinued) see page 743*

etanercept (et a NER cept)
U.S. Brand Names Enbrel®
Generic Available No
Therapeutic Category Antirheumatic, Disease Modifying
Use Reduction in signs and symptoms of moderately to severely active rheumatoid arthritis in patients who have had an inadequate response to one or more disease-modifying antirheumatic drugs (DMARDs).
Usual Dosage S.C.:
Children: 0.4 mg/kg (maximum: 25 mg dose)
Adult: 25 mg given twice weekly; if the physician determines that it is appropriate, patients may self-inject after proper training in injection technique
Dosage Forms Powder for injection: 25 mg

ethacrynic acid (eth a KRIN ik AS id)
Synonyms sodium ethacrynate
U.S. Brand Names Edecrin®
Generic Available No
Therapeutic Category Diuretic, Loop
Use Management of edema secondary to congestive heart failure; hepatic or renal disease, hypertension
Usual Dosage
Children:
Oral: 25 mg/day to start, increase by 25 mg/day at intervals of 2-3 days as needed, to a maximum of 3 mg/kg/day
I.V.: 1 mg/kg/dose, (maximum: 50 mg/dose); repeat doses not recommended
Adults:
Oral: 50-100 mg/day increased in increments of 25-50 mg at intervals of several days to a maximum of 400 mg/24 hours
I.V.: 0.5-1 mg/kg/dose (maximum: 50 mg/dose); repeat doses not recommended
Dietary Considerations This product may cause a potassium loss; your physician may prescribe a potassium supplement, another medication to help prevent the potassium loss, or recommend that you eat foods high in potassium, especially citrus fruits; do not change your diet on your own while taking this medication, especially if you are taking potassium supplements or medications to reduce potassium loss; too much potassium can be as harmful as too little
Nursing/Pharmacy Information
Tissue irritant; not to be administered I.M. or S.C.; dilute injection with 50 mL dextrose 5% or normal saline (1 mg/mL concentration resulting); may be injected without further dilution over a period of several minutes or infused over 20-30 minutes
Monitor blood pressure, serum electrolytes, renal function, hearing
Dosage Forms
Powder for injection, as ethacrynate sodium: 50 mg (50 mL)
Tablet: 25 mg, 50 mg

ethambutol (e THAM byoo tole)
U.S. Brand Names Myambutol®
Canadian Brand Names Etibi®
Generic Available No
Therapeutic Category Antimycobacterial Agent
Use Treatment of tuberculosis and other mycobacterial diseases in conjunction with other antimycobacterial agents
Usual Dosage Oral (not recommended in children <12 years of age):
Children >12 years: 15 mg/kg/day once daily
Adolescents and Adults: 15-25 mg/kg/day once daily, not to exceed 2.5 g/day
Dietary Considerations May be administered with food as absorption is not affected, may cause gastric irritation
Nursing/Pharmacy Information
Reinforce compliance
Monitor visual testing periodically in patients receiving more than 15 mg/kg/day; periodic renal, hepatic, and hematopoietic tests
Dosage Forms Tablet, as hydrochloride: 100 mg, 400 mg

♦ **Ethamolin®** *see* ethanolamine oleate *on page 248*
♦ **ETH and C** *see* terpin hydrate and codeine *on page 597*

♦ **ethanoic acid** *see* acetic acid *on page 17*
♦ **ethanol** *see* alcohol, ethyl *on page 26*

ethanolamine oleate (ETH a nol a meen OH lee ate)

U.S. Brand Names Ethamolin®
Generic Available No
Therapeutic Category Sclerosing Agent
Use Mild sclerosing agent used for bleeding esophageal varices
Usual Dosage Adults: 1.5-5 mL per varix, up to 20 mL total or 0.4 mL/kg; patients with severe hepatic dysfunction should receive less than recommended maximum dose
Nursing/Pharmacy Information Have epinephrine and resuscitative equipment nearby
Dosage Forms Injection: 5% [50 mg/mL] (2 mL)

♦ **Ethaquin®** *(Discontinued) see page 743*
♦ **Ethatab®** *(Discontinued) see page 743*

ethaverine (eth AV er een)

Generic Available Yes
Therapeutic Category Vasodilator
Use Peripheral and cerebral vascular insufficiency associated with arterial spasm
Usual Dosage Adults: Oral: 100 mg 3 times/day
Nursing/Pharmacy Information May cause dizziness or drowsiness; use caution when driving or performing other tasks requiring alertness
Dosage Forms Ethaverine hydrochloride:
Capsule: 100 mg
Tablet: 100 mg

♦ **Ethavex-100®** *(Discontinued) see page 743*

ethchlorvynol (eth klor VI nole)

U.S. Brand Names Placidyl®
Generic Available No
Therapeutic Category Hypnotic, Nonbarbiturate
Controlled Substance C-IV
Use Short-term management of insomnia
Usual Dosage Oral: 500-1000 mg at bedtime
Nursing/Pharmacy Information
Monitor cardiac and respiratory function and abuse potential
Stability: Capsules should not be crushed and should not be refrigerated
Dosage Forms Capsule: 200 mg, 500 mg, 750 mg

ethinyl estradiol (ETH in il es tra DYE ole)

U.S. Brand Names Estinyl®
Generic Available No
Therapeutic Category Estrogen Derivative
Use Atrophic vaginitis; hypogonadism; primary ovarian failure; vasomotor symptoms of menopause; prostatic carcinoma; osteoporosis prophylactic
Usual Dosage Adults: Oral:
Hypogonadism: 0.05 mg 1-3 times/day for 2 weeks
Prostatic carcinoma: 0.15-2 mg/day
Vasomotor symptoms: 0.02-0.05 mg for 21 days, off 7 days and repeat
Nursing/Pharmacy Information Administer at bedtime to minimize occurrence of adverse effects
Dosage Forms Tablet: 0.02 mg, 0.05 mg, 0.5 mg

ethinyl estradiol and desogestrel

(ETH in il es tra DYE ole & des oh JES trel)
Synonyms desogestrel and ethinyl estradiol
U.S. Brand Names Desogen®; Ortho-Cept®
Generic Available No
Therapeutic Category Contraceptive, Oral
Use Prevention of pregnancy
Usual Dosage Contraception: Oral: 1 tablet daily, beginning on day 5 of menstrual cycle (first day of menstrual flow is day 1). With 21-tablet packages, new dosing cycle begins 7 days after last tablet taken. With 28-tablet packages, dosage is 1 tablet daily without interruption; extra tablets are placebos, If next menstrual period does not begin on schedule, rule out pregnancy before starting new dosing cycle. If menstrual period begins, start new dosing cycle 7

days after last tablet was taken. if all doses have been taken on schedule and 1 menstrual period is missed, continue dosing cycle. If 2 consecutive menstrual periods are missed, pregnancy test is required before new dosing cycle is started.

One dose missed: Take as soon as remembered or take 2 tablets next day

Two doses missed: Take 2 tablets as soon as remembered or 2 tablets next 2 days

Three doses missed: Begin new compact of tablets starting on day 1 of next cycle

Dietary Considerations Should be administered with food at same time each day

Nursing/Pharmacy Information Women should inform their physicians if signs or symptoms of any of the following occur: thromboembolic or thrombotic disorders including sudden severe headache or vomiting, disturbance of vision or speech, loss of vision, numbness or weakness in an extremity, sharp or crushing chest pain, calf pain, shortness of breath, severe abdominal pain or mass, mental depression or unusual bleeding. Women should be advised that when any doses are missed, alternative contraceptive methods should be used for the next 2 days or until 2 days into the new cycle; women should discontinue taking the medication if they suspect they are pregnant or become pregnant.

Dosage Forms Tablet: Ethinyl estradiol 0.03 mg and desogestrel 0.15 mg (21s, 28s)

ethinyl estradiol and ethynodiol diacetate
(ETH in il es tra DYE ole & e thye noe DYE ole dye AS e tate)

Synonyms ethynodiol diacetate and ethinyl estradiol

U.S. Brand Names Demulen®; Zovia®

Generic Available Yes

Therapeutic Category Contraceptive, Oral

Use Prevention of pregnancy; treatment of hypermenorrhea, endometriosis, female hypogonadism

Usual Dosage

For 21-tablet cycle packs, with 21 active tablets (28-day packs have 21 active tablets and 7 inert tablets): Administer 1 tablet daily starting on the fifth day of menstrual cycle, with day 1 being the first day of menstruation; begin taking a new cycle pack on the eighth day after taking the last tablet from the previous pack

With 28-tablet packages, dosage is 1 tablet daily without interruption; extra tablets are placebos or contain iron. If next menstrual period does not begin on schedule, rule out pregnancy before starting new dosing cycle. If menstrual period begins, start new dosing cycle 7 days after last tablet was administered. If all doses have been administered on schedule and 1 menstrual period is missed, continue dosing cycle. If 2 consecutive menstrual periods are missed, pregnancy test is required before new dosing cycle is started.

One dose missed: Administer as soon as remembered or administer 2 tablets next day

Two doses missed: Administer 2 tablets as soon as remembered or 2 tablets next 2 days

Three doses missed: Begin new compact of tablets starting on day 1 of next cycle

Dietary Considerations Should be administered with food at same time each day

Nursing/Pharmacy Information Photosensitivity may occur. Inform your physician if signs or symptoms of any of the following occur: Thromboembolic or thrombotic disorders including sudden severe headache or vomiting, disturbance of vision or speech, loss of vision, numbness or weakness in an extremity, sharp or crushing chest pain, calf pain, shortness of breath, severe abdominal pain or mass, mental depression or unusual bleeding. If any doses are missed, alternative contraceptive methods should be used for the next 2 days or until 2 days into the new cycle Discontinue taking the medication if you suspect you are pregnant or become pregnant.

Dosage Forms Tablet:

1/35: Ethinyl estradiol 0.035 mg and ethynodiol diacetate 1 mg (21s, 28s)

1/50: Ethinyl estradiol 0.05 mg and ethynodiol diacetate 1 mg (21s, 28s)

ethinyl estradiol and levonorgestrel
(ETH in il es tra DYE ole & LEE voe nor jes trel)

Synonyms levonorgestrel and ethinyl estradiol

U.S. Brand Names Alesse™; Levlen®; Levlite®; Levora®; Nordette®; Preven™; Tri-Levlen®; Triphasil®

Generic Available Yes

Therapeutic Category Contraceptive, Oral

Use Prevention of pregnancy; treatment of hypermenorrhea, endometriosis, female hypogonadism

Usual Dosage Adults: Female: Oral:

Contraception: 1 tablet daily, beginning on day 5 of menstrual cycle (first day of menstrual flow is day 1). With 20-tablet and 21-tablet packages, new dosing cycle begins 7 days after last tablet taken. With 28-tablet packages, dosage is 1 tablet daily without interruption; extra tablets are placebos or contain iron. If next menstrual period does not begin on schedule, rule out pregnancy before starting new dosing cycle. If menstrual period begins, start new dosing cycle 7 days after last tablet was taken. If all doses have been taken on schedule and one menstrual period is missed, continue dosing cycle. If two consecutive menstrual periods are missed, pregnancy test is required before new dosing cycle is started.

One dose missed: Take as soon as remembered or take 2 tablets next day
Two doses missed: Take 2 tablets as soon as remembered or 2 tablets next 2 days
Three doses missed: Begin new compact of tablets starting on day 1 of next cycle

Triphasic oral contraceptive (Tri-Levlen®, Triphasil®): 1 tablet/day in the sequence specified by the manufacturer

Post-intercourse pregnancy prevention: Take 2 tablets ≤72 hours after unprotected intercourse, take second dose of 2 tablets 12 hours later

Dietary Considerations Should be administered with food at same time each day

Nursing/Pharmacy Information Inform your physician if signs or symptoms of any of the following occur: Thromboembolic or thrombotic disorders including sudden severe headache or vomiting, disturbance of vision or speech, loss of vision, numbness or weakness in an extremity, sharp or crushing chest pain, calf pain, shortness of breath, severe abdominal pain or mass, mental depression or unusual bleeding. If any doses are missed, alternative contraceptive methods should be used for the next 2 days or until 2 days into the new cycle. Discontinue taking the medication if you suspect you are pregnant or become pregnant.

Dosage Forms Tablet:

Alesse™, Levlite®: Ethinyl estradiol 0.02 mg and levonorgestrel 0.1 mg (21s, 28s)
Levlen®, Levora®, Nordette®: Ethinyl estradiol 0.03 mg and levonorgestrel 0.15 mg (21s, 28s)
Preven™: Ethinyl estradiol 0.05 mg and levonorgestrel 0.25 mg (4s)
Tri-Levlen®, Triphasil®: Phase 1 (6 brown tablets): Ethinyl estradiol 0.03 mg and levonorgestrel 0.05 mg; Phase 2 (5 white tablets): Ethinyl estradiol 0.04 mg and levonorgestrel 0.075 mg; Phase 3 (10 yellow tablets): Ethinyl estradiol 0.03 mg and levonorgestrel 0.125 mg (21s, 28s)

ethinyl estradiol and norethindrone
(ETH in il es tra DYE ole & nor eth IN drone)

Synonyms norethindrone acetate and ethinyl estradiol

U.S. Brand Names Brevicon®; Estrostep® 21; Estrostep® Fe; Genora® 0.5/35; Genora® 1/35; Jenest-28™; Loestrin®; Modicon™; N.E.E.® 1/35; Nelova™ 0.5/35E; Nelova™ 10/11; Norethin™ 1/35E; Norinyl® 1+35; Ortho-Novum® 1/35; Ortho-Novum® 7/7/7; Ortho-Novum® 10/11; Ovcon® 35; Ovcon® 50; Tri-Norinyl®

Canadian Brand Names Ortho® 0.5/35; Synphasic®

Generic Available Yes

Therapeutic Category Contraceptive, Oral

Use Prevention of pregnancy; treatment of hypermenorrhea, endometriosis, female hypogonadism

Usual Dosage

For 21-tablet cycle packs, with 21 active tablets (28-day packs have 21 active tablets and 7 inert tablets): Administer 1 tablet daily starting on the fifth day of menstrual cycle, with day 1 being the first day of menstruation; begin taking a new cycle pack on the eighth day after taking the last tablet from the previous pack

With 28-tablet packages, dosage is 1 tablet daily without interruption; extra tablets are placebos or contain iron. If next menstrual period does not begin on schedule, rule out pregnancy before starting new dosing cycle. If menstrual period begins, start new dosing cycle 7 days after last tablet was administered. If all doses have been administered on schedule and 1 menstrual period is missed, continue dosing cycle. If 2 consecutive menstrual periods are missed, pregnancy test is required before new dosing cycle is started.

One dose missed: Administer as soon as remembered or administer 2 tablets next day

Two doses missed: Administer 2 tablets as soon as remembered or 2 tablets next 2 days

Three doses missed: Begin new compact of tablets starting on day 1 of next cycle

Biphasic oral contraceptive (Ortho-Novum™ 10/11): 1 color tablet/day for 10 days, then next color tablet for 11 days

Triphasic oral contraceptive (Ortho-Novum™ 7/7/7, Tri-Norinyl®, Triphasil®): 1 tablet/day in the sequence specified by the manufacturer

Dietary Considerations Should be administered with food at same time each day

Nursing/Pharmacy Information Administer at bedtime to minimize occurrence of adverse effects

Dosage Forms Tablet:

Brevicon®, Genora® 0.5/35, Modicon™, Nelova™ 0.5/35E: Ethinyl estradiol 0.035 mg and norethindrone 0.5 mg (21s, 28s)

Estrostep®:

Triangular tablet (white): Ethinyl estradiol 0.02 mg and norethindrone acetate 1 mg

Square tablet (white): Ethinyl estradiol 0.03 mg and norethindrone acetate 1 mg

Round tablet (white): Ethinyl estradiol 0.035 mg and norethindrone acetate 1 mg

Estrostep® Fe:

Triangular tablet (white): Ethinyl estradiol 0.02 mg and norethindrone acetate 1 mg

Square tablet (white): Ethinyl estradiol 0.03 mg and norethindrone acetate 1 mg

Round tablet (white): Ethinyl estradiol 0.035 mg and norethindrone acetate 1 mg

Brown tablet: Ferrous fumarate 75 mg

Loestrin® 1.5/30: Ethinyl estradiol 0.03 mg and norethindrone acetate 1.5 mg (21s)

Loestrin® Fe 1.5/30: Ethinyl estradiol 0.03 mg and norethindrone acetate 1.5 mg with ferrous fumarate 75 mg in 7 inert tablets (28s)

Loestrin® 1/20: Ethinyl estradiol 0.02 mg and norethindrone acetate 1 mg (21s)

Loestrin® Fe 1/20: Ethinyl estradiol 0.02 mg and norethindrone acetate 1 mg with ferrous fumarate 75 mg in 7 inert tablets (28s)

Genora® 1/35, N.E.E.® 1/35, Nelova® 1/35E, Norethin™ 1/35E, Norinyl® 1+35, Ortho-Novum® 1/35: Ethinyl estradiol 0.035 mg and norethindrone 1 mg (21s, 28s)

Jenest-28™: Phase 1 (7 white tablets): Ethinyl estradiol 0.035 mg and norethindrone 0.5 mg; Phase 2 (14 peach tablets): Ethinyl estradiol 0.035 mg and norethindrone 1 mg and 7 green inert tablets (28s)

Ortho-Novum® 7/7/7: Phase 1 (7 white tablets): Ethinyl estradiol 0.035 mg and norethindrone 0.5 mg; Phase 2 (7 light peach tablets): Ethinyl estradiol 0.035 mg and norethindrone 0.75 mg; Phase 3 (7 peach tablets): Ethinyl estradiol 0.035 mg and norethindrone 1 mg (21s, 28s)

Ortho-Novum® 10/11: Phase 1 (10 white tablets): Ethinyl estradiol 0.035 mg and norethindrone 0.5 mg; Phase 2 (11 dark yellow tablets): Ethinyl estradiol 0.035 mg and norethindrone 1 mg (21s, 28s)

Ovcon® 35: Ethinyl estradiol 0.035 mg and norethindrone 0.4 mg (21s, 28s)

Ovcon® 50: Ethinyl estradiol 0.050 mg and norethindrone 1 mg (21s, 28s)

Tri-Norinyl®: Phase 1 (7 blue tablets): Ethinyl estradiol 0.035 mg and norethindrone 0.5 mg; Phase 2 (9 green tablets): Ethinyl estradiol 0.035 mg and norethindrone 1 mg; Phase 3 (5 blue tablets): Ethinyl estradiol 0.035 mg and norethindrone 0.5 mg (21s, 28s)

ethinyl estradiol and norgestimate

(ETH in il es tra DYE ole & nor JES ti mate)

Synonyms norgestimate and ethinyl estradiol

U.S. Brand Names Ortho-Cyclen®; Ortho Tri-Cyclen®

(Continued)

ethinyl estradiol and norgestimate *(Continued)*

Generic Available No

Therapeutic Category Contraceptive, Oral

Use Prevention of pregnancy

Usual Dosage

Contraception: Oral: 1 tablet daily, beginning on day 5 of menstrual cycle (first day of menstrual flow is day 1). With 21-tablet packages, new dosing cycle begins 7 days after last tablet administered. With 28-tablet packages, dosage is 1 tablet daily without interruption; extra tablets are placebos or contain iron. If next menstrual period does not begin on schedule, rule out pregnancy before starting new dosing cycle. If menstrual period begins, start new dosing cycle 7 days after last tablet was administered. If all doses have been administered on schedule and 1 menstrual period is missed, continue dosing cycle. If 2 consecutive menstrual periods are missed, pregnancy test is required before new dosing cycle is started.

One dose missed: Administer as soon as remembered or administer 2 tablets next day

Two doses missed: Administer 2 tablets as soon as remembered or 2 tablets next 2 days

Three doses missed: Begin new compact of tablets starting on day 1 of next cycle

Triphasic oral contraceptive: 1 tablet/day in the sequence specified by the manufacturer

Dietary Considerations Should be administered with food at same time each day

Nursing/Pharmacy Information Women should inform their physicians if signs or symptoms of any of the following occur: thromboembolic or thrombotic disorders including sudden severe headache or vomiting, disturbance of vision or speech, loss of vision, numbness or weakness in an extremity, sharp or crushing chest pain, calf pain, shortness of breath, severe abdominal pain or mass, mental depression or unusual bleeding. Women should be advised that when any doses are missed, alternative contraceptive methods should be used for the next 2 days or until 2 days into the new cycle; women should discontinue taking the medication if they suspect they are pregnant or become pregnant.

Dosage Forms Tablet:

Ortho-Cyclen®: Ethinyl estradiol 0.035 mg and norgestimate 0.25 mg (21s, 28s)

Ortho Tri-Cyclen®: Phase 1 (7 white tablets): Ethinyl estradiol 0.035 mg and norgestimate 0.18 mg; Phase 2 (5 light blue tablets): Ethinyl estradiol 0.035 mg and norgestimate 0.215 mg; Phase 3 (10 blue tablets): Ethinyl estradiol 0.035 mg and norgestimate 0.25 mg (21s, 28s)

ethinyl estradiol and norgestrel

(ETH in il es tra DYE ole & nor JES trel)

Synonyms norgestrel and ethinyl estradiol

U.S. Brand Names Lo/Ovral®; Ovral®

Generic Available Yes

Therapeutic Category Contraceptive, Oral

Use Prevention of pregnancy; treatment of hypermenorrhea, endometriosis, female hypogonadism

Usual Dosage Contraception: Oral: 1 tablet daily, beginning on day 5 of menstrual cycle (first day of menstrual flow is day 1). With 20-tablet and 21-tablet packages, new dosing cycle begins 7 days after last tablet administered; with 28-tablet packages, dosage is 1 tablet daily without interruption; extra tablets are placebos or contain iron. If next menstrual period does not begin on schedule, rule out pregnancy before starting new dosing cycle; if menstrual period begins, start new dosing cycle 7 days after last tablet was administered; if all doses have been administered on schedule and 1 menstrual period is missed, continue dosing cycle; if two consecutive menstrual periods are missed, pregnancy test is required before new dosing cycle is started.

One dose missed: Administer as soon as remembered or administer 2 tablets next day

Two doses missed: Administer 2 tablets as soon as remembered or 2 tablets next 2 days

Three doses missed: Begin new compact of tablets starting on day 1 of next cycle

Dietary Considerations Should be administered with food at same time each day

Nursing/Pharmacy Information Administer at bedtime to minimize occurrence of adverse effects

Dosage Forms Tablet:
Lo/Ovral®: Ethinyl estradiol 0.03 mg and norgestrel 0.3 mg (21s and 28s)
Ovral®: Ethinyl estradiol 0.05 mg and norgestrel 0.5 mg (21s and 28s)

♦ **Ethiodol®** *see* radiological/contrast media (ionic) *on page 539*
♦ **ethiofos** *see* amifostine *on page 36*

ethionamide (e thye on AM ide)
U.S. Brand Names Trecator®-SC
Generic Available No
Therapeutic Category Antimycobacterial Agent
Use In conjunction with other antituberculosis agents in the treatment of tuberculosis and other mycobacterial diseases
Usual Dosage Oral:
Children: 15-20 mg/kg/day in 2 divided doses, not to exceed 1 g/day
Adults: 500-1000 mg/day in 1-3 divided doses
Dietary Considerations Increase dietary intake of pyridoxine to prevent neurotoxic effects of ethionamide
Nursing/Pharmacy Information
Neurotoxic effects may be relieved by the administration of pyridoxine
Monitor initial and periodic serum ALT and AST
Dosage Forms Tablet, sugar coated: 250 mg

♦ **Ethmozine®** *see* moricizine *on page 422*

ethosuximide (eth oh SUKS i mide)
U.S. Brand Names Zarontin®
Generic Available Yes
Therapeutic Category Anticonvulsant
Use Management of absence (petit mal) seizures, myoclonic seizures, and akinetic epilepsy
Usual Dosage Oral:
Children 3-6 years:
Initial: 250 mg
Increment: 250 mg/day at 4- to 7-day intervals
Maintenance: 20-40 mg/kg/day
Maximum: 1500 mg/day in 2 divided doses
Children >6 years and Adults:
Initial: 500 mg/day
Increment: 250 mg/day at 4- to 7-day intervals
Maintenance: 20-40 mg/kg/day
Maximum: 1500 mg/day in 2 divided doses
Dietary Considerations Increase dietary intake of folate; may be administered with food or milk; alcohol: additive CNS depression has been reported with succinimides; avoid or limit alcohol
Nursing/Pharmacy Information Monitor CBC, platelets, liver enzymes, trough ethosuximide serum concentration; observe patient for excess sedation; maintain serum levels; monitor for bruising and bleeding
Dosage Forms
Capsule: 250 mg
Syrup (raspberry flavor): 250 mg/5 mL (473 mL)

ethotoin (ETH oh toyn)
Synonyms ethylphenylhydantoin
U.S. Brand Names Peganone®
Generic Available No
Therapeutic Category Hydantoin
Use Generalized tonic-clonic or complex-partial seizures
Usual Dosage Oral:
Children: 250 mg twice daily, up to 250 mg 4 times/day
Adults: 250 mg 4 times/day after meals, may be increased up to 3 g/day in divided doses 4 times/day
Dietary Considerations Should be administered after meals
Dosage Forms Tablet: 250 mg, 500 mg

♦ **ethoxynaphthamido penicillin sodium** *see* nafcillin *on page 428*
♦ **Ethrane®** *see* enflurane *on page 232*
♦ **ethyl aminobenzoate** *see* benzocaine *on page 79*

ethyl chloride (ETH il KLOR ide)

Synonyms chloroethane

Generic Available Yes

Therapeutic Category Local Anesthetic

Use Local anesthetic in minor operative procedures and to relieve pain caused by insect stings and burns, and irritation caused by myofascial and visceral pain syndromes

Usual Dosage Topical: Dosage varies with use

Nursing/Pharmacy Information

Spray for a few seconds to the point of frost formation when the tissue becomes white; avoid prolonged spraying of skin beyond this point

Stability: Refrigerate; store in airtight containers preferably hermetically sealed at a temperature not exceeding 15°C; protect from light

Dosage Forms Spray: 100 mL, 120 mL

ethyl chloride and dichlorotetrafluoroethane

(ETH il KLOR ide & dye klor oh te tra floo or oh ETH ane)

Synonyms dichlorotetrafluoroethane and ethyl chloride

U.S. Brand Names Fluro-Ethyl® Aerosol

Generic Available No

Therapeutic Category Local Anesthetic

Use Topical refrigerant anesthetic to control pain associated with minor surgical procedures, dermabrasion, injections, contusions, and minor strains

Usual Dosage Topical: Press gently on side of spray valve allowing the liquid to emerge as a fine mist approximately 2" to 4" from site of application

Dosage Forms Aerosol: Ethyl chloride 25% and dichlorotetrafluoroethane 75% (225 g)

♦ **ethylphenylhydantoin** *see* ethotoin *on page 253*

♦ **ethynodiol diacetate and ethinyl estradiol** *see* ethinyl estradiol and ethynodiol diacetate *on page 249*

♦ **Ethyol®** *see* amifostine *on page 36*

♦ **Etibi®** *see* ethambutol *on page 247*

etidocaine (e TI doe kane)

U.S. Brand Names Duranest®

Generic Available No

Therapeutic Category Local Anesthetic

Use Infiltration anesthesia; peripheral nerve blocks; central neural blocks

Usual Dosage Varies with procedure; use 1% for peripheral nerve block, central nerve block, lumbar peridural caudal; use 1.5% for maxillary infiltration or inferior alveolar nerve block; use 1% or 1.5% for intra-abdominal or pelvic surgery, lower limb surgery, or caesarean section

Nursing/Pharmacy Information Before injecting, withdraw syringe plunger to ensure injection is not into vein or artery; have resuscitative equipment nearby

Dosage Forms

Injection, as hydrochloride: 1% [10 mg/mL] (30 mL)

With epinephrine 1:200,000: 1% [10 mg/mL] (30 mL); 1.5% [15 mg/mL] (20 mL)

etidronate disodium (e ti DROE nate dye SOW dee um)

Synonyms EHDP; sodium etidronate

U.S. Brand Names Didronel®

Generic Available No

Therapeutic Category Bisphosphonate Derivative

Use Symptomatic treatment of Paget's disease and heterotopic ossification due to spinal cord injury; hypercalcemia associated with malignancy

Usual Dosage Adults: Oral:

Paget's disease: 5 mg/kg/day administered every day for no more than 6 months; may administer 10 mg/kg/day for up to 3 months. Daily dose may be divided if adverse GI effects occur.

Heterotopic ossification with spinal cord injury: 20 mg/kg/day for 2 weeks, then 10 mg/kg/day for 10 weeks (this dosage has been used in children, however, treatment >1 year has been associated with a rachitic syndrome)

Hypercalcemia associated with malignancy: I.V.: 7.5 mg/kg/day for 3 days

Dietary Considerations Administer with water, black coffee, tea, or fruit juice on an empty stomach; avoid administering foods/supplements with calcium, iron, or magnesium within 2 hours of drug; maintain adequate intake of calcium and vitamin D

Nursing/Pharmacy Information

Dilute I.V. dose in at least 250 mL NS, infuse over at least 2 hours, ensure adequate hydration; dosage modification required in renal insufficiency

Monitor serum calcium and phosphorous; serum creatinine and BUN

Stability: Intravenous solution diluted in ≥250 mL normal saline is stable for 48 hours at room temperature or refrigerated

Dosage Forms

Injection: 50 mg/mL (6 mL)

Tablet: 200 mg, 400 mg

etodolac (ee toe DOE lak)

Synonyms etodolic acid

U.S. Brand Names Lodine®; Lodine® XL

Mexican Brand Names Lodine® Retard

Generic Available Yes

Therapeutic Category Analgesic, Non-narcotic; Nonsteroidal Anti-inflammatory Drug (NSAID)

Use Acute and long-term use in the management of signs and symptoms of osteoarthritis and management of pain

Usual Dosage Adults: Oral:

Acute pain: 200-400 mg every 6-8 hours, as needed, not to exceed total daily doses of 1200 mg

Osteoarthritis: Initial: 800-1200 mg/day administered in divided doses: 400 mg 2 or 3 times/day; 300 mg 2, 3 or 4 times/day; 200 mg 3 or 4 times/day; total daily dose should not exceed 1200 mg; for patients weighing <60 kg, total daily dose should not exceed 20 mg/kg; extended release dose: one tablet daily

Dietary Considerations May be administered with food to decrease GI distress

Nursing/Pharmacy Information

Monitor CBC, liver enzymes; in patients receiving diuretics, monitor urine output and BUN/serum creatinine

Stability: Protect from moisture

Dosage Forms

Capsule (Lodine®): 200 mg, 300 mg

Tablet: 400 mg

Lodine®: 400 mg

Tablet, extended release (Lodine® XL): 400 mg, 500 mg, 600 mg

♦ **etodolic acid** *see* etodolac *on page 255*

etomidate (e TOM i date)

U.S. Brand Names Amidate®

Generic Available No

Therapeutic Category General Anesthetic

Use Induction of general anesthesia

Usual Dosage Children >10 years and Adults: I.V.: 0.2-0.6 mg/kg over period of 30-60 seconds

Nursing/Pharmacy Information Store in refrigerator

Dosage Forms Injection: 2 mg/mL (10 mL, 20 mL)

♦ **Etopophos®** *see* etoposide phosphate *on page 256*

♦ **Etopos** *see* etoposide *on page 255*

etoposide (e toe POE side)

Synonyms EPEG; VP-16

U.S. Brand Names Toposar® Injection; VePesid®

Mexican Brand Names Etopos; Lastet; Medsaposide; Serozide®

Generic Available Yes

Therapeutic Category Antineoplastic Agent

Use Treatment of testicular and lung carcinomas, malignant lymphoma, Hodgkin's disease, leukemias (ALL, AML), neuroblastoma; also used in the treatment of Ewing's sarcoma, rhabdomyosarcoma, Wilms' tumor, brain tumors, and as a conditioning regimen for bone marrow transplantation in patients with advanced hematologic malignancies

Usual Dosage Refer to individual protocols

Pediatric solid tumors: I.V.: 60-120 mg/m²/day for 3-5 days every 3-6 weeks

Leukemia in children: I.V.: 100-200 mg/m²/day for 5 days

Testicular cancer: I.V.: 50-100 mg/m²/day on days 1-5 or 100 mg/m²/day on days 1, 3 and 5 every 3-4 weeks for 3-4 courses

(Continued)

etoposide *(Continued)*

Small cell lung cancer:
Oral: Twice the I.V. dose rounded to the nearest 50 mg administered once daily if total dose ≤400 mg or in divided doses if >400 mg
I.V.: 35 mg/m^2/day for 4 days or 50 mg/m^2/day for 5 days every 3-4 weeks

Dietary Considerations Administration of food does not affect GI absorption with doses ≤200 mg of injection

Nursing/Pharmacy Information

I.T., I.P., and IVP administration is contraindicated; adequate airway and other supportive measures and agents for treating hypotension or anaphylactoid reactions should be present when I.V. etoposide is administered; if necessary, the injection may be used for oral administration. Mix with orange juice, apple juice, or lemonade at a final concentration not to exceed 0.4 mg/mL; administer I.V. infusion over at least 30-60 minutes to minimize the risk of hypotensive reactions at a final concentration for administration of 0.2-0.4 mg/mL in normal saline or D$_5$W

Monitor CBC with differential, platelet count, and hemoglobin, vital signs (blood pressure), bilirubin, and renal function tests

Stability: Intact vials remains stable for 2 years at room temperature; store injection at room temperature and refrigerate capsules

VP-16 should be further diluted in D$_5$W, lactated Ringer's, or normal saline for administration; stability is dependent upon the concentration of the solution at a concentration of 1 mg/mL in normal saline or D$_5$W, crystallization has occurred within 30 minutes

At room temperature in D$_5$W or normal saline in polyvinyl chloride, the concentration is stable as follows:
0.2 mg/mL: 96 hours
0.4 mg/mL: 48 hours
0.6 mg/mL: 8 hours
1 mg/mL: 2 hours
2 mg/mL: 1 hour
20 mg/mL (undiluted): 24 hours

Y-site **compatibility**: Carboplatin, cytarabine, mesna, daunorubicin

Dosage Forms
Capsule: 50 mg
Injection: 20 mg/mL (5 mL, 10 mL, 25 mL)

etoposide phosphate *(e toe POE side FOS fate)*

U.S. Brand Names Etopophos®
Generic Available No
Therapeutic Category Antineoplastic Agent
Use Treatment of refractory testicular tumors and small cell lung cancer
Usual Dosage Refer to individual protocols. Adults:

Small cell lung cancer:
I.V. (in combination with other approved chemotherapeutic drugs): **Equivalent doses of etoposide phosphate to an etoposide dosage** range of 35 mg/m^2/day for 4 days to 50 mg/m^2/day for 5 days. Courses are repeated at 3- to 4-week intervals after adequate recovery from any toxicity.

Testicular cancer:
I.V. (in combination with other approved chemotherapeutic agents): **Equivalent dose of etoposide phosphate to etoposide dosage** range of 50-100 mg/m^2/day on days 1-5 to 100 mg/m^2/day on days 1, 3, and 5. Courses are repeated at 3- to 4-week intervals after adequate recovery from any toxicity.

Dosage Forms Powder for injection, lyophilized: 119.3 mg (100 mg base)

♦ **Etrafon®** *see* amitriptyline and perphenazine *on page 40*

etretinate *(e TRET i nate)*

U.S. Brand Names Tegison®
Generic Available No
Therapeutic Category Antipsoriatic Agent
Use Treatment of severe recalcitrant psoriasis in patients intolerant of or unresponsive to standard therapies
Usual Dosage Adults: Oral (individualized): Initial: 0.75-1 mg/kg/day in divided doses up to 1.5 mg/kg/day; maintenance dose established after 8-10 weeks of therapy 0.5-0.75 mg/kg/day
Dietary Considerations May be administered with food
Dosage Forms Capsule: 10 mg, 25 mg

♦ **ETS-2%® Topical** *see* erythromycin (ophthalmic/topical) *on page 239*

- **Eudal-SR®** *see* guaifenesin and pseudoephedrine *on page 302*
- **Euflex®** *see* flutamide *on page 279*
- **Euglucon®** *see* glyburide *on page 294*
- **Eulexin®** *see* flutamide *on page 279*
- **Eumetinex** *see* amoxicillin and clavulanate potassium *on page 43*
- **Eurax® Topical** *see* crotamiton *on page 172*
- **Euthroid® Tablet** *(Discontinued) see page 743*
- **Eutirox** *see* levothyroxine *on page 367*
- **Eutron®** *see* methyclothiazide and pargyline *on page 405*
- **Evac-Q-Mag® [OTC]** *see* magnesium citrate *on page 380*
- **Evalose®** *see* lactulose *on page 359*
- **Everone® Injection** *see* testosterone *on page 598*
- **Evista®** *see* raloxifene *on page 541*
- **E-Vitamin® [OTC]** *see* vitamin E *on page 652*
- **Exact® Cream [OTC]** *see* benzoyl peroxide *on page 81*
- **Excedrin®, Extra Strength [OTC]** *see* acetaminophen, aspirin, and caffeine *on page 16*
- **Excedrin® IB [OTC]** *see* ibuprofen *on page 332*
- **Excedrin® P.M. [OTC]** *see* acetaminophen and diphenhydramine *on page 15*
- **Exelderm® Topical** *see* sulconazole *on page 584*

exemestane *New Drug* (ex e MES tane)

U.S. Brand Names Aromasin®

Therapeutic Category Antineoplastic Agent, Miscellaneous

Controlled Substance [EX196]cancer

Use Treatment of advanced breast cancer in postmenopausal women whose disease has progressed following tamoxifen therapy

Nursing/Pharmacy Information Educate the patient about getting blood pressure checked while on medicine, especially if there is a history of poor control. Encourage the patient not to drive until she sees how the medicine affects her. It can cause fatigue and dizziness. Take at a similar time every day. Take after a meal to decrease nausea and increase absorption.

Dosage Forms Tablet: 25 mg

- **Exidine® Scrub [OTC]** *see* chlorhexidine gluconate *on page 134*
- **Exna®** *see* benzthiazide *on page 82*
- **Exosurf® Neonatal™** *see* colfosceril palmitate *on page 166*
- **Exsel® Shampoo** *see* selenium sulfide *on page 562*
- **Extendryl® SR** *see* chlorpheniramine, phenylephrine, and methscopolamine *on page 141*
- **Extra Action Cough Syrup [OTC]** *see* guaifenesin and dextromethorphan *on page 300*
- **Extra Strength Doan's® [OTC]** *see* magnesium salicylate *on page 382*
- **Eye-Lube-A® Solution [OTC]** *see* artificial tears *on page 59*
- **Eye-Sed® Ophthalmic [OTC]** *see* zinc sulfate *on page 660*
- **Eyesine® Ophthalmic [OTC]** *see* tetrahydrozoline *on page 602*
- **Ezide®** *see* hydrochlorothiazide *on page 317*
- **f_3t** *see* trifluridine *on page 628*
- **Facicam** *see* piroxicam *on page 497*

factor IX complex (human) (FAK ter nyne KOM pleks HYU man)

U.S. Brand Names AlphaNine® SD; BeneFix™; Hemonyne®; Konȳne® 80; Profilnine® SD; Proplex® T

Generic Available No

Therapeutic Category Antihemophilic Agent

Use

Control bleeding in patients with factor IX deficiency (hemophilia B or Christmas disease). **Note:** Factor IX concentrate containing ONLY factor IX is also available and preferable for this indication.

Prevention/control of bleeding in hemophilia A patients with inhibitors to factor VIII

Prevention/control of bleeding in patients with factor VII deficiency

Emergency correction of the coagulopathy of warfarin excess in critical situations

Usual Dosage Factor IX deficiency (1 unit/kg raises IX levels 1%)

(Continued)

factor IX complex (human) *(Continued)*

Children and Adults: I.V.:

Hospitalized patients: 20-50 units/kg/dose; may be higher in special cases; may be administered every 24 hours or more often in special cases

Inhibitor patients: 75-100 units/kg/dose; may be administered every 6-12 hours

Nursing/Pharmacy Information

Parenteral: I.V. administration only; rate of administration should not exceed 10 mL/minute; use filter needle to draw product into syringe

Monitor levels of factors II, IX, and X

Stability: Refrigerate **unopened** vials; do not freeze; administer within 3 hours after reconstitution; do **not** refrigerate after reconstitution

Dosage Forms Injection:

AlphaNine® SD: Single dose vial

BeneFix™: 250 units, 500 units, 1000 units

Konȳne® 80: 20 mL, 40 mL

Hemonyne®: 20 mL, 40 mL

Profilnine® SD: Single dose vial

Proplex® T: 30 mL vial

♦ **factor IX purified** *see* factor IX, purified (human) *on page 258*

factor IX, purified (human)

(FAK ter nyne, PURE eh fide HYU man)

Synonyms factor IX purified; monoclonal antibody purified

U.S. Brand Names Mononine®

Generic Available No

Therapeutic Category Antihemophilic Agent

Use

Control bleeding in patients with factor IX deficiency (hemophilia B or Christmas disease)

Mononine® contains **nondetectable levels of factors II, VII, and X** (<0.0025 units per factor IX unit using standard coagulation assays) and is, therefore, **NOT INDICATED** for replacement therapy of any of these clotting factors

Mononine® is also **NOT INDICATED** in the treatment or reversal of coumarin-induced anticoagulation or in a hemorrhagic state caused by hepatitis-induced lack of production of liver dependent coagulation factors.

Usual Dosage Children and Adults: Dosage is expressed in units of factor IX activity and must be individualized. I.V. only:

Formula for units required to raise blood level %:

Number of factor IX Units Required = body weight (in kg) x desired factor IX level increase (% normal) x 1 unit/kg

For example, for a 100% level a patient who has an actual level of 20%: Number of factor IX Units needed = 70 kg x 80% x 1 Unit/kg = 5,600 Units

Dosage Forms Factor IX units listed per vial and per lot to lot variation *$0.72/* unit of factor IX

Injection: 250 units, 500 units, 1000 units

factor VIIa, recombinant *New Drug*

(factor seven ay ree KOM be nant)

Synonyms coagulation factor VIIa; rFVIIa

U.S. Brand Names Novo-Seven®

Generic Available No

Therapeutic Category Antihemophilic Agent; Blood Product Derivative

Use Treatment of bleeding episodes in patients with hemophilia A or B when inhibitors to factor VIII or factor IX are present

Usual Dosage Children and Adults: I.V. administration only: 90 mcg/kg every 2 hours until hemostasis is achieved or until the treatment is judged ineffective. The dose and interval may be adjusted based upon the severity of bleeding and the degree of hemostasis achieved. The duration of therapy following hemostasis has not been fully established; for patients experiencing severe bleeds, dosing should be continued at 3- to 6-hour intervals after hemostasis has been achieved and the duration of dosing should be minimized.

In clinical trials, dosages have ranged from 35-120 mcg/kg and a decision on the final therapeutic dosages was reached within 8 hours in the majority of patients

Dosage Forms Powder for injection: 1.2 mg, 2.4 mg, 4.8 mg

♦ **factor VIII** *see* antihemophilic factor (human) *on page 51*

♦ **factor VIII recombinant** *see* antihemophilic factor (recombinant) *on page 52*

♦ **Factrel**® *see* gonadorelin *on page 296*

famciclovir (fam SYE kloe veer)

U.S. Brand Names Famvir™
Generic Available No
Therapeutic Category Antiviral Agent
Use Management of acute herpes zoster (shingles); treatment of recurrent herpes simplex in immunocompetent patients; treatment of recurrent mucocutaneous herpes simplex infections in HIV-infected patients
Usual Dosage Adults: Oral:
Acute herpes zoster: 500 mg every 8 hours for 7 days
Recurrent herpes simplex in immunocompetent patients: 125 mg twice daily for 5 days
Herpes simplex infections in HIV-infected patients: 500 mg twice daily
Dietary Considerations May be administered with food or on an empty stomach; rate of absorption and/or conversion to penciclovir and peak concentration are reduced with food, but bioavailability is not affected
Dosage Forms Tablet: 125 mg, 250 mg, 500 mg

famotidine (fa MOE ti deen)

U.S. Brand Names Pepcid®; Pepcid® AC Acid Controller [OTC]; Pepcid RPD®
Canadian Brand Names Apo®-Famotidine; Novo-Famotidine®; Nu-Famotidine®
Mexican Brand Names Durater; Famoxal; Farmotex®; Pepcidine®; Sigafam
Generic Available Yes
Therapeutic Category Histamine H_2 Antagonist
Use Therapy and treatment of duodenal ulcer, gastric ulcer, control gastric pH in critically ill patients, symptomatic relief in gastritis, gastroesophageal reflux, active benign ulcer, and pathological hypersecretory conditions
Usual Dosage
Children: Oral, I.V.: Doses of 1-2 mg/kg/day have been used; maximum dose: 40 mg
Adults:
Oral:
Duodenal ulcer, gastric ulcer: 40 mg/day at bedtime for 4-8 weeks
Hypersecretory conditions: Initial: 20 mg every 6 hours, may increase up to 160 mg every 6 hours
GERD: 20 mg twice daily for 6 weeks
I.V.: 20 mg every 12 hours
Nursing/Pharmacy Information
Administer over 15-30 minutes; may be administered undiluted I.V. push
Stability: Reconstituted I.V. solution is stable for 48 hours at room temperature; I.V. infusion in normal saline or D_5W solution is stable for 48 hours at room temperature; reconstituted oral solution is stable for 30 days at room temperature
Dosage Forms
Infusion, premixed in NS: 20 mg (50 mL)
Injection: 10 mg/mL (2 mL, 4 mL)
Powder for oral suspension (cherry-banana-mint flavor): 40 mg/5 mL (50 mL)
Tablet, chewable (Pepcid® AC): 10 mg
Tablet, film coated: 20 mg, 40 mg
Tablet, orally disintegrating (Pepcid RPD™): 20 mg, 40 mg
Pepcid® AC Acid Controller: 10 mg

♦ **Famoxal** *see* famotidine *on page 259*

♦ **Famvir**™ *see* famciclovir *on page 259*

♦ **Fansidar**® *(Discontinued) see page 743*

♦ **Faraxen** *see* naproxen *on page 432*

♦ **Fareston**® *see* toremifene *on page 619*

♦ **Farmotex**® *see* famotidine *on page 259*

♦ **Fastin**® *(Discontinued) see page 743*

fat emulsion (fat e MUL shun)

Synonyms intravenous fat emulsion
U.S. Brand Names Intralipid®; Liposyn®; Nutrilipid®; Soyacal®
Mexican Brand Names Emulsan 20%; Lyposyn; Lipocin
Generic Available Yes
Therapeutic Category Intravenous Nutritional Therapy
(Continued)

fat emulsion *(Continued)*

Use Source of calories and essential fatty acids for patients requiring parenteral nutrition of extended duration

Usual Dosage Fat emulsion should not exceed 60% of the total daily calories
Initial dose:

Infants, premature: 0.25-0.5 g/kg/day, increase by 0.25-0.5 g/kg/day to a maximum of 3-4 g/kg/day; maximum rate of infusion: 0.15 g/kg/hour (0.75 mL/kg/hour of 20% solution)

Infants and Children: 0.5-1 g/kg/day, increase by 0.5 g/kg/day to a maximum of 3-4 g/kg/day; maximum rate of infusion: 0.25 g/kg/hour (1.25 mL/kg/hour of 20% solution)

Adolescents and Adults: 1 g/kg/day, increase by 0.5-1 g/kg/day to a maximum of 2.5 g/kg/day; maximum rate of infusion: 0.25 g/kg/hour (1.25 mL/kg/hour of 20% solution); do not exceed 50 mL/hour (20%) or 100 mL/hour (10%)

Fatty acid deficiency: Children and Adults: 8% to 10% of total caloric intake; infuse once or twice weekly

Note: At the onset of therapy, the patient should be observed for any immediate allergic reactions such as dyspnea, cyanosis, and fever. Slower initial rates of infusion may be used for the first 10-15 minutes of the infusion (eg, 0.1 mL/minute of 10% or 0.05 mL/minute of 20% solution).

Nursing/Pharmacy Information
May be simultaneously infused with amino acid dextrose mixtures by means of Y-connector located near infusion site
Monitor serum triglycerides
Stability: May be stored at room temperature; do not store partially used bottles for later use; do not use if emulsion appears to be oiling out

Dosage Forms Injection: 10% [100 mg/mL] (100 mL, 250 mL, 500 mL); 20% [200 mg/mL] (100 mL, 250 mL, 500 mL)

- **5-FC** *see* flucytosine *on page 271*
- **FC1157a** *see* toremifene *on page 619*
- **Febrin®** *see* acetaminophen *on page 13*
- **Fedahist® Expectorant [OTC]** *see* guaifenesin and pseudoephedrine *on page 302*
- **Fedahist® Expectorant Pediatric [OTC]** *see* guaifenesin and pseudoephedrine *on page 302*
- **Fedahist® Tablet [OTC]** *see* chlorpheniramine and pseudoephedrine *on page 140*
- **Feiba VH Immuno®** *see* anti-inhibitor coagulant complex *on page 52*

felbamate *(FEL ba mate)*

U.S. Brand Names Felbatol®
Generic Available No
Therapeutic Category Anticonvulsant
Use Not a first-line agent; reserved for patients who do not adequately respond to alternative agents and whose epilepsy is so severe that benefit outweighs risk of liver failure or aplastic anemia; used as monotherapy and adjunctive therapy in patients ≥14 years of age with partial seizures with and without secondary generalization; adjunctive therapy in children ≥2 years of age who have partial and generalized seizures associated with Lennox-Gastaut syndrome
Usual Dosage Oral:

Monotherapy: 1200 mg/day in divided doses 3 or 4 times/day; titrate previously untreated patients under close clinical supervision, increasing the dosage in 600 mg increments every 2 weeks to 2400 mg/day based on clinical response and thereafter to 3600 mg/day in clinically indicated

Conversion to monotherapy: Initiate at 1200 mg/day in divided doses 3 or 4 times/day, reduce the dosage of the concomitant anticonvulsant(s) by 33% at the initiation of felbamate therapy; at week 2, increase the felbamate dosage to 2400 mg/day while reducing the dosage of the other anticonvulsant(s) up to an additional 33% of their original dosage; at week 3, increase the felbamate dosage up to 3600 mg/day and continue to reduce the dosage of the other anticonvulsant(s) as clinically indicated

Adjunctive therapy:
Week 1:
Felbamate: 1200 mg/day initial dose
Concomitant anticonvulsant(s): Reduce original dosage by 20% to 33%
Week 2:
Felbamate: 2400 mg/day (Therapeutic range)

Concomitant anticonvulsant(s): Reduce original dosage by up to an additional 33%

Week 3:

Felbamate: 3600 mg/day (Therapeutic range)

Concomitant anticonvulsant(s): Reduce original dosage as clinically indicated

Dietary Considerations Food does **not** affect absorption

Nursing/Pharmacy Information

Use with caution in patients allergic to other carbamates (eg, meprobamate); antiepileptic drugs should not be suddenly discontinued because of the possibility of increasing seizure frequency; **reported 10 cases of aplastic anemia in the U.S. after 2½ to 6 months of therapy**; Carter Wallace and the FDA recommended the use of this agent be suspended unless withdrawal of the product would place a patient at greater risk as compared to the frequently fatal form of anemia

Monitor serum levels of concomitant anticonvulsant therapy

Stability: Store medication in tightly closed container at room temperature away from excessive heat

Dosage Forms

Suspension, oral: 600 mg/5 mL (240 mL, 960 mL)

Tablet: 400 mg, 600 mg

♦ **Felbatol**® *see* felbamate *on page 260*
♦ **Feldene**® *see* piroxicam *on page 497*

felodipine (fe LOE di peen)

U.S. Brand Names Plendil®

Mexican Brand Names Logimax; Munobal

Generic Available No

Therapeutic Category Calcium Channel Blocker

Use Management of angina pectoris due to coronary insufficiency, hypertension

Usual Dosage Oral:

Adults: Initial: 5 mg once daily; dosage range: 2.5-10 mg once daily; may increase dose up to a maximum of 10 mg

Elderly: Initial: 2.5 mg/day

Dietary Considerations Grapefruit juice will increase absorption

Nursing/Pharmacy Information Do not crush extended release tablets

Dosage Forms Tablet, extended release: 2.5 mg, 5 mg, 10 mg

♦ **Femara**™ *see* letrozole *on page 362*
♦ **FemCare**® *(Discontinued) see page 743*
♦ **Femcet**® *see* butalbital compound and acetaminophen *on page 99*
♦ **Femguard**® *see* sulfabenzamide, sulfacetamide, and sulfathiazole *on page 584*
♦ **Femiron**® **[OTC]** *see* ferrous fumarate *on page 264*
♦ **Femizol-M**® **[OTC]** *see* miconazole *on page 413*
♦ **Femogen**® *see* estrone *on page 246*
♦ **Femstat**® *(Discontinued) see page 743*
♦ **Fenesin**™ *see* guaifenesin *on page 299*
♦ **Fenesin**™ **DM** *see* guaifenesin and dextromethorphan *on page 300*

fenofibrate (fen oh FYE brate)

Synonyms procetofene; proctofene

U.S. Brand Names TriCor™

Generic Available No

Therapeutic Category Antihyperlipidemic Agent, Miscellaneous

Use Adjunct to dietary therapy for the treatment of adults with very high elevations of serum triglyceride levels (types IV and V hyperlipidemia) who are at risk of pancreatitis and who do not respond adequately to a determined dietary effort; its efficacy can be enhanced by combination with other hypolipidemic agents that have a different mechanism of action; safety and efficacy may be greater than that of clofibrate

Usual Dosage Adults: Oral: Initial: 67 mg/day, up to 3 capsules (201 mg)

Dosage Forms Capsule: 67 mg

fenoldopam (fe NOL doe pam)

U.S. Brand Names Corlopam®

Generic Available No

Therapeutic Category Antihypertensive Agent

(Continued)

fenoldopam *(Continued)*

Use Patients presenting with emergency hypertension and those requiring blood pressure control during hospitalization pose a challenge due to the associated risk of renal failure and end-organ compromise

Usual Dosage

Oral: 100 mg 2-4 times/day

I.V.: Severe hypertension: Initial: 0.1 mcg/kg/minute; may be increased in increments of 0.05-0.2 mcg/kg/minute; maximal infusion rate: 1.6 mcg/kg/minute

Dosage Forms Injection, as mesylate: 10 mg/mL

fenoprofen (fen oh PROE fen)

U.S. Brand Names Nalfon®

Generic Available Yes

Therapeutic Category Analgesic, Non-narcotic; Nonsteroidal Anti-inflammatory Drug (NSAID)

Use Symptomatic treatment of acute and chronic rheumatoid arthritis and osteoarthritis; relief of mild to moderate pain

Usual Dosage Oral:

Children: Juvenile arthritis: 900 mg/m^2/day, then increase over 4 weeks to 1.8 g/m^2/day

Adults:

Arthritis: 300-600 mg 3-4 times/day up to 3.2 g/day

Pain: 200 mg every 4-6 hours as needed

Dietary Considerations May be administered with food to decrease GI distress

Nursing/Pharmacy Information Monitor CBC, liver enzymes; monitor urine output and BUN/serum creatinine in patients receiving diuretics

Dosage Forms Fenoprofen calcium:

Capsule: 200 mg, 300 mg

Tablet: 600 mg

fenoterol *(Canada only)* (fen oh TER ole)

Canadian Brand Names Berotec® Forte Inhalation Aerosol; Berotec® Inhalation Aerosol; Berotec® Solution

Generic Available No

Therapeutic Category Beta$_2$-Adrenergic Agonist Agent

Use For the symptomatic relief and acute prophylaxis of bronchial obstruction in asthma and other conditions in which reversible bronchospasm is a complicating factor, such as chronic bronchitis or emphysema.

Usual Dosage Adults:

MDI: Acute symptoms: One puff will usually be adequate to relieve bronchospasm in the majority of patients, however, if required, a second puff may be taken preferably after waiting 5 minutes for the effect of the first puff to be obtained. This delay allows better assessment of the effectiveness of 1 puff and deeper penetration of the second puff. If an attack has not been relieved by 2 puffs, further puffs may be required. In these cases, patients should immediately consult the physician or the nearest hospital. If, despite other adequate maintenance therapy, regular use of beta-agonists remains necessary for the control of bronchospasm, the recommended dose is 1-2 puffs of the 100 mcg inhaler 3-4 times/day. A maximum of 8 puffs/day should not be exceeded.

Solution: Dosage should be individualized, and patient response should be monitored by the prescribing physician on an ongoing basis. Should be used only under medical supervision.

Motorized, compressed air or ultrasonic nebulizers: These nebulizers generate low pressure, low velocity aerosols. The average single dose is 0.5 to 1 mg of fenoterol. In more refractory cases, up to 2.5 mg of fenoterol may be given. Fenoterol solution should be diluted to 5 mL with preservative-free sterile sodium chloride inhalation solution, USP 0.9% (normal saline) and the total volume should be nebulized over a period of 10 to 15 minutes. Optimal deposition in the lungs is achieved with the patient breathing quietly and slowly. Treatment may be repeated every 6 hours if necessary.

Intermittent positive pressure ventilation: Fenoterol solution may be used in conjunction with Intermittent Positive Pressure Ventilation (IPPV) when such therapy is indicated. The average single dose is 0.5 to 1 mg of fenoterol. In more refractory cases, up to 2.5 mg of fenoterol may be given. Fenoterol solution should be diluted to 5 mL with preservative-free sterile sodium chloride inhalation solution, USP 0.9% and the total volume should be nebulized over a period of 10-15 minutes. The inspiratory pressure is usually 10 to 20 cm H2O and optimal deposition of the drug in the lungs is achieved with the patient breathing quietly and slowly. Treatment may be repeated every 6 hours if necessary. If a previous effective dosage regimen fails to provide the usual relief, or the effects of a dose last for less than 3 hours, medical advice should be sought immediately; this is a sign of seriously worsening asthma that requires reassessment of therapy. In accordance with the present practice for asthma treatment, concomitant anti-inflammatory therapy should be part of the regimen if fenoterol inhalation solution needs to be used on a regular daily basis.

Dosage Forms
Metered dose inhalers: 100 mcg/actuation (200 doses; 200 mcg/actuation) (100 doses)

Solution, inhalation: 1 mg/mL (20 mL)

♦ **Fentanest** *see* fentanyl *on page 263*

fentanyl (FEN ta nil)
U.S. Brand Names Actiq® Oral Transmucosal; Duragesic® Transdermal; Fentanyl Oralet®; Sublimaze® Injection

Mexican Brand Names Durogesic; Fentanest

Generic Available Injection: Yes

Therapeutic Category Analgesic, Narcotic; General Anesthetic

Controlled Substance C-II

Use Sedation; relief of pain; preoperative medication; adjunct to general or regional anesthesia; management of chronic pain (transdermal product)

Oral transmucosal: Hospital setting use only as preoperative anesthetic agent or to induce conscious sedation before procedures

Usual Dosage Doses should be titrated to appropriate effects; wide range of doses, dependent upon desired degree of analgesia/anesthesia

Children:

Sedation for minor procedures/analgesia: I.M., I.V.:

1-3 years: 2-3 mcg/kg/dose; may repeat after 30-60 minutes as required

3-12 years: 1-2 mcg/kg/dose; may repeat at 30- to 60-minute intervals as required. **Note:** Children 18-36 months of age may require 2-3 mcg/kg/dose

Continuous sedation/analgesia: Initial I.V. bolus: 1-2 mcg/kg then 1 mcg/kg/hour; titrate upward; usual: 1-3 mcg/kg/hour

Transdermal: Not recommended

Children <12 years and Adults:

Sedation for minor procedures/analgesia: 0.5-1 mcg/kg/dose; higher doses are used for major procedures

Preoperative sedation, adjunct to regional anesthesia, postoperative pain: I.M., I.V.: 50-100 mcg/dose

Adjunct to general anesthesia: I.M., I.V.: 2-50 mcg/kg

General anesthesia without additional anesthetic agents: I.V. 50-100 mcg/kg with O_2 and skeletal muscle relaxant

Transdermal: Initial: 25 mcg/hour system; if currently receiving opiates, convert to fentanyl equivalent and administer equianalgesic dosage (see package insert for further information)

Dietary Considerations
Alcohol: Additive CNS effects; avoid or limit alcohol; watch for sedation

Food: Glucose may cause hyperglycemia; monitor blood glucose concentrations

Nursing/Pharmacy Information
Patients with elevated temperature may have increased fentanyl absorption transdermally, observe for adverse effects, dosage adjustment may be needed; pharmacologic and adverse effects can be seen after discontinuation of transdermal system, observe patients for at least 12 hours after transdermal product removed; administer by slow I.V. push over 3-5 minutes or by continuous infusion

Monitor respiratory and cardiovascular status

Stability: Protect from light; **incompatible** when mixed in the same syringe with pentobarbital

Transmucosal: Store at controlled room temperature of 15°C to 30°C (59°F to 86°F)

Dosage Forms
Injection, as citrate: 0.05 mg/mL (2 mL, 5 mL, 10 mL, 20 mL, 50 mL)

Lozenge, oral transmucosal:

Fentanyl Oralet® (raspberry flavored): 200 mcg, 300 mcg, 400 mcg

(Continued)

fentanyl *(Continued)*

Actiq® Oral Transmucosal: 200 mcg, 400 mcg, 600 mcg, 800 mcg, 1200 mcg, 1600 mcg

Transdermal system: 25 mcg/hour [10 cm²]; 50 mcg/hour [20 cm²]; 75 mcg/hour [30 cm²]; 100 mcg/hour [40 cm²] (all available in 5s)

♦ **fentanyl and droperidol** *see droperidol and fentanyl on page 224*
♦ **Fentanyl Oralet®** *see fentanyl on page 263*
♦ **Feosol® [OTC]** *see ferrous sulfate on page 265*
♦ **Feostat® [OTC]** *see ferrous fumarate on page 264*
♦ **Ferancee® [OTC]** *see ferrous salt and ascorbic acid on page 265*
♦ **Feratab® [OTC]** *see ferrous sulfate on page 265*
♦ **Fergon® [OTC]** *see ferrous gluconate on page 265*
♦ **Fergon Plus®** *(Discontinued) see page 743*
♦ **Feridex I.V.®** *see ferumoxides on page 267*
♦ **Fer-in-Sol® Capsule** *(Discontinued) see page 743*
♦ **Fer-In-Sol® Drops [OTC]** *see ferrous sulfate on page 265*
♦ **Fer-Iron® [OTC]** *see ferrous sulfate on page 265*
♦ **Fermalac®** *see Lactobacillus on page 358*
♦ **Fermalox®** *(Discontinued) see page 743*
♦ **Ferndex®** *(Discontinued) see page 743*
♦ **Fero-Grad 500® [OTC]** *see ferrous salt and ascorbic acid on page 265*
♦ **Fero-Gradumet® [OTC]** *see ferrous sulfate on page 265*
♦ **Ferospace® [OTC]** *see ferrous sulfate on page 265*
♦ **Ferralet® [OTC]** *see ferrous gluconate on page 265*
♦ **Ferralyn® Lanacaps® [OTC]** *see ferrous sulfate on page 265*
♦ **Ferra-TD® [OTC]** *see ferrous sulfate on page 265*

ferric gluconate *New Drug* (FER ik GLOO koe nate)

U.S. Brand Names Ferrlecit®
Generic Available No
Therapeutic Category Iron Salt
Use Repletion of total body iron content in patients with iron deficiency anemia who are undergoing hemodialysis in conjunction with erythropoietin therapy
Usual Dosage Adults:

Test dose (recommended): 2 mL diluted in 50 mL 0.9% sodium chloride over 60 minutes

Repletion of iron in hemodialysis patients: I.V.: 125 mg (10 mL) in 100 mL 0.9% sodium chloride over 1 hour during hemodialysis. Most patients will require a cumulative dose of 1 g elemental iron over approximately 8 sequential dialysis treatments to achieve a favorable response.

Dosage Forms Injection: 12.5 mg/mL (5 mL)

♦ **Ferrlecit®** *see ferric gluconate New Drug on page 264*
♦ **Ferro-Sequels® [OTC]** *see ferrous fumarate on page 264*

ferrous fumarate (FER us FYOO ma rate)

U.S. Brand Names Femiron® [OTC]; Feostat® [OTC]; Ferro-Sequels® [OTC]; Fumasorb® [OTC]; Fumerin® [OTC]; Hemocyte® [OTC]; Ircon® [OTC]; Nephro-Fer™ [OTC]; Span-FF® [OTC]
Canadian Brand Names Palafer®
Generic Available Yes
Therapeutic Category Electrolyte Supplement, Oral
Use Prevention and treatment of iron deficiency anemias
Usual Dosage Oral:

Children: 3 mg/kg 3 times/day
Adults: 200 mg 3-4 times/day

Dietary Considerations Should be administered with water or juice on an empty stomach; may be administered with food to prevent irritation; however, not with cereals, dietary fiber, tea, coffee, eggs, or milk
Nursing/Pharmacy Information Administer 2 hours prior to or 4 hours after antacids
Dosage Forms Amount of elemental iron is listed in brackets

Capsule, controlled release (Span-FF®): 325 mg [106 mg]
Drops (Feostat®): 45 mg/0.6 mL [15 mg/0.6 mL] (60 mL)
Suspension, oral (Feostat®): 100 mg/5 mL [33 mg/5 mL] (240 mL)
Tablet: 325 mg [106 mg]
Chewable (chocolate flavor) (Feostat®): 100 mg [33 mg]
Femiron®: 63 mg [20 mg]

Fumerin®: 195 mg [64 mg]
Fumasorb®, Ircon®: 200 mg [66 mg]
Hemocyte®: 324 mg [106 mg]
Nephro-Fer™: 350 mg [115 mg]
Timed release (Ferro-Sequels®): Ferrous fumarate 150 mg [50 mg] and docusate sodium 100 mg

ferrous gluconate (FER us GLOO koe nate)

U.S. Brand Names Fergon® [OTC]; Ferralet® [OTC]; Simron® [OTC]
Canadian Brand Names Apo-Ferrous® Gluconate
Generic Available Yes
Therapeutic Category Electrolyte Supplement, Oral
Use Prevention and treatment of iron deficiency anemias
Usual Dosage Oral (dose expressed in terms of elemental iron):
Iron deficiency anemia: 3-6 Fe mg/kg/day in 3 divided doses
Maintenance:
Preterm infants:
Birthweight <1000 g: 4 Fe mg/kg/day
Birthweight 1000-1500 g: 3 Fe mg/kg/day
Birthweight 1500-2500 g: 2 Fe mg/kg/day
Term Infants and Children: 1-2 Fe mg/kg/day in 3 divided doses, up to a maximum of 18 Fe mg/day
Adults: 60-100 Fe mg/day in 3 divided doses
Dietary Considerations Should be administered with water or juice on an empty stomach; may be administered with food to prevent irritation; however not with cereals, dietary fiber, tea, coffee, eggs, or milk
Nursing/Pharmacy Information
Administer 2 hours before or 4 hours after antacids
Monitor serum iron, total iron binding capacity, reticulocyte count, hemoglobin
Dosage Forms Amount of elemental iron is listed in brackets
Capsule, soft gelatin (Simron®): 86 mg [10 mg]
Elixir (Fergon®): 300 mg/5 mL [34 mg/5 mL] with alcohol 7% (480 mL)
Tablet: 300 mg [34 mg]; 325 mg [38 mg]
Fergon®, Ferralet®: 320 mg [37 mg]
Sustained release (Ferralet® Slow Release): 320 mg [37 mg]

ferrous salt and ascorbic acid
(FER us SUL fate & a SKOR bik AS id)

Synonyms ascorbic acid and ferrous sulfate
U.S. Brand Names Ferancee® [OTC]; Fero-Grad 500® [OTC]
Generic Available Yes
Therapeutic Category Vitamin
Use Treatment of iron deficiency in nonpregnant adults; treatment and prevention of iron deficiency in pregnant adults
Usual Dosage Adults: Oral: 1 tablet daily
Dietary Considerations Should be administered with water or juice on an empty stomach; may be administered with food to prevent irritation; however, not with cereals, dietary fiber, tea, coffee, eggs or milk
Dosage Forms Amount of elemental iron is listed in brackets
Caplet, sustained release (Ferromar®): Ferrous fumarate 201.5 mg [65 mg] and ascorbic acid 200 mg
Tablet (Fero-Grad 500®): Ferrous sulfate 525 mg [105 mg] and ascorbic acid 500 mg
Chewable (Ferancee®): Ferrous fumarate 205 mg [67 mg] and ascorbic acid 150 mg

ferrous sulfate (FER us SUL fate)

Synonyms $FeSO_4$
U.S. Brand Names Feosol® [OTC]; Feratab® [OTC]; Fer-In-Sol® Drops [OTC]; Fer-Iron® [OTC]; Fero-Gradumet® [OTC]; Ferospace® [OTC]; Ferralyn® Lanacaps® [OTC]; Ferra-TD® [OTC]; Mol-Iron® [OTC]; Slow FE® [OTC]
Canadian Brand Names Apo-Ferrous® Sulfate; PMS-Ferrous Sulfate
Generic Available Yes
Therapeutic Category Electrolyte Supplement, Oral
Use Prevention and treatment of iron deficiency anemias
Usual Dosage Oral (dose expressed in terms of elemental iron):
Children:
Severe iron deficiency anemia: 4-6 mg Fe/kg/day in 3 divided doses
Mild to moderate iron deficiency anemia: 3 mg Fe/kg/day in 1-2 divided doses
(Continued)

ferrous sulfate *(Continued)*

Prophylaxis: 1-2 mg Fe/kg/day up to a maximum of 15 mg/day

Adults: Iron deficiency: 60-100 Fe/kg/day in divided doses

Dietary Considerations Should be administered with water or juice on an empty stomach; may be administered with food to prevent irritation; however not with cereals, dietary fiber, tea, coffee, eggs or milk

Nursing/Pharmacy Information

Administer 2 hours before or 4 hours after antacids

Monitor serum iron, total iron binding capacity, reticulocyte count, hemoglobin

Dosage Forms Amount of elemental iron is listed in brackets

Capsule:

Exsiccated, timed release (Feosol®): 159 mg [50 mg]

Exsiccated, timed release (Ferralyn® Lanacaps®, Ferra-TD®): 250 mg [50 mg]

Ferospace®: 250 mg [50 mg]

Drops, oral:

Fer-In-Sol®: 75 mg/0.6 mL [15 mg/0.6 mL] (50 mL)

Fer-Iron®: 125 mg/mL [25 mg/mL] (50 mL)

Elixir (Feosol®): 220 mg/5 mL [44 mg/5 mL] with alcohol 5% (473 mL, 4000 mL)

Syrup (Fer-In-Sol®): 90 mg/5 mL [18 mg/5 mL] with alcohol 5% (480 mL)

Tablet: 324 mg [65 mg]

Exsiccated (Feosol®) 200 mg [65 mg]

Exsiccated, timed release (Slow FE®): 160 mg [50 mg]

Feratab®: 300 mg [60 mg]

Mol-Iron®: 195 mg [39 mg]

Timed release (Fero-Gradumet®): 525 mg [105 mg]

ferrous sulfate, ascorbic acid, and vitamin B-complex

(FER us SUL fate, a SKOR bik AS id, & VYE ta min bee KOM pleks)

U.S. Brand Names Iberet®-Liquid [OTC]

Generic Available Yes

Therapeutic Category Vitamin

Use Treatment of conditions of iron deficiency with an increased need for B complex vitamins and vitamin C

Usual Dosage Oral:

Children 1-3 years: 5 mL twice daily after meals

Children >4 years and Adults: 10 mL 3 times/day after meals

Dietary Considerations Should be administered with water or juice on an empty stomach; may be administered with food to prevent irritation; however, not with cereals, dietary fiber, tea, coffee, eggs or milk

Nursing/Pharmacy Information Avoid concomitant administration (within 2 hours) of antacids or tetracycline, administered with plenty of water to avoid GI upset and constipation, vitamin C 200 mg/30 mg elemental iron may enhance GI absorption of iron

Dosage Forms Liquid:

Ferrous sulfate: 78.75 mg

Ascorbic acid: 375 mg

B_1: 4.5 mg

B_2: 4.5 mg

B_3: 22.5 mg

B_5: 7.5 mg

B_6: 3.75 mg

B_{12}: 18.75 mg all per 15 mL

ferrous sulfate, ascorbic acid, vitamin B-complex, and folic acid

(FER us SUL fate, a SKOR bik AS id, VYE ta min bee KOM pleks, & FOE lik AS id)

U.S. Brand Names Iberet-Folic-500®

Generic Available Yes

Therapeutic Category Vitamin

Use Treatment of iron deficiency and prevention of concomitant folic acid deficiency where there is an associated deficient intake or increased need for B complex vitamins

Usual Dosage Adults: Oral: 1 tablet daily

Dietary Considerations Should be administered with water or juice on an empty stomach; may be administered with food to prevent irritation; however, not with cereals, dietary fiber, tea, coffee, eggs, or milk

Dosage Forms Tablet, controlled release:
Ferrous sulfate: 105 mg
Ascorbic acid: 500 mg
B_1: 6 mg
B_2: 6 mg
B_3: 30 mg
B_5: 10 mg
B_6: 5 mg
B_{12}: 25 mcg
Folic acid: 800 mcg

♦ **Fertinex®** *see* urofollitropin *on page 639*
♦ **Fertinorm® H.P.** *see* urofollitropin *on page 639*

ferumoxides (fer yoo MOX ides)
U.S. Brand Names Feridex I.V.®
Generic Available No
Therapeutic Category Radiopaque Agents
Use For I.V. administration as an adjunct to MRI (in adult patients) to enhance the T2 weighted images used in the detection and evaluation of lesions of the liver
Usual Dosage Adults: 0.56 mg of iron (0.05 mL Feridex I.V.®)/kg body weight diluted in 100 mL of 5% dextrose and infused over 30 minutes; a 5-micron filter is recommended; do not administer undiluted
Dosage Forms Injection: Iron 11.2 mg and mannitol per mL (5 mL)

♦ **FeSO₄** *see* ferrous sulfate *on page 265*
♦ **Feverall™ [OTC]** *see* acetaminophen *on page 13*

fexofenadine (feks oh FEN a deen)
U.S. Brand Names Allegra®
Generic Available No
Therapeutic Category Antihistamine
Use Nonsedating antihistamine indicated for the relief of seasonal allergic rhinitis
Usual Dosage Children ≥12 years and Adults: Oral: 1 capsule (60 mg) twice daily
Dosage Forms Capsule, as hydrochloride: 60 mg

fexofenadine and pseudoephedrine
(feks oh FEN a deen & soo doe e FED rin)
U.S. Brand Names Allegra-D™
Generic Available No
Therapeutic Category Antihistamine/Decongestant Combination
Use Relief of symptoms associated with seasonal allergic rhinitis in adults and children ≥12 years. Symptoms treated effectively include sneezing, rhinorrhea, itchy nose/palate/ and/or throat, itchy/watery/red eyes, and nasal congestion.
Usual Dosage Oral: Adults: 1 tablet twice daily for adults and children ≥12 years of age. It is recommended that the administration with food should be avoided. A dose of 1 tablet once daily is recommended as the starting dose in patients with decreased renal function.
Dosage Forms Tablet, extended release: Fexofenadine hydrochloride 60 mg and pseudoephedrine hydrochloride 120 mg

♦ **Fiberall® Chewable Tablet [OTC]** *see* calcium polycarbophil *on page 107*
♦ **Fiberall® Powder [OTC]** *see* psyllium *on page 531*
♦ **Fiberall® Wafer [OTC]** *see* psyllium *on page 531*
♦ **FiberCon® Tablet [OTC]** *see* calcium polycarbophil *on page 107*
♦ **Fiber-Lax® Tablet [OTC]** *see* calcium polycarbophil *on page 107*
♦ **Fibrepur®** *see* psyllium *on page 531*

filgrastim (fil GRA stim)
Synonyms G-CSF; granulocyte colony-stimulating factor
U.S. Brand Names Neupogen®
Generic Available No
Therapeutic Category Colony-Stimulating Factor
Use To reduce the duration of neutropenia and the associated risk of infection in patients with nonmyeloid malignancies receiving myelosuppressive chemotherapeutic regimens associated with a significant incidence of severe neutropenia with fever; it has also been used in AIDS patients on zidovudine and in patients with noncancer chemotherapy-induced neutropenia
(Continued)

filgrastim *(Continued)*

Usual Dosage Children and Adults (refer to individual protocols): I.V., S.C.: 5-10 mcg/kg/day (~150-300 mcg/m^2/day) once daily for up to 14 days until ANC = 10,000/mm^3; dose escalations at 5 mcg/kg/day may be required in some individuals when response at 5 mcg/kg/day is not adequate; dosages of 0.6-120 mcg/kg/day have been used in children ranging in age from 3 months to 18 years

Nursing/Pharmacy Information

Bone pain management is usually successful with non-narcotic analgesic therapy; administer as a bolus S.C. injection, a short I.V. infusion (15-30 minutes) or a continuous infusion. If the final concentration of G-CSF in D$_5$W is <15 mcg/mL, then add 2 mg albumin/mL of I.V. fluid; the solution is stable for 24 hours; albumin acts as a carrier molecule to prevent drug adsorption to the I.V. tubing. Albumin should be added to the D$_5$W prior to addition of G-CSF; do not shake solution to avoid foaming

Monitor complete blood cell count and platelet count should be obtained twice weekly. Leukocytosis (white blood cell counts of ≥100,000/mm^3) has been observed in ~2% of patients receiving G-CSF at doses above 5 mcg/kg/day. Monitor platelets and hematocrit regularly. Monitor patients with pre-existing cardiac conditions closely as cardiac events (myocardial infarctions, arrhythmias) have been reported in premarketing clinical studies.

Stability: Store at 2°C to 8°C (36°F to 46°F); do not expose to freezing or dry ice. Prior to administration, filgrastim may be allowed to be at room temperature for a maximum of 24 hours. It may be diluted in dextrose 5% in water to a concentration of ≥15 mcg/mL for I.V. infusion administration; minimum concentration: 15 mcg/mL; concentrations <15 mcg/mL require addition of albumin (1 mL of 5%) to the bag to prevent absorption. This diluted solution is stable for 7 days under refrigeration or at room temperature. **Filgrastim is incompatible with 0.9% sodium chloride (normal saline)**.

Standard diluent: ≥375 mcg/25 mL D$_5$W

Dosage Forms Injection, preservative free: 300 mcg/mL (1 mL, 1.6 mL)

finasteride *(fi NAS teer ide)*

U.S. Brand Names Proscar®

Generic Available No

Therapeutic Category Antiandrogen

Use Early data indicate that finasteride is useful in the treatment of benign prostatic hyperplasia

Usual Dosage Benign prostatic hyperplasia: Adults: Oral: 5 mg/day as a single dose; clinical responses occur within 12 weeks to 6 months of initiation of therapy; long-term administration is recommended for maximal response

Nursing/Pharmacy Information Monitor objective and subjective signs of relief of benign prostatic hyperplasia, including improvement in urinary flow, reduction in symptoms of urgency, and relief of difficulty in micturition

Dosage Forms

Tablet, film coated:
Propecia®: 1 mg
Proscar®: 5 mg

- ♦ **Fiorgen PF®** *see* butalbital compound and aspirin *on page 99*
- ♦ **Fioricet®** *see* butalbital compound and acetaminophen *on page 99*
- ♦ **Fiorinal®** *see* butalbital compound and aspirin *on page 99*
- ♦ **Fiorinal® With Codeine** *see* butalbital compound and codeine *on page 99*
- ♦ **fisalamine** *see* mesalamine *on page 395*
- ♦ **Fisopred®** *see* prednisolone (ophthalmic) *on page 514*
- ♦ **FK506** *see* tacrolimus *on page 592*
- ♦ **Flagenase®** *see* metronidazole *on page 411*
- ♦ **Flagyl® Oral** *see* metronidazole *on page 411*
- ♦ **Flamazine®** *see* silver sulfadiazine *on page 566*
- ♦ **Flamicina** *see* ampicillin *on page 46*
- ♦ **Flanax** *see* naproxen *on page 432*
- ♦ **Flarex®** *see* fluorometholone *on page 275*
- ♦ **Flatulex® [OTC]** *see* simethicone *on page 566*
- ♦ **Flavorcee® [OTC]** *see* ascorbic acid *on page 60*

flavoxate *(fla VOKS ate)*

U.S. Brand Names Urispas®

Generic Available No

Therapeutic Category Antispasmodic Agent, Urinary

Use Antispasmodic to provide symptomatic relief of dysuria, nocturia, supra-pubic pain, urgency, and incontinence

Usual Dosage Children >12 years and Adults: Oral: 100-200 mg 3-4 times/day

Dietary Considerations Should be administered with water on an empty stomach

Nursing/Pharmacy Information Monitor I & O closely, incontinence, and PVR

Dosage Forms Tablet, film coated, as hydrochloride: 100 mg

♦ **Flaxedil®** *see* gallamine triethiodide *on page 286*

♦ **Flebocortid [Sodium Succinate]** *see* hydrocortisone (systemic) *on page 323*

flecainide (fle KAY nide)

U.S. Brand Names Tambocor™

Generic Available No

Therapeutic Category Antiarrhythmic Agent, Class I-C

Use Prevention and suppression of documented life-threatening ventricular arrhythmias (ie, sustained ventricular tachycardia); prevention of symptomatic, disabling supraventricular tachycardias in patients without structural heart disease

Usual Dosage Oral:

Children: Initial: 3 mg/kg/day in 3 divided doses; usual 3-6 mg/kg/day in 3 divided doses; up to 11 mg/kg/day for uncontrolled patients with subtherapeutic levels

Adults: Initial: 100 mg every 12 hours, increase by 100 mg/day (administer in 2 doses/day) every 4 days to maximum of 400 mg/day; for patients receiving 400 mg/day who are not controlled and have trough concentrations <0.6 mcg/mL, dosage may be increased to 600 mg/day

Dietary Considerations Dairy products (milk, infant formula, yogurt) may interfere with the absorption of flecainide in infants; there is one case report of a neonate (GA 34 weeks PNA >6 days) who required extremely large doses of oral flecainide when administered every 8 hours with feedings ("milk feeds"); changing the feedings from "milk feeds" to 5% glucose feeds alone resulted in a doubling of the flecainide serum concentration and toxicity; clearance of flecainide may be decreased in patients with strict vegetarian diets due to urinary pH ≥8

Nursing/Pharmacy Information

Administer around-the-clock rather than 4 times/day, 3 times/day, etc, (ie, 12-6-12-6, not 9-1-5-9) to promote less variation in peak and trough serum levels

Monitor EKG and serum concentrations

Dosage Forms Tablet, as acetate: 50 mg, 100 mg, 150 mg

♦ **Fleet® Babylax® Rectal [OTC]** *see* glycerin *on page 295*

♦ **Fleet® Enema [OTC]** *see* sodium phosphates *on page 573*

♦ **Fleet® Flavored Castor Oil [OTC]** *see* castor oil *on page 118*

♦ **Fleet® Laxative [OTC]** *see* bisacodyl *on page 88*

♦ **Fleet® Pain Relief [OTC]** *see* pramoxine *on page 512*

♦ **Fleet® Phospho®-Soda [OTC]** *see* sodium phosphates *on page 573*

♦ **Flemoxon** *see* amoxicillin *on page 43*

♦ **Flexaphen®** *see* chlorzoxazone *on page 146*

♦ **Flexen** *see* naproxen *on page 432*

♦ **Flexeril®** *see* cyclobenzaprine *on page 174*

♦ **Flo-Coat®** *see* radiological/contrast media (ionic) *on page 539*

floctafenine *(Canada only)* (flok ta FEN een)

Canadian Brand Names Idarac®

Generic Available No

Therapeutic Category Nonsteroidal Anti-inflammatory Drug (NSAID), Oral

Use Short-term use in acute pain of mild and moderate severity

Usual Dosage Adults: Oral: 200-400 mg every 6-8 hours as required; maximum recommended daily dose: 1200 mg

Dosage Forms Tablet: 200 mg, 400 mg

♦ **Flodine®** *see* folic acid *on page 281*

♦ **Flogen** *see* naproxen *on page 432*

♦ **Flogosan®** *see* piroxicam *on page 497*

♦ **Floian®** *see* epoprostenol *on page 236*

♦ **Flomax®** *see* tamsulosin *on page 593*

♦ **Flonase®** *see* fluticasone (nasal) *on page 279*

- **Flonase®** 9 g *(Discontinued)* see page 743
- **Florical®** [OTC] see calcium carbonate on page 103
- **Florinef®** Acetate see fludrocortisone on page 271
- **Florone®** see diflorasone on page 202
- **Florone E®** see diflorasone on page 202
- **Floropryl® Ophthalmic** see isoflurophate on page 347
- **Flovent®** see fluticasone (oral inhalation) on page 279
- **Flovent® Rotadisk®** see fluticasone (oral inhalation) on page 279
- **Floxacin®** see norfloxacin on page 448
- **Floxil** see ofloxacin on page 454
- **Floxin®** see ofloxacin on page 454
- **Floxstat** see ofloxacin on page 454

floxuridine (floks YOOR i deen)

Synonyms fluorodeoxyuridine

U.S. Brand Names FUDR®

Generic Available No

Therapeutic Category Antineoplastic Agent

Use Palliative management of carcinomas of head, neck, and brain as well as liver, gallbladder, and bile ducts

Usual Dosage Adults:

Intra-arterial infusion: 0.1-0.6 mg/kg/day for 14 days followed by heparinized saline for 14 days

Investigational: I.V.: 0.5-1 mg/kg/day for 6-15 days

Nursing/Pharmacy Information

Infused for intra-arterial use, use infusion pump, either external or implanted

Stability: Reconstituted solutions are stable for up to 14 days (refrigerated); FUDR® is stable in D_5W or normal saline

Dosage Forms

Injection, preservative free: 100 mg/mL (5 mL)

Powder for injection: 500 mg (5 mL, 10 mL)

- **Fluanxol® Depot** see flupenthixol *(Canada only)* on page 276
- **Fluanxol® Tablet** see flupenthixol *(Canada only)* on page 276
- **flubenisolone** see betamethasone (topical) on page 85

fluconazole (floo KOE na zole)

U.S. Brand Names Diflucan®

Mexican Brand Names Oxifungol; Zonal

Generic Available No

Therapeutic Category Antifungal Agent

Use Treatment of susceptible fungal infections including oropharyngeal, esophageal, and vaginal candidiasis; treatment of systemic candidal infections including urinary tract infection, peritonitis, cystitis, and pneumonia; treatment and suppression of cryptococcal meningitis; prophylaxis of candidiasis in patients undergoing bone marrow transplantation; alternative to amphotericin B in patients with pre-existing renal impairment or when requiring concomitant therapy with other potentially nephrotoxic drugs

Usual Dosage Daily dose of fluconazole is the same for oral and I.V. administration

Infants and Children: Oral, I.V.: Safety profile of fluconazole has been studied in 577 children, ages 1 day to 17 years; doses as high as 12 mg/kg/day once daily (equivalent to adult doses of 400 mg/day) have been used to treat candidiasis in immunocompromised children; 10-12 mg/kg/day doses once daily have been used prophylactically against fungal infections in pediatric bone marrow transplantation patients. Do not exceed 600 mg/day.

Adults:

Vaginal candidiasis: Oral: 150 mg single dose

Prophylaxis against fungal infections in bone marrow transplantation patients: Oral, I.V.: 400 mg/day once daily

Dietary Considerations Presence of food delays the time of peak serum concentration but it has no effect on the total amount of fluconazole absorbed

Nursing/Pharmacy Information

Parenteral fluconazole must be administered by I.V. infusion over ~1-2 hours; do not exceed 200 mg/hour when administering I.V. infusion; final concentration for administration of 2 mg/mL; do not unwrap unit until ready for use; do not use if cloudy or precipitated

Monitor periodic liver function and renal function tests; as dosage adjustments are required with significant changes in renal function

Stability: Parenteral admixture at room temperature (25°C): Manufacturer expiration dating; do not refrigerate

Dosage Forms
Injection: 2 mg/mL (100 mL, 200 mL)
Powder for oral suspension: 10 mg/mL (35 mL); 40 mg/mL (35 mL)
Tablet: 50 mg, 100 mg, 150 mg, 200 mg

flucytosine (floo SYE toe seen)
Synonyms 5-FC; 5-flurocytosine
U.S. Brand Names Ancobon®
Canadian Brand Names Ancotil®
Generic Available No
Therapeutic Category Antifungal Agent
Use In combination with amphotericin B in the treatment of serious *Candida*, *Aspergillus*, *Cryptococcus*, and *Torulopsis* infections
Usual Dosage Children and Adults: Oral: 50-150 mg/kg/day in divided doses every 6 hours
Dietary Considerations Food decreases the rate, but not the extent of absorption
Nursing/Pharmacy Information
Administer around-the-clock rather than 4 times/day, 3 times/day, etc, (ie, 12-6-12-6, not 9-1-5-9) to promote less variation in peak and trough serum levels; perform hematologic, renal and hepatic function tests
Monitor serum creatinine, BUN, alkaline phosphatase, AST, ALT, CBC; serum flucytosine concentrations
Stability: Protect from light
Dosage Forms Capsule: 250 mg, 500 mg

♦ **Fludara®** *see* fludarabine *on page 271*

fludarabine (floo DARE a been)
U.S. Brand Names Fludara®
Generic Available No
Therapeutic Category Antineoplastic Agent
Use Treatment of B-cell chronic lymphocytic leukemia unresponsive to previous therapy with an alkylating agent containing regimen. Fludarabine has been tested in patients with refractory acute lymphocytic leukemia and acute nonlymphocytic leukemia, but required a highly toxic dose to achieve response.
Usual Dosage Adults: I.V.:
Chronic lymphocytic leukemia: 25 mg/m^2/day over a 30-minute period for 5 days
Non-Hodgkin's lymphoma: Loading dose: 20 mg/m^2 followed by 30 mg/m^2/day for 48 hours
Nursing/Pharmacy Information
Parenteral: Fludarabine phosphate has been administered by intermittent I.V. infusion over 15-30 minutes and by continuous infusion; in clinical trials the loading dose has been diluted in 20 mL D$_5$W and administered over 15 minutes and the continuous infusion diluted to 240 mL in D$_5$W and administered at a constant rate of 10 mL/hour; in other clinical studies fludarabine has been diluted to a concentration of 0.25 to 1 mg/mL in D$_5$W or sodium chloride 0.9%
Monitor CBC with differential, platelet count, AST, ALT, creatinine, serum albumin, uric acid
Stability: Fludarabine should be stored under refrigeration (2°C to 8°C or 36°F to 46°F). Reconstitute with 2 mL of sterile water for injection to a final concentration of 25 mg/mL; fludarabine should be used within 8 hours of reconstitution as it contains no preservatives; however, is chemically stable 48 hours at room temperature and refrigeration.
Dosage Forms Powder for injection, as phosphate, lyophilized: 50 mg (6 mL)

fludrocortisone (floo droe KOR ti sone AS e tate)
Synonyms fluohydrocortisone; 9α-fluorohydrocortisone
U.S. Brand Names Florinef® Acetate
Generic Available No
Therapeutic Category Adrenal Corticosteroid (Mineralocorticoid)
Use Addison's disease; partial replacement therapy for adrenal insufficiency; treatment of salt-losing forms of congenital adrenogenital syndrome; has been used with increased sodium intake for the treatment of idiopathic orthostatic hypotension
(Continued)

fludrocortisone *(Continued)*

Usual Dosage Oral:
Infants and Children: 0.05-0.1 mg/day
Adults: 0.05-0.2 mg/day

Dietary Considerations Systemic use of mineralocorticoids/corticosteroids may require a diet with increased potassium, vitamins A, B_6, C, D, folate, calcium, zinc, and phosphorus, and decreased sodium; with fludrocortisone a decrease in dietary sodium is often not required as the increased retention of sodium is usually the desired therapeutic effect

Nursing/Pharmacy Information Monitor blood pressure and signs of edema when patient is on chronic therapy; very potent mineralocorticoid with high glucocorticoid activity; monitor serum electrolytes, serum renin activity, and blood pressure; monitor evidence of infection; closely monitor patients with Addison's disease and stop treatment if a significant increase in weight or blood pressure, edema or cardiac enlargement occurs

Dosage Forms Tablet, as acetate: 0.1 mg

♦ **Fluken** *see* flutamide *on page 279*

♦ **Flulem** *see* flutamide *on page 279*

♦ **Flumadine®** *see* rimantadine *on page 550*

flumazenil *(FLO may ze nil)*

U.S. Brand Names Romazicon®
Canadian Brand Names Anexate®
Mexican Brand Names Lanexat®
Generic Available No
Therapeutic Category Antidote

Use Benzodiazepine antagonist; reverses sedative effects of benzodiazepines used in general anesthesia or conscious sedation; management of benzodiazepine overdose; not indicated for ethanol, barbiturate, general anesthetic or narcotic overdose

Usual Dosage Reversal of conscious sedation or general anesthesia: 0.2 mg (2 mL) administered I.V. over 15 seconds; if desired effect is not achieved after 60 seconds, repeat in 0.2 mg (2 mL) increments every 60 seconds up to a total of 1 mg (10 mL); in event of resedation, repeat doses may be administered at 20-minute intervals with no more than 1 mg (10 mL) administered at any one time, with a maximum of 3 mg in any 1 hour

Nursing/Pharmacy Information
Parenteral: For I.V. use only; administer via freely running I.V. infusion into larger vein to decrease chance of pain, phlebitis
Monitor respiratory rate, level of sedation
Stability: For I.V. use only; **compatible** with D_5W, lactated Ringer's, or normal saline; once drawn up in the syringe or mixed with solution use within 24 hours; discard any unused solution after 24 hours

Dosage Forms Injection: 0.1 mg/mL (5 mL, 10 mL)

flunisolide *(floo NIS oh lide)*

U.S. Brand Names AeroBid®-M Oral Aerosol Inhaler; AeroBid® Oral Aerosol Inhaler; Nasalide® Nasal Aerosol; Nasarel™ Nasal Spray
Canadian Brand Names Bronalide®; Rhinalar®; Rhinaris-F®; Syn-Flunisolide®
Generic Available No
Therapeutic Category Adrenal Corticosteroid

Use Steroid-dependent asthma; nasal solution is used for seasonal or perennial rhinitis

Usual Dosage
Children:
Oral inhalation: >6 years: 2 inhalations twice daily up to 4 inhalations/day
Nasal: 6-14 years: 1 spray each nostril 2-3 times/day, not to exceed 4 sprays/day each nostril
Adults:
Oral inhalation: 2 inhalations twice daily up to 8 inhalations/day
Nasal: 2 sprays each nostril twice daily; maximum dose: 8 sprays/day in each nostril

Nursing/Pharmacy Information Shake well before administering; do not use Nasalide® orally; discard product after it has been opened for 3 months

Dosage Forms
Inhalant:
Nasal (Nasalide®): 25 mcg/actuation [200 sprays] (25 mL)
Nasal (Nasarel™): 25 mcg/actuation [200 sprays] (25 mL)

Oral:
AeroBid®: 250 mcg/actuation [100 metered doses] (7 g)
AeroBid-M® (menthol flavor): 250 mcg/actuation [100 metered doses] (7 g)
Solution, spray: 0.025% [200 actuations] (25 mL)

fluocinolone (floo oh SIN oh lone)

U.S. Brand Names Derma-Smoothe/FS® Topical; Fluonid® Topical; Flurosyn® Topical; FS Shampoo® Topical; Synalar-HP® Topical; Synalar® Topical; Synemol® Topical
Canadian Brand Names Lidemol®
Generic Available Yes
Therapeutic Category Corticosteroid, Topical
Use Relief of susceptible inflammatory dermatosis
Usual Dosage Children and Adults: Topical: Apply 2-4 times/day
Nursing/Pharmacy Information Use sparingly
Dosage Forms Fluocinolone acetonide:
Cream, topical: 0.01% (15 g, 60 g); 0.025% (15 g, 60 g)
Flurosyn®, Synalar®: 0.01% (15 g, 30 g, 60 g, 425 g)
Flurosyn®, Synalar®, Synemol®: 0.025% (15 g, 60 g, 425 g)
Synalar-HP®: 0.2% (12 g)
Ointment, topical: 0.025% (15 g, 60 g)
Flurosyn®, Synalar®: 0.025% (15 g, 30 g, 60 g, 425 g)
Oil (Derma-Smoothe/FS®): 0.01% (120 mL)
Shampoo (FS Shampoo®): 0.01% (180 mL)
Solution, topical: 0.01% (20 mL, 60 mL)
Fluonid®, Synalar®: 0.01% (20 mL, 60 mL)

fluocinonide (floo oh SIN oh nide)

U.S. Brand Names Lidex®; Lidex-E®
Canadian Brand Names Fluoderm; Lyderm®; Tiamol®; Topactin®; Topsyn®
Generic Available Yes
Therapeutic Category Corticosteroid, Topical
Use Inflammation of corticosteroid-responsive dermatoses
Usual Dosage Children and Adults: Topical: Apply thin layer to affected area 2-4 times/day depending on the severity of the condition
Nursing/Pharmacy Information Use sparingly
Dosage Forms
Cream: 0.05% (15 g, 30 g, 60 g, 120 g)
Anhydrous, emollient (Lidex®): 0.05% (15 g, 30 g, 60 g, 120 g)
Aqueous, emollient (Lidex-E®): 0.05% (15 g, 30 g, 60 g, 120 g)
Gel, topical: 0.05% (15 g, 60 g)
Lidex®: 0.05% (15 g, 30 g, 60 g, 120 g)
Ointment, topical: 0.05% (15 g, 30 g, 60 g)
Lidex®: 0.05% (15 g, 30 g, 60 g, 120 g)
Solution, topical: 0.05% (20 mL, 60 mL)
Lidex®: 0.05% (20 mL, 60 mL)

♦ **Fluoderm** see fluocinonide on page 273
♦ **Fluogen®** see influenza virus vaccine on page 338
♦ **fluohydrocortisone** see fludrocortisone on page 271
♦ **Fluonid® Topical** see fluocinolone on page 273
♦ **Fluoracaine® Ophthalmic** see proparacaine and fluorescein on page 525
♦ **Fluor-A-Day®** see fluoride on page 274
♦ **FluorCare® Neutral** see fluoride on page 274

fluorescein sodium (FLURE e seen SOW dee um)

Synonyms soluble fluorescein
U.S. Brand Names AK-Fluor Injection; Fluorescite® Injection; Fluorets® Ophthalmic Strips; Fluor-I-Strip®; Fluor-I-Strip-AT®; Flurate® Ophthalmic Solution; Fluress® Ophthalmic Solution; Ful-Glo® Ophthalmic Strips; Funduscein® Injection
Generic Available Yes
Therapeutic Category Diagnostic Agent
Use Demonstrates defects of corneal epithelium; diagnostic aid in ophthalmic angiography
Usual Dosage
Injection: Perform intradermal skin test before use to avoid possible allergic reaction
Children: 3.5 mg/lb (7.5 mg/kg) injected rapidly into antecubital vein
Adults: 500-750 mg injected rapidly into antecubital vein
(Continued)

fluorescein sodium *(Continued)*

Strips: Moisten with sterile water or irrigating solution, touch conjunctiva with moistened tip, blink several times after application

Topical solution: Instill 1-2 drops, allow a few seconds for staining, then wash out excess with sterile irrigation solution

Nursing/Pharmacy Information Avoid extravasation, results in severe local tissue damage; have epinephrine 1:1000, an antihistamine, and oxygen available

Dosage Forms

Injection (AK-Fluor, Fluorescite®, Funduscein®, Ophthifluor®): 10% [100 mg/mL] (5 mL); 25% [250 mg/mL] (2 mL, 3 mL)

Ophthalmic:

Solution: 2% [20 mg/mL] (1 mL, 2 mL, 15 mL)

Flurate®, Fluress®: 0.25% [2.5 mg/mL] with benoxinate 0.4% (5 mL)

Strip:

Ful-Glo®: 0.6 mg

Fluorets®, Fluor-I-Strip-AT®: 1 mg

Fluor-I-Strip®: 9 mg

◆ **Fluorescite® Injection** *see fluorescein sodium on page 273*

◆ **Fluorets® Ophthalmic Strips** *see fluorescein sodium on page 273*

fluoride *(FLOR ide)*

U.S. Brand Names ACT® [OTC]; FluorCare® Neutral; Fluorigard® [OTC]; Fluorinse®; Fluoritab®; Flura®; Flura-Drops®; Flura-Loz®; Gel-Kam®; Gel-Tin® [OTC]; Karidium®; Karigel®; Karigel®-N; Listermint® with Fluoride [OTC]; Lozi-Tab®; Luride®; Luride®-SF; Minute-Gel®; Pediaflor®; Pharmaflur®; Phos-Flur®; Point-Two®; Prevident®; Stop® [OTC]; Thera-Flur®; Thera-Flur-N®

Canadian Brand Names Fluor-A-Day®; Fluotic®; Pedi-Dent™

Generic Available Yes

Therapeutic Category Mineral, Oral

Use Prevention of dental caries

Usual Dosage Oral: Dental rinse or gel:

Children 6-12 years: 5-10 mL rinse or apply to teeth and spit daily after brushing

Adults: 10 mL rinse or apply to teeth and spit daily after brushing

Dietary Considerations Do not administer with milk; do **not** allow eating or drinking for 30 minutes after use

Nursing/Pharmacy Information

Avoid administering with milk or dairy products, antacids

Stability: Store in tight plastic containers (not glass)

Dosage Forms Fluoride ion content listed in brackets

Acidulated phosphate fluoride: Rinse, topical:

Minute-Gel®: 1.23% (480 mL)

Sodium fluoride:

Drops, oral:

Fluoritab®, Flura-Drops®: 0.55 mg/drop [0.25 mg/drop] (22.8 mL, 24 mL)

Karidium®, Luride®: 0.275 mg/drop [0.125 mg/drop] (30 mL, 60 mL)

Pediaflor®: 1.1 mg/mL [0.5 mg/mL] (50 mL)

Gel, topical:

Karigel®, Karigel®-N, PreviDent®: 1.1% [0.5%] (24 g, 30 g, 60 g, 120 g, 130 g, 250 g)

Rinse, topical:

ACT®, Fluorigard®: 0.05% [0.02%] (90 mL, 180 mL, 300 mL, 360 mL, 480 mL)

Fluorinse®, Point-Two®: 0.2% [0.09%] (240 mL, 480 mL, 3780 mL)

Listermint® with Fluoride: 0.02% [0.01%] (180 mL, 300 mL, 360 mL, 480 mL, 540 mL, 720 mL, 960 mL, 1740 mL)

Solution, oral, as sodium (Phos-Flur®): 0.44 mg/mL [0.2 mg/mL] (250 mL, 500 mL, 3780 mL)

Tablet:

Chewable:

Fluoritab®, Luride® Lozi-Tab®, Pharmaflur®: 1.1 mg [0.5 mg]

Fluoritab®, Karidium®, Luride® Lozi-Tab®, Luride®-SF Lozi-Tab®, Pharmaflur®: 2.2 mg [1 mg]

Oral: Flura®, Karidium®: 2.2 mg [1 mg]

Stannous fluoride: Rinse, topical:

Gel-Kam®, Gel-Tin®, Stop®: 0.4% [0.1%] (60 g, 15 g, 105 g, 120 g)

◆ **Fluorigard® [OTC]** *see fluoride on page 274*

- **Fluori-Methane® Topical Spray** *see* dichlorodifluoromethane and trichloromono-fluoromethane *on page 198*
- **Fluorinse®** *see* fluoride *on page 274*
- **Fluor-I-Strip®** *see* fluorescein sodium *on page 273*
- **Fluor-I-Strip-AT®** *see* fluorescein sodium *on page 273*
- **Fluoritab®** *see* fluoride *on page 274*
- **fluorodeoxyuridine** *see* floxuridine *on page 270*
- **9α-fluorohydrocortisone** *see* fludrocortisone *on page 271*

fluorometholone (flure oh METH oh lone)

U.S. Brand Names Flarex®; Fluor-Op®; FML®; FML® Forte
Generic Available No
Therapeutic Category Adrenal Corticosteroid
Use Inflammatory conditions of the eye, including keratitis, iritis, cyclitis, and conjunctivitis
Usual Dosage Children >2 years and Adults: Ophthalmic: 1-2 drops into conjunctival sac every hour during day, every 2 hours at night until favorable response is obtained, then use 1 drop every 4 hours; in mild or moderate inflammation: 1-2 drops into conjunctival sac 2-4 times/day. Ointment may be applied every 4 hours in severe cases or 1-3 times/day in mild to moderate cases.
Nursing/Pharmacy Information Do not discontinue without consulting physician; photosensitivity may occur; notify physician if improvement does not occur after 7-8 days
Dosage Forms Ophthalmic:
Ointment (FML®): 0.1% (3.5 g)
Suspension:
Flarex®, Fluor-Op®, FML®: 0.1% (2.5 mL, 5 mL, 10 mL)
FML® Forte: 0.25% (2 mL, 5 mL, 10 mL, 15 mL)

- **fluorometholone and sulfacetamide** *see* sulfacetamide sodium and fluorometholone *on page 586*
- **Fluor-Op®** *see* fluorometholone *on page 275*
- **Fluoroplex® Topical** *see* fluorouracil *on page 275*
- **Fluoro-uracil** *see* fluorouracil *on page 275*
- **5-fluorouracil** *see* fluorouracil *on page 275*

fluorouracil (flure oh YOOR a sil)

Synonyms 5-fluorouracil; 5-FU
U.S. Brand Names Adrucil® Injection; Efudex® Topical; Fluoroplex® Topical
Mexican Brand Names Efudix; Fluoro-uracil
Generic Available Yes: Injection
Therapeutic Category Antineoplastic Agent
Use Treatment of carcinoma of stomach, colon, rectum, breast, and pancreas; also used topically for management of multiple actinic keratoses and superficial basal cell carcinomas
Usual Dosage Children and Adults (refer to individual protocol):
I.V.: Initial: 12 mg/kg/day (maximum: 800 mg/day) for 4-5 days; maintenance: 6 mg/kg every other day for 4 doses
Single weekly bolus dose of 15 mg/kg can be administered depending on the patient's reaction to the previous course of treatment; maintenance dose of 5-15 mg/kg/week as a single dose not to exceed 1 g/week
I.V. infusion: 15 mg/kg/day (maximum daily dose: 1 g) has been administered by I.V. infusion over 4 hours for 5 days
Oral: 20 mg/kg/day for 5 days every 5 weeks for colorectal carcinoma; 15 mg/kg/week for hepatoma
Topical: 5% cream twice daily
Dietary Considerations Use of acidic solutions such as orange juice or other fruit juices to dilute 5-FU for oral administration may result in precipitation of the drug and decreased absorption; increase dietary intake of thiamine
Nursing/Pharmacy Information
Wash hands immediately after topical application of the 5% cream; grape juice improves bitter taste of solution; administer by direct I.V. push injection (50 mg/mL solution needs no further dilution) or by I.V. infusion; toxicity may be reduced by administering the drug as a constant infusion
Monitor CBC with differential and platelet count, renal function tests, liver function tests
Stability: Protect from light; slight discoloration of injection occurring during storage does not adversely affect potency or safety; but discard dark yellow solution; if precipitate forms, redissolve drug by heating to 140°F (60°C),
(Continued)

fluorouracil *(Continued)*

shake well; allow to cool to body temperature before administration; **incompatible** with cytarabine, diazepam, doxorubicin, methotrexate. Concentrations of >25 mg/mL of fluorouracil and >2 mg/mL of leucovorin are **incompatible** (precipitation occurs). **Compatible** with vincristine, methotrexate, potassium chloride, magnesium sulfate.

Dosage Forms
Cream, topical:
Efudex®: 5% (25 g)
Fluoroplex®: 1% (30 g)
Injection (Adrucil®): 50 mg/mL (10 mL, 20 mL, 50 mL, 100 mL)
Solution, topical:
Efudex®: 2% (10 mL); 5% (10 mL)
Fluoroplex®: 1% (30 mL)

♦ **fluostigmin** *see* isoflurophate *on page 347*
♦ **Fluothane®** *see* halothane *on page 309*
♦ **Fluotic®** *see* fluoride *on page 274*
♦ **Fluoxac** *see* fluoxetine *on page 276*

fluoxetine (floo OKS e teen)
U.S. Brand Names Prozac®
Mexican Brand Names Fluoxac
Generic Available No
Therapeutic Category Antidepressant, Selective Serotonin Reuptake Inhibitor
Use Treatment of major depression; preliminary studies report use for obsessive-compulsive disorders in children and adolescents
Usual Dosage Oral:
Children <18 years: Dose not established
Adults: 20 mg/day in the morning; may increase after several weeks by 20 mg/day increments; maximum: 80 mg/day; doses >20 mg should be divided into 2 daily doses
Note: Lower doses of 5 mg/day have been used for initial treatment
Dietary Considerations Should be administered in the morning without regards to meals; tryptophan supplements may increase CNS and GI adverse effects (eg, restlessness, agitation, GI problems)
Nursing/Pharmacy Information
Offer patient sugarless hard candy for dry mouth
Monitor weight gain or weight loss, nutritional intake
Dosage Forms Fluoxetine hydrochloride:
Capsule: 10 mg, 20 mg
Liquid (mint flavor): 20 mg/5 mL (120 mL)
Tablet: 10 mg

fluoxymesterone (floo oks i MES te rone)
U.S. Brand Names Halotestin®
Mexican Brand Names Stenox
Generic Available Yes
Therapeutic Category Androgen
Use Replacement of endogenous testicular hormone; in female used as palliative treatment of breast cancer, postpartum breast engorgement
Usual Dosage Adults: Oral:
Male:
Hypogonadism: 5-20 mg/day
Delayed puberty: 2.5-20 mg/day for 4-6 months
Female:
Breast carcinoma: 10-40 mg/day in divided doses for 1-3 months
Breast engorgement: 2.5 mg after delivery, 5-10 mg/day in divided doses for 4-5 days
Nursing/Pharmacy Information
In prepubertal children, perform radiographic examination of the head and wrist every 6 months
Stability: Protect from light
Dosage Forms Tablet: 2 mg, 5 mg, 10 mg

♦ **Flupazine** *see* trifluoperazine *on page 627*

flupenthixol *(Canada only)* (floo pen THIKS ol)
Canadian Brand Names Fluanxol® Depot; Fluanxol® Tablet
Generic Available No

Therapeutic Category Antipsychotic Agent; Thioxanthene Derivative

Use Maintenance therapy of chronic schizophrenic patients whose main manifestations do not include excitement, agitation, or hyperactivity

Usual Dosage

Injection: Flupenthixol is administered by deep I.M. injection, preferably in the gluteus maximus, NOT for I.V. use

Patients not previously treated with long acting depot neuroleptics should be given an initial test dose of 5 mg (0.25 mL) to 20 mg (1 mL). An initial dose of 20 mg (1 mL) is usually well tolerated; however, a 5 mg (0.25 mL) test dose is recommended in elderly, frail and cachectic patients, and in patients whose individual or family history suggests a predisposition to extrapyramidal reactions. In the subsequent 5-10 days, the therapeutic response and the appearance of extrapyramidal symptoms should be carefully monitored. Oral neuroleptic drugs may be continued, but in diminishing dosage, during this period.

Tablets: The dosage should be individualized and adjusted according to the severity of symptoms and tolerance to the drug. Initial recommended dose: 1 mg, 3 times/day. This may be increased, if necessary by 1 mg every 2-3 days until there is effective control of psychotic symptoms. The usual maintenance dosage: 3-6 mg/day in divided doses, although doses of up to 12 mg/day or more have been used in some patients.

Dosage Forms

Injection, depot: 20 mg/mL (10 mL); 100 mg/mL (2 mL)

Tablet: 0.5 mg, 3 mg

fluphenazine (floo FEN a zeen)

U.S. Brand Names Permitil® Oral; Prolixin Decanoate® Injection; Prolixin Enanthate® Injection; Prolixin® Injection; Prolixin® Oral

Canadian Brand Names Apo®-Fluphenazine; Modecate®; Modecate® Enanthate; Moditen® Hydrochloride; PMS-Fluphenazine

Generic Available Yes

Therapeutic Category Phenothiazine Derivative

Use Management of manifestations of psychotic disorders

Usual Dosage Adults:

Oral: 0.5-10 mg/day in divided doses every 6-8 hours; usual maximum dose 20 mg/day

I.M.: 2.5-10 mg/day in divided doses every 6-8 hours; usual maximum dose 10 mg/day

I.M., S.C. (Decanoate®): Oral to I.M., S.C. conversion ratio = 12.5 mg, I.M., S.C. every 3 weeks for every 10 mg of oral fluphenazine

Dietary Considerations May be administered with food or water

Nursing/Pharmacy Information

Watch for hypotension when administering I.M. or I.V.; dilute the oral concentrate with water or juice before administration; avoid skin contact with oral suspension or solution; may cause contact dermatitis

Monitor orthostatic blood pressures 3-5 days after initiation of therapy or a dose increase; observe for tremor and abnormal movement or posturing (extrapyramidal symptoms)

Dosage Forms

Fluphenazine decanoate: Injection:

Prolixin Decanoate®: 25 mg/mL (1 mL, 5 mL)

Fluphenazine enanthate: Injection:

Prolixin Enanthate®: 25 mg/mL (5 mL)

Fluphenazine hydrochloride:

Concentrate, oral:

Permitil®: 5 mg/mL with alcohol 1% (118 mL)

Prolixin®: 5 mg/mL with alcohol 14% (120 mL)

Elixir (Prolixin®): 2.5 mg/5 mL with alcohol 14% (60 mL, 473 mL)

Injection: Prolixin®: 2.5 mg/mL (10 mL)

Tablet:

Permitil®: 2.5 mg, 5 mg, 10 mg

Prolixin®: 1 mg, 2.5 mg, 5 mg, 10 mg

- ◆ **Flura®** *see* fluoride *on page 274*
- ◆ **Flura-Drops®** *see* fluoride *on page 274*
- ◆ **Flura-Loz®** *see* fluoride *on page 274*

flurandrenolide (flure an DREN oh lide)

Synonyms flurandrenolone

U.S. Brand Names Cordran®; Cordran® SP

Canadian Brand Names Drenison®

(Continued)

flurandrenolide *(Continued)*

Generic Available Yes: Lotion

Therapeutic Category Corticosteroid, Topical

Use Inflammation of corticosteroid-responsive dermatoses

Usual Dosage Topical:

Children:

Ointment or cream: Apply 1-2 times/day

Tape: Apply once daily

Adults: Cream, lotion, ointment: Apply 2-3 times/day

Nursing/Pharmacy Information A thin film of cream or ointment is effective; do not overuse; do not use tight-fitting diapers or plastic pants on children being treated in the diaper area; use only as prescribed, and for no longer than the period prescribed; apply sparingly in light film; rub in lightly; avoid contact with eyes; notify physician if condition being treated persists or worsens

Dosage Forms

Cream, emulsified base (Cordran® SP): 0.025% (30 g, 60 g); 0.05% (15 g, 30 g, 60 g)

Lotion (Cordran®): 0.05% (15 mL, 60 mL)

Ointment, topical (Cordran®): 0.025% (30 g, 60 g); 0.05% (15 g, 30 g, 60 g)

Tape, topical (Cordran®): 4 mcg/cm^2 (7.5 cm x 60 cm, 7.5 cm x 200 cm rolls)

♦ **flurandrenolone** *see* flurandrenolide *on page 277*

♦ **Flurate® Ophthalmic Solution** *see* fluorescein sodium *on page 273*

flurazepam *(flure AZ e pam)*

U.S. Brand Names Dalmane®

Canadian Brand Names Apo®-Flurazepam; Novo-Flupam®; PMS-Flupam; Somnol®; Som Pam®

Generic Available Yes

Therapeutic Category Benzodiazepine

Controlled Substance C-IV

Use Short-term treatment of insomnia

Usual Dosage Oral:

Children:

<15 years: Dose not established

>15 years: 15 mg at bedtime

Adults: 15-30 mg at bedtime

Nursing/Pharmacy Information

Provide safety measures (ie, side rails, night light, and call button); remove smoking materials from area; supervise ambulation; avoid abrupt discontinuance in patients with prolonged therapy or seizure disorders; observe for orthostasis

Monitor respiratory and cardiovascular status

Stability: Store in light-resistant containers

Dosage Forms Capsule, as hydrochloride: 15 mg, 30 mg

flurbiprofen *(flure BI proe fen)*

U.S. Brand Names Ansaid® Oral; Ocufen® Ophthalmic

Canadian Brand Names Apro-Flurbiprofen®; Froben®; Froben-SR®; Novo-Flurprofen®; Nu-Flurprofen®

Generic Available Yes

Therapeutic Category Analgesic, Non-narcotic; Nonsteroidal Anti-inflammatory Drug (NSAID)

Use

Ophthalmic: For inhibition of intraoperative trauma-induced miosis; the value of flurbiprofen for the prevention and management of postoperative ocular inflammation and postoperative cystoid macular edema remains to be determined

Systemic: Management of inflammatory disease and rheumatoid disorders; dysmenorrhea; pain

Usual Dosage

Oral: Rheumatoid arthritis and osteoarthritis: 200-300 mg/day in 2, 3, or 4 divided doses

Ophthalmic: Instill 1 drop every 30 minutes, 2 hours prior to surgery (total of 4 drops to each affected eye)

Dietary Considerations Oral product should be administered with food, milk, or antacid to decrease GI effects; food may decrease the rate but not the extent of absorption

Nursing/Pharmacy Information

Ophthalmic: Care should be taken to avoid contamination of the solution container tip

Monitor CBC, BUN, serum creatinine, liver enzymes, occult blood loss, periodic eye exams

Dosage Forms Flurbiprofen sodium:

Solution, ophthalmic (Ocufen®): 0.03% (2.5 mL, 5 mL, 10 mL)

Tablet (Ansaid®): 50 mg, 100 mg

♦ **Fluress® Ophthalmic Solution** *see* fluorescein sodium *on page 273*

♦ **5-flurocytosine** *see* flucytosine *on page 271*

♦ **Fluro-Ethyl® Aerosol** *see* ethyl chloride and dichlorotetrafluoroethane *on page 254*

♦ **Flurosyn® Topical** *see* fluocinolone *on page 273*

flutamide (FLOO ta mide)

U.S. Brand Names Eulexin®

Canadian Brand Names Euflex®

Mexican Brand Names Eulexin®; Fluken; Flulem

Generic Available No

Therapeutic Category Antiandrogen

Use In combination with LHRH agonistic analogs for the treatment of metastatic prostatic carcinoma

Usual Dosage Oral: 2 capsules every 8 hours

Nursing/Pharmacy Information

Monitor LFTs, tumor reduction, testosterone/estrogen, and phosphatase serum levels

Stability: Store at room temperature

Dosage Forms Capsule: 125 mg

♦ **Flutex® Topical** *see* triamcinolone (topical) *on page 624*

fluticasone (nasal) (floo TIK a sone)

U.S. Brand Names Flonase®

Generic Available No

Therapeutic Category Adrenal Corticosteroid

Use Management of seasonal and perennial allergic rhinitis in patients ≥12 years of age

Usual Dosage

Adolescents:

Intranasal: Initial: 1 spray (50 mcg/spray) per nostril once daily. Patients not adequately responding or patients with more severe symptoms may use 2 sprays (200 mcg) per nostril. Depending on response, dosage may be reduced to 100 mcg daily. Total daily dosage should not exceed 4 sprays (200 mcg)/day.

Adults:

Intranasal: Initial: 2 sprays (50 mcg/spray) per nostril once daily. After the first few days, dosage may be reduced to 1 spray per nostril once daily for maintenance therapy. Maximum total daily dose should not exceed 4 sprays (200 mcg)/day.

Dosage Forms Spray, intranasal: 50 mcg/actuation (16 g = 120 actuations)

fluticasone (oral inhalation) (floo TIK a sone)

U.S. Brand Names Flovent®; Flovent® Rotadisk®

Generic Available No

Therapeutic Category Adrenal Corticosteroid

Use Inhalation: Maintenance treatment of asthma as prophylactic therapy. It is also indicated for patients requiring oral corticosteroid therapy for asthma to assist in total discontinuation or reduction of total oral dose. NOT indicated for the relief of acute bronchospasm.

Usual Dosage Oral inhalation: If adequate response is not seen after 2 weeks of initial dosage, increase dosage; doses should be titrated to the lowest effective dose once asthma is controlled; Manufacturer recommendations:

Inhalation aerosol (Flovent®): Children ≥12 years and Adults:

Patients previously treated with bronchodilators only: Initial: 88 mcg twice daily; maximum dose: 440 mcg twice daily

Patients treated with an inhaled corticosteroid: Initial: 88-220 mcg twice daily; maximum dose: 440 mcg twice daily; may start doses above 88 mcg twice daily in poorly controlled patients or in those who previously required higher doses of inhaled corticosteroids

Patients previously treated with oral corticosteroids: Initial: 880 mcg twice daily; maximum dose: 880 mcg twice daily

(Continued)

fluticasone (oral inhalation) *(Continued)*

Inhalation powder (Flovent® Rotadisk®):

Children 4-11 years: Patients previously treated with bronchodilators alone or inhaled corticosteroids: Initial: 50 mcg twice daily; maximum dose: 100 mcg twice daily; may start higher initial dose in poorly controlled patients or in those who previously required higher doses of inhaled corticosteroids

Adolescents and Adults:

Patients previously treated with bronchodilators alone: Initial: 100 mcg twice daily; maximum dose: 500 mcg twice daily

Patients previously treated with inhaled corticosteroids: Initial: 100-250 mcg twice daily; maximum dose: 500 mcg twice daily; may start doses above 100 mcg twice daily in poorly controlled patients or in those who previously required higher doses of inhaled corticosteroids

Patients previously treated with oral corticosteroids: Initial: 1000 mcg twice daily; maximum dose: 1000 mcg twice daily

Dosage Forms

Powder (in 4 blisters containing 15 Rotodisks® with inhalation device): 50 mcg, 100 mcg, 250 mcg

Spray, aerosol, oral inhalation (Flovent®): 44 mcg/actuation (7.9 g = 60 actuations or 13 g = 120 actuations), 110 mcg/actuation (13 g = 120 actuations); 220 mcg/actuation (13 g = 120 actuations)

fluticasone (topical) (floo TIK a sone)

U.S. Brand Names Cutivate™

Generic Available No

Therapeutic Category Adrenal Corticosteroid; Corticosteroid, Topical

Use Relief of inflammation and pruritus associated with corticosteroid-responsive dermatoses [medium potency topical corticosteroid]

Usual Dosage

Pediatrics: Topical: Cultivate® approved for use in patients 3 months of age and older

Adolescents and Adults: Topical: Apply sparingly in a thin film twice daily. Therapy should be discontinued when control is achieved. If no improvement is seen, re-assessment of diagnosis may be necessary.

Nursing/Pharmacy Information A thin film of cream or ointment is effective; do not overuse; do not use tight-fitting diapers or plastic pants on children being treated in the diaper area; use only as prescribed, and for no longer than the period prescribed; apply sparingly in light film; rub in lightly; avoid contact with eyes; notify physician if condition being treated persists or worsens

Dosage Forms

Cream: 0.05% (15 g, 30 g, 60 g)

Ointment: 0.005% (15 g, 60 g)

fluvastatin (FLOO va sta tin)

U.S. Brand Names Lescol®

Generic Available No

Therapeutic Category HMG-CoA Reductase Inhibitor

Use Adjunct to dietary therapy to decrease elevated serum total and LDL cholesterol concentrations in primary hypercholesterolemia; slowing of progression of coronary atherosclerosis in patients with coronary heart disease as part of a treatment strategy to lower serum total and LDL cholesterol to target levels

Usual Dosage Adults: Oral: 20 mg at bedtime

Dosage Forms Capsule: 20 mg, 40 mg

♦ **Fluviral®** *see* influenza virus vaccine *on page 338*

fluvoxamine (floo VOKS ah meen)

U.S. Brand Names Luvox®

Generic Available No

Therapeutic Category Antidepressant, Selective Serotonin Reuptake Inhibitor

Use Treatment of major depression and obsessive-compulsive disorder (OCD)

Usual Dosage Adults: Initial: 50 mg at bedtime; adjust in 50 mg increments at 4- to 7-day intervals; usual dose range: 100-300 mg/day; divide total daily dose into 2 doses; administer larger portion at bedtime

Dosage Forms Tablet: 50 mg, 100 mg

♦ **Fluzone®** *see* influenza virus vaccine *on page 338*

♦ **Flynoken A** *see* leucovorin *on page 362*

♦ **FML®** *see* fluorometholone *on page 275*

- ♦ **FML® Forte** *see* fluorometholone *on page 275*
- ♦ **FML-S® Ophthalmic Suspension** *see* sulfacetamide sodium and fluorometholone *on page 586*
- ♦ **Foille® [OTC]** *see* benzocaine *on page 79*
- ♦ **Foille® Medicated First Aid [OTC]** *see* benzocaine *on page 79*
- ♦ **folacin** *see* folic acid *on page 281*
- ♦ **folate** *see* folic acid *on page 281*
- ♦ **Folex® Injection *(Discontinued)*** *see page 743*
- ♦ **Folex® PFS™** *see* methotrexate *on page 402*

folic acid (FOE lik AS id)

Synonyms folacin; folate; pteroylglutamic acid
U.S. Brand Names Folvite®
Canadian Brand Names Apo®-Folic; Flodine®; Novo-Folacid®
Mexican Brand Names A.F. Valdecasas®; Folitab
Generic Available Yes
Therapeutic Category Vitamin, Water Soluble
Use Treatment of megaloblastic and macrocytic anemias due to folate deficiency
Usual Dosage Folic acid deficiency:
    Infants: 15 mcg/kg/dose daily or 50 mcg/day
    Children: Oral, I.M., I.V., S.C.: 1 mg/day initial dosage; maintenance dose: 1-10 years: 0.1-0.3 mg/day
    Children >11 years and Adults: Oral, I.M., I.V., S.C.: 1 mg/day initial dosage; maintenance dose: 0.5 mg/day
Nursing/Pharmacy Information
    Oral, but may also be administered by deep I.M., S.C., or I.V. injection; a diluted solution for oral or for parenteral administration may be prepared by diluting 1 mL of folic acid injection (5 mg/mL), with 49 mL sterile water for injection; resulting solution is 0.1 mg folic acid per 1 mL
    Monitor hemoglobin
    Stability: **Incompatible** with oxidizing and reducing agents and heavy metal ions
Dosage Forms
    Injection, as sodium folate: 5 mg/mL (10 mL); 10 mg/mL (10 mL)
        Folvite®: 5 mg/mL (10 mL)
    Tablet: 0.1 mg, 0.4 mg, 0.8 mg, 1 mg
        Folvite®: 1 mg

- ♦ **folinic acid** *see* leucovorin *on page 362*
- ♦ **Folitab** *see* folic acid *on page 281*
- ♦ **Follistim®** *see* follitropin beta *on page 281*

follitropin alpha (foe li TRO pin AL fa)

U.S. Brand Names Gonal-F®
Generic Available No
Therapeutic Category Ovulation Stimulator
Use Induction of ovulation in the anovulatory infertile patient in whom the cause of infertility is functional and not caused by primary ovarian failure
Usual Dosage Adults (women): S.C.: Initial: 75 units/day for the first cycle; an incremental dose adjustment of up to 37.5 units may be considered after 14 days; treatment duration should not exceed 35 days unless an E2 rise indicates follicular development
Dosage Forms Injection: 75 FSH units, 150 FSH units

follitropin beta (foe li TRO pin BAY ta)

U.S. Brand Names Follistim®
Generic Available No
Therapeutic Category Ovulation Stimulator
Use The development of multiple follicles in infertility patients treated in Assisted Reproductive Technology (ART) program and for the induction of ovulation
Usual Dosage Adults (female): I.M./S.C.:
    Ovulation: In general, a sequential treatment scheme is recommended. This usually starts with daily administration of 75 int. units (International Units) FSH activity. The starting dose is maintained for at least seven days. If there is no ovarian response, the daily dose is then gradually increased until follicle growth and/or plasma estradiol levels indicate an adequate pharmacodynamic response. A daily increase in estradiol levels of 40% to 100% is considered to be optimal. The daily dose is then maintained until preovulatory conditions are reached. Preovulatory conditions are reached when
(Continued)

follitropin beta *(Continued)*

there ultrasonographic evidence of a dominant follicle of at least 18 mm in diameter and/or when plasma estradiol levels of 300-900 picograms/mL (1000-3000 pmol/L) are attained; usually, 7-14 days of treatment are sufficient to reach this state. The administration is then discontinued and ovulation can be induced by administering human chorionic gonadotropin (hCG). If the number of responding follicles is too high or estradiol levels increase too rapidly (ie, more than a daily doubling of estradiol for 2-3 consecutive days), the daily dose should be decreased. Since follicles of >14 mm may lead to pregnancies, multiple preovulatory follicles exceeding 14 mm carry the risk of multiple gestations. In that case, hCG should be withheld and pregnancy should be avoided in order to prevent multiple gestations.

ART: Various stimulation protocols are applied; starting dose of 150-225 units is recommended for at least the first four days; thereafter, the dose may be adjusted individually, based upon ovarian response. In clinical studies, it was shown that maintenance dosages ranging from 75-375 units for 6-12 days are sufficient, although longer treatment may be necessary. May be given either alone, or in combination with a GnRH agonist to prevent premature luteinization; in the latter case, a higher total treatment dose of Follistim® may be required. Ovarian response is monitored by ultrasonography and measurement of plasma estradiol levels; when ultrasonographic evaluation indicates the presence of at least three follicles of 16-20 mm, and there is evidence of a good estradiol (plasma levels of about 300-400 picogram/mL (1000-1300 pmol/L) for each follicle with a diameter >18 mm), the final phase of maturation of the follicles is induced by administration of hCG. Oocyte retrieval is performed 34-35 hours later.

Dosage Forms Injection: 75 FSH units

- ♦ **Follutein®** *see* chorionic gonadotropin *on page 149*
- ♦ **Folvite®** *see* folic acid *on page 281*

fomepizole *(foe ME pi zole)*

Synonyms 4-methylpyrazole; 4-MP
U.S. Brand Names Antizol™
Generic Available No
Therapeutic Category Antidote
Use Ethylene glycol and methanol toxicity (antifreeze); may be useful in propylene glycol; unclear whether it is useful in disulfiram-ethanol reactions
Usual Dosage Oral: 15 mg/kg followed by 5 mg/kg in 12 hours and then 10 mg/kg every 12 hours until levels of toxin are not present

One other protocol (from France) suggests an infusion of 10-20 mg/kg before dialysis and intravenous infusion of 1-1.5 mg/kg/hour during hemodialysis

META (methylpyrazole for toxic alcohol) study in U.S. (investigational): Loading I.V. dose of 15 mg/kg followed by 10 mg/kg I.V. every 12 hours for 48 hours; continue treatment until methanol or ethylene glycol levels are <20 mg/dL; supplemental doses required during dialysis; contact your local poison center regarding this study

Dosage Forms Injection: 1 g/mL (1.5 mL)

fomivirsen *New Drug* *(foe MI vir sen)*

U.S. Brand Names Vitravene™
Generic Available No
Therapeutic Category Antiviral Agent, Ophthalmic
Use Treatment of cytomegalovirus (CMV); CMV can affect one or both eyes in patients with acquired immunodeficiency syndrome (AIDS) who cannot take other treatment(s) for CMV retinitis or who did not respond to other treatments for CMV retinitis; the diagnosis should be made after a comprehensive eye exam, including indirect ophthalmoscopy
Usual Dosage Treatment with Vitravene™ consists of two phases:

Phase I (induction phase): One injection (6.6 mg) every other week for 2 doses
Phase II (maintenance phase): One injection (6.6 mg) once every 4 weeks

Dosage Forms Injection, intravitreal: 6.6 mg

- ♦ **Foradil®** *see* formoterol *(Canada only) on page 282*
- ♦ **Forane®** *see* isoflurane *on page 347*

formoterol *(Canada only)* *(for MOT ter ol)*

Canadian Brand Names Foradil®
Generic Available No
Therapeutic Category Adrenergic Agonist Agent; Beta$_2$-Adrenergic Agonist Agent; Bronchodilator

Use Long-term treatment in maintenance of asthma and in prevention of bronchospasm in patients >12 years of age with reversible obstructive airway disease

Usual Dosage Inhalation: One capsule (12 mcg) inhaled using the Aerolizer inhaler twice daily, morning and evening

Dosage Forms Capsule, for inhalation use, as fumarate: 12 mcg

- ♦ **Formula E** *see* guaifenesin *on page 299*
- ♦ **Formula Q®** *see* quinine *on page 537*
- ♦ **5-formyl tetrahydrofolate** *see* leucovorin *on page 362*
- ♦ **Fortaz®** *see* ceftazidime *on page 124*
- ♦ **Fortovase®** *see* saquinavir *on page 559*
- ♦ **Fortum** *see* ceftazidime *on page 124*
- ♦ **Fosamax®** *see* alendronate *on page 27*

foscarnet (fòs KAR net)

Synonyms PFA; phosphonoformic acid
U.S. Brand Names Foscavir®
Generic Available No
Therapeutic Category Antiviral Agent
Use Alternative to ganciclovir for treatment of CMV infections and is possibly the preferred initial agent for the treatment of CMV retinitis except for those patients with decreased renal function; treatment of acyclovir-resistant mucocutaneous herpes simplex virus infections in immunocompromised patients; and acyclovir-resistant herpes zoster infections
Usual Dosage
Induction treatment: 60 mg/kg 3 times/day for 14-21 days
Maintenance therapy: 90-120 mg/kg/day
Nursing/Pharmacy Information
Provide adequate hydration with I.V. normal saline prior to and during treatment to minimize nephrotoxicity; 24 mg/mL solution can be administered without further dilution when using a central venous catheter for infusion; for peripheral vein administration, the solution **must** be diluted to a final concentration **not to exceed** 12 mg/mL; administer by I.V. infusion at a rate **not to exceed** 60 mg/kg/dose over 1 hour or 120 mg/kg/dose over 2 hours
Monitor serum creatinine, calcium, phosphorus, potassium, magnesium; hemoglobin
Stability: Do not admix or run with other drugs, multiple incompatibilities
Dosage Forms Injection: 24 mg/mL (250 mL, 500 mL)

- ♦ **Foscavir®** *see* foscarnet *on page 283*

fosfomycin (fos foe MYE sin)

U.S. Brand Names Monurol™
Generic Available No
Therapeutic Category Antibiotic, Miscellaneous
Use Treatment of uncomplicated urinary tract infections
Usual Dosage Adults: Oral: Single dose of 3 g in 4 oz of water
Dosage Forms Powder, as tromethamine: 3 g, to be mixed in 4 oz of water

fosinopril (foe SIN oh pril)

U.S. Brand Names Monopril®
Generic Available No
Therapeutic Category Angiotensin-Converting Enzyme (ACE) Inhibitor
Use Treatment of hypertension, either alone or in combination with other antihypertensive agents
Usual Dosage Adults: Oral: 20-40 mg/day
Nursing/Pharmacy Information
May cause depression in some patients; discontinue if angioedema of the face, extremities, lips, tongue, or glottis occurs; watch for hypotensive effects within 1-3 hours of first dose or new higher dose
Monitor serum potassium
Dosage Forms Tablet: 10 mg, 20 mg

fosphenytoin (FOS fen i toyn)

U.S. Brand Names Cerebyx®
Generic Available No
Therapeutic Category Hydantoin
Use Indicated for short-term parenteral administration when other means of phenytoin administration are unavailable, inappropriate or deemed less advantageous; the safety and effectiveness of fosphenytoin in this use has not been
(Continued)

fosphenytoin *(Continued)*

systematically evaluated for more than 5 days; may be used for the control of generalized convulsive status epilepticus and prevention and treatment of seizures occurring during neurosurgery

Usual Dosage The dose, concentration in solutions, and infusion rates for fosphenytoin are expressed as phenytoin sodium equivalents; fosphenytoin should always be prescribed and dispensed in phenytoin sodium equivalents

Status epilepticus: I.V.: Adults: Loading dose: Phenytoin equivalent 15-20 mg/kg I.V. administered at 100-150 mg/minute

Nonemergent loading and maintenance dosing: I.V. or I.M.: Adults:

Loading dose: Phenytoin equivalent 10-20 mg/kg I.V. or I.M. (max I.V. rate 150 mg/minute)

Initial daily maintenance dose: Phenytoin equivalent 4-6 mg/kg/day I.V. or I.M.

I.M. or I.V. substitution for oral phenytoin therapy: May be substituted for oral phenytoin sodium at the same total daily dose, however, Dilantin® capsules are ~90% bioavailable by the oral route; phenytoin, supplied as fosphenytoin, is 100% bioavailable by both the I.M. and I.V. routes; for this reason, plasma phenytoin concentrations may increase when I.M. or I.V. fosphenytoin is substituted for oral phenytoin sodium therapy; in clinical trials I.M. fosphenytoin was administered as a single daily dose utilizing either 1 or 2 injection sites; some patients may require more frequent dosing

Nursing/Pharmacy Information I.V. administration rate should not exceed 150 mg/minute

Dosage Forms Injection, as sodium: 150 mg [equivalent to phenytoin sodium 100 mg]; 750 mg, [equivalent to phenytoin sodium 500 mg]

- ◆ **Fostex®** [OTC] *see* sulfur and salicylic acid *on page 589*
- ◆ **Fostex® 10% BPO Gel** [OTC] *see* benzoyl peroxide *on page 81*
- ◆ **Fostex® 10% Wash** [OTC] *see* benzoyl peroxide *on page 81*
- ◆ **Fostex® Bar** [OTC] *see* benzoyl peroxide *on page 81*
- ◆ **Fotexina** *see* cefotaxime *on page 122*
- ◆ **Fototar®** [OTC] *see* coal tar *on page 162*
- ◆ **Fragmin®** *see* dalteparin *on page 180*
- ◆ **Fraxiparine®** *see* nadroparin *(Canada only) on page 427*
- ◆ **Freezone® Solution** [OTC] *see* salicylic acid *on page 557*
- ◆ **Froben®** *see* flurbiprofen *on page 278*
- ◆ **Froben-SR®** *see* flurbiprofen *on page 278*
- ◆ **Froxal** *see* cefuroxime *on page 126*
- ◆ **frusemide** *see* furosemide *on page 285*
- ◆ **FS Shampoo® Topical** *see* fluocinolone *on page 273*
- ◆ **5-FU** *see* fluorouracil *on page 275*
- ◆ **Fucidin® I.V.** *see* fusidic acid *(Canada only) on page 286*
- ◆ **Fucidin® Oral Suspension** *see* fusidic acid *(Canada only) on page 286*
- ◆ **Fucidin® Tablet** *see* fusidic acid *(Canada only) on page 286*
- ◆ **FUDR®** *see* floxuridine *on page 270*
- ◆ **Ful-Glo® Ophthalmic Strips** *see* fluorescein sodium *on page 273*
- ◆ **Fulvicin® P/G** *see* griseofulvin *on page 298*
- ◆ **Fulvicin-U/F®** *see* griseofulvin *on page 298*
- ◆ **Fulvina® P/G** *see* griseofulvin *on page 298*
- ◆ **Fumasorb®** [OTC] *see* ferrous fumarate *on page 264*
- ◆ **Fumerin®** [OTC] *see* ferrous fumarate *on page 264*
- ◆ **Funduscein® Injection** *see* fluorescein sodium *on page 273*
- ◆ **Fungiquim** *see* miconazole *on page 413*
- ◆ **Fungistat** *see* terconazole *on page 597*
- ◆ **Fungistat Dual** *see* terconazole *on page 597*
- ◆ **Fungizone®** *see* amphotericin B (conventional) *on page 44*
- ◆ **Fungoid® AF Topical Solution** [OTC] *see* undecylenic acid and derivatives *on page 637*
- ◆ **Fungoid® Creme** *see* miconazole *on page 413*
- ◆ **Fungoid® Tincture** *see* miconazole *on page 413*
- ◆ **Furacin® Topical** *see* nitrofurazone *on page 444*
- ◆ **Furadantin®** *see* nitrofurantoin *on page 444*
- ◆ **Furadantina** *see* nitrofurantoin *on page 444*
- ◆ **Furalan®** *see* nitrofurantoin *on page 444*

♦ **Furan**® see nitrofurantoin *on page 444*
♦ **Furanite**® see nitrofurantoin *on page 444*

furazolidone (fyoor a ZOE li done)

U.S. Brand Names Furoxone®
Mexican Brand Names Furoxona Gotas; Furoxona Tabletas; Fuxol
Generic Available No
Therapeutic Category Antiprotozoal
Use Treatment of bacterial or protozoal diarrhea and enteritis caused by susceptible organisms: *Giardia lamblia* and *Vibrio cholerae*
Usual Dosage Oral:
   Children >1 month: 5-8.8 mg/kg/day in 3-4 divided doses for 7-10 days, not to exceed 400 mg/day
   Adults: 100 mg 4 times/day for 7-10 days
Dietary Considerations Avoid tyramine-containing foods (cheese, broad beans, dry or aged sausage, nonfresh meat, liver, salami, mortadella, concentrated yeast extracts, liquid and powdered protein supplements, fermented bean curd and soya bean, meat extract and hydrolyzed protein extracts, raspberries, Chianti wine, Kimchee or sauerkraut)
Nursing/Pharmacy Information Monitor CBC
Dosage Forms
   Liquid: 50 mg/15 mL (60 mL, 473 mL)
   Tablet: 100 mg

♦ **furazosin** see prazosin *on page 513*

furosemide (fyoor OH se mide)

Synonyms frusemide
U.S. Brand Names Lasix®
Canadian Brand Names Apo®-Furosemide; Furoside®; Lasix® Special; Novo-Semide®; Uritol®
Mexican Brand Names Edenol; Henexal
Generic Available Yes
Therapeutic Category Diuretic, Loop
Use Management of edema associated with congestive heart failure and hepatic or renal disease; used alone or in combination with antihypertensives in treatment of hypertension
Usual Dosage
   Infants and Children:
      Oral: 2 mg/kg/dose increased in increments of 1 mg/kg/dose with each succeeding dose until a satisfactory effect is achieved to a maximum of 6 mg/kg/dose no more frequently than 6 hours
      I.M., I.V.: 1 mg/kg/dose, increasing by each succeeding dose at 1 mg/kg/dose at intervals of 6-12 hours until a satisfactory response up to 6 mg/kg/dose
   Adults:
      Oral: Initial: 20-80 mg/dose, increase in increments of 20-40 mg/dose at intervals of 6-8 hours; usual maintenance dose interval is twice daily or every day
      I.M., I.V.: 20-40 mg/dose, may be repeated in 1-2 hours as needed and increased by 20 mg/dose with each succeeding dose up to 600 mg/day; usual dosing interval: 6-12 hours
Dietary Considerations This product may cause a potassium loss; your physician may prescribe a potassium supplement, another medication to help prevent the potassium loss, or recommend that you eat foods high in potassium, especially citrus fruits; do not change your diet on your own while taking this medication, especially if you are taking potassium supplements or medications to reduce potassium loss; too much potassium can be as harmful as too little; ideally, should be administered on an empty stomach; however, may be administered with food or milk if GI distress; do not mix with acidic solutions; limit intake of natural licorice
Nursing/Pharmacy Information
   I.V. injections should be administered slowly over 1-2 minutes; replace parenteral therapy with oral therapy as soon as possible; for continuous infusion furosemide in patients with severely impaired renal function, do not exceed 4 mg/minute; be alert to complaints about hearing difficulty; check the patient for orthostasis; may be administered undiluted direct I.V. at a maximum rate of 0.5 mg/kg/minute for doses <120 mg and 4 mg/minute for doses >120 mg; may also be diluted for infusion 1-2 mg/mL (maximum: 10 mg/mL) over 10-15 minutes (following maximum rate as above)
(Continued)

furosemide *(Continued)*

Monitor blood pressure, serum electrolytes, renal function; in high doses monitor hearing

Stability: Protect from light; do not dispense discolored tablets or injection; I.V. infusion solution mixed in normal saline or D_5W solution is stable for 24 hours at room temperature; do not use solutions that are yellow in color

Dosage Forms

Injection: 10 mg/mL (2 mL, 4 mL, 5 mL, 6 mL, 8 mL, 10 mL, 12 mL)

Solution, oral: 10 mg/mL (60 mL, 120 mL); 40 mg/5 mL (5 mL, 10 mL, 500 mL)

Tablet: 20 mg, 40 mg, 80 mg

♦ **Furoside®** *see* furosemide *on page 285*
♦ **Furoxona Gotas** *see* furazolidone *on page 285*
♦ **Furoxona Tabletas** *see* furazolidone *on page 285*
♦ **Furoxone®** *see* furazolidone *on page 285*

fusidic acid *(Canada only)* (fyoo SI dik AS id)

Synonyms Sodium Fusidate

Canadian Brand Names Fucidin® I.V.; Fucidin® Oral Suspension; Fucidin® Tablet

Generic Available No

Therapeutic Category Antifungal Agent, Systemic

Use The treatment of the following infections when due to susceptible strains of *S. aureus*, both penicillinase producing and nonpenicillinase producing: skin and soft tissue infections, osteomyelitis. For patients with staphylococcal infections where other antibiotics have failed (ie, patients with staphylococcal septicemia, burns, endocarditis, pneumonia, cystic fibrosis). Appropriate culture and susceptibility studies should be performed. Fucidin® may be administered to those patients in whom a staphylococcal infection is suspected. This antibiotic treatment may subsequently require modification once these results become available.

Usual Dosage Adults:

I.V.: 500 mg 3 times/day

Oral: 500 mg 3 times/day

Dosage Forms

Powder for injection: 500 mg

Suspension, oral (banana flavor): 246 mg/5 mL (50 mL)

Tablet, sodium fusidate: 250 mg (equivalent to 240 mg fusidic acid)

♦ **Fustaren Retard** *see* diclofenac *on page 198*
♦ **Fuxen** *see* naproxen *on page 432*
♦ **Fuxol** *see* furazolidone *on page 285*
♦ **G-1®** *see* butalbital compound and acetaminophen *on page 99*

gabapentin (GA ba pen tin)

U.S. Brand Names Neurontin®

Generic Available No

Therapeutic Category Anticonvulsant

Use Adjunct for treatment of drug-refractory partial and secondarily generalized seizures

Usual Dosage Adults: Oral: 900-1800 mg/day administered in 3 divided doses; therapy is initiated with a rapid titration, beginning with 300 mg on day 1, 300 mg twice daily on day 2, and 300 mg 3 times/day on day 3

Discontinuing therapy or replacing with an alternative agent should be done gradually over a minimum of 7 days

Dietary Considerations May be administered with or without food serum lipids may see increases in total cholesterol, HDL cholesterol and triglycerides; hyperlipidemia and hypercholesterolemia have been reported with gabapentin

Nursing/Pharmacy Information Administer first dose on first day at bedtime to avoid somnolence and dizziness

Dosage Forms Capsule: 100 mg, 300 mg, 400 mg

♦ **Gabitril®** *see* tiagabine *on page 611*
♦ **Galecin** *see* clindamycin *on page 156*
♦ **Galedol** *see* diclofenac *on page 198*
♦ **Galidrin** *see* ranitidine hydrochloride *on page 541*

gallamine triethiodide (GAL a meen trye eth EYE oh dide)

U.S. Brand Names Flaxedil®

Generic Available No

Therapeutic Category Skeletal Muscle Relaxant

Use Produce skeletal muscle relaxation during surgery after general anesthesia has been induced

Usual Dosage I.V.: 1 mg/kg then repeat dose of 0.5-1 mg/kg in 30-40 minutes for prolonged procedures

Nursing/Pharmacy Information Have neostigmine or edrophonium and epinephrine nearby; analgesics and sedatives are recommended

Dosage Forms Injection: 20 mg/mL (10 mL)

gallium nitrate (GAL ee um NYE trate)

U.S. Brand Names Ganite™

Generic Available No

Therapeutic Category Antidote

Use Treatment of clearly symptomatic cancer-related hypercalcemia that has not responded to adequate hydration

Usual Dosage Adults: I.V. infusion: 200 mg/m^2 for 5 consecutive days

Nursing/Pharmacy Information

Monitor serum creatinine, BUN, and serum calcium

Stability: Store at room temperature; when diluted in normal saline or D$_5$W, stable for 48 hours at room temperature or 7 days at refrigeration

Dosage Forms Injection: 25 mg/mL (20 mL)

- ♦ **Gamastan® _(Discontinued)_** see page 743
- ♦ **Gamikal** see amikacin on page 36
- ♦ **Gamimune® N** see immune globulin, intravenous on page 336
- ♦ **gamma benzene hexachloride** see lindane on page 370
- ♦ **Gammabulin Immuno** see immune globulin, intramuscular on page 335
- ♦ **Gammagard® Injection _(Discontinued)_** see page 743
- ♦ **Gammagard® S/D** see immune globulin, intravenous on page 336
- ♦ **gamma globulin** see immune globulin, intramuscular on page 335
- ♦ **gammaphos** see amifostine on page 36
- ♦ **Gammar® _(Discontinued)_** see page 743
- ♦ **Gammar®-P I.V.** see immune globulin, intravenous on page 336
- ♦ **Gamulin® Rh** see Rh$_o$(D) immune globulin (intramuscular) on page 546

ganciclovir (gan SYE kloe veer)

Synonyms DHPG sodium; GCV sodium; nordeoxyguanosine

U.S. Brand Names Cytovene®; Vitrasert®

Mexican Brand Names Cymevene

Generic Available No

Therapeutic Category Antiviral Agent

Use

Parenteral: Treatment of CMV retinitis in immunocompromised individuals, including patients with acquired immunodeficiency syndrome; prophylaxis of CMV infection in transplant patients

Oral: Alternative to the I.V. formulation for maintenance treatment of CMV retinitis in immunocompromised patients, including patients with AIDS, in whom retinitis is stable following appropriate induction therapy and for whom the risk of more rapid progression is balanced by the benefit associated with avoiding daily I.V. infusions.

Usual Dosage Slow I.V. infusion:

Retinitis: Children >3 months and Adults: Induction therapy: 5 mg/kg/dose every 12 hours for 14-21 days followed by maintenance therapy; maintenance therapy: 5 mg/kg/day as a single daily dose for 7 days/week or 6 mg/kg/day for 5 days/week

Other CMV infections: 5 mg/kg/dose every 12 hours for 14-21 days or 2.5 mg/kg/dose every 8 hours; maintenance therapy: 5 mg/kg/day as a single daily dose for 7 days/week or 6 mg/kg/day for 5 days/week

Nursing/Pharmacy Information

Handle and dispose according to guidelines issued for cytotoxic drugs; to minimize the risk of phlebitis, infuse through a large vein with adequate blood flow; maintain adequate patient hydration; administer by slow I.V. infusion over at least 1 hour at a final concentration for administration not to exceed 10 mg/mL

Monitor CBC with differential and platelet count, serum creatinine, ophthalmologic exams

Stability: Reconstituted solution is stable for 12 hours at room temperature; **do not refrigerate**; reconstitute with sterile water **not** bacteriostatic water because parabens may cause precipitation

(Continued)

ganciclovir *(Continued)*

Dosage Forms
Capsule: 250 mg, 500 mg
Implant, intravitreal: 4.5 mg released gradually over 5-8 months
Powder for injection, lyophilized: 500 mg (10 mL)

ganirelix *New Drug* (ga ni REL ix)

U.S. Brand Names Antagon™
Generic Available No
Therapeutic Category Antigonadotropic Agent
Use Inhibits premature luteinizing hormone (LH) surges in women undergoing controlled ovarian hyperstimulation in fertility clinics.
Usual Dosage Adult: S.C.: 250 mcg/day during the early to midfollicular phase after initiating follicle-stimulating hormone. Treatment should be continued daily until the day of chorionic gonadotropin administration.
Dosage Forms Injection: Prefilled glass syringe: 250 mcg/0.5 mL with 27-gauge x ½ inch needle

- ◆ **Ganite™** *see* gallium nitrate *on page 287*
- ◆ **Gantanol®** *see* sulfamethoxazole *on page 587*
- ◆ **Gantrisin®** *see* sulfisoxazole *on page 588*
- ◆ **Gantrisin® Ophthalmic** *(Discontinued) see page 743*
- ◆ **Gantrisin® Tablet** *(Discontinued) see page 743*
- ◆ **Garalen** *see* gentamicin *on page 290*
- ◆ **Garamicina®** *see* gentamicin *on page 290*
- ◆ **Garamycin®** *see* gentamicin *on page 290*
- ◆ **Garatec** *see* gentamicin *on page 290*
- ◆ **Gas-Ban DS® [OTC]** *see* aluminum hydroxide, magnesium hydroxide, and simethicone *on page 34*
- ◆ **Gastrec** *see* ranitidine hydrochloride *on page 541*
- ◆ **Gastrocrom®** *see* cromolyn sodium *on page 171*
- ◆ **Gastrografin®** *see* radiological/contrast media (ionic) *on page 539*
- ◆ **Gastrosed™** *see* hyoscyamine *on page 329*
- ◆ **Gas-X® [OTC]** *see* simethicone *on page 566*

gatifloxacin *New Drug* (ga ti FLOKS a sin)

U.S. Brand Names Tequin™
Therapeutic Category Antibiotic, Quinolone
Use Treatment of infections due to susceptible strains of the designated microorganisms in the conditions listed: Acute bacterial exacerbation of chronic bronchitis, acute sinusitis, community-acquired pneumonia, uncomplicated urinary tract infections (cystitis), complicated urinary tract infections, pyelonephritis, uncomplicated urethral and cervical gonorrhea, acute, uncomplicated rectal infections in women
Usual Dosage I.V. Oral: Adults: 400 mg given once daily, depending on infection, for 1 to 14 days
Dosage Forms
Infusion, preservative free, ready-to-use: 200 mg (100 mL); 400 mg (200 mL)
Injection, preservative free (single use vials): 200 mg (20 mL); 400 mg (40 mL)
Tablet: 200 mg, 400 mg

- ◆ **Gaviscon®-2 Tablet [OTC]** *see* aluminum hydroxide and magnesium trisilicate *on page 34*
- ◆ **Gaviscon® Liquid [OTC]** *see* aluminum hydroxide and magnesium carbonate *on page 34*
- ◆ **Gaviscon® Tablet [OTC]** *see* aluminum hydroxide and magnesium trisilicate *on page 34*
- ◆ **G-CSF** *see* filgrastim *on page 267*
- ◆ **GCV sodium** *see* ganciclovir *on page 287*
- ◆ **Gee Gee® [OTC]** *see* guaifenesin *on page 299*

gelatin, absorbable (JEL a tin, ab SORB a ble)

Synonyms absorbable gelatin sponge
U.S. Brand Names Gelfilm® Ophthalmic; Gelfoam® Topical
Generic Available No
Therapeutic Category Hemostatic Agent
Use Adjunct to provide hemostasis in surgery; also used in oral and dental surgery; in open prostatic surgery

Usual Dosage Topical: Hemostasis: Apply packs or sponges dry or saturated with sodium chloride. When applied dry, hold in place with moderate pressure. When applied wet, squeeze to remove air bubbles. Prostatectomy cones are designed for use with the Foley bag catheter. The powder is applied as a paste prepared by adding approximately 4 mL of sterile saline solution to the powder.

Nursing/Pharmacy Information
Apply dry or saturated with sodium chloride
Stability: To ensure sterility, use immediately after withdrawal from envelope

Dosage Forms
Gelfilm® (sterile)
Film: 100 mm x 125 mm (1s)
Ophthalmic: 25 mm x 50 mm (6s)
Gelfoam®
Cones, prostatectomy:
Size 13 cm (13 cm in diameter) (6s)
Size 18 cm (18 cm in diameter) (6s)
Packs:
Size 2 cm (40 cm x 2 cm) (1s)
Size 6 cm (40 cm x 6 cm) (6s)
Packs, dental:
Size 2 (10 mm x 20 mm x 7 mm) (15s)
Size 4 (20 mm x 20 mm x 7 mm) (15s)
Sponges:
Size 12-3 mm (20 mm x 60 mm x 3 mm) (4s)
Size 12-7 mm (20 mm x 60 mm x 7 mm) (4s)
Size 50 (80 mm x 62.5 mm x 10 mm) (4s)
Size 100 (80 mm x 125 mm x 10 mm) (6s)
Size 100, compressed (80 mm x 125 mm) (6s)
Size 200 (80 mm x 250 mm x 10 mm) (6s)

gelatin, pectin, and methylcellulose
(JEL a tin, PEK tin, & meth il SEL yoo lose)
U.S. Brand Names Orabase® Plain [OTC]
Generic Available No
Therapeutic Category Protectant, Topical
Use Temporary relief from minor oral irritations
Usual Dosage Oral: Press small dabs into place until the involved area is coated with a thin film; do not try to spread onto area; may be used as often as needed
Dosage Forms Paste, oral: 5 g, 15 g

♦ **Gelfilm® Ophthalmic** see gelatin, absorbable on page 288
♦ **Gelfoam® Topical** see gelatin, absorbable on page 288
♦ **Gel-Kam®** see fluoride on page 274
♦ **Gelpirin® [OTC]** see acetaminophen, aspirin, and caffeine on page 16
♦ **Gel-Tin® [OTC]** see fluoride on page 274
♦ **Gelucast®** see zinc gelatin on page 660
♦ **Gelusil® Liquid (Discontinued)** see page 743

gemcitabine (jem SIT a been)
U.S. Brand Names Gemzar®
Generic Available No
Therapeutic Category Antineoplastic Agent
Use Treatment of patients with inoperable pancreatic cancer
Usual Dosage Adults: I.V.: 1000 mg/^{2} over 30 minutes once weekly for up to 7 weeks
Dosage Forms Powder for injection, as hydrochloride, lyophilized: 20 mg/mL (10 mL, 50 mL)

gemfibrozil (jem FI broe zil)
Synonyms CI-719
U.S. Brand Names Lopid®
Canadian Brand Names Apo-Gemfibrozil®; Nu-Gemfibrozil
Generic Available Yes
Therapeutic Category Antihyperlipidemic Agent, Miscellaneous
Use Hypertriglyceridemia in types IV and V hyperlipidemia; increases HDL cholesterol
Usual Dosage Oral: 1200 mg/day in 2 divided doses, 30 minutes before breakfast and supper
Dietary Considerations Should be administered 30 minutes before meals
(Continued)

gemfibrozil *(Continued)*

Nursing/Pharmacy Information Monitor serum cholesterol; abnormal elevation of AST, ALT, LDH, bilirubin and alkaline phosphatase have occurred; if no appreciable triglyceride or cholesterol, lowering effect occurs after 3 months, the drug should be discontinued

Dosage Forms
Capsule: 300 mg
Tablet, film coated: 600 mg

- ♦ **Gemzar®** *see* gemcitabine *on page 289*
- ♦ **Genabid®** *see* papaverine *on page 469*
- ♦ **Genac® Tablet [OTC]** *see* triprolidine and pseudoephedrine *on page 632*
- ♦ **Genagesic®** *see* guaifenesin and phenylpropanolamine *on page 301*
- ♦ **Genahist® Oral** *see* diphenhydramine *on page 208*
- ♦ **Genamin® Cold Syrup [OTC]** *see* chlorpheniramine and phenylpropanolamine *on page 139*
- ♦ **Genamin® Expectorant [OTC]** *see* guaifenesin and phenylpropanolamine *on page 301*
- ♦ **Genapap® [OTC]** *see* acetaminophen *on page 13*
- ♦ **Genasoft® Plus [OTC]** *see* docusate and casanthranol *on page 215*
- ♦ **Genaspor® [OTC]** *see* tolnaftate *on page 618*
- ♦ **Genatap® Elixir [OTC]** *see* brompheniramine and phenylpropanolamine *on page 94*
- ♦ **Genatuss® [OTC]** *see* guaifenesin *on page 299*
- ♦ **Genatuss DM® [OTC]** *see* guaifenesin and dextromethorphan *on page 300*
- ♦ **Gencalc® 600 [OTC]** *see* calcium carbonate *on page 103*
- ♦ **Gen-Clobetasol** *see* clobetasol *on page 157*
- ♦ **Gen-D-phen® *(Discontinued)*** *see page 743*
- ♦ **Genebs® [OTC]** *see* acetaminophen *on page 13*
- ♦ **Genenicina®** *see* gentamicin *on page 290*
- ♦ **Geneye® Ophthalmic [OTC]** *see* tetrahydrozoline *on page 602*
- ♦ **Gen-Glybe** *see* glyburide *on page 294*
- ♦ **Gen-K®** *see* potassium chloride *on page 506*
- ♦ **Genkova** *see* gentamicin *on page 290*
- ♦ **Gen-Lac** *see* lactulose *on page 359*
- ♦ **Gen-Minoxidil** *see* minoxidil *on page 417*
- ♦ **Gen-Nifedipine** *see* nifedipine *on page 442*
- ♦ **Genoptic®** *see* gentamicin *on page 290*
- ♦ **Genora® 0.5/35** *see* ethinyl estradiol and norethindrone *on page 250*
- ♦ **Genora® 1/35** *see* ethinyl estradiol and norethindrone *on page 250*
- ♦ **Genora® 1/50** *see* mestranol and norethindrone *on page 396*
- ♦ **Genotropin®** *see* human growth hormone *on page 315*
- ♦ **Genoxal** *see* cyclophosphamide *on page 175*
- ♦ **Gen-Pindolol** *see* pindolol *on page 495*
- ♦ **Genpril® [OTC]** *see* ibuprofen *on page 332*
- ♦ **Genrex** *see* gentamicin *on page 290*
- ♦ **Gentacidin®** *see* gentamicin *on page 290*
- ♦ **Gentacin** *see* gentamicin *on page 290*
- ♦ **Gent-AK®** *see* gentamicin *on page 290*

gentamicin *(jen ta MYE sin)*

U.S. Brand Names Garamycin®; Genoptic®; Gentacidin®; Gent-AK®; Gentrasul®; G-myticin®; Jenamicin®

Canadian Brand Names Cidomycin®; Garatec; Lomicin® Ophthalmic; Ocugram®

Mexican Brand Names Garalen; Garamicina®; Genenicina®; Genkova; Genrex; Gentacin; Gentarim; Nozolon; Quilagen; Servigenta; Yectamicina

Generic Available Yes

Therapeutic Category Aminoglycoside (Antibiotic); Antibiotic, Ophthalmic; Antibiotic, Topical

Use Treatment of susceptible bacterial infections, normally due to gram-negative organisms including *Pseudomonas, Proteus, Serratia,* and gram-positive *Staphylococcus;* treatment of bone infections, CNS infections, respiratory tract infections, skin and soft tissue infections, as well as abdominal and urinary tract infections, endocarditis, and septicemia; used in combination with ampicillin as empiric therapy for sepsis in newborns; used topically to treat superficial infections of the skin or ophthalmic infections caused by susceptible bacteria

Usual Dosage Dosage should be based on an estimate of ideal body weight

Infants and Children >3 months: Intrathecal: 1-2 mg/day

Infants and Children <5 years: 2.5 mg/kg/dose every 8 hours

Children >5 years: 1.5-2.5 mg/kg/dose every 8 hours

Ophthalmic: Solution: 1-2 drops every 2-4 hours, up to 2 drops every hour for severe infections; ointment: 2-3 times/day

Topical: Apply 3-4 times/day

Adults:

I.M., I.V.: 3-5 mg/kg/day in divided doses every 8 hours

Topical: Apply 3-4 times/day

Ophthalmic: Solution: 1-2 drops every 2-4 hours; ointment: 2-3 times/day

Dietary Considerations Calcium, magnesium, potassium: Renal wasting may cause hypocalcemia, hypomagnesemia and/or hypokalemia

Nursing/Pharmacy Information

Obtain drug levels after the third dose except in neonates and patients with rapidly changing renal function in whom levels need to be measured sooner; peak levels are drawn 30 minutes after the end of a 30-minute infusion; trough levels are drawn within 30 minutes before the next dose. Administer other antibiotics such as penicillins and cephalosporins at least 1 hour before or after gentamicin; administer by I.V. slow intermittent infusion over 30 minutes; final concentration for administration should not exceed 10 mg/mL; provide optimal patient hydration and perfusion.

Monitor urinalysis, urine output, BUN, serum creatinine, peak and trough plasma gentamicin levels

Stability: I.V. infusion solutions mixed in normal saline or D_5W solution are stable for 24 hours at room temperature; **incompatible** with penicillins

Dosage Forms Gentamicin sulfate:

Cream, topical, (Garamycin®, G-myticin®): 0.1% (15 g)

Infusion, in D_5W: 60 mg, 80 mg, 100 mg

Infusion, in NS: 40 mg, 60 mg, 80 mg, 90 mg, 100 mg, 120 mg

Injection: 40 mg/mL (1 mL, 1.5 mL, 2 mL)

Pediatric: 10 mg/mL (2 mL)

Intrathecal, preservative free (Garamycin®): 2 mg/mL (2 mL)

Ointment:

Ophthalmic: 0.3% [3 mg/g] (3.5 g)

Garamycin®, Genoptic® S.O.P., Gentacidin®, Gentak®: 0.3% [3 mg/g] (3.5 g)

Topical (Garamycin®, G-myticin®): 0.1% (15 g)

Solution, ophthalmic: 0.3% (5 mL, 15 mL)

Garamycin®, Genoptic®, Gentacidin®, Gentak®: 0.3% (1 mL, 5 mL, 15 mL)

glatiramer acetate (gla TIR a mer AS e tate)

Synonyms copolymer-1

U.S. Brand Names Copaxone®

Generic Available No

Therapeutic Category Biological, Miscellaneous

(Continued)

glatiramer acetate *(Continued)*

Use Reduce the frequency of relapses in relapsing-remitting multiple sclerosis (MS)

Usual Dosage Adults: S.C.: 20 mg/day

Dosage Forms Injection: 20 mg (2 mL)

♦ **Glaucon**® *see* epinephrine *on page 234*

♦ **GlaucTabs**® *see* methazolamide *on page 400*

♦ **glibenclamide** *see* glyburide *on page 294*

♦ **Glibenil** *see* glyburide *on page 294*

gliclazide *(Canada only)* (GLYE kla zide)

Canadian Brand Names Diamicron®

Generic Available No

Therapeutic Category Antidiabetic Agent; Hypoglycemic Agent, Oral; Sulfonylurea Agent

Use Control of hyperglycemia in gliclazide responsive diabetes mellitus of stable, mild, nonketosis prone, maturity onset or adult type which cannot be controlled by proper dietary management and exercise, or when insulin therapy is not appropriate.

Usual Dosage Adults: Oral: There is no fixed dosage regimen for the management of diabetes mellitus with gliclazide or any other hypoglycemic agent. Determination of the proper dosage for gliclazide for each patient should be made on the basis of frequent determinations of blood glucose during dose titration and throughout maintenance. Recommended daily dosage: 80-320 mg. Dosage of ≥160 mg should be divided into 2 equal parts for twice daily administration. Gliclazide should be taken preferentially with meals. Recommended starting dose: 160 mg/day taken as 1 tablet twice daily with meals. Total daily dose should not exceed 320 mg.

Dosage Forms Tablet: 80 mg

glimepiride (GLYE me pye ride)

U.S. Brand Names Amaryl®

Generic Available No

Therapeutic Category Antidiabetic Agent, Oral

Use

Management of noninsulin-dependent diabetes mellitus (type II) as an adjunct to diet and exercise to lower blood glucose

In combination with insulin to lower blood glucose in patients whose hyperglycemia cannot be controlled by diet and exercise in conjunction with an oral hypoglycemic agent

Usual Dosage Oral (allow several days between dose titrations):

Adults: Initial: 1-2 mg once daily, administered with breakfast or the first main meal; usual maintenance dose: 1-4 mg once daily; after a dose of 2 mg once daily, increase in increments of 2 mg at 1- to 2-week intervals based upon the patient's blood glucose response to a maximum of 8 mg once daily

Elderly: Initial: 1 mg/day

Combination with insulin therapy (fasting glucose level for instituting combination therapy is in the range of >150 mg/dL in plasma or serum depending on the patient): 8 mg once daily with the first main meal

After starting with low-dose insulin, upward adjustments of insulin can be done approximately weekly as guided by frequent measurements of fasting blood glucose. Once stable, combination-therapy patients should monitor their capillary blood glucose on an ongoing basis, preferably daily.

Dietary Considerations Administer with breakfast or the first main meal of the day

Nursing/Pharmacy Information Patients who are NPO may need to have their dose held to avoid hypoglycemia

Dosage Forms Tablet: 1 mg, 2 mg, 4 mg

♦ **Glioten** *see* enalapril *on page 230*

glipizide (GLIP i zide)

Synonyms glydiazinamide

U.S. Brand Names Glucotrol®; Glucotrol® XL

Mexican Brand Names Minodiab

Generic Available Yes

Therapeutic Category Antidiabetic Agent, Oral

Use Management of noninsulin-dependent diabetes mellitus (type II)

Usual Dosage Adults: Oral: 2.5-40 mg/day; doses larger than 15-20 mg/day should be divided and administered twice daily

Dietary Considerations

Alcohol: A disulfiram-like reaction characterized by flushing, headache, nausea, vomiting, sweating or tachycardia; avoid alcohol

Food: Delays absorption by 40%; should be administered 30 minutes before meals to avoid erratic absorption

Glucose: Decreases blood glucose concentration; hypoglycemia may occur; educate patients how to detect and treat hypoglycemia; monitor for signs and symptoms of hypoglycemia; administer glucose if necessary; evaluate patient's diet and exercise regimen; may need to decrease or discontinue dose of sulfonylurea

Sodium: Reports of hyponatremia and SIADH; those at increased risk include patients on medications or who have medical conditions that predispose them to hyponatremia; monitor sodium serum concentration and fluid status; may need to restrict water intake

Nursing/Pharmacy Information Monitor fasting blood glucose, hemoglobin A, C, fructosamine

Dosage Forms

Tablet: 5 mg, 10 mg

Tablet, extended release: 5 mg, 10 mg

glucagon (GLOO ka gon)

Generic Available No

Therapeutic Category Antihypoglycemic Agent

Use Hypoglycemia; diagnostic aid in the radiologic examination of GI tract when a hypotonic state is needed; used with some success as a cardiac stimulant in management of severe cases of beta-adrenergic blocking agent overdosage

Usual Dosage

Hypoglycemia or insulin shock therapy: I.M., I.V., S.C.:

Children: 0.025-0.1 mg/kg/dose, not to exceed 1 mg/dose, repeated in 20 minutes as needed

Adults: 0.5-1 mg, may repeat in 20 minutes as needed

Diagnostic aid: Adults: I.M., I.V.: 0.25-2 mg 10 minutes prior to procedure

Nursing/Pharmacy Information

Parenteral: Dilute with manufacturer provided diluent resulting in 1 mg/mL; if doses exceeding 2 mg are used, dilute with sterile water instead of diluent; administer by direct I.V. injection

Monitor blood pressure, blood glucose

Stability: After reconstitution, use immediately; may be kept at 5°C for up to 48 hours if necessary

Dosage Forms Powder for injection, lyophilized: 1 mg [1 unit]; 10 mg [10 units]

♦ **Glucal** see glyburide on page 294

♦ **Glucerna™** see enteral nutritional products on page 233

♦ **glucocerebrosidase** see alglucerase on page 28

♦ **Glucophage®** see metformin on page 398

♦ **Glucophage® Forte** see metformin on page 398

glucose, instant (GLOO kose, IN stant)

U.S. Brand Names B-D Glucose® [OTC]; Glutose® [OTC]; Insta-Glucose® [OTC]

Generic Available Yes

Therapeutic Category Antihypoglycemic Agent

Use Management of hypoglycemia

Usual Dosage Oral: 10-20 g

Nursing/Pharmacy Information Monitor blood sugar closely and often until patient is stabilized; heart rate; mental status

Dosage Forms

Gel, oral (Glutose®, Insta-Glucose®): Dextrose 40% (25 g, 30.8 g, 80 g)

Tablet, chewable (B-D Glucose®): 5 g

glucose polymers (GLOO kose POL i merz)

U.S. Brand Names Moducal® [OTC]; Polycose® [OTC]; Sumacal® [OTC]

Generic Available Yes

Therapeutic Category Nutritional Supplement

Use Supplies calories for those persons not able to meet the caloric requirement with usual food intake

Usual Dosage Adults: Oral: Add to foods or beverages or mix in water

Dosage Forms

Liquid (Polycose®): 126 mL

(Continued)

glucose polymers *(Continued)*
Powder (Moducal®, Polycose®, Sumacal®): 350 g, 368 g, 400 g

♦ **Glucotrol®** *see* glipizide *on page 292*
♦ **Glucotrol® XL** *see* glipizide *on page 292*
♦ **Glukor®** *see* chorionic gonadotropin *on page 149*

glutamic acid (gloo TAM ik AS id)
Generic Available Yes
Therapeutic Category Gastrointestinal Agent, Miscellaneous
Use Treatment of hypochlorhydria and achlorhydria
Usual Dosage Adults: Oral: 340 mg to 1.02 g 3 times/day before meals or food
Dietary Considerations Should be administered before meals or food
Dosage Forms
Capsule, as hydrochloride: 340 mg
Powder: 100 g
Tablet: 500 mg

glutethimide (gloo TETH i mide)
Generic Available Yes
Therapeutic Category Hypnotic, Nonbarbiturate
Controlled Substance C-II
Use Short-term treatment of insomnia
Usual Dosage Oral:
Adults: 250-500 mg at bedtime, dose may be repeated but not less than 4
hours before intended awakening; maximum: 1 g/day
Elderly/debilitated patients: Total daily dose should not exceed 500 mg
Dosage Forms Tablet: 250 mg

♦ **Glutose® [OTC]** *see* glucose, instant *on page 293*
♦ **Glyate® [OTC]** *see* guaifenesin *on page 299*

glyburide (GLYE byoor ide)
Synonyms glibenclamide
U.S. Brand Names Diaβeta®; Glynase™ PresTab™; Micronase®
Canadian Brand Names Albert® Glyburide; Apo-Glyburide®; Euglucon®; Gen-
Glybe; Novo-Glyburide; Nu-Glyburide
Mexican Brand Names Daonil; Euglucon®; Glibenil; Glucal; Norboral
Generic Available Yes
Therapeutic Category Antidiabetic Agent, Oral
Use Management of noninsulin-dependent diabetes mellitus (type II)
Usual Dosage Oral:
Diaβeta®, Micronase®:
Adults: Initial: 1.25-5 mg, then increase at weekly intervals to 1.25-20 mg
maintenance dose/day divided in 1-2 doses
Elderly: Initial: 1.25-2.5 mg/day, increase by 1.25-2.5 mg/day every 1-3
weeks
Glynase™ PresTab™: Adults: Initial: 0.75-3 mg/day, increase by 1.5 mg/day in
weekly intervals, maximum: 12 mg/day
Dietary Considerations
Alcohol: A disulfiram-like reaction characterized by flushing, headache,
nausea, vomiting, sweating or tachycardia; avoid alcohol
Food: Does not affect absorption; glyburide may be taken with food; should be
administered before breakfast
Glucose: Decreases blood glucose concentration; hypoglycemia may occur;
educate patients how to detect and treat hypoglycemia; monitor for signs
and symptoms of hypoglycemia; administer glucose if necessary; evaluate
patient's diet and exercise regimen; may need to decrease or discontinue
dose of sulfonylurea
Sodium: Reports of hyponatremia and SIADH; those at increased risk
include patients on medications or who have medical conditions that
predispose them to hyponatremia; monitor sodium serum concentration
and fluid status; may need to restrict water intake
Nursing/Pharmacy Information
Patients who are anorexic or NPO may need to have their dose held to avoid
hypoglycemia
Monitor fasting blood glucose, hemoglobin A_{2c}, fructosamine; monitor for signs
and symptoms of hypoglycemia
Dosage Forms
Tablet (Diaβeta®, Micronase®): 1.25 mg, 2.5 mg, 5 mg
Tablet, micronized (Glynase™ PresTab™): 1.5 mg, 3 mg, 6 mg

glycerin (GLIS er in)
Synonyms glycerol
U.S. Brand Names Fleet® Babylax® Rectal [OTC]; Ophthalgan® Ophthalmic; Osmoglyn®; Sani-Supp® Suppository [OTC]
Generic Available Yes
Therapeutic Category Laxative; Ophthalmic Agent, Miscellaneous
Use Constipation; reduction of intraocular pressure; reduction of corneal edema; glycerin has been administered orally to reduce intracranial pressure
Usual Dosage
Constipation: Rectal:
Children <6 years: 1 infant suppository 1-2 times/day as needed or 2-5 mL as an enema
Children >6 years and Adults: 1 adult suppository 1-2 times/day as needed or 5-15 mL as an enema

Children and Adults:
Reduction of intraocular pressure: Oral: 1-1.8 g/kg 1-1½ hours preoperatively; additional doses may be administered at 5-hour intervals
Reduction of corneal edema: Instill 1-2 drops in eye(s) every 3-4 hours
Reduction of intracranial pressure: Oral: 1.5 g/kg/day divided every 4 hours; dose of 1 g/kg/dose every 6 hours has also been used
Nursing/Pharmacy Information
Use caution during insertion of suppository to avoid intestinal perforation, especially in neonates
Monitor blood glucose, intraocular pressure
Stability: Protect from heat; freezing should be avoided
Dosage Forms
Solution:
Ophthalmic, sterile (Ophthalgan®): Glycerin with chlorobutanol 0.55% (7.5 mL)
Oral (lime flavor)(Osmoglyn®): 50% (220 mL)
Rectal (Fleet® Babylax®): 4 mL/applicator (6s)
Suppository, rectal (Sani-Supp®): Glycerin with sodium stearate (infant and adult sizes)

glycerin, lanolin, and peanut oil
(GLIS er in, LAN oh lin, & PEE nut oyl)
U.S. Brand Names Massé® Breast Cream [OTC]
Generic Available Yes
Therapeutic Category Topical Skin Product
Use Nipple care of pregnant and nursing women
Usual Dosage Topical: Apply as often as needed
Dosage Forms Cream: 2 oz

♦ **glycerol** see glycerin on page 295
♦ **glycerol guaiacolate** see guaifenesin on page 299
♦ **Glycerol-T®** see theophylline and guaifenesin on page 604
♦ **glycerol triacetate** see triacetin on page 623
♦ **glyceryl trinitrate** see nitroglycerin on page 444
♦ **Glycofed®** see guaifenesin and pseudoephedrine on page 302

glycopyrrolate (glye koe PYE roe late)
U.S. Brand Names Robinul®; Robinul® Forte
Generic Available Yes
Therapeutic Category Anticholinergic Agent
Use Adjunct in treatment of peptic ulcer disease; inhibit salivation and excessive secretions of the respiratory tract; reversal of cholinergic agents such as neostigmine and pyridostigmine; control of upper airway secretions
Usual Dosage
Children: Control of secretions:
Oral: 40-100 mcg/kg/dose 3-4 times/day
I.M., I.V.: 4-10 mcg/kg/dose every 3-4 hours; maximum: 0.2 mg/dose or 0.8 mg/24 hours
Children:
Intraoperative: I.V.: 4 mcg/kg not to exceed 0.1 mg; repeat at 2- to 3-minute intervals as needed
Preoperative: I.M.:
<2 years: 4.4-8.8 mcg/kg 30-60 minutes before procedure
>2 years: 4.4 mcg/kg 30-60 minutes before procedure
Children and Adults: Reverse neuromuscular blockade: I.V.: 0.2 mg for each 1 mg of neostigmine or 5 mg of pyridostigmine administered
(Continued)

glycopyrrolate *(Continued)*

Adults:
Intraoperative: I.V.: 0.1 mg repeated as needed at 2- to 3-minute intervals
Peptic ulcer:
Oral: 1-2 mg 2-3 times/day
I.M., I.V.: 0.1-0.2 mg 3-4 times/day
Preoperative: I.M.: 4.4 mcg/kg 30-60 minutes before procedure

Nursing/Pharmacy Information
Dilute to a concentration of 2 mcg/mL (maximum concentration: 200 mcg/mL); infuse over 15-20 minutes; may be administered direct I.V. at a maximum rate of 20 mcg/minute
Monitor heart rate; anticholinergic effects
Stability: Unstable at pH >6; **incompatible** with secobarbital (immediate precipitation), sodium bicarbonate (gas evolves), thiopental (immediate precipitation)

Dosage Forms
Glycopyrrolate bromide:
Injection: 0.2 mg/mL (1 mL, 2 mL, 5 mL, 20 mL)
Robinul®: 0.2 mg/mL (1 mL, 2 mL, 5 mL, 20 mL)
Tablet:
Robinul®: 1 mg
Robinul® Forte: 2 mg

♦ **Glycotuss® [OTC]** *see* guaifenesin *on page 299*

♦ **Glycotuss-dM® [OTC]** *see* guaifenesin and dextromethorphan *on page 300*

♦ **glydiazinamide** *see* glipizide *on page 292*

♦ **Glynase™ PresTab™** *see* glyburide *on page 294*

♦ **Gly-Oxide® Oral [OTC]** *see* carbamide peroxide *on page 112*

♦ **Glysennid®** *see* senna *on page 563*

♦ **Glyset®** *see* miglitol *on page 416*

♦ **Glytuss® [OTC]** *see* guaifenesin *on page 299*

♦ **GM-CSF** *see* sargramostim *on page 559*

♦ **G-myticin®** *see* gentamicin *on page 290*

♦ **GnRH** *see* gonadorelin *on page 296*

♦ **Go-Evac®** *see* polyethylene glycol-electrolyte solution *on page 502*

gold sodium thiomalate *(gold SOW dee um thye oh MAL ate)*

U.S. Brand Names Aurolate®
Generic Available Yes
Therapeutic Category Gold Compound
Use Treatment of progressive rheumatoid arthritis
Usual Dosage I.M.:
Children: Initial: Test dose of 10 mg I.M. is recommended, followed by 1 mg/kg I.M. weekly for 20 weeks; not to exceed 50 mg in a single injection; maintenance: 1 mg/kg/dose at 2- to 4-week intervals thereafter for as long as therapy is clinically beneficial and toxicity does not develop. Administration for 2-4 months is usually required before clinical improvement is observed.
Adults: 10 mg first week; 25 mg second week; then 25-50 mg/week until 1 g cumulative dose has been administered. If improvement occurs without adverse reactions, administer 25-50 mg every 2-3 weeks, then every 3-4 weeks.

Nursing/Pharmacy Information
Therapy should be discontinued if platelet count falls <100,000/mm³; deep I.M. injection into the upper outer quadrant of the gluteal region; addition of 0.1 mL of 1% lidocaine to each injection may reduce the discomfort with injection; observe closely for 15 minutes after injection; vial should be thoroughly shaken before withdrawing a dose; explain the possibility of adverse reactions before initiating therapy; advise patients to report any symptoms of toxicity
Monitor for signs and symptoms of gold toxicity, serum levels, CBC, platelets, urine protein
Stability: Should not be used if solution is darker than pale yellow
Dosage Forms Injection: 25 mg/mL (1 mL); 50 mg/mL (1 mL, 2 mL, 10 mL)

♦ **GoLYTELY®** *see* polyethylene glycol-electrolyte solution *on page 502*

gonadorelin *(goe nad oh REL in)*

Synonyms GnRH; gonadotropin-releasing hormone; LHRH; LRH; luteinizing hormone-releasing hormone
U.S. Brand Names Factrel®; Lutrepulse®

Generic Available No

Therapeutic Category Diagnostic Agent; Gonadotropin

Use Evaluation of hypothalamic-pituitary gonadotropic function; used to evaluate abnormal gonadotropin regulation as in precocious puberty and delayed puberty; treatment of primary hypothalamic amenorrhea

Usual Dosage Female:

Diagnostic test: Children >12 years and Adults: I.V., S.C. hydrochloride salt: 100 mcg administered in women during early phase of menstrual cycle (day 1-7)

Primary hypothalamic amenorrhea: Adults: Acetate: I.V.: 5 mcg every 90 minutes via Lutrepulse® pump kit at treatment intervals of 21 days (pump will pulsate every 90 minutes for 7 days)

Nursing/Pharmacy Information

Parenteral: Dilute in 3 mL of normal saline; administer I.V. push over 30 seconds

Monitor LH, FSH

Stability: Prepare immediately prior to use; after reconstitution, store at room temperature and use within 1 day; discard unused portion

Dosage Forms

Injection, as acetate (Lutrepulse®): 0.8 mg, 3.2 mg

Injection, as hydrochloride (Factrel®): 100 mcg, 500 mcg

- ◆ **gonadotropin-releasing hormone** *see* gonadorelin *on page 296*
- ◆ **Gonak™ [OTC]** *see* hydroxypropyl methylcellulose *on page 328*
- ◆ **Gonal-F®** *see* follitropin alpha *on page 281*
- ◆ **Gonic®** *see* chorionic gonadotropin *on page 149*
- ◆ **gonioscopic ophthalmic solution** *see* hydroxypropyl methylcellulose *on page 328*
- ◆ **Goniosol® [OTC]** *see* hydroxypropyl methylcellulose *on page 328*
- ◆ **Goody's® Headache Powders** *see* acetaminophen, aspirin, and caffeine *on page 16*
- ◆ **Gordofilm® Liquid** *see* salicylic acid *on page 557*
- ◆ **Gormel® Creme [OTC]** *see* urea *on page 638*

goserelin (GOE se rel in)

U.S. Brand Names Zoladex® Implant

Mexican Brand Names Prozoladex

Generic Available No

Therapeutic Category Gonadotropin Releasing Hormone Analog

Use Palliative treatment of advanced prostate cancer and breast cancer

Usual Dosage Adults: S.C.:

Breast/prostatic cancer: 3.6 mg as a depot injection every 28 days into upper abdominal wall using sterile technique under the supervision of a physician. At the physician's option, local anesthesia may be used prior to injection. The injection should be repeated every 28 days as long as the patient can tolerate the side effects and there is satisfactory disease regression. While a delay of a few days is permissible, every effort should be made to adhere to the 28-day schedule.

Prostatic cancer: 10.8 mg as a depot injection every 12 weeks into upper abdominal wall using sterile technique under the supervision of a physician. At the physician's option, local anesthesia may be used prior to injection. The injection should be repeated every 12 weeks as long as the patient can tolerate the side effects and there is satisfactory disease regression. While a delay of a few days is permissible, every effort should be made to adhere to the 12-week schedule.

Nursing/Pharmacy Information

Do not try to aspirate with the goserelin syringe, if the needle is in a large vessel, blood will immediately appear in syringe chamber

Stability: Protect from light; store at room temperature

Dosage Forms Injection, implant, as acetate: 3.6 mg, 10.8 mg

- ◆ **gramicidin, neomycin, and polymyxin B** *see* neomycin, polymyxin B, and gramicidin *on page 437*
- ◆ **Graneodin-B** *see* benzocaine *on page 79*

granisetron (gra NI se tron)

U.S. Brand Names Kytril™

Generic Available No

Therapeutic Category Selective 5-HT₃ Receptor Antagonist

Use Prophylaxis and treatment of chemotherapy-related emesis

(Continued)

granisetron *(Continued)*

Usual Dosage
Oral: 1 tablet (1 mg) twice daily

I.V.:

10-40 mcg/kg for 1-3 doses; doses should be administered as a single IVPB over 5 minutes to 1 hour, administer just prior to chemotherapy (15-60 minutes before)

As intervention therapy for breakthrough nausea and vomiting, during the first 24 hours following chemotherapy, 2 or 3 repeat infusions (same dose) have been administered, separated by at least 10 minutes

Nursing/Pharmacy Information
Doses should be administered at least 15 minutes prior to initiation of chemotherapy; as a general precaution, do not mix in solution with other medications

Stability: At least 4 hours when mixed in normal saline

Dosage Forms
Injection: 1 mg/mL

Tablet: 1 mg (2s), (20s)

♦ **Granulex** *see* trypsin, balsam Peru, and castor oil *on page 635*

♦ **granulocyte colony-stimulating factor** *see* filgrastim *on page 267*

♦ **granulocyte-macrophage colony-stimulating factor** *see* sargramostim *on page 559*

♦ **Graten** *see* morphine sulfate *on page 422*

♦ **Gravol®** *see* dimenhydrinate *on page 206*

grepafloxacin *Withdrawn from U.S. market 10/27/99*
(grep a FLOX a sin)

Synonyms OPC-17116

U.S. Brand Names Raxar®

Generic Available No

Therapeutic Category Antibiotic, Quinolone

Use Treatment of acute bacterial exacerbations of chronic bronchitis caused by *Haemophilus influenzae*, *Streptococcus pneumoniae*, or *Moraxella catarrhalis*; community-acquired pneumonia caused by *Mycoplasma pneumoniae* or the organisms previously mentioned; uncomplicated gonorrhea caused by *Neisseria gonorrhoeae*, and nongonococcal cervicitis and urethritis caused by *Chlamydia trachomatis*

Usual Dosage Adults: Oral: 400-600 mg every 24 hours (given in a single dose)

Dietary Considerations May be taken with or without meals; multivitamins, antacids, or sucralfate should not be taken within 4 hours before or 4 hours after taking grepafloxacin

Dosage Forms Tablet, as hydrochloride: 200 mg, 400 mg, 600 mg

♦ **Grifulvin® V** *see* griseofulvin *on page 298*

♦ **Grisactin®** *see* griseofulvin *on page 298*

♦ **Grisactin® *(Discontinued)*** *see page 743*

♦ **Grisactin® Ultra** *see* griseofulvin *on page 298*

griseofulvin (gri see oh FUL vin)

Synonyms griseofulvin microsize; griseofulvin ultramicrosize

U.S. Brand Names Fulvicin® P/G; Fulvicin-U/F®; Grifulvin V; Grisactin®; Grisactin® Ultra; Gris-PEG®

Canadian Brand Names Grisovin®-FP

Mexican Brand Names Fulvina® P/G; Grisovin-FP

Generic Available Yes

Therapeutic Category Antifungal Agent

Use Treatment of tinea infections of the skin, hair, and nails caused by susceptible species of *Microsporum*, *Epidermophyton*, or *Trichophyton*

Usual Dosage Oral:

Children:

Microsize: 10-15 mg/kg/day in single or divided doses;

Ultramicrosize: >2 years: 5.5-7.3 mg/kg/day in single or divided doses

Adults:

Microsize: 500-1000 mg/day in single or divided doses

Ultramicrosize: 330-375 mg/day in single or divided doses; doses up to 750 mg/day have been used for infections more difficult to eradicate such as tinea unguium

Duration of therapy depends on the site of infection:
Tinea corporis: 2-4 weeks
Tinea capitis: 4-6 weeks or longer
Tinea pedis: 4-8 weeks
Tinea unguium: 3-6 months

Dietary Considerations Enhanced absorption with high fat meals; for enhanced absorption, should be administered with high fat meal; alcohol will cause "disulfiram"-type reaction consisting of flushing, headache, nausea, and in some patients, vomiting and chest and/or abdominal pain

Nursing/Pharmacy Information Monitor periodic renal, hepatic, and hematopoietic function tests

Dosage Forms
Microsize:
Capsule (Grisactin®): 125 mg, 250 mg
Suspension, oral (Grifulvin® V): 125 mg/5 mL with alcohol 0.2% (120 mL)
Tablet:
Fulvicin-U/F®, Grifulvin® V: 250 mg
Fulvicin-U/F®, Grifulvin® V, Grisactin-500®: 500 mg
Ultramicrosize:
Tablet:
Fulvicin® P/G: 165 mg, 330 mg
Fulvicin® P/G, Grisactin® Ultra, Gris-PEG®: 125 mg, 250 mg
Grisactin® Ultra: 330 mg

♦ **griseofulvin microsize** see griseofulvin on page 298
♦ **griseofulvin ultramicrosize** see griseofulvin on page 298
♦ **Grisovin®-FP** see griseofulvin on page 298
♦ **Gris-PEG®** see griseofulvin on page 298
♦ **Grunicina** see amoxicillin on page 43
♦ **Guaifed® [OTC]** see guaifenesin and pseudoephedrine on page 302
♦ **Guaifed-PD®** see guaifenesin and pseudoephedrine on page 302

guaifenesin (gwye FEN e sin)

Synonyms GG; glycerol guaiacolate

U.S. Brand Names Anti-Tuss® Expectorant [OTC]; Breonesin® [OTC]; Diabetic Tussin® EX [OTC]; Duratuss-G®; Fenesin™; Gee Gee® [OTC]; Genatuss® [OTC]; GG-Cen® [OTC]; Glyate® [OTC]; Glycotuss® [OTC]; Glytuss® [OTC]; Guaifenex® LA; GuiaCough® Expectorant [OTC]; Guiatuss® [OTC]; Halotussin® [OTC]; Humibid® L.A.; Humibid® Sprinkle; Hytuss® [OTC]; Hytuss-2X® [OTC]; Liquibid®; Medi-Tuss® [OTC]; Monafed®; Muco-Fen-LA®; Mytussin® [OTC]; Naldecon® Senior EX [OTC]; Organidin® NR; Pneumomist®; Respa-GF®; Robitussin® [OTC]; Scot-Tussin® [OTC]; Siltussin® [OTC]; Sinumist®-SR Capsulets®; Touro Ex®; Tusibron® [OTC]; Uni-tussin® [OTC]

Canadian Brand Names Balminil® Expectorant; Calmylin Expectorant

Mexican Brand Names Formula E

Generic Available Yes

Therapeutic Category Expectorant

Use Temporary control of cough due to minor throat and bronchial irritation

Usual Dosage Oral:
Children:
<2 years: 12 mg/kg/day in 6 divided doses
2-5 years: 50-100 mg (2.5-5 mL) every 4 hours, not to exceed 600 mg/day
6-11 years: 100-200 mg (5-10 mL) every 4 hours, not to exceed 1.2 g/day
Children >12 years and Adults: 200-400 mg (10-20 mL) every 4 hours to a maximum of 2.4 g/day (60 mL/day)

Nursing/Pharmacy Information
Administer with large quantity of water to ensure proper action; some products contain alcohol
Stability: Protect from light

Dosage Forms
Caplet, sustained release (Touro Ex®): 600 mg
Capsule (Breonesin®, GG-Cen®, Hytuss-2X®): 200 mg
Sustained release (Humibid® Sprinkle): 300 mg
Liquid:
Diabetic Tussin® EX, Organidin® NR, Tusibron®: 100 mg/5 mL (118 mL)
Naldecon® Senior EX: 200 mg/5 mL (118 mL, 480 mL)
Syrup (Anti-Tuss® Expectorant, Genatuss®, Glyate®, GuiaCough® Expectorant, Guiatuss®, Halotussin®, Malotuss®, Medi-Tuss®, Mytussin®, Robitussin®, Scot-Tussin®, Siltussin®, Tusibron®, Uni-Tussin®): 100 mg/5 mL with alcohol 3.5% (30 mL, 120 mL, 240 mL, 473 mL, 946 mL)
(Continued)

guaifenesin *(Continued)*

Tablet:
Duratuss-G®: 1200 mg
Gee Gee®, Glytuss®, Organidin® NR: 200 mg
Glycotuss®, Hytuss®: 100 mg
Sustained release:
Fenesin™, Guaifenex® LA, Humibid® L.A., Liquibid®, Monafed®, Muco-Fen-LA®, Pneumomist®, Respa-GF®, Sinumist®-SR Capsulets®: 600 mg

guaifenesin and codeine (gwye FEN e sin & KOE deen)

Synonyms codeine and guaifenesin

U.S. Brand Names Brontex® Liquid; Brontex® Tablet; Cheracol®; Guaituss AC®; Guiatussin® With Codeine; Mytussin® AC; Robafen® AC; Robitussin® A-C; Tussi-Organidin® NR

Generic Available Yes

Therapeutic Category Antitussive/Expectorant

Controlled Substance C-V

Use Temporary control of cough due to minor throat and bronchial irritation

Usual Dosage Oral:

Children:
2-6 years: 1-1.5 mg/kg codeine/day divided into 4 doses administered every 4-6 hours
6-12 years: 5 mL every 4 hours, not to exceed 30 mL/24 hours
>12 years: 10 mL every 4 hours, up to 60 mL/24 hours
Adults: 10 mL or 1 tablet every 6-8 hours

Dietary Considerations Codeine:
Food: Glucose may cause hyperglycemia; monitor blood glucose concentration
Alcohol: Additive CNS effects; avoid or limit alcohol; watch for sedation

Nursing/Pharmacy Information
Administer with a large quantity of fluid
The "NR" in Tussi-Organidin® NR means "Newly Reformulated"

Dosage Forms
Liquid [C-V] (Brontex®): Guaifenesin 75 mg and codeine phosphate 2.5 mg per 5 mL
Syrup [C-V] (Cheracol®, Guaituss AC®, Guiatussin® with Codeine, Mytussin® AC, Robafen® AC, Robitussin® A-C, Tussi-Organidin® NR): Guaifenesin 100 mg and codeine phosphate 10 mg per 5 mL (60 mL, 120 mL, 480 mL)
Tablet [C-III] (Brontex®): Guaifenesin 300 mg and codeine phosphate 10 mg

guaifenesin and dextromethorphan
(gwye FEN e sin & deks troe meth OR fan)

Synonyms dextromethorphan and guaifenesin

U.S. Brand Names Benylin® Expectorant [OTC]; Cheracol® D [OTC]; Clear Tussin® 30; Contac® Cough Formula Liquid [OTC]; Diabetic Tussin DM® [OTC]; Extra Action Cough Syrup [OTC]; Fenesin™ DM; Genatuss DM® [OTC]; Glycotuss-dM® [OTC]; Guaifenex® DM; GuiaCough® [OTC]; Guiatuss-DM® [OTC]; Halotussin® DM [OTC]; Humibid® DM [OTC]; Iobid DM®; Kolephrin® GG/DM [OTC]; Monafed® DM; Muco-Fen-DM®; Mytussin® DM [OTC]; Naldecon® Senior DX [OTC]; Phanatuss® Cough Syrup [OTC]; Phenadex® Senior [OTC]; Respa-DM®; Rhinosyn-DMX® [OTC]; Robaïen DM® [OTC]; Robitussin®-DM [OTC]; Safe Tussin® 30 [OTC]; Scot-Tussin® Senior Clear [OTC]; Siltussin DM® [OTC]; Synacol® CF [OTC]; Syracol-CF® [OTC]; Tolu-Sed® DM [OTC]; Tusibron-DM® [OTC]; Tuss-DM® [OTC]; Tussi-Organidin® DM NR; Uni-tussin® DM [OTC]; Vicks® 44E [OTC]; Vicks® Pediatric Formula 44E [OTC]

Generic Available Yes

Therapeutic Category Antitussive/Expectorant

Use Temporary control of cough due to minor throat and bronchial irritation

Usual Dosage Oral:

Children:
2-5 years: 2.5 mL every 6-8 hours; maximum: 10 mL/day
6-12 years: 5 mL every 6-8 hours; maximum: 20 mL/24 hours
>12 years: 10 mL every 6-8 hours; maximum: 40 mL/24 hours
Alternatively: 0.1-0.15 mL/kg/dose every 6-8 hours as needed
Adults: 10 mL every 6-8 hours

Nursing/Pharmacy Information
Administer with a large quantity of fluid
Stability: Protect from light
The "NR" in Tussi-Organidin® DM NR means "Newly Reformulated"

Dosage Forms

Syrup:

Benylin® Expectorant: Guaifenesin 100 mg and dextromethorphan hydrobromide 5 mg per 5 mL (118 mL, 236 mL)

Cheracol® D, Clear Tussin® 30, Genatuss DM®, Mytussin® DM, Robitussin®-DM, Siltussin DM®, Tolu-Sed® DM, Tussi-Organidin® DM NR: Guaifenesin 100 mg and dextromethorphan hydrobromide 10 mg per 5 mL (5 mL, 10 mL, 120 mL, 240 mL, 360 mL, 480 mL, 3780 mL)

Contac® Cough Formula Liquid: Guaifenesin 67 mg and dextromethorphan hydrobromide 10 mg per 5 mL (120 mL)

Extra Action Cough Syrup, GuiaCough®, Guiatuss DM®, Halotussin® DM, Rhinosyn-DMX®, Tusibron-DM®, Uni-tussin® DM: Guaifenesin 100 mg and dextromethorphan hydrobromide 15 mg per 5 mL (120 mL, 240 mL, 480 mL)

Kolephrin® GG/DM: Guaifenesin 150 mg and dextromethorphan hydrobromide 10 mg per 5 mL (120 mL)

Naldecon® Senior DX: Guaifenesin 200 mg and dextromethorphan hydrobromide 15 mg per 5 mL (118 mL, 480 mL)

Phanatuss®: Guaifenesin 85 mg and dextromethorphan hydrobromide 10 mg per 5 mL

Vicks® 44E: Guaifenesin 66.7 mg and dextromethorphan hydrobromide 6.7 mg per 5 mL

Tablet:

Extended release

Guaifenex DM®, Iobid DM®, Fenesin™ DM, Humibid® DM, Monafed® DM, Respa-DM®: Guaifenesin 600 mg and dextromethorphan hydrobromide 30 mg

Glycotuss-dM®: Guaifenesin 100 mg and dextromethorphan hydrobromide 10 mg

Queltuss®: Guaifenesin 100 mg and dextromethorphan hydrobromide 15 mg

Syracol-CF®: Guaifenesin 200 mg and dextromethorphan hydrobromide 15 mg

Tuss-DM®: Guaifenesin 200 mg and dextromethorphan hydrobromide 10 mg

♦ **guaifenesin and hydrocodone** see hydrocodone and guaifenesin on page 320

guaifenesin and phenylephrine (gwye FEN e sin & fen il EF rin)

Synonyms phenylephrine and guaifenesin

U.S. Brand Names Deconsal® Sprinkle®; Endal®; Sinupan®

Generic Available No

Therapeutic Category Cold Preparation

Use Symptomatic relief of those respiratory conditions where tenacious mucous plugs and congestion complicate the problem such as sinusitis, pharyngitis, bronchitis, asthma, and as an adjunctive therapy in serous otitis media

Usual Dosage Adults: Oral: 1-2 tablets/capsules every 12 hours

Dosage Forms

Capsule, sustained release:

·Deconsal® Sprinkle®: Guaifenesin 300 mg and phenylephrine hydrochloride 10 mg

Sinupan®: Guaifenesin 200 mg and phenylephrine hydrochloride 40 mg

Tablet, timed release (Endal®): Guaifenesin 300 mg and phenylephrine hydrochloride 20 mg

guaifenesin and phenylpropanolamine
(gwye FEN e sin & fen il proe pa NOLE a meen)

Synonyms phenylpropanolamine and guaifenesin

U.S. Brand Names Ami-Tex LA®; Coldlac-LA®; Conex® [OTC]; Contuss® XT; Dura-Vent®; Entex® LA; Genagesic®; Genamin® Expectorant [OTC]; Guaifenex® PPA 75; Guaipax®; Myminic® Expectorant [OTC]; Naldecon-EX® Children's Syrup [OTC]; Nolex® LA; Partuss® LA; Phenylfenesin® L.A.; Profen II®; Profen LA®; Rymed-TR®; Silaminic® Expectorant [OTC]; Sildicon-E® [OTC]; Snaplets-EX® [OTC]; Triaminic® Expectorant [OTC]; Tri-Clear® Expectorant [OTC]; Triphenyl® Expectorant [OTC]; ULR-LA®; Vicks® DayQuil® Sinus Pressure & Congestion Relief [OTC]

Generic Available Yes

Therapeutic Category Expectorant/Decongestant

Use Symptomatic relief of those respiratory conditions where tenacious mucous plugs and congestion complicate the problem such as sinusitis, pharyngitis, bronchitis, asthma, and as an adjunctive therapy in serous otitis media
(Continued)

guaifenesin and phenylpropanolamine *(Continued)*

Usual Dosage Oral:
  Children:
    2-6 years: 2.5 mL every 4 hours
    6-12 years: ½ tablet every 12 hours or 5 mL every 4 hours
    Children >12 years and Adults: 1 tablet every 12 hours or 10 mL every 4 hours
Dietary Considerations Have patient drink water after each dose
Nursing/Pharmacy Information Do not crush or chew sustained release tablet
Dosage Forms
  Caplet:
    Vicks® DayQuil® Sinus Pressure & Congestion Relief: Guaifenesin 200 mg and phenylpropanolamine hydrochloride 25 mg
    Rymed-TR®: Guaifenesin 400 mg and phenylpropanolamine hydrochloride 75 mg
  Drops:
    Sildicon-E®: Guaifenesin 30 mg and phenylpropanolamine hydrochloride 6.25 mg per mL (30 mL)
  Granules (Snaplets-EX®): Guaifenesin 50 mg and phenylpropanolamine hydrochloride 6.25 mg (pack)
  Liquid:
    Conex®, Genamin® Expectorant, Myminic® Expectorant, Silaminic® Expectorant, Triaminic® Expectorant, Tri-Clear® Expectorant, Triphenyl® Expectorant: Guaifenesin 100 mg and phenylpropanolamine hydrochloride 12.5 mg per 5 mL (120 mL, 240 mL, 480 mL, 3780 mL)
    Naldecon-EX® Children's Syrup: Guaifenesin 100 mg and phenylpropanolamine hydrochloride 6.25 mg per 5 mL (120 mL)
  Tablet, extended release:
    Ami-Tex LA®, Contuss® XT, Entex® LA, Guaipax®, Nolex® LA, Partuss® LA, Phenylfenesin® L.A., ULR-LA®: Guaifenesin 400 mg and phenylpropanolamine hydrochloride 75 mg
    Dura-Vent®, Profen LA®: Guaifenesin 600 mg and phenylpropanolamine hydrochloride 75 mg
    Coldlac-LA®, Guaifenex® PPA 75, Profen II®: Guaifenesin 600 mg and phenylpropanolamine hydrochloride 37.5 mg

guaifenesin and pseudoephedrine

(gwye FEN e sin & soo doe e FED rin)
Synonyms pseudoephedrine and guaifenesin
U.S. Brand Names Congess® Jr; Congess® Sr; Congestac®; Deconsal® II; Defen-LA®; Entex® PSE; Eudal-SR®; Fedahist® Expectorant [OTC]; Fedahist® Expectorant Pediatric [OTC]; Glycofed®; Guaifed® [OTC]; Guaifed-PD®; Guaifenex® PSE; GuaiMAX-D®; Guaitab®; Guaivent®; Guai-Vent/PSE®; Guiatuss PE® [OTC]; Halotussin® PE [OTC]; Histalet® X; Nasabid™; Respa-1st®; Respaire®-60 SR; Respaire®-120 SR; Robitussin-PE® [OTC]; Robitussin® Severe Congestion Liqui-Gels® [OTC]; Ru-Tuss® DE; Rymed®; Sinufed® Timecelles®; Touro LA®; Tuss-LA®; V-Dec-M®; Versacaps®; Zephrex®; Zephrex LA®
Generic Available Yes
Therapeutic Category Expectorant/Decongestant
Use Enhance the output of respiratory tract fluid and reduce mucosal congestion and edema in the nasal passage
Usual Dosage Oral:
  Children:
    2-6 years: 2.5 mL every 4 hours not to exceed 15 mL/24 hours
    6-12 years: 5 mL every 4 hours not to exceed 30 mL/24 hours
    Children >12 years and Adults: 10 mL every 4 hours not to exceed 60 mL/24 hours
Dosage Forms
  Capsule:
    Guaivent®: Guaifenesin 250 mg and pseudoephedrine hydrochloride 120 mg
    Robitussin® Severe Congestion Liqui-Gels®: Guaifenesin 200 mg and pseudoephedrine hydrochloride 30 mg
    Rymed®: Guaifenesin 250 mg and pseudoephedrine hydrochloride 30 mg
  Capsule, extended release:
    Congess® Jr: Guaifenesin 125 mg and pseudoephedrine hydrochloride 60 mg
    Nasabid®: Guaifenesin 250 mg and pseudoephedrine hydrochloride 90 mg
    Congess® SR, Guaifed®, Respaire®-120 SR,: Guaifenesin 250 mg and pseudoephedrine hydrochloride 120 mg

Guaifed-PD®, Sinufed® Timecelles®, Versacaps®: Guaifenesin 300 mg and pseudoephedrine hydrochloride 60 mg

Respaire®-60 SR: Guaifenesin 200 mg and pseudoephedrine hydrochloride 60 mg

Tuss-LA® Capsule: Guaifenesin 500 mg and pseudoephedrine hydrochloride 120 mg

Drops, oral (Fedahist® Expectorant Pediatric): Guaifenesin 40 mg and pseudo-ephedrine hydrochloride 7.5 mg per mL (30 mL)

Syrup:

Fedahist® Expectorant, Guaifed®: Guaifenesin 200 mg and pseudoephedrine hydrochloride 30 mg per 5 mL (120 mL, 240 mL)

Guiatuss® PE, Halotussin-PE®, Robitussin-PE®, Rymed®: Guaifenesin 100 mg and pseudoephedrine hydrochloride 30 mg per 5 mL (120 mL, 240 mL, 480 mL)

Histalet® X: Guaifenesin 200 mg and pseudoephedrine hydrochloride 45 mg per 5 mL (473 mL)

Tablet:

Congestac®, Guaitab®, Zephrex®: Guaifenesin 400 mg and pseudoephedrine hydrochloride 60 mg

Glycofed®: Guaifenesin 100 mg and pseudoephedrine hydrochloride 30 mg

Tablet, extended release:

Deconsal® II, Defen-LA®, Respa-1st®: Guaifenesin 600 mg and pseudoephedrine hydrochloride 60 mg

Entex® PSE, Guaifenex® PSE, GuaiMax-D®, Guai-Vent/PSE®, Ru-Tuss® DE, Sudex®, Zephrex LA®: Guaifenesin 600 mg and pseudoephedrine hydrochloride 120 mg

Eudal-SR®, Histalet® X, Touro LA®: Guaifenesin 400 mg and pseudoephedrine hydrochloride 120 mg

Tuss-LA® Tablet, V-Dec-M®: Guaifenesin 5mg and pseudoephedrine hydrochloride 120 mg

- **guaifenesin and theophylline** *see* theophylline and guaifenesin *on page 604*
- **guaifenesin, hydrocodone, and pseudoephedrine** *see* hydrocodone, pseudoephedrine, and guaifenesin *on page 322*

guaifenesin, phenylpropanolamine, and dextromethorphan

(gwye FEN e sin, fen il proe pa NOLE a meen, & deks troe meth OR fan)

Synonyms dextromethorphan, guaifenesin, and phenylpropanolamine; phenylpropanolamine, guaifenesin, and dextromethorphan

U.S. Brand Names Anatuss® [OTC]; Guiatuss CF® [OTC]; Naldecon® DX Adult Liquid [OTC]; Profen II DM®; Robafen® CF [OTC]; Robitussin-CF® [OTC]; Siltussin-CF® [OTC]

Generic Available Yes

Therapeutic Category Antitussive/Decongestant/Expectorant

Use Temporarily relieves nasal congestion and controls cough due to minor throat and bronchial irritation; helps loosen phlegm and thin bronchial secretions to make coughs more productive

Usual Dosage Oral:

Children:

2-6 years: 2.5 mL every 4 hours not to exceed 15 mL/24 hours

6-12 years: 5 mL every 4 hours not to exceed 30 mL/24 hours

Children >12 years and Adults: 10 mL every 4 hours not to exceed 60 mL/24 hours

Dosage Forms

Syrup:

Anatuss®: Guaifenesin 100 mg, phenylpropanolamine hydrochloride 25 mg, and dextromethorphan hydrobromide 15 mg per 5 mL (120 mL, 473 mL)

Guiatuss® CF, Robafen® CF, Robitussin-CF®: Guaifenesin 100 mg, phenylpropanolamine hydrochloride 12.5 mg, and dextromethorphan hydrobromide 10 mg per 5 mL (120 mL, 240 mL, 360 mL, 480 mL)

Naldecon® DX Adult: Guaifenesin 200 mg, phenylpropanolamine hydrochloride 12.5 mg, and dextromethorphan hydrobromide 10 mg per 5 mL (120 mL, 473 mL)

Siltussin-CF®: Guaifenesin 100 mg, phenylpropanolamine hydrochloride 12.5 mg, and dextromethorphan hydrobromide 10 mg per 5 mL

Tablet: Anatuss®: Guaifenesin 100 mg, phenylpropanolamine hydrochloride 25 mg, and dextromethorphan hydrobromide 15 mg

Timed release (Profen II DM®): Guaifenesin 600 mg, phenylpropanolamine hydrochloride 37.5 mg, and dextromethorphan hydrobromide 30 mg

guaifenesin, phenylpropanolamine, and phenylephrine

(gwye FEN e sin, fen il proe pa NOLE a meen, & fen il EF rin)

Synonyms phenylephrine, guaifenesin, and phenylpropanolamine; phenylpropanolamine, guaifenesin, and phenylephrine

U.S. Brand Names Coldloc®; Contuss®; Dura-Gest®; Enomine®; Entex®; Guaifenex®; Guiatex®

Generic Available Yes

Therapeutic Category Expectorant/Decongestant

Use Temporary relief of nasal congestion, running nose, sneezing, itching of nose and throat, and itchy, watery eyes due to common cold, hay fever, or other upper respiratory allergies

Usual Dosage Children >12 years and Adults: Oral: 1 capsule 4 times/day (every 6 hours) with food or fluid

Dietary Considerations Administer with food or fluid

Nursing/Pharmacy Information Extended release tablets may be cut in half and still maintain effective release properties, do not crush or chew

Dosage Forms

Capsule (Contuss®, Dura-Gest®, Enomine®, Entex®, Guiatex®): Guaifenesin 200 mg, phenylpropanolamine hydrochloride 45 mg, and phenylephrine hydrochloride 5 mg

Liquid (Coldloc®, Contuss®, Entex®, Guaifenex®): Guaifenesin 100 mg, phenylpropanolamine hydrochloride 20 mg, and phenylephrine hydrochloride 5 mg per 5 mL (118 mL, 480 mL)

Tablet (Respinol-G®): Guaifenesin 200 mg, phenylpropanolamine hydrochloride 45 mg, and phenylephrine hydrochloride 5 mg

guaifenesin, pseudoephedrine, and codeine

(gwye FEN e sin, soo doe e FED rin, & KOE deen)

Synonyms codeine, guaifenesin, and pseudoephedrine; pseudoephedrine, guaifenesin, and codeine

U.S. Brand Names Codafed® Expectorant; Cycofed® Pediatric; Decohistine® Expectorant; Deproist® Expectorant With Codeine; Dihistine® Expectorant; Guiatuss DAC®; Guiatussin® DAC; Halotussin® DAC; Isoclor® Expectorant; Mytussin® DAC; Nucofed®; Nucofed® Pediatric Expectorant; Nucotuss®; Phenhist® Expectorant; Robitussin®-DAC; Ryna-CX®; Tussar® SF Syrup

Generic Available Yes

Therapeutic Category Antitussive/Decongestant/Expectorant

Controlled Substance C-III; C-V

Use Temporarily relieves nasal congestion and controls cough due to minor throat and bronchial irritation; helps loosen phlegm and thin bronchial secretions to make coughs more productive

Usual Dosage Oral:

Children 6-12 years: 5 mL every 4 hours, not to exceed 40 mL/24 hours

Children >12 years and Adults: 10 mL every 4 hours, not to exceed 40 mL/24 hours

Dosage Forms Liquid:

C-III: Nucofed®, Nucotuss®: Guaifenesin 200 mg, pseudoephedrine hydrochloride 60 mg, and codeine phosphate 20 mg per 5 mL (480 mL)

C-V: Codafed® Expectorant, Decohistine® Expectorant, Deproist® Expectorant with Codeine, Dihistine® Expectorant, Guiatuss DAC®, Guiatussin® DAC, Halotussin® DAC, Isoclor® Expectorant, Mytussin® DAC, Nucofed® Pediatric Expectorant, Phenhist® Expectorant, Robitussin®-DAC, Ryna-CX®, Tussar® SF: Guaifenesin 100 mg, pseudoephedrine hydrochloride 30 mg, and codeine phosphate 10 mg per 5 mL (120 mL, 480 mL, 4000 mL)

guaifenesin, pseudoephedrine, and dextromethorphan

(gwye FEN e sin, soo doe e FED rin, & deks troe meth OR fan)

Synonyms dextromethorphan, guaifenesin, and pseudoephedrine; pseudoephedrine, dextromethorphan, and guaifenesin

U.S. Brand Names Anatuss® DM [OTC]; Dimacol® Caplets [OTC]; Rhinosyn-X® Liquid [OTC]; Ru-Tuss® Expectorant [OTC]; Sudafed® Cold & Cough Liquid Caps [OTC]

Generic Available Yes

Therapeutic Category Cold Preparation

Use Temporarily relieves nasal congestion and controls cough due to minor throat and bronchial irritation; helps loosen phlegm and thin bronchial secretions to make coughs more productive

Usual Dosage Adults: Oral: 2 capsules (caplets) or 10 mL every 4 hours

Dosage Forms

Caplets (Dimacol®): Guaifenesin 100 mg, pseudoephedrine hydrochloride 30 mg, and dextromethorphan hydrobromide 10 mg

Capsule (Sudafed® Cold & Cough Liquid Caps): Guaifenesin 100 mg, pseudoephedrine hydrochloride 30 mg, and dextromethorphan hydrobromide 10 mg

Liquid (Anatuss® DM, Rhinosyn-X® Liquid, Ru-Tuss® Expectorant): Guaifenesin 100 mg, pseudoephedrine hydrochloride 30 mg, and dextromethorphan hydrobromide 10 mg per 5 mL

♦ **Guaifenex®** see guaifenesin, phenylpropanolamine, and phenylephrine on page 304

♦ **Guaifenex® DM** see guaifenesin and dextromethorphan on page 300

♦ **Guaifenex® LA** see guaifenesin on page 299

♦ **Guaifenex® PPA 75** see guaifenesin and phenylpropanolamine on page 301

♦ **Guaifenex® PSE** see guaifenesin and pseudoephedrine on page 302

♦ **GuaiMAX-D®** see guaifenesin and pseudoephedrine on page 302

♦ **Guaipax®** see guaifenesin and phenylpropanolamine on page 301

♦ **Guaitab®** see guaifenesin and pseudoephedrine on page 302

♦ **Guaituss AC®** see guaifenesin and codeine on page 300

♦ **Guaivent®** see guaifenesin and pseudoephedrine on page 302

♦ **Guai-Vent/PSE®** see guaifenesin and pseudoephedrine on page 302

guanabenz (GWAHN a benz)

U.S. Brand Names Wytensin®

Generic Available Yes

Therapeutic Category Alpha-Adrenergic Agonist

Use Management of hypertension

Usual Dosage Adults: Oral: Initial: 4 mg twice daily, increase in increments of 4-8 mg/day every 1-2 weeks to a maximum of 32 mg twice daily

Nursing/Pharmacy Information

Do not abruptly discontinue

Monitor blood pressure, standing and sitting/supine

Stability: Protect from light

Dosage Forms Tablet, as acetate: 4 mg, 8 mg

guanadrel (GWAHN a drel)

U.S. Brand Names Hylorel®

Generic Available No

Therapeutic Category Alpha-Adrenergic Agonist

Use Step 2 agent in stepped-care treatment of hypertension, usually with a diuretic

Usual Dosage Oral: Initial: 10 mg/day (5 mg twice daily); adjust dosage until blood pressure is controlled, usual dosage: 20-75 mg/day, administered twice daily

Nursing/Pharmacy Information Monitor blood pressure, standing and sitting/supine

Dosage Forms Tablet, as sulfate: 10 mg, 25 mg

guanethidine (gwahn ETH i deen)

U.S. Brand Names Ismelin®

Canadian Brand Names Apo-Guanethidine®

Generic Available Yes

Therapeutic Category Alpha-Adrenergic Agonist

Use Treatment of moderate to severe hypertension

Usual Dosage Oral:

Children:

Initial: 0.2 mg/kg/day administered daily

Maximum dose: Up to 3 mg/kg/24 hours

Adults: Initial: 10-12.5 mg/day, then 25-50 mg/day in 3 divided doses

Nursing/Pharmacy Information

Tablet may be crushed

Monitor blood pressure, standing and sitting/supine; observe for orthostasis

Dosage Forms Tablet, as monosulfate: 10 mg, 25 mg

guanfacine (GWAHN fa seen)

U.S. Brand Names Tenex®

Generic Available No

Therapeutic Category Alpha-Adrenergic Agonist

Use Management of hypertension

(Continued)

guanfacine *(Continued)*

Usual Dosage Adults: Oral: 1 mg (usually at bedtime), may increase if needed at 3- to 4-week intervals to a maximum of 3 mg/day; 1 mg/day is most common dose

Nursing/Pharmacy Information

Administer dose at bedtime

Monitor blood pressure, standing and sitting/supine; observe for orthostasis

Dosage Forms Tablet, as hydrochloride: 1 mg, 2 mg

guanidine *(GWAHN i deen)*

Generic Available No

Therapeutic Category Cholinergic Agent

Use Reduction of the symptoms of muscle weakness associated with the myasthenic syndrome of Eaton-Lambert, not for myasthenia gravis

Usual Dosage Adults: Oral: Initial: 10-15 mg/kg/day in 3-4 divided doses, gradually increase to 35 mg/kg/day

Dosage Forms Tablet, as hydrochloride: 125 mg

- ◆ **Gugecin** *see* cinoxacin *on page 151*
- ◆ **GuiaCough® [OTC]** *see* guaifenesin and dextromethorphan *on page 300*
- ◆ **GuiaCough® Expectorant [OTC]** *see* guaifenesin *on page 299*
- ◆ **Guiatex®** *see* guaifenesin, phenylpropanolamine, and phenylephrine *on page 304*
- ◆ **Guiatuss® [OTC]** *see* guaifenesin *on page 299*
- ◆ **Guiatuss CF® [OTC]** *see* guaifenesin, phenylpropanolamine, and dextromethorphan *on page 303*
- ◆ **Guiatuss DAC®** *see* guaifenesin, pseudoephedrine, and codeine *on page 304*
- ◆ **Guiatuss-DM® [OTC]** *see* guaifenesin and dextromethorphan *on page 300*
- ◆ **Guiatussin® DAC** *see* guaifenesin, pseudoephedrine, and codeine *on page 304*
- ◆ **Guiatussin® With Codeine** *see* guaifenesin and codeine *on page 300*
- ◆ **Guiatuss PE® [OTC]** *see* guaifenesin and pseudoephedrine *on page 302*
- ◆ **gum benjamin** *see* benzoin *on page 80*
- ◆ **G-well®** *see* lindane *on page 370*
- ◆ **Gynecort® Topical [OTC]** *see* hydrocortisone (topical) *on page 324*
- ◆ **Gyne-Lotrimin® Vaginal [OTC]** *see* clotrimazole *on page 161*
- ◆ **Gynergen®** *see* ergotamine *on page 238*
- ◆ **Gyne-Sulf®** *see* sulfabenzamide, sulfacetamide, and sulfathiazole *on page 584*
- ◆ **Gyno-Daktarin** *see* miconazole *on page 413*
- ◆ **Gyno-Daktarin V** *see* miconazole *on page 413*
- ◆ **Gynogen® Injection *(Discontinued)*** *see page 743*
- ◆ **Gynogen L.A.® Injection** *see* estradiol *on page 242*
- ◆ **Gynol II® [OTC]** *see* nonoxynol 9 *on page 446*
- ◆ **H₂Oxyl®** *see* benzoyl peroxide *on page 81*
- ◆ **Habitrol™ Patch** *see* nicotine *on page 441*

Haemophilus B conjugate and hepatitis B vaccine *New Drug*

(hem OF fi lus bee KON joo gate & hep a TYE tis bee vak SEEN)

U.S. Brand Names Comvax®

Generic Available No

Therapeutic Category Vaccine, Inactivated Virus

Use For vaccination against *Haemophilus influenzae* type B and hepatitis B virus in infants 6 weeks to 15 months old of HGsAG-negative mothers

Usual Dosage Children: I.M.: 0.5 mL as a single dose should be administered

Dosage Forms Injection: *Haemophilus* B conjugate purified capsular polysaccharide 7.5 mcg and Hepatitis B vaccine surface antigen 5 mcg per 0.5 mL (0.5 mL)

Haemophilus B conjugate vaccine

(hem OF fi lus bee KON joo gate vak SEEN)

Synonyms HIB polysaccharide conjugate; PRP-D

U.S. Brand Names HibTITER®; OmniHIB™; PedvaxHIB™; ProHIBiT®

Generic Available No

Therapeutic Category Vaccine, Inactivated Bacteria

Use Immunization of children 24 months to 6 years of age against diseases caused by *H. influenzae* type b

Usual Dosage Children: I.M.: 0.5 mL as a single dose should be administered

Nursing/Pharmacy Information

Federal law requires that the date of administration, the vaccine manufacturer, lot number of vaccine, and the administering person's name, title and address be entered into the patient's permanent medical record

Stability: Store in refrigerator, may be frozen (not diluent) without affecting potency; reconstituted Hib-Imune® remains stable for only 8 hours, whereas HibVAX® remain stable for 30 days when refrigerated

Dosage Forms Injection:

HibTITER®, OmniHIB™: Capsular oligosaccharide 10 mcg and diphtheria CRM$_{197}$ protein ~25 mcg per 0.5 mL (0.5 mL, 2.5 mL, 5 mL)

PedvaxHIB™: Purified capsular polysaccharide 15 mcg and *Neisseria meningitidis* OMPC 250 mcg per dose (0.5 mL)

ProHIBiT®: Purified capsular polysaccharide 25 mcg and conjugated diphtheria toxoid protein 18 mcg per dose (0.5 mL, 2.5 mL, 5 mL)

halazepam (hal AZ e pam)
U.S. Brand Names Paxipam®
Generic Available No
Therapeutic Category Benzodiazepine
Controlled Substance C-IV
Use Management of anxiety disorders; short-term relief of the symptoms of anxiety
Usual Dosage Adults: Oral: 20-40 mg 3 or 4 times/day
Nursing/Pharmacy Information
Assist patient with ambulation
Monitor for alertness
Dosage Forms Tablet: 20 mg, 40 mg

♦ Halazone Tablet *(Discontinued)* see page 743

halcinonide (hal SIN oh nide)
U.S. Brand Names Halog®; Halog®-E
Generic Available No
Therapeutic Category Corticosteroid, Topical
Use Inflammation of corticosteroid-responsive dermatoses
Usual Dosage Children and Adults: Topical: Apply sparingly 1-3 times/day; occlusive dressing may be used for severe or resistant dermatoses
Nursing/Pharmacy Information A thin film of cream or ointment is effective; do not overuse; do not use tight-fitting diapers or plastic pants on children being treated in the diaper area; use only as prescribed, and for no longer than the period prescribed; apply sparingly in light film; rub in lightly; avoid contact with eyes; notify physician if condition being treated persists or worsens
Dosage Forms
Cream (Halog®): 0.025% (15 g, 60 g, 240 g); 0.1% (15 g, 30 g, 60 g, 240 g)
Cream, emollient base (Halog®-E) : 0.1% (15 g, 30 g, 60 g)
Ointment, topical (Halog®): 0.1% (15 g, 30 g, 60 g, 240 g)
Solution (Halog®): 0.1% (20 mL, 60 mL)

♦ Halcion® see triazolam on page 625
♦ Haldol® see haloperidol on page 308
♦ Haldol® Decanoate see haloperidol on page 308
♦ Haldrone® see paramethasone acetate on page 470
♦ Halenol® Tablet *(Discontinued)* see page 743
♦ Haley's M-O® [OTC] see magnesium hydroxide and mineral oil emulsion on page 381
♦ Halfan® see halofantrine on page 308
♦ Halfprin® [OTC] see aspirin on page 61

halobetasol (hal oh BAY ta sol)
U.S. Brand Names Ultravate™
Generic Available No
Therapeutic Category Corticosteroid, Topical
Use Relief of inflammatory and pruritic manifestations of corticosteroid-response dermatoses
Usual Dosage Children and Adults: Topical: Apply sparingly to skin twice daily; rub in gently and completely
Nursing/Pharmacy Information A thin film of cream or ointment is effective; do not overuse; do not use tight-fitting diapers or plastic pants on children
(Continued)

halobetasol *(Continued)*

being treated in the diaper area; use only as prescribed, and for no longer than the period prescribed; apply sparingly in light film; rub in lightly; avoid contact with eyes; notify physician if condition being treated persists or worsens

Dosage Forms Halobetasol propionate:
Cream: 0.05% (15 g, 45 g)
Ointment, topical: 0.05% (15 g, 45 g)

halofantrine *(ha loe FAN trin)*

U.S. Brand Names Halfan®
Generic Available No
Therapeutic Category Antimalarial Agent
Use Treatment of mild to moderate acute malaria caused by susceptible strains of *Plasmodium falciparum* and *Plasmodium vivax*
Usual Dosage Oral:
Children <40 kg: 8 mg/kg every 6 hours for 3 doses
Adults: 500 mg every 6 hours for 3 doses
Nursing/Pharmacy Information Monitor CBC, LFTs, parasite counts
Dosage Forms Halofantrine hydrochloride:
Suspension: 100 mg/5 mL
Tablet: 250 mg

♦ **Halog®** *see* halcinonide *on page 307*
♦ **Halog®-E** *see* halcinonide *on page 307*

haloperidol *(ha loe PER i dole)*

U.S. Brand Names Haldol®; Haldol® Decanoate
Canadian Brand Names Peridol
Mexican Brand Names Haloperil
Generic Available Yes
Therapeutic Category Antipsychotic Agent, Butyrophenone
Use Treatment of psychoses, Tourette's disorder, and severe behavioral problems in children
Usual Dosage
Children:
<3 years: Not recommended
3-6 years: Dose and indications are not well established
Control of agitation or hyperkinesia in disturbed children: Oral: 0.01-0.03 mg/kg/day once daily
Infantile autism: Oral: Daily doses of 0.5-4 mg have been reported to be helpful in this disorder
6-12 years: Dose not well established
I.M.: 1-3 mg/dose every 4-8 hours, up to a maximum of 0.1 mg/kg/day
Acute psychoses: Oral: Begin with 0.5-1.5 mg/day and increase gradually in increments of 0.5 mg/day, to a maintenance dose of 2-4 mg/day (0.05-0.1 mg/kg/day).
Tourette's syndrome and mental retardation with hyperkinesia: Oral: Begin with 0.5 mg/day and increase by 0.5 mg/day each day until symptoms are controlled or a maximum dose of 15 mg is reached
Children >12 years and Adults:
I.M.:
Acute psychoses: 2-5 mg/dose every 1-8 hours PRN up to a total of 10-30 mg, until control of symptoms is achieved
Mental retardation with hyperkinesia: Begin with 20 mg/day in divided doses, then increase slowly, up to a maximum of 60 mg/day; change to oral administration as soon as symptoms are controlled
Oral:
Acute psychoses: Begin with 1-15 mg/day in divided doses, then gradually increase until symptoms are controlled, up to a maximum of 100 mg/day; after control of symptoms is achieved, reduce dose to the minimal effective dose
Tourette's syndrome: Begin with 6-15 mg/day in divided doses, increase in increments of 2-10 mg/day until symptoms are controlled or adverse reactions become disabling; when symptoms are controlled, reduce to approximately 9 mg/day for maintenance
Dietary Considerations Do not mix oral concentrate with coffee or tea; should be administered with food or milk
Nursing/Pharmacy Information
Do not administer I.V.
Monitor blood pressure, heart rate, signs and symptoms and extrapyramidal effects (stiff neck, jaw pain, eye rolling, etc)

Stability: Protect oral dosage forms from light; **incompatible** when mixed in same syringe with diamorphine, heparin (precipitate in 5 minutes), or at Y-site for fluconazole, foscarnet, heparin, sargramostim

Dosage Forms
Haloperidol lactate:
Concentrate, oral: 2 mg/mL (5 mL, 10 mL, 15 mL, 120 mL, 240 mL)
Injection: 5 mg/mL (1 mL, 2 mL, 2.5 mL, 10 mL)
Haloperidol decanoate:
Injection: 50 mg/mL (1 mL, 5 mL); 100 mg/mL (1 mL, 5 mL)
Tablet: 0.5 mg, 1 mg, 2 mg, 5 mg, 10 mg, 20 mg

♦ **Haloperil** see haloperidol on page 308

haloprogin (ha loe PROE jin)
U.S. Brand Names Halotex®
Generic Available No
Therapeutic Category Antifungal Agent
Use Topical treatment of tinea pedis, tinea cruris, tinea corporis, tinea manuum caused by *Trichophyton rubrum*, *Trichophyton tonsurans*, *Trichophyton mentagrophytes*, *Microsporum canis*, or *Epidermophyton floccosum*
Usual Dosage Children and Adults: Topical: Twice daily for 2-3 weeks; intertriginous areas may require up to 4 weeks of treatment
Nursing/Pharmacy Information Avoid contact with eyes; for external use only; improvement should occur within 4 weeks; discontinue use if sensitization or irritation occur
Dosage Forms
Cream: 1% (15 g, 30 g)
Solution, topical: 1% with alcohol 75% (10 mL, 30 mL)

♦ **Halotestin**® see fluoxymesterone on page 276
♦ **Halotex**® see haloprogin on page 309

halothane (HA loe thane)
U.S. Brand Names Fluothane®
Generic Available No
Therapeutic Category General Anesthetic
Use General induction and maintenance of anesthesia (inhalation)
Usual Dosage Maintenance concentration varies from 0.5% to 1.5%
Dosage Forms Liquid: 125 mL, 250 mL

♦ **Halotussin**® [OTC] see guaifenesin on page 299
♦ **Halotussin**® **DAC** see guaifenesin, pseudoephedrine, and codeine on page 304
♦ **Halotussin**® **DM** [OTC] see guaifenesin and dextromethorphan on page 300
♦ **Halotussin**® **PE** [OTC] see guaifenesin and pseudoephedrine on page 302
♦ **Haltran**® [OTC] see ibuprofen on page 332
♦ **hamamelis water** see witch hazel on page 655
♦ **Harmonyl**® *(Discontinued)* see page 743
♦ **Havrix**® see hepatitis A vaccine on page 311
♦ **Hayfebrol**® **Liquid** [OTC] see chlorpheniramine and pseudoephedrine on page 140
♦ **H-BIG**® see hepatitis B immune globulin on page 311
♦ **HCG** see chorionic gonadotropin on page 149
♦ **HCTZ** see hydrochlorothiazide on page 317
♦ **HD 85**® see radiological/contrast media (ionic) on page 539
♦ **HD 200 Plus**® see radiological/contrast media (ionic) on page 539
♦ **HDCV** see rabies virus vaccine on page 539
♦ **HDRS** see rabies virus vaccine on page 539
♦ **Head & Shoulders**® [OTC] see pyrithione zinc on page 535
♦ **Healon**® see sodium hyaluronate on page 572
♦ **Healon**® **GV** see sodium hyaluronate on page 572
♦ **Hectorol**® see doxercalciferol New Drug on page 220
♦ **Helberina** see heparin on page 310
♦ **Helidac**™ see bismuth subsalicylate, metronidazole, and tetracycline on page 89
♦ **Helistat**® see microfibrillar collagen hemostat on page 414
♦ **Helixate**® see antihemophilic factor (recombinant) on page 52
♦ **Helminzole** see mebendazole on page 387
♦ **Hemabate**™ see carboprost tromethamine on page 115
♦ **HemFe**® *(Discontinued)* see page 743

♦ **hemiacidrin** *see citric acid bladder mixture on page 154*

hemin (HEE min)

U.S. Brand Names Panhematin®
Generic Available No
Therapeutic Category Blood Modifiers
Use Treatment of recurrent attacks of acute intermittent porphyria (AIP) only after an appropriate period of alternate therapy has been tried
Usual Dosage I.V.: 1-4 mg/kg/day administered over 10-15 minutes for 3-14 days; may be repeated no earlier than every 12 hours; not to exceed 6 mg/kg in any 24-hour period
Dosage Forms Powder for injection, preservative free: 313 mg/vial [hematin 7 mg/mL] (43 mL)

♦ **Hemocyte® [OTC]** *see ferrous fumarate on page 264*
♦ **Hemofil® M** *see antihemophilic factor (human) on page 51*
♦ **Hemonyne®** *see factor IX complex (human) on page 257*
♦ **Hemotene®** *see microfibrillar collagen hemostat on page 414*
♦ **Henexal** *see furosemide on page 285*
♦ **Hepalean®, -LOK, -LCO** *see heparin on page 310*

heparin (HEP a rin)

Synonyms heparin lock flush
U.S. Brand Names Hep-Lock®; Liquaemin®
Canadian Brand Names Calcilean® [HepCalium]; Hepalean®, -LOK, -LCO
Mexican Brand Names Dixaparine; Helberina; Inhepar
Generic Available Yes
Therapeutic Category Anticoagulant
Use Prophylaxis and treatment of thromboembolic disorders
Usual Dosage Note: For full-dose heparin (ie, nonlow-dose), the dose should be titrated according to PTT results. For anticoagulation, an APTT 1.5-2.5 times normal is usually desired. APTT is usually measured prior to heparin therapy, 6-8 hours after initiation of a continuous infusion (following a loading dose), and 6-8 hours after changes in the infusion rate; increase or decrease infusion by 2-4 units/kg/hour dependent on PTT. Continuous I.V. infusion is preferred vs I.V. intermittent injections. For intermittent I.V. injections, PTT is measured 3.5-4 hours after I.V. injection.

Children:
  Intermittent I.V.: Initial: 50-100 units/kg, then 50-100 units/kg every 4 hours
  I.V. infusion: Initial: 50 units/kg, then 15-25 units/kg/hour; increase dose by 2-4 units/kg/hour every 6-8 hours as required
Adults:
  Prophylaxis (low-dose heparin): S.C.: 5000 units every 8-12 hours
  Intermittent I.V.: Initial: 10,000 units, then 50-70 units/kg (5000-10,000 units) every 4-6 hours
  I.V. infusion: Initial: 75-100 units/kg, then 15 units/kg/hour with dose adjusted according to PTT results; usual range: 10-30 units/kg/hour
Nursing/Pharmacy Information
Do not administer I.M. due to pain, irritation, and hematoma formation
Monitor platelet counts, PTT, hemoglobin, hematocrit, signs of bleeding
Stability: Stable at room temperature; protect from freezing
Dosage Forms
Heparin sodium:
  Lock flush injection:
    Beef lung source: 10 units/mL (1 mL, 2 mL, 2.5 mL, 3 mL, 5 mL, 10 mL, 30 mL); 100 units/mL (1 mL, 2 mL, 2.5 mL, 3 mL, 5 mL, 10 mL, 30 mL)
    Porcine intestinal mucosa source: 10 units/mL (1 mL, 2 mL, 10 mL, 30 mL); 100 units/mL (1 mL, 2 mL, 10 mL, 30 mL)
    Porcine intestinal mucosa source, preservative free: 10 units/mL (1 mL); 100 units/mL (1 mL)
  Multiple-dose vial injection:
    Beef lung source, with preservative: 1000 units/mL (5 mL, 10 mL, 30 mL); 5000 units/mL (10 mL); 10,000 units/mL (4 mL, 5 mL, 10 mL); 20,000 units/mL (2 mL, 5 mL, 10 mL); 40,000 units/mL (5 mL)
    Porcine intestinal mucosa source, with preservative: 1000 units/mL (10 mL, 30 mL); 5000 units/mL (10 mL); 10,000 units/mL (4 mL); 20,000 units/mL (2 mL, 5 mL)
  Single-dose vial injection:
    Beef lung source: 1000 units/mL (1 mL); 5000 units/mL (1 mL); 10,000 units/mL (1 mL); 20,000 units/mL (1 mL); 40,000 units/mL (1 mL)

Porcine intestinal mucosa: 1000 units/mL (1 mL); 5000 units/mL (1 mL); 10,000 units/mL (1 mL); 20,000 units/mL (1 mL); 40,000 units/mL (1 mL)

Unit dose injection:

Porcine intestinal mucosa source, with preservative: 1000 units/dose (1 mL, 2 mL); 2500 units/dose (1 mL); 5000 units/dose (0.5 mL, 1 mL); 7500 units/dose (1 mL); 10,000 units/dose (1 mL); 15,000 units/dose (1 mL); 20,000 units/dose (1 mL)

Heparin sodium infusion, porcine intestinal mucosa source:

D_5W: 40 units/mL (500 mL); 50 units/mL (250 mL, 500 mL); 100 units/mL (100 mL, 250 mL)

NaCl 0.45%: 2 units/mL (500 mL, 1000 mL); 50 units/mL (250 mL); 100 units/mL (250 mL)

NaCl 0.9%: 2 units/mL (500 mL, 1000 mL); 5 units/mL (1000 mL); 50 units/mL (250 mL, 500 mL, 1000 mL)

Heparin calcium:

Unit dose injection, porcine intestinal mucosa, preservative free: 5000 units/dose (0.2 mL); 12,500 units/dose (0.5 mL); 20,000 units/dose (0.8 mL)

- ♦ **heparin cofactor I** *see* antithrombin III *on page 53*
- ♦ **heparin lock flush** *see* heparin *on page 310*

hepatitis A vaccine (hep a TYE tis aye vak SEEN)
U.S. Brand Names Havrix®
Generic Available No
Therapeutic Category Vaccine, Inactivated Virus
Use For populations desiring protection against hepatitis A or for populations at high risk of exposure to hepatitis A virus (travelers to developing countries, household and sexual contacts of persons infected with hepatitis A), child day care employees, illicit drug users, male homosexuals, institutional workers (eg, institutions for the mentally and physically handicapped persons, prisons, etc), and healthcare workers who may be exposed to hepatitis A virus (eg, laboratory employees)
Usual Dosage I.M.:
Children: 0.5 mL (360 units) on days 1 and 30, with a booster dose 6-12 months late; completion of the first 2 doses (ie, the primary series) should be accomplished at least 2 weeks before anticipated exposure to hepatitis A
Adults: 1 mL (1440 units), with a booster dose at 6-12 months
Dosage Forms
Injection: 360 ELISA units/0.5 mL (0.5 mL); 1440 ELISA units/mL (1 mL)
Injection, pediatric: 720 ELISA units/0.5 mL (0.5 mL)

hepatitis B immune globulin
(hep a TYE tis bee i MYUN GLOB yoo lin)
Synonyms HBIG
U.S. Brand Names H-BIG®; HyperHep®; Nabi-HB™
Generic Available No
Therapeutic Category Immune Globulin
Use Provide prophylactic passive immunity to hepatitis B infection to those individuals exposed. Hepatitis B immune globulin is not indicated for treatment of active hepatitis B infections and is ineffective in the treatment of chronic active hepatitis B infection.
Usual Dosage I.M.:
Newborns: Hepatitis B: 0.5 mL as soon after birth as possible (within 12 hours)
Adults: Postexposure prophylaxis: 0.06 mL/kg; usual dose: 3-5 mL; repeat at 28-30 days after exposure
Nursing/Pharmacy Information
I.M. injection only; to prevent injury from injection care should be taken when administering to patients with thrombocytopenia or bleeding disorders; do not administer I.V.
Stability: Refrigerate
Dosage Forms Injection:
H-BIG®: 4 mL, 5 mL
HyperHep®: 0.5 mL, 1 mL, 5 mL
Nabi-HB™: 1 mL, 5 mL

- ♦ **hepatitis B inactivated virus vaccine (plasma derived)** *see* hepatitis B vaccine *on page 312*
- ♦ **hepatitis B inactivated virus vaccine (recombinant DNA)** *see* hepatitis B vaccine *on page 312*

hepatitis B vaccine (hep a TYE tis bee vak SEEN)

Synonyms hepatitis B inactivated virus vaccine (plasma derived); hepatitis B inactivated virus vaccine (recombinant DNA)

U.S. Brand Names Engerix-B®; Recombivax HB®

Generic Available No

Therapeutic Category Vaccine, Inactivated Virus

Use Immunization against infection caused by all known subtypes of hepatitis B virus in individuals considered at high risk of potential exposure to hepatitis B virus or HB$_s$Ag-positive materials

Usual Dosage I.M.:

Children:

≤11 years: 2.5 mcg doses

11-19 years: 5 mcg doses

Adults >20 years: 10 mcg doses

Nursing/Pharmacy Information

I.M. injection preferred; S.C. can be used if patient cannot be given I.M. injection

Stability: Refrigerate, do not freeze

Dosage Forms Injection:

Recombinant DNA (Engerix-B®): Hepatitis B surface antigen 20 mcg/mL (1 mL)

Pediatric, recombinant DNA (Engerix-B®): Hepatitis B surface antigen 10 mcg/0.5 mL (0.5 mL)

Recombinant DNA (Recombivax HB®): Hepatitis B surface antigen 10 mcg/mL (1 mL, 3 mL)

Dialysis formulation, recombinant DNA (Recombivax HB®): Hepatitis B surface antigen 40 mcg/mL (1 mL)

♦ **Hep-B-Gammagee®** *(Discontinued)* see page 743
♦ **Hep-Lock®** see heparin on page 310
♦ **Heptalac®** see lactulose on page 359
♦ **Herceptin®** see trastuzumab on page 621
♦ **Herklin** see lindane on page 370
♦ **Herplex®** *(Discontinued)* see page 743
♦ **HES** see hetastarch on page 312
♦ **Hespan®** see hetastarch on page 312

hetastarch (HET a starch)

Synonyms HES; hydroxyethyl starch

U.S. Brand Names Hespan®

Generic Available No

Therapeutic Category Plasma Volume Expander

Use Blood volume expander used in treatment of shock or impending shock when blood or blood products are not available; does not have oxygen-carrying capacity and is not a substitute for blood or plasma; an adjunct in leukapheresis to enhance the yield of granulocytes by centrifugal means

Usual Dosage I.V.: Up to 1500 mL/day

Nursing/Pharmacy Information

I.V. only; may administer up to 1.2 g/kg/hour (20 mL/kg/hour); anaphylactoid reactions can occur, have epinephrine and resuscitative equipment available

Stability: Do not use if crystalline precipitate forms or is turbid deep brown

Dosage Forms Infusion, in sodium chloride 0.9%: 6% (500 mL)

♦ **Hetrazan®** *(Discontinued)* see page 743
♦ **Hexabrix™** see radiological/contrast media (ionic) on page 539
♦ **hexachlorocyclohexane** see lindane on page 370

hexachlorophene (heks a KLOR oh feen)

U.S. Brand Names pHisoHex®; Septisol®

Generic Available Yes

Therapeutic Category Antibacterial, Topical

Use Surgical scrub and as a bacteriostatic skin cleanser; to control an outbreak of gram-positive staphylococcal infection when other infection control procedures have been unsuccessful

Usual Dosage Children and Adults: Topical: Apply 5 mL cleanser and water to area to be cleansed; lather and rinse thoroughly under running water

Nursing/Pharmacy Information

Do not use for bathing infants; premature infants are particularly susceptible to hexachlorophene topical absorption

Stability: Store in nonmetallic container (**incompatible** with many metals)

Dosage Forms
Foam (Septisol®): 0.23% with alcohol 56% (180 mL, 600 mL)
Liquid, topical (pHisoHex®): 3% (8 mL, 150 mL, 500 mL, 3840 mL)

♦ **Hexadrol®** *see* dexamethasone (systemic) *on page 190*
♦ **Hexalen®** *see* altretamine *on page 32*
♦ **hexamethylenetetramine** *see* methenamine *on page 400*
♦ **hexamethylmelamine** *see* altretamine *on page 32*
♦ **Hexit®** *see* lindane *on page 370*

hexylresorcinol (heks il re ZOR si nole)
U.S. Brand Names Sucrets® Sore Throat [OTC]
Generic Available Yes
Therapeutic Category Local Anesthetic
Use Minor antiseptic and local anesthetic for sore throat
Usual Dosage May be used as needed, allow to dissolve slowly in mouth
Dosage Forms Lozenge: 2.4 mg

♦ **Hibiclens® [OTC]** *see* chlorhexidine gluconate *on page 134*
♦ **Hibidil® 1:2000** *see* chlorhexidine gluconate *on page 134*
♦ **Hibistat® [OTC]** *see* chlorhexidine gluconate *on page 134*
♦ **Hibitane® Skin Cleanser** *see* chlorhexidine gluconate *on page 134*
♦ **HIB polysaccharide conjugate** *see* Haemophilus B conjugate vaccine *on page 306*
♦ **HibTITER®** *see* Haemophilus B conjugate vaccine *on page 306*
♦ **Hi-Cor-1.0® Topical** *see* hydrocortisone (topical) *on page 324*
♦ **Hi-Cor-2.5® Topical** *see* hydrocortisone (topical) *on page 324*
♦ **Hidramox®** *see* amoxicillin *on page 43*
♦ **Higroton 50** *see* chlorthalidone *on page 146*
♦ **Hipokinon** *see* trihexyphenidyl *on page 628*
♦ **Hiprex®** *see* methenamine *on page 400*
♦ **Hismanal® *(Discontinued)*** *see page 743*
♦ **Histaject® *(Discontinued)*** *see page 743*
♦ **Histalet Forte® Tablet** *see* chlorpheniramine, pyrilamine, phenylephrine, and phenylpropanolamine *on page 144*
♦ **Histalet® Syrup [OTC]** *see* chlorpheniramine and pseudoephedrine *on page 140*
♦ **Histalet® X** *see* guaifenesin and pseudoephedrine *on page 302*
♦ **Histamine Phosphate Injection *(Discontinued)*** *see page 743*
♦ **Histantil** *see* promethazine *on page 522*
♦ **Histatab® Plus Tablet [OTC]** *see* chlorpheniramine and phenylephrine *on page 139*
♦ **Hista-Vadrin® Tablet** *see* chlorpheniramine, phenylephrine, and phenylpropanolamine *on page 142*
♦ **Histerone® Injection** *see* testosterone *on page 598*
♦ **Histolyn-CYL®** *see* histoplasmin *on page 313*

histoplasmin (his toe PLAZ min)
Synonyms histoplasmosis skin test antigen
U.S. Brand Names Histolyn-CYL®
Generic Available No
Therapeutic Category Diagnostic Agent
Use Diagnosing histoplasmosis; to assess cell-mediated immunity
Usual Dosage Adults: Intradermally: 0.1 mL of 1:100 dilution 5-10 cm apart into volar surface of forearm; induration of ≥5 mm in diameter indicates a positive reaction
Nursing/Pharmacy Information
Examine reaction site at 24-48 hours for cell-mediated immunity and 48-72 hours for histoplasmosis; use a $^3/_8$" to $^1/_2$" 26- or 27-gauge needle
Stability: Store in refrigerator
Dosage Forms Injection: 1:100 (0.1 mL, 1.3 mL)

♦ **histoplasmosis skin test antigen** *see* histoplasmin *on page 313*
♦ **Histor-D® Syrup** *see* chlorpheniramine and phenylephrine *on page 139*
♦ **Histor-D® Timecelles®** *see* chlorpheniramine, phenylephrine, and methscopolamine *on page 141*

histrelin (his TREL in)
U.S. Brand Names Supprelin™
Generic Available No
(Continued)

histrelin *(Continued)*

Therapeutic Category Gonadotropin Releasing Hormone Analog

Use Central idiopathic precocious puberty; also used to treat estrogen-associated gynecological disorders (ie, endometriosis, intermittent porphyria, possibly premenstrual syndrome, leiomyomata uteri [uterine fibroids])

Usual Dosage

Central idiopathic precocious puberty: S.C.: Usual dose is 10 mcg/kg/day administered as a single daily dose at the same time each day

Acute intermittent porphyria in women:

S.C.: 5 mcg/day

Intranasal: 400-800 mcg/day

Endometriosis: S.C.: 100 mcg/day

Leiomyomata uteri: S.C.: 20-50 mcg/day or 4 mcg/kg/day

Nursing/Pharmacy Information

Parenteral: S.C.: Vary the injection site daily

Monitoring for precocious puberty: Prior to initiating therapy: Height and weight, hand and wrist x-rays, total sex steroid levels, beta-hCG level, adrenal steroid level, gonadotropin-releasing hormone stimulation test, pelvic/adrenal/testicular ultrasound/head CT; during therapy monitor 3 months after initiation and then every 6-12 months; serial levels of sex steroids and gonadotropin-releasing hormone testing; physical exam; secondary sexual development; histrelin may be discontinued when the patient reaches the appropriate age for puberty

Stability: Refrigerate at 2°C to 8°C (36°F to 46°F) and protect from light; allow vial to reach room temperature before injecting contents

Dosage Forms Injection: 7-day kits of single use: 120 mcg/0.6 mL; 300 mcg/0.6 mL; 600 mcg/0.6 mL

- ◆ **Histussin D® Liquid** *see* hydrocodone and pseudoephedrine *on page 321*
- ◆ **Hi-Vegi-Lip®** *see* pancreatin *on page 467*
- ◆ **Hivid®** *see* zalcitabine *on page 657*
- ◆ **HMS Liquifilm®** *see* medrysone *on page 389*
- ◆ **HN₂** *see* mechlorethamine *on page 387*
- ◆ **Hold® DM [OTC]** *see* dextromethorphan *on page 194*

homatropine *(hoe MA troe peen)*

U.S. Brand Names AK-Homatropine® Ophthalmic; Isopto® Homatropine Ophthalmic

Generic Available Yes

Therapeutic Category Anticholinergic Agent

Use Producing cycloplegia and mydriasis for refraction; treatment of acute inflammatory conditions of the uveal tract

Usual Dosage Ophthalmic:

Children:

Mydriasis and cycloplegia for refraction: 1 drop of 2% solution immediately before the procedure; repeat at 10-minute intervals as needed

Uveitis: 1 drop of 2% solution 2-3 times/day

Adults:

Mydriasis and cycloplegia for refraction: 1-2 drops of 2% solution or 1 drop of 5% solution before the procedure; repeat at 5- to 10-minute intervals as needed

Uveitis: 1-2 drops 2-3 times/day up to every 3-4 hours as needed

Nursing/Pharmacy Information

Finger pressure should be applied to lacrimal sac for 1-2 minutes after instillation to decrease risk of absorption and systemic reactions

Stability: Protect from light

Dosage Forms Solution, ophthalmic, as hydrobromide:

2% (1 mL, 5 mL); 5% (1 mL, 2 mL, 5 mL)

AK-Homatropine®: 5% (15 mL)

Isopto® Homatropine 2% (5 mL, 15 mL); 5% (5 mL, 15 mL)

- ◆ **homatropine and hydrocodone** *see* hydrocodone and homatropine *on page 320*
- ◆ **Honvol®** *see* diethylstilbestrol *on page 201*
- ◆ **horse antihuman thymocyte gamma globulin** *see* lymphocyte immune globulin *on page 378*
- ◆ **H.P. Acthar® Gel** *see* corticotropin *on page 169*
- ◆ **Humalog®** *see* insulin preparations *on page 339*

human growth hormone (HYU man grothe HOR mone)

Synonyms somatrem; somatropin

U.S. Brand Names Genotropin®; Humatrope®; Norditropin®; Nutropin®; Nutropin® AQ; Protropin®; Saizen®; Serostim®

Generic Available No

Therapeutic Category Growth Hormone

Use Long-term treatment of growth failure from lack of adequate endogenous growth hormone secretion

Usual Dosage Children: I.M., S.C.:

Somatrem: Up to 0.1 mg (0.26 units)/kg/dose 3 times/week

Somatropin: Up to 0.06 mg (0.16 units)/kg/dose 3 times/week

Therapy should be discontinued when patient has reached satisfactory adult height, when epiphyses have fused, or when the patient ceases to respond

Nursing/Pharmacy Information

Do not shake vial when reconstituting; 1 mg = 2.6 units; a patient's booklet on mixing and administration is available; rotate injection site

Somatrem: Reconstitute each 5 mg vial with 1-5 mL bacteriostatic water for injection, USP (benzyl alcohol preserved) only; when using in newborns, reconstitute with preservative-free sterile water

Somatropin: Reconstitute each 5 mg vial with 1.5-5 mL diluent

Monitor growth curve, periodic thyroid function tests, bone age (annually), periodical urine testing for glucose, somatomedin C levels

Stability: Store in refrigerator; use reconstituted vials within 7 days (Protropin®) or 14 days (Humatrope®)

Dosage Forms Powder for injection (lyophilized):

Somatropin:

Genotropin®: 1.5 mg ~4.5 units (5 mL); 5.8 mg ~17.4 units (5 mL)

Humatrope®: 5 mg ~15 units

Norditropin®: 4 mg ~12 units; 8 mg ~24 units

Nutropin®: 5 mg ~15 units (10 mL); 10 mg ~30 units (10 mL)

Nutropin® AQ: 10 mg ~30 units (2 mL)

Saizen® (rDNA origin): 5 mg ~15 units

Serostim®: 5 mg ~15 units (5 mL); 6 mg ~18 units (5 mL)

Somatrem, Protropin®: 5 mg ~15 units (10 mL); 10 mg ~26 units (10 mL)

+ **human thyroid-stimulating hormone** *see* thyrotropin alpha *New Drug on page 610*

+ **Humatin®** *see* paromomycin *on page 471*

+ **Humatrope®** *see* human growth hormone *on page 315*

+ **Humegon™** *see* menotropins *on page 391*

+ **Humibid® DM [OTC]** *see* guaifenesin and dextromethorphan *on page 300*

+ **Humibid® L.A.** *see* guaifenesin *on page 299*

+ **Humibid® Sprinkle** *see* guaifenesin *on page 299*

+ **HuMist® Nasal Mist [OTC]** *see* sodium chloride *on page 571*

+ **Humorsol® Ophthalmic** *see* demecarium *on page 185*

+ **Humulin® 50/50** *see* insulin preparations *on page 339*

+ **Humulin® 70/30** *see* insulin preparations *on page 339*

+ **Humulin® L** *see* insulin preparations *on page 339*

+ **Humulin® N** *see* insulin preparations *on page 339*

+ **Humulin® R** *see* insulin preparations *on page 339*

+ **Humulin® U** *see* insulin preparations *on page 339*

+ **Hurricaine®** *see* benzocaine *on page 79*

+ **hyaluronic acid** *see* sodium hyaluronate *on page 572*

hyaluronidase (hye al yoor ON i dase)

U.S. Brand Names Wydase®

Generic Available No

Therapeutic Category Antidote

Use Increase the dispersion and absorption of other drugs; increase rate of absorption of parenteral fluids administered by hypodermoclysis; management of I.V. extravasations

Usual Dosage

Infants and Children:

Management of I.V. extravasation: Reconstitute the 150 unit vial of lyophilized powder with 1 mL normal saline; administer 0.1 mL of this solution and dilute with 0.9 mL normal saline to yield 15 units/mL; using a 25- or 26-gauge needle, five 0.2 mL injections are made subcutaneously or intradermally into the extravasation site at the leading edge, changing the needle after each injection

(Continued)

hyaluronidase *(Continued)*

Hypodermoclysis: S.C.: 15 units is added to each 100 mL of I.V. fluid to be administered

Adults: Absorption and dispersion of drugs: 150 units is added to the vehicle containing the drug

Nursing/Pharmacy Information
Administer hyaluronidase within the first few minutes to one hour after the extravasation is recognized

Stability: Reconstituted hyaluronidase solution remains stable for only 24 hours when stored in the refrigerator; do not use discolored solutions

Dosage Forms
Injection, stabilized solution: 150 units/mL (1 mL, 10 mL)
Powder for injection, lyophilized: 150 units, 1500 units

- **Hyate®:C** *see* antihemophilic factor (porcine) *on page 52*
- **Hybolin™ Decanoate** *see* nandrolone *on page 431*
- **Hybolin™ Improved Injection** *see* nandrolone *on page 431*
- **hycamptamine** *see* topotecan *on page 619*
- **Hycamtin™** *see* topotecan *on page 619*
- **HycoClear Tuss®** *see* hydrocodone and guaifenesin *on page 320*
- **Hycodan®** *see* hydrocodone and homatropine *on page 320*
- **Hycomine®** *see* hydrocodone and phenylpropanolamine *on page 321*
- **Hycomine® Compound** *see* hydrocodone, chlorpheniramine, phenylephrine, acetaminophen, and caffeine *on page 321*
- **Hycomine® Pediatric** *see* hydrocodone and phenylpropanolamine *on page 321*
- **Hycort® Topical** *see* hydrocortisone (topical) *on page 324*
- **Hycotuss® Expectorant Liquid** *see* hydrocodone and guaifenesin *on page 320*
- **Hydeltra-T.B.A.® *(Discontinued)*** *see page 743*
- **Hydergine®** *see* ergoloid mesylates *on page 238*
- **Hydergine® LC** *see* ergoloid mesylates *on page 238*
- **Hyderm** *see* hydrocortisone (topical) *on page 324*

hydralazine *(hye DRAL a zeen)*

U.S. Brand Names Apresoline®
Canadian Brand Names Apo®-Hydralazine; Novo-Hylazin®; Nu-Hydral®
Mexican Brand Names Apresolina
Generic Available Yes
Therapeutic Category Vasodilator
Use Management of moderate to severe hypertension, congestive heart failure, hypertension secondary to pre-eclampsia/eclampsia, primary pulmonary hypertension
Usual Dosage
Children:
Oral: Initial: 0.75-1 mg/kg/day in 2-4 divided doses, not to exceed 25 mg/dose; increase over 3-4 weeks to maximum of 7.5 mg/kg/day in 2-4 divided doses; maximum daily dose: 200 mg/day
I.M., I.V.: 0.1-0.5 mg/kg/dose (initial dose not to exceed 20 mg) every 4-6 hours as needed
Adults:
Oral: Initial: 10 mg 4 times/day, increase by 10-25 mg/dose every 2-5 days to maximum of 300 mg/day
I.M., I.V.:
Hypertensive initial: 10-20 mg/dose every 4-6 hours as needed, may increase to 40 mg/dose
Pre-eclampsia/eclampsia: 5 mg/dose then 5-10 mg every 20-30 minutes as needed
Dietary Considerations Avoid natural licorice (causes sodium and water retention and increases potassium loss); long-term use of hydralazine may cause pyridoxine deficiency resulting in numbness, tingling, and paresthesias; if symptoms develop, pyridoxine supplements may be needed
Nursing/Pharmacy Information
Do not exceed rate of 0.2 mg/kg/minute; maximum concentration for I.V. use: 20 mg/mL
Monitor blood pressure, standing and sitting/supine
Stability: Changes color after contact with a metal filter; do not store intact ampuls in refrigerator

Dosage Forms Hydralazine hydrochloride:
Injection: 20 mg/mL (1 mL)
Tablet: 10 mg, 25 mg, 50 mg, 100 mg

hydralazine and hydrochlorothiazide
(hye DRAL a zeen & hye droe klor oh THYE a zide)
Synonyms hydrochlorothiazide and hydralazine
U.S. Brand Names Apresazide®
Generic Available Yes
Therapeutic Category Antihypertensive Agent, Combination
Use Management of moderate to severe hypertension and treatment of conges-
tive heart failure
Usual Dosage Adults: Oral: 1 capsule twice daily
Dosage Forms Capsule:
25/25: Hydralazine hydrochloride 25 mg and hydrochlorothiazide 25 mg
50/50: Hydralazine hydrochloride 50 mg and hydrochlorothiazide 50 mg
100/50: Hydralazine hydrochloride 100 mg and hydrochlorothiazide 50 mg

hydralazine, hydrochlorothiazide, and reserpine
(hye DRAL a zeen, hye droe klor oh THYE a zide, & re SER peen)
Synonyms hydrochlorothiazide, hydralazine, and reserpine; reserpine, hydrala-
zine, and hydrochlorothiazide
U.S. Brand Names Hydrap-ES®; Marpres®; Ser-Ap-Es®
Generic Available Yes
Therapeutic Category Antihypertensive Agent, Combination
Use Hypertensive disorders
Usual Dosage Adults: Oral: 1-2 tablets 3 times/day
Dietary Considerations May be administered with meals
Dosage Forms Tablet: Hydralazine 25 mg, hydrochlorothiazide 15 mg, and
reserpine 0.1 mg

♦ **Hydramine®** *(Discontinued) see page 743*
♦ **Hydramyn® Syrup [OTC]** *see diphenhydramine on page 208*
♦ **Hydrap-ES®** *see hydralazine, hydrochlorothiazide, and reserpine on page 317*
♦ **Hydrate® Injection** *see dimenhydrinate on page 206*
♦ **Hydrea®** *see hydroxyurea on page 328*
♦ **Hydrobexan® Injection** *(Discontinued) see page 743*
♦ **Hydrocet®** *see hydrocodone and acetaminophen on page 319*

hydrochlorothiazide (hye droe klor oh THYE a zide)
Synonyms HCTZ
U.S. Brand Names Esidrix®; Ezide®; HydroDIURIL®; Hydro-Par®; Microzide™;
Oretic®
Canadian Brand Names Apo®-Hydro; Diuchlor®; Neo-Codema®; Novo-Hydra-
zide®; Urozide®
Mexican Brand Names Diclotride®
Generic Available Yes: Tablet
Therapeutic Category Diuretic, Thiazide
Use Management of mild to moderate hypertension; treatment of edema in
congestive heart failure and nephrotic syndrome
Usual Dosage Oral:
Children (daily dosages should be decreased if used with other antihyperten-
sives):
<6 months: 2-3 mg/kg/day in 2 divided doses
>6 months: 2 mg/kg/day in 2 divided doses
Adults: 25-50 mg/day in 1-2 doses; maximum: 200 mg/day
Dietary Considerations This product may cause a potassium loss; your
physician may prescribe a potassium supplement, another medication to help
prevent the potassium loss, or recommend that you eat foods high in potas-
sium, especially citrus fruits; do not change your diet on your own while taking
this medication, especially if you are taking potassium supplements or medica-
tions to reduce potassium loss; too much potassium can be as harmful as too
little; may be administered with food
Nursing/Pharmacy Information Monitor blood pressure, serum electrolytes,
BUN, creatinine; check patient for orthostasis
Dosage Forms
Capsule: 12.5 mg
Solution, oral (mint flavor): 50 mg/5 mL (50 mL)
Tablet: 25 mg, 50 mg, 100 mg

- **hydrochlorothiazide and amiloride** *see* amiloride and hydrochlorothiazide *on page 37*
- **hydrochlorothiazide and benazepril** *see* benazepril and hydrochlorothiazide *on page 77*
- **hydrochlorothiazide and bisoprolol** *see* bisoprolol and hydrochlorothiazide *on page 89*
- **hydrochlorothiazide and captopril** *see* captopril and hydrochlorothiazide *on page 111*
- **hydrochlorothiazide and enalapril** *see* enalapril and hydrochlorothiazide *on page 231*
- **hydrochlorothiazide and hydralazine** *see* hydralazine and hydrochlorothiazide *on page 317*
- **hydrochlorothiazide and lisinopril** *see* lisinopril and hydrochlorothiazide *on page 372*
- **hydrochlorothiazide and losartan** *see* losartan and hydrochlorothiazide *on page 377*
- **hydrochlorothiazide and methyldopa** *see* methyldopa and hydrochlorothiazide *on page 406*
- **hydrochlorothiazide and propranolol** *see* propranolol and hydrochlorothiazide *on page 528*

hydrochlorothiazide and reserpine

(hye droe klor oh THYE a zide & re SER peen)

Synonyms reserpine and hydrochlorothiazide
U.S. Brand Names Hydropres®; Hydro-Serp®; Hydroserpine®
Generic Available Yes
Therapeutic Category Antihypertensive Agent, Combination
Use Management of mild to moderate hypertension; treatment of edema in congestive heart failure and nephrotic syndrome
Usual Dosage Adults: Oral: 1-2 tablets once or twice daily
Dosage Forms Tablet:
50: Hydrochlorothiazide 50 mg and reserpine 0.125 mg

hydrochlorothiazide and spironolactone

(hye droe klor oh THYE a zide & speer on oh LAK tone)

Synonyms spironolactone and hydrochlorothiazide
U.S. Brand Names Alazide®; Aldactazide®; Spironazide®; Spirozide®
Generic Available Yes
Therapeutic Category Antihypertensive Agent, Combination
Use Management of mild to moderate hypertension; treatment of edema in congestive heart failure and nephrotic syndrome
Usual Dosage Oral:
Children: 1.66-3.3 mg/kg/day (of spironolactone) in 2-4 divided doses
Adults: 1-8 tablets in 1-2 divided doses
Dietary Considerations Food with high potassium content, natural licorice, and salt substitutes should be avoided
Nursing/Pharmacy Information
May interfere with digoxin serum assays
Monitor blood pressure, serum electrolytes, renal function
Dosage Forms Tablet:
25/25: Hydrochlorothiazide 25 mg and spironolactone 25 mg
50/50: Hydrochlorothiazide 50 mg and spironolactone 50 mg

hydrochlorothiazide and triamterene

(hye droe klor oh THYE a zide & trye AM ter een)

Synonyms triamterene and hydrochlorothiazide
U.S. Brand Names Dyazide®; Maxzide®
Canadian Brand Names Apo-Triazide®; Novo-Triamzide; Nu-Triazide
Generic Available Yes (Dyazide® strength only)
Therapeutic Category Antihypertensive Agent, Combination
Use Management of mild to moderate hypertension; treatment of edema in congestive heart failure and nephrotic syndrome
Usual Dosage Adults: Oral: 1-2 capsules twice daily after meals
Dietary Considerations Avoid excessive ingestions of foods high in potassium or use of salt substitutes; should be administered after meals
Nursing/Pharmacy Information Monitor blood pressure, serum electrolytes, BUN, creatinine, liver function tests, signs of hyperkalemia
Dosage Forms
Capsule (Dyazide®): Hydrochlorothiazide 25 mg and triamterene 37.5 mg

Tablet:
  Maxzide®-25: Hydrochlorothiazide 25 mg and triamterene 37.5 mg
  Maxzide®: Hydrochlorothiazide 50 mg and triamterene 75 mg

♦ **hydrochlorothiazide, hydralazine, and reserpine** see hydralazine, hydrochlorothiazide, and reserpine on page 317

♦ **Hydrocil® [OTC]** see psyllium on page 531

♦ **Hydro Cobex®** see hydroxocobalamin on page 326

hydrocodone and acetaminophen
(hye droe KOE done & a seet a MIN oh fen)

Synonyms acetaminophen and hydrocodone

U.S. Brand Names Anexsia®; Anodynos-DHC®; Bancap HC®; Co-Gesic®; Dolacet®; DuoCet™; Duradyne DHC®; Hydrocet®; Hydrogesic®; Hy-Phen®; Lorcet® 10/650; Lorcet®-HD; Lorcet® Plus; Lortab®; Margesic® H; Norcet®; Stagesic®; T-Gesic®; Vicodin®; Vicodin® ES; Zydone®

Canadian Brand Names Vapocet®

Generic Available Yes

Therapeutic Category Analgesic, Narcotic

Controlled Substance C-III

Use Relief of moderate to severe pain; antitussive (hydrocodone)

Usual Dosage Doses should be titrated to appropriate analgesic effect
  Adults: Oral: 1-2 tablets or capsules every 4-6 hours

Dietary Considerations Rate of absorption of acetaminophen may be decreased when administered with food high in carbohydrates

Nursing/Pharmacy Information Monitor for pain relief, respiratory and mental status, blood pressure; observe patient for excessive sedation, respiratory depression

Dosage Forms
  Capsule:
    Bancap HC®, Dolacet®, Hydrocet®, Hydrogesic®, Lorcet®-HD, Margesic® H, Medipain 5®, Norcet®, Stagesic®, T-Gesic®, Zydone®: Hydrocodone bitartrate 5 mg and acetaminophen 500 mg
  Elixir (tropical fruit punch flavor) (Lortab®): Hydrocodone bitartrate 2.5 mg and acetaminophen 167 mg per 5 mL with alcohol 7% (480 mL)
  Solution, oral (tropical fruit punch flavor) (Lortab®): Hydrocodone bitartrate 2.5 mg and acetaminophen 167 mg per 5 mL with alcohol 7% (480 mL)
  Tablet: Hydrocodone bitartrate 5 mg and acetaminophen 400 mg; hydrocodone bitartrate 7.5 mg and acetaminophen 400 mg; hydrocodone bitartrate 10 mg and acetaminophen 400 mg; hydrocodone bitartrate 5 mg and acetaminophen 500 mg; hydrocodone bitartrate 7.5 mg and acetaminophen 750 mg; hydrocodone bitartrate 7.5 mg and acetaminophen 500 mg; hydrocodone bitartrate 7.5 mg and acetaminophen 650 mg; hydrocodone bitartrate 10 mg and acetaminophen 650 mg
    Lortab® 2.5/500: Hydrocodone bitartrate 2.5 mg and acetaminophen 500 mg
    Anexsia® 5/500, Anodynos-DHC®, Co-Gesic®, DuoCet™, DHC®; Hy-Phen®, Lorcet®, Lortab®® 5/500, Vicodin®: Hydrocodone bitartrate 5 mg and acetaminophen 500 mg
    Lortab® 7.5/500: Hydrocodone bitartrate 7.5 mg and acetaminophen 500 mg
    Anexsia® 7.5/650, Lorcet® Plus: Hydrocodone bitartrate 7.5 mg and acetaminophen 650 mg
    Vicodin® ES: Hydrocodone bitartrate 7.5 mg and acetaminophen 750 mg
    Norco®: Hydrocodone bitartrate 10 mg and acetaminophen 325 mg
    Lortab® 10/500: Hydrocodone bitartrate 10 mg and acetaminophen 500 mg
    Lorcet® 10/650: Hydrocodone bitartrate 10 mg and acetaminophen 650 mg
    Vicodin® HP: Hydrocodone bitartrate 10 mg and acetaminophen 660 mg
    Zydone®: Hydrocodone bitartrate 5 mg and acetaminophen 400 mg; hydrocodone bitartrate 7.5 mg and acetaminophen 400 mg; hydrocodone bitartrate 10 mg and acetaminophen 400 mg

hydrocodone and aspirin (hye droe KOE done & AS pir in)

Synonyms aspirin and hydrocodone

U.S. Brand Names Alor® 5/500; Azdone®; Damason-P®; Lortab® ASA; Panasal® 5/500

Generic Available Yes

Therapeutic Category Analgesic, Narcotic

Controlled Substance C-III

Use Relief of moderate to moderately severe pain

Usual Dosage Adults: Oral: 1-2 tablets every 4-6 hours as needed for pain

Dietary Considerations May be administered with food or milk to minimize GI distress

(Continued)

hydrocodone and aspirin *(Continued)*

Nursing/Pharmacy Information May cause drowsiness; avoid alcohol; watch for bleeding gums or any signs of GI bleeding; notify physician if ringing in ears or persistent GI pain occurs

Dosage Forms Tablet: Hydrocodone bitartrate 5 mg and aspirin 500 mg

hydrocodone and chlorpheniramine
(hye droe KOE done & klor fen IR a meen)

Synonyms chlorpheniramine and hydrocodone

U.S. Brand Names Tussionex®

Generic Available Yes

Therapeutic Category Antihistamine/Antitussive

Controlled Substance C-III

Use Symptomatic relief of cough

Usual Dosage Oral:

Children 6-12 years: 2.5 mL every 12 hours; do not exceed 5 mL/24 hours

Adults: 5 mL every 12 hours; do not exceed 10 mL/24 hours

Nursing/Pharmacy Information Shake well before administering

Dosage Forms Syrup, alcohol free: Hydrocodone polistirex 10 mg and chlorpheniramine polistirex 8 mg per 5 mL (480 mL, 900 mL)

hydrocodone and guaifenesin
(hye droe KOE done & gwye FEN e sin)

Synonyms guaifenesin and hydrocodone

U.S. Brand Names Codiclear® DH; HycoClear Tuss®; Hycotuss® Expectorant Liquid; Kwelcof®

Generic Available Yes

Therapeutic Category Antitussive/Expectorant

Controlled Substance C-III

Use Symptomatic relief of nonproductive coughs associated with upper and lower respiratory tract congestion

Usual Dosage Oral:

Children:

<2 years: 0.3 mg/kg/day (hydrocodone) in 4 divided doses

2-12 years: 2.5 mL every 4 hours, after meals and at bedtime

>12 years: 5 mL every 4 hours, after meals and at bedtime

Adults: 5 mL every 4 hours, after meals and at bedtime, up to 30 mL/24 hours

Dietary Considerations Should be administered after meals

Dosage Forms Liquid: Hydrocodone bitartrate 5 mg and guaifenesin 100 mg per 5 mL (120 mL, 480 mL)

hydrocodone and homatropine
(hye droe KOE done & hoe MA troe peen)

Synonyms homatropine and hydrocodone

U.S. Brand Names Hycodan®; Hydromet®; Oncet®; Tussigon®

Generic Available Yes

Therapeutic Category Antitussive

Controlled Substance C-III

Use Symptomatic relief of cough

Usual Dosage Oral (based on hydrocodone component):

Children: 0.6 mg/kg/day in 3-4 divided doses; do not administer more frequently than every 4 hours

A single dose should not exceed 10 mg in children >12 years, 5 mg in children 2-12 years, and 1.25 mg in children <2 years of age

Adults: 5-10 mg every 4-6 hours, a single dose should not exceed 15 mg; do not administer more frequently than every 4 hours

Nursing/Pharmacy Information Dispense in light-resistant container; observe patient for excessive sedation, respiratory depression, implement safety measures, assist with ambulation

Dosage Forms

Syrup (Hycodan®, Hydromet®, Hydropane®, Hydrotropine®): Hydrocodone bitartrate 5 mg and homatropine methylbromide 1.5 mg per 5 mL (120 mL, 480 mL, 4000 mL)

Tablet (Hycodan®, Tussigon®): Hydrocodone bitartrate 5 mg and homatropine methylbromide 1.5 mg

hydrocodone and ibuprofen
(hye droe KOE done & eye byoo PROE fen)

Synonyms ibuprofen and hydrocodone

U.S. Brand Names Vicoprofen®

Generic Available No

Therapeutic Category Analgesic, Narcotic

Controlled Substance C-III

Use Relief of moderate to moderately severe pain (short-term, less than 10 days)

Usual Dosage Adults: Oral: 1-2 tablets every 4-6 hours as needed for pain

Dosage Forms Tablet: Hydrocodone bitartrate 7.5 mg and ibuprofen 200 mg

hydrocodone and phenylpropanolamine
(hye droe KOE done & fen il proe pa NOLE a meen)

Synonyms phenylpropanolamine and hydrocodone

U.S. Brand Names Codamine®; Codamine® Pediatric; Hycomine®; Hycomine® Pediatric; Hydrocodone PA® Syrup

Generic Available Yes

Therapeutic Category Antitussive/Decongestant

Controlled Substance C-III

Use Symptomatic relief of cough and nasal congestion

Usual Dosage Oral:
Children 6-12 years: 2.5 mL every 4 hours, up to 6 doses/24 hours
Adults: 5 mL every 4 hours, up to 6 doses/24 hours

Nursing/Pharmacy Information Dispense in a light-resistant container

Dosage Forms Syrup:
Codamine®, Hycomine®: Hydrocodone bitartrate 5 mg and phenylpropanolamine hydrochloride 25 mg per 5 mL (480 mL)
Codamine® Pediatric, Hycomine® Pediatric: Hydrocodone bitartrate 2.5 mg and phenylpropanolamine hydrochloride 12.5 mg per 5 mL (480 mL)

hydrocodone and pseudoephedrine
(hye droe KOE done & soo doe e FED rin)

U.S. Brand Names Detussin® Liquid; Entuss-D® Liquid; Histussin D® Liquid; Tyrodone® Liquid

Generic Available No

Therapeutic Category Cough and Cold Combination

Use Symptomatic relief of cough due to colds, etc

Usual Dosage Oral: Adults: 5 mL four times/day

Dosage Forms Liquid:
Entuss-D®: Hydrocodone bitartrate 5 mg and pseudoephedrine hydrochloride 30 mg per 5 mL
Detussin®, Histussin D®, Tyrodone®: Hydrocodone bitartrate 5 mg and pseudoephedrine hydrochloride 60 mg per 5 mL

hydrocodone, chlorpheniramine, phenylephrine, acetaminophen, and caffeine
(hye droe KOE done, klor fen IR a meen, fen il EF rin, a seet a MIN oh fen, & KAF een)

Synonyms acetaminophen, caffeine, hydrocodone, chlorpheniramine, and phenylephrine; caffeine, hydrocodone, chlorpheniramine, phenylephrine, and acetaminophen; chlorpheniramine, hydrocodone, phenylephrine, acetaminophen, and caffeine; phenylephrine, hydrocodone, chlorpheniramine, acetaminophen, and caffeine

U.S. Brand Names Hycomine® Compound

Generic Available Yes

Therapeutic Category Antitussive

Use Symptomatic relief of cough and symptoms of upper respiratory infections

Usual Dosage Adults: Oral: 1 tablet every 4 hours, up to 4 times/day

Dosage Forms Tablet: Hydrocodone bitartrate 5 mg, chlorpheniramine maleate 2 mg, phenylephrine hydrochloride 10 mg, acetaminophen 250 mg, and caffeine 30 mg

♦ **Hydrocodone PA® Syrup** see hydrocodone and phenylpropanolamine on page 321

hydrocodone, phenylephrine, pyrilamine, phenindamine, chlorpheniramine, and ammonium chloride

(hye droe KOE done, fen il EF rin, peer IL a meen, fen IN da meen, klor fen IR a meen, & a MOE nee um KLOR ide)

U.S. Brand Names P-V-Tussin®

Generic Available Yes

Therapeutic Category Antihistamine/Decongestant/Antitussive

Use Symptomatic relief of cough and nasal congestion

Usual Dosage Adults: Oral: 10 mL every 4-6 hours, up to 40 mL/day

Dosage Forms Syrup: Hydrocodone bitartrate 2.5 mg, phenylephrine hydrochloride 5 mg, pyrilamine maleate 6 mg, phenindamine tartrate 5 mg, chlorpheniramine maleate 2 mg, and ammonium chloride 50 mg per 5 mL with alcohol 5% (480 mL, 3780 mL)

hydrocodone, pseudoephedrine, and guaifenesin

(hye droe KOE done, soo doe e FED rin & gwye FEN e sin)

Synonyms guaifenesin, hydrocodone, and pseudoephedrine; pseudoephedrine, hydrocodone, and guaifenesin

U.S. Brand Names Cophene XP®; Detussin® Expectorant; SRC® Expectorant; Tussafin® Expectorant

Generic Available Yes

Therapeutic Category Antitussive/Decongestant/Expectorant

Controlled Substance C-III

Use Symptomatic relief of irritating, nonproductive cough associated with respiratory conditions such as bronchitis, bronchial asthma, tracheobronchitis, and the common cold

Usual Dosage Adults: Oral: 5 mL every 4-6 hours

Dosage Forms Liquid: Hydrocodone bitartrate 5 mg, pseudoephedrine hydrochloride 60 mg, and guaifenesin 200 mg per 5 mL with alcohol 12.5% (480 mL)

♦ **hydrocortisone and benzoyl peroxide** *see* benzoyl peroxide and hydrocortisone *on page 81*

♦ **hydrocortisone and clioquinol** *see* clioquinol and hydrocortisone *on page 157*

♦ **hydrocortisone and dibucaine** *see* dibucaine and hydrocortisone *on page 197*

♦ **hydrocortisone and iodoquinol** *see* iodoquinol and hydrocortisone *on page 344*

♦ **hydrocortisone and lidocaine** *see* lidocaine and hydrocortisone *on page 369*

♦ **hydrocortisone and neomycin** *see* neomycin and hydrocortisone *on page 435*

♦ **hydrocortisone and oxytetracycline** *see* oxytetracycline and hydrocortisone *on page 465*

♦ **hydrocortisone and polymyxin B** *see* polymyxin B and hydrocortisone *on page 503*

♦ **hydrocortisone and pramoxine** *see* pramoxine and hydrocortisone *on page 512*

♦ **hydrocortisone and urea** *see* urea and hydrocortisone *on page 639*

♦ **hydrocortisone, bacitracin, neomycin, and polymyxin B** *see* bacitracin, neomycin, polymyxin B, and hydrocortisone *on page 72*

♦ **hydrocortisone, colistin, and neomycin** *see* colistin, neomycin, and hydrocortisone *on page 166*

♦ **hydrocortisone, neomycin, and polymyxin B** *see* neomycin, polymyxin B, and hydrocortisone *on page 437*

hydrocortisone (rectal) (hye droe KOR ti sone)

U.S. Brand Names Anusol-HC® Suppository; Cortenema® Rectal; Cortifoam® Rectal; Proctocort™ Rectal

Canadian Brand Names Rectocort

Generic Available Yes

Therapeutic Category Adrenal Corticosteroid

Use Management of adrenocortical insufficiency; adjunctive treatment of ulcerative colitis

Usual Dosage Ulcerative colitis: Adults: Rectal: 10-100 mg 1-2 times/day for 2-3 weeks

Dosage Forms
Acetate:
  Aerosol, rectal: 10% [90 mg/applicatorful] 20 g
  Suppository, rectal: 25 mg
Base:
  Rectal: 1% (30 g)
  Suspension, rectal: 100 mg/60 mL (7s)

hydrocortisone (systemic) (hye droe KOR ti sone)

Synonyms compound F
U.S. Brand Names A-hydroCort®; Hydrocortone® Acetate; Solu-Cortef®
Mexican Brand Names Flebocortid [Sodium Succinate]; Nositrol [Sodium Succinate]
Generic Available Yes
Therapeutic Category Adrenal Corticosteroid
Use Management of adrenocortical insufficiency; relief of inflammation of corti-costeroid-responsive dermatoses
Usual Dosage Dose should be based on severity of disease and patient response
Acute adrenal insufficiency: I.M., I.V.:
  Infants and young Children: Succinate: 1-2 mg/kg/dose bolus, then 25-150 mg/day in divided doses every 6-8 hours
  Older Children: Succinate: 1-2 mg/kg bolus then 150-250 mg/day in divided doses every 6-8 hours
  Adults: Succinate: 100 mg I.V. bolus, then 300 mg/day in divided doses every 8 hours or as a continuous infusion for 48 hours; once patient is stable change to oral, 50 mg every 8 hours for 6 doses, then taper to 30-50 mg/day in divided doses
Chronic adrenal corticoid insufficiency: Adults: Oral: 20-30 mg/day

Anti-inflammatory or immunosuppressive:
  Infants and Children:
    Oral: 2.5-10 mg/kg/day **or** 75-300 mg/m^2/day every 6-8 hours
    I.M., I.V.: Succinate: 1-5 mg/kg/day **or** 30-150 mg/m^2/day divided every 12-24 hours
  Adolescents and Adults: Oral, I.M., I.V.: Succinate: 15-240 mg every 12 hours
Congenital adrenal hyperplasia: Oral: Initial: 30-36 mg/m^2/day with $^1/_3$ of dose every morning and $^2/_3$ every evening or $^1/_4$ every morning and mid-day and $^1/_2$ every evening; maintenance: 20-25 mg/m^2/day in divided doses
Physiologic replacement: Children:
  Oral: 0.5-0.75 mg/kg/day **or** 20-25 mg/m^2/day every 8 hours
  I.M.: Succinate: 0.25-0.35 mg/kg/day **or** 12-15 mg/m^2/day once daily
Shock: I.M., I.V.: Succinate:
  Children: Initial: 50 mg/kg, then repeated in 4 hours and/or every 24 hours as needed
  Adolescents and Adults: 500 mg to 2 g every 2-6 hours
Status asthmaticus: Children and Adults: I.V.: Succinate: 1-2 mg/kg/dose every 6 hours for 24 hours, then maintenance of 0.5-1 mg/kg every 6 hours
Rheumatic diseases:
  Adults: Intralesional, intra-articular, soft tissue injection: Acetate:
    Large joints: 25 mg (up to 37.5 mg)
    Small joints: 10-25 mg
  Tendon sheaths: 5-12.5 mg
  Soft tissue infiltration: 25-50 mg (up to 75 mg)
  Bursae: 25-37.5 mg
  Ganglia: 12.5-25 mg
Dermatosis: Children >2 years and Adults: Topical: Apply to affected area 3-4 times/day (Buteprate: Apply once or twice daily)
Ulcerative colitis: Adults: Rectal: 10-100 mg 1-2 times/day for 2-3 weeks
Dietary Considerations Systemic use of corticosteroids may require a diet with increased potassium, vitamins A, B$_6$, C, D, folate, calcium, zinc, phosphorus, and decreased sodium
Nursing/Pharmacy Information
I.V. bolus: Dilute to 50 mg/mL and administered over 3-5 minutes; I.V. intermittent infusion: Dilute to 1 mg/mL and administered over 20-30 minutes
Monitor blood pressure, weight, serum glucose, and electrolytes
Stability:
  Minimum volume: Concentration should not exceed 1 mg/mL
  Stability of parenteral admixture (Solu-Cortef®) at room temperature (25°C) and at refrigeration temperature (4°C) is concentration dependent
  Stability of concentration ≤1 mg/mL: 24 hours
(Continued)

hydrocortisone (systemic) *(Continued)*

Stability of concentration >1 mg/mL to <25 mg/mL: Unpredictable, 4-6 hours
Stability of concentration ≥25 mg/mL: 3 days

Dosage Forms
Injection, suspension: 25 mg/mL (5 mL, 10 mL); 50 mg/mL (5 mL, 10 mL)
Tablet: 5 mg, 10 mg, 20 mg
Suspension, oral: 10 mg/5 mL (120 mL)

hydrocortisone (topical) (hye droe KOR ti sone)

U.S. Brand Names Acticort® Topical; Aeroseb-HC® Topical; Ala-Cort® Topical; Ala-Scalp® Topical; Anusol® HC-1 Topical [OTC]; Anusol® HC-2.5% Topical [OTC]; Bactine® Hydrocortisone [OTC]; CaldeCort® Anti-Itch Topical Spray; CaldeCort® Topical [OTC]; Cetacort® Topical; Clocort® Maximum Strength [OTC]; CortaGel® Topical [OTC]; Cortaid® Maximum Strength Topical [OTC]; Cortaid® with Aloe Topical [OTC]; Cort-Dome® Topical; Cortef® Feminine Itch Topical; Cortizone®-5 Topical [OTC]; Cortizone®-10 Topical [OTC]; Delcort® Topical; Dermacort® Topical; Dermarest Dricort® Topical; Dermolate® Topical [OTC]; Dermtex® HC with Aloe Topical [OTC]; Eldecort® Topical; Gynecort® Topical [OTC]; Hi-Cor-1.0® Topical; Hi-Cor-2.5® Topical; Hycort® Topical; Hydrocort® Topical; Hydro-Tex® Topical [OTC]; Hytone® Topical; LactiCare-HC® Topical; Lanacort® Topical [OTC]; Locoid® Topical; Nutracort® Topical; Orabase® HCA Topical; Penecort® Topical; Scalpicin® Topical; S-T Cort® Topical; Synacort® Topical; Tegrin®-HC Topical [OTC]; Texacort® Topical; U-Cort™ Topical; Westcort® Topical

Canadian Brand Names Aquacort®; Cortamed®; Cortate®; Corticreme®; Cortiment®; Cortoderm; Emo-Cort™; Hyderm; Prevex™ HC

Generic Available Yes

Therapeutic Category Corticosteroid, Topical

Use Management of adrenocortical insufficiency; relief of inflammation of corticosteroid-responsive dermatoses; adjunctive treatment of ulcerative colitis

Usual Dosage Children >2 years and Adults: Topical: Apply to affected area 3-4 times/day (Buteprate: Apply once or twice daily)

Nursing/Pharmacy Information Apply sparingly

Dosage Forms
Aerosol, topical:
Cream: 0.5%, 1%, 2.5%
Gel: 0.5%
Ointment, topical: 0.5%, 1%, 2.5%
Lotion: 0.5%, 1%, 2.5%
Paste: 0.5% (5 g)
Solution, topical; 1%
Butyrate:
Cream: 0.1%
Ointment, topical: 0.1%
Solution, topical: 0.1%
Valerate:
Cream: 0.2%
Ointment, topical: 0.2%

♦ **Hydrocortone® Acetate** *see* hydrocortisone (systemic) *on page 323*
♦ **Hydrocort® Topical** *see* hydrocortisone (topical) *on page 324*
♦ **Hydro-Crysti-12®** *see* hydroxocobalamin *on page 326*
♦ **HydroDIURIL®** *see* hydrochlorothiazide *on page 317*

hydroflumethiazide (hye droe floo meth EYE a zide)

U.S. Brand Names Diucardin®; Saluron®

Generic Available Yes

Therapeutic Category Diuretic, Thiazide

Use Management of mild to moderate hypertension; treatment of edema in congestive heart failure and nephrotic syndrome

Usual Dosage Oral: 1 tablet 1-2 times/day

Nursing/Pharmacy Information Monitor blood pressure, serum electrolytes, BUN, creatinine

Dosage Forms Tablet: 50 mg

hydroflumethiazide and reserpine

(hye droe floo meth EYE a zide & re SER peen)

Synonyms reserpine and hydroflumethiazide

U.S. Brand Names Salutensin®

Generic Available Yes

Therapeutic Category Antihypertensive Agent, Combination
Use Management of hypertension
Usual Dosage Oral (determined by individual titration): Usually 1 tablet once or twice daily
Dosage Forms
Tablet (Salutensin®): Hydroflumethiazide 50 mg and reserpine 0.125 mg
Tablet (Hydro-Fluserpine®, Salutensin-Demi®): Hydroflumethiazide 25 mg and reserpine 0.125 mg

♦ **hydrogenated ergot alkaloids** see ergoloid mesylates on page 238
♦ **Hydrogesic®** see hydrocodone and acetaminophen on page 319
♦ **hydromagnesium aluminate** see magaldrate on page 380
♦ **Hydromet®** see hydrocodone and homatropine on page 320

hydromorphone (hye droe MOR fone)
Synonyms dihydromorphinone
U.S. Brand Names Dilaudid® Cough Syrup; Dilaudid-HP® Injection; Dilaudid® Injection; Dilaudid® Oral; Dilaudid® Suppository
Canadian Brand Names PMS-Hydromorphone
Generic Available Yes
Therapeutic Category Analgesic, Narcotic
Controlled Substance C-II
Use Management of moderate to severe pain; antitussive at lower doses
Usual Dosage Doses should be titrated to appropriate analgesic effects; when changing routes of administration, note that oral doses are less than half as effective as parenteral doses (may be only $1/5$ as effective)

Pain: Older Children and Adults: Oral, I.M., I.V., S.C.: 1-4 mg/dose every 4-6 hours as needed; usual adult dose: 2 mg/dose
Antitussive: Oral:
Children 6-12 years: 0.5 mg every 3-4 hours as needed
Children >12 years and Adults: 1 mg every 3-4 hours as needed
Dietary Considerations After each dose, one glass of water should be taken
Alcohol: Additive CNS effects; avoid or limit alcohol; watch for sedation
Food: Glucose may cause hyperglycemia; monitor blood glucose concentrations
Nursing/Pharmacy Information
Monitor pain relief, respiratory and mental status, blood pressure; observe patient for oversedation, respiratory depression
Stability: Protect tablets from light; do not store intact ampuls in refrigerator; a slightly yellowish discoloration has not been associated with a loss of potency; I.V. is **incompatible** when mixed with minocycline, prochlorperazine, sodium bicarbonate, tetracycline, thiopental
Dosage Forms Hydromorphone hydrochloride:
Injection:
Dilaudid®: 1 mg/mL (1 mL); 2 mg/mL (1 mL, 20 mL); 3 mg/mL (1 mL); 4 mg/mL (1 mL)
Dilaudid-HP®: 10 mg/mL (1 mL, 2 mL, 5 mL)
Liquid: 5 mg/5 mL (480 mL)
Powder for injection: (Dilaudid-HP®): 250 mg
Suppository, rectal: 3 mg (6s)
Tablet: 2 mg, 4 mg, 8 mg

♦ **Hydromox®** see quinethazone on page 536
♦ **Hydro-Par®** see hydrochlorothiazide on page 317
♦ **Hydrophed®** see theophylline, ephedrine, and hydroxyzine on page 605
♦ **Hydropres®** see hydrochlorothiazide and reserpine on page 318
♦ **Hydropres® 25 mg Tablet** *(Discontinued)* see page 743
♦ **hydroquinol** see hydroquinone on page 325

hydroquinone (HYE droe kwin one)
Synonyms hydroquinol; quinol
U.S. Brand Names Ambi® Skin Tone [OTC]; Eldopaque® [OTC]; Eldopaque Forte®; Eldoquin® [OTC]; Eldoquin® Forte®; Esoterica® Facial [OTC]; Esoterica® Regular [OTC]; Esoterica® Sensitive Skin Formula [OTC]; Esoterica® Sunscreen [OTC]; Melanex®; Porcelana® [OTC]; Porcelana® Sunscreen [OTC]; Solaquin® [OTC]; Solaquin Forte®
Canadian Brand Names Neostrata® HQ; Ultraquin™
Mexican Brand Names Crema Blanca Bustillos
Generic Available No
Therapeutic Category Topical Skin Product
(Continued)

hydroquinone *(Continued)*

Use Gradual bleaching of hyperpigmented skin conditions

Usual Dosage Topical: Apply thin layer and rub in twice daily

Nursing/Pharmacy Information Use sunscreens or clothing; do not use on irritated or denuded skin; stop using if rash or irritation develops; for external use only, avoid eye contact

Dosage Forms

Cream, topical:

Esoterica® Sensitive Skin Formula: 1.5% [OTC] (85 g)

Eldopaque®, Eldoquin®, Esoterica® Facial, Esoterica® Regular, Porcelana®: 2% [OTC] (14.2 g, 28.4 g, 60 g, 85 g, 120 g)

Eldopaque Forte®, Eldoquin® Forte®, Melquin HP®: 4% (14.2 g, 28.4 g)

Cream, topical, with sunblock:

Esoterica® Sunscreen, Porcelana®, Solaquin®: 2% [OTC] (28.4 g, 120 g)

Melpaque HP®, Nuquin HP®, Solaquin Forte®: 4% (14.2 g, 28.4 g)

Gel, topical, with sunscreen (Solaquin Forte®): 4% (14.2 g, 28.4 g)

Solution, topical (Melanex®): 3% (30 mL)

- **Hydro-Serp®** *see* hydrochlorothiazide and reserpine *on page 318*
- **Hydroserpine®** *see* hydrochlorothiazide and reserpine *on page 318*
- **Hydro-Tex® Topical [OTC]** *see* hydrocortisone (topical) *on page 324*
- **Hydroxacen®** *(Discontinued) see page 743*

hydroxocobalamin (hye droks oh koe BAL a min)

Synonyms vitamin B_{12a}

U.S. Brand Names Hydro Cobex®; Hydro-Crysti-12®; LA-12®

Canadian Brand Names Acti-B$_{12}$®

Mexican Brand Names Duradoce®

Generic Available Yes

Therapeutic Category Vitamin, Water Soluble

Use Pernicious anemia, vitamin B_{12} deficiency, increased B_{12} requirements due to pregnancy, thyrotoxicosis, hemorrhage, malignancy, liver or kidney disease

Usual Dosage

Children:

Congenital pernicious anemia (if evidence of neurologic involvement): I.M.: 1000 mcg/day for at least 2 weeks; maintenance: 50 mcg/month

Vitamin B_{12} deficiency: I.M., S.C.: 1-5 mg administered in single or S.C. doses of 100 mcg over 2 or more weeks

Adults:

Pernicious anemia: I.M., S.C.: 100 mcg/day for 6-7 days

Vitamin B_{12} deficiency:

Oral: Usually not recommended, maximum absorbed from a single oral dose is 2-3 mcg

I.M., S.C.: 30 mcg/day for 5-10 days, followed by 100-200 mcg/month

Nursing/Pharmacy Information Therapy is required throughout life; do not administer folic acid instead of B_{12} to prevent anemia

Dosage Forms Injection: 1000 mcg/mL (10 mL, 30 mL)

hydroxyamphetamine (hye droks ee am FET a meen)

U.S. Brand Names Paredrine®

Generic Available No

Therapeutic Category Adrenergic Agonist Agent

Use Produce mydriasis in diagnostic eye examination

Usual Dosage Instill 1-2 drops into conjunctival sac

Dosage Forms Solution, as hydrobromide: 1%

hydroxyamphetamine and tropicamide

(hye droks ee am FET a meen & troe PIK a mide)

U.S. Brand Names Paremyd® Ophthalmic

Generic Available No

Therapeutic Category Adrenergic Agonist Agent

Use Mydriasis with cycloplegia

Usual Dosage Adults: Ophthalmic: Instill 1-2 drops into conjunctival sac(s)

Dosage Forms Solution, ophthalmic: Hydroxyamphetamine hydrobromide 1% and tropicamide 0.25% (5 mL, 15 mL)

- **hydroxycarbamide** *see* hydroxyurea *on page 328*

hydroxychloroquine (hye droks ee KLOR oh kwin)

U.S. Brand Names Plaquenil®

Generic Available Yes

Therapeutic Category Aminoquinoline (Antimalarial)

Use Suppression or chemoprophylaxis of malaria caused by susceptible *P. vivax*, *P. ovale*, *P. malariae*, and some strains of *P. falciparum* (not active against pre-erythrocytic or exoerythrocytic tissue stages of *Plasmodium*); treatment of systemic lupus erythematosus (SLE) and rheumatoid arthritis

Usual Dosage Oral:

Children:

Chemoprophylaxis of malaria: 5 mg/kg (base) once weekly; should not exceed the recommended adult dose; begin 2 weeks before exposure; continue for 8 weeks after leaving endemic area

Acute attack: 10 mg/kg (base) initial dose; followed by 5 mg/kg in 6 hours on day 1; 5 mg/kg in 1 dose on day 2 and on day 3

Juvenile rheumatoid arthritis or SLE: 3-5 mg/kg/day divided 1-2 times/day to a maximum of 400 mg/day; not to exceed 7 mg/kg/day

Adults:

Chemoprophylaxis of malaria: 2 tablets weekly on same day each week; begin 2 weeks before exposure; continue for 6-8 weeks after leaving epidemic area

Acute attack: 4 tablets first dose day 1; 2 tablets in 6 hours day 1; 2 tablets in 1 dose day 2; and 2 tablets in 1 dose on day 3

Rheumatoid arthritis: 2-3 tablets/day to start with food or milk; increase dose until optimum response level is reached; usually after 4-12 weeks dose should be reduced by $1/2$ and a maintenance dose of 1-2 tablets/day

Lupus erythematosus: 2 tablets every day or twice daily for several weeks depending on response; 1-2 tablets/day for prolonged maintenance therapy

Dietary Considerations May be administered with food or milk

Nursing/Pharmacy Information Monitor CBC; periodic blood counts and eye examinations are recommended when patient is on chronic therapy

Dosage Forms Tablet, as sulfate: 200 mg [base 155 mg]

♦ **25-hydroxycholecalciferol** *see* calcifediol *on page 101*

♦ **hydroxydaunomycin** *see* doxorubicin *on page 220*

♦ **hydroxyethyl starch** *see* hetastarch *on page 312*

hydroxyprogesterone caproate

(hye droks ee proe JES te rone KAP roe ate)

U.S. Brand Names Hylutin®; Hyprogest® 250

Mexican Brand Names Primolut® Depot

Generic Available Yes

Therapeutic Category Progestin

Use Treatment of amenorrhea, abnormal uterine bleeding, submucous fibroids, endometriosis, uterine carcinoma, and testing of estrogen production

Usual Dosage Adults: I.M.:

Amenorrhea: 375 mg; if no bleeding, begin cyclic treatment with estradiol valerate

Endometriosis: Start cyclic therapy with estradiol valerate

Uterine carcinoma: 1 g one or more times/day (1-7 g/week) for up to 12 weeks

Test for endogenous estrogen production: 250 mg anytime; bleeding 7-14 days after injection indicate positive test

Nursing/Pharmacy Information

Patients should receive a copy of the patient labeling for the drug; administer deep I.M. only

Stability: Store at <40°C (15°C to 30°C); avoid freezing

Dosage Forms Hydroxyprogesterone caproate:

Injection: 125 mg/mL (10 mL)

Hylutin®, Hyprogest®: 250 mg/mL (5 mL)

hydroxypropyl cellulose (hye droks ee PROE pil SEL yoo lose)

U.S. Brand Names Lacrisert®

Generic Available Yes

Therapeutic Category Ophthalmic Agent, Miscellaneous

Use Dry eyes

Usual Dosage Adults: Ophthalmic: Apply once daily into the inferior cul-de-sac beneath the base of tarsus, not in apposition to the cornea nor beneath the eyelid at the level of the tarsal plate

Dosage Forms Insert, ophthalmic: 5 mg

hydroxypropyl methylcellulose
(hye droks ee PROE pil meth il SEL yoo lose)

Synonyms gonioscopic ophthalmic solution

U.S. Brand Names Gonak™ [OTC]; Goniosol® [OTC]

Generic Available No

Therapeutic Category Ophthalmic Agent, Miscellaneous

Use Ophthalmic surgical aid in cataract extraction and intraocular implantation; gonioscopic examinations

Usual Dosage Introduced into anterior chamber of eye with 20-gauge or larger cannula

Dosage Forms Solution: 2.5% (15 mL)

hydroxyurea (hye droks ee yoor EE a)

Synonyms hydroxycarbamide

U.S. Brand Names Droxia™; Hydrea®

Generic Available Yes

Therapeutic Category Antineoplastic Agent

Use CML in chronic phase; radiosensitizing agent in the treatment of primary brain tumors; head and neck tumors; uterine cervix and nonsmall cell lung cancer; psoriasis; sickle cell anemia and other hemoglobinopathies; resistant chronic myelocytic leukemia; hematologic conditions such as essential thrombocythemia, polycythemia vera, hypereosinophilia, and hyperleukocytosis due to acute leukemia. Has shown activity against renal cell cancer; malignant melanoma; metastatic or inoperable carcinoma of the ovary; head, neck, and lip cancer; and prostate cancer.

Droxia™: Approved - specifically for patients >18 years of age who have had at least three "painful crises" in the previous year - to reduce frequency of these crises and the need for blood transfusions; Droxia™ is not a cure for sickle cell disease, but it may help control the symptoms of the disease.

Unlabeled use: Thrombocythemia

Usual Dosage Adults: Oral (refer to individual protocols): Dosage based on patient's actual or ideal weight, whichever is less

Solid tumors: Intermittent therapy: 80 mg/kg as a single dose every third day; continuous therapy: 20-30 mg/kg/day given as a single dose/day

Concomitant therapy with irradiation: 80 mg/kg as a single dose every third day starting at least 7 days before initiation of irradiation

Resistant chronic myelocytic leukemia: 20-30 mg/kg/day divided daily

Sickle cell anemia: Droxia™: Initial: 15 mg/kg as a single daily dose (dose based on IBW or actual body weight whichever is less); dose may be increased by 5 mg/kg every 12 weeks to highest dose which does not produce toxic blood counts over 24 weeks, or a maximum of 35 mg/kg

Do not increase dose if counts are between acceptable and toxic; if counts are considered toxic, discontinue hydroxyurea until hematologic recovery; resume dosing at a dose which is 2.5 mg/kg/day less than the dose which resulted in toxicity; further titration should proceed at 2.5 mg/kg/day increments, adjusted every 12 weeks as above; do not attempt any dosage which results in toxicity on two occasions

Acceptable: Neutrophils ≥2500 cells/mm^3, platelets ≥95,000/mm^3, hemoglobin >5.3 g/dL and reticulocytes ≥95,000/mm^3 if the hemoglobin concentration is <9 g/dL

Toxic: Neutrophils <2000 cells/mm^3, platelets <80,000/mm^3, hemoglobin <4.5 g/dL and reticulocytes ≥80,000/mm^3 if the hemoglobin concentration is <9 g/dL

Nursing/Pharmacy Information

Monitor CBC with differential, platelets, hemoglobin, renal function and liver function tests, serum uric acid

Stability: Store capsules at room temperature; capsules may be opened and emptied into water (will not dissolve completely)

Dosage Forms

Capsule: 500 mg

Capsule (Droxia™): 200 mg, 300 mg, 400 mg

♦ **25-hydroxyvitamin D$_3$** see calcifediol on page 101

hydroxyzine (hye DROKS i zeen)

U.S. Brand Names Anxanil® Oral; Atarax® Oral; Atozine® Oral; Durrax® Oral; Hy-Pam® Oral; Hyzine-50® Injection; Neucalm-50® Injection; Quiess® Injection; Vamate® Oral; Vistacon-50® Injection; Vistaquel® Injection; Vistaril® Injection; Vistaril® Oral; Vistazine® Injection

Canadian Brand Names Apo®-Hydroxyzine; Multipax®; Novo-Hydroxyzine®; PMS-Hydroxyzine

Generic Available Yes

Therapeutic Category Antiemetic; Antihistamine

Use Treatment of anxiety; preoperative sedative; antipruritic; antiemetic

Usual Dosage

Children:
Oral: 2 mg/kg/day divided every 6-8 hours
I.M.: 0.5-1 mg/kg/dose every 4-6 hours as needed

Adults:
Antiemetic: I.M.: 25-100 mg/dose every 4-6 hours as needed
Anxiety: Oral: 25-100 mg 4 times/day; maximum dose: 600 mg/day
Preoperative sedation:
Oral: 50-100 mg
I.M.: 25-100 mg
Management of pruritus: Oral: 25 mg 3-4 times/day

Nursing/Pharmacy Information

S.C., intra-arterial, and I.V. administration **not** recommended since thrombosis and digital gangrene can occur; extravasation can result in sterile abscess and marked tissue induration; provide safety measures (ie, side rails, night light, and call button); remove smoking materials from area; supervise ambulation; for I.M. administration in children, injections should be made into the midlateral muscles of the thigh; hydroxyzine has been administered slowly I.V. to oncology patients via central venous lines without problems

Monitor for relief of symptoms, mental status

Stability: Protect from light; I.V. is **incompatible** when mixed with aminophylline, amobarbital, chloramphenicol, dimenhydrinate, heparin, penicillin G, pentobarbital, phenobarbital, phenytoin, ranitidine, sulfisoxazole, vitamin B complex with C

Dosage Forms

Hydroxyzine hydrochloride:
Injection:
Vistaril®: 25 mg/mL (1 mL, 2 mL, 10 mL)
Hyzine-50®, Neucalm®, Quiess®, Vistacon-50®, Vistaquel®, Vistaril®, Vistazine®: 50 mg/mL (1 mL, 2 mL, 10 mL)
Syrup (Atarax®): 10 mg/5 mL (120 mL, 480 mL, 4000 mL)
Tablet:
Anxanil®: 25 mg
Atarax®: 10 mg, 25 mg, 50 mg, 100 mg
Atozine®: 10 mg, 25 mg, 50 mg
Durrax®: 10 mg, 25 mg
Hydroxyzine pamoate:
Capsule:
Hy-Pam®: 25 mg, 50 mg
Vamate®: 25 mg, 50 mg, 100 mg
Vistaril®: 25 mg, 50 mg, 100 mg
Suspension, oral (Vistaril®:) 25 mg/5 mL (120 mL, 480 mL)

♦ **hydroxyzine, theophylline, and ephedrine** see theophylline, ephedrine, and hydroxyzine on page 605

♦ **Hygroton®** see chlorthalidone on page 146

♦ **Hylorel®** see guanadrel on page 305

♦ **Hylutin®** see hydroxyprogesterone caproate on page 327

♦ **hyoscine** see scopolamine on page 560

hyoscyamine (hye oh SYE a meen)

Synonyms l-Hyoscyamine sulfate

U.S. Brand Names Anaspaz®; A-Spas® S/L; Cystospaz®; Cystospaz-M®; Donnamar®; ED-SPAZ®; Gastrosed™; Levbid®; Levsin®; Levsinex®; Levsin/SL®

Generic Available Yes

Therapeutic Category Anticholinergic Agent

Use GI tract disorders caused by spasm, adjunctive therapy for peptic ulcers

Usual Dosage

Children:
<2 years: ¼ adult dosage
2-10 years: ½ adult dosage

Adults:
Oral, S.L.: 0.125-0.25 mg 3-4 times/day before meals or food and at bedtime; 0.375-0.75 mg (timed release) every 12 hours
I.M., I.V., S.C.: 0.25-0.5 mg every 6 hours

(Continued)

hyoscyamine *(Continued)*

Dietary Considerations Should be administered before meals or food
Nursing/Pharmacy Information Monitor patient for anticholinergic effects
Dosage Forms

Capsule, as sulfate, timed release (Cystospaz-M®, Levsinex®): 0.375 mg
Elixir, as sulfate (Levsin®): 0.125 mg/5 mL with alcohol 20% (480 mL)
Injection, as sulfate (Levsin®): 0.5 mg/mL (1 mL, 10 mL)
Solution, oral (Gastrosed™, Levsin®): 0.125 mg/mL (15 mL)
Tablet, as sulfate:
  Anaspaz®, Gastrosed™, Levsin®, Neoquess®: 0.125 mg
  Cystospaz®: 0.15 mg
  Extended release (Levbid®): 0.375 mg
  Sublingual (Levsin/SL®): 0.125 mg

hyoscyamine, atropine, scopolamine, and phenobarbital

(hye oh SYE a meen, A troe peen, skoe POL a meen & fee noe BAR bi tal)

Synonyms atropine, hyoscyamine, scopolamine, and phenobarbital; phenobarbital, hyoscyamine, atropine, and scopolamine; scopolamine, hyoscyamine, atropine, and phenobarbital

U.S. Brand Names Barbidonna®; Bellatal®; Donnatal®; Hyosophen®; Spasmolin®

Generic Available Yes

Therapeutic Category Anticholinergic Agent

Use Adjunct in treatment of peptic ulcer disease, irritable bowel, spastic colitis, spastic bladder, and renal colic

Usual Dosage Oral:

Children 2-12 years:
  Kinesed® dose: ¹/₂ to 1 tablet 3-4 times/day
  Donnatal®: 0.1 mL/kg/dose every 4 hours; maximum dose: 5 mL
Adults: 0.125-0.25 mg (1-2 capsules or tablets) 3-4 times/day; or 0.375-0.75 mg (1 Donnatal® Extentab®) in sustained release form every 12 hours; or 5-10 mL elixir 3-4 times/day or every 8 hours

Dietary Considerations Should be administered 30-60 minutes before meals unless otherwise directed

Nursing/Pharmacy Information Do not crush extended release tablets

Dosage Forms

Capsule (Donnatal®, Spasmolin®): Hyoscyamine sulfate 0.1037 mg, atropine sulfate 0.0194 mg, scopolamine hydrobromide 0.0065 mg, and phenobarbital 16.2 mg
Elixir (Donnatal®, Hyosophen®, Spasmophen®): Hyoscyamine sulfate 0.1037 mg, atropine sulfate 0.0194 mg, scopolamine hydrobromide 0.0065 mg, and phenobarbital 16.2 mg per 5 mL (120 mL, 480 mL, 4000 mL)
Tablet:
  Barbidonna®: Hyoscyamine hydrobromide 0.1286 mg, atropine sulfate 0.025 mg, scopolamine hydrobromide 0.0074 mg, and phenobarbital 16 mg
  Barbidonna® No. 2: Hyoscyamine hydrobromide 0.1286 mg, atropine sulfate 0.025 mg, scopolamine hydrobromide 0.0074 mg, and phenobarbital 32 mg
  Bellatal®, Donnatal®, Hyosophen®: Hyoscyamine sulfate 0.1037 mg, atropine sulfate 0.0194 mg, scopolamine hydrobromide 0.0065 mg, and phenobarbital 16.2 mg
  Long-acting (Donnatal®): Hyoscyamine sulfate 0.3111 mg, atropine sulfate 0.0582 mg, scopolamine hydrobromide 0.0195 mg, and phenobarbital 48.6 mg
  Spasmophen®: Hyoscyamine sulfate 0.1037 mg, atropine sulfate 0.0194 mg, scopolamine hydrobromide 0.0065 mg, and phenobarbital 15 mg

hyoscyamine, atropine, scopolamine, kaolin, and pectin

(hye oh SYE a meen, A troe peen, skoe POL a meen, KAY oh lin & PEK tin)

Generic Available Yes

Therapeutic Category Anticholinergic Agent

Use Antidiarrheal; also used in gastritis, enteritis, colitis, and acute gastrointestinal upsets, and nausea which may accompany any of these conditions

Usual Dosage Oral:

Children:
  10-20 lb: 2.5 mL

20-30 lb: 5 mL
>30 lb: 5-10 mL
Adults:
Diarrhea: 30 mL at once and 15-30 mL with each loose stool
Other conditions: 15 mL every 3 hours as needed
Nursing/Pharmacy Information Shake well before using
Dosage Forms Suspension, oral: Hyoscyamine sulfate 0.1037 mg, atropine sulfate 0.0194 mg, scopolamine hydrobromide 0.0065 mg, kaolin 6 g, and pectin 142.8 mg per 30 mL

hyoscyamine, atropine, scopolamine, kaolin, pectin, and opium

(hye oh SYE a meen, A troe peen, skoe POL a meen, KAY oh lin, PEK tin, & OH pee um)
U.S. Brand Names Donnapectolin-PG®; Kapectolin PG®
Generic Available Yes
Therapeutic Category Anticholinergic Agent
Controlled Substance C-V
Use Treatment of diarrhea
Usual Dosage Oral:
Children 6-12 years: Initial: 10 mL, then 5-10 mL every 3 hours thereafter
Dosage recommendations (body weight/dosage): 10 lb/2.5 mL; 20 lb/5 mL; 30 lb and over/5-10 mL; do not administer more than 4 doses in any 24-hour period
Children >12 years and Adults: Initial: 30 mL (1 fluid oz) followed by 15 mL every 3 hours
Nursing/Pharmacy Information Shake well before using; do not exceed recommended doses; report failure to respond to physician
Dosage Forms Suspension, oral: Hyoscyamine sulfate 0.1037 mg, atropine sulfate 0.0194 mg, scopolamine hydrobromide 0.0065 mg, kaolin 6 g, pectin 142.8 mg, and powdered opium 24 mg per 30 mL with alcohol 5%

- ♦ **Hyosophen®** *see* hyoscyamine, atropine, scopolamine, and phenobarbital *on page 330*
- ♦ **Hy-Pam® Oral** *see* hydroxyzine *on page 328*
- ♦ **Hypaque-Cysto®** *see* radiological/contrast media (ionic) *on page 539*
- ♦ **Hypaque® Meglumine** *see* radiological/contrast media (ionic) *on page 539*
- ♦ **Hypaque® Sodium** *see* radiological/contrast media (ionic) *on page 539*
- ♦ **Hyperab®** *see* rabies immune globulin (human) *on page 538*
- ♦ **HyperHep®** *see* hepatitis B immune globulin *on page 311*
- ♦ **Hyperstat® I.V.** *see* diazoxide *on page 197*
- ♦ **Hyper-Tet®** *see* tetanus immune globulin (human) *on page 599*
- ♦ **Hy-Phen®** *see* hydrocodone and acetaminophen *on page 319*
- ♦ **HypoTears PF Solution [OTC]** *see* artificial tears *on page 59*
- ♦ **HypoTears Solution [OTC]** *see* artificial tears *on page 59*
- ♦ **HypRho®-D** *see* Rh$_o$(D) immune globulin (intramuscular) *on page 546*
- ♦ **HypRho®-D Mini-Dose** *see* Rh$_o$(D) immune globulin (intramuscular) *on page 546*
- ♦ **Hyprogest® 250** *see* hydroxyprogesterone caproate *on page 327*
- ♦ **Hyrexin-50® Injection** *see* diphenhydramine *on page 208*
- ♦ **Hytakerol®** *see* dihydrotachysterol *on page 204*
- ♦ **Hytinic® [OTC]** *see* polysaccharide-iron complex *on page 503*
- ♦ **Hytone® Topical** *see* hydrocortisone (topical) *on page 324*
- ♦ **Hytrin®** *see* terazosin *on page 595*
- ♦ **Hytuss® [OTC]** *see* guaifenesin *on page 299*
- ♦ **Hytuss-2X® [OTC]** *see* guaifenesin *on page 299*
- ♦ **Hyzaar®** *see* losartan and hydrochlorothiazide *on page 377*
- ♦ **Hyzine-50® Injection** *see* hydroxyzine *on page 328*
- ♦ **ibenzmethyzin** *see* procarbazine *on page 519*
- ♦ **Iberet-Folic-500®** *see* ferrous sulfate, ascorbic acid, vitamin B-complex, and folic acid *on page 266*
- ♦ **Iberet®-Liquid [OTC]** *see* ferrous sulfate, ascorbic acid, and vitamin B-complex *on page 266*
- ♦ **ibidomide** *see* labetalol *on page 357*
- ♦ **Ibuprin® [OTC]** *see* ibuprofen *on page 332*

ibuprofen (eye byoo PROE fen)

Synonyms *p*-isobutylhydratropic acid

U.S. Brand Names Aches-N-Pain® [OTC]; Advil® [OTC]; Children's Advil® Suspension; Children's Motrin® Suspension [OTC]; Excedrin® IB [OTC]; Genpril® [OTC]; Haltran® [OTC]; Ibuprin® [OTC]; Ibuprohm® [OTC]; Ibu-Tab®; Junior Strength Motrin® [OTC]; Medipren® [OTC]; Menadol® [OTC]; Midol® IB [OTC]; Motrin®; Motrin® IB [OTC]; Nuprin® [OTC]; Pamprin IB® [OTC]; Pedia-Profen™; Saleto-200® [OTC]; Saleto-400®; Trendar® [OTC]; Uni-Pro® [OTC]

Mexican Brand Names Butacortelone; Dibufen; Kedvil; Proartinal; Quadrax; Tabalon

Generic Available Yes

Therapeutic Category Analgesic, Non-narcotic; Antipyretic; Nonsteroidal Anti-inflammatory Drug (NSAID)

Use Inflammatory diseases and rheumatoid disorders including juvenile rheumatoid arthritis (JRA); mild to moderate pain; fever; dysmenorrhea; gout

Usual Dosage Oral:

Children:

Antipyretic: 6 months to 12 years: Temperature <102.5°F (39°C): 5 mg/kg/dose; temperature >102.5°F: 10 mg/kg/dose administered every 6-8 hours; maximum daily dose: 40 mg/kg/day

Juvenile rheumatoid arthritis: 30-50 mg/kg/day in 4 divided doses; start at lower end of dosing range and titrate upward; maximum: 2.4 g/day

Analgesic: 4-10 mg/kg/dose every 6-8 hours

Adults:

Inflammatory disease: 400-800 mg/dose 3-4 times/day; maximum dose: 3.2 g/day

Pain/fever/dysmenorrhea: 200-400 mg/dose every 4-6 hours; maximum daily dose: 1.2 g

Dietary Considerations Food may decrease the rate but not the extent of oral absorption; may cause GI upset, bleeding, ulceration, perforation; administer with food or milk to minimize GI upset

Nursing/Pharmacy Information Monitor CBC, liver enzymes; occult blood loss and periodic liver function test; monitor urine output, serum BUN, and creatinine in patients with decreased renal function; with long-term therapy, periodic ophthalmic exams

Dosage Forms

Caplet: 100 mg

Drops, oral (berry flavor): 40 mg/mL (15 mL)

Suspension, oral: 100 mg/5 mL [OTC] (60 mL, 120 mL, 480 mL)

Drops: 40 mg/mL [OTC]

Tablet: 100 mg [OTC], 200 mg [OTC], 300 mg, 400 mg, 600 mg, 800 mg

Chewable: 50 mg, 100 mg

♦ **ibuprofen and hydrocodone** *see* hydrocodone and ibuprofen *on page 321*

♦ **Ibuprohm® [OTC]** *see* ibuprofen *on page 332*

♦ **Ibu-Tab®** *see* ibuprofen *on page 332*

ibutilide (i BYOO ti lide)

U.S. Brand Names Corvert®

Generic Available No

Therapeutic Category Antiarrhythmic Agent, Class III

Use Acute termination of atrial fibrillation or flutter of recent onset; the effectiveness of ibutilide has not been determined in patients with arrhythmias of >90 days in duration

Usual Dosage I.V.: Initial:

<60 kg: 0.01 mg/kg over 10 minutes

≥60 kg: 1 mg over 10 minutes

If the arrhythmia does not terminate within 10 minutes after the end of the initial infusion, a second infusion of equal strength may be infused over a 10-minute period

Dosage Forms Injection, as fumarate: 0.1 mg/mL (10 mL)

♦ **Icaps®** *see* vitamin, multiple (oral) *on page 654*

♦ **ICI 204, 219** *see* zafirlukast *on page 657*

♦ **ICRF-187** *see* dexrazoxane *on page 192*

♦ **Idamycin®** *see* idarubicin *on page 333*

♦ **Idamycin® PFS** *see* idarubicin *on page 333*

♦ **Idarac®** *see* floctafenine *(Canada only) on page 269*

idarubicin (eye da ROO bi sin)

Synonyms 4-demethoxydaunorubicin; 4-dmdr
U.S. Brand Names Idamycin®; Idamycin® PFS
Generic Available No
Therapeutic Category Antineoplastic Agent
Use In combination with other antineoplastic agents for treatment of acute myelogenous leukemia (AML) in adults and acute lymphocytic leukemia (ALL) in children
Usual Dosage I.V.:
 Children:
  Leukemia: 10-12 mg/m^2 once daily for 3 days and repeat every 3 weeks
  Solid tumors: 5 mg/m^2 once daily for 3 days and repeat every 3 weeks
 Adults: 12 mg/m^2/day for 3 days by slow I.V. injection (10-15 minutes) in combination with Ara-C. The Ara-C may be given as 100 mg/m^2/day by continuous infusion for 7 days or 25 mg/m^2 bolus followed by Ara-C 200 mg/m^2/day for 5 days continuous infusion.
Nursing/Pharmacy Information
 Local erythematous streaking along the vein may indicate too rapid a rate of administration; administer by intermittent infusion over 10-30 minutes into a free flowing I.V. solution of NS or D$_5$W; administer at a final concentration of 1 mg/mL
 Monitor CBC with differential, platelet count, ECHO, EKG, serum electrolytes, creatinine, uric acid, ALT, AST, bilirubin, signs of extravasation
 Stability: Parenteral: Reconstituted solutions are physically and chemically stable for at least 7 days under refrigeration at 2°C to 8°C (36°F to 46°F) and 72 hours at controlled room temperature at 15°C to 30°C (59°F to 86°F); prolonged contact with any solution of an alkaline pH will result in degradation of idarubicin; **incompatible** with fluorouracil, etoposide, dexamethasone, heparin, hydrocortisone, methotrexate, vincristine
Dosage Forms
 Injection: 1 mg/mL (5 mL, 10 mL, 20 mL)
 Powder for injection, lyophilized, as hydrochloride: 5 mg, 10 mg

♦ **Idulamine®** *see* azatadine *on page 67*
♦ **Ifex®** *see* ifosfamide *on page 333*
♦ **IFLrA** *see* interferon alfa-2a *on page 341*

ifosfamide (eye FOSS fa mide)

U.S. Brand Names Ifex®
Mexican Brand Names Ifoxan
Generic Available No
Therapeutic Category Antineoplastic Agent
Use In combination with other antineoplastics in treatment of lung cancer, Hodgkin's and non-Hodgkin's lymphoma, breast cancer, acute and chronic lymphocytic leukemia, ovarian cancer, testicular cancer, and sarcomas
Usual Dosage I.V. (refer to individual protocols):
 Children: 1800 mg/m^2/day for 3-5 days every 21-28 days or 5000 mg/m^2 as a single 24-hour infusion or 3 g/m^2/day for 2 days
 Adults: 700-2000 mg/m^2/day for 5 days or 2400 mg/m^2/day for 3 days every 21-28 days; 5000 mg/m^2 as a single dose over 24 hours
Nursing/Pharmacy Information
 Maintain adequate patient hydration; administer as a slow I.V. intermittent infusion over at least 30 minutes at a final concentration for administration not to exceed 40 mg/mL (usual concentration for administration is between 0.6-20 mg/mL) or administer as a 24-hour infusion
 Monitor CBC with differential, hemoglobin, and platelet count, urine output, urinalysis, liver function, and renal function tests
 Stability: Reconstituted solution is stable for 7 days at room temperature and 21 days when refrigerated; for I.V. infusion in normal saline or D$_5$W, solution is stable for 7 days at room temperature and 6 weeks when refrigerated; **compatible** with mesna
Dosage Forms Powder for injection: 1 g, 3 g

♦ **Ifoxan** *see* ifosfamide *on page 333*
♦ **IG** *see* immune globulin, intramuscular *on page 335*
♦ **IGIM** *see* immune globulin, intramuscular *on page 335*
♦ **IGIV** *see* immune globulin, intravenous *on page 336*
♦ **IL-11** *see* oprelvekin *on page 457*
♦ **Iletin®** *see* insulin preparations *on page 339*
♦ **Iletin® II Pork** *see* insulin preparations *on page 339*

- **Ilopan-Choline® Oral** *see* dexpanthenol *on page 192*
- **Ilopan® Injection** *see* dexpanthenol *on page 192*
- **Ilosone®** *see* erythromycin (systemic) *on page 240*
- **Iloscne® Pulvules®** *see* erythromycin (systemic) *on page 240*
- **Ilotycin®** *see* erythromycin (systemic) *on page 240*
- **Ilotycin® Ophthalmic** *see* erythromycin (ophthalmic/topical) *on page 239*
- **Ilozyme®** *see* pancrelipase *on page 467*
- **Imdur™** *see* isosorbide mononitrate *on page 349*
- **imidazole carboxamide** *see* dacarbazine *on page 179*

imiglucerase (i mi GLOO ser ace)
U.S. Brand Names Cerezyme®
Generic Available No
Therapeutic Category Enzyme
Use Long-term enzyme replacement therapy for patients with Type 1 Gaucher's disease
Usual Dosage I.V.: 2.5 units/kg 3 times/week up to as much as 60 units/kg administered as frequently as once weekly or as infrequently as every 4 weeks; 60 units/kg administered every 2 weeks is the most common dose
Dosage Forms Powder for injection, preservative free (lyophilized): 212 units [equivalent to a withdrawal dose of 200 units]

- **Imigran** *see* sumatriptan succinate *on page 590*
- **imipemide** *see* imipenem and cilastatin *on page 334*

imipenem and cilastatin (i mi PEN em & sye la STAT in)
Synonyms cilastatin and imipenem; imipemide
U.S. Brand Names Primaxin®
Mexican Brand Names Tienam®
Generic Available No
Therapeutic Category Carbapenem (Antibiotic)
Use Treatment of documented multidrug resistant gram-negative infection due to organisms proven or suspected to be susceptible to imipenem/cilastatin; treatment of multiple organism infection in which other agents have an insufficient spectrum of activity or are contraindicated due to toxic potential; therapeutic alternative for treatment of gram negative sepsis in immunocompromised patients
Usual Dosage I.V. infusion (dosage recommendation based on imipenem component):
Children: 60-100 mg/kg/day in 4 divided doses
Adults:
  Serious infection: 2-4 g/day in 3-4 divided doses
  Mild to moderate infection: 1-2 g/day in 3-4 divided doses
Nursing/Pharmacy Information
Administer by I.V. intermittent infusion; final concentration for administration should not exceed 5 mg/mL; in fluid-restricted patients, a final concentration of 7 mg/mL has been administered; infuse over 20-60 minutes; if nausea and/or vomiting occur during administration, decrease the rate of I.V. infusion
Monitor periodic renal, hepatic, and hematologic function tests
Stability: Stable for 10 hours at room temperature following reconstitution with 100 mL of 0.9% sodium chloride injection; up to 48 hours when refrigerated at 5°C. If reconstituted with 5% or 10% dextrose injection, 5% dextrose and sodium bicarbonate, 5% dextrose and 0.9% sodium chloride, is stable for 4 hours at room temperature and 24 hours when refrigerated.
Dosage Forms Powder for injection:
I.M.:
  Imipenem 500 mg and cilastatin 500 mg
  Imipenem 750 mg and cilastatin 750 mg
I.V.:
  Imipenem 250 mg and cilastatin 250 mg
  Imipenem 500 mg and cilastatin 500 mg

imipramine (im IP ra meen)
U.S. Brand Names Janimine®; Tofranil®; Tofranil-PM®
Canadian Brand Names Apo®-Imipramine; Novo-Pramine®; PMS-Imipramine
Mexican Brand Names Talpramin
Generic Available Yes: Tablet
Therapeutic Category Antidepressant, Tricyclic (Tertiary Amine)

Use Treatment of various forms of depression, often in conjunction with psychotherapy; enuresis in children; analgesic for certain chronic and neuropathic pain

Usual Dosage

Children: Oral (safety and efficacy of imipramine therapy for treatment of depression in children <12 years have not been established):

Enuresis: ≥6 years: Initial: 10-25 mg at bedtime, if inadequate response still seen after 1 week of therapy, increase by 25 mg/day; dose should not exceed 2.5 mg/kg/day or 50 mg at bedtime if 6-12 years of age or 75 mg at bedtime if ≥12 years of age

Adjunct in the treatment of cancer pain: Initial: 0.2-0.4 mg/kg at bedtime; dose may be increased by 50% every 2-3 days up to 1-3 mg/kg/dose at bedtime

Adolescents: Oral: Initial: 25-50 mg/day; increase gradually; maximum: 100 mg/day in single or divided doses

Adults:

Oral: Initial: 25 mg 3-4 times/day, increase dose gradually, total dose may be administered at bedtime; maximum: 300 mg/day

I.M.: Initial: Up to 100 mg/day in divided doses; change to oral as soon as possible

Dietary Considerations Limit caffeine; increase dietary riboflavin; may be administered with food or milk to decrease GI adverse effects

Nursing/Pharmacy Information

May increase appetite; offer patient water or hard candy for dry mouth

Monitor EKG, CBC, blood pressure, monitor weight; evaluate pressure and pulse rate prior to a during initial therapy; mental status

Stability: Solutions stable at a pH of 4-5; turns yellowish or reddish on exposure to light. Slight discoloration does not affect potency; marked discoloration is associated with loss of potency. Capsules stable for 3 years following date of manufacture.

Dosage Forms

Imipramine hydrochloride:

Injection (Tofranil®): 12.5 mg/mL (2 mL)

Tablet (Janimine®, Tofranil®): 10 mg, 25 mg, 50 mg

Imipramine pamoate: Capsule (Tofranil-PM®): 75 mg, 100 mg, 125 mg, 150 mg

imiquimod (i mi KWI mod)

U.S. Brand Names Aldara™

Generic Available No

Therapeutic Category Immune Response Modifier

Use Genital and perianal warts (condyloma acuminata)

Usual Dosage Adults: Topical: Apply 3 times/week, prior to bedtime, leave on for 6-10 hours; remove cream by washing area with mild soap and water

Nursing/Pharmacy Information Apply only to external or perianal warts; wash hands before and after application of the cream; cotton gauze or underwear may be used to manage treatment area; do not occlude treatment area; avoid sexual contact while cream is on skin; cream may weaken condoms or diaphragms, concurrent use is not recommended

Dosage Forms Cream: 5% (250 mg single dose packets)

♦ Imitrex® see sumatriptan succinate *on page 590*

♦ ImmuCyst® see BCG vaccine *on page 74*

immune globulin, intramuscular

(i MYUN GLOB yoo lin, IN tra MUS kyoo ler)

Synonyms gamma globulin; IG; IGIM; immune serum globulin; ISG

Canadian Brand Names Gammabulin Immuno

Generic Available Yes

Therapeutic Category Immune Globulin

Use Prophylaxis against hepatitis A, measles, varicella, and possibly rubella and immunoglobulin deficiency, idiopathic thrombocytopenia purpura, Kawasaki syndrome, lymphocytic leukemia

Usual Dosage I.M.:

Hepatitis A: 0.02 mL/kg

IgG: 1.3 mL/kg then 0.66 mL/kg in 3-4 weeks

Measles: 0.25 mL/kg

Rubella: 0.55 mL/kg

Varicella: 0.6-1.2 mL/kg

(Continued)

immune globulin, intramuscular *(Continued)*

Nursing/Pharmacy Information
Intramuscular injection only; do not mix with other medications; skin testing should not be performed as local irritation can occur and be misinterpreted as a positive reaction
Stability: Keep in refrigerator; do not freeze
Dosage Forms Injection: I.M.: 165±15 mg (of protein)/mL (2 mL, 10 mL)

immune globulin, intravenous

(i MYUN GLOB yoo lin, IN tra VEE nus)
Synonyms IGIV; IVIG
U.S. Brand Names Gamimune® N; Gammagard® S/D; Gammar®-P I.V.; Polygam® S/D; Sandoglobulin®; Venoglobulin®-I; Venoglobulin®-S
Mexican Brand Names Citax; Intacglobin; Sandoglobulina®
Generic Available No
Therapeutic Category Immune Globulin
Use Immunodeficiency syndrome, idiopathic thrombocytopenic purpura (ITP) and B-cell chronic lymphocytic leukemia (CLL); used in conjunction with appropriate anti-infective therapy to prevent or modify acute bacterial or viral infections in patients with iatrogenically-induced or disease-associated immunodepression; autoimmune neutropenia, bone marrow transplantation patients, Kawasaki disease, Guillain-Barré syndrome, demyelinating polyneuropathies
Usual Dosage Children and Adults: I.V. infusion:
Immunodeficiency syndrome: 100-200 mg/kg/dose every month; may increase to 400 mg/kg/dose as needed
Idiopathic thrombocytopenic purpura: 400-1000 mg/kg/dose for 2-5 consecutive days; maintenance dose: 400-1000 mg/kg/dose every 3-6 weeks based on clinical response and platelet count
Kawasaki disease: 400 mg/kg/day for 4 days or 2 g/kg as a single dose
Congenital and acquired antibody deficiency syndrome: 100-400 mg/kg/dose every 3-4 weeks
Bone marrow transplant: 500 mg/kg/week
Severe systemic viral and bacterial infections: Children: 500-1000 mg/kg/week
Nursing/Pharmacy Information
I.V. use only; for initial treatment, a lower concentration and/or a slower rate of infusion should be used
Monitor platelet count, vital signs
Stability: Dependent upon the manufacturer and brand; parenteral admixture at room temperature (25°C): 30 days; parenteral admixture at refrigeration temperature (4°C): 36 months
Dosage Forms
Injection: Gamimune® N: 5% [50 mg/mL] (10 mL, 50 mL, 100 mL); 10% [100 mg/mL] (50 mL, 100 mL, 200 mL)
Powder for injection, lyophilized:
Gammar-P®-IV: 1 g, 2.5 g, 5 g
Sandoglobulin®: 1 g, 3 g, 6 g
Venoglobulin®-I: 2.5 g, 5 g
Detergent treated:
Gammagard® S/D: 2.5 g, 5 g, 10 g
Polygam® S/D: 2.5 g, 5 g, 10 g
Venoglobulin®-S: 2.5 g, 5 g, 10 g

- **immune serum globulin** *see* immune globulin, intramuscular *on page 335*
- **Imodium®** *see* loperamide *on page 374*
- **Imodium® A-D [OTC]** *see* loperamide *on page 374*
- **Imodium® Advanced** *see* loperamide *on page 374*
- **Imogam®** *see* rabies immune globulin (human) *on page 538*
- **Imot Ofteno** *see* timolol *on page 613*
- **Imovax® Rabies I.D. Vaccine** *see* rabies virus vaccine *on page 539*
- **Imovax® Rabies Vaccine** *see* rabies virus vaccine *on page 539*
- **Imuran®** *see* azathioprine *on page 68*
- **I-Naphline® Ophthalmic** *see* naphazoline *on page 431*
- **Inapsine®** *see* droperidol *on page 223*

indapamide (in DAP a mide)

U.S. Brand Names Lozol®
Canadian Brand Names Lozide®
Generic Available Yes
Therapeutic Category Diuretic, Miscellaneous

Use Management of mild to moderate hypertension; treatment of edema in congestive heart failure and nephrotic syndrome

Usual Dosage Adults: Oral: 2.5-5 mg/day

Dietary Considerations May be administered with food or milk to decrease GI adverse effects

Nursing/Pharmacy Information Monitor blood pressure, serum electrolytes, renal function; check for orthostasis

Dosage Forms Tablet: 1.25 mg, 2.5 mg

- **Inderal®** *see* propranolol *on page 527*
- **Inderalici** *see* propranolol *on page 527*
- **Inderal® LA** *see* propranolol *on page 527*
- **Inderide®** *see* propranolol and hydrochlorothiazide *on page 528*

indinavir (in DIN a veer)
U.S. Brand Names Crixivan®

Generic Available No

Therapeutic Category Antiviral Agent

Use Treatment of HIV infection, especially advanced disease; usually administered as part of a three-drug regimen (two nucleosides plus a protease inhibitor) or double therapy (one nucleoside plus a protease inhibitor)

Usual Dosage Adults: Oral: 800 mg every 8 hours

Dietary Considerations Administer with plenty of water; drink at least 48 oz of water daily; administer 1 hour before or 2 hours after a meal

Nursing/Pharmacy Information Administer around-the-clock to avoid significant fluctuation in serum levels

Dosage Forms Capsule: 200 mg, 400 mg

- **Indocid®** *see* indomethacin *on page 337*
- **Indocin® I.V. Injection** *see* indomethacin *on page 337*
- **Indocin® Oral** *see* indomethacin *on page 337*
- **Indocin® SR Oral** *see* indomethacin *on page 337*
- **Indocollyre®** *see* indomethacin *on page 337*

indocyanine green (in doe SYE a neen green)
U.S. Brand Names Cardio-Green®

Generic Available Yes

Therapeutic Category Diagnostic Agent

Use Determining hepatic function, cardiac output and liver blood flow and for ophthalmic angiography

Usual Dosage Dilute dose in sterile water for injection or 0.9% NaCl to final volume of 1 mL if necessary doses may be repeated periodically; total dose should not exceed 2 mg/kg

Infants: 1.25 mg
Children: 2.5 mg
Adults: 5 mg

Nursing/Pharmacy Information
Do not mix with preservative, bisulfite, metabisulfite, or borohydride preparations
Stability: Reconstitute only with sterile water for injection supplied by manufacturer

Dosage Forms Injection: 25 mg, 50 mg

- **indometacin** *see* indomethacin *on page 337*

indomethacin (in doe METH a sin)
Synonyms indometacin

U.S. Brand Names Indocin® I.V. Injection; Indocin® Oral; Indocin® SR Oral

Canadian Brand Names Apo®-Indomethacin; Indocollyre®; Indotec; Novo-Methacin®; Nu-Indo®; Pro-Indo®

Mexican Brand Names Antalgin® Dialicels; Indocid®; Malival; Malival AP

Generic Available Yes (capsule and oral suspension)

Therapeutic Category Analgesic, Non-narcotic; Nonsteroidal Anti-inflammatory Drug (NSAID)

Use Management of inflammatory diseases and rheumatoid disorders; moderate pain; acute gouty arthritis; I.V. form used as alternative to surgery for closure of patent ductus arteriosus (PDA) in neonates

Usual Dosage
Patent ductus arteriosus: Neonates: I.V.: Initial: 0.2 mg/kg; followed with: 2 doses of 0.1 mg/kg at 12- to 24-hour intervals if age <48 hours at time of first dose; 0.2 mg/kg 2 times if 2-7 days old at time of first dose; or 0.25 mg/kg 2
(Continued)

indomethacin *(Continued)*

times if over 7 days at time of first dose; discontinue if significant adverse effects occur. Dose should be withheld if patient has anuria or oliguria.

Analgesia:

Children: Oral: Initial: 1-2 mg/kg/day in 2-4 divided doses; maximum: 4 mg/kg/day; not to exceed 150-200 mg/day

Adults: Oral, rectal: 25-50 mg/dose 2-3 times/day; maximum dose: 200 mg/day; extended release capsule should be administered on a 1-2 times/day schedule

Dietary Considerations Food:

Food may decrease the rate but not the extent of oral absorption; may cause GI upset, bleeding, ulceration, perforation; administer with food or milk to minimize GI upset

Potassium: Hyperkalemia has been reported; the elderly and those with renal insufficiency are at greatest risk; monitor potassium serum concentration in those at greatest risk; avoid salt substitutes

Sodium: Hyponatremia from sodium retention; suspect secondary to suppression of renal prostaglandin; monitor serum concentration and fluid status; may need to restrict fluid

Nursing/Pharmacy Information

Avoid I.V. bolus administration or infusion via an umbilical catheter into vessels near the superior mesenteric artery as these may cause vasoconstriction and can compromise blood flow to the intestines. Administer over 20-30 minutes at a concentration of 0.5-1 mg/mL in preservative free sterile water for injection or normal saline. Do not administer intra-arterially. Extended release capsules must be swallowed intact.

Monitor BUN, serum creatinine, liver enzymes, CBC; ophthalmologic exams with chronic use

Stability: Protect from light; not stable in alkaline solution; reconstitute just prior to administration; discard any unused portion; do not use preservative containing diluents for reconstitution

Dosage Forms

Capsule: 25 mg, 50 mg
Indocin®: 25 mg, 50 mg
Capsule, sustained release (Indocin® SR): 75 mg
Powder for injection, as sodium trihydrate (Indocin® I.V.): 1 mg
Suppository, rectal (Indocin®): 50 mg
Suspension, oral (Indocin®): 25 mg/5 mL (5 mL, 10 mL, 237 mL, 500 mL)

infliximab *(in FLIKS e mab)*

U.S. Brand Names Remicade®
Generic Available No
Therapeutic Category Gastrointestinal Agent, Miscellaneous
Use Treatment of moderately to severely active Crohn's disease for the reduction of the signs and symptoms in patients who have an inadequate response to conventional therapy or for the treatment of patients with fistulizing Crohn's disease for the reduction in the number of draining enterocutaneous fistula(s)

Usual Dosage

Moderately to severely active Crohn's disease: Adults: I.V.: 5 mg/kg as a single infusion over a minimum of 2 hours

Fistulizing Crohn's disease: 5 mg/kg as an infusion over a minimum of 2 hours, dose repeated at 2 and 6 weeks after the initial infusion

Dosage Forms Powder for injection: 100 mg

influenza virus vaccine *(in floo EN za VYE rus vak SEEN)*

Synonyms influenza virus vaccine (inactivated whole-virus); influenza virus vaccine (purified surface antigen); influenza virus vaccine (split-virus)
U.S. Brand Names Fluogen®; Fluzone®
Canadian Brand Names Fluviral®
Generic Available No

Therapeutic Category Vaccine, Inactivated Virus

Use Provide active immunity to influenza virus strains contained in the vaccine

Usual Dosage Annual vaccination with current vaccine; either whole- or split-virus vaccine may be used

Nursing/Pharmacy Information
Inspect for particulate matter and discoloration prior to administration; for I.M. administration only
Stability: Refrigerate

Dosage Forms Injection:
Purified surface antigen (Flu-Imune®): 5 mL
Split-virus (Fluogen®, Fluzone®): 0.5 mL, 5 mL
Whole-virus (Fluzone®): 5 mL

♦ **influenza virus vaccine (inactivated whole-virus)** see influenza virus vaccine on page 338

♦ **influenza virus vaccine (purified surface antigen)** see influenza virus vaccine on page 338

♦ **influenza virus vaccine (split-virus)** see influenza virus vaccine on page 338

♦ **INH** see isoniazid on page 347

♦ **Inhepar** see heparin on page 310

♦ **Inhibace®** see cilazapril (Canada only) on page 150

♦ **Inhibitron®** see omeprazole on page 455

♦ **Innohep®** see tinzaparin (Canada only) on page 614

♦ **Innovar®** see droperidol and fentanyl on page 224

♦ **Inocor®** see amrinone on page 47

insect sting kit (IN sekt sting kit)

U.S. Brand Names Ana-Kit®

Generic Available No

Therapeutic Category Antidote

Use Anaphylaxis emergency treatment of insect bites or stings by the sensitive patient that may occur within minutes of insect sting or exposure to an allergic substance

Usual Dosage Children and Adults:
Epinephrine:
<2 years: 0.05-0.1 mL
2-6 years: 0.15 mL
6-12 years: 0.2 mL
>12 years : 0.3 mL
Chlorpheniramine:
<6 years: 1 tablet
6-12 years: 2 tablets
>12 years: 4 tablets

Nursing/Pharmacy Information
Not intended for I.V. use (I.M. or S.C. only)
Stability: Protect from light, store at room temperature, prevent from freezing

Dosage Forms Kit: Epinephrine hydrochloride 1:1000 (1 mL syringe), chlorpheniramine maleate chewable tablet 2 mg (4), sterile alcohol pads (2), tourniquet

♦ **Insogen®** see chlorpropamide on page 145

♦ **Insta-Glucose® [OTC]** see glucose, instant on page 293

♦ **Insulina Lenta** see insulin preparations on page 339

♦ **Insulina NPH** see insulin preparations on page 339

♦ **Insulina Regular** see insulin preparations on page 339

♦ **Insulin Lente® L** see insulin preparations on page 339

insulin preparations (IN su lin prep a RAY shuns)

U.S. Brand Names Humalog®; Humulin® 50/50; Humulin® 70/30; Humulin® L; Humulin® N; Humulin® R; Humulin® U; Insulin Lente® L; Lente®; Lente® Iletin® I; Lente® Iletin® II; Novolin® 70/30; Novolin® L; Novolin® N; Novolin® R; NPH Iletin® I; NPH Insulin; NPH-N; Pork NPH; Pork Regular Iletin® II; Regular Iletin® I; Regular [Concentrated] Iletin® II U-500; Regular Insulin; Regular Purified Pork Insulin; Velosulin®; Velosulin® BR Human (Buffered)

Canadian Brand Names Iletin®; Iletin® II Pork; Novolin® ge; Novolin-Pen® II, -3

Mexican Brand Names Insulina Lenta; Insulina NPH; Insulina Regular

Generic Available Yes

Therapeutic Category Antidiabetic Agent, Parenteral
(Continued)

insulin preparations *(Continued)*

Use Treatment of insulin-dependent diabetes mellitus, also noninsulin-dependent diabetes mellitus unresponsive to treatment with diet and/or oral hypoglycemics; to assure proper utilization of glucose and reduce glucosuria in nondiabetic patients receiving parenteral nutrition whose glucosuria cannot be adequately controlled with infusion rate adjustments or those who require assistance in achieving optimal caloric intakes

Usual Dosage Dose requires continuous medical supervision; only regular insulin may be administered I.V. The daily dose should be divided up depending upon the product used and the patient's response, eg, regular insulin every 4-6 hours; NPH insulin every 8-12 hours.

Children and Adults: S.C.: 0.5-1 unit/kg/day
Adolescents (during growth spurt): S.C.: 0.8-1.2 units/kg/day

Diabetic ketoacidosis: Children: I.V. loading dose: 0.1 unit/kg, then maintenance continuous infusion: 0.1 unit/kg/hour (range: 0.05-0.2 units/kg/hour depending upon the rate of decrease of serum glucose - too rapid decrease of serum glucose may lead to cerebral edema).
Optimum rate of decrease (serum glucose): 80-100 mg/dL/hour

Note: Newly diagnosed patients with JODM presenting in DKA and patients with blood sugars <800 mg/dL may be relatively "sensitive" to insulin and should receive loading and initial maintenance doses approximately $1/2$ of those indicated above.

Note: The term "purified" refers to insulin preparations containing no more than 10 ppm proinsulin (purified and human insulins are less immunogenic)

Dietary Considerations

Alcohol: Increase in hypoglycemic effect of insulin; monitor blood glucose concentration; avoid or limit alcohol

Food:

Potassium: Shifts potassium from extracellular to intracellular space; decreases potassium serum concentration; monitor potassium serum concentration

Sodium: SIADH; water retention and dilutional hyponatremia may occur; patients at greatest risk are those with CHF or hepatic cirrhosis; monitor sodium serum concentration and fluid status

Nursing/Pharmacy Information

When mixing regular insulin with other insulin preparations, regular insulin should be drawn into the syringe first

Monitor urine sugar and acetone, serum glucose, electrolytes

Stability: Bottle in use is stable at room temperature up to 1 month; cold (freezing) causes more damage to insulin than room temperatures up to 100°F; avoid direct sunlight; cold injections should be avoided

Dosage Forms All insulins are 100 units/mL (10 mL) except where indicated:

RAPID ACTING:
Insulin lispro rDNA origin: Humalog® [*Lilly*] (1.5 mL, 10 mL)
Insulin Injection (Regular Insulin)
Beef and pork: Regular Iletin® I [*Lilly*]
Human:
rDNA: Humulin® R [*Lilly*], Novolin® R [*Novo Nordisk*]
Semisynthetic: Velosulin® Human [*Novo Nordisk*]
rDNA Human, Buffered: Velosulin® BR
Pork: Regular Insulin [*Novo Nordisk*]
Purified pork:
Pork Regular Iletin® II [*Lilly*], Regular Purified Pork Insulin [*Novo Nordisk*]
Regular (Concentrated) Iletin® II U-500 (*Lilly*): 500 units/mL

INTERMEDIATE-ACTING:
Insulin Zinc Suspension (Lente®)
Beef and pork: Lente® Iletin® I [*Lilly*]
Human, rDNA: Humulin® L [*Lilly*], Novolin® L [*Novo Nordisk*]
Purified pork: Lente® Iletin® II [*Lilly*], Lente® L [*Novo Nordisk*]

Isophane Insulin Suspension (NPH)
Beef and pork: NPH Iletin® I [*Lilly*]
Human, rDNA: Humulin® N [*Lilly*], Novolin® N [*Novo Nordisk*]
Purified pork: Pork NPH Iletin® II [*Lilly*], NPH-N [*Novo Nordisk*]

LONG-ACTING:
Insulin zinc suspension, extended (Ultralente®)
Human, rDNA: Humulin® U [*Lilly*]

COMBINATIONS:
Isophane Insulin Suspension and Insulin Injection

Isophane insulin suspension (50%) and insulin injection (50%) human (rDNA): Humulin® 50/50 [*Lilly*]

Isophane insulin suspension (70%) and insulin injection (30%) human (rDNA): Humulin® 70/30 [*Lilly*], Novolin® 70/30 [*Novo Nordisk*]

♦ **Intacglobin** *see* immune globulin, intravenous *on page 336*

♦ **Intal®** *see* cromolyn sodium *on page 171*

♦ **Intal® Inhalation Capsule** *(Discontinued) see page 743*

♦ **Integrilin®** *see* eptifibatide *on page 237*

♦ **Intercept®** *(Discontinued) see page 743*

♦ **α-2-interferon** *see* interferon alfa-2b *on page 341*

interferon alfa-2a (in ter FEER on AL fa too aye)

Synonyms IFLrA; rIFN-A

U.S. Brand Names Roferon-A®

Generic Available No

Therapeutic Category Biological Response Modulator

Use Hairy cell leukemia, AIDS-related Kaposi's sarcoma in patients >18 years of age, multiple unlabeled uses

Usual Dosage

Children: S.C.: Pulmonary hemangiomatosis: 1-3 million units/m²/day once daily

Adults >18 years:

Hairy cell leukemia: I.M., S.C.: Induction dose is 3 million units/day for 16-24 weeks; maintenance: 3 million units 3 times/week

AIDS-related Kaposi's sarcoma: I.M., S.C.: Induction dose is 36 million units for 10-12 weeks; maintenance: 36 million units 3 times/week (may begin with dose escalation from 3-9-18 million units each day over 3 consecutive days followed by 36 million units daily for the remainder of the 10-12 weeks of induction)

Nursing/Pharmacy Information

S.C. administration is suggested for those who are at risk for bleeding or are thrombocytopenic; rotate S.C. injection site; patient should be well hydrated; pretreatment with nonsteroidal anti-inflammatory drug (NSAID) or acetaminophen can decrease fever and its severity and alleviate headache

Monitor baseline chest x-ray, EKG, CBC with differential, liver function tests, electrolytes, platelets, weight; patients with pre-existing cardiac abnormalities, or in advanced stages of cancer should have EKGs taken before and during treatment

Stability: Refrigerate; reconstituted solution is stable for 24 hours at room temperature and for 1 month when refrigerated

Dosage Forms

Injection: 3 million units/mL (1 mL); 6 million units/mL (3 mL); 9 million units/mL (0.9 mL, 3 mL); 36 million units/mL (1 mL)

Powder for injection: 6 million units/mL when reconstituted

interferon alfa-2b (in ter FEER on AL fa too bee)

Synonyms INF-alpha 2; α-2-interferon; rLFN-α2

U.S. Brand Names Intron® A

Generic Available No

Therapeutic Category Biological Response Modulator

Use Induce hairy cell leukemia remission; treatment of AIDS-related Kaposi's sarcoma; condylomata acuminata; chronic hepatitis C

Usual Dosage Adults (refer to individual protocols):

Hairy cell leukemia: I.M., S.C.: 2 million units/m² 3 times/week

AIDS-related Kaposi's sarcoma: I.M., S.C.: 30 million units/m² 3 times/week or 50 million units/m² I.V. 5 days/week every other week

Condylomata acuminata: Intralesionally: 1 million units/lesion 3 times/week for 3 weeks; not to exceed 5 million units per treatment (maximum: 5 lesions at one time)

Chronic hepatitis C: I.M., S.C.: 3 million units 3 times/week for approximately a 6-month course

Nursing/Pharmacy Information

S.C. administration is suggested for those patients who are at risk for bleeding or are thrombocytopenic; rotate S.C. injection site; patient should be well hydrated; may pretreat with nonsteroidal anti-inflammatory drug (NSAID) or acetaminophen to decrease fever and its severity and to alleviate headache

Monitor baseline chest x-ray, EKG, CBC with differential, liver function tests, electrolytes, platelets, weight; patients with pre-existing cardiac abnormalities, or in advanced stages of cancer should have EKGs taken before and during treatment

(Continued)

interferon alfa-2b *(Continued)*

Stability: Refrigerate; reconstituted solution is stable for 1 month when refrigerated

Dosage Forms

Injection, albumin free: 3 million units (0.5 mL); 5 million units (0.5 mL); 10 million units (1 mL); 25 million units

Powder for injection, lyophilized: 18 million units, 50 million units

interferon alfa-2b and ribavirin combination pack

(in ter FEER on AL fa too bee)

U.S. Brand Names Rebetron™

Generic Available No

Therapeutic Category Antiviral Agent; Biological Response Modulator

Use The combination therapy is indicated for the treatment of chronic hepatitis C in patients with compensated liver disease who have relapsed following alpha interferon therapy

Usual Dosage The recommended dosage of combination therapy is 3 million int. units of Intron® A injected subcutaneously three times per week and 1000-1200 mg of Rebtrol® capsules administered orally in a divided daily (morning and evening) dose for 24 weeks; patients weighing 75 kg (165 pounds) or less should receive 1000 mg of Rebetrol® daily, while patients weighing more than 75 kg should receive 1200 mg of Rebetrol® daily

Nursing/Pharmacy Information Use acetaminophen to prevent or partially alleviate headache and fever; do not use 3, 5, and 25 million unit strengths intralesionally, solutions are hypertonic; 50 million unit strength is not for use in condylomata

Dosage Forms Combination package:

For patients ≤75 kg:

Each Rebetron™ combination package consists of:

A box containing 6 vials of Intron® A (3 million int. units in 0.5 mL per vial) and 6 syringes and alcohol swabs; two boxes containing 35 Rebetrol® capsules each for a total of 70 capsules (5 capsules per blister card)

One 18 million int. units multidose vial of Intron® A injection (22.8 million int. units per 3.8 mL; 3 million int. units/0.5 mL) and 6 syringes and alcohol swabs; two boxes containing 35 Rebetrol® capsules each for a total of 70 capsules (5 capsules per blister card)

One 18 million int. units Intron® A injection multidose pen (22.5 million int. units per 1.5 mL; 3 million int. units/0.2 mL) and 6 disposable needles and alcohol swabs; two boxes containing 35 Rebetrol® capsules each for a total of 70 capsules (5 capsules per blister card)

For patients >75 kg:

A box containing 6 vials of Intron® A injection (3 million int. units in 0.5 mL per vial) and 6 syringes and alcohol swabs; two boxes containing 42 Rebetrol® capsules each for a total of 84 capsules (6 capsules per blister card)

One 18 million int. units multidose vial of Intron® A injection (22.5 million int. units per 3.8 mL; 3 million int. units/0.5 mL) and 6 syringes and alcohol swabs; two boxes containing 42 Rebetrol® capsules each for a total of 84 capsules (6 capsules per blister card)

One 18 million int. units Intron® A injection multidose pen (22.5 million int. units per 1.5 mL; 3 million int. units/0.2 mL) and 6 disposable needles and alcohol swabs; two boxes containing 42 Rebetrol® capsules each for a total of 84 capsules (6 capsules per blister card)

For Rebetrol® dose reduction:

A box containing 6 vials of Intron® A injection (3 million int. units in 0.5 mL per vial) and 6 syringes and alcohol swabs; one box containing 42 Rebetrol® capsules (6 capsules per blister card)

One 18 million int. units multidose vial of Intron® A injection (22.8 million int. units per 3.8 mL; 3 million int. units/0.5 mL) and 6 syringes and alcohol swabs; one box containing 42 Rebetrol® capsules (6 capsules per blister card)

One 18 million int. units Introl® A injection multidose pen (22.5 million int. units per 1.5 mL; 3 million int. units/0.2 mL) and 6 disposable needles and alcohol swabs; one box containing 42 Rebetrol® capsules (6 capsules per blister card)

interferon alfa-n3 (in ter FEER on AL fa en three)

U.S. Brand Names Alferon® N

Generic Available No

Therapeutic Category Biological Response Modulator

Use Intralesional treatment of refractory or recurring genital or venereal warts; useful in patients who do not respond or are not candidates for usual treatments; indications and dosage regimens are specific for a particular brand of interferon

Usual Dosage Adults: Inject 250,000 units (0.05 mL) in each wart twice weekly for a maximum of 8 weeks; therapy should not be repeated for at least 3 months after the initial 8-week course of therapy

Nursing/Pharmacy Information
Inject into base of wart with a small 30-gauge needle
Stability: Store solution at 2°C to 8°C (36°F to 46°F); do not freeze or shake solution

Dosage Forms Injection: 5 million units (1 mL)

interferon beta-1a (in ter FEER on BAY ta won aye)
U.S. Brand Names Avonex™
Generic Available No
Therapeutic Category Biological Response Modulator
Use Treatment of relapsing forms of multiple sclerosis (MS); to slow the accumulation of physical disability and decrease the frequency of clinical exacerbations

Usual Dosage Adults >18 years: I.M.: 30 mcg once weekly

Nursing/Pharmacy Information Patient should be informed of possible side effects, especially depression, suicidal ideations, and the risk of abortion; flu-like symptoms such as chills, fever, malaise, sweating, and myalgia are common

Dosage Forms Powder for injection, lyophilized: 33 mcg [6.6 million units]

interferon beta-1b (in ter FEER on BAY ta won bee)
U.S. Brand Names Betaseron®
Mexican Brand Names Betaferon®
Generic Available No
Therapeutic Category Biological Response Modulator
Use Reduce the frequency of clinical exacerbations in ambulatory patients with relapsing-remitting multiple sclerosis

Usual Dosage Adults: S.C.: 0.25 mg every other day

Nursing/Pharmacy Information
Patient should be informed of possible side effects, especially depression, suicidal ideations, and the risk of abortion; flu-like symptoms such as chills, fever, malaise, sweating, and myalgia are common; inject 1 mL S.C. with a 27-gauge needle; may be injected into arms, thighs, hips, and abdomen
Monitor hemoglobin, liver function, and blood chemistries

Dosage Forms Powder for injection, lyophilized: 0.3 mg [9.6 million units]

interferon gamma-1b (in ter FEER on GAM ah won bee)
U.S. Brand Names Actimmune®
Generic Available No
Therapeutic Category Biological Response Modulator
Use Reduce the frequency and severity of serious infections associated with chronic granulomatous disease

Usual Dosage Adults: S.C. (dosing is based on body surface (m²)):
≤0.5: 1.5 mcg/kg/dose
>0.5: 50 mcg/m² (1.5 million units/m²) 3 times/week

Nursing/Pharmacy Information Single-dose vials only: discard unused portion

Dosage Forms Injection: 100 mcg [3 million units]

- **interleukin-2** *see* aldesleukin *on page 26*
- **interleukin-11** *see* oprelvekin *on page 457*
- **Intralipid®** *see* fat emulsion *on page 259*
- **intravenous fat emulsion** *see* fat emulsion *on page 259*
- **Intron® A** *see* interferon alfa-2b *on page 341*
- **Intropin®** *see* dopamine *on page 217*
- **Inversine®** *see* mecamylamine *on page 387*
- **Invirase®** *see* saquinavir *on page 559*
- **Iobid DM®** *see* guaifenesin and dextromethorphan *on page 300*
- **Iodex® [OTC]** *see* povidone-iodine *on page 510*
- **Iodex-p® [OTC]** *see* povidone-iodine *on page 510*

iodine (EYE oh dyne)
Generic Available Yes
Therapeutic Category Topical Skin Product
Use Topically as an antiseptic in the management of minor, superficial skin wounds and has been used to disinfect the skin preoperatively
Usual Dosage Topical: Apply as necessary to affected areas of skin
Nursing/Pharmacy Information Avoid tight bandages because iodine may cause burns on occluded skin
Dosage Forms
Solution: 2%
Tincture: 2%

♦ **iodochlorhydroxyquin and hydrocortisone** *see* clioquinol and hydrocortisone *on page 157*
♦ **Iodo-Niacin® Tablet** *(Discontinued) see page 743*
♦ **Iodopen®** *see* trace metals *on page 620*

iodoquinol (eye oh doe KWIN ole)
Synonyms diiodohydroxyquin
U.S. Brand Names Yodoxin®
Canadian Brand Names Diodoquin®
Generic Available No
Therapeutic Category Amebicide
Use Treatment of acute and chronic intestinal amebiasis due to *Entamoeba histolytica*; asymptomatic cyst passers; *Blastocystis hominis* infections; iodoquinol alone is ineffective for amebic hepatitis or hepatic abscess
Usual Dosage Oral:
Children: 30-40 mg/kg/day in 3 divided doses for 20 days; not to exceed 1.95 g/day
Adults: 650 mg 3 times/day after meals for 20 days; not to exceed 2 g/day
Dietary Considerations Should be administered after meals
Nursing/Pharmacy Information
Tablets may be crushed and mixed with applesauce or chocolate syrup
Monitor ophthalmologic exam
Dosage Forms
Powder: 25 g
Tablet: 210 mg, 650 mg

iodoquinol and hydrocortisone
(eye oh doe KWIN ole & hye droe KOR ti sone)
Synonyms hydrocortisone and iodoquinol
U.S. Brand Names Vytone® Topical
Generic Available No
Therapeutic Category Antifungal/Corticosteroid
Use Treatment of eczema; infectious dermatitis; chronic eczematoid otitis externa; mycotic dermatoses
Usual Dosage Topical: Apply 3-4 times/day
Dosage Forms Cream: Iodoquinol 1% and hydrocortisone 1% (30 g)

♦ **Iofed®** *see* brompheniramine and pseudoephedrine *on page 95*
♦ **Iofed® PD** *see* brompheniramine and pseudoephedrine *on page 95*
♦ **Ionamin®** *(Discontinued) see page 743*
♦ **Ionil-T® Plus** *see* coal tar *on page 162*
♦ **Iophen-C®** *(Discontinued) see page 743*
♦ **Iophen®** *(Discontinued) see page 743*
♦ **Iophen-DM®** *(Discontinued) see page 743*
♦ **Iophylline®** *(Discontinued) see page 743*
♦ **Iopidine®** *see* apraclonidine *on page 57*
♦ **Iotuss®** *(Discontinued) see page 743*
♦ **Iotuss-DM®** *(Discontinued) see page 743*
♦ **I-Paracaine®** *see* proparacaine *on page 524*

ipecac syrup (IP e kak SIR up)
Generic Available Yes
Therapeutic Category Antidote
Use Treatment of acute oral drug overdosage and certain poisonings
Usual Dosage Oral:
Children:
6-12 months: 5-10 mL followed by 10-20 mL/kg of water; repeat dose one time if vomiting does not occur within 20 minutes

1-12 years: 15 mL followed by 10-20 mL/kg of water; repeat dose one time if vomiting does not occur within 20 minutes

Adults: 30 mL followed by 200-300 mL of water; repeat dose one time if vomiting does not occur within 20 minutes

Dietary Considerations Milk, carbonated beverages may decrease effectiveness

Nursing/Pharmacy Information Do **not** administer to unconscious patients; patients should be kept active and moving following administration of ipecac; if vomiting does not occur after second dose, gastric lavage may be considered to remove ingested substance

Dosage Forms Syrup: 70 mg/mL (15 mL, 30 mL, 473 mL, 4000 mL)

- ♦ **I-Pentolate®** see cyclopentolate on page 174
- ♦ **I-Phrine® Ophthalmic Solution** see phenylephrine on page 487
- ♦ **I-Picamide®** see tropicamide on page 634
- ♦ **IPOL™** see poliovirus vaccine, inactivated on page 501

ipratropium (i pra TROE pee um)

U.S. Brand Names Atrovent®

Generic Available Yes

Therapeutic Category Anticholinergic Agent

Use Bronchodilator used in bronchospasm associated with asthma, COPD, bronchitis, and emphysema; nasal spray used for symptomatic relief of rhinorrhea

Usual Dosage Children >12 years and Adults: 2 inhalations 4 times/day up to 12 inhalations/24 hours

Nursing/Pharmacy Information Teach patients how to use the inhaler; shake inhaler before administering

Dosage Forms Solution, as bromide:
Inhalation: 18 mcg/actuation (14 g)
Nasal spray: 0.03% (30 mL); 0.06% (15 mL)
Nebulizing: 0.02% (2.5 mL)

ipratropium and albuterol (i pra TROE pee um & al BYOO ter ole)

U.S. Brand Names Combivent®

Generic Available No

Therapeutic Category Bronchodilator

Use Treatment of chronic obstructive pulmonary disease (COPD) in those patients that are currently on a regular bronchodilator who continue to have bronchospasms and require a second bronchodilator

Usual Dosage Adults: 2 inhalations 4 times/day, maximum of 12 inhalations/24 hours

Dosage Forms Aerosol: Ipratropium bromide 18 mcg and albuterol sulfate 103 mcg per actuation [200 doses] (14.7 g)

- ♦ **iproveratril** see verapamil on page 646
- ♦ **IPV** see poliovirus vaccine, inactivated on page 501

irbesartan (ir be SAR tan)

U.S. Brand Names Avapro®

Mexican Brand Names Aprovel

Generic Available No

Therapeutic Category Angiotensin II Antagonist

Use Treatment of hypertension alone or in combination with other antihypertensives

Usual Dosage Adults: Oral: 150 mg once daily with or without food; patients may be titrated to 300 mg once daily

Dosage Forms Tablet: 75 mg, 150 mg, 300 mg

irbesartan and hydrochlorothiazide *New Drug*
(ir be SAR tan & hye droe klor oh THYE a zide)

U.S. Brand Names Avapro® HCT

Generic Available No

Therapeutic Category Antihypertensive Agent, Combination

Use Combination therapy for the management of hypertension

Dosage Forms Tablet: Irbesartan 150 mg and hydrochlorothiazide 12.5 mg; irbesartan 300 mg and hydrochlorothiazide 12.5 mg

- ♦ **Ircon® [OTC]** see ferrous fumarate on page 264

irinotecan (eye rye no TEE kan)

U.S. Brand Names Camptosar®
Generic Available No
Therapeutic Category Antineoplastic Agent
Use Treatment of patients with metastatic carcinoma of the colon or rectum whose disease has progressed following 5-FU based therapy
Usual Dosage Adults: I.V.: The recommended starting dose is 125 mg/m^2 (I.V. infusion over 90 minutes) once a week for 4 weeks, followed by a 2-week rest period; additional 6-week cycles of treatment may be repeated indefinitely in patients who remain stable or do not develop intolerable toxicities
Dosage Forms Injection: 20 mg/mL (5 mL)

iron dextran complex (EYE ern DEKS tran KOM pleks)

U.S. Brand Names Dexferrum®; InFeD™
Mexican Brand Names Driken
Generic Available Yes
Therapeutic Category Electrolyte Supplement, Oral
Use Treatment of microcytic, hypochromic anemia resulting from iron deficiency when oral iron administration is infeasible or ineffective
Usual Dosage I.M., I.V.:
A 0.5 mL test dose (0.25 mL in infants) should be administered prior to starting iron dextran therapy
Total replacement dosage of iron dextran (mL) = 0.0476 x weight (kg) x (Hb$_n$-Hb$_o$) + 1 mL/per 5 kg body weight (up to maximum of 14 mL)
Hb$_n$ = desired hemoglobin (g/dL)
Hb$_o$ = measured hemoglobin (g/dL)
Maximum daily dose:
Infants <5 kg: 25 mg iron
Children:
5-10 kg: 50 mg iron
10-50 kg: 100 mg iron
Adults >50 kg: 100 mg iron
Nursing/Pharmacy Information
I.M.: Use Z-track technique for I.M. administration (deep into the upper outer quadrant of buttock)
I.V.: Direct I.V. push administration is **not** recommended; dilute in normal saline (250-1000 mL) and infuse over 1-6 hours at a maximum rate of 50 mg/minute; avoid dilution in dextrose due to an increased incidence of local pain and phlebitis
Monitor hemoglobin, hematocrit, reticulocyte count, serum ferritin
Stability: Commercial injection should be stored at room temperature; stability of parenteral admixture at room temperature (25°C): 3 months
Dosage Forms Injection: 50 mg/mL (2 mL, 10 mL)

- ♦ **ISD** see isosorbide dinitrate on page 349
- ♦ **ISDN** see isosorbide dinitrate on page 349
- ♦ **ISG** see immune globulin, intramuscular on page 335
- ♦ **Ismelin®** see guanethidine on page 305
- ♦ **ISMN** see isosorbide mononitrate on page 349
- ♦ **Ismo®** see isosorbide mononitrate on page 349
- ♦ **Ismotic®** see isosorbide on page 349
- ♦ **isoamyl nitrite** see amyl nitrite on page 48
- ♦ **Isobac** see co-trimoxazole on page 170
- ♦ **isobamate** see carisoprodol on page 116
- ♦ **Iso-Bid®** *(Discontinued)* see page 743
- ♦ **Isocaine® HCl** see mepivacaine on page 394
- ♦ **Isocal® [OTC]** see enteral nutritional products on page 233
- ♦ **Isocal® with Fibre** see enteral nutritional products on page 233
- ♦ **Isoclor® Expectorant** see guaifenesin, pseudoephedrine, and codeine on page 304
- ♦ **Isocom®** see acetaminophen, isometheptene, and dichloralphenazone on page 17

isoetharine (eye soe ETH a reen)

U.S. Brand Names Arm-a-Med® Isoetharine; Beta-2®; Bronkometer®; Bronkosol®; Dey-Lute® Isoetharine
Generic Available Yes
Therapeutic Category Adrenergic Agonist Agent

Use Bronchodilator used in asthma and for the reversible bronchospasm occurring with bronchitis and emphysema

Usual Dosage Treatments are usually not repeated more often than every 4 hours, except in severe cases, and may be repeated up to 5 times/day if necessary

Nebulizer: Children: 0.1-0.2 mg/kg/dose every 2-6 hours as needed; adult: 0.5 mL diluted in 2-3 mL normal saline or 4 inhalations of undiluted 1% solution

Nursing/Pharmacy Information

Instruct patient on use of nebulizer

Monitor heart rate, blood pressure, lung sounds, respiratory rate

Stability: Do not use if solution is discolored or a precipitation is present; **compatible** with sterile water, 0.45% sodium chloride, and 0.9% sodium chloride; protect from light

Dosage Forms

Isoetharine hydrochloride:

Solution, inhalation: 0.062% (4 mL); 0.08% (3.5 mL); 0.1% (2.5 mL, 5 mL); 0.125% (4 mL); 0.167% (3 mL); 0.17% (3 mL); 0.2% (2.5 mL); 0.25% (2 mL, 3.5 mL); 0.5% (0.5 mL); 1% (0.5 mL, 0.25 mL, 10 mL, 14 mL, 30 mL)

Isoetharine mesylate: Aerosol, oral: 340 mcg/metered spray

isoflurane (eye soe FLURE ane)

U.S. Brand Names Forane®

Generic Available No

Therapeutic Category General Anesthetic

Use General induction and maintenance of anesthesia (inhalation)

Usual Dosage 1.5% to 3%

Dosage Forms Solution: 100 mL, 125 mL, 250 mL

isoflurophate (eye soe FLURE oh fate)

Synonyms DFP; diisopropyl fluorophosphate; dyflos; fluostigmin

U.S. Brand Names Floropryl® Ophthalmic

Generic Available No

Therapeutic Category Cholinergic Agent

Use Treat primary open-angle glaucoma and conditions that obstruct aqueous outflow and to treat accommodative convergent strabismus

Usual Dosage Adults: Ophthalmic:

Glaucoma: Instill ¼" strip in eye every 8-72 hours

Strabismus: Instill ¼" strip to each eye every night for 2 weeks then reduce to ¼" every other night to once weekly for 2 months

Nursing/Pharmacy Information

Keep tube tightly closed to prevent absorption of moisture and loss of potency

Stability: Protect from moisture, freezing, excessive heat

Dosage Forms Ointment, ophthalmic: 0.025% in polyethylene mineral oil gel (3.5 g)

♦ **Isoket** see isosorbide dinitrate on page 349

♦ **Isollyl® Improved** see butalbital compound and aspirin on page 99

isoniazid (eye soe NYE a zid)

Synonyms INH; isonicotinic acid hydrazide

U.S. Brand Names Laniazid® Syrup

Canadian Brand Names PMS-Isoniazid

Generic Available Yes

Therapeutic Category Antitubercular Agent

Use Treatment of susceptible mycobacterial infection due to *M. tuberculosis* and prophylactically to those individuals exposed to tuberculosis

Usual Dosage Oral, I.M.:

Children: 10-20 mg/kg/day in 1-2 divided doses (maximum: 300 mg total dose)

Prophylaxis: 10 mg/kg/day administered daily (up to 300 mg total dose) for 12 months

Adults: 5 mg/kg/day administered daily (usual dose: 300 mg)

Disseminated disease: 10 mg/kg/day in 1-2 divided doses

Treatment should be continued for 9 months with rifampin or for 6 months with rifampin and pyrazinamide

Prophylaxis: 300 mg/day administered daily for 12 months

American Thoracic Society and CDC currently recommend twice weekly therapy as part of a short-course regimen which follows 1-2 months of daily treatment for uncomplicated pulmonary tuberculosis in compliant patients

Children: 20-40 mg/kg/dose (up to 900 mg) twice weekly

Adults: 15 mg/kg/dose (up to 900 mg) twice weekly

(Continued)

isoniazid *(Continued)*

Dietary Considerations Should be administered 1 hour before or 2 hours after meals on an empty stomach; avoid foods with histamine or tyramine (cheese, broad beans, dry sausage, salami, nonfresh meat, liver pate, soy bean, liquid and powdered protein supplements, wine); increase dietary intake of folate, niacin, magnesium

Nursing/Pharmacy Information

The American Academy of Pediatrics recommends that pyridoxine supplementation (1-2 mg/kg/day) should be administered to malnourished patients, children or adolescents on meat or milk-deficient diets, breast feeding infants, and those predisposed to neuritis to prevent peripheral neuropathy; administration of isoniazid syrup has been associated with diarrhea

Monitor periodic liver function tests; monitoring for prodromal signs of hepatitis

Stability: Protect oral dosage forms from light

Dosage Forms

Syrup (orange flavor): 50 mg/5 mL (473 mL)

Tablet: 50 mg, 100 mg, 300 mg

♦ **isoniazid and rifampin** *see* rifampin and isoniazid *on page 549*

♦ **isoniazid, rifampin, and pyrazinamide** *see* rifampin, isoniazid, and pyrazinamide *on page 550*

♦ **isonicotinic acid hydrazide** *see* isoniazid *on page 347*

♦ **isonipecaine** *see* meperidine *on page 392*

♦ **Isopap®** *see* acetaminophen, isometheptene, and dichloralphenazone *on page 17*

isoproterenol *(eye soe proe TER e nole)*

U.S. Brand Names Arm-a-Med® Isoproterenol; Dey-Dose® Isoproterenol; Isuprel®; Medihaler-Iso®

Generic Available Yes

Therapeutic Category Adrenergic Agonist Agent

Use Asthma or COPD (reversible airway obstruction); ventricular arrhythmias due to A-V nodal block; hemodynamically compromised bradyarrhythmias or atropine-resistant bradyarrhythmias, temporary use in third degree A-V block until pacemaker insertion; low cardiac output or vasoconstrictive shock states

Usual Dosage

Children:

Bronchodilation: Inhalation 1-2 metered doses up to 5 times/day

Nebulization: 0.01 mL/kg; minimum dose: 0.1 mL; maximum dose: 0.5 mL diluted in 2-3 mL normal saline

I.V. infusion: 0.05-2 mcg/kg/minute; rate (mL/hour) = dose (mcg/kg/minute) x weight (kg) x 60 minutes/hour divided by concentration (mcg/mL)

Adults:

Bronchodilation: 1-2 inhalations 4-6 times/day

A-V nodal block: I.V. infusion: 2-20 mcg/minute

Nursing/Pharmacy Information

Instruct patient on how to use inhaler or nebulizer; may be administered undiluted by direct I.V. injection; for continuous infusions, dilute in dextrose or normal saline to a maximum concentration of 64 mcg/mL

Monitor EKG, heart rate, respiratory rate, arterial blood gas, arterial blood pressure, CVP

Stability: Do not use discolored solutions; limit exposure to heat, light or air; stability of parenteral admixture at room temperature (25°C) and at refrigeration temperature (4°C): 24 hours; **incompatible** when mixed with aminophylline, furosemide; **incompatible** with alkaline solutions

Dosage Forms Isoprenaline hydrochloride:

Inhalation:

Aerosol: 0.2% (1:500) (15 mL, 22.5 mL); 0.25% (1:400) (15 mL)

Solution for nebulization: 0.031% (4 mL); 0.062% (4 mL); 0.25% (0.5 mL, 30 mL); 0.5% (0.5 mL, 10 mL, 60 mL); 1% (10 mL)

Injection: 0.2 mg/mL (1:5000) (1 mL, 5 mL, 10 mL)

Tablet, sublingual: 10 mg, 15 mg

isoproterenol and phenylephrine

(eye soe proe TER e nole & fen il EF rin)

Synonyms phenylephrine and isoproterenol

Generic Available No

Therapeutic Category Adrenergic Agonist Agent

Use Treatment of bronchospasm associated with acute and chronic bronchial asthma, bronchitis, pulmonary emphysema, and bronchiectasis

Usual Dosage Daily maintenance: 1-2 inhalations 4-6 times/day, no more than 2 inhalations at any one time or more than 6 in any 1 hour within 24 hours

Dosage Forms Aerosol: Each actuation releases isoproterenol hydrochloride 0.16 mg and phenylephrine bitartrate 0.24 mg (15 mL, 22.5 mL)

- ♦ **Isoptin®** *see* verapamil *on page 646*
- ♦ **Isoptin® SR** *see* verapamil *on page 646*
- ♦ **Isopto® Atropine** *see* atropine *on page 64*
- ♦ **Isopto® Carbachol Ophthalmic** *see* carbachol *on page 111*
- ♦ **Isopto® Carpine Ophthalmic** *see* pilocarpine *on page 493*
- ♦ **Isopto® Cetapred® Ophthalmic** *see* sulfacetamide and prednisolone *on page 585*
- ♦ **Isopto® Frin Ophthalmic Solution** *see* phenylephrine *on page 487*
- ♦ **Isopto® Homatropine Ophthalmic** *see* homatropine *on page 314*
- ♦ **Isopto® Hyoscine** *see* scopolamine *on page 560*
- ♦ **Isopto® P-ES** *(Discontinued) see page 743*
- ♦ **Isopto® Plain Solution [OTC]** *see* artificial tears *on page 59*
- ♦ **Isopto® Tears Solution [OTC]** *see* artificial tears *on page 59*
- ♦ **Isorbid** *see* isosorbide dinitrate *on page 349*
- ♦ **Isordil®** *see* isosorbide dinitrate *on page 349*

isosorbide (eye soe SOR bide)

U.S. Brand Names Ismotic®
Generic Available No
Therapeutic Category Diuretic, Osmotic
Use Short-term emergency treatment of acute angle-closure glaucoma
Usual Dosage Adults: Oral: Initial: 1.5 g/kg; usual range: 1-3 g/kg 2-4 times/day
Nursing/Pharmacy Information
Palatability may be improved if poured over ice and sipped
Monitor for signs of dehydration, blood pressure, renal output, intraocular pressure reduction
Dosage Forms Solution: 45% [450 mg/mL] (220 mL)

isosorbide dinitrate (eye soe SOR bide dye NYE trate)

Synonyms ISD; ISDN
U.S. Brand Names Dilatrate®-SR; Isordil®; Sorbitrate®
Canadian Brand Names Apo-ISDN®; Cedocard-SR®; Coradur®
Mexican Brand Names Isoket; Isorbid
Generic Available Yes
Therapeutic Category Vasodilator
Use Prevention and treatment of angina pectoris; for congestive heart failure; to relieve pain, dysphagia, and spasm in esophageal spasm with GE reflux
Usual Dosage Adults:
Oral: 5-30 mg 4 times/day or 40 mg every 6-12 hours in sustained-released dosage form
Chewable: 5-10 mg every 2-3 hours
Sublingual: 2.5-10 mg every 4-6 hours
Nursing/Pharmacy Information
Do not crush sustained release or sublingual drug product
Monitor blood pressure reduction for maximal effect and orthostatic hypotension
Dosage Forms
Capsule, sustained release: 40 mg
Tablet:
Chewable: 5 mg, 10 mg
Oral: 5 mg, 10 mg, 20 mg, 30 mg
Sublingual: 2.5 mg, 5 mg, 10 mg
Sustained release: 40 mg

isosorbide mononitrate (eye soe SOR bide mon oh NYE trate)

Synonyms ISMN
U.S. Brand Names Imdur™; Ismo®; Monoket®
Mexican Brand Names Elantan; Mono Mack
Generic Available Yes
Therapeutic Category Vasodilator
Use Long-acting metabolite of the vasodilator isosorbide dinitrate used for the prophylactic treatment of angina pectoris
Usual Dosage Adults: Oral:
Regular tablet: 20 mg twice daily separated by 7 hours
(Continued)

isosorbide mononitrate *(Continued)*

Extended-release tablet: 30 mg ($\frac{1}{2}$ of 60 mg tablet) or 60 mg (administered as a single tablet) once daily; after several days the dosage may be increased to 120 mg (administered as two 60 mg tablets) once daily; the daily dose should be administered in the morning upon arising

Dietary Considerations Alcohol, in particular, has been found to exhibit additive effects of this variety

Nursing/Pharmacy Information

Do not crush; monitor for orthostasis; 8- to 12-hour nitrate-free interval is needed each day to prevent tolerance; do not administer around-the-clock

Stability: Tablets should be stored in a tight container at room temperature of 15°C to 30°C (59°F to 86°F)

Dosage Forms

Tablet: 10 mg, 20 mg

Ismo®, Monoket®: 10 mg, 20 mg

Tablet, extended release: 60 mg

Imdur™: 30 mg, 60 mg, 120 mg

♦ **Isosource®** *see enteral nutritional products on page 233*

isotretinoin *(eye soe TRET i noyn)*

Synonyms 13-*cis*-retinoic acid

U.S. Brand Names Accutane®

Canadian Brand Names Isotrex®

Generic Available No

Therapeutic Category Retinoic Acid Derivative

Use Treatment of severe recalcitrant cystic and/or conglobate acne unresponsive to conventional therapy

Investigational use: Treatment of children with metastatic neuroblastoma or leukemia that does not respond to conventional therapy

Usual Dosage Oral:

Children: Maintenance therapy for neuroblastoma: 100-250 mg/m²/day in 2 divided doses has been used investigationally

Children and Adults: 0.5-2 mg/kg/day in 2 divided doses for 15-20 weeks

Dietary Considerations Increased isotretinoin bioavailability when administered with food or milk

Nursing/Pharmacy Information

Capsules can be swallowed or chewed and swallowed; the capsule may be opened with a large needle and the contents placed on apple sauce or ice cream for patients unable to swallow the capsule

Monitor CBC with differential and platelet count, baseline sedimentation rate, serum triglycerides, liver enzymes

Stability: Store at room temperature and protect from light

Dosage Forms Capsule: 10 mg, 20 mg, 40 mg

♦ **Isotrex®** *see isotretinoin on page 350*

♦ **Isovex®** *(Discontinued) see page 743*

♦ **Isovue®** *see radiological/contrast media (non-ionic) on page 540*

♦ **Isox** *see itraconazole on page 351*

isoxsuprine *(eye SOKS syoo preen)*

U.S. Brand Names Vasodilan®

Generic Available Yes

Therapeutic Category Vasodilator

Use Treatment of peripheral vascular diseases, such as arteriosclerosis obliterans and Raynaud's disease

Usual Dosage Adults: Oral: 10-20 mg 3-4 times/day

Nursing/Pharmacy Information May cause skin rash; discontinue use if rash occurs; arise slowly from prolonged sitting or lying position

Dosage Forms Tablet, as hydrochloride: 10 mg, 20 mg

isradipine *(iz RA di peen)*

U.S. Brand Names DynaCirc®

Mexican Brand Names DynaCirc SRO®

Generic Available No

Therapeutic Category Calcium Channel Blocker

Use Management of hypertension, alone or concurrently with thiazide-type diuretics

Usual Dosage Adults: Oral: Initial: 2.5 mg twice daily, if satisfactory response does not occur after 2-4 weeks the dose may be adjusted in increments of 5 mg/day at 2- to 4-week intervals up to a maximum of 20 mg/day

Nursing/Pharmacy Information Do not crush sustained release capsules

Dosage Forms Capsule: 2.5 mg, 5 mg

- ♦ **I-Sulfacet®** *see* sulfacetamide *on page 584*
- ♦ **Isuprel®** *see* isoproterenol *on page 348*
- ♦ **Isuprel® Glossets®** *(Discontinued) see page 743*
- ♦ **Italnik®** *see* ciprofloxacin *on page 151*
- ♦ **Itch-X® [OTC]** *see* pramoxine *on page 512*

itraconazole (i tra KOE na zole)

U.S. Brand Names Sporanox®

Mexican Brand Names Carexan; Isox; Itranax

Generic Available No

Therapeutic Category Antifungal Agent

Use Treatment of systemic fungal infections in immunocompromised and nonimmunocompromised patients including the treatment of susceptible blastomycosis, histoplasmosis, and aspergillosis in patients who do not respond to or cannot tolerate amphotericin B; it also has activity against *Cryptococcus*, *Coccidioides*, and sporotrichosis species; has also been used for prophylaxis against aspergillosis infection

Usual Dosage Adults: Oral: 200 mg once daily, if no obvious improvement or there is evidence of progressive fungal disease, increase the dose in 100 mg increments to a maximum of 400 mg/day; doses >200 mg/day are administered in 2 divided doses

Life-threatening: Loading dose: 200 mg administered 3 times/day (600 mg/day) should be administered for the first 3 days

Dietary Considerations Presence of food increases bioavailability of itraconazole

Nursing/Pharmacy Information Do not administer with antacids; doses >200 mg/day are administered in 2 divided doses

Dosage Forms

Capsule: 100 mg

Solution, oral: 100 mg/10 mL (150 mL)

- ♦ **Itranax** *see* itraconazole *on page 351*
- ♦ **I-Tropine®** *see* atropine *on page 64*

ivermectin (eye ver MEK tin)

U.S. Brand Names Stromectol®

Generic Available No

Therapeutic Category Antibiotic, Miscellaneous

Use Treatment of the following infections: Strongyloidiasis of the intestinal tract due the nematode parasite *Strongyloides stercoralis*. Onchocerciasis due to the nematode parasite *Onchocerca volvulus*. Note: Ivermectin is ineffective against adult *Onchocerca volvulus* parasites because they reside in subcutaneous nodules which are infrequently palpable. Surgical excision of these nodules may be considered in the management of patients with onchocerciasis.

Usual Dosage Oral:

Children >5 years: 150 mcg/kg as a single dose once every 12 months

Adults: 150 mcg/kg as a single dose; may be repeated every 6-12 **months**

Dosage Forms Tablet: 6 mg

- ♦ **IVIG** *see* immune globulin, intravenous *on page 336*
- ♦ **IvyBlock®** *see* bentoquatam *on page 77*
- ♦ **Jaa Amp®** *see* ampicillin *on page 46*
- ♦ **Jaa-Prednisone®** *see* prednisone *on page 515*
- ♦ **Janimine®** *see* imipramine *on page 334*

Japanese encephalitis virus vaccine, inactivated

(jap a NEESE en sef a LYE tis VYE rus vak SEEN, in ak ti VAY ted)

U.S. Brand Names JE-VAX®

Generic Available No

Therapeutic Category Vaccine, Inactivated Virus

Use Active immunization against Japanese encephalitis for persons spending a month or longer in endemic areas, especially if travel will include rural areas

(Continued)

Japanese encephalitis virus vaccine, inactivated
(Continued)

Usual Dosage S.C. (administered on days 0, 7, and 30):

Children 1-3 years: 3 doses of 0.5 mL; booster doses of 0.5 mL may administer 2 years after primary immunization series

Children >3 years and Adults: 3 doses of 1 mL; booster doses of 1 mL may be administered 2 years after primary immunization series

Nursing/Pharmacy Information

Adverse reactions may occur shortly after vaccination or up to 17 days (usually within 10 days) after vaccination

Stability: Refrigerate, discard 8 hours after reconstitution

Dosage Forms Powder for injection, lyophilized: 1 mL, 10 mL

- ♦ **Jenamicin®** *see* gentamicin *on page 290*
- ♦ **Jenest-28™** *see* ethinyl estradiol and norethindrone *on page 250*
- ♦ **JE-VAX®** *see* Japanese encephalitis virus vaccine, inactivated *on page 351*
- ♦ **Junior Strength Motrin® [OTC]** *see* ibuprofen *on page 332*
- ♦ **Just Tears® Solution [OTC]** *see* artificial tears *on page 59*
- ♦ **K+ 10®** *see* potassium chloride *on page 506*
- ♦ **Kabikinase®** *see* streptokinase *on page 580*
- ♦ **Kalcinate®** *see* calcium gluconate *on page 106*

kanamycin (kan a MYE sin)
U.S. Brand Names Kantrex®
Mexican Brand Names Randikan
Generic Available Yes
Therapeutic Category Aminoglycoside (Antibiotic)
Use

Oral: Preoperative bowel preparation in the prophylaxis of infections and adjunctive treatment of hepatic coma (oral kanamycin is not indicated in the treatment of systemic infections)

Parenteral: Initial therapy of severe infections where the strain is thought to be susceptible in patients allergic to other antibiotics, or in mixed staphylococcal or gram-negative infections

Usual Dosage

Children: Infections: I.M., I.V.: 15 mg/kg/day in divided doses every 8-12 hours

Adults:

Infections: I.M., I.V.: 15 mg/kg/day in divided doses every 8-12 hours

Preoperative intestinal antisepsis: Oral: 1 g every 4-6 hours for 36-72 hours

Nursing/Pharmacy Information

Aminoglycoside levels in blood taken from Silastic® central catheters can sometime give falsely high readings. Administer around-the-clock rather than 4 times/day, 3 times/day, etc, (ie, 12-6-12-6, not 9-1-5-9) to promote less variation in peak and trough serum levels; modify dosage in patients with renal impairment; I.M. doses should be administered in a large muscle mass (ie, gluteus maximus).

Monitor serum creatinine/creatine clearance

Stability: Darkening of vials does not indicate loss of potency

Dosage Forms Kanamycin sulfate:

Capsule: 500 mg

Injection:

Pediatrics: 75 mg (2 mL)

Adults: 500 mg (2 mL); 1 g (3 mL)

- ♦ **Kantrex®** *see* kanamycin *on page 352*
- ♦ **Kaochlor®** *see* potassium chloride *on page 506*
- ♦ **Kaochlor-Eff®** *see* potassium bicarbonate, potassium chloride, and potassium citrate *on page 506*
- ♦ **Kaochlor® SF** *see* potassium chloride *on page 506*
- ♦ **Kaodene® [OTC]** *see* kaolin and pectin *on page 352*

kaolin and pectin (KAY oh lin & PEK tin)
Synonyms pectin and kaolin
U.S. Brand Names Kaodene® [OTC]; Kao-Spen® [OTC]; Kapectolin® [OTC]
Canadian Brand Names Donnagel®-MB
Generic Available Yes
Therapeutic Category Antidiarrheal
Use Treatment of uncomplicated diarrhea

Usual Dosage Oral:
  Children:
    <6 years: Do not use
    6-12 years: 30-60 mL after each loose stool
  Adults: 60-120 mL after each loose stool
Nursing/Pharmacy Information Shake well
Dosage Forms Suspension, oral: Kaolin 975 mg and pectin 22 mg per 5 mL

kaolin and pectin with opium
  (KAY oh lin & PEK tin with OH pee um)
Synonyms pectin with opium and kaolin
U.S. Brand Names Parepectolin®
Generic Available Yes
Therapeutic Category Antidiarrheal
Controlled Substance C-V
Use Symptomatic relief of diarrhea
Usual Dosage Oral:
  Children:
    3-6 years: 7.5 mL with each loose bowel movement, not to exceed 30 mL in
      12 hours
    6-12 years: 5-10 mL with each loose bowel movement, not to exceed 40 mL
      in 12 hours
  Children >12 years and Adults: 15-30 mL with each loose bowel movement,
    not to exceed 120 mL in 12 hours
Nursing/Pharmacy Information
  Shake well
  Monitor for signs of opium (narcotic) action
Dosage Forms Suspension, oral: Kaolin 5.5 g, pectin 162 mg, and opium 15
  mg per 30 mL [3.7 mL paregoric] (240 mL)

- ◆ **Kenalog® Injection** *see* triamcinolone (systemic) *on page 624*
- ◆ **Kenalog® in Orabase®** *see* triamcinolone (topical) *on page 624*
- ◆ **Kenalog® Topical** *see* triamcinolone (topical) *on page 624*
- ◆ **Kenamil** *see* zidovudine *on page 658*
- ◆ **Kenaprol** *see* metoprolol *on page 410*
- ◆ **Kenoket** *see* clonazepam *on page 159*
- ◆ **Kenolan** *see* captopril *on page 110*
- ◆ **Kenonel® Topical** *see* triamcinolone (topical) *on page 624*
- ◆ **Kenopril** *see* enalapril *on page 230*
- ◆ **Kentadin** *see* pentoxifylline *on page 480*
- ◆ **Kenzoflex** *see* ciprofloxacin *on page 151*
- ◆ **Keralyt® Gel** *see* salicylic acid and propylene glycol *on page 558*
- ◆ **Kerlone® Oral** *see* betaxolol *on page 86*
- ◆ **Kestrin® Injection** *(Discontinued)* *see page 743*
- ◆ **Kestrone®** *see* estrone *on page 246*
- ◆ **Ketalar®** *see* ketamine *on page 354*

ketamine (KEET a meen)

U.S. Brand Names Ketalar®
Generic Available No
Therapeutic Category General Anesthetic
Controlled Substance C-III
Use Anesthesia, short surgical procedures, dressing changes
Usual Dosage
Children:
I.M.: 3-7 mg/kg
I.V.: Range: 0.5-2 mg/kg, use smaller doses (0.5-1 mg/kg) for sedation for
minor procedures; usual induction dosage: 1-2 mg/kg
Adults:
I.M.: 3-8 mg/kg
I.V.: Range: 1-4.5 mg/kg; usual induction dosage: 1-2 mg/kg
Children and Adults: Maintenance: Supplemental doses of $^1/_3$ to $^1/_2$ of initial
dose
Nursing/Pharmacy Information
Parenteral: I.V.: Do not exceed 0.5 mg/kg/minute or administer faster than 60
seconds; do not exceed final concentration of 2 mg/mL
Monitor cardiovascular effects, heart rate, blood pressure, respiratory rate,
transcutaneous O_2 saturation
Stability: Do not mix with barbiturates or diazepam → precipitation may occur
Dosage Forms Injection, as hydrochloride: 10 mg/mL (20 mL, 25 mL, 50 mL);
50 mg/mL (10 mL); 100 mg/mL (5 mL)

ketoconazole (kee toe KOE na zole)

U.S. Brand Names Nizoral®
Mexican Brand Names Akorazol; Conazol; Tiniazol
Generic Available Yes: Tablet
Therapeutic Category Antifungal Agent
Use Treatment of susceptible fungal infections, including candidiasis, oral
thrush, blastomycosis, histoplasmosis, coccidioidomycosis, paracoccidioido-
mycosis, chronic mucocutaneous candidiasis, as well as certain recalcitrant
cutaneous dermatophytoses; used topically for treatment of tinea corporis,
tinea cruris, tinea versicolor, and cutaneous candidiasis; shampoo is used for
dandruff
Usual Dosage
Children: Oral: 5-10 mg/kg/day divided every 12-24 hours until lesions clear
Adults:
Oral: 200-400 mg/day as a single daily dose
Topical: Rub gently into the affected area once daily to twice daily for two
weeks
Dietary Considerations May be administered with food or milk to decrease GI
adverse effects; antacids decrease absorption
Nursing/Pharmacy Information
Administer 2 hours prior to antacids or H_2 receptor antagonists to prevent
decreased ketoconazole absorption
Monitor liver function tests
Dosage Forms
Cream: 2% (15 g, 30 g, 60 g)
Shampoo: 2% (120 mL)
Tablet: 200 mg

ketoprofen (kee toe PROE fen)

U.S. Brand Names Actron® [OTC]; Orudis®; Orudis® KT [OTC]; Oruvail®

Canadian Brand Names Apo-Keto-E®; Novo-Keto-EC; Nu-Ketoprofen; Nu-Ketoprofen-E; PMS-Ketoprofen; Rhodis®; Rhodis-EC®

Mexican Brand Names Keduril®; K-Profen®; Profenid®; Profenid® 200; Profenid®-IM

Generic Available Yes

Therapeutic Category Analgesic, Non-narcotic; Nonsteroidal Anti-inflammatory Drug (NSAID)

Use Acute or long-term treatment of rheumatoid arthritis and osteoarthritis; primary dysmenorrhea; mild to moderate pain

Usual Dosage Oral:

Children 3 months to 14 years: Fever: 0.5-1 mg/kg

Children >12 years and Adults:

Rheumatoid arthritis or osteoarthritis: 50-75 mg 3-4 times/day up to a maximum of 300 mg/day

Mild to moderate pain: 25-50 mg every 6-8 hours up to a maximum of 300 mg/day

Dietary Considerations Ideally, should be administered 30 minutes before meals or 2 hours after, with full glass of water

Nursing/Pharmacy Information Dose must be lowest recommended in renal insufficiency and hypoalbuminemia. There are no clinical guidelines to predict which NSAID will give response in a particular patient. Trials with each must be initiated until response determined. Consider dose, patient convenience, and cost.

Dosage Forms

Capsule (Orudis®): 25 mg, 50 mg, 75 mg

Actron®, Orudis® KT [OTC]: 12.5 mg

Capsule, extended release: 100 mg, 150 mg, 200 mg

Oruvail®: 100 mg, 200 mg

ketorolac tromethamine (KEE toe role ak troe METH a meen)

U.S. Brand Names Acular® Ophthalmic; Toradol®

Mexican Brand Names Alidol; Dolac Inyectable; Dolac Oral

Generic Available Yes (tablet)

Therapeutic Category Analgesic, Non-narcotic; Nonsteroidal Anti-inflammatory Drug (NSAID)

Use

Oral, I.M., I.V.,: Short-term (≤5 days) management of moderate to severe pain, including postoperative pain, visceral pain associated with cancer, pain associated with trauma, acute renal colic

Ophthalmic: Ocular itch associated with seasonal allergic conjunctivitis

Usual Dosage Adults (pain relief usually begins within 10 minutes with parenteral forms):

Oral: 10 mg every 4-6 hours as needed for a maximum of 40 mg/day; on day of transition from I.M. to oral: maximum oral dose: 40 mg (or 120 mg combined oral and I.M.); maximum 5 days administration

I.M.: Initial: 30-60 mg, then 15-30 mg every 6 hours as needed for up to 5 days maximum; maximum dose in the first 24 hours: 150 mg with 120 mg/24 hours for up to 5 days total

I.V.: Initial: 30 mg, then 15-30 mg every 6 hours as needed for up to 5 days maximum; maximum daily dose: 120 mg for up to 5 days total

Ophthalmic: Instill 1 drop in eye(s) 4 times/day

Dietary Considerations May be administered with food to decrease GI distress; high-fat meals may delay time to peak (by ~1 hour) and decrease peak concentrations

Potassium: Hyperkalemia has been reported; the elderly and those with renal insufficiency are at greatest risk; monitor potassium serum concentration in those at greatest risk; avoid salt substitutes

Sodium: Hyponatremia from sodium retention; suspect secondary to suppression of renal prostaglandin; monitor serum concentration and fluid status; may need to restrict fluid

Nursing/Pharmacy Information

Monitor for excessive sedation, serum creatinine, bleeding parameters, and pain relief

Stability: Protect from light

Dosage Forms

Injection: 15 mg/mL (1 mL); 30 mg/mL (1 mL, 2 mL)

Solution, ophthalmic: 0.5% (5 mL)

Tablet: 10 mg

ketotifen *New Drug* (kee toe TYE fen)
U.S. Brand Names Zaditor™
Generic Available No
Therapeutic Category Antihistamine, H₁ Blocker, Ophthalmic
Use Temporary prevention of eye itching due to allergic conjunctivitis
Usual Dosage Adults: Ophthalmic: Instill 1 drop in the affected eye(s) every 8-12 hours
Dosage Forms Solution, ophthalmic: 0.025% (5 mL)

- **K-Profen®** *see* ketoprofen *on page 355*
- **Kristalose®** *see* lactulose *on page 359*
- **K-Tab®** *see* potassium chloride *on page 506*
- **Ku-Zyme® HP** *see* pancrelipase *on page 467*
- **K-Vescent®** *see* potassium bicarbonate and potassium citrate, effervescent *on page 506*
- **Kwelcof®** *see* hydrocodone and guaifenesin *on page 320*
- **Kwellada™** *see* lindane *on page 370*
- **Kwell® *(Discontinued)*** *see page 743*
- **Kytril™** *see* granisetron *on page 297*
- **L-3-hydroxytyrosine** *see* levodopa *on page 365*
- **LA-12®** *see* hydroxocobalamin *on page 326*

labetalol (la BET a lole)

Synonyms ibidomide
U.S. Brand Names Normodyne®; Trandate®
Mexican Brand Names Midotens
Generic Available Yes
Therapeutic Category Alpha-/Beta- Adrenergic Blocker
Use Treatment of mild to severe hypertension; I.V. for hypertensive emergencies
Usual Dosage

Children: Limited information regarding labetalol use in pediatric patients is currently available in literature. Some centers recommend initial oral doses of 4 mg/kg/day in 2 divided doses. Reported oral doses have started at 3 mg/kg/day and 20 mg/kg/day and have increased up to 40 mg/kg/day.

I.V., intermittent bolus doses of 0.3-1 mg/kg/dose have been reported

For treatment of pediatric hypertensive emergencies, initial continuous infusions of 0.4-1 mg/kg/hour with a maximum of 3 mg/kg/hour have been used.

Due to limited documentation of its use, labetalol should be initiated cautiously in pediatric patients with careful dosage adjustment and blood pressure monitoring

Adults:
Oral: Initial: 100 mg twice daily, may increase as needed every 2-3 days by 100 mg until desired response is obtained; usual dose: 200-400 mg twice daily; not to exceed 2.4 g/day
I.V.: 20 mg or 1-2 mg/kg whichever is lower, IVP over 2 minutes, may administer 40-80 mg at 10-minute intervals, up to 300 mg total dose
I.V. infusion: Initial: 2 mg/minute; titrate to response

Dietary Considerations Avoid natural licorice (causes sodium and water retention and increases potassium loss); food may increase bioavailability
Nursing/Pharmacy Information

Instruct patient regarding compliance; do **not** abruptly withdraw medication in patients with ischemic heart disease; IVP: Administer over 2-3 minutes
Monitor blood pressure, standing and sitting/supine; pulse
Stability: Stable in D_5W, saline for 24 hours; **incompatible** with $NaHCO_3$; use only solutions that are clear or slightly yellow; may cause a precipitate if exposed to alkaline admixture; protect from light; **incompatible** with alkaline solutions
Stability of parenteral admixture at room temperature (25°C) and at refrigeration temperature (4°C): 24 hours

Dosage Forms Labetalol hydrochloride:
Injection: 5 mg/mL (20 mL, 40 mL, 60 mL)
Tablet: 100 mg, 200 mg, 300 mg

- **Lac-Hydrin®** *see* lactic acid with ammonium hydroxide *on page 358*
- **Lacril® Ophthalmic Solution [OTC]** *see* artificial tears *on page 59*
- **Lacrisert®** *see* hydroxypropyl cellulose *on page 327*
- **LactAid® [OTC]** *see* lactase *on page 357*

lactase (LAK tase)

U.S. Brand Names Dairy Ease® [OTC]; LactAid® [OTC]; Lactrase® [OTC]
Generic Available No
Therapeutic Category Nutritional Supplement
Use Help digest lactose in milk for patients with lactose intolerance
Usual Dosage Oral:

Capsule: 1-2 capsules administered with milk or meal; pretreat milk with 1-2 capsules per quart of milk
(Continued)

lactase *(Continued)*

Liquid: 5-15 drops per quart of milk
Tablet: 1-3 tablets with meals
Dietary Considerations May be administered with meals
Dosage Forms
Caplet: 3000 FCC lactase units
Capsule: 250 mg
Liquid: 1250 neutral lactase units/5 drops
Tablet, chewable: 3300 FCC lactase units

♦ **Lacteol® Fort** *see* Lactobacillus *on page 358*
♦ **lactic acid and salicylic acid** *see* salicylic acid and lactic acid *on page 557*

lactic acid and sodium-PCA

(LAK tik AS id & SOW dee um-pee see aye)
Synonyms sodium-pca and lactic acid
U.S. Brand Names LactiCare® [OTC]
Generic Available No
Therapeutic Category Topical Skin Product
Use Lubricate and moisturize the skin counteracting dryness and itching
Usual Dosage Topical: Apply as needed
Dosage Forms Lotion, topical: Lactic acid 5% and sodium-PCA 2.5% (240 mL)

lactic acid with ammonium hydroxide

(LAK tik AS id with a MOE nee um hye DROKS ide)
Synonyms ammonium lactate
U.S. Brand Names Lac-Hydrin®
Generic Available No
Therapeutic Category Topical Skin Product
Use Treatment of moderate to severe xerosis and ichthyosis vulgaris
Usual Dosage Topical: Shake well; apply to affected areas, use twice daily, rub in well
Dosage Forms Lotion: Lactic acid 12% with ammonium hydroxide (150 mL)

♦ **LactiCare® [OTC]** *see* lactic acid and sodium-PCA *on page 358*
♦ **LactiCare-HC® Topical** *see* hydrocortisone (topical) *on page 324*
♦ **Lactinex® [OTC]** *see* Lactobacillus *on page 358*

Lactobacillus (lak toe ba SIL us)

Synonyms *Lactobacillus acidophilus*; *Lactobacillus acidophilus* and *Lactobacillus bulgaricus*
U.S. Brand Names Bacid® [OTC]; Lactinex® [OTC]; More-Dophilus® [OTC]
Canadian Brand Names Fermalac®
Mexican Brand Names Lacteol® Fort; Sinuberase®
Generic Available No
Therapeutic Category Gastrointestinal Agent, Miscellaneous
Use Uncomplicated diarrhea particularly that caused by antibiotic therapy; reestablish normal physiologic and bacterial flora of the intestinal tract
Usual Dosage Children >3 years and Adults: Oral:
Capsules: 2 capsules 2-4 times/day
Granules: 1 packet added to or taken with cereal, food, milk, fruit juice, or water, 3-4 times/day
Powder: 1/4-1 teaspoonful 1-3 times/daily with liquid
Tablet, chewable: 4 tablets 3-4 times/day; may follow each dose with a small amount of milk, fruit juice, or water
Dietary Considerations Granules or contents of capsules may be added to or administered with cereal, food, milk, fruit juice, or water
Nursing/Pharmacy Information Stability: Store in refrigerator
Dosage Forms
Capsule:
Bacid®: *Lactobacillus acidophilus* cultured strain ≥500 million viable (50s, 100s)
Pro-Bionate®: *Lactobacillus acidophilus* strain NAS 2 billion units/g
Granules (Lactinex®): *Lactobacillus acidophilus* and *Lactobacillus bulgaricus* mixed culture (1 g/packet-12s)
Powder:
MoreDophilus®: Acidophilus-carrot derivative 4 billion units/g
Pro-Bionate®: *Lactobacillus acidophilus* strain NAS 2 billion units/g
Tablet, chewable (Lactinex®): *Lactobacillus acidophilus* and *Lactobacillus bulgaricus* mixed culture (50s)

- **Lactobacillus acidophilus** *see* Lactobacillus *on page 358*
- **Lactobacillus acidophilus** and **Lactobacillus bulgaricus** *see* Lactobacillus *on page 358*
- **lactoflavin** *see* riboflavin *on page 548*
- **Lactrase® [OTC]** *see* lactase *on page 357*
- **Lactulax** *see* lactulose *on page 359*

lactulose (LAK tyoo lose)

U.S. Brand Names Cephulac®; Cholac®; Chronulac®; Constilac®; Constulose®; Duphalac®; Enulose®; Evalose®; Heptalac®; Kristalose®; Lactulose PSE®

Canadian Brand Names Acilac; Comalose-R; Gen-Lac; Lactulax; Laxilose; PMS-Lactulose

Generic Available Yes

Therapeutic Category Ammonium Detoxicant; Laxative

Use Adjunct in the prevention and treatment of portal-systemic encephalopathy (PSE); treatment of chronic constipation

Usual Dosage Oral:

Infants: 2.5-10 mL/day divided 3-4 times/day

Children: 40-90 mL/day divided 3-4 times/day

Adults:

Acute episodes of portal systemic encephalopathy: 30-45 mL at 1- to 2-hour intervals until laxative effect observed

Chronic therapy: 30-45 mL/dose 3-4 times/day; titrate dose to produce 2-3 soft stools per day

Rectal: 300 mL diluted with 700 mL of water or normal saline, and administered via a rectal balloon catheter and retained for 30-60 minutes; may administer every 4-6 hours

Dietary Considerations Contraindicated in patients on galactose-restricted diet; may be mixed with fruit juice, milk, water, or citrus-flavored carbonated beverages

Nursing/Pharmacy Information

Dilute lactulose in water, usually 60-120 mL, prior to administering through a gastric or feeding tube; monitor serum ammonia in hepatic disease

Monitor blood pressure, standing/supine; serum potassium, bicarbonate

Stability: Keep solution at room temperature to reduce viscosity; discard solution if cloudy or very dark

Dosage Forms Syrup: 10 g/15 mL (15 mL, 30 mL, 237 mL, 473 mL, 946 mL, 1890 mL)

- **Lactulose PSE®** *see* lactulose *on page 359*
- **ladakamycin** *see* azacitidine *on page 67*
- **Ladogal** *see* danazol *on page 181*
- **L-AmB** *see* amphotericin B liposomal *on page 46*
- **Lamictal®** *see* lamotrigine *on page 360*
- **Lamisil® Cream** *see* terbinafine, topical *on page 596*
- **Lamisil® Oral** *see* terbinafine, oral *on page 596*

lamivudine (la MI vyoo deen)

Synonyms 3TC

U.S. Brand Names Epivir®; Epivir®-HBV™

Canadian Brand Names 3TC®

Generic Available No

Therapeutic Category Antiviral Agent

Use

Epivir®: In combination with zidovudine for treatment of HIV infection when therapy is warranted based on clinical and/or immunological evidence of disease progression

Epivir®-HBV™: Treatment of chronic hepatitis B associated with evidence of hepatitis B viral replication and active liver inflammation

Usual Dosage Oral:

Hepatitis B virus (HBV): 100 mg once daily

HIV:

Adolescents 12-16 years and Adults: 150 mg twice daily with zidovudine

Adults <50 kg: 2 mg/kg twice daily with zidovudine

Dosage Forms

Solution, oral: 10 mg/mL (240 mL)

Tablet: 150 mg

lamotrigine (la MOE tri jeen)
Synonyms LTG
U.S. Brand Names Lamictal®
Generic Available No
Therapeutic Category Anticonvulsant
Use Adjunctive treatment of partial seizures, with or without secondary generalized seizures; investigations for absence, generalized tonic-clonic, atypical absence, myoclonic seizures, and Lennox-Gastaut syndrome are in progress
Usual Dosage Oral:
Initial dose: 50-100 mg/day then titrate to daily maintenance dose of 100-400 mg/day in 1-2 divided daily doses
With concomitant valproic acid therapy: Start initial dose at 25 mg/day then titrate to maintenance dose of 50-200 mg/day in 1-2 divided daily doses
Dietary Considerations Absorption is not affected by food; may cause GI upset; administer without regard to meals
Nursing/Pharmacy Information Low water solubility
Dosage Forms Tablet: 25 mg, 100 mg, 150 mg, 200 mg

- ♦ **Lampicin** *see* ampicillin *on page 46*
- ♦ **Lamprene®** *see* clofazimine *on page 158*
- ♦ **Lamprene® 100 mg (Discontinued)** *see page 743*
- ♦ **Lanacane® [OTC]** *see* benzocaine *on page 79*
- ♦ **Lanacort® Topical [OTC]** *see* hydrocortisone (topical) *on page 324*
- ♦ **Lanaphilic® Topical [OTC]** *see* urea *on page 638*
- ♦ **Lanexat®** *see* flumazenil *on page 272*
- ♦ **Laniazid® Syrup** *see* isoniazid *on page 347*
- ♦ **Laniazid® Tablet (Discontinued)** *see page 743*

lanolin, cetyl alcohol, glycerin, and petrolatum
(LAN oh lin, SEE til AL koe hol, GLIS er in, & pe troe LAY tum)
U.S. Brand Names Lubriderm® [OTC]
Generic Available Yes
Therapeutic Category Topical Skin Product
Use Treatment of dry skin
Usual Dosage Topical: Apply to skin as necessary
Nursing/Pharmacy Information For external use only; if irritation develops, discontinue use and consult a physician
Dosage Forms Lotion: 480 mL

- ♦ **Lanorinal®** *see* butalbital compound and aspirin *on page 99*
- ♦ **Lanoxicaps®** *see* digoxin *on page 203*
- ♦ **Lanoxin®** *see* digoxin *on page 203*

lansoprazole (lan SOE pra zole)
U.S. Brand Names Prevacid®
Generic Available No
Therapeutic Category Gastric Acid Secretion Inhibitor
Use Short-term treatment (up to 4 weeks) for healing and symptom relief of active duodenal ulcers (should not be used for maintenance therapy of duodenal ulcers); up to 8 weeks of treatment for all grades of erosive esophagitis (8 additional weeks can be given for incompletely healed esophageal erosions or for recurrence); and long-term treatment of pathological hypersecretory conditions, including Zollinger-Ellison syndrome
Usual Dosage
Duodenal or gastric ulcer:
Treatment: 15 mg once daily for 4 weeks
Maintenance (healed): 15 mg once daily
Erosive esophagitis:
Treatment: 30 mg once daily for up to 8 weeks; may give for additional 8 weeks for patients who do not heal with the first 8 weeks; if recurrence or erosive esophagitis, consider an additional 8-week course
Maintenance (healing): 15 mg once daily
Hypersecretory conditions: 30-180 mg once daily, titrated to reduce acid secretion to <10 mEq/hour (5 mEq/hour in patients with prior gastric surgery)
Dietary Considerations Administer before eating
Dosage Forms Capsule, delayed release: 15 mg, 30 mg

- ♦ **Lanvis®** *see* thioguanine *on page 607*
- ♦ **Largactil®** *see* chlorpromazine *on page 144*
- ♦ **Lariam®** *see* mefloquine *on page 390*

- **Larodopa®** *see* levodopa *on page 365*
- **Lasan® HP-1 Topical** *(Discontinued) see page 743*
- **Lasan® Topical** *(Discontinued) see page 743*
- **Lasix®** *see* furosemide *on page 285*
- **Lasix® Special** *see* furosemide *on page 285*
- **Lassar's zinc paste** *see* zinc oxide *on page 660*
- **Lastet** *see* etoposide *on page 255*

latanoprost (la TAN oh prost)

U.S. Brand Names Xalatan®
Generic Available No
Therapeutic Category Prostaglandin
Use Prostaglandin analog to reduce intraocular pressure that occurs in patients with glaucoma who cannot tolerate or have not responded to any other available treatments
Usual Dosage Ophthalmic:
   Children: Not recommended
   Adults: 1 drop in affected eye(s) once daily in the evening
Dosage Forms Solution, ophthalmic: 0.005% (2.5 mL)

- **Latotryd®** *see* erythromycin (systemic) *on page 240*
- ***Latrodectus mactans* antivenin** *see* antivenin (*Latrodectus mactans*) *on page 54*
- **Lauricin** *see* erythromycin (systemic) *on page 240*
- **Lavacol® [OTC]** *see* alcohol, ethyl *on page 26*
- **Laxilose** *see* lactulose *on page 359*
- **l-bunolol** *see* levobunolol *on page 364*
- **l-carnitine** *see* levocarnitine *on page 365*
- **LCD** *see* coal tar *on page 162*
- **LCR** *see* vincristine *on page 648*
- **l-deprenyl** *see* selegiline *on page 562*
- **l-dopa** *see* levodopa *on page 365*
- **Lectopam®** *see* bromazepam *(Canada only) on page 93*
- **Ledercillin VK®** *(Discontinued) see page 743*
- **Ledercort** *see* triamcinolone (systemic) *on page 624*
- **Ledermicina** *see* demeclocycline *on page 185*
- **Lederpax** *see* erythromycin (systemic) *on page 240*
- **Lederplex® [OTC]** *see* vitamin B complex *on page 651*
- **Ledertrexate** *see* methotrexate *on page 402*
- **Ledoxina** *see* cyclophosphamide *on page 175*

leflunomide (le FLU no mide)

U.S. Brand Names Arava™
Generic Available No
Therapeutic Category Anti-inflammatory Agent
Use Treatment of active rheumatoid arthritis to reduce signs and symptoms and to retard structural damage as evidenced by X-ray erosions and joint space narrowing
Usual Dosage Oral:
   Adults: Initial: 100 mg/day for 3 days, followed by 20 mg/day; dosage may be decreased to 10 mg/day in patients who have difficulty tolerating the 20 mg dose. Due to the long half-life of the active metabolite, plasma levels may require a prolonged period to decline after dosage reduction.

   Guidelines for dosage adjustment or discontinuation based on the severity and persistence of ALT elevation have been developed. For ALT elevations >2 times the upper limit of normal, dosage reduction to 10 mg/day may allow continued administration. Cholestyramine 8 g 3 times/day for 1-3 days may be administered to decrease plasma levels. If elevations >2 times but less than or equal to 3 times the upper limit of normal persist, liver biopsy is recommended. If elevations >3 times the upper limit of normal persist despite cholestyramine administration and dosage reduction, leflunomide should be discontinued and drug elimination should be enhanced with additional cholestyramine as indicated.

   Elderly: Although hepatic function may decline with age, no specific dosage adjustment is recommended; patients should be monitored closely for adverse effects which may require dosage adjustment
Dosage Forms Tablet: 10 mg, 20 mg, 100 mg

- **Lemblastine** *see* vinblastine *on page 648*

- **Lenoltec® No.1, 2, 3, 4** *see* acetaminophen and codeine *on page 14*
- **Lenpryl** *see* captopril *on page 110*
- **Lente®** *see* insulin preparations *on page 339*
- **Lente® Iletin® I** *see* insulin preparations *on page 339*
- **Lente® Iletin® II** *see* insulin preparations *on page 339*
- **Lentopenil** *see* penicillin G, parenteral, aqueous *on page 475*

lepirudin (leh puh ROO din)

U.S. Brand Names Refludan®

Generic Available No

Therapeutic Category Anticoagulant

Use Indicated for anticoagulation in patient with heparin-induced thrombocytopenia (HIT) and associated thromboembolic disease in order to prevent further thromboembolic complications

Usual Dosage Maximum dose: Do not exceed 0.21 mg/kg/hour unless an evaluation of coagulation abnormalities limiting response has been completed; dosing is weight-based, however patients weighing >110 kg should not receive doses greater than the recommended dose for a patient weighing 110 kg (44 mg bolus and initial maximal infusion rate of 16.5 mg/hour)

Use in patients with heparin-induced thrombocytopenia: Bolus dose: 0.4 mg/kg IVP (over 15-20 seconds), followed by continuous infusion at 0.15 mg/kg/hour; bolus and infusion must be reduced in renal insufficiency

Concomitant use with thrombolytic therapy: Bolus dose: 0.2 mg/kg IVP (over 15-20 seconds), followed by continuous infusion at 0.1 mg/kg/hour

Dosing adjustments during infusions: Monitor first APTT 4 hours after the start of the infusion; subsequent determinations of APTT should be obtained at least once daily during treatment; more frequent monitoring is recommended in renally impaired patients; any APTT out of range should be confirmed prior to adjusting dose, unless a clinical need for immediate reaction exists; if the APTT is below target range, increase infusion by 20%; if the APTT is in excess of the target range, decrease infusion rate by 50%; a repeat APTT should be obtained 4 hours after any dosing change

Dosage Forms Injection: 50 mg

- **Leponex®** *see* clozapine *on page 162*
- **Leptilan®** *see* valproic acid and derivatives *on page 641*
- **Leptopsique** *see* perphenazine *on page 482*
- **Lertamine** *see* loratadine *on page 375*
- **Lescol®** *see* fluvastatin *on page 280*

letrozole (LET roe zole)

U.S. Brand Names Femara™

Generic Available No

Therapeutic Category Antineoplastic Agent, Hormone (Antiestrogen)

Use Treatment of advanced breast cancer in postmenopausal women with disease progression following tamoxifen therapy. Patients with ER-negative disease and patients who did not respond to tamoxifen therapy rarely responded to anastrozole.

Usual Dosage Adults: Oral: 2.5 mg once/day, without regard to meals

Dosage Forms Tablet: 2.5 mg

- **Leucomax®** *see* sargramostim *on page 559*

leucovorin (loo koe VOR in)

Synonyms citrovorum factor; folinic acid; 5-formyl tetrahydrofolate

U.S. Brand Names Wellcovorin®

Mexican Brand Names Dalisol; Flynoken A; Medsavorin

Generic Available Yes

Therapeutic Category Folic Acid Derivative

Use Antidote for folic acid antagonists; treatment of folate deficient megaloblastic anemias of infancy, sprue, pregnancy; nutritional deficiency when oral folate therapy is not possible

Usual Dosage Children and Adults:

Adjunctive therapy with antimicrobial agents (pyrimethamine): Oral: 2-15 mg/day for 3 days or until blood counts are normal or 5 mg every 3 days; doses of 6 mg/day are needed for patients with platelet counts <100,000/mm^3

Folate-deficient megaloblastic anemia: I.M.: 1 mg/day

Megaloblastic anemia secondary to congenital deficiency of dihydrofolate reductase: I.M.: 3-6 mg/day

Rescue dose: I.V.: 10 mg/m^2 to start, then 10 mg/m^2 every 6 hours orally for 72 hours; if serum creatinine 24 hours after methotrexate is elevated 50% or more **or** the serum MTX concentration is >5 x 10^{-6}M, increase dose to 100 mg/m^2/dose every 3 hours until serum methotrexate level is less than 1 x 10^{-8}M

Nursing/Pharmacy Information

Parenteral: Reconstitute 50 mg or 100 mg powder for injection vials with 5-10 mL concentration (350 mg vial requires 17 mL diluent resulting in 20 mg/mL); infuse at a maximum rate of 160 mg/minute

Monitor plasma MTX concentration as a therapeutic guide to high-dose MTX therapy with leucovorin factor rescue. Leucovorin is continued until the plasma MTX level is <1 x 10^{-7} molar.

Stability: Protect from light; store intact vials at room temperature

Stability of parenteral admixture at room temperature (25°C): 24 hours

Stability of parenteral admixture at refrigeration temperature (4°C): 7 days

Reconstituted I.V. solutions are stable 24 hours at room temperature

Concentrations of >2 mg/mL of leucovorin and >25 mg/mL of fluorouracil are **incompatible** (precipitation occurs); **incompatible** with sodium bicarbonate, foscarnet, droperidol

Dosage Forms Leucovorin calcium:

Injection: 3 mg/mL (1 mL)

Powder for injection: 25 mg, 50 mg, 100 mg, 350 mg

Powder for oral solution: 1 mg/mL (60 mL)

Tablet: 5 mg, 10 mg, 15 mg, 25 mg

♦ **Leukeran®** see chlorambucil on page 132
♦ **Leukine™** see sargramostim on page 559
♦ **Leunase** see asparaginase on page 60

leuprolide acetate (loo PROE lide AS e tate)

U.S. Brand Names Lupron®; Lupron Depot®; Lupron Depot-3® Month; Lupron Depot-4® Month; Lupron Depot-Ped®

Mexican Brand Names Lucrin; Lucrin Depot

Generic Available Yes

Therapeutic Category Antineoplastic Agent; Luteinizing Hormone-Releasing Hormone Analog

Use Treatment of precocious puberty; palliative treatment of advanced prostate carcinoma

Usual Dosage

Children: S.C.: Precocious puberty: 20-45 mcg/kg/day

Adults:

Advanced prostatic carcinoma:

S.C.: 1 mg/day **or**

I.M. (suspension): 7.5 mg/dose administered monthly

Endometriosis: ≥18 years: I.M.: 3.75 mg/month for 6 months

Nursing/Pharmacy Information

Rotate S.C. injection sites frequently

Monitor serum estradiol, FSH, LH levels; closely monitor patients with prostatic carcinoma for weakness, paresthesias, and urinary tract obstruction in first few weeks of therapy; serum levels of testosterone, acid phosphatase; bone density in high-risk patients (osteoporosis, use of Depot® leuprolide)

Stability: Store unopened vials in refrigerator, vial in use can be kept at room temperature for several months with minimal loss of potency; upon reconstitution, the suspension is stable for 24 hours, however the product does not contain a preservative; protect from light

Dosage Forms Leuprolide acetate:

Injection: 5 mg/mL (2.8 mL)

Powder for injection (depot):

Depot®: 3.75 mg, 7.5 mg

Depot-3® Month: 11.25 mg, 22.5 mg

Depot-Ped™: 7.5 mg, 11.25 mg, 15 mg

♦ **leurocristine** see vincristine on page 648
♦ **Leustatin™** see cladribine on page 154

levalbuterol *New Drug* (leve al BYOO ter ole)

Synonyms R-albuterol

U.S. Brand Names Xopenex™

Generic Available No

Therapeutic Category Adrenergic Agonist Agent; Beta$_2$-Adrenergic Agonist Agent; Bronchodilator

(Continued)

levalbuterol *New Drug* (Continued)

Use Treatment or prevention of bronchospasm in adults and adolescents 12 years of age and older with reversible obstructive airway disease.

Usual Dosage

Pediatric: Safety and efficacy in patients <12 years of age not established.

Children >12 years and Adults: Inhalation: 0.63 mg 3 times/day at intervals of 6-8 hours, via nebulization. Dosage may be increased to 1.25 mg 3 times/day with close monitoring for adverse effects. Most patients gain optimal benefit from regular use

Elderly: Only a small number of patients have been studied. Although greater sensitivity of some elderly patients cannot be ruled out, no overall differences in safety or effectiveness were observed. An initial dose of 0.63 mg should be used in all patients >65 years of age.

Dosage Forms Solution, inhalation: 0.63 mg/3 mL, 1.25 mg/3 mL

levamisole (lee VAM i sole)

U.S. Brand Names Ergamisol®

Mexican Brand Names Decaris

Generic Available No

Therapeutic Category Immune Modulator

Use Adjuvant treatment with fluorouracil in Dukes stage C colon cancer

Usual Dosage Oral: Initial: 50 mg every 8 hours for 3 days, then 50 mg every 8 hours for 3 days every 2 weeks (fluorouracil is always administered concomitantly)

Nursing/Pharmacy Information Monitor CBC with platelets prior to therapy and weekly prior to treatment; LFTs every 3 months

Dosage Forms Tablet, as base: 50 mg

- ◆ **Levaquin**™ *see* levofloxacin *on page 366*
- ◆ **Levate**® *see* amitriptyline *on page 40*
- ◆ **Levatol**® *see* penbutolol *on page 473*
- ◆ **Levbid**® *see* hyoscyamine *on page 329*
- ◆ **Levlen**® *see* ethinyl estradiol and levonorgestrel *on page 250*
- ◆ **Levlite**® *see* ethinyl estradiol and levonorgestrel *on page 250*

levobunolol (lee voe BYOO noe lole)

Synonyms l-bunolol

U.S. Brand Names AKBeta® Ophthalmic; Betagan® Liquifilm® Ophthalmic

Canadian Brand Names Optho-Bunolol®

Generic Available Yes

Therapeutic Category Beta-Adrenergic Blocker

Use To lower intraocular pressure in chronic open-angle glaucoma or ocular hypertension

Usual Dosage Adults: Ophthalmic: 1-2 drops of 0.5% solution in eye(s) once daily or 1-2 drops of 0.25% solution twice daily

Nursing/Pharmacy Information

Apply finger pressure over nasolacrimal duct to decrease systemic absorption

Monitor intraocular pressure, heart rate, funduscopic exam, visual field testing

Dosage Forms Solution, ophthalmic, as hydrochloride: 0.25% (5 mL, 10 mL, 15 mL); 0.5% (2 mL, 5 mL, 10 mL, 15 mL)

levobupivacaine *New Drug* (LEE voe byoo PIV a kane)

U.S. Brand Names Chirocaine®

Generic Available No

Therapeutic Category Local Anesthetic, Amide Derivative; Local Anesthetic, Injectable

Use Production of local or regional anesthesia for surgery and obstetrics, and for postoperative pain management

Usual Dosage Adults: **Note:** Rapid injection of a large volume of local anesthetic solution should be avoided. Fractional (incremental) doses are recommended.

Maximum dosage: Epidural doses up to 375 mg have been administered incrementally to patients during a surgical procedure

Intraoperative block and postoperative pain: 695 mg in 24 hours

Postoperative epidural infusion over 24 hours: 570 mg

Single-fractionated injection for brachial plexus block: 300 mg

Dosage Forms Injection: 2.5 mg/mL (10 mL, 30 mL); 5 mg/mL (10 mL, 30 mL); 7.5 mg/mL (10 mL, 30 mL)

levocabastine (LEE voe kab as teen)

U.S. Brand Names Livostin®
Generic Available No
Therapeutic Category Antihistamine
Use Temporary relief of the signs and symptoms of seasonal allergic conjunctivitis
Usual Dosage Adults: Ophthalmic: Instill 1 drop in affected eye 4 times/day for up to 2 weeks
Nursing/Pharmacy Information Shake well before using
Dosage Forms Suspension, ophthalmic, as hydrochloride: 0.05% (2.5 mL, 5 mL, 10 mL)

levocarnitine (lee voe KAR ni teen)

Synonyms l-carnitine
U.S. Brand Names Carnitor® Injection; Carnitor® Oral; VitaCarn® Oral
Generic Available Yes
Therapeutic Category Dietary Supplement
Use Treatment of primary or secondary carnitine deficiency
Usual Dosage Oral:
  Children: 50-100 mg/kg/day divided 2-3 times/day, maximum: 3 g/day; dosage must be individualized based upon patient response; higher dosages have been used
  Adults: 1-3 g/day for 50 kg subject; start at 1 g/day, increase slowly assessing tolerance and response
Nursing/Pharmacy Information
  Parenteral: May be administered by direct I.V. infusion over 2-3 minutes or as continuous infusion
  Monitor serum triglycerides, fatty acids, and carnitine levels
  Stability: Protect from light
Dosage Forms
  Capsule: 250 mg
  Injection: 1 g/5 mL (5 mL)
  Liquid (cherry flavor): 100 mg/mL (10 mL)
  Tablet: 330 mg

levodopa (lee voe DOE pa)

Synonyms L-3-hydroxytyrosine; l-dopa
U.S. Brand Names Dopar®; Larodopa®
Generic Available No
Therapeutic Category Diagnostic Agent; Dopaminergic Agent (Anti-Parkinson's)
Use Diagnostic agent for growth hormone deficiency
Usual Dosage Children: Oral (administered as a single dose to evaluate growth hormone deficiency): 0.5 g/m^2
    or
    <30 lbs: 125 mg
    30-70 lbs: 250 mg
    >70 lbs: 500 mg
Dietary Considerations High protein diets may decrease the efficacy of levodopa when used for parkinsonism via competition with amino acids in crossing the blood-brain barrier
Nursing/Pharmacy Information Monitor serum growth hormone concentration
Dosage Forms
  Capsule: 100 mg, 250 mg, 500 mg
  Tablet: 100 mg, 250 mg, 500 mg

levodopa and carbidopa (lee voe DOE pa & kar bi DOE pa)

Synonyms carbidopa and levodopa
U.S. Brand Names Sinemet®
Mexican Brand Names Racovel
Generic Available Yes
Therapeutic Category Anti-Parkinson's Agent; Dopaminergic Agent (Anti-Parkinson's)
Use Treatment of Parkinsonian's syndrome
Usual Dosage Adults: Oral (carbidopa/levodopa): 75/300 to 150/1500 mg/day in 3-4 divided doses; can increase up to 200/2000 mg/day
Dietary Considerations Avoid vitamin products containing vitamin B6 (pyridoxine), which reduces the effectiveness of this medication; avoid or limit the
(Continued)

levodopa and carbidopa *(Continued)*

intake of these food products that contain high quantities of pyridoxine (ie, avocado, bacon, beans, beef liver, dry skim milk, oatmeal, peas, pork, sweet potato, and tuna); this is not an absolute contraindication, check with physician about how much of these foods to eat while you are taking this medication

Nursing/Pharmacy Information
Space doses evenly over the waking hours; do not crush sustained release product
Monitor blood pressure, standing and sitting/supine; symptoms of parkinsonism, dyskinesias, mental status

Dosage Forms Tablet:
10/100: Carbidopa 10 mg and levodopa 100 mg
25/100: Carbidopa 25 mg and levodopa 100 mg
25/250: Carbidopa 25 mg and levodopa 250 mg
Sustained release: Carbidopa 25 mg and levodopa 100 mg; carbidopa 50 mg and levodopa 200 mg

♦ **Levo-Dromoran®** *see* levorphanol *on page 367*

levofloxacin (lee voe FLOKS a sin)
U.S. Brand Names Levaquin™
Mexican Brand Names Elequine; Tavanic
Generic Available No
Therapeutic Category Quinolone
Use Treatment of bacterial respiratory tract infections
Usual Dosage Adults: Oral, I.V.: 500 mg every 24 hours for at least 7 days (dose and duration varies with indication); at least 2 hours before or 2 hours after antacids containing magnesium or aluminum
Nursing/Pharmacy Information Administer oral dose at least 2 hours before or 2 hours after antacids containing magnesium or aluminum, metal cations such as iron or zinc, as well as sucralfate
Dosage Forms
Infusion, in D_5W: 5 mg/mL (50 mL, 100 mL)
Injection: 25 mg/mL (20 mL)
Tablet: 250 mg, 500 mg

♦ **levomepromazine** *see* methotrimeprazine *on page 403*

levomethadyl acetate hydrochloride
(lee voe METH a dil AS e tate hye droe KLOR ide)
U.S. Brand Names ORLAAM®
Generic Available No
Therapeutic Category Analgesic, Narcotic
Controlled Substance C-II
Use Management of opiate dependence
Usual Dosage Adults: Oral: 20-40 mg 3 times/week; range: 10 mg to as high as 140 mg 3 times/week
Nursing/Pharmacy Information Monitor patient adherence with regimen and avoidance of illicit substances; random drug testing is recommended
Dosage Forms Solution, oral: 10 mg/mL (474 mL)

levonorgestrel (LEE voe nor jes trel)
U.S. Brand Names Norplant® Implant
Mexican Brand Names Microlut®
Generic Available No
Therapeutic Category Contraceptive, Implant (Progestin); Contraceptive, Progestin Only
Use Prevention of pregnancy
Usual Dosage Each Norplant® silastic capsule releases 80 mcg of drug/day for 6-18 months, following which a rate of release of 25-30 mcg/day is maintained for ≤5 years
Nursing/Pharmacy Information The net cumulative 5-year pregnancy rate for levonorgestrel implant use has been reported to be from 1.5-3.9 pregnancies/100 users. This compares to a cumulative rate of 4.9 pregnancies/100 women with an IUD after 5 years. At the end of the first year of use, the pregnancy rate with levonorgestrel implants has been reported to be from 0.2-0.6 pregnancies/100 users. This compares quite favorably with the 2.3 pregnancies/100 users of oral contraceptives during the first year of use and 2.4 pregnancies/100 women with an IUD during the first year. Norplant® is a very efficient, yet reversible, method of contraception. The long duration of action

may be particularly advantageous in women who desire an extended period of contraceptive protection without sacrificing the possibility of future fertility.

Dosage Forms Capsule, subdermal implantation: 36 mg (6s)

♦ **levonorgestrel and ethinyl estradiol** *see* ethinyl estradiol and levonorgestrel *on page 250*

♦ **Levophed®** *see* norepinephrine *on page 447*

♦ **Levoprome®** *see* methotrimeprazine *on page 403*

♦ **Levora®** *see* ethinyl estradiol and levonorgestrel *on page 250*

levorphanol (lee VOR fa nole)

U.S. Brand Names Levo-Dromoran®
Generic Available No
Therapeutic Category Analgesic, Narcotic
Controlled Substance C-II
Use Relief of moderate to severe pain; also used parenterally for preoperative sedation and an adjunct to nitrous oxide/oxygen anesthesia
Usual Dosage Adults: Oral, S.C.: 2 mg, up to 3 mg if necessary
Dietary Considerations
Alcohol: Additive CNS effects; avoid or limit alcohol; watch for sedation
Food: Glucose may cause hyperglycemia; monitor blood glucose concentrations
Nursing/Pharmacy Information
Monitor pain relief, respiratory and mental status, blood pressure
Stability: Store at room temperature, protect from freezing; I.V. is **incompatible** when mixed with aminophylline, barbiturates, heparin, methicillin, phenytoin, sodium bicarbonate
Dosage Forms Levorphanol tartrate:
Injection: 2 mg/mL (1 mL, 10 mL)
Tablet: 2 mg

♦ **Levo-T™** *see* levothyroxine *on page 367*

♦ **Levothroid®** *see* levothyroxine *on page 367*

levothyroxine (lee voe thye ROKS een)

Synonyms *l*-thyroxine; t_4 thyroxine
U.S. Brand Names Eltroxin®; Levo-T™; Levothroid®; Levoxyl®; Synthroid®
Canadian Brand Names PMS-Levothyroxine Sodium
Mexican Brand Names Eutirox; Tiroidine
Generic Available Yes
Therapeutic Category Thyroid Product
Use Replacement or supplemental therapy in hypothyroidism; management of nontoxic goiter, chronic lymphocytic thyroiditis, as an adjunct to thyrotoxicosis
Usual Dosage
Children:
Oral:
0-6 months: 8-10 mcg/kg/day
6-12 months: 6-8 mcg/kg/day
1-5 years: 5-6 mcg/kg/day
6-12 years: 4-5 mcg/kg/day
>12 years: 2-3 mcg/kg/day
I.M., I.V.: 75% of the oral dose
Adults:
Oral: 12.5-50 mcg/day to start, then increase by 25-50 mcg/day at intervals of 2-4 weeks; average adult dose: 100-200 mcg/day
I.M., I.V.: 50% of the oral dose
Myxedema coma or stupor: I.V.: 200-500 mcg one time, then 100-300 mcg the next day if necessary
Dietary Considerations Should be administered on an empty stomach; limit intake of goitrogenic foods (asparagus, cabbage, peas, turnip greens, broccoli, spinach, Brussel sprouts, lettuce, soybeans)
Nursing/Pharmacy Information
Parenteral: Dilute vial with 5 mL normal saline; use immediately after reconstitution; administer by direct I.V. infusion over 2- to 3-minute period
Monitor thyroid function test (serum thyroxine, thyrotropin concentrations), resin triiodothyronine uptake (RT_3U), free thyroxine index (FTI), T_4, TSH, heart rate, blood pressure, clinical signs of hypo- and hyperthyroidism; TSH is the most reliable guide for evaluating adequacy of thyroid replacement dosage. TSH may be elevated during the first few months of thyroid replacement despite patients being clinically euthyroid. In cases where T_4 remains
(Continued)

levothyroxine *(Continued)*

low and TSH is within normal limits, an evaluation of "free" (unbound) T_4 is needed to evaluate further increase in dosage

Stability: Protect tablets from light; do not mix I.V. solution with other I.V. infusion solutions; reconstituted solutions should be used immediately and any unused portions discarded

Dosage Forms

Powder for injection, as sodium, lyophilized: 200 mcg/vial (6 mL, 10 mL); 500 mcg/vial (6 mL, 10 mL)

Tablet, as sodium: 25 mcg, 50 mcg, 75 mcg, 88 mcg, 100 mcg, 112 mcg, 125 mcg, 137 mcg, 150 mcg, 175 mcg, 200 mcg, 300 mcg

- **Levoxyl®** *see* levothyroxine *on page 367*
- **Levsin®** *see* hyoscyamine *on page 329*
- **Levsinex®** *see* hyoscyamine *on page 329*
- **Levsin/SL®** *see* hyoscyamine *on page 329*
- **levulose, dextrose and phosphoric acid** *see* phosphorated carbohydrate solution *on page 492*
- **Lexxel™** *see* enalapril and felodipine *on page 231*
- **LHRH** *see* gonadorelin *on page 296*
- **l-hyoscyamine sulfate** *see* hyoscyamine *on page 329*
- **Librax®** *see* clidinium and chlordiazepoxide *on page 156*
- **Libritabs®** *see* chlordiazepoxide *on page 134*
- **Libritabs® 5 mg** *(Discontinued) see page 743*
- **Librium®** *see* chlordiazepoxide *on page 134*
- **Lice-Enz® Shampoo [OTC]** *see* pyrethrins and piperonyl butoxide *on page 533*
- **Lida-Mantle HC® Topical** *see* lidocaine and hydrocortisone *on page 369*
- **Lidemol®** *see* fluocinolone *on page 273*
- **Lidex®** *see* fluocinonide *on page 273*
- **Lidex-E®** *see* fluocinonide *on page 273*

lidocaine *(LYE doe kane)*

Synonyms lignocaine

U.S. Brand Names Anestacon® Topical Solution; Dilocaine® Injection; Duo-Trach® Injection; LidoPen® I.M. Injection Auto-Injector; Nervocaine® Injection; Solarcaine® Topical; Xylocaine® HCl I.V. Injection for Cardiac Arrhythmias; Xylocaine® Oral; Xylocaine® Topical Ointment; Xylocaine® Topical Solution; Xylocaine® Topical Spray

Canadian Brand Names Lidodan®; PMS-Lidocaine Viscous; Xylocard®

Mexican Brand Names Pisacaina; Xylocaina

Generic Available Yes

Therapeutic Category Analgesic, Topical; Antiarrhythmic Agent, Class I-B; Local Anesthetic

Use Drug of choice for ventricular ectopy, ventricular tachycardia (VT), ventricular fibrillation (VF); for pulseless VT or VF preferably administer **after** defibrillation and epinephrine; control of premature ventricular contractions, wide-complex PSVT; local anesthetic

Usual Dosage

Topical: Apply to affected area as needed; maximum: 3 mg/kg/dose; do not repeat within 2 hours

Injectable local anesthetic: Varies with procedure, degree of anesthesia needed, vascularity of tissue, duration of anesthesia required, and physical condition of patient; maximum: 4.5 mg/kg/dose; do not repeat within 2 hours

Children: Endotracheal, I.O., I.V.: Loading dose: 1 mg/kg; may repeat in 10-15 minutes to a maximum total dose of 5 mg/kg; after loading dose, start I.V. continuous infusion 20-50 mcg/kg/minute. Use 20 mcg/kg/minute in patients with shock, hepatic disease, mild congestive heart failure (CHF); moderate to severe CHF may require $\frac{1}{2}$ loading dose and lower infusion rates to avoid toxicity. Endotracheal doses should be diluted to 1-2 mL with normal saline prior to endotracheal administration and may need 2-3 times the I.V. dose.

Adults: Antiarrhythmic:

Endotracheal: Total dose: 5 mg/kg; follow with 0.5 mg/kg in 10 minutes if effective

I.M.: 300 mg may be repeated in 1-1½ hours

I.V.: Loading dose: 1 mg/kg/dose, then 50-100 mg bolus over 2-3 minutes; may repeat in 5-10 minutes up to 200-300 mg in a 1-hour period; continuous infusion of 20-50 mcg/kg/minute or 1-4 mg/minute; decrease the dose in patients with CHF, shock, or hepatic disease

Nursing/Pharmacy Information

Multiple products and concentrations exist

Endotracheal doses should be diluted to 1-2 mL with normal saline prior to E.T. administration

I.V.: Solutions of 40-200 mg/mL must be diluted for I.V. use; final concentration not to exceed 20 mg/mL for I.V. push or 8 mg/mL for I.V. infusion; I.V. push rate of administration should not exceed 0.7 mg/kg/minute or 50 mg/minute, whichever is less

Monitor EKG continuously; serum concentrations with continuous infusion; I.V. site (local thrombophlebitis may occur with prolonged infusions)

Stability: I.V. infusion solutions admixed in D_5W are stable for a minimum of 24 hours

Dosage Forms Lidocaine hydrochloride:

Cream: 2% (56 g)

Injection: 0.5% [5 mg/mL] (50 mL); 1% [10 mg/mL] (2 mL, 5 mL, 10 mL, 20 mL, 30 mL, 50 mL); 1.5% [15 mg/mL] (20 mL); 2% [20 mg/mL] (2 mL, 5 mL, 10 mL, 20 mL, 30 mL, 50 mL); 4% [40 mg/mL] (5 mL); 10% [100 mg/mL] (10 mL); 20% [200 mg/mL] (10 mL, 20 mL)

Injection:

I.M. use: 10% [100 mg/mL] (3 mL, 5 mL)

Direct I.V.: 1% [10 mg/mL] (5 mL, 10 mL); 20 mg/mL (5 mL)

I.V. admixture, preservative free: 4% [40 mg/mL] (25 mL, 30 mL); 10% [100 mg/mL] (10 mL); 20% [200 mg/mL] (5 mL, 10 mL)

I.V. infusion, in D_5W: 0.2% [2 mg/mL] (500 mL); 0.4% [4 mg/mL] (250 mL, 500 mL, 1000 mL); 0.8% [8 mg/mL] (250 mL, 500 mL)

Gel, topical: 2% (30 mL); 2.5% (15 mL)

Liquid:

Topical: 2.5% (7.5 mL)

Viscous: 2% (20 mL, 100 mL)

Ointment, topical: 2.5% [OTC], 5% (35 g)

Solution, topical: 2% (15 mL, 240 mL); 4% (50 mL)

lidocaine and epinephrine (LYE doe kane & ep i NEF rin)

Synonyms epinephrine and lidocaine

U.S. Brand Names Octocaine®; Xylocaine® With Epinephrine

Generic Available Yes

Therapeutic Category Local Anesthetic

Use Local infiltration anesthesia

Usual Dosage Children (dosage varies with the anesthetic procedure): Use lidocaine concentrations of 0.5% or 1% (or even more dilute) to decrease possibility of toxicity; lidocaine dose should not exceed 4.5 mg/kg/dose; do not repeat within 2 hours

Nursing/Pharmacy Information

Contains metabisulfites

Stability: Solutions with epinephrine should be protected from light

Dosage Forms Injection with epinephrine:

Epinephrine 1:200,000: Lidocaine hydrochloride 0.5% [5 mg/mL] (50 mL); 1% [10 mg/mL] (30 mL); 1.5% [15 mg/mL] (5 mL, 10 mL, 30 mL); 2% [20 mg/mL] (20 mL)

Epinephrine 1:100,000: Lidocaine hydrochloride 1% [10 mg/mL] (20 mL, 50 mL); 2% [20 mg/mL] (1.8 mL, 20 mL, 50 mL)

Epinephrine 1:50,000: Lidocaine hydrochloride 2% [20 mg/mL] (1.8 mL)

lidocaine and hydrocortisone

(LYE doe kane & hye droe KOR ti sone)

Synonyms hydrocortisone and lidocaine

U.S. Brand Names Lida-Mantle HC® Topical

Generic Available No

Therapeutic Category Anesthetic/Corticosteroid

Use Topical anti-inflammatory and anesthetic for skin disorders

Usual Dosage Topical: Apply 2-4 times/day

Dosage Forms Cream: Lidocaine 3% and hydrocortisone 0.5% (15 g, 30 g)

lidocaine and prilocaine (LYE doe kane & PRIL oh kane)

Synonyms prilocaine and lidocaine

U.S. Brand Names EMLA®

Generic Available No

Therapeutic Category Analgesic, Topical

Use Topical anesthetic for use on normal intact skin to provide local analgesia for minor procedures such as I.V. cannulation or venipuncture; has also been used for painful procedures such as lumbar puncture and skin graft harvesting (Continued)

lidocaine and prilocaine *(Continued)*

Usual Dosage Children and Adults: Topical: Apply a thick layer of cream to intact skin and cover with an occlusive dressing; for minor procedures, apply 2.5 g/site for at least 60 minutes; for painful procedures, apply 2 g/10 cm² of skin and leave on for at least 2 hours

Nursing/Pharmacy Information

In small infants and children, an occlusive bandage should be placed over the EMLA® cream to prevent the child from placing the cream in his mouth

Monitor patients to ensure that dressing is intact and not leaking; a secondary protective dressing of conforming cotton bandage may be applied when necessary

Stability: Store at room temperature

Dosage Forms Cream: Lidocaine 2.5% and prilocaine 2.5% [2 Tegaderm® dressings] (5 g, 30 g)

- **Lidodan®** *see lidocaine on page 368*
- **LidoPen® I.M. Injection Auto-Injector** *see lidocaine on page 368*
- **Lifenal** *see diclofenac on page 198*
- **lignocaine** *see lidocaine on page 368*
- **Limbitrol® DS 10-25** *see amitriptyline and chlordiazepoxide on page 40*
- **Lincocin®** *see lincomycin on page 370*

lincomycin *(lin koe MYE sin)*

U.S. Brand Names Lincocin®; Lincorex® Injection

Generic Available No

Therapeutic Category Macrolide (Antibiotic)

Use Treatment of susceptible bacterial infections, mainly those caused by streptococci and staphylococci

Usual Dosage

Children >1 month:

Oral: 30-60 mg/kg/day in 3-4 divided doses

I.M.: 10 mg/kg every 12-24 hours

I.V.: 10-20 mg/kg/day in divided doses 2-3 times/day

Adults:

Oral: 500 mg every 6-8 hours

I.M.: 600 mg every 12-24 hours

I.V.: 600-1 g every 8-12 hours up to 8 g/day

Dietary Considerations Decreased absorption with food; should be administered on empty stomach with water

Nursing/Pharmacy Information Administer oral dosage form with a full glass of water to minimize esophageal ulceration; administer around-the-clock to promote less variation in peak and trough serum levels

Dosage Forms Lincomycin hydrochloride:

Capsule: 250 mg, 500 mg

Injection: 300 mg/mL (2 mL, 10 mL)

- **Lincorex® Injection** *see lincomycin on page 370*
- **Linctus Codeine Blac** *see codeine on page 164*
- **Linctus With Codeine Phosphate** *see codeine on page 164*

lindane *(LIN dane)*

Synonyms benzene hexachloride; gamma benzene hexachloride; hexachlorocyclohexane

U.S. Brand Names G-well®

Canadian Brand Names Hexit®; Kwellada™; PMS-Lindane

Mexican Brand Names Herklin; Scabisan Shampoo

Generic Available Yes

Therapeutic Category Scabicides/Pediculicides

Use Treatment of scabies (*Sarcoptes scabiei*), *Pediculus capitis* (head lice), and *Pediculus pubis* (crab lice)

Usual Dosage Children and Adults: Topical:

Scabies: Apply a thin layer of lotion and massage it on skin from the neck to the toes. For adults, bathe and remove the drug after 8-12 hours; for children, wash off 6 hours after application.

Pediculosis: 15-30 mL of shampoo is applied and lathered for 4-5 minutes; rinse hair thoroughly and comb with a fine tooth comb to remove nits; repeat treatment in 7 days if lice or nits are still present

Nursing/Pharmacy Information Lindane lotion should be applied to dry, cool skin

Dosage Forms
Cream: 1% (60 g, 454 g)
Lotion: 1% (60 mL, 473 mL, 4000 mL)
Shampoo: 1% (60 mL, 473 mL, 4000 mL)

♦ **Lioresal®** *see* baclofen *on page 72*

liothyronine (lye oh THYE roe neen)

Synonyms *l*-triiodothyronine; t_3 thyronine
U.S. Brand Names Cytomel® Oral; Triostat™ Injection
Generic Available Yes
Therapeutic Category Thyroid Product
Use Replacement or supplemental therapy in hypothyroidism, management of nontoxic goiter, chronic lymphocytic thyroiditis, as an adjunct in thyrotoxicosis and as a diagnostic aid; levothyroxine is recommended for chronic therapy; (if rapid correction of thyroid is needed, T_3 is preferred, but use cautiously and with lower recommended doses)
Usual Dosage
Mild hypothyroidism: 25 mcg/day; daily dosage may then be increased by 12.5 or 25 mcg/day every 1 or 2 weeks; maintenance: 25-75 mcg/day
Myxedema: 5mcg/day; may be increased by 5-10 mcg/day every 1-2 weeks; when 25 mcg is reached, dosage may often be increased by 12.5 or 25 mcg every 1 or 2 weeks; maintenance: 50-100 mcg/day
Cretinism: 5 mcg/day with a 5 mcg increment every 3-4 days until the desired response is achieved
Simple (nontoxic) goiter: 5 mcg/day; may be increased every week or two by 5 or 10 mcg; when 25 mcg/day is reached, dosage may be increased every week or two by 12.5 or 25 mcg; maintenance: 75 mcg/day
T_3 suppression test: I^{131} thyroid uptake is in the borderline-high range, administer 75-100 mcg/day for 7 days then repeat I^{131} thyroid uptake test

Children and Elderly: Start therapy with 5 mcg/day; increase only by 5 mcg increments at the recommended intervals
Dietary Considerations Limit intake of goitrogenic foods (asparagus, cabbage, peas, turnip greens, broccoli, spinach, Brussel sprouts, lettuce, soybeans)
Nursing/Pharmacy Information
I.V. form must be prepared immediately prior to administration; dilute 200 mcg/mL vial with 2 mL of 0.9% sodium chloride injection and shake well until a clear solution is obtained; should not be admixed with other solutions
Monitor T_4, TSH, heart rate, blood pressure, clinical signs of hypo- and hyperthyroidism; TSH is the most reliable guide for evaluating adequacy of thyroid replacement dosage. TSH may be elevated during the first few months of thyroid replacement despite patients being clinically euthyroid. In cases where T_4 remains low and TSH is within normal limits, an evaluation of "free" (unbound) T_4 is needed to evaluate further increase in dosage
Stability: Store between 2°C and 8°C (36°F to 46°F)
Dosage Forms Liothyronine sodium:
Injection: 10 mcg/mL (1 mL)
Tablet: 5 mcg, 25 mcg, 50 mcg

liotrix (LYE oh triks)

Synonyms t_3/t_4 liotrix
U.S. Brand Names Thyrolar®
Generic Available No
Therapeutic Category Thyroid Product
Use Replacement or supplemental therapy in hypothyroidism
Usual Dosage Congenital hypothyroidism: Oral:
Children (dose/day):
0-6 months: 8-10 mcg/kg
6-12 months: 6-8 mcg/kg
1-5 years: 5-6 mcg/kg
6-12 years: 4-5 mcg/kg
>12 years: 2-3 mcg/kg
Adults: 30 mg/day, increasing by 15 mg/day at 2- to 3-week intervals to a maximum of 180 mg/day
Nursing/Pharmacy Information Monitor T_4, TSH, heart rate, blood pressure, clinical signs of hypo- and hyperthyroidism; TSH is the most reliable guide for evaluating adequacy of thyroid replacement dosage. TSH may be elevated during the first few months of thyroid replacement despite patients being clinically euthyroid. In cases where T_4 remains low and TSH is within normal limits, (Continued)

liotrix *(Continued)*

an evaluation of "free" (unbound) T_4 is needed to evaluate further increase in dosage

Dosage Forms Tablet: 30 mg, 60 mg, 120 mg, 180 mg [thyroid equivalent]

- ◆ **lipancreatin** *see* pancrelipase *on page 467*
- ◆ **lipase, protease, and amylase** *see* pancrelipase *on page 467*
- ◆ **Lipitor®** *see* atorvastatin *on page 64*
- ◆ **Lipocin** *see* fat emulsion *on page 259*
- ◆ **Liposyn®** *see* fat emulsion *on page 259*
- ◆ **Lipovite® [OTC]** *see* vitamin B complex *on page 651*
- ◆ **Liquaemin®** *see* heparin *on page 310*
- ◆ **Liquibid®** *see* guaifenesin *on page 299*
- ◆ **Liqui-Char® [OTC]** *see* charcoal *on page 131*
- ◆ **liquid antidote** *see* charcoal *on page 131*
- ◆ **Liquid Barosperse®** *see* radiological/contrast media (ionic) *on page 539*
- ◆ **Liquid Pred®** *see* prednisone *on page 515*
- ◆ **Liqui-E®** *see* tocophersolan *on page 616*
- ◆ **Liquifilm® Forte Solution [OTC]** *see* artificial tears *on page 59*
- ◆ **Liquifilm® Tears Solution [OTC]** *see* artificial tears *on page 59*
- ◆ **Liquipake®** *see* radiological/contrast media (ionic) *on page 539*
- ◆ **Liquiprin® [OTC]** *see* acetaminophen *on page 13*
- ◆ **Liroken** *see* diclofenac *on page 198*

lisinopril *(lyse IN oh pril)*

U.S. Brand Names Prinivil®; Zestril®
Generic Available No
Therapeutic Category Angiotensin-Converting Enzyme (ACE) Inhibitor
Use Treatment of hypertension, either alone or in combination with other antihypertensive agents
Usual Dosage Adults: Oral: 10-40 mg/day in a single dose
Nursing/Pharmacy Information Watch for hypotensive effect within 1-3 hours of first dose or new higher dose; monitor serum potassium
Dosage Forms Tablet: 2.5 mg, 5 mg, 10 mg, 20 mg, 40 mg

lisinopril and hydrochlorothiazide

(lyse IN oh pril & hye droe klor oh THYE a zide)
Synonyms hydrochlorothiazide and lisinopril
U.S. Brand Names Prinzide®; Zestoretic®
Generic Available No
Therapeutic Category Antihypertensive Agent, Combination
Use Treatment of hypertension
Usual Dosage Adults: Oral: Dosage is individualized; see each component for appropriate dosing suggestions
Dosage Forms Tablet:
Lisinopril 10 mg and hydrochlorothiazide 12.5 mg
[12.5]-Lisinopril 20 mg and hydrochlorothiazide 12.5 mg
[25]-Lisinopril 20 mg and hydrochlorothiazide 25 mg

- ◆ **Listerex® Scrub *(Discontinued)*** *see page 743*
- ◆ **Listermint® with Fluoride [OTC]** *see* fluoride *on page 274*
- ◆ **Lithane®** *see* lithium *on page 372*
- ◆ **Lithellm® 300** *see* lithium *on page 372*

lithium *(LITH ee um)*

U.S. Brand Names Eskalith®; Lithane®; Lithobid®; Lithonate®; Lithotabs®
Canadian Brand Names Carbolith™; Duralith®
Mexican Brand Names Carbolit®; Lithellm® 300
Generic Available Yes
Therapeutic Category Antimanic Agent
Use Management of acute manic episodes, bipolar disorders, and depression
Usual Dosage Oral: Monitor serum concentrations and clinical response (efficacy and toxicity) to determine proper dose

Children: 15-60 mg/kg/day in 3-4 divided doses; dose not to exceed usual adult dosage
Adults: 300 mg 3-4 times/day; usual maximum maintenance dose: 2.4 g/day

Dietary Considerations May be administered with meals to avoid GI upset; avoid changes in sodium content of diet; limit caffeine; food increases absorption; have patient drink 2-3 L of water daily; avoid changes in sodium content of diet (reduction in sodium intake can increase lithium toxicity), sodium is exchanged with lithium which may lead to elevated lithium levels; syrup may precipitate in tube feedings

Nursing/Pharmacy Information
Avoid dehydration
Monitor lithium levels, fluid status, serum electrolytes, renal function, thyroid function, mental status, EKG

Dosage Forms
Lithium carbonate:
  Capsule: 150 mg, 300 mg, 600 mg
  Tablet: 300 mg
  Tablet, controlled release: 450 mg (Eskalith CR®)
  Tablet, slow release: 300 mg (Lithobid®)
Lithium citrate:
  Syrup: 300 mg/5 mL (5 mL, 10 mL, 480 mL)

♦ **Lithobid®** see lithium on page 372
♦ **Lithonate®** see lithium on page 372
♦ **Lithostat®** see acetohydroxamic acid on page 18
♦ **Lithotabs®** see lithium on page 372
♦ **Livostin®** see levocabastine on page 365
♦ **LKV-Drops® [OTC]** see vitamin, multiple (pediatric) on page 654

l-lysine (el LYE seen)
U.S. Brand Names Enisyl® [OTC]; Lycolan® Elixir [OTC]
Generic Available Yes
Therapeutic Category Dietary Supplement
Use Improves utilization of vegetable proteins
Usual Dosage Adults: Oral: 334-1500 mg/day
Dosage Forms l-lysine hydrochloride:
  Capsule: 500 mg
  Elixir: 100 mg/15 mL with glycine 1800 mg/15 mL and alcohol 12%
  Tablet: 312 mg, 334 mg, 500 mg, 1000 mg

♦ **8-l-lysine vasopressin** see lypressin on page 379
♦ **LMD®** see dextran on page 192
♦ **LoCHOLEST®** see cholestyramine resin on page 147
♦ **LoCHOLEST® Light** see cholestyramine resin on page 147
♦ **Locoid® Topical** see hydrocortisone (topical) on page 324
♦ **Lodimol** see dipyridamole on page 212
♦ **Lodine®** see etodolac on page 255
♦ **Lodine® Retard** see etodolac on page 255
♦ **Lodine® XL** see etodolac on page 255
♦ **Lodosyn®** see carbidopa on page 113

lodoxamide tromethamine (loe DOKS a mide troe METH a meen)
U.S. Brand Names Alomide® Ophthalmic
Generic Available No
Therapeutic Category Mast Cell Stabilizer
Use Symptomatic treatment of vernal keratoconjunctivitis, vernal conjunctivitis, and vernal keratitis
Usual Dosage Children >2 years and Adults: Ophthalmic: Instill 1-2 drops in eye(s) 4 times/day for up to 3 months
Dosage Forms Solution, ophthalmic: 0.1% (10 mL)

♦ **Loestrin®** see ethinyl estradiol and norethindrone on page 250
♦ **Logen®** see diphenoxylate and atropine on page 209
♦ **Logesic** see diclofenac on page 198
♦ **Logimax** see felodipine on page 261
♦ **Lomanate®** see diphenoxylate and atropine on page 209

lomefloxacin (loe me FLOKS a sin)
U.S. Brand Names Maxaquin®
Generic Available No
Therapeutic Category Quinolone
Use Quinolone antibiotic for skin and skin structure, lower respiratory and urinary tract infections, and sexually transmitted diseases
(Continued)

lomefloxacin *(Continued)*

Usual Dosage Adults: Oral: 400 mg once daily for 10-14 days

Nursing/Pharmacy Information Monitor signs and symptoms of infection, urinalysis, appropriate cultures, and sensitivities; patients receiving warfarin concurrent therapy should have protimes/INR monitored

Dosage Forms Tablet, as hydrochloride: 400 mg

♦ **Lomicin® Ophthalmic** *see* gentamicin *on page 290*
♦ **Lomotil®** *see* diphenoxylate and atropine *on page 209*

lomustine *(loe MUS teen)*

Synonyms CCNU
U.S. Brand Names CeeNU®
Generic Available No
Therapeutic Category Antineoplastic Agent

Use Treatment of brain tumors, Hodgkin's and non-Hodgkin's lymphomas, melanoma, renal carcinoma, lung cancer, colon cancer

Usual Dosage Oral (refer to individual protocol):

Children: 75-150 mg/m^2 as a single dose every 6 weeks. Subsequent doses are readjusted after initial treatment according to platelet and leukocyte counts

Adults: 100-130 mg/m^2 as a single dose every 6 weeks; readjust after initial treatment according to platelet and leukocyte counts

Dietary Considerations Should be administered with fluids on an empty stomach; no food or drink for 2 hours after administration to decrease nausea

Nursing/Pharmacy Information

Monitor CBC with differential and platelet count, hepatic and renal function tests, pulmonary function tests

Stability: Refrigerate (<40°C, <104°F)

Dosage Forms

Capsule: 10 mg, 40 mg, 100 mg
Dose Pack: 10 mg (2s); 100 mg (2s); 40 mg (2s)

♦ **Loniten® Oral** *see* minoxidil *on page 417*
♦ **Lonox®** *see* diphenoxylate and atropine *on page 209*
♦ **Lo/Ovral®** *see* ethinyl estradiol and norgestrel *on page 252*

loperamide *(loe PER a mide)*

U.S. Brand Names Diar-aid® [OTC]; Imodium®; Imodium® A-D [OTC]; Imodium® Advanced; Kaopectate® II [OTC]; Pepto® Diarrhea Control [OTC]
Canadian Brand Names PMS-Loperamine
Mexican Brand Names Acanol; Pramidal; Raxedin
Generic Available Yes
Therapeutic Category Antidiarrheal

Use Treatment of acute diarrhea and chronic diarrhea associated with inflammatory bowel disease; chronic functional diarrhea (idiopathic), chronic diarrhea caused by bowel resection or organic lesions; to decrease the volume of ileostomy discharge

Usual Dosage Oral:

Children:

Acute diarrhea: 0.4-0.8 mg/kg/day divided every 6-12 hours, maximum: 2 mg/dose

Chronic diarrhea: 0.08-0.24 mg/kg/day divided 2-3 times/day, maximum: 2 mg/dose

Adults: Initial: 4 mg (2 capsules), followed by 2 mg after each loose stool, up to 16 mg/day (8 capsules)

Nursing/Pharmacy Information

Therapy for chronic diarrhea should not exceed 10 days; if diarrhea persists longer than 48 hours for acute diarrhea, etiology should be examined

Monitor stool frequency and consistency

Dosage Forms Loperamide hydrochloride:

Caplet: 2 mg
Capsule: 2 mg
Liquid, oral: 1 mg/5 mL (60 mL, 90 mL, 120 mL)
Tablet: 2 mg

♦ **Lopid®** *see* gemfibrozil *on page 289*
♦ **lopremone** *see* protirelin *on page 529*
♦ **Lopresor** *see* metoprolol *on page 410*
♦ **Lopressor®** *see* metoprolol *on page 410*
♦ **Loprox®** *see* ciclopirox *on page 149*

♦ Lorabid™ *see* loracarbef *on page 375*

loracarbef (lor a KAR bef)
U.S. Brand Names Lorabid™
Mexican Brand Names Carbac
Generic Available No
Therapeutic Category Antibiotic, Carbacephem
Use Treatment of mild to moderate community-acquired infections of the respiratory tract, skin and skin structure, and urinary tract that are caused by susceptible *S. pneumoniae, H. influenzae, B. catarrhalis, S. aureus,* and *E. coli*
Usual Dosage Oral:
Acute otitis media: Children: 15 mg/kg twice a day for 10 days
Urinary tract infections: Women: 200 mg once a day for 7 days
Dietary Considerations Should be administered on an empty stomach at least 1 hour before or 2 hours after meals; administration with food decreases and delays the peak plasma concentration
Nursing/Pharmacy Information
Finish all medication
Stability: Suspension may be kept at room temperature for 14 days
Dosage Forms
Capsule: 200 mg, 400 mg
Suspension, oral: 100 mg/5 mL (50 mL, 100 mL); 200 mg/5 mL (50 mL, 100 mL)

loratadine (lor AT a deen)
U.S. Brand Names Claritin®; Claritin® RediTab®
Mexican Brand Names Clarityne®; Lertamine; Lowadina; Sensibit
Generic Available No
Therapeutic Category Antihistamine
Use Perennial and seasonal allergic rhinitis and other allergic symptoms including urticaria
Usual Dosage Adults: Oral: 10 mg/day on an empty stomach
Nursing/Pharmacy Information Drink plenty of water; may cause dry mouth, sedation, drowsiness, and can impair judgment and coordination
Dosage Forms
Solution, oral: 1 mg/mL
Tablet: 10 mg
Rapid-disintegrating tablets: 10 mg (RediTabs®)

loratadine and pseudoephedrine
(lor AT a deen & soo doe e FED rin)
Synonyms pseudoephedrine and loratadine
U.S. Brand Names Claritin-D®; Claritin-D® 24-Hour
Generic Available No
Therapeutic Category Antihistamine/Decongestant Combination
Use Temporary relief of symptoms of seasonal and perennial allergic rhinitis, and vasomotor rhinitis, including nasal obstruction
Usual Dosage Adults: Oral: 1 tablet every 12 hours
Dosage Forms
Tablet: Loratadine 5 mg and pseudoephedrine sulfate 120 mg
Tablet, extended release: Loratadine 10 mg and pseudoephedrine sulfate 240 mg

lorazepam (lor A ze pam)
U.S. Brand Names Ativan®
Canadian Brand Names Apo®-Lorazepam; Novo-Lorazepam®; Nu-Loraz®; PMS-Lorazepam; Pro-Lorazepam®
Generic Available Yes
Therapeutic Category Benzodiazepine
Controlled Substance C-IV
Use Management of anxiety; status epilepticus; preoperative sedation and amnesia
Usual Dosage
Anxiety and sedation:
Infants and Children: Oral, I.V.: Usual: 0.05 mg/kg/dose (range: 0.02-0.09 mg/kg) every 4-8 hours
Adults: Oral: 1-10 mg/day in 2-3 divided doses; usual dose: 2-6 mg/day in divided doses
Insomnia: Adults: Oral: 2-4 mg at bedtime
(Continued)

lorazepam *(Continued)*

Preoperative: Adults:

I.M.: 0.05 mg/kg administered 2 hours before surgery; maximum: 4 mg/dose
I.V.: 0.044 mg/kg 15-20 minutes before surgery; usual maximum: 2 mg/dose

Operative amnesia: Adults: I.V.: up to 0.05 mg/kg; maximum: 4 mg/dose

Status epilepticus: I.V.:

Infants and Children: 0.1 mg/kg slow I.V. over 2-5 minutes, do not exceed 4 mg/single dose; may repeat second dose of 0.05 mg/kg slow I.V. in 10-15 minutes if needed

Adolescents: 0.07 mg/kg slow I.V. over 2-5 minutes; maximum: 4 mg/dose; may repeat in 10-15 minutes

Adults: 4 mg/dose administered slowly over 2-5 minutes; may repeat in 10-15 minutes; usual maximum dose: 8 mg

Dietary Considerations Alcohol: Additive CNS depression; has been reported with benzodiazepines; avoid or limit alcohol

Nursing/Pharmacy Information

Keep injectable form in the refrigerator; inadvertent intra-arterial injection may produce arteriospasm resulting in gangrene which may require amputation; emergency resuscitative equipment should be available when administering by I.V.; prior to I.V. use, Ativan® injection must be diluted with an equal amount of compatible diluent; injection must be made slowly with repeated aspiration to make sure the injection is not intra-arterial and that perivascular extravasation has not occurred; do not exceed 2 mg/minute, if administered faster, lorazepam may cause respiratory depression; provide safety measures (ie, side rails, night light, and call button); remove smoking materials from area; supervise ambulation

Monitor respiratory and cardiovascular status

Stability: Intact vials should be refrigerated, protect from light; may be stored at room temperature for up to 2 weeks; do not use discolored or precipitate containing solutions; stability of parenteral admixture at room temperature (25°C): 4 hours; I.V. is **incompatible** when administered in the same line with foscarnet, ondansetron, sargramostim

Dosage Forms

Injection: 2 mg/mL (1 mL, 10 mL); 4 mg/mL (1 mL, 10 mL)
Solution, oral concentrated, alcohol and dye free: 2 mg/mL (30 mL)
Tablet: 0.5 mg, 1 mg, 2 mg

♦ **Lorcet® 10/650** *see* hydrocodone and acetaminophen *on page 319*
♦ **Lorcet®** *(Discontinued) see page 743*
♦ **Lorcet®-HD** *see* hydrocodone and acetaminophen *on page 319*
♦ **Lorcet® Plus** *see* hydrocodone and acetaminophen *on page 319*
♦ **Lorelco®** *(Discontinued) see page 743*
♦ **Loroxide® [OTC]** *see* benzoyl peroxide *on page 81*
♦ **Lortab®** *see* hydrocodone and acetaminophen *on page 319*
♦ **Lortab® ASA** *see* hydrocodone and aspirin *on page 319*

losartan *(loe SAR tan)*

Synonyms DuP 753; MK594
U.S. Brand Names Cozaar®
Generic Available No
Therapeutic Category Angiotensin II Antagonist
Use Treatment of hypertension alone or in combination with other antihypertensives; in considering the use of monotherapy with Cozaar®, it should be noted that in controlled trials Cozaar® had an effect on blood pressure that was notably less in black patients than in nonblacks, a finding similar to the small effect of ACE inhibitors in blacks

Usual Dosage Adults: Oral: Initial: 50 mg once daily, with 25 mg used in patients with possible depletion of intravascular volume (eg, patients treated with diuretics) and patients with a history of hepatic impairment; can be administered once or twice daily with total daily doses ranging from 25-100 mg; if the antihypertensive effect measured at trough using once daily dosing is inadequate, a twice daily regimen at the same total daily dose or an increase in dose may give a more satisfactory response; if blood pressure is not controlled by Cozaar® alone, a low dose of a diuretic may be added; hydrochlorothiazide has been shown to have an additive effect

Nursing/Pharmacy Information Cozaar® may be administered with other antihypertensive agents; may be administered with or without food

Dosage Forms Tablet, film coated, as potassium: 25 mg, 50 mg

losartan and hydrochlorothiazide
(loe SAR tan & hye droe klor oh THYE a zide)
Synonyms hydrochlorothiazide and losartan
U.S. Brand Names Hyzaar®
Generic Available No
Therapeutic Category Antihypertensive Agent, Combination
Use Treatment of hypertension
Usual Dosage Adults: Oral: 1 tablet daily
Dosage Forms Tablet: Losartan potassium 50 mg and hydrochlorothiazide 12.5 mg; losartan potassium 100 mg and hydrochlorothiazide 25 mg

- ♦ **Losec®** *see* omeprazole *on page 455*
- ♦ **Lotemax®** *see* loteprednol *on page 377*
- ♦ **Lotensin®** *see* benazepril *on page 77*
- ♦ **Lotensin® HCT** *see* benazepril and hydrochlorothiazide *on page 77*

loteprednol (loe te PRED nol)
U.S. Brand Names Alrex™; Lotemax®
Generic Available No
Therapeutic Category Corticosteroid, Ophthalmic
Use Temporary relief of signs and symptoms of seasonal allergic conjunctivitis
Usual Dosage Adults: Ophthalmic: Instill 1 drop in eye(s) 4 times/day
Dosage Forms Suspension, ophthalmic, as etabonate: 0.2% (2.5 mL, 5 mL, 10 mL)

- ♦ **Lotrel®** *see* amlodipine and benazepril *on page 41*
- ♦ **Lotrimin® AF Powder [OTC]** *see* miconazole *on page 413*
- ♦ **Lotrimin® AF Spray Liquid [OTC]** *see* miconazole *on page 413*
- ♦ **Lotrimin® AF Spray Powder [OTC]** *see* miconazole *on page 413*
- ♦ **Lotrimin AF® Topical [OTC]** *see* clotrimazole *on page 161*
- ♦ **Lotrimin® Topical** *see* clotrimazole *on page 161*
- ♦ **Lotrisone®** *see* betamethasone and clotrimazole *on page 84*

lovastatin (LOE va sta tin)
Synonyms mevinolin; monacolin k
U.S. Brand Names Mevacor®
Generic Available No
Therapeutic Category HMG-CoA Reductase Inhibitor
Use Adjunct to dietary therapy to decrease elevated serum total and LDL cholesterol concentrations in primary hypercholesterolemia
Usual Dosage Adults: Oral: Initial: 20 mg with evening meal, then adjust at 4-week intervals; maximum dose: 80 mg/day
Dietary Considerations May be administered with meals; food maximizes absorption and increases bioavailability
Nursing/Pharmacy Information Monitor plasma triglycerides, cholesterol, and liver function tests
Dosage Forms Tablet: 10 mg, 20 mg, 40 mg

- ♦ **Lovenox®** *see* enoxaparin *on page 232*
- ♦ **Lowadina** *see* loratadine *on page 375*
- ♦ **Loxapac®** *see* loxapine *on page 377*

loxapine (LOKS a peen)
Synonyms oxilapine
U.S. Brand Names Loxitane®
Canadian Brand Names Loxapac®
Generic Available Yes
Therapeutic Category Antipsychotic Agent, Dibenzoxazepine
Use Management of psychotic disorders
Usual Dosage Adults:
Oral: 10 mg twice daily, increase dose until psychotic symptoms are controlled; usual dose range: 60-100 mg/day in divided doses 2-4 times/day; dosages >250 mg/day are not recommended
I.M.: 12.5-50 mg every 4-6 hours or longer as needed and change to oral therapy as soon as possible
Dietary Considerations May be administered with food or water
Nursing/Pharmacy Information
Injectable is for I.M. use only; dilute the oral concentrate with water or juice before administration; avoid skin contact with oral suspension or solution; may cause contact dermatitis
(Continued)

loxapine *(Continued)*

Monitor orthostatic blood pressures 3-5 days after initiation of therapy or a dose increase; observe for tremor and abnormal movement or posturing (extrapyramidal symptoms)

Dosage Forms

Loxapine hydrochloride:
Concentrate, oral: 25 mg/mL (120 mL dropper bottle)
Injection: 50 mg/mL (1 mL)
Loxapine succinate:
Capsule: 5 mg, 10 mg, 25 mg, 50 mg

- ♦ **Loxitane®** *see loxapine on page 377*
- ♦ **Lozide®** *see indapamide on page 336*
- ♦ **Lozi-Tab®** *see fluoride on page 274*
- ♦ **Lozol®** *see indapamide on page 336*
- ♦ **l-PAM** *see melphalan on page 390*
- ♦ **LRH** *see gonadorelin on page 296*
- ♦ **l-sarcolysin** *see melphalan on page 390*
- ♦ **LTG** *see lamotrigine on page 360*
- ♦ **l-thyroxine** *see levothyroxine on page 367*
- ♦ **l-triiodothyronine** *see liothyronine on page 371*
- ♦ **Lubriderm® [OTC]** *see lanolin, cetyl alcohol, glycerin, and petrolatum on page 360*
- ♦ **LubriTears® Solution [OTC]** *see artificial tears on page 59*
- ♦ **Lucrin** *see leuprolide acetate on page 363*
- ♦ **Lucrin Depot** *see leuprolide acetate on page 363*
- ♦ **Ludiomil®** *see maprotiline on page 384*
- ♦ **Lufyllin®** *see dyphylline on page 226*
- ♦ **Lugol's solution** *see potassium iodide on page 509*
- ♦ **Luminal®** *see phenobarbital on page 485*
- ♦ **Lupron®** *see leuprolide acetate on page 363*
- ♦ **Lupron Depot®** *see leuprolide acetate on page 363*
- ♦ **Lupron Depot-3® Month** *see leuprolide acetate on page 363*
- ♦ **Lupron Depot-4® Month** *see leuprolide acetate on page 363*
- ♦ **Lupron Depot-Ped®** *see leuprolide acetate on page 363*
- ♦ **Lurdex** *see albendazole on page 24*
- ♦ **Luride®** *see fluoride on page 274*
- ♦ **Luride®-SF** *see fluoride on page 274*
- ♦ **Luritran®** *see erythromycin (systemic) on page 240*
- ♦ **luteinizing hormone-releasing hormone** *see gonadorelin on page 296*
- ♦ **Lutrepulse®** *see gonadorelin on page 296*
- ♦ **Luvox®** *see fluvoxamine on page 280*
- ♦ **LY170053** *see olanzapine on page 454*
- ♦ **Lycolan® Elixir [OTC]** *see l-lysine on page 373*
- ♦ **Lyderm®** *see fluocinonide on page 273*

Lyme disease vaccine *(LIME dee seas vak SEEN)*

U.S. Brand Names LYMErix®
Generic Available No
Therapeutic Category Vaccine
Use Active immunization against Lyme disease in individuals between 15-70 years of age
Usual Dosage Adults: I.M.: Vaccination with three doses of 30 mcg (0.5 mL), administered at 0, 1 and 12 months, is recommended for optimal protection
Dosage Forms Injection:
Vial: 30 mcg/0.5 mL
Prefilled syringe (Tip-Lok™): 30 mcg/0.5 mL

- ♦ **LYMErix®** *see Lyme disease vaccine on page 378*
- ♦ **Lymphazurin®** *see radiological/contrast media (ionic) on page 539*

lymphocyte immune globulin

(LIM foe site i MYUN GLOB yoo lin)

Synonyms antithymocyte globulin (equine); ATG; horse antihuman thymocyte gamma globulin
U.S. Brand Names Atgam®
Generic Available No
Therapeutic Category Immunosuppressant Agent

Use Prevention and treatment of acute allograft rejection; treatment of moderate to severe aplastic anemia in patients not considered suitable candidates for bone marrow transplantation; prevention of graft-vs-host disease following bone marrow transplantation

Usual Dosage An intradermal skin test is recommended prior to administration of the initial dose of ATG. Use 0.1 mL of a 1:1000 dilution of ATG in normal saline

Aplastic anemia protocol: I.V.: 10-20 mg/kg/day for 8-14 days, then administer every other day for 7 more doses

Rejection prevention: Children and Adults: I.V.: 15 mg/kg/day for 14 days, then administer every other day for 7 more doses; initial dose should be administered within 24 hours before or after transplantation

Rejection treatment: Children and Adults: I.V. 10-15 mg/kg/day for 14 days, then administer every other day for 7 more doses

Nursing/Pharmacy Information

Patient may need to be pretreated with an antipyretic, antihistamine, and/or corticosteroid to prevent chills and fever; administer via central line; use of high flow veins will minimize the occurrence of phlebitis and thrombosis; administer by slow I.V. infusion through an inline filter with pore size of 0.2-1 micrometer over 4-8 hours at a final concentration not to exceed 4 mg ATG/mL

Monitor lymphocyte profile, CBC with differential and platelet count, vital signs during administration

Stability: Ampuls must be stored in refrigerator; dilute in 0.45% or 0.9% sodium chloride; use of dextrose solutions is not recommended; ATG infusion solution is stable for 24 hours at room temperature or refrigeration; precipitation can occur in solutions with a low salt concentration (ie, D_5W). Concentration should not exceed 1 mg/mL for a peripheral line or 4 mg/mL for a central line.

Dosage Forms Injection: 50 mg/mL (5 mL)

♦ **Lyphocin® Injection** *see* vancomycin *on page 642*

♦ **Lyposyn** *see* fat emulsion *on page 259*

lypressin (lye PRES in)

Synonyms 8-*l*-lysine vasopressin

U.S. Brand Names Diapid® Nasal Spray

Generic Available No

Therapeutic Category Antidiuretic Hormone Analog

Use Control or prevent signs and complications of neurogenic diabetes insipidus

Usual Dosage Children and Adults: Nasal: 1-2 sprays into one or both nostrils 4 times/day; approximately 2 USP posterior pituitary pressor units per spray

Nursing/Pharmacy Information Approximately 2 USP posterior pituitary pressor units per spray

Dosage Forms Spray: 0.185 mg/mL (equivalent to 50 USP posterior pituitary units/mL) (8 mL)

♦ **Lysatec-rt-PA®** *see* alteplase *on page 31*

♦ **Lysodren®** *see* mitotane *on page 418*

♦ **Maalox® [OTC]** *see* aluminum hydroxide and magnesium hydroxide *on page 34*

♦ **Maalox Anti-Gas® [OTC]** *see* simethicone *on page 566*

♦ **Maalox® Plus [OTC]** *see* aluminum hydroxide, magnesium hydroxide, and simethicone *on page 34*

♦ **Maalox® Therapeutic Concentrate [OTC]** *see* aluminum hydroxide and magnesium hydroxide *on page 34*

♦ **Macrobid®** *see* nitrofurantoin *on page 444*

♦ **Macrodantin®** *see* nitrofurantoin *on page 444*

♦ **Macrodantina** *see* nitrofurantoin *on page 444*

♦ **Macrodex®** *see* dextran *on page 192*

♦ **Madel** *see* phenazopyridine *on page 483*

mafenide (MA fe nide)

Synonyms succinate mafenide acetate

U.S. Brand Names Sulfamylon® Topical

Generic Available No

Therapeutic Category Antibacterial, Topical

Use Adjunct in the treatment of second and third degree burns to prevent septicemia caused by susceptible organisms such as *Pseudomonas aeruginosa*

(Continued)

mafenide *(Continued)*

Usual Dosage Children and Adults: Topical: Apply once or twice daily with a sterile gloved hand; apply to a thickness of approximately 16 mm; the burned area should be covered with cream at all times

Nursing/Pharmacy Information
For external use only
Monitor acid base balance

Dosage Forms Cream, topical, as acetate: 85 mg/g (56.7 g, 113.4 g, 411 g)

magaldrate (MAG al drate)

Synonyms hydromagnesium aluminate

U.S. Brand Names Riopan® [OTC]

Generic Available Yes

Therapeutic Category Antacid

Use Symptomatic relief of hyperacidity associated with peptic ulcer, gastritis, peptic esophagitis and hiatal hernia

Usual Dosage Adults: Oral: 540-1080 mg between meals and at bedtime

Dietary Considerations Should be administered on empty stomach

Nursing/Pharmacy Information
Administer 1-2 hours apart from oral drugs; shake suspensions well
Monitor for constipation, fecal impaction, diarrhea, and hypophosphatemia

Dosage Forms Suspension, oral: 540 mg/5 mL (360 mL)

magaldrate and simethicone (MAG al drate & sye METH i kone)

Synonyms simethicone and magaldrate

U.S. Brand Names Riopan Plus® [OTC]

Generic Available Yes

Therapeutic Category Antacid; Antiflatulent

Use Relief of hyperacidity associated with peptic ulcer, gastritis, peptic esophagitis and hiatal hernia which are accompanied by symptoms of gas

Usual Dosage Adults: Oral: 5-10 mL between meals and at bedtime

Dietary Considerations Should be administered on empty stomach

Nursing/Pharmacy Information
Administer 1-2 hours apart from oral drugs; shake suspensions well
Monitor for constipation, fecal impaction, diarrhea, and hypophosphatemia

Dosage Forms Suspension, oral: Magaldrate 540 mg and simethicone 40 mg per 5 mL (360 mL)

- ♦ **Magalox Plus® [OTC]** *see* aluminum hydroxide, magnesium hydroxide, and simethicone *on page 34*
- ♦ **Magan®** *see* magnesium salicylate *on page 382*
- ♦ **Maglucate™** *see* magnesium gluconate *on page 381*
- ♦ **Magnacal® [OTC]** *see* enteral nutritional products *on page 233*
- ♦ **magnesia magma** *see* magnesium hydroxide *on page 381*

magnesium chloride (mag NEE zhum KLOR ide)

U.S. Brand Names Slow-Mag® [OTC]

Generic Available Yes

Therapeutic Category Electrolyte Supplement, Oral

Use Correct or prevent hypomagnesemia

Usual Dosage I.V. in TPN:
Children: 2-10 mEq/day; the usual recommended pediatric maintenance intake of magnesium ranges from 0.2-0.6 mEq/kg/day. The dose of magnesium may also be based on the caloric intake; on that basis, 3-10 mEq/day of magnesium are needed; maximum maintenance dose: 8-16 mEq/day
Adults: 8-24 mEq/day

Nursing/Pharmacy Information Monitor serum magnesium level, respiratory rate, deep tendon reflex, renal function

Dosage Forms
Injection: 200 mg/mL [1.97 mEq/mL] (30 mL, 50 mL)
Tablet: Elemental magnesium 64 mg

magnesium citrate (mag NEE zhum SIT rate)

Synonyms citrate of magnesia

U.S. Brand Names Evac-Q-Mag® [OTC]

Generic Available Yes

Therapeutic Category Laxative

Use Evacuation of bowel prior to certain surgical and diagnostic procedures

Usual Dosage Cathartic: Oral:

Children:
    <6 years: 2-4 mL/kg administered as a single daily dose or in divided doses
    6-12 years: $^1/_3$ to $^1/_2$ bottle
Children ≥12 years and Adults: $^1/_2$ to 1 full bottle
Nursing/Pharmacy Information To increase palatability, manufacturer suggests chilling the solution prior to administration
Dosage Forms Solution, oral: 300 mL

magnesium gluconate (mag NEE zhum GLOO koe nate)
U.S. Brand Names Magonate® [OTC]
Canadian Brand Names Maglucate™
Generic Available Yes
Therapeutic Category Electrolyte Supplement, Oral
Use Dietary supplement for treatment of magnesium deficiencies
Usual Dosage The recommended dietary allowance (RDA) of magnesium is 4.5 mg/kg which is a total daily allowance of 350-400 mg for adult men and 280-300 mg for adult women. During pregnancy the RDA is 300 mg and during lactation the RDA is 355 mg. Average daily intakes of dietary magnesium have declined in recent years due to processing of food. The latest estimate of the average American dietary intake was 349 mg/day.

Dietary supplement: Oral:
    Children: 3-6 mg/kg/day in divided doses 3-4 times/day; maximum: 400 mg/day
    Adults: 27-54 mg 2-3 times/day or 100 mg 4 times/day
Dosage Forms Tablet: 500 mg [elemental magnesium 27 mg]

magnesium hydroxide (mag NEE zhum hye DROKS ide)
Synonyms magnesia magma; milk of magnesia; MOM
U.S. Brand Names Phillips'® Milk of Magnesia [OTC]
Generic Available Yes
Therapeutic Category Antacid; Electrolyte Supplement, Oral; Laxative
Use Short-term treatment of occasional constipation and symptoms of hyperacidity
Usual Dosage Oral:
Laxative:
    <2 years: 0.5 mL/kg/dose
    2-5 years: 5-15 mL/day or in divided doses
    6-12 years: 15-30 mL/day or in divided doses
    ≥12 years: 30-60 mL/day or in divided doses
Antacid:
    Children: 2.5-5 mL as needed
    Adults: 5-15 mL as needed
Dietary Considerations May be administered with fluids, taste can be improved by following each dose with citrus fruit juice
Nursing/Pharmacy Information
MOM concentrate is 3 times as potent as regular strength product
Monitor toxicity in patients with decreased renal function
Dosage Forms
Liquid: 390 mg/5 mL (10 mL, 15 mL, 20 mL, 30 mL, 100 mL, 120 mL, 180 mL, 360 mL, 720 mL)
Liquid, concentrate: 10 mL equivalent to 30 mL milk of magnesia USP (3 times as potent as regular strength product)
Suspension, oral: 2.5 g/30 mL (10 mL, 15 mL, 30 mL)
Tablet: 300 mg, 600 mg

♦ **magnesium hydroxide and aluminum hydroxide** *see* aluminum hydroxide and magnesium hydroxide *on page 34*

magnesium hydroxide and mineral oil emulsion
(mag NEE zhum hye DROKS ide & MIN er al oyl e MUL shun)
Synonyms mom/mineral oil emulsion
U.S. Brand Names Haley's M-O® [OTC]
Generic Available Yes
Therapeutic Category Laxative
Use Short-term treatment of occasional constipation
Usual Dosage Adults: Oral: 5-45 mL at bedtime
Nursing/Pharmacy Information Shake well; administer with full glass of water; report persistent diarrhea or abdominal pains with incidence of blood in stool or vomit
Dosage Forms Suspension, oral: Equivalent to magnesium hydroxide 24 mL/mineral oil emulsion 6 mL (30 mL unit dose)

magnesium oxide (mag NEE zhum OKS ide)

U.S. Brand Names Mag-Ox® 400 [OTC]; Maox® [OTC]; Uro-Mag® [OTC]
Generic Available Yes
Therapeutic Category Antacid; Electrolyte Supplement, Oral; Laxative
Use Treatment of magnesium deficiencies, short-term treatment of occasional constipation, and symptoms of hyperacidity
Usual Dosage Oral:
Antacid: 250 mg to 1.5 g with water or milk 4 times/day after meals and at bedtime
Laxative: 2-4 g at bedtime with full glass of water
Dietary Considerations Should be administered after meals
Nursing/Pharmacy Information Monitor for diarrhea and signs of hypermagnesemia
Dosage Forms
Capsule: 140 mg
Tablet: 400 mg, 420 mg, 500 mg

magnesium salicylate (mag NEE zhum sa LIS i late)

U.S. Brand Names Doan's®, Original [OTC]; Extra Strength Doan's® [OTC]; Magan®; Magsal®; Mobidin®
Generic Available Yes
Therapeutic Category Nonsteroidal Anti-inflammatory Drug (NSAID)
Use Mild to moderate pain, fever, various inflammatory conditions
Usual Dosage Adults: Oral: 650 mg 4 times/day or 1090 mg 3 times/day; may increase to 3.6-4.8 mg/day in 3-4 divided doses
Dosage Forms
Caplet:
Doan's®, Original: 325 mg
Extra Strength Doan's®: 500 mg
Tablet:
Magan®: 545 mg
Magsal®: 600 mg
Mobidin®: 600 mg

magnesium sulfate (mag NEE zhum SUL fate)

Synonyms epsom salts
Generic Available Yes
Therapeutic Category Anticonvulsant; Electrolyte Supplement, Oral; Laxative
Use Treatment and prevention of hypomagnesemia; hypertension; encephalopathy and seizures associated with acute nephritis in children; also used as a cathartic
Usual Dosage Dose represented as $MgSO_4$ unless stated otherwise
Hypomagnesemia:
Children:
I.M., I.V.: 25-50 mg/kg/dose (0.2-0.4 mEq/kg/dose) every 4-6 hours for 3-4 doses, maximum single dose: 2000 mg (16 mEq), may repeat if hypomagnesemia persists (higher dosage up to 100 mg/kg/dose $MgSO_4$ I.V. has been used)
Oral: 100-200 mg/kg/dose 4 times/day
Maintenance: I.V.: 30-60 mg/kg/day (0.25-0.5 mEq/kg/day)
Adults: I.M., I.V.: 1 g every 6 hours for 4 doses or 250 mg/kg over a 4-hour period; for severe hypomagnesemia: 8-12 g $MgSO_4$/day in divided doses has been used; Oral: 3 g every 6 hours for 4 doses as needed
Management of seizures and hypertension: Children: I.M., I.V.: 20-100 mg/kg/dose every 4-6 hours as needed; in severe cases doses as high as 200 mg/kg/dose have been used
Cathartic: Oral:
Children: 0.25 g/kg/dose
Adults: 10-30 g
Dietary Considerations $MgSO_4$ oral solution: Mix with water and administered on an empty stomach
Nursing/Pharmacy Information
Dilute to a maximum concentration of 100 mg/mL and infuse over 2-4 hours; do not exceed 125 mg/kg/hour (1 mEq/kg/hour)
Monitor arrhythmias, hypotension, diarrhea, respiratory and CNS depression during rapid I.V. administration; monitor serum magnesium level to avoid overdosages
Stability: Refrigeration of intact ampuls may result in precipitation or crystallization

Stability of parenteral admixture at room temperature (25°C): 60 days

I.V. is **incompatible** when mixed with fat emulsion (flocculation), calcium gluceptate, clindamycin, dobutamine, hydrocortisone (same syringe), poly-myxin B, procaine hydrochloride, nafcillin, tetracyclines, thiopental

Dosage Forms
Granules: ~40 mEq magnesium/5 g (240 g)
Injection: 100 mg/mL (20 mL); 125 mg/mL (8 mL); 250 mg/mL (150 mL); 500 mg/mL (2 mL, 5 mL, 10 mL, 30 mL, 50 mL)
Solution, oral: 50% [500 mg/mL] (30 mL)

- ◆ **Magnevist®** *see* radiological/contrast media (ionic) *on page 539*
- ◆ **Magonate® [OTC]** *see* magnesium gluconate *on page 381*
- ◆ **Mag-Ox® 400 [OTC]** *see* magnesium oxide *on page 382*
- ◆ **Magsal®** *see* magnesium salicylate *on page 382*
- ◆ **Malatal®** *(Discontinued) see page 743*

malathion (mal a THYE on)
U.S. Brand Names Ovide™ Topical
Generic Available No
Therapeutic Category Scabicides/Pediculicides
Use Treatment of head lice and their ova
Usual Dosage Topical: Sprinkle Ovide™ lotion on dry hair and rub gently until the scalp is thoroughly moistened; pay special attention to the back of the head and neck. Allow to dry naturally, use no heat and leave uncovered. After 8-12 hours, the hair should be washed with a nonmedicated shampoo; rinse and use a fine-toothed comb to remove dead lice and eggs. If required, repeat with second application in 7-9 days. Further treatment is generally not necessary. Other family members should be evaluated to determine if infested and if so, receive treatment.
Nursing/Pharmacy Information Topical use only
Dosage Forms Lotion: 0.5% (59 mL)

- ◆ **Malival** *see* indomethacin *on page 337*
- ◆ **Malival AP** *see* indomethacin *on page 337*
- ◆ **Mallamint® [OTC]** *see* calcium carbonate *on page 103*
- ◆ **Mallazine® Eye Drops [OTC]** *see* tetrahydrozoline *on page 602*
- ◆ **Mallisol® [OTC]** *see* povidone-iodine *on page 510*
- ◆ **Malotuss® Syrup** *(Discontinued) see page 743*
- ◆ **Maltlevol®** *see* vitamin, multiple (oral) *on page 654*

malt soup extract (malt soop EKS trakt)
U.S. Brand Names Maltsupex® [OTC]
Generic Available No
Therapeutic Category Laxative
Use Short-term treatment of constipation
Usual Dosage Oral:
Infants >1 month:
Breast fed: 1-2 teaspoonfuls in 2-4 oz of water or fruit juice 1-2 times/day
Bottle fed: $1/2$ to 2 tablespoonfuls/day in formula for 3-4 days, then 1-2 teaspoonfuls/day
Children 2-11 years: 1-2 tablespoonfuls 1-2 times/day
Adults ≥12 years: 2 tablespoonfuls twice daily for 3-4 days, then 1-2 table-spoonfuls every evening
Nursing/Pharmacy Information Add to warm water and stir; then add milk, water, or fruit juice until dissolved
Dosage Forms
Liquid: Nondiastatic barley malt extract 16 g/15 mL
Powder: Nondiastatic barley malt extract 16 g/heaping tablespoonful
Tablet: Nondiastatic barley malt extract 750 mg

- ◆ **Maltsupex® [OTC]** *see* malt soup extract *on page 383*
- ◆ **Mandelamine®** *see* methenamine *on page 400*
- ◆ **Mandelamine® Tablet** *(Discontinued) see page 743*
- ◆ **Mandol®** *see* cefamandole *on page 119*
- ◆ **mandrake** *see* podophyllum resin *on page 501*
- ◆ **manganese injection** *see* trace metals *on page 620*

mannitol (MAN i tole)
Synonyms *d*-mannitol
U.S. Brand Names Osmitrol® Injection; Resectisol® Irrigation Solution
Generic Available Yes
(Continued)

mannitol *(Continued)*

Therapeutic Category Diuretic, Osmotic

Use Reduction of increased intracranial pressure (ICP) associated with cerebral edema; promotion of diuresis in the prevention and/or treatment of oliguria or anuria due to acute renal failure; reduction of increased intraocular pressure; promotion of urinary excretion of toxic substances

Usual Dosage

Children:

Test dose (to assess adequate renal function): 200 mg/kg over 3-5 minutes to produce a urine flow of at least 1 mL/kg/hour for 1-3 hours

Initial: 0.5-1 g/kg

Maintenance: 0.25-0.5 g/kg/hour administered every 4-6 hours

Adults:

Test dose: 12.5 g (200 mg/kg) over 3-5 minutes to produce a urine flow of at least 30-50 mL of urine per hour over the next 2-3 hours

Initial: 0.5-1 g/kg

Maintenance: 0.25-0.5 g/kg every 4-6 hours

Nursing/Pharmacy Information

Avoid extravasation; crenation and agglutination of red blood cells may occur if administered with whole blood; in-line 5 micron filter set should always be used for mannitol infusion with concentrations of 20% or greater; administer test dose (for oliguria) I.V. push over 3-5 minutes; for cerebral edema or elevated ICP, administer over 20-30 minutes

Monitor renal function, daily fluid I & O, serum electrolytes, serum and urine osmolality; for treatment of elevated intracranial pressure, maintain serum osmolality 310-320 mOsm/kg

Stability: Should be stored at room temperature (15°C to 30°C) and protected from freezing; crystallization may occur at low temperatures; do not use solutions that contain crystals, heating in a hot water bath and vigorous shaking may be utilized for resolubilization; cool solutions to body temperature before using

Dosage Forms

Injection: 5% [50 mg/mL] (1000 mL); 10% [100 mg/mL] (500 mL, 1000 mL); 15% [150 mg/mL] (150 mL, 500 mL); 20% [200 mg/mL] (150 mL, 250 mL, 500 mL); 25% [250 mg/mL] (50 mL)

Solution, urogenital: 0.54% [5.4 mg/mL] (2000 mL)

- **Mantadil® Cream *(Discontinued)* see page 743**
- **Mantoux** see tuberculin tests on page 635
- **Maolate®** see chlorphenesin on page 138
- **Maox® [OTC]** see magnesium oxide on page 382
- **Mapap® [OTC]** see acetaminophen on page 13
- **Mapluxin®** see digoxin on page 203

maprotiline *(ma PROE ti leen)*

U.S. Brand Names Ludiomil®

Generic Available Yes

Therapeutic Category Antidepressant, Tetracyclic

Use Treatment of depression and anxiety associated with depression

Usual Dosage Oral:

Children 6-14 years: 10 mg/day, increase to a maximum daily dose of 75 mg

Adults: 75 mg/day to start, increase by 25 mg every 2 weeks up to 150-225 mg/day; administered in 3 divided doses or in a single daily dose

Dietary Considerations May be administered with food to decrease GI distress

Nursing/Pharmacy Information

Offer patient sugarless hard candy for dry mouth

Monitor blood pressure and pulse rate prior to and during initial therapy; evaluate mental status; monitor weight and appetite

Dosage Forms Tablet, as hydrochloride: 25 mg, 50 mg, 75 mg

- **Maranox® [OTC]** see acetaminophen on page 13
- **Marax®** see theophylline, ephedrine, and hydroxyzine on page 605
- **Marcaine®** see bupivacaine on page 97
- **Marcillin®** see ampicillin on page 46
- **Marezine® Injection *(Discontinued)* see page 743**
- **Marezine® Oral [OTC]** see cyclizine on page 174
- **Margesic® H** see hydrocodone and acetaminophen on page 319
- **Marinol®** see dronabinol on page 223
- **Marmine® Injection** see dimenhydrinate on page 206

- **Marmine® Oral [OTC]** *see* dimenhydrinate *on page 206*
- **Marovilina®** *see* ampicillin *on page 46*
- **Marplan® (Discontinued)** *see page 743*
- **Marpres®** *see* hydralazine, hydrochlorothiazide, and reserpine *on page 317*
- **Marthritic®** *see* salsalate *on page 559*

masoprocol (ma SOE pro kole)
U.S. Brand Names Actinex® Topical
Generic Available Yes
Therapeutic Category Topical Skin Product
Use Treatment of actinic keratosis
Usual Dosage Adults: Topical: Wash and dry area; gently massage into affected area every morning and evening for 28 days
Nursing/Pharmacy Information For external use only; may stain clothing or fabrics; avoid eyes and mucous membranes; do not use occlusive dressings; transient local burning sensation may occur immediately after application; contact physician if oozing or blistering occurs; wash hands immediately after use.
Dosage Forms Cream: 10% (30 g)

- **Massé® Breast Cream [OTC]** *see* glycerin, lanolin, and peanut oil *on page 295*
- **Massengill® Medicated Douche w/Cepticin [OTC]** *see* povidone-iodine *on page 510*
- **Materna®** *see* vitamin, multiple (oral) *on page 654*
- **Matulane®** *see* procarbazine *on page 519*
- **Mavik®** *see* trandolapril *on page 620*
- **Maxair™ Inhalation Aerosol** *see* pirbuterol *on page 497*
- **Maxalt®** *see* rizatriptan *on page 552*
- **Maxalt-MLT™** *see* rizatriptan *on page 552*
- **Maxaquin®** *see* lomefloxacin *on page 373*
- **Max-Caro® (Discontinued)** *see page 743*
- **Maxeran®** *see* metoclopramide *on page 409*
- **Maxidex®** *see* dexamethasone (ophthalmic) *on page 189*
- **Maxiflor®** *see* diflorasone *on page 202*
- **Maximum Strength Anbesol® [OTC]** *see* benzocaine *on page 79*
- **Maximum Strength Desenex® Antifungal Cream [OTC]** *see* miconazole *on page 413*
- **Maximum Strength Dex-A-Diet® [OTC]** *see* phenylpropanolamine *on page 489*
- **Maximum Strength Dexatrim® [OTC]** *see* phenylpropanolamine *on page 489*
- **Maximum Strength Nytol® [OTC]** *see* diphenhydramine *on page 208*
- **Maximum Strength Orajel® [OTC]** *see* benzocaine *on page 79*
- **Maxipime®** *see* cefepime *on page 120*
- **Maxitrol®** *see* neomycin, polymyxin B, and dexamethasone *on page 436*
- **Maxivate® Topical** *see* betamethasone (topical) *on page 85*
- **Maxolon®** *see* metoclopramide *on page 409*
- **Maxzide®** *see* hydrochlorothiazide and triamterene *on page 318*
- **may apple** *see* podophyllum resin *on page 501*
- **Mazanor®** *see* mazindol *on page 385*
- **Mazepine®** *see* carbamazepine *on page 112*

mazindol (MAY zin dole)
U.S. Brand Names Mazanor®; Sanorex®
Generic Available No
Therapeutic Category Anorexiant
Controlled Substance C-IV
Use Short-term adjunct in exogenous obesity
Usual Dosage Adults: Oral:
Initial: 1 mg once daily; adjust to patient response
Usual dose: 1 mg 3 times/day one hour before meals, or 2 mg once daily one hour before lunch; administer with meals to avoid GI discomfort
Dosage Forms Tablet:
Mazanor®: 1 mg
Sanorex®: 1 mg, 2 mg

- **MCH** *see* microfibrillar collagen hemostat *on page 414*

m-cresyl acetate (em-KREE sil AS e tate)
U.S. Brand Names Cresylate®
Generic Available No
Therapeutic Category Otic Agent, Anti-infective
Use Provides an acid medium; for external otitis infections caused by susceptible bacteria or fungus
Usual Dosage Otic: Instill 2-4 drops as required
Dosage Forms Solution: 25% with isopropanol 25%, chlorobutanol 1%, benzyl alcohol 1%, and castor oil 5% in propylene glycol (15 mL dropper bottle)

♦ **MCT Oil® [OTC]** see medium chain triglycerides on page 388
♦ **MD-Gastroview®** see radiological/contrast media (ionic) on page 539

measles and rubella vaccines, combined
(MEE zels & roo BEL a vak SEENS, kom BINED)
Synonyms rubella and measles vaccines, combined
U.S. Brand Names M-R-VAX® II
Generic Available No
Therapeutic Category Vaccine, Live Virus
Use Simultaneous immunization against measles and rubella
Usual Dosage S.C.: Inject into outer aspect of upper arm
Nursing/Pharmacy Information
Federal law requires that the date of administration, the vaccine manufacturer, lot number of vaccine, and the administering person's name, title and address be entered into the patient's permanent medical record
Stability: Refrigerate prior to use, use as soon as possible; discard if not used within 8 hours of reconstitution
Dosage Forms Injection: 1000 $TCID_{50}$ each of live attenuated measles virus vaccine and live rubella virus vaccine

measles, mumps and rubella vaccines, combined
(MEE zels, mumpz & roo BEL a vak SEENS, kom BINED)
Synonyms MMR
U.S. Brand Names M-M-R® II
Generic Available No
Therapeutic Category Vaccine, Live Virus
Use Measles, mumps, and rubella prophylaxis
Usual Dosage S.C.: Inject in outer aspect of the upper arm to children ≥15 months of age; each dose contains 1000 $TCID_{50}$ (tissue culture infectious doses) of live attenuated measle virus vaccine, 5000 $TCID_{50}$ of live mumps virus vaccine and 1000 $TCID_{50}$ of live rubella virus vaccine
Nursing/Pharmacy Information
Federal law requires that the date of administration, the vaccine manufacturer, lot number of vaccine, and the administering person's name, title and address be entered into the patient's permanent medical record
Stability: Refrigerate, protect from light prior to reconstitution; use as soon as possible; discard 8 hours after reconstitution
Dosage Forms Injection: 1000 $TCID_{50}$ each of measles virus vaccine and rubella virus vaccine, 5000 $TCID_{50}$ mumps virus vaccine

measles virus vaccine, live (MEE zels VYE rus vak SEEN, live)
Synonyms more attenuated enders strain; rubeola vaccine
U.S. Brand Names Attenuvax®
Generic Available No
Therapeutic Category Vaccine, Live Virus
Use Immunization against measles (rubeola) in persons ≥15 months of age
Usual Dosage Children >15 months and Adults: S.C.: 0.5 mL in outer aspect of the upper arm
Nursing/Pharmacy Information
Vaccine should not be administered I.V.; S.C. injection preferred with a 25-gauge ⅝" needle; federal law requires that the date of administration, the vaccine manufacturer, lot number of vaccine, and the administering person's name, title and address be entered into the patient's permanent medical record
Stability: Refrigerate
Dosage Forms Injection: 1000 $TCID_{50}$ per dose

♦ **Measurin® [OTC]** see aspirin on page 61
♦ **Mebaral®** see mephobarbital on page 393

mebendazole (me BEN da zole)
U.S. Brand Names Vermox®
Mexican Brand Names Helminzole; Mebensole; Revapol; Soltric; Vermicol
Generic Available Yes
Therapeutic Category Anthelmintic
Use Treatment of enterobiasis (pinworm infection), trichuriasis (whipworm infections), ascariasis (roundworm infection), and hookworm infections caused by *Necator americanus* or *Ancylostoma duodenale*; drug of choice in the treatment of capillariasis
Usual Dosage Children and Adults: Oral:
Pinworms: Single chewable tablet; may need to repeat after 2 weeks
Whipworms, roundworms, hookworms: 1 tablet twice daily, morning and evening on 3 consecutive days; if patient is not cured within 3-4 weeks, a second course of treatment may be administered
Dietary Considerations Tablet can be crushed and mixed with food, swallowed whole, or chewed; food increases mebendazole absorption
Nursing/Pharmacy Information Monitor for helminth ova in feces within 3-4 weeks following the initial therapy
Dosage Forms Tablet, chewable: 100 mg

♦ **Mebensole** *see* mebendazole *on page 387*

mecamylamine (mek a MIL a meen)
U.S. Brand Names Inversine®
Generic Available No
Therapeutic Category Ganglionic Blocking Agent
Use Treatment of moderately severe to severe hypertension and in uncomplicated malignant hypertension
Usual Dosage Adults: Oral: 2.5 mg twice daily after meals for 2 days; increased by increments of 2.5 mg at intervals of ≥2 days until desired blood pressure response is achieved
Dietary Considerations Should be administered after meals
Nursing/Pharmacy Information
Aid with ambulation
Monitor frequently for orthostatic hypotension
Dosage Forms Tablet, as hydrochloride: 2.5 mg

mechlorethamine (me klor ETH a meen)
Synonyms HN_2; mustine; nitrogen mustard
U.S. Brand Names Mustargen® Hydrochloride
Generic Available No
Therapeutic Category Antineoplastic Agent
Use Combination therapy of Hodgkin's disease, brain tumors, non-Hodgkin's lymphoma, and malignant lymphomas; palliative treatment of bronchogenic, breast, and ovarian carcinoma; sclerosing agent in intracavitary therapy of pleural, pericardial, and other malignant effusions
Usual Dosage Refer to individual protocols
Children: MOPP: I.V.: 6 mg/m^2 on days 1 and 8 of a 28-day cycle
Adults:
I.V.: 0.4 mg/kg or 12-16 mg/m^2 for one dose or divided into 0.1 mg/kg/day for 4 days
Intracavitary: 10-20 mg or 0.2-0.4 mg/kg
Nursing/Pharmacy Information
Avoid extravasation or contact with skin and eyes since mechlorethamine is a potent vesicant; sodium thiosulfate is the specific antidote for nitrogen mustard extravasations; administer I.V. push through a free flowing I.V. over 1-3 minutes at a concentration not to exceed 1 mg/mL
Monitor CBC with differential, hemoglobin and platelet count
Stability: Prepare solution immediately before each injection, since decomposition will occur upon standing; highly unstable in neutral or alkaline solutions; discard any unused drug after 15 minutes
Dosage Forms Powder for injection, as hydrochloride: 10 mg

♦ **Meclan® Topical** *see* meclocycline *on page 388*

meclizine (MEK li zeen)
Synonyms meclozine
U.S. Brand Names Antivert®; Antrizine®; Bonine® [OTC]; Dizmiss® [OTC]; Dramamine® II [OTC]; Meni-D®; Nico-Vert® [OTC]; Ru-Vert-M®; Vergon® [OTC]
Canadian Brand Names Bonamine®
Generic Available Yes
(Continued)

meclizine *(Continued)*

Therapeutic Category Antihistamine
Use Prevention and treatment of motion sickness; management of vertigo
Usual Dosage Children >12 years and Adults: Oral:
Motion sickness: 25-50 mg 1 hour before travel, repeat dose every 24 hours if needed
Vertigo: 25-100 mg/day in divided doses
Dietary Considerations May be administered with food
Nursing/Pharmacy Information May impair ability to perform hazardous tasks
Dosage Forms Meclizine hydrochloride:
Capsule: 15 mg, 25 mg, 30 mg
Tablet: 12.5 mg, 25 mg, 50 mg
Tablet:
Chewable: 25 mg
Film coated: 25 mg

meclocycline *(me kloe SYE kleen)*

U.S. Brand Names Meclan® Topical
Generic Available No
Therapeutic Category Antibiotic, Topical
Use Topical treatment of inflammatory acne vulgaris
Usual Dosage Topical: Apply to affected areas twice daily
Nursing/Pharmacy Information Apply generously until skin is wet; avoid contact with eyes, nose, and mouth; stinging may occur with application, but soon stops; if skin is discolored yellow, washing will remove the color
Dosage Forms Cream, topical, as sulfosalicylate: 1% (20 g, 45 g)

meclofenamate *(me kloe fen AM ate)*

Generic Available Yes
Therapeutic Category Analgesic, Non-narcotic; Nonsteroidal Anti-inflammatory Drug (NSAID)
Use Treatment of inflammatory disorders
Usual Dosage Adults: Oral: 200-300 mg 3-4 times/day
Dietary Considerations May be administered with food, milk, or antacids
Dosage Forms Capsule, as sodium: 50 mg, 100 mg

- **Meclomen®** *(Discontinued)* see page 743
- **Meclomid** see metoclopramide on page 409
- **meclozine** see meclizine on page 387
- **Meda-Cap®** [OTC] see acetaminophen on page 13
- **Meda® Tab** [OTC] see acetaminophen on page 13
- **medicinal carbon** see charcoal on page 131
- **Medigesic®** see butalbital compound and acetaminophen on page 99
- **Medihaler-Epi®** *(Discontinued)* see page 743
- **Medihaler Ergotamine®** *(Discontinued)* see page 743
- **Medihaler-Iso®** see isoproterenol on page 348
- **Medilium®** see chlordiazepoxide on page 134
- **Medimet®** see methyldopa on page 406
- **Mediplast® Plaster** [OTC] see salicylic acid on page 557
- **Medipren®** [OTC] see ibuprofen on page 332
- **Medi-Quick® Topical Ointment** [OTC] see bacitracin, neomycin, and polymyxin B on page 71
- **Meditran®** see meprobamate on page 394
- **Medi-Tuss®** [OTC] see guaifenesin on page 299

medium chain triglycerides

(mee DEE um chane trye GLIS er ides)
Synonyms triglycerides, medium chain
U.S. Brand Names MCT Oil® [OTC]
Generic Available No
Therapeutic Category Nutritional Supplement
Use Dietary supplement for those who cannot digest long chain fats; malabsorption associated with disorders such as pancreatic insufficiency, bile salt deficiency, and bacterial overgrowth of the small bowel; induce ketosis as a prevention for seizures (akinetic, clonic, and petit mal)
Usual Dosage Oral: 15 mL 3-4 times/day
Dietary Considerations May be administered with meals

Nursing/Pharmacy Information
Dilute with at least an equal volume of water or mix with some other vehicle such as fruit juice (flavoring may be added); mixture should be sipped slowly; administer no more than 15-20 mL at any one time (up to 100 mL may be administered in divided doses in a 24-hour period); formulas should not be cold; since the powdered formula diet provides a high osmolar load, it should be administered slowly by patients with previous gastric surgery
Possible gastrointestinal side effects from medication can be prevented if therapy is initiated with small supplements at meals and gradually increased according to patient's tolerance
Dosage Forms Oil: 14 g/15 mL (960 mL)

♦ **Medralone® Injection** see methylprednisolone on page 407
♦ **Medrapred® (Discontinued)** see page 743
♦ **Medrol® Acetate Topical (Discontinued)** see page 743
♦ **Medrol® Oral** see methylprednisolone on page 407
♦ **Medrol® Veriderm® Cream** see methylprednisolone on page 407

medroxyprogesterone acetate
(me DROKS ee proe JES te rone AS e tate)
Synonyms acetoxymethylprogesterone; methylacetoxyprogesterone
U.S. Brand Names Amen® Oral; Curretab® Oral; Cycrin® Oral; Depo-Provera® Injection; Provera® Oral
Generic Available Yes
Therapeutic Category Contraceptive, Progestin Only; Progestin
Use Secondary amenorrhea or abnormal uterine bleeding due to hormonal imbalance
Usual Dosage
Adolescents and Adults: Oral:
Amenorrhea: 5-10 mg/day for 5-10 days or 2.5 mg/day
Abnormal uterine bleeding: 5-10 mg for 5-10 days starting on day 16 or 21 of cycle
Accompanying cyclic estrogen therapy, postmenopausal: 2.5-10 mg the last 10-13 days of estrogen dosing each month
Adults:
Contraception: Deep I.M.: 150 mg every 3 months or 450 mg every 6 months
Endometrial or renal carcinoma: I.M.: 400-1000 mg/week
Nursing/Pharmacy Information Patients should receive a copy of the patient labeling for the drug; in diabetics, glucose tolerance may be decreased
Dosage Forms Medroxyprogesterone acetate:
Injection, suspension: 150 mg/mL (1 mL); 400 mg/mL (1 mL, 2.5 mL, 10 mL)
Tablet: 2.5 mg, 5 mg, 10 mg

♦ **medroxyprogesterone and estrogens** see estrogens and medroxyprogesterone on page 244

medrysone (ME dri sone)
U.S. Brand Names HMS Liquifilm®
Generic Available No
Therapeutic Category Adrenal Corticosteroid
Use Treatment of allergic conjunctivitis, vernal conjunctivitis, episcleritis, ophthalmic epinephrine sensitivity reaction
Usual Dosage Children and Adults: Ophthalmic: 1 drop in conjunctival sac 2-4 times/day up to every 4 hours; may use every 1-2 hours during first 1-2 days
Nursing/Pharmacy Information
Shake well before using; do not touch dropper to the eye
Monitor intraocular pressure and periodic examination of lens (with prolonged use)
Dosage Forms Solution, ophthalmic: 1% (5 mL, 10 mL)

♦ **Medsaplatin** see cisplatin on page 153
♦ **Medsaposide** see etoposide on page 255
♦ **Medsavorin** see leucovorin on page 362

mefenamic acid (me fe NAM ik AS id)
U.S. Brand Names Ponstel®
Canadian Brand Names Ponstan®
Generic Available No
Therapeutic Category Analgesic, Non-narcotic; Nonsteroidal Anti-inflammatory Drug (NSAID)
Use Short-term relief of mild to moderate pain including primary dysmenorrhea
(Continued)

mefenamic acid *(Continued)*

Usual Dosage Children >14 years and Adults: Oral: 500 mg to start then 250 mg every 4 hours as needed; maximum therapy: 1 week

Dietary Considerations May be administered with food, milk, or antacids

Nursing/Pharmacy Information Extended release capsules must be swallowed intact

Dosage Forms Capsule: 250 mg

mefloquine *(ME floe kwin)*

U.S. Brand Names Lariam®

Generic Available No

Therapeutic Category Antimalarial Agent

Use Treatment of acute malarial infections and prevention of malaria

Usual Dosage Adults: Oral:

Mild to moderate malaria infection: 5 tablets (1250 mg) as a single dose with at least 8 oz of water

Malaria prophylaxis: 1 tablet (250 mg) weekly starting 1 week before travel, continuing weekly during travel and for 4 weeks after leaving endemic area

Nursing/Pharmacy Information Monitor LFTS; ocular examination

Dosage Forms Tablet, as hydrochloride: 250 mg

♦ **Mefoxin®** *see* cefoxitin *on page 123*

♦ **Mega B® [OTC]** *see* vitamin B complex *on page 651*

♦ **Megace®** *see* megestrol acetate *on page 390*

♦ **Megacillin® Susp** *see* penicillin G benzathine *on page 474*

♦ **Megaton™ [OTC]** *see* vitamin B complex *on page 651*

megestrol acetate *(me JES trole AS e tate)*

U.S. Brand Names Megace®

Generic Available Yes

Therapeutic Category Antineoplastic Agent; Progestin

Use Palliative treatment of breast and endometrial carcinomas, appetite stimulation and promotion of weight gain in cachexia

Usual Dosage Adults: Oral:

Breast carcinoma: 40 mg 4 times/day

Endometrial: 40-320 mg/day in divided doses

Nursing/Pharmacy Information Monitor tumor response; observe for signs of thromboembolic phenomena

Dosage Forms Megestrol acetate:

Suspension, oral: 40 mg/mL with alcohol 0.06% (240 mL)

Tablet: 20 mg, 40 mg

♦ **Melanex®** *see* hydroquinone *on page 325*

♦ **Melfiat-105® Unicelles®** *see* phendimetrazine *on page 484*

♦ **Melfiat® Tablet *(Discontinued)*** *see page 743*

♦ **Mellaril®** *see* thioridazine *on page 608*

♦ **Mellaril-S®** *see* thioridazine *on page 608*

melphalan *(MEL fa lan)*

Synonyms l-PAM; l-sarcolysin; phenylalanine mustard

U.S. Brand Names Alkeran®

Generic Available No

Therapeutic Category Antineoplastic Agent

Use Palliative treatment of multiple myeloma and nonresectable epithelial ovarian carcinoma; neuroblastoma, rhabdomyosarcoma, breast cancer, sarcoma; I.V. formulation: Use in patients in whom oral therapy is not appropriate

Usual Dosage Refer to individual protocols

Children: I.V. (investigational, distributed under the auspices of the NCI for authorized studies):

Pediatric rhabdomyosarcoma: 10-35 mg/m^2 bolus every 21-28 days

Chemoradiotherapy supported by marrow infusions for neuroblastoma: 70-140 mg/m^2 on day 7 and 6 before BMT

Adults: Oral:

Multiple myeloma: 6 mg/day or 10 mg/day for 7-10 days, or 0.15 mg/kg/day for 7 days

Ovarian carcinoma: 0.2 mg/kg/day for 5 days, repeat in 4-5 weeks

Dietary Considerations Food interferes with oral absorption

Nursing/Pharmacy Information

Protect tablets from light; reconstitute injection with special diluent 50 mg vial with special diluent to yield a 5 mg/mL solution; filter through a 0.45 µM Millex-HV filter; dilute the reconstituted solution with normal saline to a final concentration not to exceed 2 mg/mL; administer by I.V. infusion at a rate not to exceed 10 mg/minute but total infusion should be administered within 1 hour

Monitor CBC with differential and platelet count, serum electrolytes, serum uric acid; observe for infections and bleeding

Stability: Dilute I.V. formulation with diluent (to 5 mg/mL), then immediately further dilute to ≤0.45 mg/mL with 0.9% sodium chloride injection in a glass bottle and administer within 60 minutes; store at room temperature; protect from light; do not refrigerate reconstituted product; use within 1 hour of reconstitution

Dosage Forms

Powder for injection: 50 mg
Tablet: 2 mg

* **Menadol® [OTC]** *see* ibuprofen *on page 332*
* **Menest®** *see* estrogens, esterified *on page 246*
* **Meni-D®** *see* meclizine *on page 387*

meningococcal polysaccharide vaccine, groups A, C, Y and W-135

(me NIN joe kok al pol i SAK a ride vak SEEN groops aye, see, why & dubl yoo won thur tee fyve)

U.S. Brand Names Menomune®-A/C/Y/W-135
Generic Available No
Therapeutic Category Vaccine, Live Bacteria
Use Immunization against infection caused by *Neisseria meningitidis* groups A,C,Y, and W-135 in persons ≥2 years
Usual Dosage S.C.: 0.5 mL; do not inject intradermally or I.V.
Nursing/Pharmacy Information

Epinephrine 1:1000 should be available to control allergic reaction
Stability: Discard remainder of vaccine within 5 days after reconstitution; store reconstituted vaccine in refrigerator

Dosage Forms Injection: 10 dose, 50 dose

* **Menomune®-A/C/Y/W-135** *see* meningococcal polysaccharide vaccine, groups A, C, Y and W-135 *on page 391*

menotropins (men oh TROE pins)

U.S. Brand Names Humegon™; Pergonal®; Repronex™
Generic Available Yes
Therapeutic Category Gonadotropin
Use Sequentially with hCG to induce ovulation and pregnancy in the infertile woman with functional anovulation or in patients who have previously received pituitary suppression; used with hCG in men to stimulate spermatogenesis in those with primary hypogonadotropic hypogonadism
Usual Dosage Adults: I.M.:

Male: Following pretreatment with hCG, 1 ampul 3 times/week and hCG 2000 units twice weekly until sperm is detected in the ejaculate (4-6 months) then may be increased to 2 ampuls of menotropins (150 units FSH/150 units LH) 3 times/week

Female: 1 ampul/day (75 units of FSH and LH) for 9-12 days followed by 10,000 units hCG 1 day after the last dose; repeated at least twice at same level before increasing dosage to 2 ampuls (150 units FSH/150 units LH)

Repronex™: I.M., S.C.:

Infertile patients with oligo-anovulation: Initial: 150 int. units daily for the first 5 days of treatment. Adjustments should not be made more frequently than once every 2 days and should not exceed 75-150 int. units per adjustment. Maximum daily dose should not exceed 450 int. units and dosing beyond 12 days is not recommended. If patient's response to Repronex™ is appropriate, hCG 5000-10,000 units should be given one day following the last dose of Repronex™.

Assisted reproductive technologies: Initial (in patients who have received GnRH agonist or antagonist pituitary suppression): 225 int. units; adjustments in dose should not be made more frequently than once every 2 days and should not exceed more than 75-50 int. units per adjustment. The maximum daily doses of Repronex™ given should not exceed 450 int. units and dosin beyond 12 days is not recommended. Once adequate follicular

(Continued)

menotropins *(Continued)*

development is evident, hCG (5000-10,000 units) should be administered to induce final follicular maturation in preparation for oocyte retrieval.

Nursing/Pharmacy Information
I.M. administration only
Stability: Lyophilized powder may be refrigerated or stored at room temperature; after reconstitution inject immediately, discard any unused portion
Dosage Forms Injection: Follicle stimulating hormone activity 75 units and luteinizing hormone activity 75 units per 2 mL ampul; follicle-stimulating hormone activity 150 units and luteinizing hormone activity 150 units per 2 mL ampul

♦ **Mentax®** *see* butenafine *on page 100*

mepenzolate *(me PEN zoe late)*

U.S. Brand Names Cantil®
Generic Available No
Therapeutic Category Anticholinergic Agent
Use Management of peptic ulcer disease; inhibit salivation and excessive secretions in respiratory tract preoperatively
Usual Dosage Adults: Oral: 25-50 mg 4 times/day with meals and at bedtime
Dietary Considerations May be administered with meals
Dosage Forms Tablet, as bromide: 25 mg

♦ **Mepergan®** *see* meperidine and promethazine *on page 392*

meperidine *(me PER i deen)*

Synonyms isonipecaine; pethidine
U.S. Brand Names Demerol®
Generic Available Yes
Therapeutic Category Analgesic, Narcotic
Controlled Substance C-II
Use Management of moderate to severe pain; adjunct to anesthesia and preoperative sedation
Usual Dosage Doses should be titrated to appropriate analgesic effect; when changing route of administration, note that oral doses are about half as effective as parenteral dose

Oral, I.M., I.V., S.C.:
Children: 1-1.5 mg/kg/dose every 3-4 hours as needed; 1-2 mg/kg as a single dose preoperative medication may be used; maximum 100 mg/dose
Adults: 50-150 mg/dose every 3-4 hours as needed
Dietary Considerations
Alcohol: Additive CNS effects; avoid or limit alcohol; watch for sedation
Food: Glucose may cause hyperglycemia; monitor blood glucose concentrations
Nursing/Pharmacy Information
If I.V. administration is required, inject very slowly using a diluted solution; administer over at least 5 minutes; intermittent infusion: dilute to 1 mg/mL and administer over 15-30 minutes; dilute to ≤10 mg/mL for intermittent I.V. use
Monitor for pain relief, respiratory and mental status, blood pressure; observe patient for excessive sedation, CNS depression, seizures
Stability: Protect oral dosage forms from light; **incompatible** with aminophylline, heparin, phenobarbital, phenytoin, and sodium bicarbonate
Dosage Forms Meperidine hydrochloride:
Injection:
Multiple-dose vials: 50 mg/mL (30 mL); 100 mg/mL (20 mL)
Single dose: 10 mg/mL (5 mL, 10 mL, 30 mL); 25 mg/dose (0.5 mL, 1 mL); 50 mg/dose (1 mL); 75 mg/dose (1 mL, 1.5 mL); 100 mg/dose (1 mL)
Syrup: 50 mg/5 mL (500 mL)
Tablet: 50 mg, 100 mg

meperidine and promethazine

(me PER i deen & proe METH a zeen)
Synonyms promethazine and meperidine
U.S. Brand Names Mepergan®
Generic Available No
Therapeutic Category Analgesic, Narcotic
Use Management of moderate to severe pain
Usual Dosage Adults:
Oral: 1 capsule every 4-6 hours

I.M.: 1-2 mL every 3-4 hours

Nursing/Pharmacy Information Monitor for CNS depression, seizures, respiratory depression, constipation, urine retention; assist with ambulation

Dosage Forms

Capsule: Meperidine hydrochloride 50 mg and promethazine hydrochloride 25 mg

Injection: Meperidine hydrochloride 25 mg and promethazine hydrochloride 25 per mL (2 mL, 10 mL)

mephentermine (me FEN ter meen)

U.S. Brand Names Wyamine® Sulfate

Generic Available No

Therapeutic Category Adrenergic Agonist Agent

Use Treatment of hypotension secondary to ganglionic blockade or spinal anesthesia; may be used as an emergency measure to maintain blood pressure until whole blood replacement becomes available

Usual Dosage

Hypotension: I.M., I.V.:

Children: 0.4 mg/kg

Adults: 0.5 mg/kg

Hypotensive emergency: I.V. infusion: 20-60 mg

Dosage Forms Injection, as sulfate: 15 mg/mL (2 mL, 10 mL); 30 mg/mL (10 mL)

mephenytoin (me FEN i toyn)

Synonyms methoin; methylphenylethylhydantoin; phenantoin

U.S. Brand Names Mesantoin®

Generic Available No

Therapeutic Category Anticonvulsant

Use Treatment of tonic-clonic and partial seizures in patients who are uncontrolled with less toxic anticonvulsants

Usual Dosage Oral:

Children: 3-15 mg/kg/day in 3 divided doses; usual maintenance dose: 100-400 mg/day in 3 divided doses

Adults: Initial dose: 50-100 mg/day administered daily; increase by 50-100 mg at weekly intervals; usual maintenance dose: 200-600 mg/day in 3 divided doses; maximum: 800 mg/day

Dietary Considerations

Alcohol: Additive CNS depression; has been reported with hydantoins; avoid or limit alcohol

Food:

Fresh fruits containing vitamin C: Displaces drug from binding sites, resulting in increased urinary excretion of hydantoin; education patients regarding the potential for decreased anticonvulsant effect of hydantoins with consumption of foods high in vitamin C

Glucose: Hyperglycemia and glycosuria may occur in patients receiving high-dose therapy; monitor blood glucose concentration, especially in patients with impaired renal function

Nursing/Pharmacy Information Monitor CBC and platelet

Dosage Forms Tablet: 100 mg

mephobarbital (me foe BAR bi tal)

Synonyms methylphenobarbital

U.S. Brand Names Mebaral®

Generic Available No

Therapeutic Category Barbiturate

Controlled Substance C-IV

Use Treatment of generalized tonic-clonic and simple partial seizures

Usual Dosage Epilepsy: Oral:

Children: 4-10 mg/kg/day in 2-4 divided doses

Adults: 200-600 mg/day in 2-4 divided doses

Dietary Considerations High doses of pyridoxine may decrease drug effect; barbiturates may increase the metabolism of vitamin D & K; dietary requirements of vitamin D, K, C, B_{12}, folate and calcium may be increased with long-term use

Nursing/Pharmacy Information High doses of pyridoxine may decrease drug effect

Dosage Forms Tablet: 32 mg, 50 mg, 100 mg

♦ **Mephyton® Oral** see phytonadione on page 493

mepivacaine (me PIV a kane)
U.S. Brand Names Carbocaine®; Isocaine® HCl; Polocaine®
Generic Available Yes
Therapeutic Category Local Anesthetic
Use Local anesthesia by nerve block; infiltration in dental procedures
Usual Dosage
   Injectable local anesthetic: Varies with procedure, degree of anesthesia needed, vascularity of tissue, duration of anesthesia required, and physical condition of patient
   Topical: Apply to affected area as needed
Nursing/Pharmacy Information Before injecting, withdraw syringe plunger to ensure injection is not into vein or artery; solution is acidic
Dosage Forms Injection, as hydrochloride: 1% [10 mg/mL] (30 mL, 50 mL); 1.5% [15 mg/mL] (30 mL); 2% [20 mg/mL] (20 mL, 50 mL); 3% [30 mg/mL] (1.8 mL)

meprobamate (me proe BA mate)
U.S. Brand Names Equanil®; Miltown®; Neuramate®
Canadian Brand Names Apo-Meprobamate®; Meditran®; Novo-Mepro®
Generic Available Yes
Therapeutic Category Antianxiety Agent, Miscellaneous
Controlled Substance C-IV
Use Management of anxiety disorders
Usual Dosage Oral:
   Children 6-12 years: 100-200 mg 2-3 times/day
      Sustained release: 200 mg twice daily
   Adults: 400 mg 3-4 times/day, up to 2400 mg/day
      Sustained release: 400-800 mg twice daily
Nursing/Pharmacy Information
   Assist with ambulation
   Monitor mental status
Dosage Forms
   Capsule, sustained release: 200 mg, 400 mg
   Tablet: 200 mg, 400 mg, 600 mg

♦ **meprobamate and aspirin** see aspirin and meprobamate on page 62

♦ **Mepron™** see atovaquone on page 64

♦ **Meprospan®** *(Discontinued)* see page 743

merbromin (mer BROE min)
U.S. Brand Names Mercurochrome®
Generic Available Yes
Therapeutic Category Topical Skin Product
Use Topical antiseptic
Usual Dosage Topical: Apply freely, until injury has healed
Dosage Forms Solution, topical: 2%

mercaptopurine (mer kap toe PYOOR een)
Synonyms 6-mercaptopurine; 6-MP
U.S. Brand Names Purinethol®
Generic Available No
Therapeutic Category Antineoplastic Agent
Use Treatment of acute leukemias (ALL, CML)
Usual Dosage Oral (refer to individual protocols):
   Induction: 2.5 mg/kg/day for several weeks or more; if, after 4 weeks there is no improvement and no myelosuppression, increase dosage up to 5 mg/kg/day
   Maintenance: 1.5-2.5 mg/kg/day
Dietary Considerations Should not be administered with meals
Nursing/Pharmacy Information
   Adjust dosage in patients with renal insufficiency to lowest recommended dose; monitor dose response with WBC and platelet counts; observe for signs of infection and bleeding or bruising; further dilute the 10 mg/mL reconstituted solution in normal saline or D_5W to a final concentration for administration of 1-2 mg/mL; administer by slow I.V. continuous infusion
   Monitor CBC with differential and platelet count, liver function tests, uric acid, urinalysis
   Stability: Store at room temperature
Dosage Forms Tablet: 50 mg

♦ **6-mercaptopurine** see mercaptopurine on page 394

♦ **mercapturic acid** *see* acetylcysteine *on page 19*

mercuric oxide (mer KYOOR ik OKS ide)
Synonyms yellow mercuric oxide
Generic Available Yes
Therapeutic Category Antibiotic, Ophthalmic
Use Treatment of irritation and minor infections of the eyelids
Usual Dosage Ophthalmic: Apply small amount to inner surface of lower eyelid once or twice daily
Dosage Forms Ointment, ophthalmic: 1%, 2% [OTC]

♦ **Mercurochrome**® *see* merbromin *on page 394*
♦ **Meridia**™ *see* sibutramine *on page 565*

meropenem (mer oh PEN em)
U.S. Brand Names Merrem® I.V.
Generic Available No
Therapeutic Category Carbapenem (Antibiotic)
Use Meropenem is indicated as single agent therapy for the treatment of intra-abdominal infections including complicated appendicitis and peritonitis in adults and bacterial meningitis in pediatric patients >3 months of age caused by *S. pneumoniae*, *H. influenzae*, and *N. meningitidis* (penicillin-resistant pneumococci have not been studied in clinical trials); it is better tolerated than imipenem and highly effective against a broad range of bacteria
Usual Dosage
  Children:
    Intra-abdominal infections: 20 mg/kg every 8 hours (maximum dose: 1 g every 8 hours)
    Meningitis: 40 mg/kg every 8 hours (maximum dose: 2 g every 8 hours)
  Adults: 1 g every 8 hours
Dosage Forms
  Infusion: 500 mg (100 mL); 1 g (100 mL)
  Infusion, ADD-vantage®: 500 mg (15 mL); 1 g (15 mL)
  Injection: 25 mg/mL (20 mL); 33.3 mg/mL (30 mL)

♦ **Merrem**® **I.V.** *see* meropenem *on page 395*
♦ **Mersol**® **[OTC]** *see* thimerosal *on page 607*
♦ **Merthiolate**® **[OTC]** *see* thimerosal *on page 607*
♦ **Meruvax**® **II** *see* rubella virus vaccine, live *on page 556*

mesalamine (me SAL a meen)
Synonyms 5-aminosalicylic acid; 5-ASA; fisalamine; mesalazine
U.S. Brand Names Asacol® Oral; Pentasa® Oral; Rowasa® Rectal
Generic Available No
Therapeutic Category 5-Aminosalicylic Acid Derivative
Use Treatment of ulcerative colitis, proctosigmoiditis, and proctitis
Usual Dosage Adults (usual course of therapy is 3-6 weeks): Oral: 800 mg 3 times/day
  Retention enema: 60 mL (4 g) at bedtime, retained overnight, approximately 8 hours
  Rectal suppository: Insert 1 suppository in rectum twice daily
Nursing/Pharmacy Information
  Provide patient with copy of mesalamine administration instructions
  Stability: Unstable in presence of water or light; once foil has been removed, unopened bottles have an expiration of 1 year following the date of manufacture
Dosage Forms
  Capsule, controlled release (Pentasa®): 250 mg
  Suppository, rectal (Rowasa®): 500 mg
  Suspension, rectal (Rowasa®): 4 g/60 mL (7s)
  Tablet, enteric coated (Asacol®): 400 mg

♦ **mesalazine** *see* mesalamine *on page 395*
♦ **Mesantoin**® *see* mephenytoin *on page 393*
♦ **M-Eslon**® *see* morphine sulfate *on page 422*

mesna (MES na)
Synonyms sodium 2-mercaptoethane sulfonate
U.S. Brand Names Mesnex™
Generic Available No
Therapeutic Category Antidote
  (Continued)

mesna *(Continued)*

Use Detoxifying agent used as a protectant against hemorrhagic cystitis induced by ifosfamide and cyclophosphamide

Usual Dosage Children and Adults (refer to individual protocols):

Ifosfamide: I.V.: 20% W/W of ifosfamide dose at time of administration and 4 and 8 hours after each dose of ifosfamide

Cyclophosphamide: I.V.: 20% W/W of cyclophosphamide dose prior to administration and 3, 6, 9, 12 hours after cyclophosphamide dose (total daily dose: 120% to 180% of cyclophosphamide dose)

Oral dose: 40% W/W of the antineoplastic agent dose in 3 doses at 4-hour intervals

Nursing/Pharmacy Information

Used concurrent with and/or following high-dose ifosfamide or cyclophosphamide; mesna also has been administered orally with carbonated beverages or juice (most palatable in grape juice); administer by I.V. infusion over 15-30 minutes or per protocol; mesna can be diluted in D_5W or NS to a final concentration of 1-20 mg/mL

Monitor urinalysis

Stability: Diluted solutions are chemically and physically stable for 24 hours at room temperature; however, it is recommended that solutions be refrigerated and used within 6 hours; **incompatible** with cisplatin; **compatible** with cyclophosphamide, etoposide, lorazepam, potassium chloride, bleomycin, dexamethasone

Dosage Forms Injection: 100 mg/mL (2 mL, 4 mL, 10 mL)

♦ **Mesnex™** *see mesna on page 395*

mesoridazine *(mez oh RID a zeen)*

U.S. Brand Names Serentil®

Generic Available No

Therapeutic Category Phenothiazine Derivative

Use Symptomatic management of psychotic disorders, including schizophrenia, behavioral problems, alcoholism as well as reducing anxiety and tension occurring in neurosis

Usual Dosage Initial: 25 mg for most patients; may repeat dose in 30-60 minutes, if necessary; usual optimum dosage range: 25-200 mg/day. Concentrate may be diluted just prior to administration with distilled water, acidified tap water, orange or grape juice; do not prepare and store bulk dilutions.

Dietary Considerations May be administered with food, milk, or water

Nursing/Pharmacy Information

Dilute oral concentrate with water or juice before administration; avoid skin contact with oral suspension or solution; may cause contact dermatitis; monitor orthostatic blood pressures 3-5 days after initiation of therapy or a dose increase

Monitor orthostatic blood pressures; tremors, gait changes, abnormal movement in trunk, neck, buccal area or extremities; monitor target behaviors for which the agent is administered; monitor hepatic function (especially if fever with flu-like symptoms); watch for hypotension when administering I.M. or I.V.

Dosage Forms Mesoridazine besylate:

Injection: 25 mg/mL (1 mL)

Liquid, oral: 25 mg/mL (118 mL)

Tablet: 10 mg, 25 mg, 50 mg, 100 mg

♦ **Mestatin®** *see nystatin on page 452*

♦ **Mestinon® Injection** *see pyridostigmine on page 533*

♦ **Mestinon® Oral** *see pyridostigmine on page 533*

mestranol and norethindrone *(MES tra nole & nor eth IN drone)*

Synonyms norethindrone and mestranol

U.S. Brand Names Genora® 1/50; Nelova® 1/50M; Norethin 1/50M; Norinyl® 1+50; Ortho-Novum® 1/50

Generic Available Yes

Therapeutic Category Contraceptive, Oral

Use Prevention of pregnancy; treatment of hypermenorrhea, endometriosis, female hypogonadism

Usual Dosage Contraception: Oral: 1 tablet daily, beginning on day 5 of menstrual cycle (first day of menstrual flow is day 1). With 20-tablet and 21-tablet packages, new dosing cycle begins 7 days after last tablet taken; with 28-tablet packages, dosage is 1 tablet daily without interruption; extra tablets are placebos or contain iron. If next menstrual period does not begin on schedule, rule out pregnancy before starting new dosing cycle; if menstrual period begins, start new dosing cycle 7 days after last tablet was taken. If all doses have been taken on schedule and 1 menstrual period is missed, continue dosing cycle; if 2 consecutive menstrual periods are missed, pregnancy test is required before new dosing cycle is started.

Dietary Considerations Should be administered with food at same time each day

Nursing/Pharmacy Information 80 mcg of mestranol is approximately equivalent to 50 mcg of ethinyl estradiol

Dosage Forms Tablet: Mestranol 0.05 mg and norethindrone 1 mg (21s and 28s)

♦ **metacortandralone** *see* prednisolone (systemic) *on page 514*
♦ **Metahydrin®** *see* trichlormethiazide *on page 626*
♦ **Metamucil® [OTC]** *see* psyllium *on page 531*
♦ **Metamucil® Instant Mix [OTC]** *see* psyllium *on page 531*
♦ **Metaprel® Aerosol** *(Discontinued) see page 743*
♦ **Metaprel® Inhalation Solution** *(Discontinued) see page 743*
♦ **Metaprel® Syrup** *see* metaproterenol *on page 397*
♦ **Metaprel® Tablet** *(Discontinued) see page 743*

metaproterenol (met a proe TER e nol)

Synonyms orciprenaline
U.S. Brand Names Alupent®; Arm-a-Med® Metaproterenol; Dey-Dose® Metaproterenol; Metaprel® Syrup; Prometa®
Generic Available Yes (except inhaler)
Therapeutic Category Adrenergic Agonist Agent
Use Bronchodilator in reversible airway obstruction due to asthma or COPD
Usual Dosage
Oral:
Children:
<2 years: 0.4 mg/kg/dose administered 3-4 times/day; in infants, the dose can be administered every 8-12 hours
2-6 years: 1-2.6 mg/kg/day divided every 6-8 hours
6-9 years: 10 mg/dose administered 3-4 times/day
Children >9 years and Adults: 20 mg/dose administered 3-4 times/day
Inhalation: Children >12 years and Adults: 2-3 inhalations every 3-4 hours, up to 12 inhalations in 24 hours
Nebulizer:
Infants: 6 mg/dose administered over 5 minutes
Children <12 years: 0.01-0.02 mL/kg of 5% solution; diluted in 2-3 mL normal saline every 4-6 hours (may be administered more frequently according to need), maximum dose: 15 mg/dose every 4-6 hours
Adolescents and Adults: 5-20 breaths of full strength 5% metaproterenol **or** 0.2-0.3 mL of 5% metaproterenol in 2.5-3 mL normal saline nebulized every 4-6 hours (can be administered more frequently according to need)
Nursing/Pharmacy Information
Before using, the inhaler must be shaken well; assess lung sounds, pulse, and blood pressure before administration and during peak of medication; observe patient for wheezing after administration, if this occurs, call physician
Monitor for improvement of respirations, heart rate, blood pressure
Stability: Store in tight, light-resistant container
Dosage Forms Metaproterenol sulfate:
Aerosol, oral: 0.65 mg/dose (5 mL, 10 mL)
Solution for inhalation, preservative free: 0.4% [4 mg/mL] (2.5 mL); 0.6% [6 mg/mL] (2.5 mL); 5% [50 mg/mL] (10 mL, 30 mL)
Syrup: 10 mg/5 mL (480 mL)
Tablet: 10 mg, 20 mg

metaraminol (met a RAM i nole)

U.S. Brand Names Aramine®
Generic Available Yes
Therapeutic Category Adrenergic Agonist Agent
Use Acute hypotensive crisis in the treatment of shock
Usual Dosage Adults:
Prevention of hypotension: I.M., S.C.: 2-10 mg
Adjunctive treatment of hypotension: I.V.: 15-100 mg in 250-500 mL NS or 5% dextrose in water
Severe shock: I.V.: 0.5-5 mg direct I.V. injection then use I.M. dose
Nursing/Pharmacy Information
Monitor blood pressure, EKG, PCWP, CVP, pulse, and urine output
(Continued)

metaraminol (Continued)

Stability: Infusion solutions are stable for 24 hours; I.V. metaraminol is **incompatible** when mixed with amphotericin B, dexamethasone, erythromycin, hydrocortisone, methicillin, penicillin G, prednisolone, thiopental

Dosage Forms Injection, as bitartrate: 10 mg/mL (10 mL)

♦ **Metasep®** [OTC] see parachlorometaxylenol on page 469

♦ **Metastron®** see strontium-89 on page 582

metaxalone (me TAKS a lone)

U.S. Brand Names Skelaxin®

Generic Available No

Therapeutic Category Skeletal Muscle Relaxant

Use Relief of discomfort associated with acute, painful musculoskeletal conditions

Usual Dosage Children >12 years and Adults: Oral: 800 mg 3-4 times/day

Nursing/Pharmacy Information Avoid alcohol and other CNS depressants; may cause drowsiness, impairment of judgment, or coordination; notify physician of dark urine, pale stools, yellowing of eyes, severe nausea, vomiting, or abdominal pain

Dosage Forms Tablet: 400 mg

metformin (met FOR min)

U.S. Brand Names Glucophage®

Canadian Brand Names Novo-Metformin

Mexican Brand Names Dabex; Glucophage® Forte

Generic Available No

Therapeutic Category Antidiabetic Agent, Oral

Use Management of noninsulin-dependent diabetes mellitus (type II) as monotherapy when hyperglycemia cannot be managed on diet alone. May be used concomitantly with a sulfonylurea when diet and metformin or sulfonylurea alone do not result in adequate glycemic control.

Usual Dosage Oral (allow 1-2 weeks between dose titrations):

Adults:

500 mg tablets: Initial: 500 mg twice daily (administered with the morning and evening meals). Dosage increases should be made in increments of one tablet every week, administered in divided doses, up to a maximum of 2,500 mg/day. Doses of up to 2000 mg/day may be administered twice daily. If a dose of 2,500 mg/day is required, it may be better tolerated 3 times/day (with meals).

850 mg tablets: Initial: 850 mg once daily (administered with the morning meal). Dosage increases should be made in increments of one tablet every OTHER week, administered in divided doses, up to a maximum of 2550 mg/day. The usual maintenance dose is 850 mg twice daily (with the morning and evening meals). Some patients may be administered 850 mg 3 times/day (with meals).

Elderly patients: The initial and maintenance dosing should be conservative, due to the potential for decreased renal function. Generally, elderly patients should not be titrated to the maximum dose of metformin.

Transfer from other antidiabetic agents: No transition period is generally necessary except when transferring from chlorpropamide. When transferring from chlorpropamide, care should be exercised during the first 2 weeks because of the prolonged retention of chlorpropamide in the body, leading to overlapping drug effects and possible hypoglycemia.

Concomitant metformin and oral sulfonylurea therapy: If patients have not responded to 4 weeks of the maximum dose of metformin monotherapy, consideration to a gradually addition of an oral sulfonylurea while continuing metformin at the maximum dose, even if prior primary or secondary failure to a sulfonylurea has occurred.

Dietary Considerations

Alcohol: Incidence of lactic acidosis may be increased; avoid or limit alcohol

Food: Decreases the extent and slightly delays the absorption; may cause GI upset; administer with food to decrease GI upset

Glucose: Decreases blood glucose concentration; hypoglycemia does not usually occur unless a patient is predisposed; monitor blood glucose concentration; exercise caution with administration in patients predisposed to hypoglycemia (eg, cases of reduced caloric intake, strenuous exercise without repletion of calories, alcohol ingestion or when metformin is combined with another oral antidiabetic agent)

Vitamin B$_{12}$: Decreases absorption of Vitamin B$_{12}$; monitor for signs and symptoms of Vitamin B$_{12}$ deficiency

Folic acid: Decreases absorption of folic acid; monitor for signs and symptoms of folic acid deficiency

Nursing/Pharmacy Information May be used in combination with oral sulfonylureas if indicated for glycemic control; patients who are NPO may need to have their dose held to avoid hypoglycemia

Dosage Forms Tablet, as hydrochloride: 500 mg, 850 mg

methacholine (meth a KOLE leen)

U.S. Brand Names Provocholine®

Generic Available No

Therapeutic Category Diagnostic Agent

Use Diagnosis of bronchial airway hyperactivity in subjects who do not have clinically apparent asthma

Usual Dosage The table is a suggested schedule for administration of methacholine challenge. Calculate cumulative units by multiplying number of breaths by concentration given. Total cumulative units is the sum of cumulative units for each concentration given.

Vial	Serial Concentration (mg/mL)	No. of Breaths	Cumulative Units per Concentration	Total Cumulative Units
E	0.025	5	0.125	0.125
D	0.25	5	1.25	1.375
C	2.5	5	12.5	13.88
B	10	5	50	63.88
A	25	5	125	188.88

Nursing/Pharmacy Information Stability: Store unreconstituted powder at 59°F to 86°F; store dilutions in refrigerator (36°F to 46°F) for up to 2 weeks

Dosage Forms Powder for reconstitution, inhalation, as chloride: 100 mg/5 mL

methadone (METH a done)

U.S. Brand Names Dolophine®

Canadian Brand Names Methadose®

Generic Available Yes

Therapeutic Category Analgesic, Narcotic

Controlled Substance C-II

Use Management of severe pain, used in narcotic detoxification maintenance programs and for the treatment of iatrogenic narcotic dependency

Usual Dosage Doses should be titrated to appropriate effects:

Children: Analgesia:

Oral, I.M., S.C.: 0.7 mg/kg/24 hours divided every 4-6 hours as needed or 0.1-0.2 mg/kg every 4-12 hours as needed; maximum: 10 mg/dose

I.V.: Initial: 0.1 mg/kg every 4 hours for 2-3 doses, then every 6-12 hours as needed; maximum: 10 mg/dose

Adults:

Analgesia: Oral, I.M., S.C.: 2.5-10 mg every 3-8 hours as needed, up to 5-20 mg every 6-8 hours

Detoxification: Oral: 15-40 mg/day

Maintenance of opiate dependence: Oral: 20-120 mg/day

Dietary Considerations

Alcohol: Additive CNS effects; avoid or limit alcohol; watch for sedation

Food: Glucose may cause hyperglycemia; monitor blood glucose concentrations; may be administered with juice or water

Nursing/Pharmacy Information

Implement safety measures, assist with ambulation

Monitor for pain relief, respiratory and mental status, blood pressure; observe patient for excessive sedation, respiratory depression

Stability: Highly **incompatible** with all other I.V. agents when mixed together

Dosage Forms Methadone hydrochloride:

Injection: 10 mg/mL (1 mL, 10 mL, 20 mL)

Solution:

Oral: 5 mg/5 mL (5 mL, 500 mL); 10 mg/5 mL (500 mL)

Oral, concentrate: 10 mg/mL (30 mL)

Tablet: 5 mg, 10 mg

Tablet, dispersible: 40 mg

♦ **Methadose®** see methadone on page 399

♦ **methaminodiazepoxide** *see* chlordiazepoxide *on page 134*

methamphetamine (meth am FET a meen)

Synonyms desoxyephedrine
U.S. Brand Names Desoxyn®
Generic Available No
Therapeutic Category Amphetamine
Controlled Substance C-II
Use Narcolepsy; exogenous obesity; abnormal behavioral syndrome in children (minimal brain dysfunction)
Usual Dosage Oral:
Attention deficit disorder: Children >6 years: 2.5-5 mg 1-2 times/day, may increase by 5 mg increments weekly until optimum response is achieved, usually 20-25 mg/day
Exogenous obesity: Children >12 years and Adults: 5 mg, 30 minutes before each meal, 10-15 mg in morning; treatment duration should not exceed a few weeks
Dietary Considerations Should be administered 30 minutes before meals
Nursing/Pharmacy Information Monitor heart rate, respiratory rate, blood pressure, and CNS activity
Dosage Forms Methamphetamine hydrochloride:
Tablet: 5 mg
Tablet, extended release (Gradumet®): 5 mg, 10 mg, 15 mg

methantheline (meth AN tha leen)

Synonyms methanthelinium
U.S. Brand Names Banthine®
Generic Available No
Therapeutic Category Anticholinergic Agent
Use Adjunctive treatment of peptic ulcer, irritable bowel syndrome, pancreatitis, ureteral and urinary bladder spasm; to reduce duodenal motility during diagnostic radiologic procedures and treatment of an uninhibited neurogenic bladder
Usual Dosage Oral:
Children:
<1 year: 12.5-25 mg 4 times/day
>1 year: 12.5-50 mg 4 times/day
Adults: 50-100 mg every 6 hours
Dosage Forms Tablet, as bromide: 50 mg

♦ **methanthelinium** *see* methantheline *on page 400*

methazolamide (meth a ZOE la mide)

U.S. Brand Names GlaucTabs®; Neptazane®
Generic Available Yes
Therapeutic Category Carbonic Anhydrase Inhibitor
Use Adjunctive treatment of open-angle or secondary glaucoma; short-term therapy of narrow-angle glaucoma when delay of surgery is desired
Usual Dosage Adults: Oral: 50-100 mg 2-3 times/day
Nursing/Pharmacy Information May cause an alteration in taste, especially when drinking carbonated beverages
Dosage Forms Tablet: 25 mg, 50 mg

methenamine (meth EN a meen)

Synonyms hexamethylenetetramine
U.S. Brand Names Hiprex®; Mandelamine®; Urex®
Canadian Brand Names Dehydral™; Urasal®
Generic Available Yes
Therapeutic Category Antibiotic, Miscellaneous
Use Prophylaxis or suppression of recurrent urinary tract infections
Usual Dosage Oral:
Children:
Hippurate: 6-12 years: 25-50 mg/kg/day divided every 12 hours
Mandelate: 50-75 mg/kg/day divided every 6 hours
Adults:
Hippurate: 1 g twice daily
Mandelate: 1 g 4 times/day after meals and at bedtime
Dietary Considerations Foods/diets which alkalinize urine pH >5.5 decrease activity of methenamine; cranberry juice can be used to acidify urine and increase activity of methenamine

Nursing/Pharmacy Information
Urine should be acidic, pH <5.5 for maximum effect
Monitor urinalysis, periodic liver function tests in patients
Stability: Protect from excessive heat
Dosage Forms
Methenamine hippurate:
Tablet, (Hiprex®, Urex®): 1 g (Hiprex® contains tartrazine dye)
Methenamine mandelate:
Tablet, enteric coated: 500 mg, 1 g

♦ **Methergine®** *see* methylergonovine *on page 407*

methimazole (meth IM a zole)
Synonyms thiamazole
U.S. Brand Names Tapazole®
Generic Available No
Therapeutic Category Antithyroid Agent
Use Palliative treatment of hyperthyroidism, to return the hyperthyroid patient to a normal metabolic state prior to thyroidectomy, and to control thyrotoxic crisis that may accompany thyroidectomy
Usual Dosage Oral:
Children: Initial: 0.4 mg/kg/day in 3 divided doses; maintenance: 0.2 mg/kg/day in 3 divided doses
Adults: Initial: 10 mg every 8 hours; maintenance dose ranges from 5-30 mg/day
Dietary Considerations Should be administered consistently in relation to meals every day
Nursing/Pharmacy Information
Monitor for signs of hypothyroidism, hyperthyroidism, T_4, T_3, CBC with differential, liver function (baseline and as needed), serum thyroxine, free thyroxine index
Stability: Protect from light
Dosage Forms Tablet: 5 mg, 10 mg

methionine (me THYE oh neen)
U.S. Brand Names Pedameth®
Generic Available Yes
Therapeutic Category Dietary Supplement
Use Treatment of diaper rash and control of odor, dermatitis and ulceration caused by ammoniacal urine
Usual Dosage Oral:
Children: Control of diaper rash: 75 mg in formula or other liquid 3-4 times/day for 3-5 days
Adults:
Control of odor in incontinent adults: 200-400 mg 3-4 times/day
Dietary supplement: 500 mg/day
Nursing/Pharmacy Information Mix with formula, milk, or other liquid
Dosage Forms
Capsule: 200 mg, 300 mg, 500 mg
Liquid: 75 mg/5 mL (473 mL)
Tablet: 500 mg

methocarbamol (meth oh KAR ba mole)
U.S. Brand Names Robaxin®
Generic Available Yes
Therapeutic Category Skeletal Muscle Relaxant
Use Treatment of muscle spasm associated with acute painful musculoskeletal conditions; supportive therapy in tetanus
Usual Dosage
Children: Recommended **only** for use in tetanus I.V.: 15 mg/kg/dose or 500 mg/m²/dose, may repeat every 6 hours if needed; maximum dose: 1.8 g/m²/day for 3 days only
Adults: Muscle spasm:
Oral: 1.5 g 4 times/day for 2-3 days, then decrease to 4-4.5 g/day in 3-6 divided doses
I.M., I.V.: 1 g every 8 hours if oral not possible
Dietary Considerations Tablets may be crushed and mixed with food or liquid if needed
Nursing/Pharmacy Information
Avoid infiltration, extremely irritating to tissues; may be injected directly without dilution at a maximum rate of 180 mg/m²/minute; may also be diluted in
(Continued)

methocarbamol *(Continued)*

normal saline or 5% dextrose to a concentration of 4 mg/mL and infused more slowly; patient should be in the recumbent position during and for 10-15 minutes after I.V. administration

Stability: Injection when diluted to 4 mg/mL in sterile water, 5% dextrose, or 0.9% saline is stable for 6 days at room temperature; do **not** refrigerate after dilution

Dosage Forms
Injection: 100 mg/mL in polyethylene glycol 50% (10 mL)
Tablet: 500 mg, 750 mg

methocarbamol and aspirin *(meth oh KAR ba mole & AS pir in)*

Synonyms aspirin and methocarbamol
U.S. Brand Names Robaxisal®
Generic Available Yes
Therapeutic Category Skeletal Muscle Relaxant
Use Adjunct to rest, physical therapy, and other measures for the relief of discomfort associated with acute, painful musculoskeletal disorders
Usual Dosage Children >12 years and Adults: Oral: 2 tablets 4 times/day
Dietary Considerations May be administered with food to minimize GI upset
Dosage Forms Tablet: Methocarbamol 400 mg and aspirin 325 mg

methohexital *(meth oh HEKS i tal)*

U.S. Brand Names Brevital® Sodium
Canadian Brand Names Brietal Sodium®
Generic Available No
Therapeutic Category Barbiturate
Controlled Substance C-IV
Use Induction and maintenance of general anesthesia for short procedures
Usual Dosage Doses must be titrated to effect
Children:
I.M.: Preop: 5-10 mg/kg/dose
I.V.: Induction: 1-2 mg/kg/dose
Rectal: Preop/induction: 20-35 mg/kg/dose; usual: 25 mg/kg/dose; administer as 10% aqueous solution
Adults: I.V.: Induction: 50-120 mg to start; 20-40 mg every 4-7 minutes
Nursing/Pharmacy Information
Avoid extravasation or intra-arterial administration; dilute to a maximum concentration of 1% for I.V. use
Monitor blood pressure, heart rate, respiratory rate
Stability: Do not dilute with solutions containing bacteriostatic agents; solutions are alkaline (pH 9.5-11) and **incompatible** with acids (eg, atropine sulfate, succinylcholine, silicone), also **incompatible** with phenol-containing solutions and silicone
Dosage Forms Injection, as sodium: 500 mg, 2.5 g, 5 g

♦ **methoin** *see* mephenytoin *on page 393*

methotrexate *(meth oh TREKS ate)*

Synonyms amethopterin; MTX
U.S. Brand Names Folex® PFS™; Rheumatrex®
Mexican Brand Names Ledertrexate
Generic Available Yes
Therapeutic Category Antineoplastic Agent
Use Treatment of trophoblastic neoplasms, leukemias, osteosarcoma, non-Hodgkin's lymphoma; psoriasis, rheumatoid arthritis
Usual Dosage Refer to individual protocols
Children:
High-dose MTX for acute lymphocytic leukemia: I.V.: Loading dose of 200 mg/m^2 and a 24-hour infusion of 1200 mg/m^2/day
Induction of remission in acute lymphoblastic leukemias: Oral, I.M., I.V.: 3.3 mg/m^2/day for 4-6 weeks
Leukemia: Remission maintenance: Oral, I.M.: 20-30 mg/m^2 2 times/week
Juvenile rheumatoid arthritis: Oral: 5-15 mg/m^2/week as a single dose or as 3 divided doses administered 12 hours apart
Osteosarcoma:
I.T.: 10-15 mg/m^2 (maximum dose: 15 mg) by protocol
I.V.: <12 years: 12 g/m^2 (12-18 g); >12 years: 8 g/m^2 (maximum dose: 18 g)
Non-Hodgkin's lymphoma: I.V.: 200-300 mg/m^2

Adults:
Trophoblastic neoplasms: Oral, I.M.: 15-30 mg/day for 5 days, repeat in 7 days for 3-5 courses
Rheumatoid arthritis: Oral: 7.5 mg once weekly or 2.5 mg every 12 hours for 3 doses/week; not to exceed 20 mg/week

Dietary Considerations Milk-rich foods may decrease MTX absorption; folate may decrease drug response

Nursing/Pharmacy Information
For intrathecal use, mix methotrexate without preservatives with normal saline or lactated Ringer's to a concentration no greater than 2 mg/mL; can be administered I.V. push, I.V. intermittent infusion, or I.V. continuous infusion at a concentration <25 mg/mL; doses >100-300 mg/m^2 are usually administered by I.V. continuous infusion and are followed by a course of leucovorin rescue

Monitor CBC with differential and platelet count, creatinine clearance, serum creatinine, BUN, and hepatic function tests, LFTs every 3-4 months, chest x-ray; for prolonged use (especially rheumatoid arthritis, psoriasis) a baseline liver biopsy, repeated at each 1-1.5 g cumulative dose interval, should be performed

Stability: Store intact vials at room temperature; intrathecal solutions should be diluted immediately prior to use; reconstituted solutions remain stable for 4 weeks at room temperature and 3 months when refrigerated; protect from light

Dosage Forms Methotrexate sodium:
Injection: 2.5 mg/mL (2 mL); 25 mg/mL (2 mL, 4 mL, 8 mL, 10 mL)
Injection, preservative free: 25 mg (2 mL, 4 mL, 8 mL, 10 mL)
Powder, for injection: 20 mg, 25 mg, 50 mg, 100 mg, 250 mg, 1 g
Tablet: 2.5 mg
Tablet, dose pack: 2.5 mg (4 cards with 2, 3, 4, 5, or 6 tablets each)

methotrimeprazine (meth oh trye MEP ra zeen)

Synonyms levomepromazine
U.S. Brand Names Levoprome®
Generic Available No
Therapeutic Category Analgesic, Non-narcotic
Use Relief of moderate to severe pain in nonambulatory patients; for analgesia and sedation when respiratory depression is to be avoided, as in obstetrics; preanesthetic for producing sedation, somnolence and relief of apprehension and anxiety
Usual Dosage Adults: I.M.:
Sedation analgesia: 10-20 mg every 4-6 hours as needed
Preoperative medication: 2-20 mg, 45 minutes to 3 hours before surgery
Postoperative analgesia: 2.5-7.5 mg every 4-6 hours is suggested as necessary since residual effects of anesthetic may be present
Pre- and postoperative hypotension: I.M.: 5-10 mg
Nursing/Pharmacy Information May cause drowsiness, rise slowly after sitting or lying after administration
Dosage Forms Injection, as hydrochloride: 20 mg/mL (10 mL)

methoxamine (meth OKS a meen)

U.S. Brand Names Vasoxyl®
Generic Available No
Therapeutic Category Adrenergic Agonist Agent
Use Treatment of hypotension occurring during general anesthesia; to terminate episodes of supraventricular tachycardia; treatment of shock
Usual Dosage Adults:
Emergencies: I.V.: 3-5 mg
Supraventricular tachycardia: I.V.: 10 mg
During spinal anesthesia: I.M.: 10-20 mg
Dosage Forms Injection, as hydrochloride: 20 mg/mL (1 mL)

methoxsalen (meth OKS a len)

Synonyms methoxypsoralen
U.S. Brand Names Oxsoralen-Ultra®
Canadian Brand Names Ultramop™
Generic Available No
Therapeutic Category Psoralen
Use Symptomatic control of severe, recalcitrant, disabling psoriasis in conjunction with long wave ultraviolet radiation; induce repigmentation in vitiligo topical
(Continued)

methoxsalen *(Continued)*

repigmenting agent in conjunction with controlled doses of ultraviolet A (UVA) or sunlight

Usual Dosage

Psoriasis: Adults: Oral: 10-70 mg 1½-2 hours before exposure to ultraviolet light, 2-3 times at least 48 hours apart; dosage is based upon patient's body weight and skin type

Vitiligo: Children >12 years and Adults:

Oral: 20 mg 2-4 hours before exposure to UVA light or sunlight

Topical: Apply lotion 1-2 hours before exposure to UVA light, no more than once weekly

Dietary Considerations To reduce nausea, oral drug can be administered with food or milk or in 2 divided doses 30 minutes apart; avoid furocoumarin-containing foods (limes, figs, parsley, celery, cloves, lemon, mustard, carrots)

Nursing/Pharmacy Information If burning or blistering or intractable pruritus occurs, discontinue therapy until effects subside. Do not sunbathe for at least 24 hours prior to therapy or 48 hours after PUVA therapy. Avoid direct and indirect sunlight for 8 hours after oral and 12-48 hours after topical therapy. **If sunlight cannot be avoided, protective clothing and/or sunscreens must be worn.** Following oral therapy, wraparound sunglasses with UVA-absorbing properties must be worn for 24 hours. do not exceed prescribed dose or exposure times.

Dosage Forms

Capsule: 10 mg

Lotion: 1% (30 mL)

methoxycinnamate and oxybenzone

(meth OKS ee SIN a mate & oks i BEN zone)

Synonyms sunscreen (paba-free)

U.S. Brand Names PreSun® 29 [OTC]; Ti-Screen® [OTC]

Generic Available Yes

Therapeutic Category Sunscreen

Use Reduce the chance of premature aging of the skin and skin cancer from overexposure to the sun

Usual Dosage Adults: Topical: Apply liberally to all exposed areas at least 30 minutes prior to sun exposure

Dosage Forms Lotion:

SPF 15: 120 mL

SPF 29: 120 mL

methoxyflurane *(meth oks ee FLOO rane)*

U.S. Brand Names Penthrane®

Generic Available No

Therapeutic Category General Anesthetic

Use Adjunct to provide anesthesia procedures <4 hours in duration

Usual Dosage 0.3% to 0.8% for analgesia and anesthesia, with 0.1% to 2% for maintenance when used with nitrous oxide

Dosage Forms Liquid: 15 mL, 125 mL

♦ **methoxypsoralen** *see methoxsalen on page 403*

methscopolamine *(meth skoe POL a meen)*

U.S. Brand Names Pamine®

Generic Available No

Therapeutic Category Anticholinergic Agent

Use Adjunctive therapy in the treatment of peptic ulcer

Usual Dosage Oral: 2.5 mg 30 minutes before meals or food and 2.5-5 mg at bedtime

Dietary Considerations Should be administered 30 minutes before meals or food

Dosage Forms Tablet, as bromide: 2.5 mg

methsuximide *(meth SUKS i mide)*

U.S. Brand Names Celontin®

Generic Available No

Therapeutic Category Anticonvulsant

Use Control of absence (petit mal) seizures; useful adjunct in refractory, partial complex (psychomotor) seizures

Usual Dosage Oral:
Children: Initial: 10-15 mg/kg/day in 3-4 divided doses; increase weekly up to maximum of 30 mg/kg/day
Adults: 300 mg/day for the first week; may increase by 300 mg/day at weekly intervals up to 1.2 g in 2-4 divided doses/day
Nursing/Pharmacy Information
Monitor CBC, hepatic function tests, urinalysis
Stability: Protect from high temperature
Dosage Forms Capsule: 150 mg, 300 mg

methyclothiazide (meth i kloe THYE a zide)
U.S. Brand Names Aquatensen®; Enduron®
Generic Available Yes
Therapeutic Category Diuretic, Thiazide
Use Management of mild to moderate hypertension; treatment of edema in congestive heart failure and nephrotic syndrome
Usual Dosage Adults: Oral:
Edema: 2.5-10 mg/day
Hypertension: 2.5-5 mg/day
Nursing/Pharmacy Information Monitor blood pressure, fluids, weight loss, serum potassium
Dosage Forms Tablet: 2.5 mg, 5 mg

methyclothiazide and deserpidine
(meth i kloe THYE a zide & de SER pi deen)
Synonyms deserpidine and methyclothiazide
U.S. Brand Names Enduronyl®; Enduronyl® Forte
Generic Available No
Therapeutic Category Antihypertensive Agent, Combination
Use Management of mild to moderately severe hypertension
Usual Dosage Oral: Individualized, normally 1-4 tablets/day
Dietary Considerations May be administered with food
Dosage Forms Tablet: Methyclothiazide 5 mg and deserpidine 0.25 mg; methyclothiazide 5 mg and deserpidine 0.5 mg

methyclothiazide and pargyline
(meth i kloe THYE a zide & PAR gi leen)
Synonyms pargyline and methyclothiazide
U.S. Brand Names Eutron®
Generic Available No
Therapeutic Category Antihypertensive Agent, Combination
Use Management of hypertension
Usual Dosage Oral: Individualized, normally 1-4 tablets/day
Dosage Forms Tablet: Methyclothiazide 5 mg and pargyline hydrochloride 25 mg

♦ **methylacetoxyprogesterone** see medroxyprogesterone acetate on page 389

methylbenzethonium chloride
(meth il ben ze THOE nee um KLOR ide)
U.S. Brand Names Diaparene® [OTC]; Puri-Clens™ [OTC]; Sween Cream® [OTC]
Generic Available No
Therapeutic Category Topical Skin Product
Use Treatment of diaper rash and ammonia dermatitis
Usual Dosage Topical: Apply to area as needed
Nursing/Pharmacy Information Notify physician if condition worsens or fails to improve within 4 days
Dosage Forms
Cream: 0.1% (30 g, 60 g, 120 g)
Ointment, topical: 0.1% (30 g, 60 g, 120 g)
Powder: 0.055% (120 g, 270 g, 420 g)

methylcellulose (meth il SEL yoo lose)
U.S. Brand Names Citrucel® [OTC]
Generic Available Yes
Therapeutic Category Laxative
Use Adjunct in treatment of constipation
Usual Dosage Oral:
Children: 5-10 mL 1-2 times/day
(Continued)

methylcellulose *(Continued)*
Adults: 5-20 mL 3 times/day
Dosage Forms Powder: 105 mg/g

methyldopa (meth il DOE pa)
U.S. Brand Names Aldomet®
Canadian Brand Names Apo®-Methyldopa; Dopamet®; Medimet®; Novo-Medopa®; Nu-Medopa®
Generic Available Yes
Therapeutic Category Alpha-Adrenergic Blocking Agent
Use Management of moderate to severe hypertension
Usual Dosage
Children:
Oral: Initial: 10 mg/kg/day in 2-4 divided doses; increase every 2 days as needed to maximum dose of 65 mg/kg/day; do not exceed 3 g/day
I.V.: 5-10 mg/kg/dose every 6-8 hours
Adults:
Oral: Initial: 250 mg 2-3 times/day; increase every 2 days as needed; usual dose 1-1.5 g/day in 2-4 divided doses; maximum dose: 3 g/day
I.V.: 250-1000 mg every 6-8 hours
Dietary Considerations Avoid natural licorice (causes sodium and water retention and increases potassium loss); dietary requirements for vitamin B_{12} and folate may be increased with high doses of methyldopa
Nursing/Pharmacy Information
May cause urine discoloration; infuse I.V. dose slowly over 30-60 minutes at a concentration ≤10 mg/mL
Monitor blood pressure, standing and sitting/lying down
Stability: Injectable dosage form is most stable at acid to neutral pH; stability of parenteral admixture at room temperature (25°C): 24 hours
Dosage Forms
Suspension, oral: 250 mg/5 mL (5 mL, 473 mL)
Tablet: 125 mg, 250 mg, 500 mg
Methyldopate hydrochloride: Injection: 50 mg/mL (5 mL, 10 mL)

♦ **methyldopa and chlorothiazide** *see* chlorothiazide and methyldopa *on page 137*

methyldopa and hydrochlorothiazide
(meth il DOE pa & hye droe klor oh THYE a zide)
Synonyms hydrochlorothiazide and methyldopa
U.S. Brand Names Aldoril®
Generic Available Yes
Therapeutic Category Antihypertensive Agent, Combination
Use Management of moderate to severe hypertension
Usual Dosage Oral: 1 tablet 2-3 times/day for first 48 hours, then decrease or increase at intervals of not less than 2 days until an adequate response is achieved
Dosage Forms Tablet:
15: Methyldopa 250 mg and hydrochlorothiazide 15 mg
25: Methyldopa 250 mg and hydrochlorothiazide 25 mg
D30: Methyldopa 500 mg and hydrochlorothiazide 30 mg
D50: Methyldopa 500 mg and hydrochlorothiazide 50 mg

methylene blue (METH i leen bloo)
U.S. Brand Names Urolene Blue®
Generic Available Yes
Therapeutic Category Antidote
Use Antidote for cyanide poisoning and drug-induced methemoglobinemia, indicator dye, bacteriostatic genitourinary antiseptic
Usual Dosage
Children:
NADH-methemoglobin reductase deficiency: Oral: 1.5-5 mg/kg/day (maximum: 300 mg/day) administered with 5-8 mg/kg/day of ascorbic acid
Methemoglobinemia: I.V.: 1-2 mg/kg over several minutes
Adults:
Genitourinary antiseptic: Oral: 55-130 mg 3 times/day (maximum: 390 mg/day)
Methemoglobinemia: I.V.: 1-2 mg/kg over several minutes; may be repeated in 1 hour if necessary
Nursing/Pharmacy Information Parenteral: Administer undiluted by direct I.V. injection over several minutes

Dosage Forms
Injection: 10 mg/mL (1 mL, 10 mL)
Tablet: 65 mg

methylergonovine (meth il er goe NOE veen)
U.S. Brand Names Methergine®
Generic Available No
Therapeutic Category Ergot Alkaloid and Derivative
Use Prevention and treatment of postpartum and postabortion hemorrhage caused by uterine atony or subinvolution
Usual Dosage Adults:
Oral: 0.2-0.4 mg every 6-12 hours for 2-7 days
I.M., I.V.: 0.2 mg every 2-4 hours for 5 doses then change to oral dosage
Nursing/Pharmacy Information Ampuls containing discolored solution should not be used
Dosage Forms Methylergonovine maleate:
Injection: 0.2 mg/mL (1 mL)
Tablet: 0.2 mg

♦ **methylmorphine** see codeine on page 164

methylphenidate (meth il FEN i date)
U.S. Brand Names Ritalin®; Ritalin-SR®
Canadian Brand Names PMS-Methylphenidate
Generic Available Yes
Therapeutic Category Central Nervous System Stimulant, Nonamphetamine
Controlled Substance C-II
Use Attention-deficit/hyperactivity disorder (ADHD); narcolepsy
Usual Dosage Oral:
Children ≥6 years: Attention deficit disorder: Initial: 0.3 mg/kg/dose or 2.5-5 mg/dose administered before breakfast and lunch; increase by 0.1 mg/kg/dose or by 5-10 mg/day at weekly intervals; usual dose: 0.5-1 mg/kg/day; maximum dose: 2 mg/kg/day or 60 mg/day
Adults: Narcolepsy: 10 mg 2-3 times/day, up to 60 mg/day
Dietary Considerations Food may increase oral absorption
Nursing/Pharmacy Information Do not crush or allow patient to chew sustained release dosage form; last daily dose should be administered several hours before retiring
Dosage Forms Methylphenidate hydrochloride:
Tablet: 5 mg, 10 mg, 20 mg
Tablet, sustained release: 20 mg

♦ **methylphenobarbital** see mephobarbital on page 393
♦ **methylphenylethylhydantoin** see mephenytoin on page 393
♦ **methylphenyl isoxazolyl penicillin** see oxacillin on page 459
♦ **methylphytyl napthoquinone** see phytonadione on page 493

methylprednisolone (meth il pred NIS oh lone)
Synonyms 6-α-methylprednisolone
U.S. Brand Names Adlone® Injection; A-methaPred® Injection; depMedalone® Injection; Depoject® Injection; Depo-Medrol® Injection; Depopred® Injection; D-Med® Injection; Duralone® Injection; Medralone® Injection; Medrol® Oral; M-Prednisol® Injection; Solu-Medrol® Injection
Canadian Brand Names Medrol® Veriderm® Cream
Mexican Brand Names Cryosolona
Generic Available Yes
Therapeutic Category Adrenal Corticosteroid
Use Anti-inflammatory or immunosuppressant agent in the treatment of a variety of diseases including those of hematologic, allergic, inflammatory, neoplastic, and autoimmune origin
Usual Dosage Methylprednisolone sodium succinate is highly soluble and has a rapid effect by I.M. and I.V. routes. Methylprednisolone acetate has a low solubility and has a sustained I.M. effect.

Children:
Anti-inflammatory or immunosuppressive: Oral, I.M., I.V. (sodium succinate): 0.16-0.8 mg/kg/day or 5-25 mg/m²/day in divided doses every 6-12 hours
Status asthmaticus: I.V. (sodium succinate): Loading dose: 2 mg/kg/dose, then 0.5-1 mg/kg/dose every 6 hours for up to 5 days
Lupus nephritis: I.V. (sodium succinate): 30 mg/kg every other day for 6 doses
(Continued)

methylprednisolone *(Continued)*

Adults:

Anti-inflammatory or immunosuppressive: Oral: 4-48 mg/day to start, followed by gradual reduction in dosage to the lowest possible level consistent with maintaining an adequate clinical response

I.M. (sodium succinate): 10-80 mg/day once daily

I.M. (acetate): 40-120 mg every 1-2 weeks

I.V. (sodium succinate): 10-40 mg over a period of several minutes and repeated I.V. or I.M. at intervals depending on clinical response; when high dosages are needed, administer 30 mg/kg over a period of 10-20 minutes and may be repeated every 4-6 hours for 48 hours

Status asthmaticus: I.V. (sodium succinate): Loading dose: 2 mg/kg/dose, then 0.5-1 mg/kg/dose every hours for up to 5 days

Lupus nephritis:

I.V. (sodium succinate): 1 g/day for 3 days

Intra-articular (acetate):

Large joints: 20-80 mg

Small joints: 4-10 mg

Intralesional (acetate): 20-60 mg

Dietary Considerations Should be administered after meals or with food or milk; limit caffeine; need diet rich in pyridoxine, vitamin C, vitamin D, folate, calcium, phosphorus, and protein

Nursing/Pharmacy Information

Do **not** administer acetate form I.V.; Succinate: I.V. push over 1-15 minutes; intermittent infusion over 15-60 minutes; maximum concentration: IVP: 125 mg/mL; I.V. infusion: 2.5 mg/mL

Monitor blood pressure, blood glucose, electrolytes

Stability: Parenteral admixture (Solu-Medrol®) at room temperature (25°C) or at refrigeration (4°C): 24 hours

Dosage Forms

Injection:

As acetate: 20 mg/mL (5 mL, 10 mL); 40 mg/mL (1 mL, 5 mL, 10 mL); 80 mg/mL (1 mL, 5 mL)

As sodium succinate: 40 mg (1 mL, 3 mL); 125 mg (2 mL, 5 mL); 500 mg (1 mL, 4 mL, 8 mL, 20 mL); 1000 mg (1 mL, 8 mL, 50 mL); 2000 mg (30.6 mL)

Tablet: 2 mg, 4 mg, 8 mg, 16 mg, 24 mg, 32 mg

Dose pack: 4 mg (21s)

♦ **6-α-methylprednisolone** *see* methylprednisolone *on page 407*

♦ **4-methylpyrazole** *see* fomepizole *on page 282*

methyltestosterone *(meth il tes TOS te rone)*

U.S. Brand Names Android®; Oreton® Methyl; Testred®; Virilon®

Generic Available Yes

Therapeutic Category Androgen

Use

Male: Hypogonadism; delayed puberty; impotence and climacteric symptoms

Female: Palliative treatment of metastatic breast cancer; postpartum breast pain and/or engorgement

Usual Dosage Adults:

Male:

Oral: 10-40 mg/day

Buccal: 5-20 mg/day

Female:

Breast pain/engorgement:

Oral: 80 mg/day for 3-5 days

Buccal: 40 mg/day for 3-5 days

Breast cancer:

Oral: 200 mg/day

Buccal: 100 mg/day

Nursing/Pharmacy Information In prepubertal children, perform radiographic examination of the hand and wrist every 6 months to determine the rate of bone maturation and to assess the effect of treatment on the epiphyseal centers

Dosage Forms

Capsule: 10 mg

Tablet: 10 mg, 25 mg

Buccal: 5 mg, 10 mg

methysergide (meth i SER jide)

U.S. Brand Names Sansert®

Generic Available No

Therapeutic Category Ergot Alkaloid and Derivative

Use Prophylaxis of vascular headache

Usual Dosage Oral: 4-8 mg/day with meals; if no improvement is noted after 3 weeks, drug is unlikely to be beneficial; must not be administered continuously for longer than 6 months, and a drug-free interval of 3-4 weeks must follow each 6-month course; dosage should be tapered over the 2- to 3-week period before drug discontinuation to avoid rebound headaches

Dietary Considerations May be administered with food or milk

Nursing/Pharmacy Information Advise patient to make position changes slowly

Dosage Forms Tablet, as maleate: 2 mg

♦ **Meticorten®** see prednisone on page 515

♦ **Metimyd® Ophthalmic** see sulfacetamide and prednisolone on page 585

metipranolol (met i PRAN oh lol)

U.S. Brand Names OptiPranolol® Ophthalmic

Generic Available No

Therapeutic Category Beta-Adrenergic Blocker

Use Agent for lowering intraocular pressure

Usual Dosage Adults: Ophthalmic: 1 drop in the affected eye(s) twice daily

Nursing/Pharmacy Information Monitor for systemic effect of beta blockade

Dosage Forms Solution, ophthalmic, as hydrochloride: 0.3% (5 mL, 10 mL)

♦ **Metizol® Tablet (Discontinued)** see page 743

metoclopramide (met oh kloe PRA mide)

U.S. Brand Names Clopra®; Maxolon®; Octamide®; Reglan®

Canadian Brand Names Apo®-Metoclop; Maxeran®

Mexican Brand Names Carnotprim Primperan®; Carnotprim Primperan® Retard; Meclomid; Plasil; Pramotil

Generic Available Yes

Therapeutic Category Gastrointestinal Agent, Prokinetic

Use Gastroesophageal reflux; prevention of nausea associated with chemotherapy; facilitates intubation of the small intestine and symptomatic treatment of diabetic gastric stasis

Usual Dosage

Children:

Gastroesophageal reflux: Oral: 0.1 mg/kg/dose up to 4 times/day; efficacy of continuing metoclopramide beyond 12 weeks in reflux has not been determined; total daily dose should not exceed 0.5 mg/kg/day

Gastrointestinal hypomotility: Oral, I.M., I.V.: 0.1 mg/kg/dose up to 4 times/day, not to exceed 0.5 mg/kg/day

Antiemetic: I.V.: 1-2 mg/kg 30 minutes before chemotherapy and every 2-4 hours

Facilitate intubation: I.V.: <6 years: 0.1 mg/kg; 6-14 years: 2.5-5 mg

Adults:

Stasis/reflux: Oral: 10-15 mg/dose up to 4 times/day 30 minutes before meals or food and at bedtime; efficacy of continuing metoclopramide beyond 12 weeks in reflux has not been determined

Gastrointestinal hypomotility: Oral, I.M., I.V.: 10 mg 30 minutes before each meal and at bedtime

Antiemetic: I.V.: 1-2 mg/kg 30 minutes before chemotherapy and every 2-4 hours

Facilitate intubation: I.V.: 10 mg

Dietary Considerations Should be administered 30 minutes before meals and at bedtime

Nursing/Pharmacy Information

Parenteral doses of up to 10 mg should be administered I.V. push over 1-2 minutes; rapid boluses cause transient anxiety and restlessness followed by drowsiness; higher doses to be administered IVPB; dilute to 0.2 mg/mL (maximum concentration: 5 mg/mL) and infuse over 15-30 minutes (maximum rate of infusion: 5 mg/minute); rapid I.V. administration is associated with a transient but intense feeling of anxiety and restlessness, followed by drowsiness

Monitor periodic renal function test

(Continued)

metoclopramide *(Continued)*

Stability: Dilutions do not require light protection if used within 24 hours; stability of parenteral admixture at room temperature (25°C) and at refrigeration temperature (4°C): 2 days

Dosage Forms
Injection: 5 mg/mL (2 mL, 10 mL, 30 mL, 50 mL, 100 mL)
Solution, oral, concentrated: 10 mg/mL (10 mL, 30 mL)
Syrup, sugar free: 5 mg/5 mL (10 mL, 480 mL)
Tablet: 5 mg, 10 mg

metocurine iodide *(met oh KYOOR een EYE oh dide)*

Synonyms dimethyl tubocurarine iodide
U.S. Brand Names Metubine® Iodide
Generic Available No
Therapeutic Category Skeletal Muscle Relaxant
Use Adjunct to anesthesia to induce skeletal muscle relaxation
Usual Dosage I.V.:
Children:
Chronic respiratory paralysis in neonates: Start 0.25-0.5 mg/kg/dose (repeat once if paralysis is not achieved in 3 minutes); maintenance: repeat previous dose as soon as movement is observed. The dose should be titrated to achieve a dosage interval of 3-4 hours, then plateau at 10-20 mg/kg/24 hours
Neuromuscular blockade for surgery: Initial: 0.2-0.4 mg/kg/dose; maintenance: 0.1-0.25 mg/kg/dose every 25-90 minutes
Adults:
Surgery: Initial: 0.2-0.4 mg/kg; supplement dose: 0.5-1 mg; use of anesthetics that potentiate effect of neuromuscular blocking drug requires less metocurine
Electric shock therapy: 1.75-5.5 mg
Nursing/Pharmacy Information
Less histaminic release or ganglionic blockade than other curares, otherwise comparable
Stability: Unstable in alkaline solutions; may precipitate if mixed with barbiturates
Dosage Forms Injection: 2 mg/mL (20 mL)

metolazone *(me TOLE a zone)*

U.S. Brand Names Mykrox®; Zaroxolyn®
Generic Available No
Therapeutic Category Diuretic, Miscellaneous
Use Management of mild to moderate hypertension; treatment of edema in congestive heart failure, nephrotic syndrome, and impaired renal function
Usual Dosage Oral:
Children: 0.2-0.4 mg/kg/day divided every 12-24 hours
Adults:
Edema: 5-20 mg/dose every 24 hours
Hypertension: 2.5-5 mg/dose every 24 hours
Dietary Considerations This product may cause a potassium loss; your physician may prescribe a potassium supplement, another medication to help prevent the potassium loss, or recommend that you eat foods high in potassium, especially citrus fruits; do not change your diet on your own while taking this medication, especially if you are taking potassium supplements or medications to reduce potassium loss; too much potassium can be as harmful as too little; avoid natural licorice; should be administered after breakfast
Nursing/Pharmacy Information Monitor serum electrolytes; check patient for orthostasis
Dosage Forms Tablet:
Zaroxolyn® (slow acting): 2.5 mg, 5 mg, 10 mg
Mykrox® (rapidly acting): 0.5 mg

♦ **Metopirone® Tablet *(Discontinued)* see page 743**

metoprolol *(me toe PROE lole)*

U.S. Brand Names Lopressor®; Toprol XL®
Canadian Brand Names Apo-Metoprolol®; Betaloc®; Betaloc Durules®; Novo-Metoprolol®; Nu-Metop
Mexican Brand Names Kenaprol; Lopresor; Proken M; Prolaken; Ritmolol; Seloken; Selopres
Generic Available Yes

Therapeutic Category Beta-Adrenergic Blocker

Use Treatment of hypertension and angina pectoris; prevention of myocardial infarction; selective inhibitor of beta$_1$-adrenergic receptors

Usual Dosage Safety and efficacy in children have not been established.

Children: Oral: 1-5 mg/kg/24 hours divided twice daily; allow 3 days between dose adjustments

Adults:

Oral: 100-450 mg/day in 2-3 divided doses, begin with 50 mg twice daily and increase doses at weekly intervals to desired effect

I.V.: 5 mg every 2 minutes for 3 doses in early treatment of myocardial infarction; thereafter administer 50 mg orally every 6 hours 15 minutes after last I.V. dose and continue for 48 hours; then administer a maintenance dose of 100 mg twice daily

Dietary Considerations Should be administered with food, as food increases absorption

Nursing/Pharmacy Information Monitor hemodynamic status carefully after acute MI, monitor orthostatic blood pressures, apical and peripheral pulse and mental status changes (ie, confusion, depression)

Dosage Forms

Metoprolol succinate:

Tablet, sustained release: 50 mg, 100 mg, 200 mg

Metoprolol tartrate:

Injection: 1 mg/mL (5 mL)

Tablet: 50 mg, 100 mg

- ♦ **Metoxiprim** *see* co-trimoxazole *on page 170*
- ♦ **Metra®** *(Discontinued) see page 743*
- ♦ **Metreton® Ophthalmic** *see* prednisolone (ophthalmic) *on page 514*
- ♦ **Metrocream™** *see* metronidazole *on page 411*
- ♦ **Metrodin®** *see* urofollitropin *on page 639*
- ♦ **MetroGel® Topical** *see* metronidazole *on page 411*
- ♦ **MetroGel®-Vaginal** *see* metronidazole *on page 411*
- ♦ **Metro I.V.® Injection** *see* metronidazole *on page 411*

metronidazole (me troe NI da zole)

U.S. Brand Names Flagyl® Oral; MetroGel® Topical; MetroGel®-Vaginal; Metro I.V.® Injection; Protostat® Oral

Canadian Brand Names Apo®-Metronidazole; Metrocream™; Nidagel™; Noritate®; Novo-Nidazol®; TriKacide®

Mexican Brand Names Ameblin; Flagenase®; Milezzol; Otrozol; Vatrix-S; Vertisal

Generic Available Yes

Therapeutic Category Amebicide; Antibiotic, Topical; Antibiotic, Miscellaneous; Antiprotozoal

Use Treatment of susceptible anaerobic bacterial and protozoal infections in the following conditions: amebiasis (liver abscess, dysentery), giardiasis, symptomatic and asymptomatic trichomoniasis; skin and skin structure infections, CNS infections, intra-abdominal infections, and systemic anaerobic bacterial infections; topically for the treatment of acne rosacea; treatment of antibiotic-associated pseudomembranous colitis (AAPC) caused by *C. difficile*; bacterial vaginosis

Usual Dosage

Infants and Children:

Amebiasis: Oral: 35-50 mg/kg/day in divided doses every 8 hours

Other parasitic Infections: Oral: 15-30 mg/kg/day in divided doses every 8 hours

Anaerobic infections: Oral, I.V.: 30 mg/kg/day in divided doses every 6 hours

Clostridium difficile (antibiotic-associated colitis): Oral: 20 mg/kg/day divided every 6 hours

Maximum dose: 2 g/day

Adults:

Amebiasis: Oral: 500-750 mg every 8 hours

Other parasitic infections: Oral: 250 mg every 8 hours or 2 g as a single dose

Anaerobic infections: Oral, I.V.: 30 mg/kg/day in divided doses every 6 hours; not to exceed 4 g/day

AAPC: Oral: 250-500 mg 3-4 times/day for 10-14 days

Topical: Apply a thin film twice daily to affected areas

Vaginal: One applicatorful in vagina each morning and evening or given once daily at bedtime

Dietary Considerations May be administered with food because of gastric irritation, however, there is delayed absorption with food; alcohol will cause (Continued)

metronidazole *(Continued)*

"disulfiram"-type reaction consisting of flushing, headache, nausea, and in some patients, vomiting and chest and/or abdominal pain

Nursing/Pharmacy Information

Avoid contact between the drug and aluminum in the infusion set; administer I.V. by slow intermittent infusion over 30-60 minutes at a final concentration for administration of 5-8 mg/mL

Monitor WBC count

Stability: Reconstituted solution is stable for 96 hours when refrigerated; for I.V. infusion in normal saline or D_5W and neutralized (with sodium bicarbonate), solution is stable for 24 hours at room temperature; do not refrigerate neutralized solution because a precipitate will occur

Dosage Forms

Capsule: 375 mg

Cream: 0.75% (45 g); 1% (30 g)

Gel, topical: 0.75% [7.5 mg/mL] (30 g)

Gel, vaginal: 0.75% (5 g applicator delivering 37.5 mg in 70 g tube)

Injection, ready to use: 5 mg/mL (100 mL)

Lotion: 0.75%

Powder for injection, as hydrochloride: 500 mg

Tablet: 250 mg, 500 mg

Tablet, extended release: 750 mg

♦ **Metubine® Iodide** *see* metocurine iodide *on page 410*

metyrapone *(me TEER a pone)*

Generic Available No

Therapeutic Category Diagnostic Agent

Use Diagnostic test for hypothalamic-pituitary ACTH function

Usual Dosage Oral:

Children: 15 mg/kg every 4 hours for 6 doses; minimum dose: 250 mg

Adults: 750 mg every 4 hours for 6 doses

Dosage Forms Capsule, as tartrate: 250 mg

metyrosine *(me TYE roe seen)*

Synonyms AMPT; OGMT

U.S. Brand Names Demser®

Generic Available No

Therapeutic Category Tyrosine Hydroxylase Inhibitor

Use Short-term management of pheochromocytoma before surgery, long-term management when surgery is contraindicated or when malignant

Usual Dosage Children >12 years and Adults: Oral: Initial: 250 mg 4 times/day, increased by 250-500 mg/day up to 4 g/day; maintenance: 2-3 g/day in 4 divided doses; for preoperative preparation, administer optimum effective dosage for 5-7 days

Nursing/Pharmacy Information Administer plenty of fluids each day; may cause drowsiness, impair coordination and judgment; notify physician if drooling, tremors, speech difficulty, or diarrhea occurs; avoid alcohol and central nervous system depressants

Dosage Forms Capsule: 250 mg

♦ **Mevacor®** *see* lovastatin *on page 377*

♦ **Meval®** *see* diazepam *on page 196*

♦ **mevinolin** *see* lovastatin *on page 377*

mexiletine *(MEKS i le teen)*

U.S. Brand Names Mexitil®

Generic Available Yes

Therapeutic Category Antiarrhythmic Agent, Class I-B

Use Management of serious ventricular arrhythmias; suppression of PVCs

Unlabeled use: Diabetic neuropathy

Usual Dosage Oral:

Children: Range: 1.4-5 mg/kg/dose (mean: 3.3 mg/kg/dose) administered every 8 hours; start with lower initial dose and increase according to effects and serum concentrations

Adults: Initial: 200 mg every 8 hours (may load with 400 mg if necessary); adjust dose every 2-3 days; usual dose: 200-300 mg every 8 hours; maximum dose: 1.2 g/day (some patients respond to every 12-hour dosing)

Dietary Considerations Food may decrease the rate, but not the extent of oral absorption; diets which affect urine pH can increase or decrease excretion of mexiletine; avoid dietary changes that alter urine pH

Nursing/Pharmacy Information Administer around-the-clock rather than 4 times/day, 3 times/day, etc, (ie, 12-6-12-6, not 9-1-5-9) to promote less variation in peak and trough serum levels

Dosage Forms Capsule: 150 mg, 200 mg, 250 mg

♦ **Mexitil®** *see* mexiletine *on page 412*

♦ **Mezlin®** *see* mezlocillin *on page 413*

mezlocillin (mez loe SIL in)

U.S. Brand Names Mezlin®

Generic Available No

Therapeutic Category Penicillin

Use Treatment of infections caused by susceptible gram-negative aerobic bacilli (*Klebsiella, Proteus, Escherichia coli, Enterobacter, Pseudomonas aeruginosa, Serratia*) involving the skin and skin structure, bone and joint, respiratory tract, urinary tract, gastrointestinal tract, as well as septicemia

Usual Dosage I.M., I.V.:

Children: 200-300 mg/kg/day divided every 4-6 hours; maximum: 24 g/day

Adults:

Uncomplicated urinary tract infection: 1.5-2 g every 6 hours

Serious infections: 3-4 g every 4-6 hours

Nursing/Pharmacy Information

Administer around-the-clock rather than 4 times/day, 3 times/day, etc, (ie, 12-6-12-6, not 9-1-5-9) to promote less variation in peak and trough serum levels; dosage modification required in patients with impaired renal function; administer I.M. injections in large muscle mass, not more than 2 g/injection. I.M. injections administered over 12-15 seconds will be less painful. Administer IVP over 3-5 minutes at a final concentration for administration not to exceed 100 mg/mL or administer by I.V. intermittent infusion over 15-30 minutes at a concentration of 10-20 mg/mL; maximum concentration for administration in a fluid-restricted patient: 178 mg/mL

Monitor serum electrolytes; periodic renal, hepatic, and hematologic function tests

Stability: Reconstituted solution is stable for 48 hours at room temperature and 7 days when refrigerated; for I.V. infusion in normal saline or D_5W solution is stable for 48 hours at room temperature, 7 days when refrigerated or 28 days when frozen; after freezing, thawed solution is stable for 48 hours at room temperature or 7 days when refrigerated; if precipitation occurs under refrigeration, warm in water bath (37°C) for 20 minutes and shake well

Dosage Forms Powder for injection, as sodium: 1 g, 2 g, 3 g, 4 g, 20 g

♦ **Miacalcin®** *see* calcitonin *on page 102*

♦ **Miacalcin® Nasal Spray** *see* calcitonin *on page 102*

♦ **Micanol® Cream** *see* anthralin *on page 50*

♦ **Micardis®** *see* telmisartan *on page 594*

♦ **Micatin® Topical [OTC]** *see* miconazole *on page 413*

miconazole (mi KON a zole)

U.S. Brand Names Absorbine® Antifungal Foot Powder [OTC]; Breezee® Mist Antifungal [OTC]; Femizol-M® [OTC]; Fungoid® Creme; Fungoid® Tincture; Lotrimin® AF Powder [OTC]; Lotrimin® AF Spray Liquid [OTC]; Lotrimin® AF Spray Powder [OTC]; Maximum Strength Desenex® Antifungal Cream [OTC]; Micatin® Topical [OTC]; Monistat-Derm™ Topical; Monistat i.v.™ Injection; Monistat™ Vaginal; M-Zole® 7 Dual Pack [OTC]; Ony-Clear® Spray; Prescription Strength Desenex® [OTC]; Zeasorb-AF® Powder [OTC]

Mexican Brand Names Aloid; Daktarin; Dermifun; Fungiquim; Gyno-Daktarin; Gyno-Daktarin V; Neomicol®

Generic Available Yes

Therapeutic Category Antifungal Agent

Use

I.V.: Treatment of severe systemic fungal infections and fungal meningitis due to susceptible *Cryptococcus* neoformans, *Candida albicans, Candida tropicalis, Candida parapsilosis, Coccidioides immitis*, and *Histoplasma capsulatum* that are refractory to standard treatment

Topical: Treatment of vulvovaginal candidiasis; topical treatment of superficial fungal infections

Usual Dosage

Children:

I.V.: 20-40 mg/kg/day divided every 8 hours

Topical: Apply twice daily for 2-4 weeks

(Continued)

miconazole *(Continued)*

Vaginal: Insert contents of one applicator of vaginal cream or 100 mg suppository at bedtime for 7 days, or 200 mg suppository at bedtime for 3 days

Adults:

I.T.: 20 mg every 3-7 days

I.V.: Candidiasis: 600-1800 mg/day divided every 8 hours

Topical: Apply twice daily for 2-4 weeks

Vaginal: Insert contents of one applicator of vaginal cream or 100 mg suppository at bedtime for 7 days, or 200 mg suppository at bedtime for 3 days

Coccidioidomycosis: 1800-3600 mg/day divided every 8 hours

Cryptococcosis: 1200-2400 mg/day divided every 8 hours

Paracoccidioidomycosis: 200-1200 mg/day divided every 8 hours

Nursing/Pharmacy Information

I.V. administration over 2 hours may minimize the potential for arrhythmias or anaphylactoid reactions; diphenhydramine may help to reduce pruritus; an antihistamine or antiemetic prior to miconazole administration, or dosage reduction, or slowing the I.V. rate and avoiding administration at mealtime may decrease nausea and vomiting

Monitor hematocrit, hemoglobin, serum electrolytes and lipids

Stability: Protect from heat; darkening of solution indicates deterioration; stability of parenteral admixture at room temperature (25°C): 2 days

Dosage Forms Miconazole nitrate:

Cream:

Topical: 2% (15 g, 30 g, 56.7 g, 85 g)

Vaginal: 2% (45 g is equivalent to 7 doses)

Injection: 1% [10 mg/mL] (20 mL)

Lotion: 2% (30 mL, 60 mL)

Powder, topical: 2% (45 g, 90 g, 113 g)

Spray, topical: 2% (105 mL)

Suppository, vaginal: 100 mg (7s); 200 mg (3s)

Tincture: 2% with alcohol (7.39 mL, 29.57 mL)

- ♦ **Micostatin** *see* nystatin *on page 452*
- ♦ **Micostyl** *see* econazole *on page 227*
- ♦ **MICRhoGAM™** *see* Rh₀(D) immune globulin (intramuscular) *on page 546*

microfibrillar collagen hemostat

(mye kro FI bri lar KOL la jen HEE moe stat)

Synonyms MCH

U.S. Brand Names Avitene®; Helistat®; Hemotene®

Generic Available No

Therapeutic Category Hemostatic Agent

Use Adjunct to hemostasis when control of bleeding by ligature is ineffective or impractical

Usual Dosage Apply dry directly to source of bleeding

Nursing/Pharmacy Information Fragments of MCH may pass through filters of blood-scavenging systems; avoid reintroduction of blood from operative sites treated with MCH

Dosage Forms

Fibrous: 1 g, 5 g

Nonwoven web: 70 mm x 70 mm x 1 mm; 70 mm x 35 mm x 1 mm

Sponge: 1" x 2" (10s); 3" x 4" (10s); 9" x 10" (5s)

- ♦ **Micro-K® 10** *see* potassium chloride *on page 506*
- ♦ **Micro-K® 10 Extencaps®** *see* potassium chloride *on page 506*
- ♦ **Micro-K® LS** *see* potassium chloride *on page 506*
- ♦ **Microlipid™ [OTC]** *see* enteral nutritional products *on page 233*
- ♦ **Microlut®** *see* levonorgestrel *on page 366*
- ♦ **Micronase®** *see* glyburide *on page 294*
- ♦ **microNefrin® [OTC]** *see* epinephrine *on page 234*
- ♦ **Micronor®** *see* norethindrone *on page 447*
- ♦ **Microrgan®** *see* ciprofloxacin *on page 151*
- ♦ **Microtid** *see* ranitidine hydrochloride *on page 541*
- ♦ **Microzide™** *see* hydrochlorothiazide *on page 317*
- ♦ **Midamor®** *see* amiloride *on page 37*

midazolam (MID aye zoe lam)
Synonyms midazolam hydrochloride
U.S. Brand Names Versed®
Mexican Brand Names Dormicum
Generic Available No
Therapeutic Category Benzodiazepine
Controlled Substance C-IV
Use Preoperative sedation; conscious sedation prior to diagnostic or radiographic procedures
Usual Dosage
Preoperative sedation: Children:
Oral:
<5 years: 0.5 mg/kg;
>5 years: 0.4-0.5 mg/kg; doses as high as 0.5-0.75 mg/kg have provided effective preanesthetic sedation
I.M.: 0.07-0.08 mg/kg 30 minutes to 1 hour before surgery; range: 0.05-0.1 mg/kg
I.V.: 0.035 mg/kg/dose, repeat over several minutes as required to achieve the desired sedative effect up to a total dose of 0.1-0.2 mg/kg or 5 mg total

Conscious sedation during mechanical ventilation:
Neonates: I.V. continuous infusion: 0.15-1 mcg/kg/minute
Children:
I.V.: 0.1-0.2 mg/kg; follow loading dose with a 1-2 mcg/kg/minute continuous infusion; titrate to the desired effect; range: 0.4-6 mcg/kg/minute
I.V. intermittent infusion: 0.05-0.2 mg/kg every 1-2 hours as needed

Conscious sedation for procedures:
Children:
Oral: 0.2-0.4 mg/kg; dose as high as 1 mg/kg have been used in younger (6 months to <6 years of age) and less cooperative patients; (maximum: 20 mg) 30-45 minutes before the procedure
Intranasal: 0.2-0.4 mg/kg (use undiluted 5 mg/mL injectable drug for intranasal administration)
I.V.: 0.05-0.1 mg/kg 3 minutes before procedure

Adolescents >12 years:
Sedation for procedure: I.V.: 0.5 mg every 3-4 minutes until effect achieved
Preoperative sedation: I.M.: 0.07-0.08 mg/kg 30-60 minutes before surgery; usual dose: 5 mg
Conscious sedation: I.V.: Initial: 0.5-2 mg; slowly titrate to effect by repeating doses every 2-3 minutes; usual total dose: 2.5-5 mg
Adults, healthy <60 years: Some patients respond to doses as low as 1 mg; no more than 2.5 mg should be administered over a period of 2 minutes. Additional doses of midazolam may be administered after a 2-minute waiting period and evaluation of sedation after each dose increment. A total dose >5 mg is generally not needed. If narcotics or other CNS depressants are administered concomitantly, the midazolam dose should be reduced by 30%.
Nursing/Pharmacy Information
Parenteral: Infuse I.V. doses over 2-3 minutes
Monitor respiratory and cardiovascular status
Stability: Admixtures do not require protection from light for short-term storage; **compatible** with normal saline, D_5W
Dosage Forms
Injection, as hydrochloride: 1 mg/mL (2 mL, 5 mL, 10 mL); 5 mg/mL (1 mL, 2 mL, 5 mL, 10 mL)
Syrup, as hydrochloride: 2 mg/mL (118 mL)

♦ **midazolam hydrochloride** *see* midazolam *on page 415*
♦ **Midchlor®** *see* acetaminophen, isometheptene, and dichloralphenazone *on page 17*

midodrine (MI doe dreen)
U.S. Brand Names ProAmatine
Generic Available No
Therapeutic Category Alpha-Adrenergic Agonist
Use Treatment of symptomatic orthostatic hypotension in patients whose lives are considerably impaired despite standard clinical care.
Usual Dosage Adults: Oral: 10 mg 3 times/day (every 3-4 hours); dosing should take place during daytime hours when the patient needs to be upright, pursuing activities of daily living; a suggested dosing schedule is as follows:
Dose 1: Shortly before or upon rising in the morning
Dose 2: At midday
(Continued)

midodrine (Continued)

Dose 3: In the late afternoon (not later than 6 PM)

Nursing/Pharmacy Information Patients should be told that certain over-the-counter products, such as cold remedies and diet aids, can elevate blood pressure, and therefore, should be used cautiously, as they may enhance or potentiate the pressor effects. Patients should be made aware of the possibility of supine hypertension and told to avoid taking their dose if they are to be supine for any length of time (ie, they should take their last daily dose 3-4 hours before bedtime to minimize nighttime supine hypertension).

Dosage Forms Tablet, as hydrochloride: 2.5 mg, 5 mg

♦ **Midol® IB [OTC]** see ibuprofen on page 332

♦ **Midol® PM [OTC]** see acetaminophen and diphenhydramine on page 15

♦ **Midotens** see labetalol on page 357

♦ **Midrin®** see acetaminophen, isometheptene, and dichloralphenazone on page 17

♦ **Miflex® Tablet (Discontinued)** see page 743

miglitol (MIG li tol)

U.S. Brand Names Glyset®

Generic Available No

Therapeutic Category Antidiabetic Agent, Oral

Use As an adjunct to diet to lower blood glucose in patients with noninsulin-dependent diabetes mellitus (NIDDM)

Usual Dosage Adults: Oral: 25 mg 3 times/day with the first bite of food at each meal; dose may be increased to 50 mg 3 times/day after 4-8 weeks; maximum recommended dose: 100 mg 3 times/day

Dosage Forms Tablet: 25 mg, 50 mg, 100 mg

♦ **Migranal® Nasal Spray** see dihydroergotamine on page 204

♦ **Migratine®** see acetaminophen, isometheptene, and dichloralphenazone on page 17

♦ **MIH** see procarbazine on page 519

♦ **Miles Nervine® Caplets [OTC]** see diphenhydramine on page 208

♦ **Milezzol** see metronidazole on page 411

♦ **milk of magnesia** see magnesium hydroxide on page 381

♦ **Milontin®** see phensuximide on page 487

♦ **Milophene®** see clomiphene on page 158

♦ **Milprem® (Discontinued)** see page 743

milrinone (MIL ri none)

U.S. Brand Names Primacor®

Generic Available No

Therapeutic Category Cardiovascular Agent, Other

Use Short-term I.V. therapy of congestive heart failure

Usual Dosage Adults: I.V.: Loading dose: 50 mcg/kg administered over 10 minutes, then 0.375-0.75 mcg/kg/min as a continuous infusion for a total daily dose of 0.59-1.13 mg/kg

Nursing/Pharmacy Information Monitor serum potassium

Dosage Forms Injection, as lactate: 1 mg/mL (5 mL, 10 mL, 20 mL)

♦ **Miltown®** see meprobamate on page 394

♦ **Minidyne® [OTC]** see povidone-iodine on page 510

♦ **Mini-Gamulin® Rh** see Rh₀(D) immune globulin (intramuscular) on page 546

♦ **Minims® Pilocarpine** see pilocarpine on page 493

♦ **Minipress®** see prazosin on page 513

♦ **Minirin** see desmopressin acetate on page 188

♦ **Minitran® Patch** see nitroglycerin on page 444

♦ **Minizide®** see prazosin and polythiazide on page 513

♦ **Minocin®** see minocycline on page 416

♦ **Minocin® IV Injection** see minocycline on page 416

♦ **Minocin® Tablet (Discontinued)** see page 743

minocycline (mi noe SYE kleen)

U.S. Brand Names Dynacin® Oral; Minocin®; Minocin® IV Injection; Vectrin®

Canadian Brand Names Apo-Minocycline®; Syn-Minocycline®

Generic Available Yes

Therapeutic Category Tetracycline Derivative

Use Treatment of susceptible bacterial infections of both gram-negative and gram-positive organisms; acne

Usual Dosage
Children 8-12 years: 4 mg/kg stat, then 4 mg/kg/day (maximum: 200 mg/day) in divided doses every 12 hours
Adults:
Infection: Oral, I.V.: 200 mg stat, 100 mg every 12 hours
Acne: Oral: 50 mg 1-3 times/day

Dietary Considerations May be administered with food or milk

Nursing/Pharmacy Information Infuse I.V. minocycline over 1 hour

Dosage Forms Minocycline hydrochloride:
Capsule: 50 mg, 100 mg
Capsule (Dynacin®): 50 mg, 100 mg
Capsule, pellet-filled (Minocin®): 50 mg, 100 mg
Injection (Minocin® IV): 100 mg
Suspension, oral (Minocin®): 50 mg/5 mL (60 mL)

♦ **Minodiab** see glipizide on page 292
♦ **Minofen®** see acetaminophen on page 13

minoxidil (mi NOKS i dil)
U.S. Brand Names Loniten® Oral; Rogaine® Topical
Canadian Brand Names Apo®-Gain; Gen-Minoxidil; Minoxigaine™
Generic Available Yes
Therapeutic Category Topical Skin Product; Vasodilator
Use Management of severe hypertension; topically for management of alopecia or male pattern alopecia

Usual Dosage
Children <12 years: Hypertension: Oral: Initial: 0.1-0.2 mg/kg once daily; maximum: 5 mg/day; increase gradually every 3 days; usual dosage: 0.25-1 mg/kg/day in 1-2 divided doses; maximum: 50 mg/day
Adults:
Hypertension: Oral: Initial: 5 mg once daily, increase gradually every 3 days; usual dose: 10-40 mg/day in 1-2 divided doses; maximum: 100 mg/day
Alopecia: Topical: Apply twice daily

Dietary Considerations Avoid natural licorice (causes sodium and water retention and increases potassium loss)

Nursing/Pharmacy Information
May cause hirsutism or hypertrichosis
Monitor blood pressure, standing and sitting/supine

Dosage Forms
Solution, topical: 2% = 20 mg/metered dose (60 mL); 5% = 50 mg/metered dose (60 mL)
Tablet: 2.5 mg, 10 mg

♦ **Minoxigaine™** see minoxidil on page 417
♦ **Mintezol®** see thiabendazole on page 605
♦ **Minute-Gel®** see fluoride on page 274
♦ **Miocarpine®** see pilocarpine on page 493
♦ **Miochol® (Discontinued)** see page 743
♦ **Miochol-E®** see acetylcholine on page 19
♦ **Miostat® Intraocular** see carbachol on page 111
♦ **Miradon®** see anisotropine on page 50
♦ **Mirapex®** see pramipexole on page 511

mirtazapine (mir TAZ a peen)
U.S. Brand Names Remeron®
Generic Available No
Therapeutic Category Antidepressant, Selective Serotonin Reuptake Inhibitor
Use Treatment of depression, works through noradrenergic and serotonergic pharmacologic action
Usual Dosage Adults: Oral: Initial: 15 mg/day, then 15-45 mg/day
Dosage Forms Tablet: 15 mg, 30 mg

misoprostol (mye soe PROST ole)
U.S. Brand Names Cytotec®
Generic Available No
Therapeutic Category Prostaglandin
Use Prevention of NSAID-induced gastric ulcers
Usual Dosage Oral: 200 mcg 4 times/day with food
(Continued)

misoprostol *(Continued)*

Dietary Considerations Incidence of diarrhea may be lessened by having patient take dose right after meals and at bedtime

Dosage Forms Tablet: 100 mcg, 200 mcg

- ♦ **misoprostol and diclofenac** *see* diclofenac and misoprostol *on page 199*
- ♦ **Misostol** *see* mitoxantrone *on page 418*
- ♦ **Mithracin®** *see* plicamycin *on page 499*
- ♦ **mithramycin** *see* plicamycin *on page 499*

mitomycin *(mye toe MYE sin)*

Synonyms mitomycin-c; MTC

U.S. Brand Names Mutamycin®

Generic Available Yes

Therapeutic Category Antineoplastic Agent

Use Therapy of disseminated adenocarcinoma of stomach, colon, or pancreas in combination with other approved chemotherapeutic agents; bladder cancer, breast cancer

Usual Dosage Children and Adults (refer to individual protocols): I.V.: 10-20 mg/m^2/dose every 6-8 weeks, or 2 mg/m^2/day for 5 days, stop for 2 days then repeat; subsequent doses should be adjusted to platelet and leukocyte response

Nursing/Pharmacy Information

Care should be taken to avoid extravasation since ulceration and tissue sloughing can occur; administer by short I.V. infusion over 30-60 minutes or by slow I.V. push over 5-10 minutes via a running I.V.; short I.V. infusions are usually administered at a final concentration of 20-40 mcg/mL (in 50-250 mL of D$_5$W or NS) or I.V. slow push can be administered at a concentration not to exceed 0.5 mg/mL

Monitor platelet count, CBC with differential, hemoglobin, prothrombin time, renal and pulmonary function tests

Stability: Reconstituted solution (with sterile water) is stable for 7 days at room temperature and 14 days when refrigerated; **incompatible** with D$_5$W

Dosage Forms Powder for injection: 5 mg, 20 mg, 40 mg

- ♦ **mitomycin-c** *see* mitomycin *on page 418*

mitotane *(MYE toe tane)*

Synonyms o,p'-DDD

U.S. Brand Names Lysodren®

Generic Available No

Therapeutic Category Antineoplastic Agent

Use Treatment of inoperable adrenal cortical carcinoma

Usual Dosage Adults: Oral: 8-10 g/day in 3-4 divided doses; dose is changed based on side effects with aim of administering as high a dose as tolerated

Nursing/Pharmacy Information

Patients should be warned that mitotane may impair ability to operate hazardous equipment or drive; avoid alcohol and other CNS depressants; notify physician if rash or darkening of skin, severe nausea, vomiting, depression, flushing, or fever occurs; contraceptive measures are recommended during therapy

Stability: Protect from light, store at room temperature

Dosage Forms Tablet: 500 mg

mitoxantrone *(mye toe ZAN trone)*

Synonyms DHAD

U.S. Brand Names Novantrone®

Mexican Brand Names Novantrone®; Misostol

Generic Available No

Therapeutic Category Antineoplastic Agent

Use FDA approved for remission-induction therapy of acute nonlymphocytic leukemia (ANLL); mitoxantrone is also active against other various leukemias, lymphoma, and breast cancer, and moderately active against pediatric sarcoma

Usual Dosage I.V. (refer to individual protocols):

Leukemias:

Children ≤2 years: 0.4 mg/kg/day once daily for 3-5 days

Children >2 years and Adults: 8-12 mg/m^2/day once daily for 5 days or 12 mg/m^2/day once daily for 3 days

Solid tumors:

Children: 18-20 mg/m^2 every 3-4 weeks

Adults: 12-14 mg/m^2 every 3-4 weeks

Nursing/Pharmacy Information

Mitoxantrone is a nonvesicant; if extravasation occurs, the drug should be discontinued and restarted in another vein; **Do not** administer I.V. bolus over <3 minutes; can be administered I.V. intermittent infusion over 15-30 minutes at a concentration of 0.02 to 0.5 mg/mL in D$_5$W or normal saline

Monitor CBC, serum uric acid, liver function tests, ECHO

Stability: **Incompatible** with heparin and hydrocortisone; after penetration of the stopper, undiluted mitoxantrone solution is stable for 7 days at room temperature or 14 days when refrigerated

Dosage Forms Injection, as base: 2 mg/mL (10 mL, 12.5 mL, 15 mL)

♦ **Mitran® Oral** *see* chlordiazepoxide *on page 134*
♦ **Mitroken** *see* ciprofloxacin *on page 151*
♦ **Mitrolan® Chewable Tablet [OTC]** *see* calcium polycarbophil *on page 107*
♦ **Mivacron®** *see* mivacurium *on page 419*

mivacurium (mye va KYOO ree um)

U.S. Brand Names Mivacron®
Generic Available No
Therapeutic Category Skeletal Muscle Relaxant
Use Short-acting nondepolarizing neuromuscular blocking agent; an adjunct to general anesthesia; facilitates endotracheal intubation; provides skeletal muscle relaxation during surgery or mechanical ventilation
Usual Dosage I.V.:

Children 2-12 years: 0.2 mg/kg over 5-15 seconds; continuous infusion: 14 mcg/kg

Adults: Initial: 0.15 mg/kg administered over 5-15 seconds

Nursing/Pharmacy Information Use with caution in patients in whom histamine release would be detrimental (eg, patients with severe cardiovascular disease or asthma); Children require higher mivacurium infusion rates than adults; during opioid/nitrous oxide/oxygen anesthesia, the infusion rate required to maintain 89% to 99% neuromuscular block averages 14 mcg/kg/minute (range: 5-31). For adults and children, the amount of infusion solution required per hour depends upon the clinical requirements of the patient, the concentration of mivacurium in the infusion solution, and the patient's weight. The contribution of the infusion solution to the fluid requirements of the patient must be considered.

Dosage Forms Mivacurium chloride:

Infusion, in D$_5$W: 0.5 mg/mL (50 mL)
Injection: 2 mg/mL (5 mL, 10 mL)

♦ **MK594** *see* losartan *on page 376*
♦ **MMR** *see* measles, mumps and rubella vaccines, combined *on page 386*
♦ **M-M-R® II** *see* measles, mumps and rubella vaccines, combined *on page 386*
♦ **Moban®** *see* molindone *on page 420*
♦ **Mobenol®** *see* tolbutamide *on page 617*
♦ **Mobidin®** *see* magnesium salicylate *on page 382*
♦ **Moctanin®** *see* monoctanoin *on page 421*

modafinil (moe DAF i nil)

U.S. Brand Names Provigil®
Generic Available No
Therapeutic Category Central Nervous System Stimulant, Nonamphetamine
Controlled Substance C-IV
Use Indicated to improve wakefulness in patients with excessive daytime sleepiness associated with narcolepsy
Usual Dosage Adults: Oral: Initial: 200 mg as a single daily dose
Dosage Forms Tablet: 100 mg, 200 mg

♦ **Modane® Bulk [OTC]** *see* psyllium *on page 531*
♦ **Modane® Soft [OTC]** *see* docusate *on page 214*
♦ **Modecate®** *see* fluphenazine *on page 277*
♦ **Modecate® Enanthate** *see* fluphenazine *on page 277*
♦ **Modicon™** *see* ethinyl estradiol and norethindrone *on page 250*
♦ **modified Dakin's solution** *see* sodium hypochlorite solution *on page 572*
♦ **Moditen® Hydrochloride** *see* fluphenazine *on page 277*
♦ **Moducal® [OTC]** *see* glucose polymers *on page 293*
♦ **Modulon®** *see* trimebutine *(Canada only) on page 629*
♦ **Moduretic®** *see* amiloride and hydrochlorothiazide *on page 37*

moexipril (mo EKS i pril)

U.S. Brand Names Univasc®

Generic Available No

Therapeutic Category Angiotensin-Converting Enzyme (ACE) Inhibitor

Use Treatment of hypertension, alone or in combination with thiazide diuretics

Usual Dosage Oral:

Patients not receiving diuretics: Initial: 7.5 mg 1 hour prior to meals once daily; if antihypertensive effect diminishes toward end of dosing interval, increase or divide dose; maintenance dose of 7.5-30 mg/day in 1 or 2 divided doses

Patients receiving diuretics: Discontinue diuretic 2-3 days before starting moexipril to avoid symptomatic hypotension; if blood pressure is not controlled, resume diuretic therapy; if diuretic cannot be held, initiate moexipril at 3.75 mg/day

Dietary Considerations Administer on an empty stomach

Nursing/Pharmacy Information Do not interrupt therapy without consulting physician; notify physician if any of the following occur: sore throat, fever, swelling of hands or feet, difficulty swallowing, excessive perspiration; may cause dizziness, fainting, lightheadedness; avoid sudden postural changes; may cause skin rash or altered taste perception; do not use salt substitutes containing potassium without consulting physician; consult physician if you develop a persistent dry cough

Dosage Forms Tablet, as hydrochloride: 7.5 mg, 15 mg

moexipril and hydrochlorothiazide

(mo EKS i pril & hye droe klor oh THYE a zide)

U.S. Brand Names Uniretic™

Generic Available No

Therapeutic Category Angiotensin-Converting Enzyme (ACE) Inhibitor; Diuretic, Thiazide

Use Treatment of hypertension

Usual Dosage Adults: Oral: 7.5-30 mg of moexipril, taken either in a single or divided dose one hour before meals

Dosage Forms Tablet: Moexipril hydrochloride 7.5 mg and hydrochlorothiazide 12.5 mg; moexipril hydrochloride 15 mg and hydrochlorothiazide 25 mg

♦ **Moi-Stir® Solution [OTC]** *see* saliva substitute *on page 558*

♦ **Moi-Stir® Swabsticks [OTC]** *see* saliva substitute *on page 558*

♦ **Moisturel® Lotion (Discontinued)** *see page 743*

♦ **Moisture® Ophthalmic Drops [OTC]** *see* artificial tears *on page 59*

molindone (moe LIN done)

U.S. Brand Names Moban®

Generic Available No

Therapeutic Category Antipsychotic Agent, Dihydroindoline

Use Management of psychotic disorder

Usual Dosage Oral: 50-75 mg/day; up to 225 mg/day

Dietary Considerations May be administered with glass of water or milk to decrease GI distress

Nursing/Pharmacy Information Monitor orthostatic blood pressures 3-5 days after initiation of therapy or after a dose increase; observe for tremor and abnormal movement or posturing (extrapyramidal symptoms)

Dosage Forms Molindone hydrochloride:

Concentrate, oral: 20 mg/mL (120 mL)

Tablet: 5 mg, 10 mg, 25 mg, 50 mg, 100 mg

♦ **Mol-Iron® [OTC]** *see* ferrous sulfate *on page 265*

♦ **Mollifene® Ear Wax Removing Formula [OTC]** *see* carbamide peroxide *on page 112*

♦ **molybdenum injection** *see* trace metals *on page 620*

♦ **Molypen®** *see* trace metals *on page 620*

♦ **MOM** *see* magnesium hydroxide *on page 381*

mometasone furoate (moe MET a sone FYOOR oh ate)

U.S. Brand Names Elocon®; Nasonex®

Canadian Brand Names Elocom

Generic Available No

Therapeutic Category Corticosteroid, Topical

Use Relief of inflammatory and pruritic manifestations of corticosteroid-responsive dermatoses

Usual Dosage Topical: Apply to area once daily, do not use occlusive dressings

Nursing/Pharmacy Information Use sparingly

Dosage Forms Mometasone furoate:
Cream: 0.1% (15 g, 45 g)
Lotion: 0.1% (30 mL, 60 mL)
Ointment, topical: 0.1% (15 g, 45 g)

♦ **mom/mineral oil emulsion** *see* magnesium hydroxide and mineral oil emulsion *on page 381*

♦ **monacolin k** *see* lovastatin *on page 377*

♦ **Monafed®** *see* guaifenesin *on page 299*

♦ **Monafed® DM** *see* guaifenesin and dextromethorphan *on page 300*

♦ *Monilia* **skin test** *see* Candida albicans (Monilia) *on page 109*

♦ **Monistat-Derm™ Topical** *see* miconazole *on page 413*

♦ **Monistat i.v.™ Injection** *see* miconazole *on page 413*

♦ **Monistat™ Vaginal** *see* miconazole *on page 413*

♦ **Monitan®** *see* acebutolol *on page 13*

monobenzone (mon oh BEN zone)
U.S. Brand Names Benoquin®
Generic Available No
Therapeutic Category Topical Skin Product
Use Final depigmentation in extensive vitiligo
Usual Dosage Adults: Topical: Apply 2-3 times/day
Dosage Forms Cream: 20% (35.4 g)

♦ **Monocete® Topical Liquid** *(Discontinued) see page 743*

♦ **Monocid®** *see* cefonicid *on page 121*

♦ **Monocidur** *see* cefonicid *on page 121*

♦ **monoclonal antibody** *see* muromonab-CD3 *on page 425*

♦ **monoclonal antibody purified** *see* factor IX, purified (human) *on page 258*

monoctanoin (mon OK ta noyn)
Synonyms monooctanoin
U.S. Brand Names Moctanin®
Generic Available No
Therapeutic Category Gallstone Dissolution Agent
Use Solubilize cholesterol gallstones that are retained in the biliary tract after cholecystectomy
Usual Dosage Administer via T-tube into common bile duct at rate of 3-5 mL/hour at pressure of 10 mL water for 7-21 days
Nursing/Pharmacy Information Solution must be diluted prior to use; do not administer I.M. or I.V.
Dosage Forms Solution: 120 mL

♦ **Monodox®** *see* doxycycline *on page 222*

♦ **Mono-Gesic®** *see* salsalate *on page 559*

♦ **Monoket®** *see* isosorbide mononitrate *on page 349*

♦ **Mono Mack** *see* isosorbide mononitrate *on page 349*

♦ **Mononine®** *see* factor IX, purified (human) *on page 258*

♦ **monooctanoin** *see* monoctanoin *on page 421*

♦ **Monopril®** *see* fosinopril *on page 283*

montelukast (mon te LOO kast)
U.S. Brand Names Singulair®
Generic Available No
Therapeutic Category Leukotriene Receptor Antagonist
Use Prophylaxis and chronic treatment of asthma in adults and children ≥6 years
Usual Dosage Oral:
Children 6-14 years: 5 mg once daily
Children >14 years and Adults: 10 mg once daily
Dosage Forms Montelukast sodium:
Tablet: 10 mg
Tablet, chewable: 5 mg

♦ **Monurol™** *see* fosfomycin *on page 283*

♦ **more attenuated enders strain** *see* measles virus vaccine, live *on page 386*

♦ **More-Dophilus® [OTC]** *see* Lactobacillus *on page 358*

moricizine (mor EYE siz een)

U.S. Brand Names Ethmozine®

Generic Available No

Therapeutic Category Antiarrhythmic Agent, Class I

Use Treatment of ventricular tachycardia and life-threatening ventricular arrhythmias; a Class I antiarrhythmic agent

Usual Dosage Adults: Oral: 200-300 mg every 8 hours, adjust dosage at 150 mg/day at 3-day intervals

Dietary Considerations Food delays absorption; best if taken on an empty stomach

Nursing/Pharmacy Information Administering 30 minutes after a meal delays the rate of absorption, resulting in lower peak plasma concentrations

Dosage Forms Tablet, as hydrochloride: 200 mg, 250 mg, 300 mg

♦ **Morphine-HP®** *see* morphine sulfate *on page 422*

morphine sulfate (MOR feen SUL fate)

Synonyms MS

U.S. Brand Names Astramorph™ PF Injection; Duramorph® Injection; MS Contin® Oral; MSIR® Oral; OMS® Oral; Oramorph SR™ Oral; RMS® Rectal; Roxanol™ Oral; Roxanol SR™ Oral

Canadian Brand Names Epimorph®; M-Eslon®; Morphine-HP®; MS-IR®; Statex®

Mexican Brand Names Graten; MST Continus

Generic Available Yes

Therapeutic Category Analgesic, Narcotic

Controlled Substance C-II

Use Relief of moderate to severe acute and chronic pain; pain of myocardial infarction; relieves dyspnea of acute left ventricular failure and pulmonary edema; preanesthetic medication

Usual Dosage Doses should be titrated to appropriate effect; when changing routes of administration in chronically treated patients, please note that oral doses are approximately $1/6$ as effective as parenteral dose

Infants and Children:
  Oral: Tablet and solution (prompt-release): 0.2-0.5 mg/kg/dose every 4-6 hours as needed; tablet (controlled-release): 0.3-0.6 mg/kg/dose every 12 hours
  I.M., I.V., S.C.: 0.1-0.2 mg/kg/dose every 2-4 hours as needed; usual maximum: 15 mg/dose; may initiate at 0.05 mg/kg/dose
  I.V., S.C. continuous infusion: Sickle cell or cancer pain: 0.025-2 mg/kg/hour; postoperative pain: 0.01-0.04 mg/kg/hour
  Sedation/analgesia for procedures: I.V.: 0.05-0.1 mg/kg 5 minutes before the procedure
  Adolescents >12 years: Sedation/analgesia for procedures: I.V.: 3-4 mg and repeat in 5 minutes if necessary
Adults:
  Oral: Prompt-release: 10-30 mg every 4 hours as needed; controlled release: 15-30 mg every 8-12 hours
  I.M., I.V., S.C.: 2.5-20 mg/dose every 2-6 hours as needed; usual: 10 mg/dose every 4 hours as needed
  I.V., S.C. continuous infusion: 0.8-10 mg/hour; may increase depending on pain relief/adverse effects; usual range up to 80 mg/hour
  Epidural: Initial: 5 mg in lumbar region; if inadequate pain relief within 1 hour, administer 1-2 mg, maximum dose: 10 mg/24 hours
  Intrathecal ($1/10$ of epidural dose): 0.2-1 mg/dose; repeat doses **not** recommended

Dietary Considerations
  Alcohol: Additive CNS effects; avoid or limit alcohol; watch for sedation
  Food:
    Glucose may cause hyperglycemia; monitor blood glucose concentrations
    Administration of oral morphine solution with food may increase bioavailability (ie, a report of 34% increase in morphine AUC when morphine oral solution followed a high-fat meal); morphine may cause GI upset; be consistent when taking morphine with or without meals; administer with food if GI upset

Nursing/Pharmacy Information
  Do not crush controlled release drug product; do not administer rapidly I.V.; administer I.V. push over at least 5 minutes at a final concentration of 0.5-5 mg/mL; administer intermittent infusion over 15-30 minutes; continuous I.V. infusion concentration: 0.1-1 mg/mL in D_5W

Monitor for pain relief, respiratory and mental status, blood pressure

Stability: Refrigerate suppositories; do not freeze; degradation depends on pH and presence of oxygen; relatively stable in pH 4 and below; darkening of solutions indicate degradation; usual concentration for continuous I.V. infusion = 0.1-1 mg/mL in D_5W

Dosage Forms

Capsule (MSIR®): 15 mg, 30 mg

Capsule, sustained release (Kadian™): 20 mg, 50 mg, 100 mg

Injection: 0.5 mg/mL (10 mL); 1 mg/mL (10 mL, 30 mL, 60 mL); 2 mg/mL (1 mL, 2 mL, 60 mL); 3 mg/mL (50 mL); 4 mg/mL (1 mL, 2 mL); 5 mg/mL (1 mL, 30 mL); 8 mg/mL (1 mL, 2 mL); 10 mg/mL (1 mL, 2 mL, 10 mL); 15 mg/mL (1 mL, 2 mL, 20 mL); 25 mg/mL (4 mL, 10 mL, 20 mL, 40 mL); 50 mg/mL (10 mL, 20 mL, 40 mL)

Injection:

Preservative free (Astramorph™ PF, Duramorph®): 0.5 mg/mL (2 mL, 10 mL); 1 mg/mL (2 mL, 10 mL); 10 mg/mL (20 mL); 25 mg/mL (20 mL)

I.V. via PCA pump: 1 mg/mL (10 mL, 30 mL, 60 mL); 5 mg/mL (30 mL)

I.V. infusion preparation: 25 mg/mL (4 mL, 10 mL, 20 mL)

Solution, oral: 10 mg/5 mL (5 mL, 10 mL, 100 mL, 120 mL, 500 mL); 20 mg/5 mL (5 mL, 100 mL, 120 mL, 500 mL)

MSIR®: 10 mg/5 mL (5 mL, 120 mL, 500 mL); 20 mg/5 mL (5 mL 120 mL, 500 mL); 20 mg/mL (30 mL, 120 mL)

MS/L®: 100 mg/5 mL (120 mL) 20 mg/5 mL

OMS®: 20 mg/mL (30 mL, 120 mL)

Roxanol™: 10 mg/2.5 mL (2.5 mL); 20 mg/mL (1 mL, 1.5 mL, 30 mL, 120 mL, 240 mL)

Suppository, rectal: 5 mg, 10 mg, 20 mg, 30 mg

MS/S®, RMS®, Roxanol™: 5 mg, 10 mg, 20 mg, 30 mg

Tablet: 15 mg, 30 mg

MSIR®: 15 mg, 30 mg

Controlled release:

MS Contin®: 15 mg, 30 mg, 60 mg, 100 mg, 200 mg

Roxanol™ SR: 30 mg

Soluble: 10 mg, 15 mg, 30 mg

Sustained release (Oramorph SR™): 30 mg, 60 mg, 100 mg

morrhuate sodium (MOR yoo ate SOW dee um)

U.S. Brand Names Scleromate™

Generic Available No

Therapeutic Category Sclerosing Agent

Use Treatment of small, uncomplicated varicose veins of the lower extremities

Usual Dosage I.V.:

Children 1-18 years: Esophageal hemorrhage: 2, 3, or 4 mL of 5% solution repeated every 3-4 days until bleeding is controlled, then every 6 weeks until varices obliterated

Adults: 50-250 mg, repeat at 5- to 7-day intervals (50-100 mg for small veins, 150-250 mg for large veins)

Nursing/Pharmacy Information

For I.V. use only, avoid extravasation; use only clear solutions, solution should become clear when warmed

Stability: Refrigerate

Dosage Forms Injection: 50 mg/mL (30 mL)

- ♦ **Motilium®** see domperidone *(Canada only) on page 217*
- ♦ **Motofen®** see difenoxin and atropine *on page 201*
- ♦ **Motrin®** see ibuprofen *on page 332*
- ♦ **Motrin® IB [OTC]** see ibuprofen *on page 332*
- ♦ **Motrin® IB Sinus [OTC]** see pseudoephedrine and ibuprofen *on page 531*
- ♦ **Mouthkote® Solution [OTC]** see saliva substitute *on page 558*
- ♦ **Moxam® Injection** *(Discontinued)* see *page 743*
- ♦ **4-MP** see fomepizole *on page 282*
- ♦ **6-MP** see mercaptopurine *on page 394*
- ♦ **M-Prednisol® Injection** see methylprednisolone *on page 407*
- ♦ **M-R-VAX® II** see measles and rubella vaccines, combined *on page 386*
- ♦ **MS** see morphine sulfate *on page 422*
- ♦ **MS Contin® Oral** see morphine sulfate *on page 422*
- ♦ **MSD® Enteric Coated ASA** see aspirin *on page 61*
- ♦ **MS-IR®** see morphine sulfate *on page 422*
- ♦ **MSIR® Oral** see morphine sulfate *on page 422*
- ♦ **MSTA** see mumps skin test antigen *on page 424*

- **MST Continus** *see* morphine sulfate *on page 422*
- **MTC** *see* mitomycin *on page 418*
- **M.T.E.-4®** *see* trace metals *on page 620*
- **M.T.E.-5®** *see* trace metals *on page 620*
- **M.T.E.-6®** *see* trace metals *on page 620*
- **MTX** *see* methotrexate *on page 402*
- **Muco-Fen-DM®** *see* guaifenesin and dextromethorphan *on page 300*
- **Muco-Fen-LA®** *see* guaifenesin *on page 299*
- **Mucomyst®** *see* acetylcysteine *on page 19*
- **Mucoplex® [OTC]** *see* vitamin B complex *on page 651*
- **Mucosil™** *see* acetylcysteine *on page 19*
- **MulTE-PAK-4®** *see* trace metals *on page 620*
- **MulTE-PAK-5®** *see* trace metals *on page 620*
- **Multipax®** *see* hydroxyzine *on page 328*
- **multiple sulfonamides** *see* sulfadiazine, sulfamethazine, and sulfamerazine *on page 586*
- **Multitest CMI®** *see* skin test antigens, multiple *on page 568*
- **multivitamins/fluoride** *see* vitamin, multiple (pediatric) *on page 654*
- **Multi Vit® Drops [OTC]** *see* vitamin, multiple (pediatric) *on page 654*

mumps skin test antigen (mumpz skin test AN ti jen)

Synonyms MSTA
Generic Available No
Therapeutic Category Diagnostic Agent
Use Assess the status of cell-mediated immunity
Usual Dosage Children and Adults: 0.1 mL intradermally into flexor surface of the forearm; examine reaction site in 24-48 hours; a positive reaction is ≥1.5 mm diameter induration
Nursing/Pharmacy Information Administer intradermally only into the flexor surface of the forearm only
Dosage Forms Injection: 1 mL (10 tests)

- **Mumpsvax®** *see* mumps virus vaccine, live, attenuated *on page 424*

mumps virus vaccine, live, attenuated
(mumpz VYE rus vak SEEN, live, a ten YOO ate ed)
U.S. Brand Names Mumpsvax®
Generic Available No
Therapeutic Category Vaccine, Live Virus
Use Immunization against mumps in children ≥12 months and adults
Usual Dosage S.C.: 1 vial (5000 units) in outer aspect of the upper arm
Nursing/Pharmacy Information
Federal law requires that the date of administration, the vaccine manufacturer, lot number of vaccine, and the administering person's name, title and address be entered into the patient's permanent medical record
Stability: Refrigerate
Dosage Forms Injection: Single dose

- **Munobal** *see* felodipine *on page 261*
- **Mupiban** *see* mupirocin *on page 424*

mupirocin (myoo PEER oh sin)

Synonyms pseudomonic acid A
U.S. Brand Names Bactroban®; Bactroban® Nasal
Mexican Brand Names Mupiban
Generic Available No
Therapeutic Category Antibiotic, Topical
Use Topical treatment of impetigo caused by *Staphylococcus aureus* and *Streptococcus pyogenes*; also effective for the topical treatment of folliculitis, furunculosis, minor wounds, burns, and ulcers caused by susceptible organisms; used as a prophylactic agent applied to intravenous catheter exit sites; used for eradication of *S. aureus* from nasal and perineal carriage sites
Usual Dosage
Children and Adults: Topical: Apply small amount to affected area 2-5 times/day for 5-14 days
Children ≥12 years and Adults: Intranasal: ~1/2 of a single use tube (0.5 g) to each nostril twice daily for 5 days
Nursing/Pharmacy Information
Not for treatment of pressure sores in elderly patients; contains polyethylene glycol vehicle

Stability: Do not mix with Aquaphor®, coal tar solution, or salicylic acid
Dosage Forms Mupirocin calcium: Ointment:
Intranasal: 2% (1 g single use tube)
Topical: 2% (15 g)

♦ **Murine® Ear Drops [OTC]** *see* carbamide peroxide *on page 112*
♦ **Murine® Plus Ophthalmic [OTC]** *see* tetrahydrozoline *on page 602*
♦ **Murine® Solution [OTC]** *see* artificial tears *on page 59*
♦ **Muro 128® Ophthalmic [OTC]** *see* sodium chloride *on page 571*
♦ **Murocel® Ophthalmic Solution [OTC]** *see* artificial tears *on page 59*
♦ **Murocoll-2® Ophthalmic** *see* phenylephrine and scopolamine *on page 489*

muromonab-CD3 (myoo roe MOE nab see dee three)
Synonyms monoclonal antibody; OKT3
U.S. Brand Names Orthoclone® OKT3
Mexican Brand Names Orthoclone OKT3
Generic Available No
Therapeutic Category Immunosuppressant Agent
Use Treatment of acute allograft rejection in renal transplant patients; effective in reversing acute hepatic, cardiac, and bone marrow transplant rejection episodes resistant to conventional treatment
Usual Dosage I.V. (refer to individual protocols):
Children <30 kg: 2.5 mg/day once daily for 10-14 days
Adults: 5 mg/day once daily for 10-14 days
Children and Adults: Methylprednisolone sodium succinate 1 mg/kg I.V. administered prior to first muromonab-CD3 administration and I.V. hydrocortisone sodium succinate 50-100 mg administered 30 minutes after administration are strongly recommended to decrease the incidence of reactions to the first dose; patient temperature should not exceed 37.8°C (100°F) at time of administration
Nursing/Pharmacy Information
Inform patient of expected first dose effects which are markedly reduced with subsequent doses; monitor patient closely for 48 hours after the first dose; acetaminophen and antihistamines can be administered concomitantly with OKT3 to reduce early reactions; filter each dose through a low protein-binding 0.22 micron filter (Millex GV) before administration; administer I.V. push over <1 minute at a final concentration of 1 mg/mL
Monitor chest x-ray, weight gain, CBC with differential, temperature, vital signs (blood pressure, temperature, pulse, respiration); immunologic monitoring of T cells, serum levels of OKT3
Stability: Store in refrigerator; do not freeze or shake; OKT3 must not be used if left out of refrigerator for >4 hours
Dosage Forms Injection: 5 mg/5 mL

♦ **Muroptic-5® [OTC]** *see* sodium chloride *on page 571*
♦ **Muse® Pellet** *see* alprostadil *on page 30*
♦ **Mus-Lax® (Discontinued)** *see page 743*
♦ **Mustargen® Hydrochloride** *see* mechlorethamine *on page 387*
♦ **mustine** *see* mechlorethamine *on page 387*
♦ **Mutamycin®** *see* mitomycin *on page 418*
♦ **M.V.C.® 9 + 3** *see* vitamin, multiple (injectable) *on page 652*
♦ **M.V.I.®-12** *see* vitamin, multiple (injectable) *on page 652*
♦ **M.V.I.® Concentrate** *see* vitamin, multiple (injectable) *on page 652*
♦ **M.V.I.® Pediatric** *see* vitamin, multiple (injectable) *on page 652*
♦ **Myambutol®** *see* ethambutol *on page 247*
♦ **Myapap® [OTC]** *see* acetaminophen *on page 13*
♦ **Mycelex®-G Topical** *see* clotrimazole *on page 161*
♦ **Mycelex®-G Vaginal [OTC]** *see* clotrimazole *on page 161*
♦ **Mycelex® Troche** *see* clotrimazole *on page 161*
♦ **Mycifradin® Sulfate** *see* neomycin *on page 435*
♦ **Myciguent®** *see* neomycin *on page 435*
♦ **Mycinettes® [OTC]** *see* benzocaine *on page 79*
♦ **Mycitracin® Topical [OTC]** *see* bacitracin, neomycin, and polymyxin B *on page 71*
♦ **Myclo-Derm®** *see* clotrimazole *on page 161*
♦ **Myclo-Gyne®** *see* clotrimazole *on page 161*
♦ **Mycobutin®** *see* rifabutin *on page 548*
♦ **Mycogen II Topical** *see* nystatin and triamcinolone *on page 452*
♦ **Mycolog®-II Topical** *see* nystatin and triamcinolone *on page 452*

♦ **Myconel® Topical** *see nystatin and triamcinolone on page 452*

mycophenolate (mye koe FEN oh late)
U.S. Brand Names CellCept®
Generic Available No
Therapeutic Category Immunosuppressant Agent
Use Immunosuppressant used with corticosteroids and cyclosporine to prevent organ rejection in patients receiving allogenic renal transplants
Usual Dosage Adults: I.V./Oral: 1 g twice daily (2 g daily dose), administered within 72 hours of transplantation, when administered in combination with corticosteroids and cyclosporine
Nursing/Pharmacy Information Increased risk for infection and development of lymphoproliferative disorders. Patients should be monitored appropriately and given supportive treatment should these conditions occur. Increased toxicity in patients with renal impairment.
Dosage Forms
Capsule, as mofetil: 250 mg
Powder for injection, as hydrochloride: 500 mg
Tablet, as mofetil: 500 mg

♦ **Mycostatin®** *see nystatin on page 452*

♦ **Myco-Triacet® II** *see nystatin and triamcinolone on page 452*

♦ **Mydfrin® Ophthalmic Solution** *see phenylephrine on page 487*

♦ **Mydriacyl®** *see tropicamide on page 634*

♦ **Mykrox®** *see metolazone on page 410*

♦ **Mylanta® [OTC]** *see aluminum hydroxide, magnesium hydroxide, and simethicone on page 34*

♦ **Mylanta Gas® [OTC]** *see simethicone on page 566*

♦ **Mylanta® Gelcaps®** *see calcium carbonate and magnesium carbonate on page 104*

♦ **Mylanta®-II [OTC]** *see aluminum hydroxide, magnesium hydroxide, and simethicone on page 34*

♦ **Mylaxen® Injection *(Discontinued)*** *see page 743*

♦ **Myleran®** *see busulfan on page 98*

♦ **Mylicon® [OTC]** *see simethicone on page 566*

♦ **Mylosar®** *see azacitidine on page 67*

♦ **Myminic® Expectorant [OTC]** *see guaifenesin and phenylpropanolamine on page 301*

♦ **Myochrysine® *(Discontinued)*** *see page 743*

♦ **Myoflex® [OTC]** *see triethanolamine salicylate on page 627*

♦ **Myotonachol™** *see bethanechol on page 86*

♦ **Myphetane DC®** *see brompheniramine, phenylpropanolamine, and codeine on page 95*

♦ **Mysoline®** *see primidone on page 517*

♦ **Mytelase® Caplets®** *see ambenonium on page 35*

♦ **Mytrex® F Topical** *see nystatin and triamcinolone on page 452*

♦ **Mytussin® [OTC]** *see guaifenesin on page 299*

♦ **Mytussin® AC** *see guaifenesin and codeine on page 300*

♦ **Mytussin® DAC** *see guaifenesin, pseudoephedrine, and codeine on page 304*

♦ **Mytussin® DM [OTC]** *see guaifenesin and dextromethorphan on page 300*

♦ **M-Zole® 7 Dual Pack [OTC]** *see miconazole on page 413*

♦ **Nabi-HB™** *see hepatitis B immune globulin on page 311*

nabilone (NA bi lone)
U.S. Brand Names Cesamet®
Generic Available No
Therapeutic Category Antiemetic
Use Treatment of nausea and vomiting associated with cancer chemotherapy
Usual Dosage Oral:
Children >4 years:
<18 kg: 0.5 mg twice daily
18-30 kg: 1 mg twice daily
>30 kg: 1 mg 3 times/day
Adults: 1-2 mg twice daily beginning 1-3 hours before chemotherapy is administered and continuing around-the-clock until 1 dose after chemotherapy is completed; maximum daily dose: 6 mg divided in 3 doses
Dosage Forms Capsule: 1 mg

nabumetone (na BYOO me tone)

U.S. Brand Names Relafen®

Generic Available Yes

Therapeutic Category Analgesic, Non-narcotic; Nonsteroidal Anti-inflammatory Drug (NSAID)

Use Management of osteoarthritis and rheumatoid arthritis

Usual Dosage Adults: Oral: 1000 mg/day; an additional 500-1000 mg may be needed in some patients to obtain more symptomatic relief; may be administered once or twice daily

Dietary Considerations Food increases the rate but not the extent of oral absorption; administer without regard to meals OR administer with food or milk to minimize GI upset

Nursing/Pharmacy Information Advise patient to inform physician if stomach disturbances, blurred vision, or other eye symptoms, rash, weight gain, edema, or passing of dark-colored or tarry stools occurs; concomitant use of alcohol should be avoided if possible since it may add to the irritant action of nabumetone in the stomach; aspirin should be avoided

Dosage Forms Tablet: 500 mg, 750 mg

♦ **NAC** *see* acetylcysteine *on page 19*

♦ **N-acetylcysteine** *see* acetylcysteine *on page 19*

♦ **N-acetyl-L-cysteine** *see* acetylcysteine *on page 19*

♦ **n-acetyl-p-aminophenol** *see* acetaminophen *on page 13*

♦ **NaCl** *see* sodium chloride *on page 571*

nadolol (nay DOE lole)

U.S. Brand Names Corgard®

Canadian Brand Names Apo®-Nadol; Syn-Nadolol®

Generic Available Yes

Therapeutic Category Beta-Adrenergic Blocker

Use Treatment of hypertension and angina pectoris; prevention of myocardial infarction; prophylaxis of migraine headaches

Usual Dosage Adults: Oral: Initial: 40 mg once daily; increase gradually; usual dosage: 40-80 mg/day; may need up to 240-320 mg/day; doses as high as 640 mg/day have been used

Dietary Considerations May be administered without regard to meals; avoid natural licorice (causes sodium and water retention and increases potassium loss)

Nursing/Pharmacy Information
Advise against abrupt withdrawal
Monitor blood pressure, heart rate, fluid I & O, apical and peripheral pulse; mental status changes (ie, confusion, depression)

Dosage Forms Tablet: 20 mg, 40 mg, 80 mg, 120 mg, 160 mg

♦ **Nadopen-V®** *see* penicillin V potassium *on page 476*

♦ **Nadostine®** *see* nystatin *on page 452*

nadroparin *(Canada only)* (nad roe PA rin)

Canadian Brand Names Fraxiparine®

Generic Available No

Therapeutic Category Low Molecular Weight Heparin

Use Prevention of clotting during hemodialysis; Prophylaxis of thromboembolic disorders (particularly deep vein thrombosis and pulmonary embolism) in general surgery and in orthopedic surgery; treatment of deep vein thrombosis

Usual Dosage Adult: S.C.:
Thromboembolism prophylaxis: 0.3 mL daily S.C for 7 days.
Orthopaedic surgery: 0.2-0.4 mL daily for 3 days then 0.3-0.6 mL daily; doses should be adjusted for bodyweight.
Thromboembolism treatment: 0.4-0.9 mL twice daily for 10 days. Doses should be adjusted for bodyweight.
Hemodialysis: 0.3-0.6 mL into the arterial line at start of 4 hour session. Dose should be adjusted for bodyweight.
Child: Hemodialysis: 60-120 int. units/kg at the start of 4 hour session. Duration of therapy should be determined by the clinical need. Dosage should be individualized.

Dosage Forms Injection, as calcium: in pre-filled syringes or graduated syringes: 9500 int. units anti-Xa/mL (0.2mL, 0.3 mL, 0.4 mL, 0.6 mL, 0.8 mL, 1 mL)

nafarelin (NAF a re lin)
U.S. Brand Names Synarel®
Generic Available No
Therapeutic Category Hormone, Posterior Pituitary
Use Treatment of endometriosis, including pain and reduction of lesions; treatment of central precocious puberty (gonadotropin-dependent precocious puberty) in children of both sexes
Usual Dosage Adults: 1 spray in one nostril each morning and evening for 6 months
Nursing/Pharmacy Information
Each spray delivers 200 mcg
Stability: Store at room temperature; protect from light
Dosage Forms Solution, nasal, as acetate: 2 mg/mL (10 mL)

- **Nafazair® Ophthalmic** *see* naphazoline *on page 431*
- **Nafcil® (Discontinued)** *see page 743*

nafcillin (naf SIL in)
Synonyms ethoxynaphthamido penicillin sodium
U.S. Brand Names Nallpen®
Generic Available Yes
Therapeutic Category Penicillin
Use Treatment of bacterial infections such as osteomyelitis, septicemia, endocarditis, and CNS infections due to susceptible penicillinase-producing strains of *Staphylococcus*
Usual Dosage
Children: I.M., I.V.:
Mild to moderate infections: 50-100 mg/kg/day in divided doses every 6 hours
Severe infections: 100-200 mg/kg/day in divided doses every 4-6 hours
Maximum dose: 12 g/day
Oral: 50-100 mg/kg/day divided every 6 hours
Adults:
Oral: 250-500 mg every 4-6 hours, up to 1 g every 4-6 hours for more severe infections
I.M.: 500 mg every 4-6 hours
I.V.: 500-2000 mg every 4-6 hours
Dietary Considerations Should be administered on an empty stomach, as there is decreased absorption with food
Nursing/Pharmacy Information
Extravasation may cause tissue sloughing and necrosis; hyaluronidase infiltration may help avoid injury; can be administered by I.V. push over 5-10 minutes or by I.V. intermittent infusion over 15-60 minutes at a final concentration not to exceed 40 mg/mL; in fluid-restricted patients, a maximum concentration of 100 mg/mL can be administered
Monitor periodic CBC, urinalysis, BUN, serum creatinine, AST and ALT
Stability: Refrigerate oral solution after reconstitution; discard after 7 days; reconstituted parenteral solution is stable for 3 days at room temperature and 7 days when refrigerated or 12 weeks when frozen; for I.V. infusion in normal saline or D_5W, solution is stable for 24 hours at room temperature and 96 hours when refrigerated
Dosage Forms Nafcillin sodium:
Capsule: 250 mg
Powder for injection: 500 mg, 1 g, 2 g, 4 g, 10 g
Solution: 250 mg/5 mL (100 mL)
Tablet: 500 mg

naftifine (NAF ti feen)
U.S. Brand Names Naftin®
Generic Available No
Therapeutic Category Antifungal Agent
Use Topical treatment of tinea cruris and tinea corporis
Usual Dosage Adults: Topical: Apply twice daily
Nursing/Pharmacy Information External use only; avoid eyes, mouth, and other mucous membranes; do not use occlusive dressings unless directed to do so; discontinue if irritation or sensitivity develops; wash hands after application
Dosage Forms Naftifine hydrochloride:
Cream: 1% (15 g, 30 g, 60 g)
Gel, topical: 1% (20 g, 40 g, 60 g)

♦ **Naftin®** *see* naftifine *on page 428*

♦ **NaHCO₃** *see* sodium bicarbonate *on page 570*

nalbuphine (NAL byoo feen)
U.S. Brand Names Nubain®
Mexican Brand Names Bufigen
Generic Available Yes
Therapeutic Category Analgesic, Narcotic
Use Relief of moderate to severe pain
Usual Dosage I.M., I.V., S.C.: 10 mg/70 kg every 3-6 hours
Dietary Considerations Alcohol: Additive CNS effects; avoid or limit alcohol; watch for sedation
Nursing/Pharmacy Information
Implement safety measures, assist with ambulation
Monitor relief of pain, respiratory and mental status, blood pressure; observe patient for excessive sedation, respiratory depression, observe for narcotic withdrawal
Dosage Forms Injection, as hydrochloride: 10 mg/mL (1 mL, 10 mL); 20 mg/mL (1 mL, 10 mL)

♦ **Naldecon®** *see* chlorpheniramine, phenyltoloxamine, phenylpropanolamine, and phenylephrine *on page 143*

♦ **Naldecon® DX Adult Liquid [OTC]** *see* guaifenesin, phenylpropanolamine, and dextromethorphan *on page 303*

♦ **Naldecon-EX® Children's Syrup [OTC]** *see* guaifenesin and phenylpropanolamine *on page 301*

♦ **Naldecon® Senior DX [OTC]** *see* guaifenesin and dextromethorphan *on page 300*

♦ **Naldecon® Senior EX [OTC]** *see* guaifenesin *on page 299*

♦ **Naldelate®** *see* chlorpheniramine, phenyltoloxamine, phenylpropanolamine, and phenylephrine *on page 143*

♦ **Nalfon®** *see* fenoprofen *on page 262*

♦ **Nalfon® Tablet** *(Discontinued) see page 743*

♦ **Nalgest®** *see* chlorpheniramine, phenyltoloxamine, phenylpropanolamine, and phenylephrine *on page 143*

nalidixic acid (nal i DIKS ik AS id)
Synonyms nalidixinic acid
U.S. Brand Names NegGram®
Generic Available Yes
Therapeutic Category Quinolone
Use Lower urinary tract infections due to susceptible gram-negative organisms including *E. coli, Enterobacter, Klebsiella,* and *Proteus* (inactive against *Pseudomonas*)
Usual Dosage Oral:
Children: 55 mg/kg/day divided every 6 hours; suppressive therapy is 33 mg/kg/day divided every 6 hours
Adults: 1 g 4 times/day for 2 weeks; then suppressive therapy of 500 mg 4 times/day
Dietary Considerations Should be administered 1 hour before meals; can administer with food to minimize GI
Nursing/Pharmacy Information
Administer around-the-clock rather than 4 times/day, 3 times/day, etc, (ie, 12-6-12-6, not 9-1-5-9) to promote less variation in peak and trough serum levels
Monitor urinalysis, urine culture; CBC, renal and hepatic function tests
Dosage Forms
Suspension, oral (raspberry flavor): 250 mg/5 mL (473 mL)
Tablet: 250 mg, 500 mg, 1 g

♦ **nalidixinic acid** *see* nalidixic acid *on page 429*

♦ **Nallpen®** *see* nafcillin *on page 428*

♦ **n-allylnoroxymorphone** *see* naloxone *on page 430*

nalmefene (NAL me feen)
U.S. Brand Names Revex®
Generic Available No
Therapeutic Category Antidote
Use Complete or partial of opioid drug effects; management of known or suspected opioid overdose
(Continued)

nalmefene (Continued)

Usual Dosage Titrate to reverse the undesired effects of opioids; once adequate reversal has been established, additional administration is not required and may actually be harmful due to unwanted reversal of analgesia or precipitated withdrawal; the recommended initial dose for nonopioid dependent patient is 0.5 mg/70 kg, a second dose of 1 mg/70 kg 2-5 minutes later may be administered, after a total dose of 1.5 mg/70 kg has been administered with no clinical response, additional nalmefene is not likely to have an effect

Dosage Forms Injection, as hydrochloride: 100 mcg/mL [blue label] (1 mL); 1000 mcg/mL [green label] (2 mL)

naloxone (nal OKS one)

Synonyms n-allylnoroxymorphone

U.S. Brand Names Narcan®

Generic Available Yes

Therapeutic Category Antidote

Use Reverses CNS and respiratory depression in suspected narcotic overdose; neonatal opiate depression; coma of unknown etiology

Investigational use: Shock, phencyclidine, and alcohol ingestion

Usual Dosage I.M., I.V. (preferred), intratracheal, S.C. (administer undiluted injection):

Infants and Children:

Postanesthesia narcotic reversal: 0.01 mg/kg; may repeat every 2-3 minutes as needed based on response

Opiate intoxication:

Birth (including premature infants) to 5 years or <20 kg: 0.1 mg/kg; repeat every 2-3 minutes if needed; may need to repeat doses every 20-60 minutes

>5 years or ≥20 kg: 2 mg/dose; if no response, repeat every 2-3 minutes; may need to repeat doses every 20-60 minutes

Children and Adults: Continuous infusion: I.V.: If continuous infusion is required, calculate dosage/hour based on effective intermittent dose used and duration of adequate response seen, titrate dose

Adults: 0.4-2 mg every 2-3 minutes as needed; may need to repeat doses every 20-60 minutes; if no response is observed for a total of 10 mg, re-evaluate patient for possibility of a drug or disease process unresponsive to naloxone. **Note:** Use 0.1-0.2 mg increments in patients who are opioid dependent and in postoperative patients to avoid large cardiovascular changes

Nursing/Pharmacy Information

Use of neonatal naloxone (0.02 mg/mL) is no longer recommended because unacceptable fluid volumes may result, especially in small neonates; the 0.4 mg/mL preparation is available and can be accurately dosed with appropriately sized syringes (1 mL)

Endotracheal: Dilute to 1-2 mL with normal saline

I.V. push: Administer over 30 seconds as undiluted preparation

I.V. continuous infusion: Dilute to 4 mcg/mL in D_5W or normal saline

Monitor respiratory rate, heart rate, blood pressure

Stability: Protect from light; stable in 0.9% sodium chloride and D_5W at 4 mcg/mL for 24 hours; do not mix with alkaline solutions

Dosage Forms Injection, as hydrochloride: 0.4 mg/mL (1 mL, 2 mL, 10 mL)

♦ **Nalspan®** see chlorpheniramine, phenyltoloxamine, phenylpropanolamine, and phenylephrine on page 143

naltrexone (nal TREKS one)

U.S. Brand Names Depade®; ReVia®

Generic Available Yes

Therapeutic Category Antidote

Use Adjunct to the maintenance of an opioid-free state in detoxified individual

Usual Dosage Do not administer until patient is opioid-free for 7-10 days as required by urine analysis

Adults: Oral: 25 mg; if no withdrawal signs within 1 hour administer another 25 mg; maintenance regimen is flexible, variable and individualized (50 mg/day to 100-150 mg 3 times/week)

Nursing/Pharmacy Information Monitor for narcotic withdrawal

Dosage Forms Tablet, as hydrochloride: 50 mg

♦ **Nandrobolic® Injection (Discontinued)** see page 743

nandrolone (NAN droe lone)

U.S. Brand Names Anabolin®; Androlone®; Androlone®-D; Deca-Durabolin®; Hybolin™ Decanoate; Hybolin™ Improved Injection; Neo-Durabolic

Generic Available Yes

Therapeutic Category Androgen

Controlled Substance C-III

Use Control of metastatic breast cancer; management of anemia of renal insufficiency

Usual Dosage
Children 2-13 years: 25-50 mg every 3-4 weeks
Adults:
Male: 100-200 mg/week
Female: 50-100 mg/week

Nursing/Pharmacy Information Inject deeply I.M., preferably into the gluteal muscle

Dosage Forms
Nandrolone phenpropionate: Injection in oil: 25 mg/mL (5 mL); 50 mg/mL (2 mL)
Nandrolone decanoate:
Injection in oil: 50 mg/mL (1 mL, 2 mL); 100 mg/mL (1 mL, 2 mL); 200 mg/mL (1 mL)
Injection, repository: 50 mg/mL (2 mL); 100 mg/mL (2 mL); 200 mg/mL (2 mL)

naphazoline (naf AZ oh leen)

U.S. Brand Names AK-Con® Ophthalmic; Albalon® Liquifilm® Ophthalmic; Allerest® Eye Drops [OTC]; Clear Eyes® [OTC]; Comfort® Ophthalmic [OTC]; Degest® 2 Ophthalmic [OTC]; Estivin® II Ophthalmic [OTC]; I-Naphline® Ophthalmic; Nafazair® Ophthalmic; Naphcon Forte® Ophthalmic; Naphcon® Ophthalmic [OTC]; Opcon® Ophthalmic; Privine® Nasal [OTC]; VasoClear® Ophthalmic [OTC]; Vasocon Regular® Ophthalmic

Canadian Brand Names Red Away®

Generic Available Yes

Therapeutic Category Adrenergic Agonist Agent

Use Topical ocular vasoconstrictor (to soothe, refresh, moisturize, and relieve redness due to minor eye irritation); temporarily relieves nasal congestion associated with rhinitis, sinusitis, hay fever, or the common cold

Usual Dosage
Nasal:
Children:
<6 years: Not recommended (especially infants) due to CNS depression
6-12 years: 1 spray of 0.05% into each nostril, repeat in 3 hours if necessary
Children >12 years and Adults: 0.05%, instill 2 drops or sprays every 3-6 hours if needed; therapy should not exceed 3-5 days or more frequently than every 3 hours
Ophthalmic:
Children <6 years: Not recommended for use due to CNS depression (especially in infants)
Children >6 years and Adults: Instill 1-2 drops into conjunctival sac of affected eye(s) every 3-4 hours; therapy generally should not exceed 3-4 days

Nursing/Pharmacy Information
Rebound congestion can result with continued use beyond 3 days
Stability: Store in tight, light-resistant containers; do not use if solution changes color or becomes cloudy

Dosage Forms Solution, as hydrochloride:
Nasal:
Drops: 0.05% (20 mL)
Spray: 0.05% (15 mL)
Ophthalmic: 0.012% (7.5 mL, 30 mL); 0.02% (15 mL); 0.03% (15 mL); 0.1% (15 mL)

naphazoline and antazoline (naf AZ oh leen & an TAZ oh leen)

U.S. Brand Names Albalon-A® Ophthalmic; Antazoline-V® Ophthalmic; Vasocon-A® [OTC] Ophthalmic

Generic Available No

Therapeutic Category Antihistamine/Decongestant Combination

Use Topical ocular congestion, irritation, and itching

Usual Dosage Ophthalmic: 1-2 drops every 3-4 hours

(Continued)

naphazoline and antazoline *(Continued)*
Nursing/Pharmacy Information
Do not use discolored solutions
Stability: Store in tight, light-resistant containers
Dosage Forms Solution: Naphazoline hydrochloride 0.05% and antazoline phosphate 0.5% (15 mL)

naphazoline and pheniramine (naf AZ oh leen & fen NIR a meen)
Synonyms pheniramine and naphazoline
U.S. Brand Names Naphcon-A® Ophthalmic [OTC]
Generic Available No
Therapeutic Category Antihistamine/Decongestant Combination
Use Topical ocular vasoconstrictor
Usual Dosage Ophthalmic: 1-2 drops every 3-4 hours
Nursing/Pharmacy Information Discontinue drug and consult physician if ocular pain or visual changes occur, ocular redness or irritation, or condition worsens or persists more than 72 hours
Dosage Forms Solution, ophthalmic: Naphazoline hydrochloride 0.025% and pheniramine 0.3% (15 mL)

- **Naphcon-A® Ophthalmic [OTC]** *see* naphazoline and pheniramine *on page 432*
- **Naphcon Forte® Ophthalmic** *see* naphazoline *on page 431*
- **Naphcon® Ophthalmic [OTC]** *see* naphazoline *on page 431*
- **Naprodil** *see* naproxen *on page 432*
- **Naprosyn®** *see* naproxen *on page 432*

naproxen (na PROKS en)
U.S. Brand Names Aleve® [OTC]; Anaprox®; Naprosyn®
Canadian Brand Names Apo®-Naproxen; Naxen®; Novo-Naprox®; Nu-Naprox®; Synflex®
Mexican Brand Names Artron; Atiflan; Atiquim®; Dafloxen®; Faraxen; Flanax; Flexen; Flogen; Fuxen; Naprodil; Naxen®; Naxil; Pactens; Pronaxil; Supradol®; Velsay
Generic Available Yes
Therapeutic Category Analgesic, Non-narcotic; Antipyretic; Nonsteroidal Anti-inflammatory Drug (NSAID)
Use Management of inflammatory disease and rheumatoid disorders (including juvenile rheumatoid arthritis); acute gout; mild to moderate pain; dysmenorrhea; fever
Usual Dosage Oral (as naproxen):
Children >2 years:
Antipyretic or analgesic: 5-7 mg/kg/dose every 8-12 hours
Juvenile rheumatoid arthritis: 10 mg/kg/day, up to a maximum of 1000 mg/day divided twice daily
Adults:
Rheumatoid arthritis, osteoarthritis, and ankylosing spondylitis: 500-1000 mg/day in 2 divided doses
Mild to moderate pain or dysmenorrhea: Initial: 500 mg, then 250 mg every 6-8 hours; maximum: 1250 mg/day
Dietary Considerations
Alcohol: Additive impairment of mental alertness and physical coordination; avoid or limit alcohol
Food may decrease the rate but not the extent of oral absorption; may cause GI upset, bleeding, ulceration, perforation; administer with food or milk to minimize GI upset
Nursing/Pharmacy Information Monitor occult blood loss, periodic liver function test, hemoglobin, CBC, BUN, serum creatinine
Dosage Forms
Suspension, oral: 125 mg/5 mL (15 mL, 30 mL, 480 mL)
Tablet:
Aleve®: 200 mg
Naprosyn®: 250 mg, 375 mg, 500 mg
Tablet, controlled release (Naprelan®): 375 mg, 500 mg

Naproxen sodium:
Tablet, as sodium: 220 mg (200 mg base)
Anaprox®: 220 mg (200 mg base); 275 mg (250 mg base); 550 mg (500 mg base)

- **Naqua®** *see* trichlormethiazide *on page 626*

naratriptan (NAR a trip tan)

U.S. Brand Names Amerge®

Generic Available No

Therapeutic Category Antimigraine Agent; Serotonin Agonist

Use Acute treatment of migraine with or without aura

Usual Dosage Oral: Adults: 1 mg or 2.5 mg (maximum dose: 5 mg); if no response, dose may be repeated in 4 hours

Dosage Forms Tablet, as hydrochloride: 1 mg, 2.5 mg

♦ **Narcan®** see naloxone on page 430
♦ **Narcan® 1 mg/mL Injection (Discontinued)** see page 743
♦ **Nardil®** see phenelzine on page 484
♦ **Naropin™** see ropivacaine on page 554
♦ **Nasabid™** see guaifenesin and pseudoephedrine on page 302
♦ **Nasacort®** see triamcinolone (inhalation, nasal) on page 623
♦ **Nasacort® AQ** see triamcinolone (inhalation, nasal) on page 623
♦ **Nasahist B®** see brompheniramine on page 94
♦ **NaSal™ [OTC]** see sodium chloride on page 571
♦ **Nasalcrom® [OTC]** see cromolyn sodium on page 171
♦ **Nasalide® Nasal Aerosol** see flunisolide on page 272
♦ **Nasal Moist® [OTC]** see sodium chloride on page 571
♦ **Nasarel™ Nasal Spray** see flunisolide on page 272
♦ **Nasonex®** see mometasone furoate on page 420
♦ **Natabec® [OTC]** see vitamin, multiple (prenatal) on page 654
♦ **Natabec® FA [OTC]** see vitamin, multiple (prenatal) on page 654
♦ **Natabec® Rx** see vitamin, multiple (prenatal) on page 654
♦ **Natacyn®** see natamycin on page 433
♦ **Natalins® [OTC]** see vitamin, multiple (prenatal) on page 654
♦ **Natalins® Rx** see vitamin, multiple (prenatal) on page 654

natamycin (na ta MYE sin)

Synonyms pimaricin

U.S. Brand Names Natacyn®

Generic Available No

Therapeutic Category Antifungal Agent

Use Treatment of blepharitis, conjunctivitis, and keratitis caused by susceptible fungi (*Aspergillus, Candida*), *Cephalosporium, Curvularia, Fusarium, Penicillium, Microsporum, Epidermophyton, Blastomyces dermatitidis, Coccidioides immitis, Cryptococcus neoformans, Histoplasma capsulatum, Sporothrix schenckii, Trichomonas vaginalis*

Usual Dosage Adults: Ophthalmic: 1 drop in conjunctival sac every 1-2 hours, after 3-4 days dose may be reduced to one drop 6-8 times/day; usual course of therapy: 2-3 weeks

Nursing/Pharmacy Information
Shake suspension before using
Stability: Protect from excessive heat and light; do not freeze

Dosage Forms Suspension, ophthalmic: 5% (15 mL)

♦ **Natulan®** see procarbazine on page 519
♦ **natural lung surfactant** see beractant on page 83
♦ **Nature's Tears® Solution [OTC]** see artificial tears on page 59
♦ **Naturetin®** see bendroflumethiazide on page 77
♦ **Naus-A-Way® [OTC]** see phosphorated carbohydrate solution on page 492
♦ **Nausetrol® [OTC]** see phosphorated carbohydrate solution on page 492
♦ **Navane® Capsule** see thiothixene on page 609
♦ **Navane® Concentrate & Injection (Discontinued)** see page 743
♦ **Navelbine®** see vinorelbine on page 649
♦ **Naxen®** see naproxen on page 432
♦ **Naxifelar** see cephalexin on page 128
♦ **Naxil** see naproxen on page 432
♦ **Naxodol (Carisoprodol With Naproxen)** see carisoprodol on page 116
♦ **N-B-P® Ointment (Discontinued)** see page 743
♦ **ND-Stat®** see brompheniramine on page 94
♦ **Nebcin® Injection** see tobramycin on page 615
♦ **NebuPent™ Inhalation** see pentamidine on page 477

nedocromil (inhalation) (ne doe KROE mil, in hil LA shun)
U.S. Brand Names Tilade® Inhalation Aerosol
Generic Available No
Therapeutic Category Mast Cell Stabilizer
Use Maintenance therapy in patients with mild to moderate bronchial asthma
Usual Dosage Adults: Inhalation: 2 inhalations 4 times/day
Nursing/Pharmacy Information
   Nedocromil is **not** a bronchodilator and, therefore, should not be used for reversal of acute bronchospasm; has no known therapeutic systemic activity when delivered by inhalation
   Stability: Do not freeze
Dosage Forms Aerosol, as sodium: 1.75 mg/activation (16.2 g)

nedocromil (ophthalmic) *New Drug*
   (ne doe KROE mil, op THAL mik)
U.S. Brand Names Alocril™
Therapeutic Category Mast Cell Stabilizer
Use Treatment of itching associated with allergic conjunctivitis
Usual Dosage Adults: Ophthalmic: 1-2 drops in eye(s) twice daily
Dosage Forms Solution, ophthalmic, as sodium: 2% (5 mL)

♦ **N.E.E.® 1/35** *see* ethinyl estradiol and norethindrone *on page 250*

nefazodone (nef AY zoe done)
U.S. Brand Names Serzone®
Generic Available No
Therapeutic Category Antidepressant, Miscellaneous
Use Treatment of depression
Usual Dosage Adults: Oral: Initial: 200 mg/day administered in two divided doses with a range of 300-600 mg/day in two divided doses thereafter
Dosage Forms Tablet, as hydrochloride: 100 mg, 150 mg, 200 mg, 250 mg

♦ **NegGram®** *see* nalidixic acid *on page 429*

nelfinavir (nel FIN a veer)
U.S. Brand Names Viracept®
Generic Available No
Therapeutic Category Antiviral Agent
Use As monotherapy or preferably in combination with nucleoside analogs in the treatment of HIV infection, in adults and children, when antiretroviral therapy is warranted
Usual Dosage Oral:
   Children 2-13 years: 20-30 mg/kg 3 times/day with a meal or light snack; if tablets are unable to be taken, use oral powder in small amount of water, milk, formula, or dietary supplements; do not use acidic food/juice or store for >6 hours
   Adults: 750 mg 3 times/day with meals
Dosage Forms Nelfinavir mesylate:
   Powder, oral: 50 mg/g [144 g] (contains 11.2 mg phenylalanine)
   Tablet: 250 mg

♦ **Nelova™ 0.5/35E** *see* ethinyl estradiol and norethindrone *on page 250*
♦ **Nelova® 1/50M** *see* mestranol and norethindrone *on page 396*
♦ **Nelova™ 10/11** *see* ethinyl estradiol and norethindrone *on page 250*
♦ **Nembutal®** *see* pentobarbital *on page 479*
♦ **Neo-Calglucon® [OTC]** *see* calcium glubionate *on page 105*
♦ **Neo-Castaderm** *(Discontinued) see page 743*
♦ **Neo-Codema®** *see* hydrochlorothiazide *on page 317*
♦ **Neo-Cortef® Ophthalmic** *see* neomycin and hydrocortisone *on page 435*
♦ **Neo-Cortef® Topical** *(Discontinued) see page 743*
♦ **NeoDecadron® Ophthalmic** *see* neomycin and dexamethasone *on page 435*
♦ **NeoDecadron® Topical** *(Discontinued) see page 743*
♦ **Neo-Dexameth® Ophthalmic** *see* neomycin and dexamethasone *on page 435*
♦ **Neodol** *see* acetaminophen *on page 13*
♦ **Neo-Durabolic** *see* nandrolone *on page 431*
♦ **Neo-Estrone®** *see* estrone *on page 246*
♦ **Neofed® [OTC]** *see* pseudoephedrine *on page 530*
♦ **Neo-fradin®** *see* neomycin *on page 435*

♦ **Neoloid®** [OTC] *see* castor oil *on page 118*
♦ **Neo-Medrol® Acetate Topical** *(Discontinued)* *see page 743*
♦ **Neomicol®** *see* miconazole *on page 413*
♦ **Neomixin® Topical** *see* bacitracin, neomycin, and polymyxin B *on page 71*

neomycin (nee oh MYE sin)

U.S. Brand Names Mycifradin® Sulfate; Neo-fradin®; Neo-Tabs®
Canadian Brand Names Myciguent®
Generic Available Yes
Therapeutic Category Aminoglycoside (Antibiotic); Antibiotic, Topical
Use Administered orally to prepare GI tract for surgery; treat minor skin infections; treat diarrhea caused by *E. coli*; adjunct in the treatment of hepatic encephalopathy
Usual Dosage
Children: Oral:
Preoperative intestinal antisepsis: 90 mg/kg/day divided every 4 hours for 2 days; or 25 mg/kg at 1 PM, 2 PM, and 11 PM on the day preceding surgery as an adjunct to mechanical cleansing of the intestine and in combination with erythromycin base
Hepatic coma: 50-100 mg/kg/day in divided doses every 6-8 hours or 2.5-7 g/m²/day divided every 4-6 hours for 5-6 days not to exceed 12 g/day
Children and Adults: Topical: Apply ointment 1-4 times/day; topical solutions containing 0.1% to 1% neomycin have been used for irrigation
Adults: Oral:
Preoperative intestinal antisepsis: 1 g each hour for 4 doses then 1 g every 4 hours for 5 doses; or 1 g at 1 PM, 2 PM, and 11 PM on day preceding surgery as an adjunct to mechanical cleansing of the bowel and oral erythromycin; or 6 g/day divided every 4 hours for 2-3 days
Hepatic coma: 500-2000 mg every 6-8 hours or 4-12 g/day divided every 4-6 hours for 5-6 days
Chronic hepatic insufficiency: Oral: 4 g/day for an indefinite period
Nursing/Pharmacy Information
Monitor renal function tests
Stability: Use reconstituted parenteral solutions within 7 days of mixing, when refrigerated
Dosage Forms Neomycin sulfate:
Cream: 0.5% (15 g)
Ointment, topical: 0.5% (15 g, 30 g, 120 g)
Solution, oral: 125 mg/5 mL (480 mL)
Tablet: 500 mg [base 300 mg]

neomycin and dexamethasone
(nee oh MYE sin & deks a METH a sone)
Synonyms dexamethasone and neomycin
U.S. Brand Names AK-Neo-Dex® Ophthalmic; NeoDecadron® Ophthalmic; Neo-Dexameth® Ophthalmic
Generic Available No
Therapeutic Category Antibiotic/Corticosteroid, Ophthalmic; Antibiotic/Corticosteroid, Topical
Use Treatment of steroid responsive inflammatory conditions of the palpebral and bulbar conjunctiva, lid, cornea, and anterior segment of the globe
Usual Dosage
Ophthalmic: Instill 1-2 drops in eye(s) every 3-4 hours
Topical: Apply thin coat 3-4 times/day until favorable response is observed, then reduce dose to one application/day
Nursing/Pharmacy Information
May cause sensitivity to light, can minimize by wearing sunglasses
Stability: Store in tight, light-resistant container
Dosage Forms
Cream: Neomycin sulfate 0.5% [5 mg/g] and dexamethasone 0.1% [1 mg/g] (15 g, 30 g)
Ointment, ophthalmic: Neomycin sulfate 0.35% [3.5 mg/g] and dexamethasone 0.05% [0.5 mg/g] (3.5 g)
Solution, ophthalmic: Neomycin sulfate 0.35% [3.5 mg/mL] and dexamethasone 0.1% [1 mg/mL] (5 mL)

neomycin and hydrocortisone
(nee oh MYE sin & hye droe KOR ti sone)
Synonyms hydrocortisone and neomycin
U.S. Brand Names Neo-Cortef® Ophthalmic
(Continued)

neomycin and hydrocortisone *(Continued)*

Generic Available No

Therapeutic Category Antibiotic/Corticosteroid, Ophthalmic; Antibiotic/Corticosteroid, Topical

Use Treatment of susceptible topical bacterial infections with associated inflammation

Usual Dosage Topical: Apply to area in a thin film 2-4 times/day

Dosage Forms

Cream: Neomycin sulfate 0.5% and hydrocortisone 1% (20 g)

Ointment, topical: Neomycin sulfate 0.5% and hydrocortisone 0.5% (20 g); neomycin sulfate 0.5% and hydrocortisone 1% (20 g)

Solution, ophthalmic: Neomycin sulfate 0.5% and hydrocortisone 0.5% (5 mL)

neomycin and polymyxin B *(nee oh MYE sin & pol i MIKS in bee)*

Synonyms polymyxin B and neomycin

U.S. Brand Names Neosporin® Cream [OTC]; Neosporin® G.U. Irrigant

Generic Available Yes

Therapeutic Category Antibiotic, Topical; Genitourinary Irrigant

Use Short-term use as a continuous irrigant or rinse in the urinary bladder to prevent bacteriuria and gram-negative rod septicemia associated with the use of indwelling catheters; to help prevent infection in minor cuts, scrapes, and burns

Usual Dosage Children and Adults:

Topical: Apply cream 2-4 times/day

Bladder irrigation: Continuous irrigant or rinse in the urinary bladder for up to 10 days where 1 mL is added to 1 L of normal saline with administration rate adjusted to patient's urine output; usually no more than 1 L of irrigant is used per day

Nursing/Pharmacy Information

Do not inject irrigant solution; connect irrigation container to the inflow lumen of a 3-way catheter to permit continuous irrigation of the urinary bladder

Monitor urinalysis

Stability: Aseptic prepared dilutions (1 mL/1 L) should be stored in the refrigerator and discarded after 48 hours

Dosage Forms

Cream: Neomycin sulfate 3.5 mg and polymyxin B sulfate 10,000 units per g (0.94 g, 15 g)

Solution, irrigant: Neomycin sulfate 40 mg and polymyxin B sulfate 200,000 units per mL (1 mL, 20 mL)

♦ **neomycin, bacitracin, and polymyxin B** *see* bacitracin, neomycin, and polymyxin B *on page 71*

♦ **neomycin, bacitracin, polymyxin B, and hydrocortisone** *see* bacitracin, neomycin, polymyxin B, and hydrocortisone *on page 72*

♦ **neomycin, colistin, and hydrocortisone** *see* colistin, neomycin, and hydrocortisone *on page 166*

neomycin, colistin, hydrocortisone, and thonzonium

(nee oh MYE sin, koe LIS tin, hye droe KOR ti sone, & thon ZOE nee um)

U.S. Brand Names Cortisporin®-TC Otic Suspension

Generic Available No

Therapeutic Category Antibiotic/Corticosteroid, Otic

Use Treatment of superficial and susceptible bacterial infections of the external auditory canal; for treatment of susceptible bacterial infections of mastoidectomy and fenestration cavities

Usual Dosage

Children: 4 drops in affected ear 3-4 times/day

Adults: 5 drops in affected ear 3-4 times/day

Dosage Forms Suspension, otic: Neomycin sulfate 3.3 mg, colistin sulfate 3 mg, hydrocortisone acetate 1%, and thonzonium bromide 0.5 mg per mL (10 mL)

neomycin, polymyxin B, and dexamethasone

(nee oh MYE sin, pol i MIKS in bee, & deks a METH a sone)

Synonyms dexamethasone, neomycin, and polymyxin B; polymyxin B, neomycin, and dexamethasone

U.S. Brand Names AK-Trol®; Dexacidin®; Dexasporin®; Maxitrol®

Generic Available Yes

Therapeutic Category Antibiotic/Corticosteroid, Ophthalmic

Use Steroid-responsive inflammatory ocular conditions in which a corticosteroid is indicated and where bacterial infection or a risk of bacterial infection exists

Usual Dosage Children and Adults: Ophthalmic:

Ointment: Place a small amount (~½") in the affected eye 3-4 times/day or apply at bedtime as an adjunct with drops

Solution: Instill 1-2 drops into affected eye(s) every 4-6 hours; in severe disease, drops may be used hourly and tapered to discontinuation

Nursing/Pharmacy Information

Shake well before using

Monitor intraocular pressure with use >10 days

Dosage Forms

Ointment, ophthalmic: Neomycin sulfate 3.5 mg, polymyxin B sulfate 10,000 units, and dexamethasone 0.1% per g (3.5 g)

Suspension, ophthalmic: Neomycin sulfate 3.5 mg, polymyxin B sulfate 10,000 units, and dexamethasone 0.1% per mL (5 mL)

neomycin, polymyxin B, and gramicidin

(nee oh MYE sin, pol i MIKS in bee, & gram i SYE din)

Synonyms gramicidin, neomycin, and polymyxin B; polymyxin B, neomycin, and gramicidin

U.S. Brand Names AK-Spore® Ophthalmic Solution; Neosporin® Ophthalmic Solution

Mexican Brand Names Neosporin® Oftalmico

Generic Available Yes

Therapeutic Category Antibiotic, Ophthalmic

Use Treatment of superficial ocular infection, infection prophylaxis in minor skin abrasions

Usual Dosage Ophthalmic: Drops: 1-2 drops 4-6 times/day or more frequently as required for severe infections

Nursing/Pharmacy Information Tilt head back, place medication in conjunctival sac, and close eyes; apply finger pressure on lacrimal sac for 1 minute following instillation

Dosage Forms Solution, ophthalmic: Neomycin sulfate 1.75 mg, polymyxin B sulfate 10,000 units, and gramicidin 0.025 mg per mL (2 mL, 10 mL)

neomycin, polymyxin B, and hydrocortisone

(nee oh MYE sin, pol i MIKS in bee, & hye droe KOR ti sone)

Synonyms hydrocortisone, neomycin, and polymyxin B; polymyxin B, neomycin, and hydrocortisone

U.S. Brand Names AK-Spore® H.C. Ophthalmic Suspension; AK-Spore® H.C. Otic; AntibiOtic® Otic; Cortatrigen® Otic; Cortisporin® Ophthalmic Suspension; Cortisporin® Otic; Cortisporin® Topical Cream; Octicair® Otic; Otic-Care® Otic; Otocort® Otic; Otosporin® Otic; Pediotic® Otic; UAD Otic®

Generic Available Yes

Therapeutic Category Antibiotic/Corticosteroid, Ophthalmic; Antibiotic/Corticosteroid, Otic; Antibiotic/Corticosteroid, Topical

Use Steroid-responsive inflammatory condition for which a corticosteroid is indicated and where bacterial infection or a risk of bacterial infection exists

Usual Dosage Duration of use should be limited to 10 days unless otherwise directed by the physician

Ophthalmic: Adults and Children:

Ointment: Apply to the affected eye every 3-4 hours

Suspension: 1 drop every 3-4 hours

Otic: Solution/suspension:

Children: 3 drops into affected ear 3-4 times/day

Adults: 4 drops into affected ear 3-4 times/day

Nursing/Pharmacy Information Otic suspension is the preferred otic preparation; otic suspension can be used for the treatment of infections of mastoidectomy and fenestration cavities caused by susceptible organisms; otic solution is used **only** for superficial infections of the external auditory canal (ie, swimmer's ear)

Dosage Forms

Cream, topical: Neomycin sulfate 5 mg, polymyxin B sulfate 10,000 units, and hydrocortisone 10 mg per mL (7.5 g)

Solution, otic: Neomycin sulfate 5 mg, polymyxin B sulfate 10,000 units, and hydrocortisone 10 mg per mL (10 mL)

Suspension:

Ophthalmic: Neomycin sulfate 5 mg, polymyxin B sulfate 10,000 units, and hydrocortisone 10 mg per mL (7.5 mL)

(Continued)

neomycin, polymyxin B, and hydrocortisone
(Continued)

Otic: Neomycin sulfate 5 mg, polymyxin B sulfate 10,000 units, and hydro-cortisone 10 mg per mL (10 mL)

neomycin, polymyxin B, and prednisolone
(nee oh MYE sin, pol i MIKS in bee, & pred NIS oh lone)

Synonyms polymyxin B, neomycin, and prednisolone; prednisolone, neomycin, and polymyxin B

U.S. Brand Names Poly-Pred® Ophthalmic Suspension

Generic Available Yes

Therapeutic Category Antibiotic/Corticosteroid, Ophthalmic

Use Steroid-responsive inflammatory ocular condition in which bacterial infection or a risk of bacterial ocular infection exists

Usual Dosage Children and Adults: Ophthalmic: Instill 1-2 drops every 3-4 hours; acute infections may require every 30-minute instillation initially with frequency of administration reduced as the infection is brought under control. To treat the lids: Instill 1-2 drops every 3-4 hours, close the eye and rub the excess on the lids and lid margins.

Nursing/Pharmacy Information Shake suspension before using

Dosage Forms Suspension, ophthalmic: Neomycin sulfate 0.35%, polymyxin B sulfate 10,000 units, and prednisolone acetate 0.5% per mL (5 mL, 10 mL)

♦ **neonatal trace metals** *see* trace metals *on page 620*

♦ **Neopap® [OTC]** *see* acetaminophen *on page 13*

♦ **Neoquess® Injection *(Discontinued)*** *see page 743*

♦ **Neoquess® Tablet *(Discontinued)*** *see page 743*

♦ **Neoral®** *see* cyclosporine *on page 176*

♦ **Neosar®** *see* cyclophosphamide *on page 175*

♦ **Neosporin® Cream [OTC]** *see* neomycin and polymyxin B *on page 436*

♦ **Neosporin® G.U. Irrigant** *see* neomycin and polymyxin B *on page 436*

♦ **Neosporin® Oftalmico** *see* neomycin, polymyxin B, and gramicidin *on page 437*

♦ **Neosporin® Ophthalmic Ointment** *see* bacitracin, neomycin, and polymyxin B *on page 71*

♦ **Neosporin® Ophthalmic Solution** *see* neomycin, polymyxin B, and gramicidin *on page 437*

♦ **Neosporin® Topical Ointment [OTC]** *see* bacitracin, neomycin, and polymyxin B *on page 71*

neostigmine (nee oh STIG meen)

U.S. Brand Names Prostigmin®

Generic Available Yes

Therapeutic Category Cholinergic Agent

Use Treatment of myasthenia gravis; prevention and treatment of postoperative bladder distention and urinary retention; reversal of the effects of nondepolarizing neuromuscular blocking agents after surgery

Usual Dosage
Myasthenia gravis: Diagnosis: I.M.:
  Children: 0.04 mg/kg as a single dose
  Adults: 0.02 mg/kg as a single dose
Myasthenia gravis: Treatment:
  Children:
    Oral: 2 mg/kg/day divided every 3-4 hours
    I.M., I.V., S.C.: 0.01-0.04 mg/kg every 2-4 hours
  Adults:
    Oral: 15 mg/dose every 3-4 hours
    I.M., I.V., S.C.: 0.5-2.5 mg every 1-3 hours
Reversal of nondepolarizing neuromuscular blockade after surgery in conjunction with atropine or glycopyrrolate: I.V.:
  Infants: 0.025-0.1 mg/kg/dose
  Children: 0.025-0.08 mg/kg/dose
  Adults: 0.5-2.5 mg; total dose not to exceed 5 mg
Bladder atony: Adults: I.M., S.C.:
  Prevention: 0.25 mg every 4-6 hours for 2-3 days
  Treatment: 0.5-1 mg every 3 hours for 5 doses after bladder has emptied

Nursing/Pharmacy Information
Parenteral: May be administered undiluted by slow I.V. injection over several minutes

Monitor muscle strength, heart rate, respiratory rate

Dosage Forms

Injection, as methylsulfate: 0.25 mg/mL (1 mL); 0.5 mg/mL (1 mL, 10 mL); 1 mg/mL (10 mL)

Tablet, as bromide: 15 mg

♦ **Neostrata® HQ** *see* hydroquinone *on page 325*

♦ **Neo-Synalar® Topical** *(Discontinued) see page 743*

♦ **Neo-Synephrine® 12 Hour Nasal Solution [OTC]** *see* oxymetazoline *on page 463*

♦ **Neo-Synephrine® 12 Hour Nasal Solution** *(Discontinued) see page 743*

♦ **Neo-Synephrine® Nasal Solution [OTC]** *see* phenylephrine *on page 487*

♦ **Neo-Synephrine® Ophthalmic Solution** *see* phenylephrine *on page 487*

♦ **Neo-Tabs®** *see* neomycin *on page 435*

♦ **Neotopic®** *see* bacitracin, neomycin, and polymyxin B *on page 71*

♦ **Neotrace-4®** *see* trace metals *on page 620*

♦ **Neotricin HC® Ophthalmic Ointment** *see* bacitracin, neomycin, polymyxin B, and hydrocortisone *on page 72*

♦ **NeoVadrin® [OTC]** *see* vitamin, multiple (oral) *on page 654*

♦ **NeoVadrin® B Complex [OTC]** *see* vitamin B complex *on page 651*

♦ **Nephro-Calci® [OTC]** *see* calcium carbonate *on page 103*

♦ **Nephrocaps®** *see* vitamin B complex with vitamin C and folic acid *on page 652*

♦ **Nephro-Fer™ [OTC]** *see* ferrous fumarate *on page 264*

♦ **Nephronex®** *see* nitrofurantoin *on page 444*

♦ **Nephrox Suspension [OTC]** *see* aluminum hydroxide *on page 33*

♦ **Neptazane®** *see* methazolamide *on page 400*

♦ **Nervocaine® Injection** *see* lidocaine *on page 368*

♦ **Nesacaine®** *see* chloroprocaine *on page 136*

♦ **Nesacaine®-MPF** *see* chloroprocaine *on page 136*

♦ **Nestrex®** *see* pyridoxine *on page 534*

♦ **1-n-ethyl sisomicin** *see* netilmicin *on page 439*

netilmicin (ne til MYE sin)

Synonyms 1-n-ethyl sisomicin

U.S. Brand Names Netromycin®

Generic Available No

Therapeutic Category Aminoglycoside (Antibiotic)

Use Short-term treatment of serious or life-threatening infections including septicemia, peritonitis, intra-abdominal abscess, lower respiratory tract infections, urinary tract infections, skin, bone and joint infections caused by sensitive *Pseudomonas aeruginosa*, *Escherichia coli*, *Proteus*, *Klebsiella*, *Serratia*, *Enterobacter*, *Citrobacter*, and *Staphylococcus*

Usual Dosage I.M., I.V.:

Children 6 weeks to 12 years: 1-2.5 mg/kg/dose every 8 hours

Children >12 years and Adults: 1.5-2 mg/kg/dose every 8-12 hours

Nursing/Pharmacy Information Aminoglycoside levels measured in blood taken from Silastic® central catheters can sometimes give falsely high readings

Dosage Forms Injection, as sulfate: 100 mg/mL (1.5 mL)

♦ **Netromycin®** *see* netilmicin *on page 439*

♦ **Neucalm-50® Injection** *see* hydroxyzine *on page 328*

♦ **Neugal** *see* ranitidine hydrochloride *on page 541*

♦ **Neugeron** *see* carbamazepine *on page 112*

♦ **Neuleptil®** *see* pericyazine *(Canada only) on page 481*

♦ **Neumega®** *see* oprelvekin *on page 457*

♦ **Neupogen®** *see* filgrastim *on page 267*

♦ **Neuramate®** *see* meprobamate *on page 394*

♦ **Neurontin®** *see* gabapentin *on page 286*

♦ **Neurosine** *see* buspirone *on page 98*

♦ **Neut®** *see* sodium bicarbonate *on page 570*

♦ **Neutra-Phos® Capsule** *(Discontinued) see page 743*

♦ **Neutra-Phos®-K** *see* potassium phosphate *on page 509*

♦ **Neutrexin®** *see* trimetrexate glucuronate *on page 630*

♦ **Neutrogena® Acne Mask [OTC]** *see* benzoyl peroxide *on page 81*

♦ **Neutrogena® T/Derm** *see* coal tar *on page 162*

nevirapine (ne VYE ra peen)
U.S. Brand Names Viramune®
Generic Available No
Therapeutic Category Antiviral Agent
Use In combination therapy with nucleoside antiretroviral agents in HIV-1 infected adults previously treated for whom current therapy is deemed inadequate
Usual Dosage Adults: Oral: 200 mg once daily for 2 weeks followed by 200 mg twice daily
Dosage Forms
Suspension, oral: 50 mg/5 mL (240 mL)
Tablet: 200 mg

♦ **New Decongestant®** *see* chlorpheniramine, phenyltoloxamine, phenylpropanolamine, and phenylephrine *on page 143*

♦ **N.G.T.® Topical** *see* nystatin and triamcinolone *on page 452*

♦ **Niac®** *(Discontinued) see page 743*

♦ **Niacels®** *(Discontinued) see page 743*

niacin (NYE a sin)
Synonyms nicotinic acid; vitamin B_3
U.S. Brand Names Niaspan®; Nicobid® [OTC]; Nicolar® [OTC]; Nicotinex [OTC]; Slo-Niacin® [OTC]
Generic Available Yes
Therapeutic Category Vitamin, Water Soluble
Use Adjunctive treatment of hyperlipidemias; peripheral vascular disease and circulatory disorders; treatment of pellagra; dietary supplement
Usual Dosage
Children: Pellagra: Oral, I.M., I.V.: 50-100 mg/dose 3 times/day
Oral: Recommended daily allowances:
0-1 year: 6-8 mg/day
2-6 years: 9-11 mg/day
7-10 years: 16 mg/day
>10 years: 15-18 mg/day
Adults: Oral:
Hyperlipidemia: 1.5-6 g/day in 3 divided doses with or after meals
Pellagra: 50 mg 3-10 times/day, maximum: 500 mg/day
Niacin deficiency: 10-20 mg/day, maximum: 100 mg/day
Dietary Considerations Should be administered after meals
Nursing/Pharmacy Information
If dizziness occurs, avoid sudden changes in posture
Monitor blood glucose, liver function tests, serum cholesterol
Dosage Forms
Capsule, timed release: 125 mg, 250 mg, 300 mg, 400 mg, 500 mg
Elixir: 50 mg/5 mL (473 mL, 4000 mL)
Injection: 100 mg/mL (30 mL)
Tablet: 25 mg, 50 mg, 100 mg, 250 mg, 500 mg
Extended release: 500 mg, 750 mg, 1000 mg
Timed release: 150 mg, 250 mg, 500 mg, 750 mg

niacinamide (nye a SIN a mide)
Synonyms nicotinamide
Generic Available Yes
Therapeutic Category Vitamin, Water Soluble
Use Prophylaxis and treatment of pellagra
Usual Dosage Oral:
Children: Pellagra: 100-300 mg/day
Adults: 50 mg 3-10 times/day
Pellagra: 300-500 mg/day
Hyperlipidemias: 1-2 g 3 times/day
Dosage Forms Tablet: 50 mg, 100 mg, 125 mg, 250 mg, 500 mg

♦ **Niaspan®** *see* niacin *on page 440*

nicardipine (nye KAR de peen)
U.S. Brand Names Cardene®; Cardene® SR
Mexican Brand Names Ridene
Generic Available Yes: Capsule
Therapeutic Category Calcium Channel Blocker
Use Chronic stable angina; management of essential hypertension

Usual Dosage Adults:

Oral: 40 mg 3 times/day (allow 3 days between dose increases)

Oral, sustained release: Initial: 30 mg twice daily, titrate up to 60 mg twice daily

I.V.: (Dilute to 0.1 mg/mL) Initial: 5 mg/hour increased by 2.5 mg/hour every 15 minutes to a maximum of 15 mg/hour

Oral to I.V. dose:

20 mg every 8 hours = I.V. 0.5 mg/hour

30 mg every 8 hours = I.V. 1.2 mg/hour

40 mg every 8 hours = I.V. 2.2 mg/hour

Nursing/Pharmacy Information

Do not crush sustained release capsules

Stability: I.V. dilution stable for 24 hours at room temperature in D_5W or normal saline

Dosage Forms Nicardipine hydrochloride:

Capsule: 20 mg, 30 mg

Capsule, sustained release: 30 mg, 45 mg, 60 mg

Injection: 2.5 mg/mL (10 mL)

- ♦ **N'ice®** *see* ascorbic acid *on page 60*
- ♦ **Niclocide®** *(Discontinued) see page 743*
- ♦ **Nicobid® [OTC]** *see* niacin *on page 440*
- ♦ **Nicoderm® Patch** *see* nicotine *on page 441*
- ♦ **Nicolan** *see* nicotine *on page 441*
- ♦ **Nicolar® [OTC]** *see* niacin *on page 440*
- ♦ **Nicorette® DS Gum** *see* nicotine *on page 441*
- ♦ **Nicorette® Gum** *see* nicotine *on page 441*
- ♦ **Nicorette® Plus** *see* nicotine *on page 441*
- ♦ **nicotinamide** *see* niacinamide *on page 440*

nicotine (nik oh TEEN)

U.S. Brand Names Habitrol™ Patch; Nicoderm® Patch; Nicorette® DS Gum; Nicorette® Gum; Nicotrol® Inhaler; Nicotrol® NS Nasal Spray; Nicotro!® Patch [OTC]; ProStep® Patch

Canadian Brand Names Nicorette® Plus

Mexican Brand Names Nicolan; Nicotinell TTS

Generic Available No

Therapeutic Category Smoking Deterrent

Use Treatment aid to giving up smoking while participating in a behavioral modification program, under medical supervision

Usual Dosage

Gum: Chew 1 piece of gum when urge to smoke, up to 30 pieces/day; most patients require 10-12 pieces of gum/day

Inhaler: Usually 6 to 16 cartridges per day; best effect was achieved by frequent continuous puffing (20 minutes); recommended duration of treatment is 3 months, after which patients may be weaned from the inhaler by gradual reduction of the daily dose over 6-12 weeks

Transdermal patch (patients should be advised to completely stop smoking upon initiation of therapy): Apply new patch every 24 hours to nonhairy, clean, dry skin on the upper body or upper outer arm; each patch should be applied to a different site

Initial starting dose: 21 mg/day for 4-8 weeks for most patients

First weaning dose: 14 mg/day for 2-4 weeks

Second weaning dose: 7 mg/day for 2-4 weeks

Initial starting dose for patients <100 pounds, smoke <10 cigarettes/day, have a history of cardiovascular disease: 14 mg/day for 4-8 weeks followed by 7 mg/day for 2-4 weeks

In patients who are receiving >600 mg/day of cimetidine: Decrease to the next lower patch size

Benefits of use of nicotine transdermal patches beyond 3 months have not been demonstrated

Spray: 1-2 sprays/hour; do not exceed more than 5 doses (10 sprays) per hour; each dose (2 sprays) contains 1 mg of nicotine. **Warning:** A dose of 40 mg can cause fatalities

Nursing/Pharmacy Information Patients should be instructed to chew slowly to avoid jaw ache and to maximize benefit

Dosage Forms

Inhaler, oral (cartridge): 10 mg [delivering 4 mg] (42s); each unit consists of one mouthpiece, 7 storage trays each containing 6 cartridges and one storage case

Patch, transdermal:

Habitrol™: 21 mg/day; 14 mg/day; 7 mg/day (30 systems/box)

(Continued)

nicotine *(Continued)*

    Nicoderm®: 21 mg/day; 14 mg/day; 7 mg/day (14 systems/box)
    Nicotrol® [OTC]: 15 mg/day (gradually released over 16 hours)
    ProStep®: 22 mg/day; 11 mg/day (7 systems/box)
    Pieces, chewing gum, as polacrilex: 2 mg/square [OTC] (96 pieces/box); 4 mg/square (96 pieces/box)
    Spray, nasal: 0.5 mg/actuation [10 mg/mL - 200 actuations] (10 mL)

◆ **Nicotinell TTS** *see nicotine on page 441*
◆ **Nicotinex [OTC]** *see niacin on page 440*
◆ **nicotinic acid** *see niacin on page 440*
◆ **Nicotrol® Inhaler** *see nicotine on page 441*
◆ **Nicotrol® NS Nasal Spray** *see nicotine on page 441*
◆ **Nicotrol® Patch [OTC]** *see nicotine on page 441*

nicoumalone *(Canada only)* (nye KYOO ma lone)

Canadian Brand Names Sintrom®
Generic Available No
Therapeutic Category Anticoagulant
Use Prophylaxis and treatment of venous thrombosis and its extension, the treatment of atrial fibrillation with embolization, the prophylaxis and treatment of pulmonary embolism and as an adjunct in the treatment of coronary occlusion and transient cerebral ischemic attacks
Usual Dosage Adults: Oral:
    First day: 8-12 mg
    Second day: 4-8 mg; if the thromboplastin time is initially abnormal, treatment must be commenced with great caution
    Maintenance therapy and coagulation tests: In view of the marked individual differences encountered, the maintenance dose should be established and adjusted by reference to the results of periodically performed laboratory tests to determine the patient's blood coagulation time.
Dosage Forms Tablet: 1 mg, 4 mg

◆ **Nico-Vert® [OTC]** *see meclizine on page 387*
◆ **Nidagel™** *see metronidazole on page 411*
◆ **Nidryl® *(Discontinued)* see page 743**

nifedipine (nye FED i peen)

U.S. Brand Names Adalat®; Adalat® CC; Procardia®; Procardia XL®
Canadian Brand Names Adalat PA®; Apo®-Nifed; Gen-Nifedipine; Novo-Nifedin®; Nu-Nifedin®
Mexican Brand Names Adalat® Oros; Adalat® Retard; Corogal; Corotrend; Corotrend Retard; Dilafed; Nifedipres; Noviken-N
Generic Available Yes: Capsule
Therapeutic Category Calcium Channel Blocker
Use Angina, hypertrophic cardiomyopathy, hypertension
Usual Dosage
    Children: Oral:
        Hypertensive emergencies: 0.25-0.5 mg/kg/dose
        Hypertrophic cardiomyopathy: 0.6-0.9 mg/kg/24 hours in 3-4 divided doses
    Adults: Initial: 10 mg 3 times/day as capsules or 30-60 mg once daily as sustained release tablet; maintenance: 10-30 mg 3-4 times/day (capsules); maximum: 180 mg/24 hours (capsules) or 120 mg/day (sustained release)
Dietary Considerations Capsule is rapidly absorbed orally if it is administered without food but may result in vasodilator side effects; administration with low-fat meals may decrease flushing; grapefruit juice may increase the oral bioavailability of nifedipine tablets; food may decrease the rate but not the extent of absorption of Procardia XL®
Nursing/Pharmacy Information
    Do not crush or break sustained release tablets
    Monitor blood pressure
Dosage Forms
    Capsule, liquid-filled (Adalat®, Procardia®): 10 mg, 20 mg
    Tablet, extended release (Adalat® CC): 30 mg, 60 mg, 90 mg
    Tablet, sustained release (Procardia XL®): 30 mg, 60 mg, 90 mg

◆ **Nifedipres** *see nifedipine on page 442*
◆ **Niferex® [OTC]** *see polysaccharide-iron complex on page 503*
◆ **Niferex Forte® *(Discontinued)* see page 743**
◆ **Niferex®-PN** *see vitamin, multiple (oral) on page 654*
◆ **Nilandron™** *see nilutamide on page 443*

♦ **Niloric®** *(Discontinued) see page 743*
♦ **Nilstat®** *see* nystatin *on page 452*

nilutamide (ni LU ta mide)
U.S. Brand Names Nilandron™
Canadian Brand Names Anandron®
Generic Available No
Therapeutic Category Antineoplastic Agent
Use With orchiectomy (surgical castration) for the treatment of metastatic prostate cancer
Usual Dosage Adults: Oral: 300 mg (6-50 mg tablets) once daily for 30 days, then 150 mg (3-50 mg tablets) once daily; starting on the same day or day after surgical castration
Dosage Forms Tablet: 50 mg

♦ **Nimbex®** *see* cisatracurium *on page 153*

nimodipine (nye MOE di peen)
U.S. Brand Names Nimotop®
Generic Available No
Therapeutic Category Calcium Channel Blocker
Use Improvement of neurological deficits due to spasm following subarachnoid hemorrhage from ruptured congenital intracranial aneurysms who are in good neurological condition postictus
Usual Dosage Adults: Oral: 60 mg every 4 hours for 21 days, start therapy within 96 hours after subarachnoid hemorrhage
Nursing/Pharmacy Information If capsules cannot be swallowed, the liquid may be removed by making a hole in each end of the capsule with an 18-gauge needle and extracting the contents into a syringe; if administered via NG tube, follow with a flush of 30 mL NS
Dosage Forms Capsule, liquid-filled: 30 mg

♦ **Nimotop®** *see* nimodipine *on page 443*
♦ **Nipent™** *see* pentostatin *on page 480*
♦ **Nipride® Injection** *(Discontinued) see page 743*
♦ **Nisaval®** *(Discontinued) see page 743*

nisoldipine (NYE sole di peen)
U.S. Brand Names Sular®
Mexican Brand Names Syscor
Generic Available No
Therapeutic Category Calcium Channel Blocker
Use Management of hypertension, may be used alone or in combination with other antihypertensive agents
Usual Dosage Adults: Oral: Initial: 20 mg once daily, then increase by 10 mg per week (or longer intervals) to attain adequate control of blood pressure; doses >60 mg once daily are not recommended
Dietary Considerations Do not administer with a high-fat meal, best administered on an empty stomach; avoid grapefruit products before and after dosing
Nursing/Pharmacy Information Doses are administered orally once daily; administration with a high fat meal can lead to excessive peak drug concentration and should be avoided
Dosage Forms Tablet, extended release: 10 mg, 20 mg, 30 mg, 40 mg

♦ **Nistaken** *see* propafenone *on page 524*
♦ **Nistaquim** *see* nystatin *on page 452*
♦ **Nitalapram** *see* citalopram *on page 153*
♦ **Nitoman®** *see* tetrabenazine *(Canada only) on page 600*
♦ **Nitradisc** *see* nitroglycerin *on page 444*
♦ **Nitro-Bid® I.V. Injection** *see* nitroglycerin *on page 444*
♦ **Nitro-Bid® Ointment** *see* nitroglycerin *on page 444*
♦ **Nitro-Bid® Oral** *(Discontinued) see page 743*
♦ **Nitrocine® Oral** *(Discontinued) see page 743*
♦ **Nitroderm TTS** *see* nitroglycerin *on page 444*
♦ **Nitrodisc® Patch** *see* nitroglycerin *on page 444*
♦ **Nitro-Dur® Patch** *see* nitroglycerin *on page 444*
♦ **nitrofural** *see* nitrofurazone *on page 444*

nitrofurantoin (nye troe fyoor AN toyn)

U.S. Brand Names Furadantin®; Furalan®; Furan®; Furanite®; Macrobid®; Macrodantin®

Canadian Brand Names Apo®-Nitrofurantoin; Nephronex®; Novo-Furan®

Mexican Brand Names Furadantina; Macrodantina

Generic Available Yes: Tablet and suspension

Therapeutic Category Antibiotic, Miscellaneous

Use Prevention and treatment of urinary tract infections caused by susceptible gram-negative and some gram-positive organisms including *E. coli*, *Klebsiella*, *Enterobacter*, *Enterococa*, and *S. aureus*; *Pseudomonas*, *Serratia*, and most species of *Proteus* are generally resistant to nitrofurantoin

Usual Dosage Oral:

Children >1 month: 5-7 mg/kg/day divided every 6 hours; maximum: 400 mg/day

Chronic therapy: 1-2 mg/kg/day in divided doses every 12-24 hours; maximum dose: 400 mg/day

Adults: 50-100 mg/dose every 6 hours (not to exceed 400 mg/24 hours)

Prophylaxis: 50-100 mg/dose at bedtime

Dietary Considerations Should be administered with meals to slow the rate of absorption and thus decrease adverse effects; do not administer with alcohol; ensure diet adequate in protein and vitamin B complex

Nursing/Pharmacy Information

Higher peak serum levels may cause increased GI upset; administer around-the-clock rather than 4 times/day, 3 times/day, etc, (ie, 12-6-12-6, not 9-1-5-9) to promote less variation in peak and trough serum levels; therapeutic concentrations of nitrofurantoin are not attained in the urine of patients with Cl_{cr} <40 mL/minute

Monitor for signs of pulmonary reaction, signs of numbness or tingling of the extremities, periodic liver function tests

Dosage Forms

Capsule: 50 mg, 100 mg

Capsule:

Macrocrystal: 25 mg, 50 mg, 100 mg

Macrocrystal/monohydrate: 100 mg

Suspension, oral: 25 mg/5 mL (470 mL)

nitrofurazone (nye troe FYOOR a zone)

Synonyms nitrofural

U.S. Brand Names Furacin® Topical

Generic Available Yes

Therapeutic Category Antibacterial, Topical

Use Antibacterial agent used in second- and third-degree burns and skin grafting

Usual Dosage Children and Adults: Topical: Apply once daily or every few days to lesion or place on gauze

Nursing/Pharmacy Information

Discoloration does not appreciably affect potency of the drug

Stability: Avoid exposure to direct sunlight; excessive heat, strong fluorescent lighting, and alkaline materials

Dosage Forms

Cream: 0.2% (4 g, 28 g)

Ointment, soluble dressing: 0.2% (28 g, 56 g, 454 g, 480 g)

Solution, topical: 0.2% (480 mL, 3780 mL)

♦ **Nitrogard® Buccal** *see* nitroglycerin *on page 444*

♦ **nitrogen mustard** *see* mechlorethamine *on page 387*

nitroglycerin (nye troe GLI ser in)

Synonyms glyceryl trinitrate; nitroglycerol; NTG

U.S. Brand Names Deponit® Patch; Minitran® Patch; Nitro-Bid® I.V. Injection; Nitro-Bid® Ointment; Nitrodisc® Patch; Nitro-Dur® Patch; Nitrogard® Buccal; Nitroglyn® Oral; Nitrolingual® Translingual Spray; Nitrol® Ointment; Nitrong® Oral Tablet; Nitrostat® Sublingual; Transdermal-NTG® Patch; Transderm-Nitro® Patch; Tridil® Injection

Canadian Brand Names Nitrong® SR

Mexican Brand Names Anglix; Cardinit; Nitradisc; Nitroderm TTS

Generic Available Yes

Therapeutic Category Vasodilator

Use Angina pectoris; I.V. for congestive heart failure (especially when associated with acute myocardial infarction); pulmonary hypertension; hypertensive emergencies occurring perioperatively (especially during cardiovascular surgery)

Usual Dosage Note: Hemodynamic and antianginal tolerance often develops within 24-48 hours of continuous nitrate administration

Children: Pulmonary hypertension: Continuous infusion: Start 0.25-0.5 mcg/kg/minute and titrate by 1 mcg/kg/minute at 20- to 60-minute intervals to desired effect; usual dose: 1-3 mcg/kg/minute; maximum: 5 mcg/kg/minute

Adults:

Oral: 2.5-9 mg 2-4 times/day (up to 26 mg 4 times/day)

I.V.: 5 mcg/minute, increase by 5 mcg/minute every 3-5 minutes to 20 mcg/minute; if no response at 20 mcg/minute increase by 10 mcg/minute every 3-5 minutes, up to 200 mcg/minute

Sublingual: 0.2-0.6 mg every 5 minutes for maximum of 3 doses in 15 minutes; may also use prophylactically 5-10 minutes prior to activities which may provoke an attack

Ointment: 1" to 2" every 8 hours up to 4" to 5" every 4 hours

Patch, transdermal: 0.2-0.4 mg/hour initially and titrate to doses of 0.4-0.8 mg/hour; tolerance is minimized by using a patch on period of 12-14 hours and patch off period of 10-12 hours

Translingual: 1-2 sprays into mouth under tongue every 3-5 minutes for maximum of 3 doses in 15 minutes, may also be used 5-10 minutes prior to activities which may provoke an attack prophylactically

Buccal: Initial: 1 mg every 3-5 hours while awake (3 times/day); titrate dosage upward if angina occurs with tablet in place

May need to use nitrate-free interval (10-12 hours/day) to avoid tolerance development; tolerance may possibly be reversed with acetylcysteine; gradually decrease dose in patients receiving NTG for prolonged period to avoid withdrawal reaction

Nursing/Pharmacy Information

I.V. must be prepared in glass bottles and special sets intended for nitroglycerin must be used; transdermal patches labeled as mg/hour; do not crush sublingual or buccal drug product; I.V. continuous infusion: Dilute in D_5W or normal saline to 50-100 mcg/mL; maximum concentration not to exceed 400 mcg/mL

Monitor blood pressure, heart rate

Stability: I.V. infusion solution in normal saline or D_5W is stable for 48 hours at room temperature, mixed and stored in glass containers; maximum concentration not to exceed 400 mcg/mL; do not mix with other drugs; store sublingual tablets and ointment in tightly closed container; store at 15°C to 30°C

Dosage Forms

Capsule, sustained release: 2.5 mg, 6.5 mg, 9 mg

Injection: 0.5 mg/mL (10 mL); 0.8 mg/mL (10 mL); 5 mg/mL (1 mL, 5 mL, 10 mL, 20 mL); 10 mg/mL (5 mL, 10 mL)

Ointment, topical (Nitrol®): 2% [20 mg/g] (30 g, 60 g)

Patch, transdermal, topical: Systems designed to deliver 2.5, 5, 7.5, 10, or 15 mg NTG over 24 hours

Spray, translingual: 0.4 mg/metered spray (13.8 g)

Tablet:

Buccal, controlled release: 1 mg, 2 mg, 3 mg

Sublingual (Nitrostat®): 0.3 mg, 0.4 mg, 0.6 mg

Sustained release: 2.6 mg, 6.5 mg, 9 mg

- ♦ **nitroglycerol** *see* nitroglycerin *on page 444*
- ♦ **Nitroglyn® Oral** *see* nitroglycerin *on page 444*
- ♦ **Nitrolingual® Translingual Spray** *see* nitroglycerin *on page 444*
- ♦ **Nitrol® Ointment** *see* nitroglycerin *on page 444*
- ♦ **Nitrong® Oral Tablet** *see* nitroglycerin *on page 444*
- ♦ **Nitrong® SR** *see* nitroglycerin *on page 444*
- ♦ **Nitropress®** *see* nitroprusside *on page 445*

nitroprusside (nye troe PRUS ide)

Synonyms sodium nitroferricyanide

U.S. Brand Names Nitropress®

Generic Available Yes

Therapeutic Category Vasodilator

Use Management of hypertensive crises; congestive heart failure; used for controlled hypotension during anesthesia

(Continued)

nitroprusside *(Continued)*

Usual Dosage I.V.:

Children: Continuous infusion:

Initial: 1 mcg/kg/minute by continuous I.V. infusion; increase in increments of 1 mcg/kg/minute at intervals of 20-60 minutes; titrating to the desired response

Usual dose: 3 mcg/kg/minute; rarely need >4 mcg/kg/minute

Maximum: 10 mcg/kg/minute. Dilute 15 mg x weight (kg) to 250 mL D_5W, then dose in mcg/kg/minute = infusion rate in mL/hour

Adults: Begin at 5 mcg/kg/minute; increase in increments of 5 mcg/kg/minute (up to 20 mcg/kg/minute), then in increments of 10-20 mcg/kg/minute; titrating to the desired hemodynamic effect or the appearance of headache or nausea. When >500 mcg/kg is administered by prolonged infusion of faster than 2 mcg/kg/minute, cyanide is generated faster than an unaided patient can handle.

Nursing/Pharmacy Information

I.V. continuous infusion only via controlled infusion device; not for direct injection; solution should be protected from light, but not necessary to wrap administration set or I.V. tubing. Do not add other medications to nitroprusside solutions.

Monitor for signs of cyanide toxicity and thiocyanate levels; blood pressure, cardiac status

Stability: Discard solution 24 hours after reconstitution and dilution in D_5W; promptly wrap in aluminum foil or other opaque material to protect from light; reconstituted solution should be very faint brown, discard if highly colored (blue, green, or red); store powder in carton until use

Dosage Forms Injection, as sodium: 10 mg/mL (5 mL); 25 mg/mL (2 mL)

♦ **Nitrostat® 0.15 mg Tablet *(Discontinued)*** see page 743
♦ **Nitrostat® Sublingual** see nitroglycerin *on page 444*
♦ **Nivoflox** see ciprofloxacin *on page 151*
♦ **Nix™ Creme Rinse** see permethrin *on page 482*
♦ **Niyaplat** see cisplatin *on page 153*

nizatidine (ni ZA ti deen)

U.S. Brand Names Axid®; Axid® AR [OTC]
Generic Available No
Therapeutic Category Histamine H_2 Antagonist
Use Treatment and maintenance of duodenal ulcer; treatment of gastroesophageal reflux disease (GERD)
Usual Dosage Adults: Active duodenal ulcer: Oral:

Treatment: 300 mg at bedtime or 150 mg twice daily

Maintenance: 150 mg/day

Nursing/Pharmacy Information Administering a dose at 6 PM may more effectively suppress nocturnal acid secretion than administering a dose at 10 PM

Dosage Forms

Capsule: 150 mg, 300 mg

Tablet: 75 mg

♦ **Nizoral®** see ketoconazole *on page 354*
♦ **n-methylhydrazine** see procarbazine *on page 519*
♦ **Nobesine®** see diethylpropion *on page 201*
♦ **Noctec® *(Discontinued)*** see page 743
♦ **Nolahist® [OTC]** see phenindamine *on page 484*
♦ **Nolamine®** see chlorpheniramine, phenindamine, and phenylpropanolamine *on page 141*
♦ **Nolex® LA** see guaifenesin and phenylpropanolamine *on page 301*
♦ **Noludar® *(Discontinued)*** see page 743
♦ **Nolvadex®** see tamoxifen *on page 592*

nonoxynol 9 (non OKS i nole nine)

U.S. Brand Names Because® [OTC]; Delfen® [OTC]; Emko® [OTC]; Encare® [OTC]; Gynol II® [OTC]; Koromex® [OTC]; Ramses® [OTC]; Semicid® [OTC]; Shur-Seal® [OTC]
Generic Available Yes
Therapeutic Category Spermicide
Use Spermatocide in contraception
Usual Dosage Insert into vagina at least 15 minutes before intercourse

Nursing/Pharmacy Information Use product prior to intercourse, but not more than 1 hour in advance; reapply each time intercourse takes place; wait 6 hours after intercourse to use cleansing douche; burning of the vagina or penis has been reported, discontinue use if this occurs

Dosage Forms Vaginal:
Cream: 2% (103.5 g)
Foam: 12.5% (60 g)
Jelly: 2% (81 g, 126 g)

- **No Pain-HP® [OTC]** *see* capsaicin *on page 110*
- **noradrenaline acid tartrate** *see* norepinephrine *on page 447*
- **Norboral** *see* glyburide *on page 294*
- **Norcet®** *see* hydrocodone and acetaminophen *on page 319*
- **Norciden** *see* danazol *on page 181*
- **Norcuron®** *see* vecuronium *on page 645*
- **nordeoxyguanosine** *see* ganciclovir *on page 287*
- **Nordette®** *see* ethinyl estradiol and levonorgestrel *on page 250*
- **Norditropin®** *see* human growth hormone *on page 315*
- **Nordryl® Injection** *see* diphenhydramine *on page 208*
- **Nordryl® Oral** *see* diphenhydramine *on page 208*

norepinephrine (nor ep i NEF rin)

Synonyms noradrenaline acid tartrate
U.S. Brand Names Levophed®
Generic Available No
Therapeutic Category Adrenergic Agonist Agent
Use Treatment of shock which persists after adequate fluid volume replacement; severe hypotension; cardiogenic shock
Usual Dosage Note: Dose stated in terms of norepinephrine base. I.V.:
Children: Initial: 0.05-0.1 mcg/kg/minute, titrate to desired effect; rate (mL/hour) = dose (mcg/kg/minute) x weight (kg) x 60 minutes/hour divided by concentration (mcg/mL)
Adults: 8-12 mcg/minute as an infusion; initiate at 4 mcg/minute and titrate to desired response
Nursing/Pharmacy Information
Parenteral: Administer into large vein to avoid the potential for extravasation; standard concentration: 4 mg/500 mL but 8 mg/500 mL has been used
Monitor blood pressure, heart rate, urine output, peripheral perfusion
Stability: Readily oxidized, protect from light, do not use if brown coloration; dilute with D_5W or DS/NS, but not recommended to dilute in normal saline; not stable with alkaline solutions
Stability of parenteral admixture at room temperature (25°C): 24 hours
Dosage Forms Injection, as bitartrate: 1 mg/mL (4 mL)

- **Norethin™ 1/35E** *see* ethinyl estradiol and norethindrone *on page 250*
- **Norethin 1/50M** *see* mestranol and norethindrone *on page 396*

norethindrone (nor eth IN drone)

Synonyms norethisterone
U.S. Brand Names Aygestin®; Micronor®; NOR-QD®
Mexican Brand Names Syngestal
Generic Available No
Therapeutic Category Contraceptive, Progestin Only; Progestin
Use Treatment of amenorrhea; abnormal uterine bleeding; endometriosis
Usual Dosage Adolescents and Adults: Oral:
Amenorrhea and abnormal uterine bleeding: 2.5-10 mg on days 5-25 of menstrual cycle
Endometriosis: 5 mg/day for 14 days; increase at increments of 2.5 mg/day every 2 weeks up to 15 mg/day
Dietary Considerations Limit caffeine; high-dose vitamin C (1 g/day) may increase adverse effects; increase dietary intake of folate and pyridoxine; should be taken with food at same time each day
Nursing/Pharmacy Information Norethindrone acetate is ~2 times as potent as norethindrone
Dosage Forms
Tablet: 0.35 mg, 5 mg
Tablet, as acetate: 5 mg

- **norethindrone acetate and ethinyl estradiol** *see* ethinyl estradiol and norethindrone *on page 250*

- **norethindrone and mestranol** *see* mestranol and norethindrone *on page 396*
- **norethisterone** *see* norethindrone *on page 447*
- **Norfenon®** *see* propafenone *on page 524*
- **Norflex™** *see* orphenadrine *on page 458*

norfloxacin (nor FLOKS a sin)

U.S. Brand Names Chibroxin™ Ophthalmic; Noroxin® Oral
Mexican Brand Names Floxacin®; Oranor
Generic Available No
Therapeutic Category Quinolone
Use Complicated and uncomplicated urinary tract infections caused by susceptible gram-negative and gram-positive bacteria
Usual Dosage
Children >1 year and Adults: Ophthalmic: Instill 1-2 drops in affected eye(s) 4 times/day for up to 7 days
Adults: Oral: 400 mg twice daily for 7-21 days depending on infection
Dietary Considerations Decreases absorption with food; should be administered on an empty stomach with water
Nursing/Pharmacy Information Hold antacids for 2-4 hours before and after administering dose
Dosage Forms
Solution, ophthalmic: 0.3% [3 mg/mL] (5 mL)
Tablet: 400 mg

- **Norgesic™** *see* orphenadrine, aspirin, and caffeine *on page 458*
- **Norgesic™ Forte** *see* orphenadrine, aspirin, and caffeine *on page 458*
- **norgestimate and ethinyl estradiol** *see* ethinyl estradiol and norgestimate *on page 251*

norgestrel (nor JES trel)

U.S. Brand Names Ovrette®
Generic Available No
Therapeutic Category Contraceptive, Progestin Only
Use Prevention of pregnancy; treatment of hypermenorrhea, endometriosis, female hypogonadism
Usual Dosage Oral: Administer daily, starting the first day of menstruation, administer one tablet at the same time each day, every day of the year. If one dose is missed, administer as soon as remembered, then next tablet at regular time; if two doses are missed, administer one tablet and discard the other, then administer daily at usual time; if three doses are missed, use an additional form of birth control until menses or pregnancy is ruled out
Dietary Considerations Should be administered with food at same time each day
Nursing/Pharmacy Information Patients should receive a copy of the patient labeling
Dosage Forms Tablet: 0.075 mg

- **norgestrel and ethinyl estradiol** *see* ethinyl estradiol and norgestrel *on page 252*
- **Norinyl® 1+35** *see* ethinyl estradiol and norethindrone *on page 250*
- **Norinyl® 1+50** *see* mestranol and norethindrone *on page 396*
- **Noritate®** *see* metronidazole *on page 411*
- **Norlutate® *(Discontinued)*** *see page 743*
- **Norlutin® *(Discontinued)*** *see page 743*
- **normal saline** *see* sodium chloride *on page 571*
- **Normiflo®** *see* ardeparin *on page 58*
- **Normodyne®** *see* labetalol *on page 357*
- **Noroxin® Oral** *see* norfloxacin *on page 448*
- **Norpace®** *see* disopyramide *on page 213*
- **Norpace® CR** *see* disopyramide *on page 213*
- **Norplant® Implant** *see* levonorgestrel *on page 366*
- **Norpramin®** *see* desipramine *on page 187*
- **NOR-QD®** *see* norethindrone *on page 447*
- **Nor-tet® Oral** *see* tetracycline *on page 601*
- **North American coral snake antivenin** *see* antivenin (*Micrurus fulvius*) *on page 55*
- **North and South American antisnake-bite serum** *see* antivenin (*Crotalidae*) polyvalent *on page 54*

nortriptyline (nor TRIP ti leen)

U.S. Brand Names Aventyl® Hydrochloride; Pamelor®

Generic Available Yes

Therapeutic Category Antidepressant, Tricyclic (Secondary Amine)

Use Treatment of various forms of depression, often in conjunction with psychotherapy; nocturnal enuresis

Usual Dosage Oral:

Adults: 25 mg 3-4 times/day up to 150 mg/day

Adolescents and Elderly: 30-50 mg/day in divided doses

Dietary Considerations May be administered with food to decrease GI distress; riboflavin dietary requirements may be increased

Nursing/Pharmacy Information

Monitor blood pressure and pulse rate prior to and during initial therapy; evaluate mental status; monitor weight, may increase appetite and possibly a craving for sweets

Stability: Protect from light

Dosage Forms Nortriptyline hydrochloride:

Capsule: 10 mg, 25 mg, 50 mg, 75 mg

Solution: 10 mg/5 mL (473 mL)

- ♦ **Norvas** *see* amlodipine *on page 41*
- ♦ **Norvasc®** *see* amlodipine *on page 41*
- ♦ **Norvir®** *see* ritonavir *on page 552*
- ♦ **Nositrol [Sodium Succinate]** *see* hydrocortisone (systemic) *on page 323*
- ♦ **Nōstrilla® [OTC]** *see* oxymetazoline *on page 463*
- ♦ **Nostril® Nasal Solution [OTC]** *see* phenylephrine *on page 487*
- ♦ **Novacef** *see* cefixime *on page 121*
- ♦ **Novacet® Topical** *see* sulfur and sulfacetamide *on page 589*
- ♦ **Novafed® *(Discontinued)*** *see page 743*
- ♦ **Novahistine®** *see* phenylephrine *on page 487*
- ♦ **Novahistine DH® Liquid *(Discontinued)*** *see page 743*
- ♦ **Novahistine DMX® Liquid *(Discontinued)*** *see page 743*
- ♦ **Novahistine® Elixir *(Discontinued)*** *see page 743*
- ♦ **Novahistine® Expectorant *(Discontinued)*** *see page 743*
- ♦ **Novamoxin®** *see* amoxicillin *on page 43*
- ♦ **Novantrone®** *see* mitoxantrone *on page 418*
- ♦ **Nova Rectal®** *see* pentobarbital *on page 479*
- ♦ **Novasen** *see* aspirin *on page 61*
- ♦ **Noviken-N** *see* nifedipine *on page 442*
- ♦ **Novo-Aloprazol®** *see* alprazolam *on page 30*
- ♦ **Novo-Atenol®** *see* atenolol *on page 63*
- ♦ **Novo-AZT®** *see* zidovudine *on page 658*
- ♦ **Novo-Butamide®** *see* tolbutamide *on page 617*
- ♦ **Novocain®** *see* procaine *on page 518*
- ♦ **Novo-Captopril®** *see* captopril *on page 110*
- ♦ **Novo-Carbamaz®** *see* carbamazepine *on page 112*
- ♦ **Novo-Chlorhydrate®** *see* chloral hydrate *on page 132*
- ♦ **Novo-Chlorpromazine®** *see* chlorpromazine *on page 144*
- ♦ **Novo-Cimetidine®** *see* cimetidine *on page 150*
- ♦ **Novo-Clobetasol** *see* clobetasol *on page 157*
- ♦ **Novo-Clonidine®** *see* clonidine *on page 159*
- ♦ **Novo-Clopate®** *see* clorazepate *on page 160*
- ♦ **Novo-Cloxin®** *see* cloxacillin *on page 161*
- ♦ **Novo-Cromolyn®** *see* cromolyn sodium *on page 171*
- ♦ **Novo-Cycloprine®** *see* cyclobenzaprine *on page 174*
- ♦ **Novo-Difenac®** *see* diclofenac *on page 198*
- ♦ **Novo-Difenac-SR®** *see* diclofenac *on page 198*
- ♦ **Novo-Diflunisal** *see* diflunisal *on page 202*
- ♦ **Novo-Digoxin®** *see* digoxin *on page 203*
- ♦ **Novo-Diltazem®** *see* diltiazem *on page 205*
- ♦ **Novo-Dipam®** *see* diazepam *on page 196*
- ♦ **Novo-Dipiradol®** *see* dipyridamole *on page 212*
- ♦ **Novo-Doxepin®** *see* doxepin *on page 219*
- ♦ **Novo-Doxylin®** *see* doxycycline *on page 222*
- ♦ **Novo-Famotidine®** *see* famotidine *on page 259*
- ♦ **Novo-Fibrate®** *see* clofibrate *on page 158*

- **Novo-Flupam®** *see* flurazepam *on page 278*
- **Novo-Flurprofen®** *see* flurbiprofen *on page 278*
- **Novo-Folacid®** *see* folic acid *on page 281*
- **Novo-Furan®** *see* nitrofurantoin *on page 444*
- **Novo-Gesic-C8®** *see* acetaminophen and codeine *on page 14*
- **Novo-Gesic-C15®** *see* acetaminophen and codeine *on page 14*
- **Novo-Gesic-C30®** *see* acetaminophen and codeine *on page 14*
- **Novo-Glyburide** *see* glyburide *on page 294*
- **Novo-Hexidyl®** *see* trihexyphenidyl *on page 628*
- **Novo-Hydrazide®** *see* hydrochlorothiazide *on page 317*
- **Novo-Hydroxyzine®** *see* hydroxyzine *on page 328*
- **Novo-Hylazin®** *see* hydralazine *on page 316*
- **Novo-Keto-EC** *see* ketoprofen *on page 355*
- **Novo-Lexin®** *see* cephalexin *on page 128*
- **Novolin® 70/30** *see* insulin preparations *on page 339*
- **Novolin® ge** *see* insulin preparations *on page 339*
- **Novolin® L** *see* insulin preparations *on page 339*
- **Novolin® N** *see* insulin preparations *on page 339*
- **Novolin-Pen® II, -3** *see* insulin preparations *on page 339*
- **Novolin® R** *see* insulin preparations *on page 339*
- **Novo-Lorazepam®** *see* lorazepam *on page 375*
- **Novo-Medopa®** *see* methyldopa *on page 406*
- **Novo-Mepro®** *see* meprobamate *on page 394*
- **Novo-Metformin** *see* metformin *on page 398*
- **Novo-Methacin®** *see* indomethacin *on page 337*
- **Novo-Metoprolol®** *see* metoprolol *on page 410*
- **Novo-Mucilax®** *see* psyllium *on page 531*
- **Novo-Naprox®** *see* naproxen *on page 432*
- **Novo-Nidazol®** *see* metronidazole *on page 411*
- **Novo-Nifedin®** *see* nifedipine *on page 442*
- **Novo-Oxazepam®** *see* oxazepam *on page 460*
- **Novo-Pen-VK®** *see* penicillin V potassium *on page 476*
- **Novo-Pindol** *see* pindolol *on page 495*
- **Novo-Piroxicam®** *see* piroxicam *on page 497*
- **Novo-Poxide®** *see* chlordiazepoxide *on page 134*
- **Novo-Pramine®** *see* imipramine *on page 334*
- **Novo-Prazin®** *see* prazosin *on page 513*
- **Novo-Prednisolone®** *see* prednisolone (systemic) *on page 514*
- **Novo-Prednisone®** *see* prednisone *on page 515*
- **Novo-Propamide®** *see* chlorpropamide *on page 145*
- **Novo-Propoxyn®** *see* propoxyphene *on page 526*
- **Novo-purol®** *see* allopurinol *on page 29*
- **Novo-Pyrazone** *see* sulfinpyrazone *on page 588*
- **Novo-Ranidine®** *see* ranitidine hydrochloride *on page 541*
- **Novo-Reserpine®** *see* reserpine *on page 544*
- **Novo-Ridazine®** *see* thioridazine *on page 608*
- **Novo-Rythro Encap** *see* erythromycin (systemic) *on page 240*
- **Novo-Salmol®** *see* albuterol *on page 25*
- **Novo-Secobarb®** *see* secobarbital *on page 561*
- **Novo-Selegiline** *see* selegiline *on page 562*
- **Novo-Semide®** *see* furosemide *on page 285*
- **Novo-Seven®** *see* factor VIIa, recombinant *New Drug on page 258*
- **Novo-Soxazole®** *see* sulfisoxazole *on page 588*
- **Novo-Spiroton®** *see* spironolactone *on page 578*
- **Novo-Sucralate®** *see* sucralfate *on page 583*
- **Novo-Sundac®** *see* sulindac *on page 589*
- **Novo-Tamoxifen** *see* tamoxifen *on page 592*
- **Novo-Terfenadine®** *see* terfenadine *on page 597*
- **Novo-Tetra®** *see* tetracycline *on page 601*
- **Novo-Thalidone®** *see* chlorthalidone *on page 146*
- **Novo-Timol®** *see* timolol *on page 613*
- **Novo-Tolmetin®** *see* tolmetin *on page 617*
- **Novo-Triamzide** *see* hydrochlorothiazide and triamterene *on page 318*
- **Novo-Trimel®** *see* co-trimoxazole *on page 170*

- **Novo-Triolam®** *see* triazolam *on page 625*
- **Novo-Tripramine** *see* trimipramine *on page 630*
- **Novo-Tryptin®** *see* amitriptyline *on page 40*
- **Novo-Veramil®** *see* verapamil *on page 646*
- **Novo-Zolamide®** *see* acetazolamide *on page 17*
- **Nozolon** *see* gentamicin *on page 290*
- **NP-27®** [OTC] *see* tolnaftate *on page 618*
- **NPH Iletin® I** *see* insulin preparations *on page 339*
- **NPH Insulin** *see* insulin preparations *on page 339*
- **NPH-N** *see* insulin preparations *on page 339*
- **NTG** *see* nitroglycerin *on page 444*
- **NTZ® Long Acting Nasal Solution** [OTC] *see* oxymetazoline *on page 463*
- **Nu-Alprax®** *see* alprazolam *on page 30*
- **Nu-Amoxi** *see* amoxicillin *on page 43*
- **Nu-Ampi** *see* ampicillin *on page 46*
- **Nu-Atenol®** *see* atenolol *on page 63*
- **Nubain®** *see* nalbuphine *on page 429*
- **Nu-Capto®** *see* captopril *on page 110*
- **Nu-Carbamazepine®** *see* carbamazepine *on page 112*
- **Nu-Cephalex®** *see* cephalexin *on page 128*
- **Nu-Cimet®** *see* cimetidine *on page 150*
- **Nu-Clonidine®** *see* clonidine *on page 159*
- **Nu-Cloxi®** *see* cloxacillin *on page 161*
- **Nucofed®** *see* guaifenesin, pseudoephedrine, and codeine *on page 304*
- **Nucofed® Pediatric Expectorant** *see* guaifenesin, pseudoephedrine, and codeine *on page 304*
- **Nu-Cotrimox®** *see* co-trimoxazole *on page 170*
- **Nucotuss®** *see* guaifenesin, pseudoephedrine, and codeine *on page 304*
- **Nu-Diclo®** *see* diclofenac *on page 198*
- **Nu-Diflunisal** *see* diflunisal *on page 202*
- **Nu-Diltiaz®** *see* diltiazem *on page 205*
- **Nu-Doxycycline®** *see* doxycycline *on page 222*
- **Nu-Famotidine®** *see* famotidine *on page 259*
- **Nu-Flurprofen®** *see* flurbiprofen *on page 278*
- **Nu-Gemfibrozil** *see* gemfibrozil *on page 289*
- **Nu-Glyburide** *see* glyburide *on page 294*
- **Nu-Hydral®** *see* hydralazine *on page 316*
- **Nu-Indo®** *see* indomethacin *on page 337*
- **Nu-Iron®** [OTC] *see* polysaccharide-iron complex *on page 503*
- **Nu-Ketoprofen** *see* ketoprofen *on page 355*
- **Nu-Ketoprofen-E** *see* ketoprofen *on page 355*
- **Nullo®** [OTC] *see* chlorophyll *on page 135*
- **Nu-Loraz®** *see* lorazepam *on page 375*
- **NuLYTELY®** *see* polyethylene glycol-electrolyte solution *on page 502*
- **Nu-Medopa®** *see* methyldopa *on page 406*
- **Nu-Metop** *see* metoprolol *on page 410*
- **Numorphan®** *see* oxymorphone *on page 464*
- **Numzitdent®** [OTC] *see* benzocaine *on page 79*
- **Numzit Teething®** [OTC] *see* benzocaine *on page 79*
- **Nu-Naprox®** *see* naproxen *on page 432*
- **Nu-Nifedin®** *see* nifedipine *on page 442*
- **Nu-Pen-VK®** *see* penicillin V potassium *on page 476*
- **Nupercainal®** [OTC] *see* dibucaine *on page 197*
- **Nu-Pindol** *see* pindolol *on page 495*
- **Nu-Pirox®** *see* piroxicam *on page 497*
- **Nu-Prazo®** *see* prazosin *on page 513*
- **Nuprin®** [OTC] *see* ibuprofen *on page 332*
- **Nu-Prochlor®** *see* prochlorperazine *on page 519*
- **Nu-Propranolol®** *see* propranolol *on page 527*
- **Nu-Ranit®** *see* ranitidine hydrochloride *on page 541*
- **Nuromax®** *see* doxacurium *on page 219*
- **Nursoy®** *(Discontinued)* *see* page 743
- **Nu-Sulfinpyrazone** *see* sulfinpyrazone *on page 588*
- **Nu-Tears®** II Solution [OTC] *see* artificial tears *on page 59*

- **Nu-Tears® Solution [OTC]** *see* artificial tears *on page 59*
- **Nu-Tetra®** *see* tetracycline *on page 601*
- **Nu-Timolol®** *see* timolol *on page 613*
- **Nutracort® Topical** *see* hydrocortisone (topical) *on page 324*
- **Nutraplus® Topical [OTC]** *see* urea *on page 638*
- **Nu-Triazide** *see* hydrochlorothiazide and triamterene *on page 318*
- **Nu-Triazo®** *see* triazolam *on page 625*
- **Nutrilipid®** *see* fat emulsion *on page 259*
- **Nu-Trimipramine®** *see* trimipramine *on page 630*
- **Nutrisource™** *see* enteral nutritional products *on page 233*
- **Nutropin®** *see* human growth hormone *on page 315*
- **Nutropin® AQ** *see* human growth hormone *on page 315*
- **Nu-Verap®** *see* verapamil *on page 646*
- **Nyaderm** *see* nystatin *on page 452*
- **Nydrazid® Injection** *(Discontinued)* see page 743

nystatin (nye STAT in)

U.S. Brand Names Mycostatin®; Nilstat®; Nystat-Rx®; Nystex®; O-V Staticin®
Canadian Brand Names Candistatin®; Mestatin®; Nadostine®; Nilstat®; Nyaderm; PMS-Nystatin
Mexican Brand Names Micostatin; Nistaquim
Generic Available Yes
Therapeutic Category Antifungal Agent
Use Treatment of susceptible cutaneous, mucocutaneous, oral cavity and vaginal fungal infections normally caused by the *Candida* species
Usual Dosage
Oral candidiasis:
  Infants: 200,000 units 4 times/day or 100,000 units to each side of mouth 4 times/day
  Children and Adults: 400,000-600,000 units 4 times/day; troche: 200,000-400,000 units 4-5 times/day
Cutaneous candidal infections: Children and Adults: Topical: Apply 3-4 times/day
Intestinal infections: Adults: Oral: 500,000-1,000,000 units every 8 hours
Vaginal infections: Adults: Vaginal tablets: Insert 1-2 tablets/day at bedtime for 2 weeks
Nursing/Pharmacy Information
Administer around-the-clock rather than 4 times/day, 3 times/day, etc, (ie, 12-6-12-6, not 9-1-5-9) to promote less variation in peak and trough serum levels
Stability: Keep vaginal inserts in refrigerator; protect from temperature extremes, moisture, and light
Dosage Forms
Cream: 100,000 units/g (15 g, 30 g)
Ointment, topical: 100,000 units/g (15 g, 30 g)
Powder, for preparation of oral suspension: 50 million units, 1 billion units, 2 billion units, 5 billion units
Powder, topical: 100,000 units/g (15 g)
Suspension, oral: 100,000 units/mL (5 mL, 60 mL, 480 mL)
Tablet:
  Oral: 500,000 units
  Vaginal: 100,000 units (15 and 30/box with applicator)
Troche: 200,000 units

nystatin and triamcinolone (nye STAT in & trye am SIN oh lone)

Synonyms triamcinolone and nystatin
U.S. Brand Names Mycogen II Topical; Mycolog®-II Topical; Myconel® Topical; Myco-Triacet® II; Mytrex® F Topical; N.G.T.® Topical; Tri-Statin® II Topical
Generic Available Yes
Therapeutic Category Antifungal/Corticosteroid
Use Treatment of cutaneous candidiasis
Usual Dosage Topical: Apply twice daily
Nursing/Pharmacy Information External use only; do not use on open wounds; apply sparingly to occlusive dressings; should not be used in the presence of open or weeping lesions
Dosage Forms
Cream: Nystatin 100,000 units and triamcinolone acetonide 0.1% (15 g, 30 g, 45 g, 60 g, 240 g)

Ointment, topical: Nystatin 100,000 units and triamcinolone acetonide 0.1% (15 g, 30 g, 60 g, 120 g)

♦ **Nystat-Rx®** *see* nystatin *on page 452*
♦ **Nystex®** *see* nystatin *on page 452*
♦ **Nytol® Oral [OTC]** *see* diphenhydramine *on page 208*
♦ **Obe-Nix® 30** *(Discontinued) see page 743*
♦ **Obephen®** *(Discontinued) see page 743*
♦ **Obermine®** *(Discontinued) see page 743*
♦ **Obestin-30®** *(Discontinued) see page 743*
♦ **Occlucort®** *see* betamethasone (topical) *on page 85*
♦ **Occlusal®-HP Liquid** *see* salicylic acid *on page 557*
♦ **Ocean Nasal Mist [OTC]** *see* sodium chloride *on page 571*
♦ **OCL®** *see* polyethylene glycol-electrolyte solution *on page 502*
♦ **Octamide®** *see* metoclopramide *on page 409*
♦ **Octicair® Otic** *see* neomycin, polymyxin B, and hydrocortisone *on page 437*
♦ **Octocaine®** *see* lidocaine and epinephrine *on page 369*
♦ **Octostim®** *see* desmopressin acetate *on page 188*

octreotide (ok TREE oh tide)

U.S. Brand Names Sandostatin®; Sandostatin LAR®
Mexican Brand Names Sandostatina®
Generic Available No
Therapeutic Category Somatostatin Analog
Use Control of symptoms in patients with metastatic carcinoid and vasoactive intestinal peptide-secreting tumors (VIPomas); acromegaly, insulinomas, Zollinger-Ellison syndrome, pancreatic tumors, gastrinoma, postgastrectomy dumping syndrome, bleeding esophageal varices, small bowel fistulas, AIDS-associated secretory diarrhea, chemotherapy-induced diarrhea, GVHD-induced diarrhea, control of bleeding of esophageal varices; depot suspension is indicated for long term maintenance therapy in acromegalic patients for whom medical treatment is appropriate and who have been shown to respond to and can tolerate the injection
Usual Dosage Adults: S.C.: Initial: 50 mcg 1-2 times/day and titrate dose based on patient tolerance and response

Carcinoid: 100-600 mcg/day in 2-4 divided doses
VIPomas: 200-300 mcg/day in 2-4 divided doses
Diarrhea: Initial: I.V.: 50-100 mcg every 8 hours; increase by 100 mcg/dose at 48-hour intervals; maximum dose: 500 mcg every 8 hours
Dietary Considerations Schedule injections between meals to decrease GI effects
Nursing/Pharmacy Information
Parenteral: For I.V. infusion, dilute in 50-100 mL NS or D_5W and infuse over 20-30 minutes; in emergency situations, may be administered by direct I.V. push over 3 minutes
Monitor baseline and periodic ultrasound evaluations for cholelithiasis, blood sugar, baseline and periodic thyroid function tests, fluid and electrolyte balance; for carcinoid, monitor 5-HIAA, plasma serotonin, plasma substance P; for VIPoma, monitor VIP
Stability: For prolonged storage, keep in refrigerator; for ampuls that will be used within 24 hours, refrigeration is not required; **compatible** with normal saline or D_5W
Dosage Forms
Injection: 0.05 mg/mL (1 mL); 0.1 mg/mL (1 mL); 0.2 mg/mL (5 mL); 0.5 mg/mL (1 mL); 1 mg/mL (5 mL)
Injection, suspension, depot: 10 mg (5 mL); 20 mg (5 mL); 30 mg (5 mL)

♦ **Ocu-Carpine® Ophthalmic** *see* pilocarpine *on page 493*
♦ **OcuClear® Ophthalmic [OTC]** *see* oxymetazoline *on page 463*
♦ **OcuCoat® Ophthalmic Solution [OTC]** *see* artificial tears *on page 59*
♦ **OcuCoat® PF Ophthalmic Solution [OTC]** *see* artificial tears *on page 59*
♦ **Ocufen® Ophthalmic** *see* flurbiprofen *on page 278*
♦ **Ocuflox™ Ophthalmic** *see* ofloxacin *on page 454*
♦ **Ocugram®** *see* gentamicin *on page 290*
♦ **Ocupress® Ophthalmic** *see* carteolol *on page 117*
♦ **Ocusert Pilo-20® Ophthalmic** *see* pilocarpine *on page 493*
♦ **Ocusert Pilo-40® Ophthalmic** *see* pilocarpine *on page 493*
♦ **Ocutricin® Topical Ointment** *see* bacitracin, neomycin, and polymyxin B *on page 71*

- **Ocuvite™** *see* vitamin, multiple (oral) *on page 654*
- **Oestrillin®** *see* estrone *on page 246*
- **Oestrogel** *see* estradiol *on page 242*

ofloxacin (oh FLOKS a sin)

U.S. Brand Names Floxin®; Ocuflox™ Ophthalmic
Mexican Brand Names Bactocin; Floxil; Floxstat
Generic Available No
Therapeutic Category Antibiotic, Ophthalmic; Antibiotic, Otic; Quinolone
Use Quinolone antibiotic for skin and skin structure, lower respiratory and urinary tract infections, and sexually transmitted diseases; bacterial conjunctivitis caused by susceptible organisms; otitis externa in adults and pediatric ≥1 year of age caused by susceptible organisms; otitis media in patients ≥12 years of age with perforated tympanic membranes caused by susceptible organisms; acute otitis media in pediatric patients ≥1 year of age with tympanostomy tubes caused by susceptible organisms

Usual Dosage
Children >1 year and Adults: Ophthalmic: Instill 1-2 drops in affected eye(s) every 2-4 hours for the first 2 days, then use 4 times/day for an additional 5 days
Children >1 year to 12 years: Otic: Instill 5 drops in affected ear(s) twice daily for 10 days
Children ≥12 years: Otic: Instill 10 drops in affected ear(s) twice daily for 10 days
Adults: Oral, I.V.: 200-400 mg every 12 hours for 7-10 days for most infections or for 6 weeks for prostatitis

Nursing/Pharmacy Information Hold antacids for 2-4 hours before and after administering dose
Dosage Forms
Injection: 200 mg (50 mL); 400 mg (10 mL, 20 mL, 100 mL)
Solution:
Ophthalmic: 0.3% (5 mL)
Otic: 0.3% (5 mL)
Tablet: 200 mg, 300 mg, 400 mg

- **Ogen® Oral** *see* estropipate *on page 246*
- **Ogen® Vaginal** *see* estropipate *on page 246*
- **OGMT** *see* metyrosine *on page 412*
- **OKT3** *see* muromonab-CD3 *on page 425*

olanzapine (oh LAN za peen)

Synonyms LY170053
U.S. Brand Names Zyprexa™
Generic Available No
Therapeutic Category Antipsychotic Agent
Use Treatment of schizophrenia
Usual Dosage Adults: Oral: Usual starting dose: 10 mg/day, up to a maximum of 20 mg/day
Dosage Forms Tablet: 2.5 mg, 5 mg, 7.5 mg, 10 mg

- **old tuberculin** *see* tuberculin tests *on page 635*
- **oleovitamin A** *see* vitamin A *on page 650*
- **oleum ricini** *see* castor oil *on page 118*

olopatadine (oh LOP ah tah deen)

U.S. Brand Names Patanol®
Generic Available No
Therapeutic Category Antihistamine
Use Allergic conjunctivitis
Usual Dosage Adults: Ophthalmic: 1 drop in affected eye(s) every 6-8 hours (twice daily)
Dosage Forms Solution, ophthalmic: 0.1% (5 mL)

olsalazine (ole SAL a zeen)

U.S. Brand Names Dipentum®
Generic Available No
Therapeutic Category 5-Aminosalicylic Acid Derivative
Use Maintenance of remission of ulcerative colitis in patients intolerant to sulfasalazine
Usual Dosage Adults: Oral: 1 g daily in 2 divided doses

Dietary Considerations Administer with food, increase residence of drug in body

Nursing/Pharmacy Information Monitor stool frequency

Dosage Forms Capsule, as sodium: 250 mg

omeprazole (oh ME pray zol)

U.S. Brand Names Prilosec™

Canadian Brand Names Losec®

Mexican Brand Names Inhibitron®; Ozoken; Prazidec; Ulsen

Generic Available No

Therapeutic Category Gastric Acid Secretion Inhibitor

Use Short-term (4-8 weeks) treatment of erosive esophagitis (grade 2 or above), diagnosed by endoscopy; maintain healing of erosive esophagitis; short-term treatment of symptomatic gastroesophageal reflux disease (GERD) poorly responsive to customary medical treatment; short-term treatment of active duodenal ulcer; long-term treatment of pathological hypersecretory conditions

Usual Dosage Adults: Oral:

Duodenal ulcer: 20 mg/day for 4-8 weeks

GERD or erosive esophagitis: 20 mg/day for 4-8 weeks

Maintenance of healing erosive esophagitis: 20 mg/day

Pathological hypersecretory conditions: 60 mg once daily initially; doses up to 120 mg 3 times/day have been administered; administer daily doses >80 mg in divided doses; patients with Zollinger-Ellison syndrome have been treated continuously for over 5 years

Dietary Considerations Food delays absorption, administer on an empty stomach

Nursing/Pharmacy Information

Capsule should be swallowed whole; not chewed, crushed, or opened; administration via NG tube should be in an acidic juice

Stability: Omeprazole stability is a function of pH; it is rapidly degraded in acidic media, but has acceptable stability under alkaline conditions. Prilosec™ is supplied as capsules for oral administration; each capsule contains 20 mg of omeprazole in the form of enteric coated granules to inhibit omeprazole degradation by gastric acidity; therefore, cannot recommend the extemporaneous preparation of an oral liquid form of Prilosec™ for administration into the stomach through an NG tube.

Dosage Forms Capsule, delayed release: 10 mg, 20 mg

- ♦ **Omifin** *see* clomiphene *on page 158*
- ♦ **Omnicef®** *see* cefdinir *on page 120*
- ♦ **OmniHIB™** *see* Haemophilus B conjugate vaccine *on page 306*
- ♦ **Omnipaque®** *see* radiological/contrast media (non-ionic) *on page 540*
- ♦ **Omnipen®** *see* ampicillin *on page 46*
- ♦ **Omnipen®-N** *see* ampicillin *on page 46*
- ♦ **OMS® Oral** *see* morphine sulfate *on page 422*
- ♦ **Oncaspar®** *see* pegaspargase *on page 472*
- ♦ **Oncet®** *see* hydrocodone and homatropine *on page 320*
- ♦ **Oncovin®** *see* vincristine *on page 648*

ondansetron (on DAN se tron)

U.S. Brand Names Zofran®; Zofran® ODT

Generic Available No

Therapeutic Category Selective 5-HT$_3$ Receptor Antagonist

Use Prevention of nausea and vomiting associated with initial and repeat courses of emetogenic cancer chemotherapy and prevention of postoperative nausea and vomiting; prevent postoperative nausea/vomiting (I.M.)

Usual Dosage

Oral:

Children 4-11 years: 4 mg 30 minutes before chemotherapy; repeat 4 and 8 hours after initial dose

Children >11 years and Adults: 8 mg 30 minutes before chemotherapy; repeat 4 and 8 hours after initial dose or every 8 hours for a maximum of 48 hours

I.V.: Administer either three 0.15 mg/kg doses or a single 32 mg dose; with the 3-dose regimen, the initial dose is given 30 minutes prior to chemotherapy with subsequent doses administered 4 and 8 hours after the first dose. With the single-dose regimen 32 mg is infused over 15 minutes beginning 30

(Continued)

ondansetron *(Continued)*

minutes before the start of emetogenic chemotherapy. Dosage should be calculated based on weight:

Children: Pediatric dosing should follow the manufacturer's guidelines for 0.15 mg/kg/dose administered 30 minutes prior to chemotherapy, 4 and 8 hours after the first dose. While not as yet FDA-approved, literature supports the day's total dose administered as a single dose 30 minutes prior to chemotherapy.

Adults:
>80 kg: 12 mg IVPB
45-80 kg: 8 mg IVPB
<45 kg: 0.15 mg/kg/dose IVPB

Dietary Considerations
Food increases the extent of absorption; the C_{max} and T_{max} does not change much; administer without regard to meals
Potassium: Hypokalemia; monitor potassium serum concentration

Nursing/Pharmacy Information
First dose should be administered 30 minutes prior to starting chemotherapy treatment; if injected undiluted, administer over a 2- to 5-minute period; dilute in 50 mL I.V. fluid (maximum concentration: 0.64 mg/mL) and infuse over 15 minutes
Stability: The injection may be stored between 36°F and 86°F; stable when mixed in 5% dextrose or 0.9% sodium chloride for 48 hours at room temperature; does not need protection from light

Dosage Forms Ondansetron hydrochloride:
Injection: 2 mg/mL (2 mL, 20 mL); 32 mg (single-dose vials)
Tablet: 4 mg, 8 mg

- ◆ **Ontak®** *see* denileukin deftitox *New Drug on page 186*
- ◆ **Ony-Clear® Nail** *see* triacetin *on page 623*
- ◆ **Ony-Clear® Spray** *see* miconazole *on page 413*
- ◆ **Onyvul®** *see* urea *on page 638*
- ◆ **OPC-17116** *see* grepafloxacin *Withdrawn from U.S. market 10/27/99 on page 298*
- ◆ **OP-CCK** *see* sincalide *on page 567*
- ◆ **Opcon® Ophthalmic** *see* naphazoline *on page 431*
- ◆ **o,p'-DDD** *see* mitotane *on page 418*
- ◆ **Operand® [OTC]** *see* povidone-iodine *on page 510*
- ◆ **Ophthacet®** *see* sulfacetamide *on page 584*
- ◆ **Ophthaine® *(Discontinued)*** *see page 743*
- ◆ **Ophthalgan® Ophthalmic** *see* glycerin *on page 295*
- ◆ **Ophthetic®** *see* proparacaine *on page 524*
- ◆ **Ophthochlor® Ophthalmic** *see* chloramphenicol *on page 133*
- ◆ **Ophthocort® *(Discontinued)*** *see page 743*
- ◆ **Ophtho-tate®** *see* prednisolone (ophthalmic) *on page 514*

opium alkaloids (OH pee um AL ka loyds)

U.S. Brand Names Pantopon®
Generic Available Yes
Therapeutic Category Analgesic, Narcotic
Controlled Substance C-II
Use For relief of severe pain
Usual Dosage Adults: I.M., S.C.: 5-20 mg every 4-5 hours
Nursing/Pharmacy Information Observe patient for excessive sedation, respiratory depression, implement safety measures, assist with ambulation
Dosage Forms Injection: 20 mg/mL (1 mL)

- ◆ **opium and belladonna** *see* belladonna and opium *on page 76*

opium tincture (OH pee um TINGK chur)

Synonyms deodorized opium tincture; DTO
Generic Available Yes
Therapeutic Category Analgesic, Narcotic
Controlled Substance C-II
Use Treatment of diarrhea or relief of pain; **a 25-fold dilution with water** (final concentration 0.4 mg/mL morphine) can be used to treat neonatal abstinence syndrome (opiate withdrawal)
Usual Dosage Oral:
Children:
Diarrhea: 0.005-0.01 mL/kg/dose every 3-4 hours

Analgesia: 0.01-0.02 mL/kg/dose every 3-4 hours
Adults: 0.6 mL 4 times/day

Nursing/Pharmacy Information Monitor patient for excessive sedation, respiratory depression, implement safety measures, assist with ambulation

Dosage Forms Liquid: 10% [0.6 mL equivalent to morphine 6 mg] with alcohol 19%

oprelvekin (oh PREL ve kin)

Synonyms IL-11; interleukin-11; recombinant human interleukin-11; recombinant interleukin-11; rhIL-11; rIL-11

U.S. Brand Names Neumega®

Generic Available No

Therapeutic Category Platelet Growth Factor

Use Prevention and treatment of severe thrombocytopenia following myelosuppressive chemotherapy

Usual Dosage Refer to individual protocols
Children: 75-100 mcg/kg/day for 10-21 days (until platelet count >50,000/mm^3)
Adults: 50 mcg/kg/day for 10-21 days (until platelet count >50,000/mm^3)

Dosage Forms Powder for injection, lyophilized: 5 mg

- ♦ **Opthaflox** *see* ciprofloxacin *on page 151*
- ♦ **Optho-Bunolol®** *see* levobunolol *on page 364*
- ♦ **Optho-Dipivefrin™** *see* dipivefrin *on page 211*
- ♦ **Opticrom®** *see* cromolyn sodium *on page 171*
- ♦ **Optifast® 900** *see* enteral nutritional products *on page 233*
- ♦ **Optigene® Ophthalmic [OTC]** *see* tetrahydrozoline *on page 602*
- ♦ **Optimine®** *see* azatadine *on page 67*
- ♦ **Optimoist® Solution [OTC]** *see* saliva substitute *on page 558*
- ♦ **OptiPranolol® Ophthalmic** *see* metipranolol *on page 409*
- ♦ **Optiray®** *see* radiological/contrast media (non-ionic) *on page 540*
- ♦ **OPV** *see* poliovirus vaccine, live, trivalent, oral *on page 501*
- ♦ **Orabase®-B [OTC]** *see* benzocaine *on page 79*
- ♦ **Orabase® HCA Topical** *see* hydrocortisone (topical) *on page 324*
- ♦ **Orabase®-O [OTC]** *see* benzocaine *on page 79*
- ♦ **Orabase® Plain [OTC]** *see* gelatin, pectin, and methylcellulose *on page 289*
- ♦ **Orabase® With Benzocaine [OTC]** *see* benzocaine, gelatin, pectin, and sodium carboxymethylcellulose *on page 80*
- ♦ **Oradex-C®** ***(Discontinued)*** *see page 743*
- ♦ **Oragrafin® Calcium** *see* radiological/contrast media (ionic) *on page 539*
- ♦ **Oragrafin® Sodium** *see* radiological/contrast media (ionic) *on page 539*
- ♦ **Orajel® Brace-Aid Oral Anesthetic [OTC]** *see* benzocaine *on page 79*
- ♦ **Orajel® Maximum Strength [OTC]** *see* benzocaine *on page 79*
- ♦ **Orajel® Mouth-Aid [OTC]** *see* benzocaine *on page 79*
- ♦ **Orajel® Perioseptic® [OTC]** *see* carbamide peroxide *on page 112*
- ♦ **Oramorph SR™ Oral** *see* morphine sulfate *on page 422*
- ♦ **Oranor** *see* norfloxacin *on page 448*
- ♦ **Orap™** *see* pimozide *on page 494*
- ♦ **Orasept® [OTC]** *see* benzocaine *on page 79*
- ♦ **Orasol® [OTC]** *see* benzocaine *on page 79*
- ♦ **Orasone®** *see* prednisone *on page 515*
- ♦ **Oratect®** ***(Discontinued)*** *see page 743*
- ♦ **Orazinc® Oral [OTC]** *see* zinc sulfate *on page 660*
- ♦ **Orbenin®** *see* cloxacillin *on page 161*
- ♦ **orciprenaline** *see* metaproterenol *on page 397*
- ♦ **Ordrine AT® Extended Release Capsule** *see* caramiphen and phenylpropanolamine *on page 111*
- ♦ **Oretic®** *see* hydrochlorothiazide *on page 317*
- ♦ **Oreticyl®** ***(Discontinued)*** *see page 743*
- ♦ **Oreton® Methyl** *see* methyltestosterone *on page 408*
- ♦ **Orexin® [OTC]** *see* vitamin B complex *on page 651*
- ♦ **Organidin®** ***(Discontinued)*** *see page 743*
- ♦ **Organidin® NR** *see* guaifenesin *on page 299*
- ♦ **Orgaran®** *see* danaparoid *on page 181*
- ♦ **ORG NC 45** *see* vecuronium *on page 645*
- ♦ **Orifer® F** *see* vitamin, multiple (oral) *on page 654*
- ♦ **Orimune®** *see* poliovirus vaccine, live, trivalent, oral *on page 501*

♦ **Orinase® Diagnostic Injection** *see* tolbutamide *on page 617*

♦ **Orinase® Oral** *see* tolbutamide *on page 617*

♦ **ORLAAM®** *see* levomethadyl acetate hydrochloride *on page 366*

orlistat *New Drug* (OR li stat)
U.S. Brand Names Xenical®
Generic Available No
Therapeutic Category Lipase Inhibitor
Use Management of obesity, including weight loss and weight management when used in conjunction with a reduced-calorie diet; reduce the risk of weight regain after prior weight loss; indicated for obese patients with an initial body mass index (BMI) ≥30 kg/m^2 or ≥27 kg/m^2 in the presence of other risk factors
Usual Dosage Adults: Oral: 120 mg 3 times/day with each main meal containing fat (during or up to 1 hour after the meal); omit dose if meal is occasionally missed or contains no fat
Dosage Forms Capsule: 120 mg

♦ **Ormazine®** *see* chlorpromazine *on page 144*

♦ **Ornade® Spansule®** *see* chlorpheniramine and phenylpropanolamine *on page 139*

♦ **Ornex® No Drowsiness [OTC]** *see* acetaminophen and pseudoephedrine *on page 15*

♦ **Ornidyl®** *see* eflornithine *on page 229*

♦ **Oro-Clense** *see* chlorhexidine gluconate *on page 134*

orphenadrine (or FEN a dreen)
U.S. Brand Names Norflex™
Generic Available Yes
Therapeutic Category Skeletal Muscle Relaxant
Use Treatment of muscle spasm associated with acute painful musculoskeletal conditions; supportive therapy in tetanus
Usual Dosage Adults:
Oral: 100 mg twice daily
I.M., I.V.: 60 mg every 12 hours
Nursing/Pharmacy Information Do not crush sustained release drug product; raise bed rails, institute safety measures, assist with ambulation
Dosage Forms Orphenadrine citrate:
Injection: 30 mg/mL (2 mL, 10 mL)
Tablet: 100 mg
Tablet, sustained release: 100 mg

orphenadrine, aspirin, and caffeine
(or FEN a dreen, AS pir in, & KAF een)
Synonyms aspirin, orphenadrine, and caffeine; caffeine, orphenadrine, and aspirin
U.S. Brand Names Norgesic™; Norgesic™ Forte
Generic Available Yes
Therapeutic Category Analgesic, Non-narcotic; Skeletal Muscle Relaxant
Use Relief of discomfort associated with skeletal muscular conditions
Usual Dosage Oral: 1-2 tablets 3-4 times/day
Dosage Forms
Tablet: Orphenadrine citrate 25 mg, aspirin 385 mg, and caffeine 30 mg
Tablet (Norgesic® Forte): Orphenadrine citrate 50 mg, aspirin 770 mg, and caffeine 60 mg

♦ **Ortho® 0.5/35** *see* ethinyl estradiol and norethindrone *on page 250*

♦ **Ortho-Cept®** *see* ethinyl estradiol and desogestrel *on page 248*

♦ **Ortho-Chloram®** *see* chloramphenicol *on page 133*

♦ **Orthoclone OKT3** *see* muromonab-CD3 *on page 425*

♦ **Ortho-Cyclen®** *see* ethinyl estradiol and norgestimate *on page 251*

♦ **Ortho®-Dienestrol Vaginal** *see* dienestrol *on page 200*

♦ **Ortho-Est® Oral** *see* estropipate *on page 246*

♦ **Ortho-Novum® 1/35** *see* ethinyl estradiol and norethindrone *on page 250*

♦ **Ortho-Novum® 1/50** *see* mestranol and norethindrone *on page 396*

♦ **Ortho-Novum® 7/7/7** *see* ethinyl estradiol and norethindrone *on page 250*

♦ **Ortho-Novum® 10/11** *see* ethinyl estradiol and norethindrone *on page 250*

♦ **Ortho Tri-Cyclen®** *see* ethinyl estradiol and norgestimate *on page 251*

♦ **Or-Tyl® Injection** *see* dicyclomine *on page 199*

♦ **Orudis®** *see* ketoprofen *on page 355*

♦ **Orudis® KT [OTC]** *see* ketoprofen *on page 355*

♦ **Oruvail®** *see* ketoprofen *on page 355*
♦ **Os-Cal® 500 [OTC]** *see* calcium carbonate *on page 103*

oseltamivir *New Drug* (o sel TAM e veer)
U.S. Brand Names Tamiflu™
Generic Available No
Therapeutic Category Antiviral Agent, Oral
Controlled Substance [FS100]influenza
Use Treatment of uncomplicated influenza in adults whose flu symptoms have not lasted more than two days; approved to treat Type A and B influenza
Usual Dosage Oral: Adults: 1 capsule (75 mg) twice daily for 5 days; may be taken with or without food
Dosage Forms Capsule, as phosphate: 75 mg

♦ **Osmitrol® Injection** *see* mannitol *on page 383*
♦ **Osmoglyn®** *see* glycerin *on page 295*
♦ **Osmolite® HN [OTC]** *see* enteral nutritional products *on page 233*
♦ **Osteocalcin®** *see* calcitonin *on page 102*
♦ **Ostoforte®** *see* ergocalciferol *on page 237*
♦ **Otic-Care® Otic** *see* neomycin, polymyxin B, and hydrocortisone *on page 437*
♦ **Otic Domeboro®** *see* aluminum acetate and acetic acid *on page 32*
♦ **Otic Tridesilon® *(Discontinued)*** *see page 743*
♦ **Otobiotic® Otic** *see* polymyxin B and hydrocortisone *on page 503*
♦ **Otocort® Otic** *see* neomycin, polymyxin B, and hydrocortisone *on page 437*
♦ **Otosporin® Otic** *see* neomycin, polymyxin B, and hydrocortisone *on page 437*
♦ **Otrivin® Nasal [OTC]** *see* xylometazoline *on page 656*
♦ **Otrozol** *see* metronidazole *on page 411*
♦ **Ovcon® 35** *see* ethinyl estradiol and norethindrone *on page 250*
♦ **Ovcon® 50** *see* ethinyl estradiol and norethindrone *on page 250*
♦ **Ovide™ Topical** *see* malathion *on page 383*
♦ **Ovol®** *see* simethicone *on page 566*
♦ **Ovral®** *see* ethinyl estradiol and norgestrel *on page 252*
♦ **Ovrette®** *see* norgestrel *on page 448*
♦ **O-V Staticin®** *see* nystatin *on page 452*

oxacillin (oks a SIL in)
Synonyms methylphenyl isoxazolyl penicillin
Generic Available Yes
Therapeutic Category Penicillin
Use Treatment of bacterial infections such as osteomyelitis, septicemia, endocarditis, and CNS infections due to susceptible penicillinase-producing strains of *Staphylococcus*
Usual Dosage
Infants and Children:
I.M., I.V.: 150-200 mg/kg/day in divided doses every 6 hours; maximum dose: 12 g/day
Oral: 50-100 mg/kg/day divided every 6 hours
Adults:
Oral: 500-1000 mg every 4-6 hours for at least 5 days
I.M., I.V.: 250 mg to 2 g/dose every 4-6 hours
Dietary Considerations Should be administered orally on an empty stomach 1 hour before meals or 2 hours after meals; presence of food decreases GI absorption of oxacillin
Nursing/Pharmacy Information
Administer around-the-clock rather than 4 times/day, 3 times/day, etc, (ie, 12-6-12-6, not 9-1-5-9) to promote less variation in peak and trough serum levels; I.M. injections should be administered deep into a large muscle mass such as the gluteus maximus; can be administered by I.V. push over 10 minutes at a maximum concentration of 100 mg/mL or by I.V. intermittent infusion over 15-30 minutes at a final concentration ≤40 mg/mL
Monitor periodic CBC, urinalysis, BUN, serum creatinine, AST and ALT
Stability: Reconstituted parenteral solution is stable for 3 days at room temperature and 7 days when refrigerated; for I.V. infusion in normal saline or D_5W, solution is stable for 6 hours at room temperature
Dosage Forms Oxacillin sodium:
Capsule: 250 mg, 500 mg
Powder for injection: 250 mg, 500 mg, 1 g, 2 g, 4 g, 10 g
Powder for oral solution: 250 mg/5 mL (100 mL)

oxamniquine (oks AM ni kwin)
U.S. Brand Names Vansil™
Generic Available No
Therapeutic Category Anthelmintic
Use Treat all stages of *Schistosoma mansoni* infection
Usual Dosage Oral:
  Children <30 kg: 20 mg/kg in 2 divided doses of 10 mg/kg at 2- to 8-hour intervals
  Adults: 12-15 mg/kg as a single dose
Dietary Considerations May be administered with food
Dosage Forms Capsule: 250 mg

♦ **Oxandrin®** *see* oxandrolone *on page 460*

oxandrolone (oks AN droe lone)
U.S. Brand Names Oxandrin®
Generic Available No
Therapeutic Category Androgen
Controlled Substance C-III
Use Treatment of catabolic or tissue-depleting processes
Usual Dosage Adults: Oral: 2.5 mg 2-4 times/day
Dosage Forms Tablet: 2.5 mg

oxaprozin (oks a PROE zin)
U.S. Brand Names Daypro™
Generic Available No
Therapeutic Category Analgesic, Non-narcotic; Nonsteroidal Anti-inflammatory Drug (NSAID)
Use Acute and long-term use in the management of signs and symptoms of osteoarthritis and rheumatoid arthritis
Usual Dosage Adults: Oral (individualize the dosage to the lowest effective dose to minimize adverse effects):
  Osteoarthritis: 600-1200 mg once daily
  Rheumatoid arthritis: 1200 mg once daily
  Maximum dose: 1800 mg/day or 26 mg/kg (whichever is lower) in divided doses
Nursing/Pharmacy Information Monitor blood, hepatic, renal, and ocular function
Dosage Forms Tablet: 600 mg

oxazepam (oks A ze pam)
U.S. Brand Names Serax®
Canadian Brand Names Apo-Oxazepam®; Novo-Oxazepam®; Oxpam®; PMS-Oxazepam; Zapex®
Generic Available Yes
Therapeutic Category Anticonvulsant; Benzodiazepine
Controlled Substance C-IV
Use Treatment of anxiety and management of alcohol withdrawal; may also be used as an anticonvulsant in management of simple partial seizures
Usual Dosage Oral:
  Children: 1 mg/kg/day has been administered
  Adults:
    Anxiety: 10-30 mg 3-4 times/day
    Alcohol withdrawal: 15-30 mg 3-4 times/day
    Hypnotic: 15-30 mg
Dietary Considerations May be administered with food or water
Nursing/Pharmacy Information
  Assist patient with ambulation
  Monitor respiratory and cardiovascular status, monitor for alertness
Dosage Forms
  Capsule: 10 mg, 15 mg, 30 mg
  Tablet: 15 mg

♦ **Oxicanol** *see* piroxicam *on page 497*

oxiconazole (oks i KON a zole)
U.S. Brand Names Oxistat® Topical
Generic Available No
Therapeutic Category Antifungal Agent
Use Treatment of tinea pedis, tinea cruris, and tinea corporis

Usual Dosage Topical: Apply once daily to affected areas for 2 weeks to 1 month

Nursing/Pharmacy Information External use only; discontinue if sensitivity or chemical irritation occurs, contact physician if condition fails to improve in 3-4 days

Dosage Forms Oxiconazole nitrate:
Cream: 1% (15 g, 30 g, 60 g)
Lotion: 1% (30 mL)

- ♦ **Oxifungol** *see* fluconazole *on page 270*
- ♦ **Oxiken** *see* dobutamine *on page 214*
- ♦ **oxilapine** *see* loxapine *on page 377*
- ♦ **Oxistat® Topical** *see* oxiconazole *on page 460*
- ♦ **Oxitopisa** *see* oxytocin *on page 465*
- ♦ **Oxitraklin** *see* oxytetracycline *on page 464*
- ♦ **Oxpam®** *see* oxazepam *on page 460*
- ♦ **oxpentifylline** *see* pentoxifylline *on page 480*

oxprenolol *(Canada only)* (ox PREN oh lole)
Canadian Brand Names Trasicor®
Generic Available No
Therapeutic Category Beta-Adrenergic Blocker
Use Treatment of mild to moderate hypertension
Usual Dosage Adults: Oral: Start with 20 mg three times/day, titrated upward to a maximum dose of 480 mg/day
Dosage Forms Tablet: 40 mg, 80 mg

- ♦ **Oxsoralen® Oral** *(Discontinued)* *see page 743*
- ♦ **Oxsoralen-Ultra®** *see* methoxsalen *on page 403*

oxtriphylline (oks TRYE fi lin)
Synonyms choline theophyllinate
Generic Available Yes
Therapeutic Category Theophylline Derivative
Use Bronchodilator in symptomatic treatment of asthma and reversible broncho-spasm
Usual Dosage Oral:
Children:
1-9 years: 6.2 mg/kg/dose every 6 hours
9-16 years: 4.7 mg/kg/dose every 6 hours
Adults: 4.7 mg/kg every 8 hours; sustained release: administer every 12 hours
Dietary Considerations Should be administered with water 1 hour before or 2 hours after meals
Nursing/Pharmacy Information
Administer oral administration around-the-clock rather than 4 times/day, 3 times/day, etc, (ie, 12-6-12-6, not 9-1-5-9) to promote less variation in peak and trough serum levels; do not crush sustained release drug products; encourage patient to drink adequate fluids (2 L/day) to decrease mucous viscosity in airways
Monitor heart rate, vital signs, serum concentrations, CNS effects (insomnia, irritability); respiratory rate (COPD patients often have resting controlled respiratory rates in the low 20s)
Dosage Forms
Elixir: 100 mg/5 mL (5 mL, 10 mL, 473 mL)
Syrup: 50 mg/5 mL (473 mL)
Tablet: 100 mg, 200 mg
Sustained release: 400 mg, 600 mg

- ♦ **Oxy-5® Advanced Formula for Sensitive Skin [OTC]** *see* benzoyl peroxide *on page 81*
- ♦ **Oxy-5® Tinted [OTC]** *see* benzoyl peroxide *on page 81*
- ♦ **Oxy-10® Advanced Formula for Sensitive Skin [OTC]** *see* benzoyl peroxide *on page 81*
- ♦ **Oxy 10® Wash [OTC]** *see* benzoyl peroxide *on page 81*

oxybutynin (oks i BYOO ti nin)
U.S. Brand Names Ditropan®; Ditropan® XL
Generic Available Yes
Therapeutic Category Antispasmodic Agent, Urinary
Use Relief of bladder spasms associated with voiding in patients with uninhibited and reflex neurogenic bladder
(Continued)

oxybutynin *(Continued)*

Usual Dosage Oral:
Children:
1-5 years: 0.2 mg/kg/dose 2-4 times/day
>5 years: 5 mg twice daily, up to 5 mg 3 times/day
Adults: 5 mg 2-3 times/day up to 5 mg 4 times/day maximum
Dietary Considerations Should be administered on an empty stomach with water
Nursing/Pharmacy Information Monitor incontinence episodes, postvoid residual (PVR)
Dosage Forms Oxybutynin chloride:
Syrup: 5 mg/5 mL (473 mL)
Tablet: 5 mg
Tablet, extended release: 5 mg, 10 mg

♦ **Oxycel®** *see* cellulose, oxidized *on page 127*

oxychlorosene (oks i KLOR oh seen)

U.S. Brand Names Clorpactin® WCS-90
Generic Available No
Therapeutic Category Antibiotic, Topical
Use Treating localized infections
Usual Dosage Topical (0.1% to 0.5% solutions): Apply by irrigation, instillation, spray, soaks, or wet compresses
Nursing/Pharmacy Information Refrigerate
Dosage Forms Powder for solution, as sodium: 2 g, 5 g

♦ **Oxycocet®** *see* oxycodone and acetaminophen *on page 462*
♦ **Oxycodan®** *see* oxycodone and aspirin *on page 463*

oxycodone (oks i KOE done)

Synonyms dihydrohydroxycodeinone
U.S. Brand Names OxyContin®; OxyIR™; Percolone™; Roxicodone™
Generic Available Yes
Therapeutic Category Analgesic, Narcotic
Controlled Substance C-II
Use Management of moderate to severe pain, normally used in combination with non-narcotic analgesics
Usual Dosage Oral:
Children:
6-12 years: 1.25 mg every 6 hours as needed
>12 years: 2.5 mg every 6 hours as needed
Adults: 5 mg every 6 hours as needed
Nursing/Pharmacy Information Monitor for pain relief, respiratory and mental status, blood pressure, and constipation
Dosage Forms
Capsule, as hydrochloride, immediate release (OxyIR™): 5 mg
Liquid, oral, as hydrochloride: 5 mg/5 mL (500 mL)
Solution, oral concentrate, as hydrochloride: 20 mg/mL (30 mL)
Tablet, as hydrochloride: 5 mg
Percolone™: 5 mg
Tablet, controlled release, as hydrochloride (OxyContin®): 10 mg, 20 mg, 40 mg, 80 mg

oxycodone and acetaminophen

(oks i KOE done & a seet a MIN oh fen)
Synonyms acetaminophen and oxycodone
U.S. Brand Names Endocet®; Percocet®; Roxicet® 5/500; Roxilox®; Tylox®
Canadian Brand Names Endocet®; Oxycocet®; Percocet®-Demi
Generic Available Yes
Therapeutic Category Analgesic, Narcotic
Controlled Substance C-II
Use Management of moderate to severe pain
Usual Dosage Oral (doses should be titrated to appropriate analgesic effects):
Children: Oxycodone: 0.05-0.15 mg/kg/dose to 5 mg/dose (maximum) every 4-6 hours as needed
Adults: 1-2 tablets every 4-6 hours as needed for pain
Maximum daily dose of acetaminophen: 4 g/day
Dietary Considerations Rate of absorption of acetaminophen may be decreased when administered with food high in carbohydrates

Oxycodone: Alcohol: Additive CNS effects; avoid or limit alcohol; watch for sedation

Oxycodone: Food: Glucose may cause hyperglycemia; monitor blood glucose concentrations

Nursing/Pharmacy Information Monitor for pain relief, respiratory and mental status, blood pressure, constipation

Dosage Forms

Caplet: Oxycodone hydrochloride 5 mg and acetaminophen 500 mg

Capsule: Oxycodone hydrochloride 5 mg and acetaminophen 500 mg

Solution, oral: Oxycodone hydrochloride 5 mg and acetaminophen 325 mg per 5 mL (5 mL, 500 mL)

Tablet: Oxycodone hydrochloride 5 mg and acetaminophen 325 mg

oxycodone and aspirin (oks i KOE done & AS pir in)

Synonyms aspirin and oxycodone

U.S. Brand Names Codoxy®; Percodan®; Percodan®-Demi; Roxiprin®

Canadian Brand Names Endodan®; Oxycodan®

Generic Available Yes

Therapeutic Category Analgesic, Narcotic

Controlled Substance C-II

Use Relief of moderate to moderately severe pain

Usual Dosage Oral (based on oxycodone combined salts):

Children: 0.05-0.15 mg/kg/dose every 4-6 hours as needed; maximum: 5 mg/dose (1 tablet Percodan® or 2 tablets Percodan®-Demi/dose) **or**

Alternatively:

6-12 years: Percodan®-Demi: $^1/_4$ tablet every 6 hours as needed for pain

>12 years: $^1/_2$ tablet every 6 hours as needed for pain

Adults: Percodan®: 1 tablet every 6 hours as needed for pain or Percodan®-Demi: 1-2 tablets every 6 hours as needed for pain

Dietary Considerations May be administered with food or water; aspirin may increase renal excretion of vitamin C and may decrease serum folate levels

Nursing/Pharmacy Information Monitor for pain relief, respiratory and mental status, blood pressure, constipation

Dosage Forms Tablet: Oxycodone hydrochloride 4.5 mg, oxycodone terephthalate 0.38 mg, and aspirin 325 mg; oxycodone hydrochloride 2.25 mg, oxycodone terephthalate 0.19 mg, and aspirin 325 mg

♦ **OxyContin®** *see* oxycodone *on page 462*

♦ **Oxyderm™ 5%, 10%, 20%** *see* benzoyl peroxide *on page 81*

♦ **OxyIR™** *see* oxycodone *on page 462*

oxymetazoline (oks i met AZ oh leen)

U.S. Brand Names Afrin® Children's Nose Drops [OTC]; Afrin® Nasal Solution [OTC]; Allerest® 12 Hour Nasal Solution [OTC]; Chlorphed®-LA Nasal Solution [OTC]; Dristan® Long Lasting Nasal Solution [OTC]; Duramist Plus® [OTC]; Duration® Nasal Solution [OTC]; Neo-Synephrine® 12 Hour Nasal Solution [OTC]; Nōstrilla® [OTC]; NTZ® Long Acting Nasal Solution [OTC]; OcuClear® Ophthalmic [OTC]; Sinarest® 12 Hour Nasal Solution; Sinex® Long-Acting [OTC]; Twice-A-Day® Nasal Solution [OTC]; Visine® L.R. Ophthalmic [OTC]; 4-Way® Long Acting Nasal Solution [OTC]

Canadian Brand Names Drixoral® Nasal

Generic Available Yes

Therapeutic Category Adrenergic Agonist Agent

Use Symptomatic relief of nasal mucosal congestion associated with acute or chronic rhinitis, the common cold, sinusitis, hay fever, or other allergies

Usual Dosage

Intranasal:

Children 2-5 years: 0.025% solution: Instill 2-3 drops in each nostril twice daily

Children ≥6 years and Adults: 0.05% solution: Instill 2-3 drops or 2-3 sprays into each nostril twice daily

Ophthalmic: Adults: Instill 1-2 drops into affected eye(s) every 6 hours

Nursing/Pharmacy Information

Spray/drops should not be used for >3 days without direct physician supervision

Stability: Do not use if solution changes colors or becomes cloudy

Dosage Forms Oxymetazoline hydrochloride:

Ophthalmic solution (OcuClear®, Visine® L.R.): 0.025% (15 mL, 30 mL)

Solution, nasal:

Drops:

Afrin® Children's Nose Drops: 0.025% (20 mL)

(Continued)

oxymetazoline *(Continued)*

Afrin®, NTZ® Long Acting Nasal Solution: 0.05% (15 mL, 20 mL)
Spray: Afrin® Sinus, Allerest® 12 Hours, Chlorphed®-LA, Dristan® Long Lasting, Duration®, 4-Way® Long Acting, Genasal®, Nasal Relief®, Nŏstrilla®, NTZ® Long Acting Nasal Solution, Sinex® Long-Acting, Twice-A-Day®: 0.05% (15 mL, 30 mL)

oxymetholone (oks i METH oh lone)
U.S. Brand Names Anadrol®
Canadian Brand Names Anapolon®
Generic Available No
Therapeutic Category Anabolic Steroid
Controlled Substance C-III
Use Anemias caused by the administration of myelotoxic drugs
Usual Dosage Erythropoietic effects: 1-5 mg/kg/day as a single dose; maximum: 100 mg/day
Nursing/Pharmacy Information Monitor liver function tests
Dosage Forms Tablet: 50 mg

oxymorphone (oks i MOR fone)
U.S. Brand Names Numorphan®
Generic Available No
Therapeutic Category Analgesic, Narcotic
Controlled Substance C-II
Use Management of moderate to severe pain and preoperatively as a sedative and a supplement to anesthesia
Usual Dosage Adults:
I.M., S.C.: Initial: 0.5 mg, then 1-1.5 mg every 4-6 hours as needed
I.V.: Initial: 0.5 mg
Rectal: 5 mg every 4-6 hours
Nursing/Pharmacy Information
Monitor respiratory rate, heart rate, blood pressure, CNS activity
Stability: Refrigerate suppository
Dosage Forms Oxymorphone hydrochloride:
Injection: 1 mg (1 mL); 1.5 mg/mL (1 mL, 10 mL)
Suppository, rectal: 5 mg

oxyphenbutazone (oks i fen BYOO ta zone)
Generic Available Yes
Therapeutic Category Analgesic, Non-narcotic; Nonsteroidal Anti-inflammatory Drug (NSAID)
Use Management of inflammatory disorders, as an analgesic in the treatment of mild to moderate pain and as an antipyretic; I.V. form used as an alternate to surgery in management of patent ductus arteriosus in premature neonates; acute gouty arthritis
Usual Dosage Adults: Oral:
Rheumatoid arthritis: 100-200 mg 3-4 times/day until desired effect, then reduce dose to ≤400 mg/day
Acute gouty arthritis: Initial: 400 mg then 100 mg every 4 hours until acute attack subsides
Nursing/Pharmacy Information Warn patients not to exceed recommended dosage; do not crush tablet
Dosage Forms Tablet: 100 mg

oxytetracycline (oks i tet ra SYE kleen)
U.S. Brand Names Terramycin® I.M. Injection; Terramycin® Oral
Mexican Brand Names Oxitraklin; Terramicina
Generic Available Yes
Therapeutic Category Tetracycline Derivative
Use Treatment of susceptible bacterial infections; both gram-positive and gram-negative, as well as *Rickettsia* and *Mycoplasma* organisms
Usual Dosage
Oral:
Children: 40-50 mg/kg/day in divided doses every 6 hours (maximum: 2 g/24 hours)
Adults: 250-500 mg/dose every 6 hours
I.M.:
Children >8 years: 15-25 mg/kg/day (maximum: 250 mg/dose) in divided doses every 8-12 hours

Adults: 250-500 mg every 24 hours or 300 mg/day divided every 8-12 hours

Nursing/Pharmacy Information Injection for intramuscular use only; reduce dose in renal insufficiency

Dosage Forms Oxytetracycline hydrochloride:
Capsule: 250 mg
Injection with lidocaine 2%: 5% [50 mg/mL] (2 mL, 10 mL); 12.5% [125 mg/mL] (2 mL)

oxytetracycline and hydrocortisone
(oks i tet ra SYE kleen & hye droe KOR ti sone)

Synonyms hydrocortisone and oxytetracycline

U.S. Brand Names Terra-Cortril® Ophthalmic Suspension

Generic Available Yes

Therapeutic Category Antibiotic/Corticosteroid, Ophthalmic

Use Treatment of susceptible ophthalmic bacterial infections with associated inflammation

Usual Dosage Ophthalmic: Adults: Instill 1-2 drops in eye(s) every 3-4 hours

Dosage Forms Suspension, ophthalmic: Oxytetracycline hydrochloride 0.5% and hydrocortisone 0.5% (5 mL)

oxytetracycline and polymyxin B
(oks i tet ra SYE kleen & pol i MIKS in bee)

Synonyms polymyxin B and oxytetracycline

U.S. Brand Names Terak® Ophthalmic Ointment; Terramycin® Ophthalmic Ointment; Terramycin® w/Polymyxin B Ophthalmic Ointment

Generic Available No

Therapeutic Category Antibiotic, Ophthalmic

Use Treatment of superficial ocular infections involving the conjunctiva and/or cornea

Usual Dosage Ophthalmic: Apply ½" of ointment onto the lower lid of affected eye 2-4 times/day

Dosage Forms
Ointment, ophthalmic/otic: Oxytetracycline hydrochloride 5 mg and polymyxin B 10,000 units per g (3.5 g)
Tablet, vaginal: Oxytetracycline hydrochloride 100 mg and polymyxin B 100,000 units (10s)

oxytocin (oks i TOE sin)

Synonyms PIT

U.S. Brand Names Pitocin®

Canadian Brand Names Toesen®

Mexican Brand Names Oxitopisa; Syntocinon®; Xitocin

Generic Available Yes

Therapeutic Category Oxytocic Agent

Use Induce labor at term; control postpartum bleeding

Usual Dosage Adults:
Induction of labor: I.V.: 0.001-0.002 unit/minute; increase by 0.001-0.002 units every 15-30 minutes until contraction pattern has been established
Postpartum bleeding: I.V.: 0.001-0.002 unit/minute as needed

Nursing/Pharmacy Information
Monitor fluid intake and output during administration; fetal monitoring
Stability: Store at room temperature, protect from freezing

Dosage Forms Injection: 10 units/mL (1 mL, 10 mL)

- ◆ **Oyst-Cal 500 [OTC]** *see* calcium carbonate *on page 103*
- ◆ **Oystercal® 500** *see* calcium carbonate *on page 103*
- ◆ **Ozoken** *see* omeprazole *on page 455*
- ◆ **P-071** *see* cetirizine *on page 130*
- ◆ **Pacerone®** *see* amiodarone *on page 39*
- ◆ **Pacis™** *see* BCG vaccine *on page 74*

paclitaxel (PAK li taks el)

U.S. Brand Names Paxene®; Taxol®

Generic Available No

Therapeutic Category Antineoplastic Agent

Use Treatment of metastatic carcinoma of the ovary after failure of first-line or subsequent chemotherapy; treatment for AIDS-related Kaposi's sarcoma

Usual Dosage Adults: I.V.: 135 mg/m² over 24 hours every 3 weeks

Nursing/Pharmacy Information
Monitor hypersensitivity reactions
(Continued)

paclitaxel *(Continued)*

Stability: Vials must be stored under refrigeration 2°C to 8°C (36°F to 46°F) and protected from light. Dilute to a final concentration of 0.3-1.2 mg/mL in 0.9% sodium chloride injection, dextrose 5% in water, dextrose 5% in 0.9% sodium chloride, or dextrose 5% in Ringer's injection. These solutions are physically and chemically stable for up to 27 hours at ambient temperature (25°C) and room light; formulated in a vehicle known as Cremophor® EL (polyoxyethylated castor oil). Cremophor® EL has been found to leach the plasticizer DEHP from polyvinyl chloride infusion bags or administration sets. Taxol® solutions should be stored in glass bottles or polypropylene/polyolefin (Excel®) bags and administered through nonpolyvinyl chloride (ie, polyethylene-lined) administration sets; administer through I.V. tubing containing an in-line (0.22 micron) filter; administration through IVEX-2® filters (which incorporate short inlet and outlet polyvinyl chloride-coated tubing) has not resulted in significant leaching of DEHP.

Dosage Forms Injection: 6 mg/mL (5 mL, 16.7 mL)

♦ **Pactens** *see* naproxen *on page 432*
♦ **Palafer®** *see* ferrous fumarate *on page 264*

palivizumab *(pah li VIZ u mab)*

U.S. Brand Names Synagis®
Generic Available No
Therapeutic Category Monoclonal Antibody
Use Prevention of serious lower respiratory tract disease caused by respiratory syncytial virus (RSV) in pediatric patients at high risk of RSV disease; safety and efficacy were established in infants with bronchopulmonary dysplasia (BPD) and infants with a history of prematurity ≤35 weeks gestational age
Usual Dosage Children: I.M.: 15 mg/kg of body weight, monthly throughout RSV season (First dose administered prior to commencement of RSV season)
Dosage Forms Injection, lyophilized: 100 mg

♦ **Palmitate-A® 5000 [OTC]** *see* vitamin A *on page 650*
♦ **Palmocare®** *see* enteral nutritional products *on page 233*
♦ **PALS® [OTC]** *see* chlorophyll *on page 135*
♦ **2-PAM** *see* pralidoxime *on page 511*
♦ **Pamelor®** *see* nortriptyline *on page 449*

pamidronate *(pa mi DROE nate)*

U.S. Brand Names Aredia™
Generic Available No
Therapeutic Category Bisphosphonate Derivative
Use Symptomatic treatment of Paget's disease; hypercalcemia associated with malignancy
Usual Dosage Drug must be diluted properly before administration and infused slowly (at least over 2 hours)

Adults: I.V.:
Moderate cancer-related hypercalcemia (12-13 mg/dL): 60-90 mg administered as a slow infusion over 2-24 hours
Severe cancer-related hypercalcemia (>13.5 mg/dL): 90 mg as a slow infusion over 2-24 hours
A period of 7 days should elapse before the use of second course; repeat infusions every 2-3 weeks have been suggested, however, could be administered every 2-3 months according to the degree and of severity of hypercalcemia and/or the type of malignancy
Paget's disease: 60 mg as a single 2- to 24-hour infusion

Nursing/Pharmacy Information
Parenteral: Dilute in 1000 mL D_5W; infuse over 24 hours
Monitor serum calcium, phosphate, magnesium, potassium, serum creatinine, CBC with differential
Stability: Reconstitute by adding 10 mL of sterile water for injection, USP, to each 30 mg vial of lyophilized pamidronate disodium powder, the resulting solution will be 30 mg/10 mL; **incompatible** with calcium-containing infusion solutions such as Ringer's injection; may be diluted in 1000 mL of 0.45% or 0.9% sodium chloride, USP, or 5% dextrose; stable under refrigeration at 36°F to 46°F (2°C to 8°C) for 24 hours

Dosage Forms Powder for injection, lyophilized, as disodium: 30 mg, 60 mg, 90 mg

♦ **Pamine®** *see* methscopolamine *on page 404*
♦ **Pamprin IB® [OTC]** *see* ibuprofen *on page 332*

♦ **Panadol®** [OTC] *see* acetaminophen *on page 13*
♦ **Panasal® 5/500** *see* hydrocodone and aspirin *on page 319*
♦ **Pan-B antibodies** *see* rituximab *on page 552*
♦ **Pancrease®** *see* pancrelipase *on page 467*
♦ **Pancrease® MT** *see* pancrelipase *on page 467*

pancreatin (PAN kree a tin)

U.S. Brand Names Creon®; Digepepsin®; Donnazyme®; Hi-Vegi-Lip®
Generic Available No
Therapeutic Category Enzyme
Use Replacement therapy in symptomatic treatment of malabsorption syndrome caused by pancreatic insufficiency
Usual Dosage Enteric coated microspheres: The following dosage recommendations are only an approximation for initial dosages. The actual dosage will depend on the digestive requirements of the individual patient.

Oral:
Children:
<1 year: 2000 units of lipase with meals/feedings
1-6 years: 4000-8000 units of lipase with meals and 4000 units with snacks
7-12 years: 4000-12,000 units of lipase with meals and snacks
Adults: 4000-16,000 units of lipase with meals and with snacks
Dietary Considerations May be administered with food
Nursing/Pharmacy Information Monitor stool fat content
Dosage Forms
Capsule, enteric coated microspheres (Creon®): Lipase 8000 units, amylase 30,000 units, protease 13,000 units and pancreatin 300 mg
Tablet:
Digepepsin®: Pancreatin 300 mg, pepsin 250 mg, and bile salts 150 mg
Donnazyme®: Lipase 1000 units, amylase 12,500 units, protease 12,500 units and pancreatin 500 mg
Hi-Vegi-Lip®: Lipase 4800 units, amylase 60,000 units, protease 60,000 units and pancreatin 2400 mg

♦ **Pancrecarb®** *see* pancrelipase *on page 467*

pancrelipase (pan kre LI pase)

Synonyms lipancreatin; lipase, protease, and amylase
U.S. Brand Names Cotazym®; Cotazym-S®; Creon® 10; Creon® 20; Ilozyme®; Ku-Zyme® HP; Pancrease®; Pancrease® MT; Pancrecarb®; Protilase®; Ultrase® MT; Viokase®; Zymase®
Canadian Brand Names Digess®8000
Generic Available Yes
Therapeutic Category Enzyme
Use Replacement therapy in symptomatic treatment of malabsorption syndrome caused by pancreatic insufficiency
Usual Dosage Oral:
Powder: Actual dose depends on the digestive requirements of the patient
Children <1 year: Start with 1/8 teaspoonful with feedings
Enteric coated microspheres and microtablets: The following dosage recommendations are only an approximation for initial dosages. The actual dosage will depend on the digestive requirements of the individual patient.
Children:
<1 year: 2000 units of lipase with meals/feedings
1-6 years: 4000-8000 units of lipase with meals and 4000 units with snacks
7-12 years: 4000-12,000 units of lipase with meals and snacks
Adults: 4000-16,000 units of lipase with meals and with snacks
Dietary Considerations Avoid taking with alkaline food (pH >5.5); may impair oral iron absorption; should be administered with meals
Nursing/Pharmacy Information Monitor stool fat content
Dosage Forms
Capsule:
Cotazym®: Lipase 8000 units, protease 30,000 units, amylase 30,000 units
Ku-Zyme® HP: Lipase 8000 units, protease 30,000 units, amylase 30,000 units
Ultrase® MT12: Lipase 12,000 units, protease 39,000 units, amylase 39,000 units
Ultrase® MT20: Lipase 20,000 units, protease 65,000 units, amylase 65,000 units
Enteric coated microspheres (Pancrease®): Lipase 4000 units, protease 25,000 units, amylase 20,000 units
(Continued)

467

pancrelipase *(Continued)*

Enteric coated microtablets:

Pancrease® MT 4: Lipase 4500 units, protease 12,000 units, amylase 12,000 units

Pancrease® MT 10: Lipase 10,000 units, protease 30,000 units, amylase 30,000 units

Pancrease® MT 16: Lipase 16,000 units, protease 48,000 units, amylase 48,000 units

Pancrease® MT 20: Lipase 20,000 units, protease 44,000 units, amylase 56,000 units

Enteric coated spheres:

Cotazym-S®: Lipase 5000 units, protease 20,000 units, amylase 20,000 units

Pancrelipase, Protilase®: Lipase 4000 units, protease 25,000 units, amylase 20,000 units

Zymase®: Lipase 12,000 units, protease 24,000 units, amylase 24,000 units

Delayed release:

Creon® 10: Lipase 10,000 units, protease 37,500 units, amylase 33,200 units

Creon® 20: Lipase 20,000 units, protease 75,000 units, amylase 66,400 units

Powder (Viokase®): Lipase 16,800 units, protease 70,000 units, amylase 70,000 units per 0.7 g

Tablet:

Ilozyme®: Lipase 11,000 units, protease 30,000 units, amylase 30,000 units

Viokase®: Lipase 8000 units, protease 30,000 units, amylase 30,000 units

pancuronium *(pan kyoo ROE nee um)*

U.S. Brand Names Pavulon®

Generic Available Yes

Therapeutic Category Skeletal Muscle Relaxant

Use Produces skeletal muscle relaxation during surgery after induction of general anesthesia, increases pulmonary compliance during assisted mechanical respiration, facilitates endotracheal intubation

Usual Dosage Infants >1 month, Children, and Adults: I.V.: 0.04-0.1 mg/kg; maintenance dose: 0.02-0.1 mg/kg/dose every 30-60 minutes as needed

Nursing/Pharmacy Information

Does not alter the patient's state of consciousness; addition of sedation and analgesia are recommended; may be administered undiluted by rapid I.V. injection

Monitor respiratory rate, heart rate, blood pressure, and CNS activity

Stability: Refrigerate; however, is stable for up to 6 months at room temperature; I.V. form is **incompatible** when mixed with diazepam at a Y-site injection

Dosage Forms Injection, as bromide: 1 mg/mL (10 mL); 2 mg/mL (2 mL, 5 mL)

- ♦ **Panhematin®** see hemin *on page 310*
- ♦ **Panmycin® Oral** see tetracycline *on page 601*
- ♦ **PanOxyl®-AQ** see benzoyl peroxide *on page 81*
- ♦ **PanOxyl® Bar [OTC]** see benzoyl peroxide *on page 81*
- ♦ **Panretin™** see alitretinoin *New Drug on page 28*
- ♦ **Panscol® Lotion [OTC]** see salicylic acid *on page 557*
- ♦ **Panscol® Ointment [OTC]** see salicylic acid *on page 557*
- ♦ **Panthoderm® Cream [OTC]** see dexpanthenol *on page 192*
- ♦ **Pantoloc™** see pantoprazole *(Canada only) on page 468*
- ♦ **Pantomicina** see erythromycin (systemic) *on page 240*
- ♦ **Pantopon®** see opium alkaloids *on page 456*

pantoprazole *(Canada only)* *(pan TOE pra zole)*

Canadian Brand Names Pantoloc™

Generic Available No

Therapeutic Category Proton Pump Inhibitor

Use Treatment of acute gastric and duodenal ulcer; severe gastroesophageal reflux disease (GERD)

Usual Dosage Adults: Oral: 40 mg once daily in the morning

Dosage Forms Tablet, enteric coated: 40 mg

pantothenic acid (pan toe THEN ik AS id)
Synonyms calcium pantothenate; vitamin B$_5$
Generic Available Yes
Therapeutic Category Vitamin, Water Soluble
Use Pantothenic acid deficiency
Usual Dosage Adults: Oral: Recommended daily dose: 4-7 mg/day
Dosage Forms Tablet: 25 mg, 50 mg, 100 mg, 218 mg, 250 mg, 500 mg, 545 mg, 1000 mg

♦ **pantothenyl alcohol** *see* dexpanthenol *on page 192*
♦ **Panwarfarin®** *(Discontinued) see page 743*

papaverine (pa PAV er een)
U.S. Brand Names Genabid®; Pavabid®; Pavatine®
Generic Available Yes
Therapeutic Category Vasodilator
Use Relief of peripheral and cerebral ischemia associated with arterial spasm

Investigational use: Prophylaxis of migraine headache
Usual Dosage Adults:
Oral: 100-300 mg 3-5 times/day
Oral, sustained release: 150-300 mg every 12 hours
Dietary Considerations May be administered with food
Nursing/Pharmacy Information
Rapid I.V. administration may result in arrhythmias and fatal apnea; administer slow I.V. over 1-2 minutes
Stability: Protect from heat or freezing; not do refrigerate injection; solutions should be clear to pale yellow; precipitates with lactated Ringer's
Dosage Forms Papaverine hydrochloride:
Capsule, sustained release: 150 mg
Tablet: 30 mg, 60 mg, 100 mg, 150 mg, 200 mg, 300 mg
Tablet, timed release: 200 mg

♦ **Paplex®** *(Discontinued) see page 743*
♦ **parabromdylamine** *see* brompheniramine *on page 94*
♦ **paracetaldehyde** *see* paraldehyde *on page 469*
♦ **paracetamol** *see* acetaminophen *on page 13*

parachlorometaxylenol (PAIR a klor oh met a ZYE le nol)
Synonyms PCMX
U.S. Brand Names Metasep® [OTC]
Generic Available No
Therapeutic Category Antiseborrheic Agent, Topical
Use Aid in relief of dandruff and associated conditions
Usual Dosage Massage to a foamy lather, allow to remain on hair for 5 minutes, rinse thoroughly and repeat
Dosage Forms Shampoo: 2% with isopropyl alcohol 9%

♦ **Paradione®** *(Discontinued) see page 743*
♦ **Paraflex®** *see* chlorzoxazone *on page 146*
♦ **Parafon Forte™ DSC** *see* chlorzoxazone *on page 146*
♦ **Para-Hist AT®** *(Discontinued) see page 743*
♦ **Paral®** *see* paraldehyde *on page 469*

paraldehyde (par AL de hyde)
Synonyms paracetaldehyde
U.S. Brand Names Paral®
Generic Available Yes
Therapeutic Category Anticonvulsant
Controlled Substance C-IV
Use Treatment of status epilepticus and tetanus-induced seizures; has been used as a sedative/hypnotic and in the treatment of alcohol withdrawal symptoms
Usual Dosage Dilute in milk or iced fruit juice to mask taste and odor
Oral, rectal:
Children: 0.15-0.3 mL/kg
Adults:
Hypnotic: 10-30 mL
Sedative: 5-10 mL
Rectal: Mix paraldehyde 2:1 with oil (cottonseed or olive)
(Continued)

paraldehyde *(Continued)*

Nursing/Pharmacy Information

Discard unused contents of any container which has been opened for more than 24 hours; do **not** use discolored solution or solutions with strong smell of acetic acid (vinegar); dilute in milk or iced fruit juice; Do **not** use any plastic equipment for administration, use glass syringes and rubber tubing; outdated preparations can be toxic

Rectal: Mix paraldehyde 2:1 with oil (cottonseed or olive)

Stability: Decomposes with exposure to air and light to acetaldehyde which then oxidizes to acetic acid; store in tightly closed containers; protect from light

Dosage Forms Liquid, oral or rectal: 1 g/mL (30 mL)

paramethasone acetate *(par a METH a sone AS e tate)*

U.S. Brand Names Haldrone®; Stemex®

Generic Available No

Therapeutic Category Adrenal Corticosteroid

Use Treatment of variety of diseases including those of hematologic, allergic, inflammatory, neoplastic, and autoimmune in origin

Usual Dosage Oral: 2-24 mg/day

Nursing/Pharmacy Information Likely to inhibit maturation and growth in adolescents; at high doses (>15 mg/d) increased urinary excretion of nitrogen and calcium will occur

Dosage Forms Tablet: 1 mg

♦ **Paraplatin®** *see* carboplatin *on page 114*

♦ **Parathar™** *see* teriparatide *on page 597*

♦ **Paraxin** *see* chloramphenicol *on page 133*

♦ **Par Decon®** *see* chlorpheniramine, phenyltoloxamine, phenylpropanolamine, and phenylephrine *on page 143*

♦ **Paredrine®** *see* hydroxyamphetamine *on page 326*

paregoric *(par e GOR ik)*

Synonyms camphorated tincture of opium

Generic Available Yes

Therapeutic Category Analgesic, Narcotic

Controlled Substance C-III

Use Treatment of diarrhea or relief of pain; neonatal abstinence syndrome (neonatal opiate withdrawal)

Usual Dosage Oral:

Neonatal opiate withdrawal: 3-6 drops every 3-6 hours as needed, or initially 0.2 mL every 3 hours; increase dosage by approximately 0.05 mL every 3 hours until withdrawal symptoms are controlled; it is rare to exceed 0.7 mL/ dose. Stabilize withdrawal symptoms for 3-5 days, then gradually decrease dosage over a 2- to 4-week period.

Children: 0.25-0.5 mL/kg 1-4 times/day

Adults: 5-10 mL 1-4 times/day

Dietary Considerations May be administered with food

Nursing/Pharmacy Information

Monitor respiratory rate, blood pressure, heart rate, level of sedation

Stability: Store in light-resistant, tightly closed container

Dosage Forms Liquid: 2 mg morphine equivalent/5 mL [equivalent to 20 mg opium powder] (5 mL, 60 mL, 473 mL, 4000 mL)

♦ **Paremyd® Ophthalmic** *see* hydroxyamphetamine and tropicamide *on page 326*

♦ **Parepectolin®** *see* kaolin and pectin with opium *on page 353*

♦ **Pargen Fortified®** *(Discontinued) see page 743*

♦ **Par Glycerol®** *(Discontinued) see page 743*

♦ **pargyline and methyclothiazide** *see* methyclothiazide and pargyline *on page 405*

paricalcitol *(par eh CAL ci tol)*

U.S. Brand Names Zemplar™

Generic Available No

Therapeutic Category Vitamin D Analog

Use Prevention and treatment of secondary hyperparathyroidism associated with chronic renal failure

Usual Dosage Adults: I.V.: 0.04-0.1 mcg/kg (2.8-7 mcg) given as a bolus dose no more frequently than every other day at any time during dialysis; doses as high as 0.24 mcg/kg (16.8 mcg) have been administered safely

Dosage Forms Injection: 5 mcg/mL (1 mL, 2 mL, 5 mL)

♦ **pariprazole** *see* rabeprazole *New Drug on page 538*

♦ **Parlodel**® *see* bromocriptine *on page 93*

♦ **Parmine**® *(Discontinued) see page 743*

♦ **Parnate**® *see* tranylcypromine *on page 621*

paromomycin (par oh moe MYE sin)

U.S. Brand Names Humatin®

Generic Available No

Therapeutic Category Amebicide

Use Treatment of acute and chronic intestinal amebiasis due to susceptible *Entamoeba histolytica* (not effective in the treatment of extraintestinal amebiasis); tapeworm infestations; adjunctive management of hepatic coma; treatment of cryptosporidial diarrhea

Usual Dosage Oral:

Intestinal amebiasis: Children and Adults: 25-35 mg/kg/day in 3 divided doses for 5-10 days

Tapeworm (fish, dog, bovine, porcine):

Children: 11 mg/kg every 15 minutes for 4 doses

Adults: 1 g every 15 minutes for 4 doses

Hepatic coma: Adults: 4 g/day in 2-4 divided doses for 5-6 days

Dwarf tapeworm: Children and Adults: 45 mg/kg/dose every day for 5-7 days

Dietary Considerations Paromomycin may cause malabsorption of xylose, sucrose, and fats

Nursing/Pharmacy Information Monitor hearing loss before and during therapy

Dosage Forms Capsule, as sulfate: 250 mg

paroxetine (pa ROKS e teen)

U.S. Brand Names Paxil™

Generic Available No

Therapeutic Category Antidepressant, Selective Serotonin Reuptake Inhibitor

Use Treatment of depression, obsessive compulsive disorder (OCD) and panic disorder (PD)

Usual Dosage Adults: Oral: 20 mg once daily, preferably in the morning

Nursing/Pharmacy Information Monitor hepatic and renal function tests, blood pressure, heart rate

Dosage Forms

Suspension, oral: 10 mg/5 mL

Tablet: 10 mg, 20 mg, 30 mg, 40 mg

♦ **Parsidol**® *(Discontinued) see page 743*

♦ **Partuss**® LA *see* guaifenesin and phenylpropanolamine *on page 301*

♦ **Parvolex**® *see* acetylcysteine *on page 19*

♦ **PAS** *see* aminosalicylate sodium *on page 39*

♦ **Patanol**® *see* olopatadine *on page 454*

♦ **Pathilon**® *see* tridihexethyl *on page 626*

♦ **Pathocil**® *see* dicloxacillin *on page 199*

♦ **Pavabid**® *see* papaverine *on page 469*

♦ **Pavabid HP**® *(Discontinued) see page 743*

♦ **Pavasule**® *(Discontinued) see page 743*

♦ **Pavatine**® *see* papaverine *on page 469*

♦ **Pavatym**® *(Discontinued) see page 743*

♦ **Paveral Stanley Syrup With Codeine Phosphate** *see* codeine *on page 164*

♦ **Pavesed**® *(Discontinued) see page 743*

♦ **Pavulon**® *see* pancuronium *on page 468*

♦ **Paxene**® *see* paclitaxel *on page 465*

♦ **Paxil**™ *see* paroxetine *on page 471*

♦ **Paxipam**® *see* halazepam *on page 307*

♦ **PBZ**® *see* tripelennamine *on page 631*

♦ **PBZ**® Elixir *(Discontinued) see page 743*

♦ **PBZ-SR**® *see* tripelennamine *on page 631*

♦ **PCE**® *see* erythromycin (systemic) *on page 240*

- **PCMX** *see* parachlorometaxylenol *on page 469*
- **Pebegal** *see* benzonatate *on page 80*
- **pectin and kaolin** *see* kaolin and pectin *on page 352*
- **pectin with opium and kaolin** *see* kaolin and pectin with opium *on page 353*
- **Pedameth**® *see* methionine *on page 401*
- **PediaCare**® **Oral** *see* pseudoephedrine *on page 530*
- **Pediacof**® *see* chlorpheniramine, phenylephrine, and codeine *on page 141*
- **Pediaflor**® *see* fluoride *on page 274*
- **Pedialyte**® **[OTC]** *see* enteral nutritional products *on page 233*
- **PediaPatch Transdermal Patch [OTC]** *see* salicylic acid *on page 557*
- **Pediapred**® **Oral** *see* prednisolone (systemic) *on page 514*
- **Pedia-Profen**™ *see* ibuprofen *on page 332*
- **Pediasure**™ *see* enteral nutritional products *on page 233*
- **Pediatric Triban**® *see* trimethobenzamide *on page 629*
- **Pediatrix**® *see* acetaminophen *on page 13*
- **Pediazole**® *see* erythromycin and sulfisoxazole *on page 239*
- **Pedi-Boro**® **[OTC]** *see* aluminum acetate and calcium acetate *on page 32*
- **Pedi-Cort V**® **Creme** *see* clioquinol and hydrocortisone *on page 157*
- **Pedi-Dent**™ *see* fluoride *on page 274*
- **Pediotic**® **Otic** *see* neomycin, polymyxin B, and hydrocortisone *on page 437*
- **Pedi-Pro Topical [OTC]** *see* undecylenic acid and derivatives *on page 637*
- **Pedituss**® *see* chlorpheniramine, phenylephrine, and codeine *on page 141*
- **PedTE-PAK-4**® *see* trace metals *on page 620*
- **Pedtrace-4**® *see* trace metals *on page 620*
- **PedvaxHIB**™ *see* Haemophilus B conjugate vaccine *on page 306*

pegademase (bovine) (peg A de mase BOE vine)

U.S. Brand Names Adagen™
Generic Available No
Therapeutic Category Enzyme
Use Enzyme replacement therapy for adenosine deaminase (ADA) deficiency in patients with severe combined immunodeficiency disease (SCID) who can not benefit from bone marrow transplant
Usual Dosage Children: I.M.: Dose administered every 7 days, 10 units/kg the first dose, 15 units/kg the second dose, and 20 units/kg the third; maintenance dose: 20 units/kg/week is recommended depending on patient's ADA level
Nursing/Pharmacy Information
   Not a cure for SCID; unlike bone marrow transplants, injections must be used the rest of the child's life; frequent blood tests are necessary to monitor effect and adjust the dose as needed
   Stability: Refrigerate at 2°C to 8°C (36°F to 46°F); do not freeze
Dosage Forms Injection: 250 units/mL (1.5 mL)

- **Peganone**® *see* ethotoin *on page 253*

pegaspargase (peg AS par jase)

Synonyms PEG-L-asparaginase
U.S. Brand Names Oncaspar®
Generic Available No
Therapeutic Category Antineoplastic Agent
Use Induction treatment of acute lymphoblastic leukemia in combination with other chemotherapeutic agents in patients who have developed hypersensitivity to native forms of asparaginase derived from *E. coli* and/or *Erwinia chrysanthem*, treatment of lymphoma
Usual Dosage Refer to individual protocols; I.M. administration may decrease the risk of anaphylaxis; dose must be individualized based upon clinical response and tolerance of the patient
   I.M., I.V.: 2000 units/m^2 every 14 days
Nursing/Pharmacy Information
   Parenteral: I.M. route is the preferred route of administration because of the lower incidence of hepatotoxicity, coagulopathy, and GI and renal disorders compared to the I.V. route; in the I.M. administration, limit the volume at a single injection site to 2 mL, if the volume to be administered is >2mL, use multiple injection sites; may be administered as an I.V. infusion in 100 mL of D$_5$W or NS over a period of 1-2 hours, through an infusion that is already running
   Stability: Avoid excessive agitation, do not shake; do not freeze; do not administer if there is any indication that the drug has been frozen

Dosage Forms Injection, preservative free: 750 units/mL

♦ **PEG-ES** see polyethylene glycol-electrolyte solution on page 502

♦ **PEG-L-asparaginase** see pegaspargase on page 472

♦ **Peglyte™** see polyethylene glycol-electrolyte solution on page 502

pemoline (PEM oh leen)
Synonyms phenylisohydantoin; PIO
U.S. Brand Names Cylert®
Generic Available No
Therapeutic Category Central Nervous System Stimulant, Nonamphetamine
Controlled Substance C-IV
Use Treatment of attention-deficit/hyperactivity disorder (ADHD); narcolepsy
Usual Dosage Oral:
Children <6 years: Not recommended
Children ≥6 years and Adults: Initial: 37.5 mg administered once daily in the morning, increase by 18.75 mg/day at weekly intervals; effective dose range: 56.25-75 mg/day; maximum: 112.5 mg/day; dosage range: 0.5-3 mg/kg/24 hours
Nursing/Pharmacy Information
Administer medication in the morning
Monitor liver enzymes
Dosage Forms
Tablet: 18.75 mg, 37.5 mg, 75 mg
Tablet, chewable: 37.5 mg

penbutolol (pen BYOO toe lole)
U.S. Brand Names Levatol®
Generic Available No
Therapeutic Category Beta-Adrenergic Blocker
Use Treatment of mild to moderate arterial hypertension
Usual Dosage Adults: Oral: Initial: 20 mg once daily, full effect of a 20 or 40 mg dose is seen by the end of a 2-week period, doses of 40-80 mg have been tolerated but have shown little additional antihypertensive effects
Nursing/Pharmacy Information
Advise against abrupt withdrawal
Monitor orthostatic blood pressures, apical and peripheral pulse and mental status changes (ie, confusion, depression)
Dosage Forms Tablet, as sulfate: 20 mg

penciclovir (pen SYE kloe veer)
U.S. Brand Names Denavir™
Generic Available No
Therapeutic Category Antiviral Agent
Use Antiviral cream for the treatment of recurrent herpes labialis (cold sores) in adults
Usual Dosage Apply cream at the first sign or symptom of cold sore (eg, tingling, swelling); apply every 2 hours during waking hours for 4 days
Dosage Forms Cream: 1% [10 mg/g] (2 g)

♦ **Penecort® Topical** see hydrocortisone (topical) on page 324

♦ **Penetrex™** see enoxacin on page 232

♦ **Penicil** see penicillin G procaine on page 476

penicillamine (pen i SIL a meen)
Synonyms d-3-mercaptovaline; β,β-dimethylcysteine; d-penicillamine
U.S. Brand Names Cuprimine®; Depen®
Mexican Brand Names Adalken®
Generic Available No
Therapeutic Category Chelating Agent
Use Treatment of Wilson's disease, cystinuria, adjunct in the treatment of severe rheumatoid arthritis; lead poisoning, primary biliary cirrhosis
Usual Dosage Oral:
Rheumatoid arthritis:
Children: Initial: 3 mg/kg/day (≤250 mg/day) for 3 months, then 6 mg/kg/day (≤500 mg/day) in divided doses twice daily for 3 months to a maximum of 10 mg/kg/day in 3-4 divided doses
Adults: 125-250 mg/day, may increase dose at 1- to 3-month intervals up to 1-1.5 g/day
(Continued)

penicillamine *(Continued)*

Wilson's disease (doses titrated to maintain urinary copper excretion >1 mg/day):
Infants <6 months: 250 mg/dose once daily
Children <12 years: 250 mg/dose 2-3 times/day
Adults: 250 mg 4 times/day
Cystinuria:
Children: 30 mg/kg/day in 4 divided doses
Adults: 1-4 g/day in divided doses every 6 hours
Lead poisoning (continue until blood lead level is <60 mcg/dL):
Children: 25-40 mg/kg/day in 3 divided doses
Adults: 250 mg/dose every 8-12 hours
Primary biliary cirrhosis: 250 mg/day to start, increase by 250 mg every 2 weeks up to a maintenance dose of 1 g/day, usually administered 250 mg 4 times/day
Arsenic poisoning: Children: 100 mg/kg/day in divided doses every 6 hours for 5 days; maximum: 1 g/day

Dietary Considerations Should be administered at least 1 hour before a meal on an empty stomach; do not administer with milk; iron and zinc may decrease drug action; increase dietary intake of pyridoxine; for Wilson's disease, decrease copper in diet and omit chocolate, nuts, shellfish, mushrooms, liver, raisins, broccoli, and molasses; for lead poisoning, decrease calcium in diet Patients unable to swallow capsules may mix contents of capsule with fruit juice or chilled pureed fruit; limit alcohol

Nursing/Pharmacy Information
Monitor urinalysis, CBC with differential, hemoglobin, platelet count, liver function tests
Stability: Store in tight, well-closed containers

Dosage Forms
Capsule: 125 mg, 250 mg
Tablet: 250 mg

penicillin G benzathine *(pen i SIL in jee BENZ a theen)*

Synonyms benzathine benzylpenicillin; benzathine penicillin g; benzylpenicillin benzathine
U.S. Brand Names Bicillin® L-A; Permapen®
Canadian Brand Names Megacillin® Susp
Mexican Brand Names Benzetacil; Benzilfan
Generic Available No
Therapeutic Category Penicillin
Use Active against most gram-positive organisms and some spirochetes; used only for the treatment of mild to moderately severe infections (ie, *Streptococcus* pharyngitis) caused by organisms susceptible to low concentrations of penicillin G, or for prophylaxis of infections caused by these organisms such as rheumatic fever prophylaxis
Usual Dosage I.M.: Administer undiluted injection, very slowly released from site of injection, providing uniform levels over 2-4 weeks; higher doses result in more sustained rather than higher levels. Use a penicillin G benzathine-penicillin G procaine combination to achieve early peak levels in acute infections

Infants and Children:
Group A streptococcal upper respiratory infection: 25,000 units/kg as a single dose; maximum: 1.2 million units
Prophylaxis of recurrent rheumatic fever: 25,000 units/kg every 3-4 weeks; maximum: 1.2 million units/dose
Early syphilis: 50,000 units/kg as a single injection; maximum: 2.4 million units
Syphilis of more than 1-year duration: 50,000 units/kg every week for 3 doses; maximum: 2.4 million units/dose
Adults:
Group A streptococcal upper respiratory infection: 1.2 million units as a single dose
Prophylaxis of recurrent rheumatic fever: 1.2 million units every 3-4 weeks or 600,000 units twice monthly; a single dose of 600,000 to 1,2000,000 units is effective in the prevention of rheumatic fever secondary to streptococcal pharyngitis
Early syphilis: 2.4 million units as a single dose
Syphilis of more than 1-year duration: 2.4 million units once weekly for 3 doses

Nursing/Pharmacy Information

Administer undiluted injection; administer by deep I.M. injection in the upper outer quadrant of the buttock; do **not** administer I.V., intra-arterially or S.C.; inadvertent I.V. administration has resulted in thrombosis, severe neurovascular damage, cardiac arrest, and death; in infants and children, I.M. injections should be made into the midlateral muscle of the thigh

Monitor CBC, urinalysis, renal function tests

Stability: Store in refrigerator

Dosage Forms Injection: 300,000 units/mL (10 mL); 600,000 units/mL (1 mL, 2 mL, 4 mL)

penicillin G benzathine and procaine combined

(pen i SIL in jee BENZ a theen & PROE kane KOM bined)

Synonyms penicillin G procaine and benzathine combined

U.S. Brand Names Bicillin® C-R; Bicillin® C-R 900/300

Generic Available No

Therapeutic Category Penicillin

Use Active against most gram-positive organisms, mostly streptococcal and pneumococcal

Usual Dosage I.M.:

Children:

<30 lb: 600,000 units in a single dose

30-60 lb: 900,000 units to 1.2 million units in a single dose

Children >60 lb and Adults: 2.4 million units in a single dose

Nursing/Pharmacy Information

Administer by deep I.M. injection in the upper outer quadrant of the buttock; do **not** administer I.V., intravascularly, or intra-arterially

Stability: Store in the refrigerator

Dosage Forms

Injection:

300,000 units [150,000 units each of penicillin G benzathine and penicillin G procaine] (10 mL)

600,000 units [300,000 units each penicillin G benzathine and penicillin G procaine] (1 mL)

1,200,000 units [600,000 units each penicillin G benzathine and penicillin G procaine] (2 mL)

2,400,000 units [1,200,000 units each penicillin G benzathine and penicillin G procaine] (4 mL)

Injection: Penicillin G benzathine 900,000 units and penicillin G procaine 300,000 units per dose (2 mL)

penicillin G, parenteral, aqueous

(pen i SIL in jee, pa REN ter al, AYE kwee us)

Synonyms benzylpenicillin; crystalline penicillin

U.S. Brand Names Pfizerpen®

Mexican Brand Names Benzanil; Lentopenil

Generic Available Yes

Therapeutic Category Penicillin

Use Active against most gram-positive organisms except *Staphylococcus aureus*; some gram-negative such as *Neisseria gonorrhoeae* and some anaerobes and spirochetes; although ceftriaxone is now the drug of choice for Lyme disease and gonorrhea

Usual Dosage I.M., I.V.:

Infants and Children (sodium salt is preferred in children): 100,000-250,000 units/kg/day in divided doses every 4 hours; maximum: 4.8 million units/24 hours

Severe infections: Up to 400,000 units/kg/day in divided doses every 4 hours; maximum dose: 24 million units/day

Adults: 2-24 million units/day in divided doses every 4 hours

Nursing/Pharmacy Information

Dosage modification required in patients with renal insufficiency; administer around-the-clock rather than 4 times/day to avoid variations in peak and trough concentrations

Stability: Reconstituted parenteral solution is stable for 7 days when refrigerated; for I.V. infusion in normal saline or D_5W, solution is stable for 24 hours at room temperature; thawed solutions stable for 24 hours at room temperature or 14 days at refrigeration

Dosage Forms Injection:

Penicillin G potassium:

Frozen premixed: 1 million units, 2 million units, 3 million units

Powder: 1 million units, 5 million units, 10 million units, 20 million units

(Continued)

penicillin G, parenteral, aqueous (Continued)

Penicillin G sodium: 5 million units

penicillin G procaine (pen i SIL in jee PROE kane)

Synonyms APPG; aqueous procaine penicillin G; procaine benzylpenicillin; procaine penicillin G

U.S. Brand Names Crysticillin® A.S.; Wycillin®

Canadian Brand Names Ayercillin®

Mexican Brand Names Penicil; Penipot; Penprocilina

Generic Available Yes

Therapeutic Category Penicillin

Use Moderately severe infections due to *Neisseria gonorrhoeae*, *Treponema pallidum*, and other penicillin G-sensitive microorganisms that are susceptible to low but prolonged serum penicillin concentrations

Usual Dosage I.M.:

Newborns: 50,000 units/kg/day administered every day (avoid using in this age group since sterile abscesses and procaine toxicity occur more frequently with neonates than older patients)

Children: 25,000-50,000 units/kg/day in divided doses 1-2 times/day; not to exceed 4.8 million units/24 hours

Gonorrhea: 100,000 units/kg one time (in 2 injection sites) along with probenecid 25 mg/kg (maximum: 1 g) orally 30 minutes prior to procaine penicillin

Adults: 0.6-4.8 million units/day in divided doses 1-2 times/day

Uncomplicated gonorrhea: 1 g probenecid orally, then 4.8 million units procaine penicillin divided into 2 injection sites 30 minutes later. When used in conjunction with an aminoglycoside for the treatment of endocarditis caused by susceptible *S. viridans*: 1.2 million units every 6 hours for 2-4 weeks

Nursing/Pharmacy Information

Procaine suspension for deep I.M. injection only; administer around-the-clock rather than 4 times/day, 3 times/day, etc, (ie, 12-6-12-6, not 9-1-5-9) to promote less variation in peak and trough serum levels; when doses are repeated, rotate the injection site; administer into the gluteus maximus or into the midlateral muscles of the thigh; in infants and children it is preferable to administer I.M. into the midlateral muscles of the thigh; avoid I.V., intravascular, or intra-arterial administration of penicillin G procaine since severe and/or permanent neurovascular damage may occur; renal and hematologic systems should be evaluated periodically during prolonged therapy

Monitor periodic renal and hematologic function tests with prolonged therapy

Stability: Store in refrigerator

Dosage Forms Injection, suspension: 300,000 units/mL (10 mL); 500,000 units/mL (1.2 mL); 600,000 units/mL (1 mL, 2 mL, 4 mL)

♦ **penicillin G procaine and benzathine combined** *see* penicillin G benzathine and procaine combined *on page 475*

penicillin V potassium (pen i SIL in vee poe TASS ee um)

Synonyms pen VK; phenoxymethyl penicillin

U.S. Brand Names Beepen-VK®; Pen.Vee® K; Veetids®

Canadian Brand Names Apo®-Pen VK; Nadopen-V®; Novo-Pen-VK®; Nu-Pen-VK®; Pen-Vee®; PVF® K

Mexican Brand Names Anapenil; Pen-Vi-K

Generic Available Yes

Therapeutic Category Penicillin

Use Treatment of mild to moderately severe susceptible bacterial infections involving the upper respiratory tract, skin, and urinary tract; prophylaxis of pneumococcal infections and rheumatic fever

Usual Dosage Oral:

Systemic infections:

Children <12 years: 25-50 mg/kg/day in divided doses every 6-8 hours; maximum dose: 3 g/day

Children >12 years and Adults: 125-500 mg every 6-8 hours

Prophylaxis of pneumococcal infections:

Children <5 years: 125 mg twice daily

Children ≥5 years: 250 mg twice daily

Prophylaxis of recurrent rheumatic fever:

Children <5 years: 125 mg

Children ≥5 years and Adults: 250 mg twice daily

Dietary Considerations May be administered with water on an empty stomach 1 hour before or 2 hours after meals or may be administered with food, however, peak concentration may be delayed

Nursing/Pharmacy Information

Administer around-the-clock rather than 4 times/day, 3 times/day, etc, (ie, 12-6-12-6, not 9-1-5-9) to promote less variation in peak and trough serum levels; dosage modification required in patients with renal insufficiency

Monitor periodic renal and hematologic function tests during prolonged therapy

Stability: Refrigerate suspension after reconstitution; discard after 14 days

Dosage Forms

Powder for oral solution: 125 mg/5 mL (3 mL, 100 mL, 150 mL, 200 mL); 250 mg/5 mL (100 mL, 150 mL, 200 mL)

Tablet: 125 mg, 250 mg, 500 mg

♦ **penicilloyl-polylysine** *see* benzylpenicilloyl-polylysine *on page 82*

♦ **Penipot** *see* penicillin G procaine *on page 476*

♦ **Penprocilina** *see* penicillin G procaine *on page 476*

♦ **Penta/3B® Plus** *see* vitamin, multiple (oral) *on page 654*

♦ **Pentacarinat®** *see* pentamidine *on page 477*

♦ **Pentacarinat® Injection** *see* pentamidine *on page 477*

pentaerythritol tetranitrate (pen ta er ITH ri tole te tra NYE trate)

Synonyms PETN

U.S. Brand Names Duotrate®; Peritrate®; Peritrate® SA

Generic Available Yes

Therapeutic Category Vasodilator

Use Prophylactic long-term management of angina pectoris

Usual Dosage Oral: 10-20 mg 4 times/day (160 mg/day) up to 40 mg 4 times/day before or after meals and at bedtime; administer sustained-release preparation every 12 hours; maximum daily dose: 240 mg

Dietary Considerations Should be administered with glass of water on an empty stomach

Nursing/Pharmacy Information

Do not crush sustained release drug product

Monitor blood pressure reduction for maximal effect and orthostatic hypotension

Dosage Forms

Capsule: sustained release: 15 mg, 30 mg

Tablet: 10 mg, 20 mg, 40 mg

Sustained release: 80 mg

pentagastrin (pen ta GAS trin)

U.S. Brand Names Peptavlon®

Generic Available No

Therapeutic Category Diagnostic Agent

Use Evaluate gastric acid secretory function in pernicious anemia, gastric carcinoma; in suspected duodenal ulcer or Zollinger-Ellison tumor

Usual Dosage Adults: S.C.: 6 mcg/kg

Dietary Considerations Patient should fast from food and liquids overnight and be instructed not to take antacids on the morning of the test nor drugs that inhibit gastric secretion

Nursing/Pharmacy Information Refrigerate

Dosage Forms Injection: 0.25 mg/mL (2 mL)

♦ **Pentam-300® Injection** *see* pentamidine *on page 477*

pentamidine (pen TAM i deen)

U.S. Brand Names NebuPent™ Inhalation; Pentacarinat® Injection; Pentam-300® Injection

Mexican Brand Names Pentacarinat®

Generic Available No

Therapeutic Category Antiprotozoal

Use Treatment and prevention of pneumonia caused by *Pneumocystis carinii* in patients who cannot tolerate co-trimoxazole or who fail to respond to this drug; treatment of African trypanosomiasis; treatment of visceral leishmaniasis caused by *L. donovani*

Usual Dosage

Children:

Treatment: I.M., I.V. (I.V. preferred): 4 mg/kg/day once daily for 14-21 days

Prevention:

I.M., I.V.: 4 mg/kg monthly or biweekly

(Continued)

pentamidine *(Continued)*

Inhalation (aerosolized pentamidine in children ≥5 years): 300 mg/dose administered every 3 weeks or monthly via Respirgard® II inhaler (8 mg/kg dose has also been used in children <5 years)

Treatment of trypanosomiasis: I.V.: 4 mg/kg/day once daily for 10 days

Adults:

Treatment: I.M., I.V. (I.V. preferred): 4 mg/kg/day once daily for 14 days

Prevention: Inhalation: 300 mg every 4 weeks via Respirgard® II nebulizer

Dietary Considerations Avoid alcohol

Nursing/Pharmacy Information

Patients should receive parenteral pentamidine while lying down and blood pressure should be monitored closely during administration and after completion of the infusion until blood pressure is stabilized; may administer deep I.M. or by slow I.V. infusion; rapid I.V. administration can cause severe hypotension; infuse I.V. slowly over a period of at least 60 minutes at a final concentration for administration not to exceed 6 mg/mL

Monitor liver function tests, renal function tests, blood glucose, serum potassium and calcium, EKG, blood pressure

Stability: Reconstituted solution is stable for 24 hours at room temperature; do not refrigerate due to the possibility of crystallization; do not use normal saline as a diluent; normal saline is **incompatible** with pentamidine

Dosage Forms Pentamidine isethionate:

Inhalation: 300 mg

Powder for injection, lyophilized: 300 mg

♦ **Pentamycetin®** *see* chloramphenicol *on page 133*

♦ **Pentasa® Oral** *see* mesalamine *on page 395*

♦ **Pentaspan®** *see* pentastarch *on page 478*

pentastarch *(PEN ta starch)*

U.S. Brand Names Pentaspan®

Generic Available No

Therapeutic Category Blood Modifiers

Use Adjunct in leukapheresis to improve the harvesting and increase the yield of leukocytes by centrifugal means

Usual Dosage 250-700 mL to which citrate anticoagulant has been added is administered by adding to the input line of the centrifugation apparatus at a ratio of 1:8-1:13 to venous whole blood

Dosage Forms Injection, in NS: 10%

pentazocine *(pen TAZ oh seen)*

U.S. Brand Names Talwin®; Talwin® NX

Generic Available No

Therapeutic Category Analgesic, Narcotic

Controlled Substance C-IV

Use Relief of moderate to severe pain; a sedative prior to surgery; supplement to surgical anesthesia

Usual Dosage

Children: I.M., S.C.:

5-8 years: 15 mg

8-14 years: 30 mg

Children >12 years and Adults: Oral: 50 mg every 3-4 hours; may increase to 100 mg/dose if needed, but should not exceed 600 mg/day

Adults:

I.M., S.C.: 30-60 mg every 3-4 hours, not to exceed total daily dose of 360 mg

I.V.: 30 mg every 3-4 hours

Nursing/Pharmacy Information

Rotate injection site for I.M., S.C. use; avoid intra-arterial injection; implement safety measures, assist with ambulation

Monitor for relief of pain, respiratory and mental status, blood pressure; observe patient for excessive sedation; observe for narcotic withdrawal

Stability: Store at room temperature, protect from heat and from freezing; I.V. form is **incompatible** with aminophylline, amobarbital (and all other I.V. barbiturates), glycopyrrolate (same syringe), heparin (same syringe), nafcillin (Y-site)

Dosage Forms

Injection, as lactate: 30 mg/mL (1 mL, 1.5 mL, 2 mL, 10 mL)

Tablet: Pentazocine hydrochloride 50 mg and naloxone hydrochloride 0.5 mg

pentazocine compound (pen TAZ oh seen KOM pownd)
U.S. Brand Names Talacen®; Talwin® Compound
Generic Available No
Therapeutic Category Analgesic, Narcotic
Use Relief of moderate to severe pain; has also been used as a sedative prior to surgery and as a supplement to surgical anesthesia
Usual Dosage Adults: Oral: 2 tablets 3-4 times/day
Nursing/Pharmacy Information Observe patient for excessive sedation, respiratory depression, implement safety measures, assist with ambulation; observe for narcotic withdrawal
Dosage Forms Tablet:
Talacen®: Pentazocine hydrochloride 25 mg and acetaminophen 650 mg
Talwin® Compound: Pentazocine hydrochloride 12.5 mg and aspirin 325 mg

♦ **Penthrane®** *see* methoxyflurane *on page 404*
♦ **Pentids® (all Forms) (Discontinued)** *see page 743*

pentobarbital (pen toe BAR bi tal)
U.S. Brand Names Nembutal®
Canadian Brand Names Nova Rectal®
Generic Available Yes
Therapeutic Category Barbiturate
Controlled Substance C-II
Use Short-term treatment of insomnia; preoperative sedation; high-dose barbiturate coma for treatment of increased intracranial pressure or status epilepticus unresponsive to other therapy
Usual Dosage
Children:
Sedative: Oral: 2-6 mg/kg/day divided in 3 doses; maximum: 100 mg/day
Hypnotic: I.M.: 2-6 mg/kg; maximum: 100 mg/dose
Rectal:
2 months to 1 year (10-20 lb): 30 mg
1-4 years (20-40 lb): 30-60 mg
5-12 years (40-80 lb): 60 mg
12-14 years (80-110 lb): 60-120 mg **or**
<4 years: 3-6 mg/kg/dose
>4 years: 1.5-3 mg/kg/dose
Preoperative/preprocedure sedation: ≥6 months:
Oral, I.M., rectal: 2-6 mg/kg; maximum: 100 mg/dose
I.V.: 1-3 mg/kg to a maximum of 100 mg until asleep
Children 5-12 years: Conscious sedation prior to a procedure: I.V.: 2 mg/kg 5-10 minutes before procedures, may repeat one time
Adolescents: Conscious sedation: Oral, I.V.: 100 mg prior to a procedure

Children and Adults: Barbiturate coma in head injury patients: I.V.:
Loading dose: 5-10 mg/kg administered slowly over 1-2 hours; monitor blood pressure and respiratory rate
Maintenance infusion: Initial: 1 mg/kg/hour; may increase to 2-3 mg/kg/hour; maintain burst suppression on EEG
Adults:
Hypnotic:
Oral: 100-200 mg at bedtime or 20 mg 3-4 times/day for daytime sedation
I.M.: 150-200 mg
I.V.: Initial: 100 mg, may repeat every 1-3 minutes up to 200-500 mg total dose
Rectal: 120-200 mg at bedtime
Preoperative sedation: I.M.: 150-200 mg
Dietary Considerations Food may decrease the rate but not the extent of oral absorption; high doses of pyridoxine may decrease drug effect; barbiturates may increase the metabolism of vitamins D and K; dietary requirements of vitamins D, K, C, B_{12}, folate, and calcium may be increased with long-term use
Nursing/Pharmacy Information
Suppositories should not be divided; parenteral solutions are very alkaline; avoid extravasation; avoid intra-arterial injection; do not inject >50 mg/minute; rapid I.V. injection may cause respiratory depression, apnea, laryngospasm, bronchospasm, and hypotension, administer over 10-30 minutes; maximum concentration: 50 mg/mL for slow I.V. push
Monitor respiratory status (for conscious sedation, includes pulse oximetry), cardiovascular status
(Continued)

479

pentobarbital *(Continued)*

Stability: Protect from light; aqueous solutions are not stable, commercially available vehicle (containing propylene glycol) is more stable; low pH may cause precipitate; use only clear solution

Dosage Forms Pentobarbital sodium:
Capsule (C-II): 50 mg, 100 mg
Elixir (C-II): 18.2 mg/5 mL (473 mL, 4000 mL)
Injection (C-II): 50 mg/mL (1 mL, 2 mL, 20 mL, 50 mL)
Suppository, rectal (C-III): 30 mg, 60 mg, 120 mg, 200 mg

pentosan polysulfate sodium

(PEN toe san pol i SUL fate SOW dee um)
Synonyms PPS
U.S. Brand Names Elmiron®
Generic Available No
Therapeutic Category Analgesic, Urinary
Use Bladder pain relief or discomfort associated with interstitial cystitis
Usual Dosage Adults: Oral: 100 mg capsule 3 times/day; administer with water at least 1 hour before meals or 2 hours after meals
Dosage Forms Capsule: 100 mg

pentostatin (PEN toe stat in)

Synonyms DCF; 2′-deoxycoformycin
U.S. Brand Names Nipent™
Generic Available No
Therapeutic Category Antineoplastic Agent
Use Treatment of adult patients with alpha-interferon-refractory hairy cell leukemia; significant antitumor activity in various lymphoid neoplasms has been demonstrated; pentostatin also is known as 2′-deoxycoformycin; it is a purine analogue capable of inhibiting adenosine deaminase
Usual Dosage Refractory hairy cell leukemia: Adults: I.V.: 4 mg/m^2 every other week
Nursing/Pharmacy Information Stability: Vials are stable under refrigeration at 2°C to 8°C; reconstituted vials, or further dilutions, may be stored at room temperature exposed to ambient light; diluted solutions are stable for 24 hours in D$_5$W or 48 hours in normal saline or lactated Ringer's at room temperature; infusion with 5% dextrose injection USP or 0.9% sodium chloride injection USP does not interact with PVC-containing administration sets or containers
Dosage Forms Powder for injection: 10 mg/vial

◆ **Pentothal® Sodium** *see* thiopental *on page 607*

pentoxifylline (pen toks I fi leen)

Synonyms oxpentifylline
U.S. Brand Names Trental®
Mexican Brand Names Kentadin; Peridane; Sufisal
Generic Available Yes
Therapeutic Category Blood Viscosity Reducer Agent
Use Symptomatic management of peripheral vascular disease, mainly intermittent claudication

Investigational use: AIDS patients with increased tumor necrosis factor, cerebrovascular accidents, cerebrovascular diseases, new onset type I diabetes mellitus, diabetic atherosclerosis, diabetic neuropathy, gangrene, cutaneous polyarteritis nodosa, hemodialysis shunt thrombosis, cerebral malaria, septic shock, sepsis in premature neonates, sickle cell syndromes, vasculitis, Kawasaki disease, Raynaud's syndrome, cystic fibrosis, and persistent pulmonary hypertension of the newborn (case report)

Usual Dosage Adults: Oral: 400 mg 3 times/day with meals; may reduce to 400 mg twice daily if GI or CNS side effects occur
Dietary Considerations May be administered with meals or food; food may decrease rate but not extent of absorption
Nursing/Pharmacy Information Do not crush or chew
Dosage Forms Tablet, controlled release: 400 mg

◆ **Pentrax® [OTC]** *see* coal tar *on page 162*
◆ **Pentrexyl** *see* ampicillin *on page 46*
◆ **Pen-Vee®** *see* penicillin V potassium *on page 476*
◆ **Pen.Vee® K** *see* penicillin V potassium *on page 476*
◆ **Pen-Vi-K** *see* penicillin V potassium *on page 476*
◆ **pen VK** *see* penicillin V potassium *on page 476*

- **Pepcid®** *see* famotidine *on page 259*
- **Pepcid® AC Acid Controller [OTC]** *see* famotidine *on page 259*
- **Pepcidine®** *see* famotidine *on page 259*
- **Pepcid RPD®** *see* famotidine *on page 259*
- **Peptavlon®** *see* pentagastrin *on page 477*
- **Pepto-Bismol® [OTC]** *see* bismuth subsalicylate *on page 88*
- **Pepto® Diarrhea Control [OTC]** *see* loperamide *on page 374*
- **Peptol®** *see* cimetidine *on page 150*
- **Perchloracap®** *see* radiological/contrast media (ionic) *on page 539*
- **Percocet®** *see* oxycodone and acetaminophen *on page 462*
- **Percocet®-Demi** *see* oxycodone and acetaminophen *on page 462*
- **Percodan®** *see* oxycodone and aspirin *on page 463*
- **Percodan®-Demi** *see* oxycodone and aspirin *on page 463*
- **Percogesic® [OTC]** *see* acetaminophen and phenyltoloxamine *on page 15*
- **Percolone™** *see* oxycodone *on page 462*
- **Perdiem® Plain [OTC]** *see* psyllium *on page 531*
- **Perfectoderm® Gel [OTC]** *see* benzoyl peroxide *on page 81*

pergolide (PER go lide)
U.S. Brand Names Permax®
Generic Available No
Therapeutic Category Anti-Parkinson's Agent; Dopaminergic Agent (Anti-Parkinson's); Ergot Alkaloid and Derivative
Use Adjunctive treatment to levodopa/carbidopa in the management of Parkinson's Disease
Usual Dosage Adults: Oral: Initial: 0.05 mg/day for 2 days, then increase dosage by 0.1 or 0.15 mg/day every 3 days over next 12 days, increase dose by 0.25 mg/day every 3 days until optimal therapeutic dose is achieved
Nursing/Pharmacy Information
Raise bed rails and institute safety measures, aid patient with ambulation; may cause postural hypotension and drowsiness
Monitor blood pressure (both sitting/supine and standing), symptoms of parkinsonism, dyskinesias, mental status
Dosage Forms Tablet, as mesylate: 0.05 mg, 0.25 mg, 1 mg

- **Pergonal®** *see* menotropins *on page 391*
- **Periactin®** *see* cyproheptadine *on page 177*
- **Peri-Colace® [OTC]** *see* docusate and casanthranol *on page 215*

pericyazine *(Canada only)* (per ee CYE ah zeen)
Canadian Brand Names Neuleptil®
Generic Available No
Therapeutic Category Phenothiazine Derivative
Use As adjunctive medication in some psychotic patients, for the control of residual prevailing hostility, impulsiveness and aggressiveness
Usual Dosage Oral:
Children and adolescents (5 years of age and over): 2.5-10 mg in the morning and 5-30 mg in the evening. These dosages approximate a daily dosage range of 1-3 mg/year of age.
Adults: 5-20 mg in the morning and 10-40 mg in the evening. For maintenance therapy, the dosage should be reduced to the minimum effective dose. Lower doses of 2.5-15 mg in the morning, and 5-30 mg in the evening have been suggested. For elderly patients the initial total daily dosage should be in the order of 5 mg and increased gradually as tolerated, until an adequate response is obtained. A daily dosage of more than 30 mg will rarely be needed. Children and adolescents (5 years of age and over): 2.5-10 mg in the morning and 5-30 mg in the evening. These dosages approximate a daily dosage range of 1-3 mg/year of age.
Dosage Forms
Capsule: 5 mg, 10 mg, 20 mg
Drops, oral: 10 mg/mL (100 mL)

- **Peridane** *see* pentoxifylline *on page 480*
- **Peridex®** *see* chlorhexidine gluconate *on page 134*
- **Peridol** *see* haloperidol *on page 308*

perindopril erbumine (per IN doe pril er BYOO meen)
U.S. Brand Names Aceon®
Canadian Brand Names Coversyl®
Generic Available No
(Continued)

perindopril erbumine *(Continued)*
Therapeutic Category Miscellaneous Product
Use Treatment of hypertension
Usual Dosage Adults: Oral: 4 mg once daily; usual range: 4-8 mg/day; maximum: 16 mg/day
Dosage Forms Tablet: 2 mg, 4 mg, 8 mg

♦ **Periochip**® *see* chlorhexidine gluconate *on page 134*
♦ **PerioGard**® *see* chlorhexidine gluconate *on page 134*
♦ **Peritrate**® *see* pentaerythritol tetranitrate *on page 477*
♦ **Peritrate**® **SA** *see* pentaerythritol tetranitrate *on page 477*
♦ **Permapen**® *see* penicillin G benzathine *on page 474*
♦ **Permax**® *see* pergolide *on page 481*

permethrin *(per METH rin)*
U.S. Brand Names Acticin® Cream; Elimite™ Cream; Nix™ Creme Rinse
Generic Available Yes
Therapeutic Category Scabicides/Pediculicides
Use Single application treatment of infestation with *Pediculus humanus capitis* (head louse) and its nits, or *Sarcoptes scabiei* (scabies)
Usual Dosage
Head lice: Children >2 months and Adults: Topical: After hair has been washed with shampoo, rinsed with water and towel-dried, apply a sufficient volume to saturate the hair and scalp. Leave on hair for 10 minutes before rinsing off with water; remove remaining nits.
Scabies: Apply cream from head to toe; leave on for 8-14 hours before washing off with water
Nursing/Pharmacy Information Because scabies and lice are so contagious, use caution to avoid spreading or infecting oneself; wear gloves when applying
Dosage Forms
Cream: 5% (60 g)
Creme rinse: 1% (60 mL with comb)

♦ **Permitil**® **Oral** *see* fluphenazine *on page 277*
♦ **Pernox**® **[OTC]** *see* sulfur and salicylic acid *on page 589*
♦ **Peroxin A5**® *see* benzoyl peroxide *on page 81*
♦ **Peroxin A10**® *see* benzoyl peroxide *on page 81*

perphenazine *(per FEN a zeen)*
U.S. Brand Names Trilafon®
Mexican Brand Names Leptopsique
Generic Available Yes
Therapeutic Category Phenothiazine Derivative
Use Symptomatic management of psychotic disorders, as well as severe nausea and vomiting
Usual Dosage
Children:
Psychoses: Oral:
1-6 years: 4-6 mg/day in divided doses
6-12 years: 6 mg/day in divided doses
>12 years: 4-16 mg 2-4 times/day
I.M.: 5 mg every 6 hours
Nausea/vomiting: I.M.: 5 mg every 6 hours
Adults:
Psychoses:
Oral: 4-16 mg 2-4 times/day not to exceed 64 mg/day
I.M.: 5 mg every 6 hours up to 15 mg/day in ambulatory patients and 30 mg/day in hospitalized patients
Nausea/vomiting:
Oral: 8-16 mg/day in divided doses up to 24 mg/day
I.M.: 5-10 mg every 6 hours as necessary up to 15 mg/day in ambulatory patients and 30 mg/day in hospitalized patients
I.V. (severe): 1 mg at 1- to 2-minute intervals up to a total of 5 mg
Dietary Considerations May be administered with food
Nursing/Pharmacy Information
Dilute oral concentration to at least 2 oz with water, juice, or milk; for I.V. use, injection should be diluted to at least 0.5 mg/mL with NS and administered at a rate of 1 mg/minute

Monitor hypotension when administering I.M. or I.V.; orthostatic hypotension 3-5 days after initiation of therapy or a dose increase; observe for tremor and abnormal movement or posturing.

Dosage Forms
Concentrate, oral: 16 mg/5 mL (118 mL)
Injection: 5 mg/mL (1 mL)
Tablet: 2 mg, 4 mg, 8 mg, 16 mg

- **perphenazine and amitriptyline** *see* amitriptyline and perphenazine *on page 40*
- **Persa-Gel®** *see* benzoyl peroxide *on page 81*
- **Persantine®** *see* dipyridamole *on page 212*
- **Pertussin® CS [OTC]** *see* dextromethorphan *on page 194*
- **Pertussin® ES [OTC]** *see* dextromethorphan *on page 194*
- **pethidine** *see* meperidine *on page 392*
- **PETN** *see* pentaerythritol tetranitrate *on page 477*
- **PFA** *see* foscarnet *on page 283*
- **Pfizerpen®** *see* penicillin G, parenteral, aqueous *on page 475*
- **Pfizerpen-AS® *(Discontinued)*** *see page 743*
- **PGE₁** *see* alprostadil *on page 30*
- **PGE₂** *see* dinoprostone *on page 207*
- **PGF₂ₐ** *see* dinoprost tromethamine *on page 207*
- **Phanatuss® Cough Syrup [OTC]** *see* guaifenesin and dextromethorphan *on page 300*
- **Pharmacal®** *see* calcium carbonate *on page 103*
- **Pharmaflur®** *see* fluoride *on page 274*
- **Phazyme® [OTC]** *see* simethicone *on page 566*
- **Phenadex® Senior [OTC]** *see* guaifenesin and dextromethorphan *on page 300*
- **Phenahist-TR®** *see* chlorpheniramine, phenylephrine, phenylpropanolamine, and belladonna alkaloids *on page 142*
- **Phenameth® DM** *see* promethazine and dextromethorphan *on page 523*
- **phenantoin** *see* mephenytoin *on page 393*
- **Phenaphen®/Codeine #4 *(Discontinued)*** *see page 743*
- **Phenaphen® *(Discontinued)*** *see page 743*
- **Phenaseptic® *(Discontinued)*** *see page 743*
- **Phenazine® Injection** *see* promethazine *on page 522*
- **Phenazo** *see* phenazopyridine *on page 483*

phenazopyridine (fen az oh PEER i deen)

Synonyms phenylazo diamino pyridine hydrochloride
U.S. Brand Names Azo-Standard®; Baridium®; Geridium®; Prodium® [OTC]; Pyridiate®; Pyridium®; Urodine®; Urogesic®
Canadian Brand Names Phenazo; Pyronium®; Vito Reins®
Mexican Brand Names Azo Wintomylon; Madel; Urovalidin
Generic Available Yes
Therapeutic Category Analgesic, Urinary
Use Symptomatic relief of urinary burning, itching, frequency and urgency in association with urinary tract infection, or following urologic procedures
Usual Dosage Oral:
Children 6-12 years: 12 mg/kg/day in 3 divided doses administered after meals for 2 days
Adults: 100-200 mg 3-4 times/day for 2 days
Dietary Considerations Should be administered after meals
Nursing/Pharmacy Information Colors urine orange or red; stains clothing and is difficult to remove
Dosage Forms Phenazopyridine hydrochloride: Tablet:
Azo-Standard®, Prodium®: 95 mg
Baridium®, Geridium®, Pyridiate®, Pyridium®, Urodine®, Urogesic®: 100 mg
Geridium®, Phenazodine®, Pyridium®, Urodine®: 200 mg

- **phenazopyridine and sulfamethoxazole** *see* sulfamethoxazole and phenazopyridine *on page 587*
- **phenazopyridine and sulfisoxazole** *see* sulfisoxazole and phenazopyridine *on page 589*
- **Phencen-50® *(Discontinued)*** *see page 743*
- **Phenchlor® S.H.A.** *see* chlorpheniramine, phenylephrine, phenylpropanolamine, and belladonna alkaloids *on page 142*

phendimetrazine (fen dye ME tra zeen)

Synonyms phendimetrazine tartrate
U.S. Brand Names Bontril PDM®; Bontril® Slow-Release; Dital®; Dyrexan-OD®; Melfiat-105® Unicelles®; Plegine®; Prelu-2®; Rexigen Forte®
Generic Available Yes
Therapeutic Category Anorexiant
Controlled Substance C-III
Use Appetite suppressant during the first few weeks of dieting to help establish new eating habits; its effectiveness lasts only for short periods 3-12 weeks
Usual Dosage Adults: Oral:
  Regular capsule or tablet: 35 mg 2-3 times/day one hour before meals
  Sustained release: 105 mg once daily in the morning before breakfast
Dosage Forms
  Capsule, as tartrate: 35 mg
  Capsule, as tartrate, sustained release (Adipost®, Bontril® Slow-Release, Dital®, Dyrexan-OD®, Melfiat-105® Unicelles®, Prelu-2®; Rexigen Forte®): 105 mg
  Tablet, as tartrate (Bontril PDM®, Plegine®): 35 mg

♦ **phendimetrazine tartrate** *see* phendimetrazine *on page 484*
♦ **Phendry® Oral [OTC]** *see* diphenhydramine *on page 208*

phenelzine (FEN el zeen)

U.S. Brand Names Nardil®
Generic Available No
Therapeutic Category Antidepressant, Monoamine Oxidase Inhibitor
Use Symptomatic treatment of atypical, nonendogenous or neurotic depression
Usual Dosage Adults: Oral: 15 mg 3 times/day; may increase to 60-90 mg/day during early phase of treatment, then reduce to dose for maintenance therapy slowly after maximum benefit is obtained; takes 2-4 weeks for a significant response to occur
Dietary Considerations This medication may cause sudden and severe high blood pressure when taken with food high in tyramine: cheeses, sour cream, yogurt, pickled herring, chicken liver, canned figs, raisins, bananas, avocados, soy sauce, broad bean pods, yeast extracts, meats prepared with tenderizers, and many foods aged to improve flavor; beer and wine (Chianti and hearty red); small amounts of caffeine may produce irregular heartbeat or high blood pressure and can interact with this medication for up to 2 weeks after stopping its use
Nursing/Pharmacy Information
  Check for dietary and drug restriction
  Monitor blood pressure, LFTs, CBC; watch for postural hypotension; monitor blood pressure carefully, especially at therapy onset or if other CNS drugs or cardiovascular drugs are added
  Stability: Protect from light
Dosage Forms Tablet, as sulfate: 15 mg

♦ **Phenerbel-S®** *see* belladonna, phenobarbital, and ergotamine tartrate *on page 76*
♦ **Phenerbel-S®** *see* ergotamine *on page 238*
♦ **Phenergan® Injection** *see* promethazine *on page 522*
♦ **Phenergan® Oral** *see* promethazine *on page 522*
♦ **Phenergan® Rectal** *see* promethazine *on page 522*
♦ **Phenergan® VC Syrup** *see* promethazine and phenylephrine *on page 523*
♦ **Phenergan® VC With Codeine** *see* promethazine, phenylephrine, and codeine *on page 523*
♦ **Phenergan® With Codeine** *see* promethazine and codeine *on page 522*
♦ **Phenergan® With Dextromethorphan** *see* promethazine and dextromethorphan *on page 523*
♦ **Phenetron®** *(Discontinued) see page 743*
♦ **Phenhist® Expectorant** *see* guaifenesin, pseudoephedrine, and codeine *on page 304*

phenindamine (fen IN dah meen)

U.S. Brand Names Nolahist® [OTC]
Generic Available Yes
Therapeutic Category Antihistamine
Use Treatment of perennial and seasonal allergic rhinitis and chronic urticaria
Usual Dosage Oral:
  Children <6 years: As directed by physician

Children 6 to <12 years: 12.5 mg every 4-6 hours, up to 75 mg/24 hours
Adults: 25 mg every 4-6 hours, up to 150 mg/24 hours
Dosage Forms Tablet, as tartrate: 25 mg

♦ **pheniramine and naphazoline** see naphazoline and pheniramine on page 432

pheniramine, phenylpropanolamine, and pyrilamine
(fen EER a meen, fen il proe pa NOLE a meen, & peer IL a meen)
U.S. Brand Names Triaminic® Oral Infant Drops
Generic Available Yes
Therapeutic Category Antihistamine/Decongestant Combination
Use Symptomatic relief of nasal congestion and postnasal drip as well as allergic rhinitis
Usual Dosage Infants <1 year: Drops: 0.05 mL/kg/dose 4 times/day
Dosage Forms Drops: Pheniramine maleate 10 mg, phenylpropanolamine hydrochloride 20 mg, and pyrilamine maleate 10 mg per mL (15 mL)

phenobarbital (fee noe BAR bi tal)
Synonyms phenobarbitone; phenylethylmalonylurea
U.S. Brand Names Barbita®; Luminal®; Solfoton®
Canadian Brand Names Barbilixir®
Mexican Brand Names Alepsal
Generic Available Yes
Therapeutic Category Anticonvulsant; Barbiturate
Controlled Substance C-IV
Use Management of generalized tonic-clonic (grand mal) and partial seizures; neonatal seizures; febrile seizures in children; sedation; may also be used for prevention and treatment of neonatal hyperbilirubinemia and lowering of bilirubin in chronic cholestasis
Usual Dosage
Children:
  Sedation: Oral: 2 mg/kg 3 times/day
  Hypnotic: I.M., I.V., S.C.: 3-5 mg/kg at bedtime
  Hyperbilirubinemia: <12 years: Oral: 3-8 mg/kg/day in 2-3 divided doses; doses up to 12 mg/kg/day have been used
  Preoperative sedation: Oral, I.M., I.V.: 1-3 mg/kg 1-1.5 hours before procedure
Adults:
  Sedation: Oral, I.M.: 30-120 mg/day in 2-3 divided doses
  Hypnotic: Oral, I.M., I.V., S.C.: 100-320 mg at bedtime
  Hyperbilirubinemia: Oral: 90-180 mg/day in 2-3 divided doses
  Preoperative sedation: I.M.: 100-200 mg 1-1½ hours before procedure

Anticonvulsant: Status epilepticus: **Loading dose:** I.V.:
  Infants, Children, and Adults: 15-18 mg/kg in a single or divided dose; usual maximum loading dose: 20 mg/kg; in select patients may administer additional 5 mg/kg/dose every 15-30 minutes until seizure is controlled or a total dose of 30 mg/kg is reached
Anticonvulsant: Maintenance dose: Oral, I.V.:
  Infants: 5-6 mg/kg/day in 1-2 divided doses
  Children:
    1-5 years: 6-8 mg/kg/day in 1-2 divided doses
    5-12 years: 4-6 mg/kg/day in 1-2 divided doses
  Children >12 years and Adults: 1-3 mg/kg/day in divided doses
Dietary Considerations Food:
  Protein-deficient diets: Increases duration of action of barbiturates; should not restrict or delete protein from diet unless discussed with physician; be consistent with protein intake during therapy with barbiturates
  Fresh fruits containing vitamin C: Displaces drug from binding sites, resulting in increased urinary excretion of barbiturate; educate patients regarding the potential for a decreased anticonvulsant effect of barbiturates with consumption of foods high in vitamin C
  Vitamin D: Loss in vitamin D due to malabsorption; increase intake of foods rich in vitamin D; supplementation of vitamin D may be necessary
Nursing/Pharmacy Information
  Parenteral solutions are very alkaline; high dose pyridoxine >80 mg may decrease drug effect; do not inject I.V. faster than 1 mg/kg/minute (50 mg/minute for patients >60 kg); do not administer intra-arterially; avoid extravasation; use only powder for injection for S.C. use, not solutions for injection
  Monitor phenobarbital serum concentrations, mental status, CBC, LFTs, seizure activity
  (Continued)

phenobarbital *(Continued)*

Stability: Protect elixir from light; not stable in aqueous solutions; use only clear solutions; do not add to acidic solutions, precipitation may occur; I.V. form is **incompatible** with benzquinamide (in syringe), cephalothin, chlorpromazine, hydralazine, hydrocortisone, hydroxyzine, insulin, levorphanol, meperidine, methadone, morphine, norepinephrine, pentazocine, prochlorperazine, promazine, promethazine, ranitidine (in syringe), vancomycin

Dosage Forms Phenobarbital sodium:
Capsule: 16 mg
Elixir: 15 mg/5 mL (5 mL, 10 mL, 20 mL); 20 mg/5 mL (3.75 mL, 5 mL, 7.5 mL, 120 mL, 473 mL, 946 mL, 4000 mL)
Injection: 30 mg/mL (1 mL); 60 mg/mL (1 mL); 65 mg/mL (1 mL); 130 mg/mL (1 mL)
Powder for injection: 120 mg
Tablet: 8 mg, 15 mg, 16 mg, 30 mg, 32 mg, 60 mg, 65 mg, 100 mg

♦ **phenobarbital, belladonna, and ergotamine tartrate** *see* belladonna, phenobarbital, and ergotamine tartrate *on page 76*

♦ **phenobarbital, hyoscyamine, atropine, and scopolamine** *see* hyoscyamine, atropine, scopolamine, and phenobarbital *on page 330*

♦ **phenobarbital, theophylline, and ephedrine** *see* theophylline, ephedrine, and phenobarbital *on page 605*

♦ **phenobarbitone** *see* phenobarbital *on page 485*

phenol *(FEE nol)*
Synonyms carbolic acid
U.S. Brand Names Baker's P&S Topical [OTC]; Cēpastat® [OTC]; Chloraseptic® Oral [OTC]; Ulcerease® [OTC]
Generic Available Yes
Therapeutic Category Pharmaceutical Aid
Use Relief of sore throat pain, mouth, gum, and throat irritations
Usual Dosage Oral: Allow to dissolve slowly in mouth; may be repeated every 2 hours as needed
Nursing/Pharmacy Information Monitor CBC, electrolytes, glucose, BUN
Dosage Forms
Liquid:
Oral, sugar free (Ulcerease®): 6% with glycerin (180 mL)
Topical (Baker's P&S): 1% with sodium chloride, liquid paraffin oil and water (120 mL, 240 mL)
Lozenge:
Cēpastat®: 1.45% with menthol and eucalyptus oil
Cēpastat® Cherry: 0.72% with menthol and eucalyptus oil
Chloraseptic®: 32.5 mg total phenol, sugar, corn syrup
Mouthwash (Chloraseptic®): 1.4% with thymol, sodium borate, menthol, and glycerin (180 mL)
Solution (Liquified Phenol): 88% [880 mg/mL]
Aqueous: 6% [60 mg/mL]

♦ **phenol red** *see* phenolsulfonphthalein *on page 486*

phenolsulfonphthalein *(fee nol sul fon THAY leen)*
Synonyms phenol red; PSP
Generic Available Yes
Therapeutic Category Diagnostic Agent
Use Evaluation of renal blood flow to aid in the determination of renal function
Usual Dosage I.M., I.V.: 6 mg
Dosage Forms Injection: 6 mg/mL (1 mL)

♦ **Phenoxine® [OTC]** *see* phenylpropanolamine *on page 489*

phenoxybenzamine *(fen oks ee BEN za meen)*
U.S. Brand Names Dibenzyline®
Generic Available No
Therapeutic Category Alpha-Adrenergic Blocking Agent
Use Symptomatic management of hypertension and sweating in patients with pheochromocytoma
Usual Dosage Oral:
Children: Initial: 0.2 mg/kg (maximum: 10 mg) once daily, increase by 0.2 mg/kg increments; usual maintenance dose: 0.4-1.2 mg/kg/day every 6-8 hours, maximum single dose: 10 mg
Adults: 10-40 mg every 8-12 hours
Nursing/Pharmacy Information Monitor blood pressure, heart rate

Dosage Forms Capsule, as hydrochloride: 10 mg

♦ **phenoxymethyl penicillin** *see* penicillin V potassium *on page 476*

phensuximide (fen SUKS i mide)

U.S. Brand Names Milontin®
Generic Available No
Therapeutic Category Anticonvulsant
Use Control of absence (petit mal) seizures
Usual Dosage Children and Adults: Oral: 0.5-1 g 2-3 times/day
Dietary Considerations May be administered with food
Nursing/Pharmacy Information Do not discontinue abruptly; may cause drowsiness and impair judgment
Dosage Forms Capsule: 500 mg

phentolamine (fen TOLE a meen)

U.S. Brand Names Regitine®
Canadian Brand Names Rogitine®
Generic Available No
Therapeutic Category Alpha-Adrenergic Blocking Agent; Diagnostic Agent
Use Diagnosis of pheochromocytoma; treatment of hypertension associated with pheochromocytoma or other causes of excess sympathomimetic amines; local treatment of dermal necrosis after extravasation of drugs with alpha-adrenergic effects (dobutamine, dopamine, epinephrine, metaraminol, norepinephrine, phenylephrine)
Usual Dosage
Treatment of extravasation: Infiltrate area S.C. with small amount of solution made by diluting 5-10 mg in 10 mL 0.9% NaCl within 12 hours of extravasation; for children, use 0.1-0.2 mg/kg up to a maximum of 10 mg

Children: I.M., I.V.:
Diagnosis of pheochromocytoma: 0.05-0.1 mg/kg/dose, maximum single dose: 5 mg
Hypertension: 0.05-0.1 mg/kg/dose administered 1-2 hours before procedure; repeat as needed until hypertension is controlled; maximum single dose: 5 mg
Adults: I.M., I.V.:
Diagnosis of pheochromocytoma: 5 mg
Hypertension: 5 mg administered 1-2 hours before procedure
Nursing/Pharmacy Information
Parenteral: Treatment of extravasation: Infiltrate area of extravasation with multiple small injections; use 27- or 30-gauge needles and change needle between each skin entry
Monitor blood pressure, heart rate
Stability: Reconstituted solution is stable for 48 hours at room temperature and 1 week when refrigerated
Dosage Forms Injection, as mesylate: 5 mg/mL (1 mL)

♦ **Phentrol®** *(Discontinued) see page 743*
♦ **Phenurone®** *(Discontinued) see page 743*
♦ **phenylalanine mustard** *see* melphalan *on page 390*
♦ **phenylazo diamino pyridine hydrochloride** *see* phenazopyridine *on page 483*
♦ **Phenyldrine® [OTC]** *see* phenylpropanolamine *on page 489*

phenylephrine (fen il EF rin)

U.S. Brand Names AK-Dilate® Ophthalmic Solution; AK-Nefrin® Ophthalmic Solution; Alconefrin® Nasal Solution [OTC]; Doktors® Nasal Solution [OTC]; I-Phrine® Ophthalmic Solution; Isopto® Frin Ophthalmic Solution; Mydfrin® Ophthalmic Solution; Neo-Synephrine® Nasal Solution [OTC]; Neo-Synephrine® Ophthalmic Solution; Nostril® Nasal Solution [OTC]; Prefrin™ Prefrin™ Ophthalmic Solution; Relief® Ophthalmic Solution; Rhinall® Nasal Solution [OTC]; Sinarest® Nasal Solution [OTC]; St. Joseph® Measured Dose Nasal Solution [OTC]; Vicks® Sinex® Nasal Solution [OTC]
Canadian Brand Names Dionephrine; Novahistine®; Prefrin™ Liquifilm®
Generic Available Yes
Therapeutic Category Adrenergic Agonist Agent
Use Treatment of hypotension and vascular failure in shock; supraventricular tachycardia; as a vasoconstrictor in regional analgesia; symptomatic relief of nasal and nasopharyngeal mucosal congestion; as a mydriatic in ophthalmic procedures and treatment of wide-angle glaucoma
(Continued)

phenylephrine *(Continued)*

Usual Dosage

Ophthalmic procedures:

Infants <1 year: Instill 1 drop of 2.5% 15-30 minutes before procedures

Children and Adults: Instill 1 drop of 2.5% or 10% solution, may repeat in 10-60 minutes as needed

Nasal decongestant:

Children:

2-6 years: Instill 1 drop every 2-4 hours of 0.125% solution as needed

6-12 years: Instill 1-2 sprays or instill 1-2 drops every 4 hours of 0.25% solution as needed

Children >12 years and Adults: Instill 1-2 sprays or instill 1-2 drops every 4 hours of 0.25% to 0.5% solution as needed; 1% solution may be used in adult in cases of extreme nasal congestion; do not use nasal solutions more than 3 days

Hypotension/shock:

Children:

I.M., S.C.: 0.1 mg/kg/dose every 1-2 hours as needed (maximum: 5 mg)

I.V. bolus: 5-20 mcg/kg/dose every 10-15 minutes as needed

I.V. infusion: 0.1-0.5 mcg/kg/minute; the concentration and rate of infusion can be calculated using the following formulas: Dilute 0.6 mg x weight (kg) to 100 mL; then the dose in mcg/kg/minute = 0.1 x the infusion rate in mL/hour

Adults:

I.M., S.C.: 2-5 mg/dose every 1-2 hours as needed (initial dose should not exceed 5 mg)

I.V. bolus: 0.1-0.5 mg/dose every 10-15 minutes as needed (initial dose should not exceed 0.5 mg)

I.V. infusion: 10 mg in 250 mL D_5W or NS (1:25,000 dilution) (40 mcg/mL); start at 100-180 mcg/minute (2-5 mL/minute; 50-90 drops/minute) initially. When blood pressure is stabilized, maintenance rate: 40-60 mcg/minute (20-30 drops/minute)

Paroxysmal supraventricular tachycardia: I.V.:

Children: 5-10 mcg/kg/dose over 20-30 seconds

Adults: 0.25-0.5 mg/dose over 20-30 seconds

Nursing/Pharmacy Information

May cause extravasation; avoid I.V. infiltration; for direct I.V. administration, dilute to 1 mg/mL by adding 1-9 mL of sterile water; the specific dosage may be administered by direct I.V. injection over 20-30 seconds; continuous infusion concentrations are usually 20-60 mcg/mL by adding 5 mg to 250 mL I.V. solution (20 mcg/mL) or 15 mg to 250 mL (60 mcg/mL)

Monitor blood pressure, heart rate, EKG

Stability: Stable for 48 hours in 5% dextrose in water at pH 3.5-7.5; do not use brown colored solutions

Dosage Forms

Phenylephrine hydrochloride:

Injection (Neo-Synephrine®): 1% [10 mg/mL] (1 mL)

Nasal solution:

Drops:

Neo-Synephrine®: 0.125% (15 mL)

Alconefrin® 12: 0.16% (30 mL)

Alconefrin® 25, Neo-Synephrine®, Children's Nostril®, Rhinall®: 0.25% (15 mL, 30 mL, 40 mL)

Alconefrin®, Neo-Synephrine®: 0.5% (15 mL, 30 mL)

Spray:

Alconefrin® 25, Neo-Synephrine®, Rhinall®: 0.25% (15 mL, 30 mL, 40 mL)

Neo-Synephrine®, Nostril®, Sinex®: 0.5% (15 mL, 30 mL)

Neo-Synephrine®: 1% (15 mL)

Ophthalmic solution:

AK-Nefrin®, Isopto® Frin, Prefrin™ Liquifilm®, Relief®: 0.12% (0.3 mL, 15 mL, 20 mL)

AK-Dilate®, Mydfrin®, Neo-Synephrine®, Phenoptic®: 2.5% (2 mL, 3 mL, 5 mL, 15 mL)

AK-Dilate®, Neo-Synephrine®, Neo-Synephrine® Viscous: 10% (1 mL, 2 mL, 5 mL, 15 mL)

♦ **phenylephrine and chlorpheniramine** *see* chlorpheniramine and phenylephrine *on page 139*

♦ **phenylephrine and cyclopentolate** *see* cyclopentolate and phenylephrine *on page 175*

♦ **phenylephrine and guaifenesin** *see* guaifenesin and phenylephrine *on page 301*

♦ **phenylephrine and isoproterenol** *see* isoproterenol and phenylephrine *on page 348*

♦ **phenylephrine and promethazine** *see* promethazine and phenylephrine *on page 523*

phenylephrine and scopolamine
(fen il EF rin & skoe POL a meen)

Synonyms scopolamine and phenylephrine

U.S. Brand Names Murocoll-2® Ophthalmic

Generic Available Yes

Therapeutic Category Anticholinergic/Adrenergic Agonist

Use Mydriasis, cycloplegia and to break posterior synechiae in iritis

Usual Dosage Ophthalmic: Instill 1-2 drops into eye(s); repeat in 5 minutes

Dosage Forms Solution, ophthalmic: Phenylephrine hydrochloride 10% and scopolamine hydrobromide 0.3% (7.5 mL)

♦ **phenylephrine and sulfacetamide** *see* sulfacetamide and phenylephrine *on page 585*

phenylephrine and zinc sulfate (fen il EF rin & zingk SUL fate)

U.S. Brand Names Zincfrin® Ophthalmic [OTC]

Generic Available Yes

Therapeutic Category Adrenergic Agonist Agent

Use Soothe, moisturize, and remove redness due to minor eye irritation

Usual Dosage Ophthalmic: Instill 1-2 drops in eye(s) 2-4 times/day as needed

Dosage Forms Solution, ophthalmic: Phenylephrine hydrochloride 0.12% and zinc sulfate 0.25% (15 mL)

♦ **phenylephrine, chlorpheniramine, phenylpropanolamine, and belladonna alkaloids** *see* chlorpheniramine, phenylephrine, phenylpropanolamine, and belladonna alkaloids *on page 142*

♦ **phenylephrine, guaifenesin, and phenylpropanolamine** *see* guaifenesin, phenylpropanolamine, and phenylephrine *on page 304*

♦ **phenylephrine, hydrocodone, chlorpheniramine, acetaminophen, and caffeine** *see* hydrocodone, chlorpheniramine, phenylephrine, acetaminophen, and caffeine *on page 321*

♦ **phenylephrine, promethazine, and codeine** *see* promethazine, phenylephrine, and codeine *on page 523*

♦ **phenylethylmalonylurea** *see* phenobarbital *on page 485*

♦ **Phenylfenesin® L.A.** *see* guaifenesin and phenylpropanolamine *on page 301*

♦ **phenylisohydantoin** *see* pemoline *on page 473*

phenylpropanolamine (fen il proe pa NOLE a meen)

Synonyms *dl*-norephedrine; PPA

U.S. Brand Names Acutrim® 16 Hours [OTC]; Acutrim® II, Maximum Strength [OTC]; Acutrim® Late Day [OTC]; Control® [OTC]; Dexatrim® Pre-Meal [OTC]; Maximum Strength Dex-A-Diet® [OTC]; Maximum Strength Dexatrim® [OTC]; Phenoxine® [OTC]; Phenyldrine® [OTC]; Propagest® [OTC]; Unitrol® [OTC]

Generic Available Yes

Therapeutic Category Adrenergic Agonist Agent

Use Anorexiant and nasal decongestant

Usual Dosage Oral:

Children: Decongestant:

2-6 years: 6.25 mg every 4 hours

6-12 years: 12.5 mg every 4 hours not to exceed 75 mg/day

Adults:

Decongestant: 25 mg every 4 hours or 50 mg every 8 hours, not to exceed 150 mg/day

Anorexic: 25 mg 3 times/day 30 minutes before meals or 75 mg (timed release) once daily in the morning

Precision release: 75 mg after breakfast

Dietary Considerations Should be administered 30 minutes before meals

Nursing/Pharmacy Information Monitor blood pressure, heart rate

Dosage Forms Phenylpropanolamine hydrochloride:

Capsule: 37.5 mg

Capsule, timed release: 25 mg, 75 mg

Tablet: 25 mg, 50 mg

Tablet:

Precision release: 75 mg

Timed release: 75 mg

♦ **phenylpropanolamine and brompheniramine** *see* brompheniramine and phenylpropanolamine *on page 94*

♦ **phenylpropanolamine and caramiphen** *see* caramiphen and phenylpropanolamine *on page 111*

♦ **phenylpropanolamine and chlorpheniramine** *see* chlorpheniramine and phenylpropanolamine *on page 139*

♦ **phenylpropanolamine and guaifenesin** *see* guaifenesin and phenylpropanolamine *on page 301*

♦ **phenylpropanolamine and hydrocodone** *see* hydrocodone and phenylpropanolamine *on page 321*

♦ **phenylpropanolamine, brompheniramine, and codeine** *see* brompheniramine, phenylpropanolamine, and codeine *on page 95*

♦ **phenylpropanolamine, chlorpheniramine, phenylephrine, and belladonna alkaloids** *see* chlorpheniramine, phenylephrine, phenylpropanolamine, and belladonna alkaloids *on page 142*

♦ **phenylpropanolamine, guaifenesin, and dextromethorphan** *see* guaifenesin, phenylpropanolamine, and dextromethorphan *on page 303*

♦ **phenylpropanolamine, guaifenesin, and phenylephrine** *see* guaifenesin, phenylpropanolamine, and phenylephrine *on page 304*

phenyltoloxamine, phenylpropanolamine, and acetaminophen

(fen il tol OKS a meen, fen il proe pa NOLE a meen, & a seet a MIN oh fen)

U.S. Brand Names Sinubid®

Generic Available Yes

Therapeutic Category Antihistamine/Decongestant/Analgesic

Use Intermittent symptomatic treatment of nasal congestion in sinus or other frontal headache; allergic rhinitis, vasomotor rhinitis, coryza; facial pain and pressure of acute and chronic sinusitis

Usual Dosage Oral:
Children 6-12 years: ¹/₂ tablet every 12 hours (twice daily)
Adults: 1 tablet every 12 hours (twice daily)

Dosage Forms Tablet: Phenyltoloxamine citrate 22 mg, phenylpropanolamine hydrochloride 25 mg, and acetaminophen 325 mg

phenyltoloxamine, phenylpropanolamine, pyrilamine, and pheniramine

(fen il tol OKS a meen, fen il proe pa NOLE a meen, peer IL a meen, & fen IR a meen)

U.S. Brand Names Poly-Histine-D® Capsule

Generic Available Yes

Therapeutic Category Cold Preparation

Use Treatment of nasal congestion

Usual Dosage Adults: Oral: 1 capsule every 8-12 hours

Dosage Forms Capsule: Phenyltoloxamine citrate 16 mg, phenylpropanolamine hydrochloride 50 mg, pyrilamine maleate 16 mg, and pheniramine maleate 16 mg

phenytoin (FEN i toyn)

Synonyms diphenylhydantoin; DPH

U.S. Brand Names Dilantin®; Diphenylan Sodium®

Canadian Brand Names Tremytoine®

Generic Available Yes

Therapeutic Category Antiarrhythmic Agent, Class I-B; Hydantoin

Use Management of generalized tonic-clonic (grand mal), simple partial and complex partial seizures; prevention of seizures following head trauma/neurosurgery; ventricular arrhythmias, including those associated with digitalis intoxication, prolonged Q-T interval and surgical repair of congenital heart diseases in children; epidermolysis bullosa

Usual Dosage
Status epilepticus: I.V.:
Infants and Children: Loading dose: 15-18 mg/kg in a single or divided dose; maintenance, anticonvulsant: Initial: 5 mg/kg/day in 2 divided doses, usual doses:
6 months to 3 years: 8-10 mg/kg/day
4-6 years: 7.5-9 mg/kg/day
7-9 years: 7-8 mg/kg/day

10-16 years: 6-7 mg/kg/day, some patients may require every 8 hours dosing

Adults: Loading dose: 15-18 mg/kg in a single or divided dose; maintenance, anticonvulsant: usual: 300 mg/day or 5-6 mg/kg/day in 3 divided doses or 1-2 divided doses using extended release

Anticonvulsant: Children and Adults: Oral: Loading dose: 15-20 mg/kg; based on phenytoin serum concentrations and recent dosing history; administer oral loading dose in 3 divided doses administered every 2-4 hours to decrease GI adverse effects and to ensure complete oral absorption; maintenance dose: same as I.V.

Arrhythmias:

Children and Adults: Loading dose: I.V.: 1.25 mg/kg IVP every 5 minutes may repeat up to total loading dose: 15 mg/kg

Children: Maintenance dose: Oral, I.V.: 5-10 mg/kg/day in 2 divided doses

Adults: Maintenance dose: Oral: 250 mg 4 times/day for 1 day, 250 mg twice daily for 2 days, then maintenance at 300-400 mg/day in divided doses 1-4 times/day

Dietary Considerations Charcoal-broiled foods will increase metabolism requiring higher doses

Alcohol: Additive CNS depression; has been reported with hydantoins

Alcohol (acute use): Inhibits metabolism of phenytoin; avoid or limit alcohol; watch for sedation

Alcohol (chronic use): Stimulates metabolism of phenytoin; avoid or limit alcohol

Food:

Folic acid: Low erythrocyte and CSF folate concentrations; phenytoin may decrease mucosal uptake of folic acid; to avoid folic acid deficiency and megaloblastic anemia, some clinicians recommend giving patients on anticonvulsants prophylactic doses of folic acid and cyanocobalamin

Calcium: Hypocalcemia has been reported in patients taking prolonged high-dose therapy with an anticonvulsant; phenytoin may decrease calcium absorption; monitor calcium serum concentration and for bone disorders (eg, rickets, osteomalacia); some clinicians have given an additional 4,000 Units/week of vitamin D (especially in those receiving poor nutrition and getting no sun exposure) to prevent hypocalcemia

Vitamin D: Phenytoin interferes with vitamin D metabolism and osteomalacia may result; may need to supplement with vitamin D

Glucose: Hyperglycemia and glycosuria may occur in patients receiving high-dose therapy; monitor blood glucose concentration, especially in patients with impaired renal function

Tube Feedings: Tube feedings decrease phenytoin bioavailability; to avoid decreased serum levels with continuous NG feeds, hold feedings for 2 hours prior to and 2 hours after phenytoin administration, if possible; there is a variety of opinions on how to administer phenytoin with enteral feedings; BE CONSISTENT throughout therapy

Nursing/Pharmacy Information

Maintenance doses usually start 12 hours after loading dose; shake oral suspension well prior to each dose; do not exceed I.V. infusion rate of 1-3 mg/kg/minute or 50 mg/minute; I.V. injections should be followed by normal saline flushes through the same needle or I.V. catheter to avoid local irritation of the vein; avoid extravasation; avoid I.M. use due to erratic absorption, pain on injection, and precipitation of drug at injection site

Monitor blood pressure, vital signs (with I.V. use), plasma level monitoring, CBC, liver function tests

Stability: Parenteral solution may be used as long as there is no precipitate and it is not hazy; slightly yellowed solution may be used; refrigeration may cause precipitate, sometimes the precipitate is resolved by allowing the solution to reach room temperature again; drug may precipitate with pH ≤11.5; do not mix with other medications; may dilute with normal saline for I.V. infusion, but must be diluted to concentration of 1-10 mg/mL, stable for 4 hours. I.V. form is highly **incompatible** with many drugs and solutions such as dextrose in water, some saline solutions, amikacin, bretylium, dobutamine, cephapirin, insulin, levorphanol, lidocaine, meperidine, metaraminol, morphine, norepinephrine, heparin, potassium chloride, vitamin B complex with C

Dosage Forms Phenytoin sodium:

Capsule, extended release: 30 mg, 100 mg

Capsule, prompt: 30 mg, 100 mg

Injection: 50 mg/mL (2 mL, 5 mL)

Suspension, oral: 125 mg/5 mL (5 mL, 240 mL)

Tablet, chewable: 50 mg

- **Pherazine® VC w/ Codeine** *see* promethazine, phenylephrine, and codeine *on page 523*
- **Pherazine® w/DM** *see* promethazine and dextromethorphan *on page 523*
- **Pherazine® With Codeine** *see* promethazine and codeine *on page 522*
- **Phicon® [OTC]** *see* pramoxine *on page 512*
- **Phillips'® Milk of Magnesia [OTC]** *see* magnesium hydroxide *on page 381*
- **pHisoHex®** *see* hexachlorophene *on page 312*
- **Phos-Ex® 62.5** *(Discontinued) see page 743*
- **Phos-Ex® 125** *(Discontinued) see page 743*
- **Phos-Ex® 167** *(Discontinued) see page 743*
- **Phos-Ex® 250** *(Discontinued) see page 743*
- **Phos-Flur®** *see* fluoride *on page 274*
- **PhosLo®** *see* calcium acetate *on page 103*
- **pHos-pHaid®** *(Discontinued) see page 743*
- **Phosphaljel®** *(Discontinued) see page 743*
- **Pholine Iodide® Ophthalmic** *see* echothiophate iodide *on page 227*
- **phosphonoformic acid** *see* foscarnet *on page 283*

phosphorated carbohydrate solution
(FOS for ate ed kar boe HYE drate soe LOO shun)

Synonyms dextrose, levulose and phosphoric acid; levulose, dextrose and phosphoric acid; phosphoric acid, levulose and dextrose

U.S. Brand Names Emecheck® [OTC]; Emetrol® [OTC]; Naus-A-Way® [OTC]; Nausetrol® [OTC]

Generic Available Yes

Therapeutic Category Antiemetic

Use Relief of nausea associated with upset stomach that occurs with intestinal flu, pregnancy, food indiscretions, and emotional upsets

Usual Dosage Oral:

Morning sickness: 15-30 mL on arising; repeat every 3 hours or when nausea threatens

Motion sickness and vomiting due to drug therapy: 5 mL doses for young children; 15 mL doses for older children and adults

Regurgitation in infants: 5 or 10 mL, 10-15 minutes before each feeding; in refractory cases: 10-15 mL, 30 minutes before each feeding

Vomiting due to psychogenic factors:

Children: 5-10 mL; repeat dose every 15 minutes until distress subsides; do not take for more than 1 hour

Adults: 15-30 mL; repeat dose every 15 minutes until distress subsides; do not take for more than 1 hour

Nursing/Pharmacy Information Never dilute or drink fluids of any kind immediately before or after taking dose

Dosage Forms Liquid, oral: Fructose, dextrose, and orthophosphoric acid (120 mL, 480 mL, 4000 mL)

- **phosphoric acid, levulose and dextrose** *see* phosphorated carbohydrate solution *on page 492*
- **Photofrin®** *see* porfimer *on page 504*
- **Phrenilin®** *see* butalbital compound and acetaminophen *on page 99*
- **Phrenilin® Forte** *see* butalbital compound and acetaminophen *on page 99*
- **p-hydroxyampicillin** *see* amoxicillin *on page 43*
- **Phyllocontin®** *see* aminophylline *on page 38*
- **phylloquinone** *see* phytonadione *on page 493*

physostigmine (fye zoe STIG meen)

U.S. Brand Names Antilirium®

Generic Available Yes: Ophthalmic

Therapeutic Category Cholinesterase Inhibitor

Use Reverse toxic CNS and cardiac effects caused by anticholinergics and tricyclic antidepressants; ophthalmic solution is used to treat open-angle glaucoma

Usual Dosage

Children: Reserve for life-threatening situations only: I.V.: 0.01-0.03 mg/kg/ dose; may repeat after 15-20 minutes to a maximum total dose of 2 mg

Adults:

I.M., I.V., S.C.: 0.5-2 mg to start, repeat every 20 minutes until response occurs or adverse effect occurs

I.M., I.V. to reverse the anticholinergic effects of atropine or scopolamine administered as preanesthetic medications: Administer twice the dose, on a weight basis of the anticholinergic drug

Ophthalmic: 1-2 drops of 0.25% or 0.5% solution every 4-8 hours (up to 4 times/day); the ointment can be instilled at night

Nursing/Pharmacy Information
Too rapid administration (I.V. rate not to exceed 1 mg/minute) can cause bradycardia, hypersalivation leading to respiratory difficulties and seizures

Monitor heart rate, respiratory rate

Stability: Do not use solution if cloudy or dark brown

Dosage Forms
Injection, as salicylate: 1 mg/mL (2 mL)

Ointment, ophthalmic, as sulfate: 0.25% (3.5 g, 3.7 g)

♦ **phytomenadione** see phytonadione on page 493

phytonadione (fye toe na DYE one)
Synonyms methylphytyl napthoquinone; phylloquinone; phytomenadione; vitamin K_1

U.S. Brand Names AquaMEPHYTON® Injection; Konakion® Injection; Mephyton® Oral

Generic Available Yes

Therapeutic Category Vitamin, Fat Soluble

Use Prevention and treatment of hypoprothrombinemia caused by vitamin K deficiency or anticoagulant-induced hypoprothrombinemia; hemorrhagic disease of the newborn

Usual Dosage I.V. route should be restricted for emergency use only

Hemorrhagic disease of the newborn:
Prophylaxis: I.M., S.C.: 0.5-1 mg within 1 hour of birth
Treatment: I.M., S.C.: 1-2 mg/dose/day

Oral anticoagulant overdose:
Infants: I.M., I.V., S.C.: 1-2 mg/dose every 4-8 hours
Children and Adults: Oral, I.M., I.V., S.C.: 2.5-10 mg/dose; rarely up to 25-50 mg has been used; may repeat in 6-8 hours if administered by I.M., I.V., S.C. route; may repeat 12-48 hours after oral route

Vitamin K deficiency: Due to drugs, malabsorption or decreased synthesis of vitamin K

Infants and Children:
Oral: 2.5-5 mg/24 hours
I.M., I.V.: 1-2 mg/dose as a single dose

Adults:
Oral: 5-25 mg/24 hours
I.M., I.V.: 10 mg

Minimum daily requirement: Not well established
Infants: 1-5 mcg/kg/day
Adults: 0.03 mcg/kg/day

Nursing/Pharmacy Information
I.V. administration: Dilute in normal saline, D_5W or D_5NS and infuse slowly; rate of infusion should not exceed 1 mg/minute. **This route should be used only if administration by another route is not feasible for phytonadione;** I.V. administration should not exceed 1 mg/minute; for I.V. infusion, dilute in PF (preservative free) D_5W or normal saline.

Monitor PT

Stability: Protect injection from light at all times; may be autoclaved

Dosage Forms
Injection:
Aqueous colloidal: 2 mg/mL (0.5 mL); 10 mg/mL (1 mL, 2.5 mL, 5 mL)
Aqueous (I.M. only): 2 mg/mL (0.5 mL); 10 mg/mL (1 mL)
Tablet: 5 mg

♦ **Pilagan® Ophthalmic** see pilocarpine on page 493

♦ **Pilocar® Ophthalmic** see pilocarpine on page 493

pilocarpine (pye loe KAR peen)
U.S. Brand Names Adsorbocarpine® Ophthalmic; Akarpine® Ophthalmic; Isopto® Carpine Ophthalmic; Ocu-Carpine® Ophthalmic; Ocusert Pilo-20® Ophthalmic; Ocusert Pilo-40® Ophthalmic; Pilagan® Ophthalmic; Pilocar® Ophthalmic; Pilopine HS® Ophthalmic; Piloptic® Ophthalmic; Pilostat® Ophthalmic; Salagen® Oral

Canadian Brand Names Diocarpine; Minims® Pilocarpine; Miocarpine®

Mexican Brand Names Pilogrin

Generic Available Yes: Hydrochloride Solution

(Continued)

pilocarpine *(Continued)*

Therapeutic Category Cholinergic Agent

Use

Ophthalmic: Management of chronic simple glaucoma, chronic and acute angle-closure glaucoma; counter effects of cycloplegics

Oral: Symptomatic treatment of xerostomia caused by salivary gland hypofunction resulting from radiotherapy for cancer of the head and neck

Usual Dosage Adults:

Oral: 5 mg 3 times/day, titration up to 10 mg 3 times/day may be considered for patients who have not responded adequately

Ophthalmic:

Nitrate solution: Shake well before using; instill 1-2 drops 2-4 times/day

Hydrochloride solution:

Instill 1-2 drops up to 6 times/day; adjust the concentration and frequency as required to control elevated intraocular pressure

To counteract the mydriatic effects of sympathomimetic agents: Instill 1 drop of a 1% solution in the affected eye

Gel: Instill 0.5" ribbon into lower conjunctival sac once daily at bedtime

Ocular systems: Systems are labeled in terms of mean rate of release of pilocarpine over 7 days; begin with 20 mcg/hour at night and adjust based on response

Nursing/Pharmacy Information

Following topical administration, finger pressure should be applied on the lacrimal sac for 1-2 minutes

Monitor intraocular pressure, funduscopic exam, visual field testing

Stability: Refrigerate gel; store solution at room temperature of 8°C to 30°C (46°F to 86°F) and protect from light

Dosage Forms

Ocular therapeutic system (Ocusert® Pilo): Releases 20 or 40 mcg/hour for 1 week (8s)

Tablet: 5 mg

Pilocarpine hydrochloride:

Gel, ophthalmic (Pilopine HS®): 4% (3.5 g)

Solution, ophthalmic (Adsorbocarpine®, Akarpine®, Isopto® Carpine, Pilagan®, Pilocar®, Piloptic®, Pilostat®): 0.25% (15 mL); 0.5% (15 mL, 30 mL); 1% (1 mL, 2 mL, 15 mL, 30 mL); 2% (1 mL, 2 mL, 15 mL, 30 mL); 3% (15 mL, 30 mL); 4% (1 mL, 2 mL, 15 mL, 30 mL); 5% (15 mL); 6% (15 mL, 30 mL); 8% (2 mL); 10% (15 mL)

Pilocarpine nitrate: Solution, ophthalmic (Pilagan®): 1% (15 mL); 2% (15 mL); 4% (15 mL)

pilocarpine and epinephrine *(pye loe KAR peen & ep i NEF rin)*

Synonyms epinephrine and pilocarpine

U.S. Brand Names E-Pilo-x® Ophthalmic; P$_x$E$_x$® Ophthalmic

Generic Available No

Therapeutic Category Cholinergic Agent

Use Treatment of glaucoma; counter effect of cycloplegics

Usual Dosage Ophthalmic: Instill 1-2 drops up to 6 times/day

Nursing/Pharmacy Information

Usually causes difficulty in dark adaptation; advise patients to use caution while night driving or performing hazardous tasks in poor illumination

Stability: Store at 8°C to 30°C (46°F to 86°F); keep tightly closed; do not use solution if it is brown or contains a precipitate; protect from heat and light

Dosage Forms Solution, ophthalmic: Epinephrine bitartrate 1% and pilocarpine hydrochloride 1%, 2%, 3%, 4%, 6% (15 mL)

♦ **Pilogrin** *see* pilocarpine *on page 493*
♦ **Pilopine HS® Ophthalmic** *see* pilocarpine *on page 493*
♦ **Piloptic® Ophthalmic** *see* pilocarpine *on page 493*
♦ **Pilostat® Ophthalmic** *see* pilocarpine *on page 493*
♦ **Pima®** *see* potassium iodide *on page 509*
♦ **pimaricin** *see* natamycin *on page 433*

pimozide *(PI moe zide)*

U.S. Brand Names Orap™

Generic Available No

Therapeutic Category Neuroleptic Agent

Use Suppression of severe motor and phonic tics in patients with Tourette's disorder

Usual Dosage Children >12 years and Adults: Oral: Initial: 1-2 mg/day, then increase dosage as needed every other day; range: 7-16 mg/day, maximum dose: 20 mg/day or 0.3 mg/kg/day should not be exceeded

Nursing/Pharmacy Information Perform EKG at baseline and periodically thereafter, and with dose increases; use in patients receiving macrolide antibiotics such as clarithromycin, erythromycin, azithromycin, and dirithromycin may predispose those patients to fatal cardiac arrhythmias

Dosage Forms Tablet: 2 mg

pinaverium *(Canada only)* (pin ah VEER ee um)
Canadian Brand Names Dicetel®
Generic Available No
Therapeutic Category Calcium Antagonist; Gastrointestinal Agent, Miscellaneous
Use For the treatment and relief of symptoms associated with irritable bowel syndrome (IBS): abdominal pain, bowel disturbances and intestinal discomfort; treatment of symptoms related to functional disorders of the biliary tract
Usual Dosage Adults: Oral: Three 50 mg tablets (1 tablet 3 times a day). In exceptional cases, the dosage may be increased up to 6 tablets a day (2 tablets 3 times/day). It is recommended that the tablet be taken with a glass of water during meals or snacks. The tablet should not be swallowed when in the lying position or just before bedtime.
Dosage Forms Tablet, as bromide: 50 mg

♦ Pindac® *(Discontinued) see page 743*

pindolol (PIN doe lole)
U.S. Brand Names Visken®
Canadian Brand Names Apo-Pindol®; Gen-Pindolol; Novo-Pindol; Nu-Pindol; Syn-Pindol®
Generic Available Yes
Therapeutic Category Beta-Adrenergic Blocker
Use Management of hypertension
Usual Dosage Oral: 5 mg twice daily
Dietary Considerations May be administered without regard to meals
Nursing/Pharmacy Information
Do not discontinue abruptly
Monitor blood pressure, standing and sitting/supine; pulse
Dosage Forms Tablet: 5 mg, 10 mg

♦ Pin-Rid® [OTC] *see pyrantel pamoate on page 532*
♦ Pin-X® [OTC] *see pyrantel pamoate on page 532*
♦ PIO *see pemoline on page 473*

pioglitazone *New Drug* (pye oh GLI ta zone)
U.S. Brand Names Actos™
Generic Available No
Therapeutic Category Antidiabetic Agent; Thiazolidinedione Derivative
Use
Type 2 diabetes, monotherapy: Adjunct to diet and exercise, to improve glycemic control
Type 2 diabetes, combination therapy with sulfonylurea, metformin, or insulin: When diet, exercise, and a single agent alone does not result in adequate glycemic control
Usual Dosage Adults: Oral:
Monotherapy: Initial: 15-30 mg once daily; if response is inadequate, the dosage may be increased in increments up to 45 mg once daily; maximum recommended dose: 45 mg once daily
Combination therapy:
With sulfonylureas: Initial: 15-30 mg once daily; dose of sulfonylurea should be reduced if the patient reports hypoglycemia
With metformin: Initial: 15-30 mg once daily; it is unlikely that the dose of metformin will need to be reduced due to hypoglycemia
With insulin: Initial: 15-30 mg once daily; dose of insulin should be reduced by 10% to 25% if the patient reports hypoglycemia or if the plasma glucose falls to below 100 mg/dL. Doses greater than 30 mg/day have not been evaluated in combination regimens.
A 1-week washout period is recommended in patients with normal liver enzymes who are changed from troglitazone to pioglitazone therapy.
Dosage Forms Tablet: 15 mg, 30 mg, 45 mg

pipecuronium (pi pe kur OH nee um)

U.S. Brand Names Arduan®
Generic Available No
Therapeutic Category Skeletal Muscle Relaxant
Use Adjunct to general anesthesia, to provide skeletal muscle relaxation during surgery and to provide skeletal muscle relaxation for endotracheal intubation; recommended only for procedures anticipated to last 90 minutes or longer
Usual Dosage I.V.:

Children:

3 months to 1 year: Adult dosage

1-14 years: May be less sensitive to effects

Adults: Dose is individualized based on ideal body weight, ranges are 85-100 mcg/kg initially to a maintenance dose of 5-25 mcg/kg

Nursing/Pharmacy Information Not recommended for dilution into or administration from large volume I.V. solutions
Dosage Forms Injection, as bromide: 10 mg (10 mL)

piperacillin (pi PER a sil in)

U.S. Brand Names Pipracil®
Generic Available No
Therapeutic Category Penicillin •
Use Treatment of serious infections caused by susceptible strains of gram-positive, gram-negative, and anaerobic bacilli; mixed aerobic-anaerobic bacterial infections or empiric antibiotic therapy in granulocytopenic patients. Its primary use is in the treatment of serious carbenicillin-resistant or ticarcillin-resistant *Pseudomonas aeruginosa* infections susceptible to piperacillin.
Usual Dosage

Infants and Children: I.M., I.V.: 200-300 mg/kg/day in divided doses every 4-6 hours; maximum dose: 24 g/day

Higher doses have been used in cystic fibrosis: 350-500 mg/kg/day in divided doses every 4 hours

Adults:

I.M.: 2-3 g/dose every 6-12 hours I.M.; maximum 24 g/24 hours

I.V.: 3-4 g/dose every 4-6 hours; maximum 24 g/24 hours

Nursing/Pharmacy Information

Administer one hour apart from aminoglycosides; extended spectrum includes *Pseudomonas aeruginosa*; dosage modification required in patients with impaired renal function; can be administered I.V. push over 3-5 minutes at a maximum concentration of 200 mg/mL or I.V. intermittent infusion over 30-60 minutes at a final concentration ≤20 mg/mL

Monitor serum electrolytes, bleeding time especially in patients with renal impairment, periodic tests of renal, hepatic and hematologic function

Stability: Reconstituted solution is stable (I.V. infusion) in normal saline or D_5W for 24 hours at room temperature, 7 days when refrigerated or 4 weeks when frozen; after freezing, thawed solution is stable for 24 hours at room temperature or 48 hours when refrigerated; 40 g bulk vial should **not** be frozen after reconstitution; **incompatible** with aminoglycosides

Dosage Forms Powder for injection, as sodium: 2 g, 3 g, 4 g, 40 g

piperacillin and tazobactam sodium

(pi PER a sil in & ta zoe BAK tam SOW dee um)
Synonyms tazobactam and piperacillin
U.S. Brand Names Zosyn™
Canadian Brand Names Tacozin®
Generic Available No
Therapeutic Category Penicillin
Use Treatment of infections caused by piperacillin-resistant, beta-lactamase producing strains that are piperacillin/tazobactam susceptible involving the lower respiratory tract, urinary tract, skin and skin structures, gynecologic, intra-abdominal, and septicemia. Tazobactam expands activity of piperacillin to include beta-lactamase producing strains of *S. aureus*, *H. influenzae*, *B. fragilis*, *Klebsiella*, *E. coli*, and *Acinetobacter*.
Usual Dosage Adults: I.V.: 3.375 g (3 g piperacillin/0.375 g tazobactam) every 6 hours
Nursing/Pharmacy Information

Administer 1 hour apart from aminoglycosides; administer around-the-clock (ie, 6-12-6-12)

Stability: Store at controlled room temperature; after reconstitution, stable for 24 hours at room temperature and 1 week when refrigerated; unused portions should be discarded after 24 hours at room temperature and 48 hours when refrigerated

Dosage Forms Injection: Piperacillin sodium 2 g and tazobactam sodium 0.25 g; piperacillin sodium 3 g and tazobactam sodium 0.375 g; piperacillin sodium 4 g and tazobactam sodium 0.5 g (vials at an 8:1 ratio of piperacillin sodium to tazobactam sodium)

♦ **piperazine estrone sulfate** *see* estropipate *on page 246*

♦ **piperonyl butoxide and pyrethrins** *see* pyrethrins and piperonyl butoxide *on page 533*

pipobroman (pi poe BROE man)
Generic Available No
Therapeutic Category Antineoplastic Agent
Use Treat polycythemia vera; chronic myelocytic leukemia
Usual Dosage Children >15 years and Adults: Oral:
Polycythemia: 1 mg/kg/day for 30 days; may increase to 1.5-3 mg/kg until hematocrit reduced to 50% to 55%; maintenance: 0.1-0.2 mg/kg/day
Myelocytic leukemia: 1.5-2.5 mg/kg/day until WBC drops to 10,000 mm^3 then start maintenance 7-175 mg/day; stop if WBC falls below 3000/mm^3 or platelets fall below 150,000/mm^3
Nursing/Pharmacy Information Monitor CBC, liver and kidney function tests
Dosage Forms Tablet: 25 mg

♦ **Pipracil®** *see* piperacillin *on page 496*

pirbuterol (peer BYOO ter ole)
U.S. Brand Names Maxair™ Inhalation Aerosol
Generic Available No
Therapeutic Category Adrenergic Agonist Agent
Use Prevention and treatment of reversible bronchospasm including asthma
Usual Dosage Children >12 years and Adults: 2 inhalations every 4-6 hours for prevention; 2 inhalations at an interval of at least 1-3 minutes, followed by a third inhalation in treatment of bronchospasm, not to exceed 12 inhalations/day
Nursing/Pharmacy Information
Before using, the inhaler must be shaken well; assess lung sounds, pulse, and blood pressure before administration and during peak of medication; observe patient for wheezing after administration, if this occurs, call physician
Monitor respiratory rate, heart rate, and blood pressure
Dosage Forms
Aerosol, oral, as acetate: 0.2 mg per actuation (25.6 g (300 inhalations))
Autohaler™: 0.2 mg per actuation (2.8 g (80 inhalations); 14 g (400 inhalations))

♦ **Piroxan** *see* piroxicam *on page 497*
♦ **Piroxen** *see* piroxicam *on page 497*

piroxicam (peer OKS i kam)
U.S. Brand Names Feldene®
Canadian Brand Names Apo®-Piroxicam; Novo-Piroxicam®; Nu-Pirox®; Pro-Piroxicam®
Mexican Brand Names Artyflam; Citoken; Dixonal; Facicam; Flogosan®; Oxicanol; Piroxan; Piroxen; Rogal
Generic Available Yes
Therapeutic Category Analgesic, Non-narcotic; Nonsteroidal Anti-inflammatory Drug (NSAID)
Use Management of inflammatory disorders; symptomatic treatment of acute and chronic rheumatoid arthritis, osteoarthritis, and ankylosing spondylitis; also used to treat sunburn; dysmenorrhea
Usual Dosage Oral:
Children: 0.2-0.3 mg/kg/day once daily; maximum dose: 15 mg/day
Adults: 10-20 mg/day once daily; although associated with increases in GI adverse effects, doses >20 mg/day have been used (ie, 30-40 mg/day)
Therapeutic efficacy of the drug should not be assessed for at least 2 weeks after initiation of therapy or adjustment of dosage
Dietary Considerations May be administered with food to decrease GI adverse effect
Nursing/Pharmacy Information Monitor occult blood loss, hemoglobin, hematocrit, and periodic renal and hepatic function tests; periodic ophthalmologic exams with chronic use
Dosage Forms Capsule: 10 mg, 20 mg

♦ **Pisacaina** *see* lidocaine *on page 368*

- *p*-isobutylhydratropic acid *see* ibuprofen *on page 332*
- **PIT** *see* oxytocin *on page 465*
- **Pitocin®** *see* oxytocin *on page 465*
- **Pitressin®** *see* vasopressin *on page 645*
- **Pitrex®** *see* tolnaftate *on page 618*
- **pit vipers antivenin** *see* antivenin (*Crotalidae*) polyvalent *on page 54*

pivampicillin *(Canada only)* (piv am pi SIL in)

Canadian Brand Names Pondocillin®
Generic Available No
Therapeutic Category Antibiotic, Penicillin
Use For the treatment of respiratory tract infections (including acute bronchitis, acute exacerbations of chronic bronchitis and pneumonia); ear, nose and throat infections; gynecological infections; urinary tract infections (including acute uncomplicated gonococcal urethritis) when caused by nonpenicillinase-producing susceptible strains of the following organisms: gram-positive organisms, ie, streptococci, pneumococci and staphylococci; gram-negative organisms, ie, *H. influenzae*, *N. gonorrhoeae*, *E. coli*, *P. mirabilis*.
Usual Dosage Oral
Suspension:
Infants 3 to 12 months: 40-60 mg/kg body weight daily divided into 2 equal doses
Children:
1 to 3 years: 5 mL (175 mg) twice daily
4 to 6 years: 7.5 mL (262.5 mg) twice daily
7 to 10 years: 10 mL (350 mg) twice daily
In children 10 years of age or less the dosage range is 25 to 35 mg/kg/day and should not exceed the recommended adult dose of 500 mg twice daily
Children over 10 years and adults: 15 mL (525 mg) twice daily. For severe infections: Dosage may be doubled.
Tablet: Adults and children over 10 years: 500 mg twice daily; double in severe infections
In gonococcal urethritis: 1.5 g as a single dose with 1 g probenecid concurrently
Dosage Forms
Suspension, oral: 35 mg/5 mL (100 mL, 150 mL, 200 mL)
Tablet: 500 mg (equivalent to ampicillin 377 mg)

- **pix carbonis** *see* coal tar *on page 162*
- **Placidyl®** *see* ethchlorvynol *on page 248*

plague vaccine (plaig vak SEEN)

Generic Available No
Therapeutic Category Vaccine, Inactivated Bacteria
Use Vaccination of persons at high risk exposure to plaque
Usual Dosage Three I.M. doses: First dose 1 mL, second dose (0.2 mL) 1 month later, third dose (0.2 mL) 5 months after the second dose; booster doses (0.2 mL) at 1- to 2-year intervals if exposure continues
Nursing/Pharmacy Information Federal law requires that the date of administration, the vaccine manufacturer, lot number of vaccine, and the administering person's name, title and address be entered into the patient's permanent medical record
Dosage Forms Injection: 2 mL, 20 mL

- **plantago seed** *see* psyllium *on page 531*
- **plantain seed** *see* psyllium *on page 531*
- **Plaquenil®** *see* hydroxychloroquine *on page 327*
- **Plasbumin®** *see* albumin *on page 24*
- **Plasil** *see* metoclopramide *on page 409*
- **Plasmanate®** *see* plasma protein fraction *on page 498*
- **Plasma-Plex®** *see* plasma protein fraction *on page 498*

plasma protein fraction (PLAS mah PROE teen FRAK shun)

U.S. Brand Names Plasmanate®; Plasma-Plex®; Plasmatein®; Protenate®
Generic Available No
Therapeutic Category Blood Product Derivative
Use Plasma volume expansion and maintenance of cardiac output in the treatment of certain types of shock or impending shock
Usual Dosage I.V.: 250-1500 mL/day
Nursing/Pharmacy Information 5% albumin and 5% plasma protein fraction can usually be used interchangeably

Dosage Forms Injection: 5% (50 mL, 250 mL, 500 mL)

- ◆ **Plasmatein®** see plasma protein fraction on page 498
- ◆ **Platinol®** see cisplatin on page 153
- ◆ **Platinol®-AQ** see cisplatin on page 153
- ◆ **Plavix®** see clopidogrel on page 160
- ◆ **Plegine®** see phendimetrazine on page 484
- ◆ **Plendil®** see felodipine on page 261
- ◆ **Pletal®** see cilostazol New Drug on page 150

plicamycin (plye kay MYE sin)

Synonyms mithramycin

U.S. Brand Names Mithracin®

Generic Available No

Therapeutic Category Antidote; Antineoplastic Agent

Use Malignant testicular tumors; treatment of hypercalcemia and hypercalciuria of malignancy not responsive to conventional treatment; chronic myelogenous leukemia in blast phase; Paget's disease

Usual Dosage Refer to individual protocols. Adults: I.V. (dose based on ideal body weight):

Testicular cancer: 25-50 mcg/kg/day or every other day for 5-10 days

Blastic chronic granulocytic leukemia: 25 mcg/kg over 2-4 hours every other day for 3 weeks

Paget's disease: 15 mcg/kg/day once daily for 10 days

Hypercalcemia:

25 mcg/kg single dose which may be repeated in 48 hours if no response occurs

or 25 mcg/kg/day for 3-4 days

or 25-50 mcg/kg/dose every other day for 3-8 doses

Nursing/Pharmacy Information

Rapid I.V. infusion has been associated with an increased incidence of nausea and vomiting; an antiemetic administered prior to and during plicamycin infusion may be helpful. Avoid extravasation since plicamycin is a strong vesicant. For adults, the dose should be diluted in 1 L of D_5W or NS and administered as an I.V. infusion over 4-6 hours; bolus or short infusion over 30-60 minutes in 100-150 mL D_5W is an alternative method of administration

Monitor hepatic and renal function tests, CBC, platelet count, prothrombin time, serum electrolytes

Stability: Refrigeration is recommended but drug remains stable for up to 3 months unrefrigerated; drug is unstable at a pH <4; reconstituted solution is stable for 24 hours at room temperature and 48 hours when refrigerated

Dosage Forms Powder for injection: 2.5 mg

- ◆ **PMS-Amantadine** see amantadine on page 35
- ◆ **PMS-Baclofen** see baclofen on page 72
- ◆ **PMS-Benztropine** see benztropine on page 82
- ◆ **PMS-Bethanechol Chloride** see bethanechol on page 86
- ◆ **PMS-Bisacodyl** see bisacodyl on page 88
- ◆ **PMS-Carbamazepine** see carbamazepine on page 112
- ◆ **PMS-Chloral Hydrate** see chloral hydrate on page 132
- ◆ **PMS-Cholestyramine** see cholestyramine resin on page 147
- ◆ **PMS-Clonazepam** see clonazepam on page 159
- ◆ **PMS-Cyproheptadine** see cyproheptadine on page 177
- ◆ **PMS-Desipramine** see desipramine on page 187
- ◆ **PMS-Diazepam** see diazepam on page 196
- ◆ **PMS-Dimenhydrinate** see dimenhydrinate on page 206
- ◆ **PMS-Docusate Calcium** see docusate on page 214
- ◆ **PMS-Erythromycin** see erythromycin (systemic) on page 240
- ◆ **PMS-Ferrous Sulfate** see ferrous sulfate on page 265
- ◆ **PMS-Flupam** see flurazepam on page 278
- ◆ **PMS-Fluphenazine** see fluphenazine on page 277
- ◆ **PMS-Hydromorphone** see hydromorphone on page 325
- ◆ **PMS-Hydroxyzine** see hydroxyzine on page 328
- ◆ **PMS-Imipramine** see imipramine on page 334
- ◆ **PMS-Isoniazid** see isoniazid on page 347
- ◆ **PMS-Ketoprofen** see ketoprofen on page 355
- ◆ **PMS-Lactulose** see lactulose on page 359
- ◆ **PMS-Levothyroxine Sodium** see levothyroxine on page 367
- ◆ **PMS-Lidocaine Viscous** see lidocaine on page 368

- ♦ **PMS-Lindane** *see* lindane *on page 370*
- ♦ **PMS-Loperamine** *see* loperamide *on page 374*
- ♦ **PMS-Lorazepam** *see* lorazepam *on page 375*
- ♦ **PMS-Methylphenidate** *see* methylphenidate *on page 407*
- ♦ **PMS-Nystatin** *see* nystatin *on page 452*
- ♦ **PMS-Opium & Beladonna** *see* belladonna and opium *on page 76*
- ♦ **PMS-Oxazepam** *see* oxazepam *on page 460*
- ♦ **PMS-Prochlorperazine** *see* prochlorperazine *on page 519*
- ♦ **PMS-Procyclidine** *see* procyclidine *on page 520*
- ♦ **PMS-Progesterone** *see* progesterone *on page 520*
- ♦ **PMS-Propranolol®** *see* propranolol *on page 527*
- ♦ **PMS-Pseudoephedrine** *see* pseudoephedrine *on page 530*
- ♦ **PMS-Pyrazinamide** *see* pyrazinamide *on page 532*
- ♦ **PMS-Sodium Cromoglycate** *see* cromolyn sodium *on page 171*
- ♦ **PMS-Sulfasalazine** *see* sulfasalazine *on page 587*
- ♦ **PMS-Thioridazine** *see* thioridazine *on page 608*
- ♦ **PMS-Trihexyphenidyl** *see* trihexyphenidyl *on page 628*
- ♦ **pneumococcal polysaccharide vaccine** *see* pneumococcal vaccine *on page 500*

pneumococcal vaccine (noo moe KOK al vak SEEN)

Synonyms pneumococcal polysaccharide vaccine
U.S. Brand Names Pneumovax® 23; Pnu-Imune® 23
Generic Available No
Therapeutic Category Vaccine, Inactivated Bacteria
Use Immunity to pneumococcal lobar pneumonia and bacteremia in individuals ≥2 years of age who are at high risk of morbidity and mortality from pneumococcal infection
Usual Dosage Children >2 years and Adults: I.M., S.C.: 0.5 mL
  Revaccination should be considered if ≥6 years since initial vaccination; revaccination is recommended in patients who received 14-valent pneumococcal vaccine and are at highest risk (asplenic) for fatal infection, or at ≥6 years in patients with nephrotic syndrome, renal failure, or transplant recipients, or 3-5 years in children with nephrotic syndrome, asplenia, or sickle cell disease
Nursing/Pharmacy Information
  Do not inject I.V., avoid intradermal, administer S.C. or I.M. (deltoid muscle or lateral midthigh); no dilution or reconstitution necessary
  Stability: Refrigerate
Dosage Forms Injection: 25 mcg each of 23 polysaccharide isolates/0.5 mL dose (0.5 mL, 1 mL, 5 mL)

- ♦ **Pneumomist®** *see* guaifenesin *on page 299*
- ♦ **Pneumovax® 23** *see* pneumococcal vaccine *on page 500*
- ♦ **Pnu-Imune® 23** *see* pneumococcal vaccine *on page 500*
- ♦ **Pod-Ben-25®** *see* podophyllum resin *on page 501*
- ♦ **Podocon-25™** *see* podophyllum resin *on page 501*
- ♦ **Podofilm®** *see* podophyllum resin *on page 501*

podofilox (po do FIL oks)

U.S. Brand Names Condylox®
Generic Available No
Therapeutic Category Keratolytic Agent
Use Treatment of external genital warts
Usual Dosage Adults: Topical: Apply twice daily (morning and evening) for 3 consecutive days, then withhold use for 4 consecutive days; cycle may be repeated up to 4 times until there is no visible wart tissue
Nursing/Pharmacy Information Apply to warts with a cotton-tipped applicator supplied with the drug, dispose carefully after use; allow the solution to dry before allowing the return of opposing skin surfaces to their normal positions; wash hands after application
Dosage Forms Solution, topical: 0.5% (3.5 mL)

- ♦ **Podofin®** *see* podophyllum resin *on page 501*

podophyllin and salicylic acid
  (po DOF fil um & sal i SIL ik AS id)
Synonyms salicylic acid and podophyllin
U.S. Brand Names Verrex-C&M®
Generic Available No

Therapeutic Category Keratolytic Agent

Use Topical treatment of benign growths including external genital and perianal warts, papillomas, fibroids

Usual Dosage Topical: Apply daily with applicator, allow to dry; remove necrotic tissue before each application

Dosage Forms Solution, topical: Podophyllum 10% and salicylic acid 30% with penederm 0.5% (7.5 mL)

podophyllum resin (po DOF fil um REZ in)

Synonyms mandrake; may apple

U.S. Brand Names Pod-Ben-25®; Podocon-25™; Podofin®

Canadian Brand Names Podofilm®

Generic Available Yes

Therapeutic Category Keratolytic Agent

Use Topical treatment of benign growths including external genital and perianal warts (condylomata acuminata), papillomas, fibroids

Usual Dosage Topical:

Children and Adults: 10% to 25% solution in compound benzoin tincture; apply drug to dry surface, use 1 drop at a time allowing drying between drops until area is covered; total volume should be limited to <0.5 mL per treatment session

Condylomata acuminatum: 25% solution is applied daily; use a 10% solution when applied to or near mucous membranes

Verrucae: 25% solution is applied 3-5 times/day directly to the wart

Nursing/Pharmacy Information Shake well before using; solution should be washed off within 1-4 hours for genital and perianal warts and within 1-2 hours for accessible meatal warts; use protective occlusive dressing around warts to prevent contact with unaffected skin

Dosage Forms Liquid, topical: 25% in benzoin tincture (5 mL, 7.5 mL, 30 mL)

- ◆ **Point-Two®** *see* fluoride *on page 274*
- ◆ **Poladex®** *see* dexchlorpheniramine *on page 191*
- ◆ **Polaramine®** *see* dexchlorpheniramine *on page 191*
- ◆ **Polargen®** *(Discontinued) see page 743*
- ◆ **poliomyelitis vaccine** *see* poliovirus vaccine, inactivated *on page 501*
- ◆ **Poliovax®** Injection *(Discontinued) see page 743*

poliovirus vaccine, inactivated

(POE lee oh VYE rus vak SEEN, in ak ti VAY ted)

Synonyms IPV; poliomyelitis vaccine; Salk vaccine

U.S. Brand Names IPOL™

Generic Available No

Therapeutic Category Vaccine, Live Virus and Inactivated Virus

Use Active immunization for the prevention of poliomyelitis

Usual Dosage

S.C.: 3 doses of 0.5 mL; the first 2 doses should be administered at an interval of 8 weeks; the third dose should be administered at least 6 and preferably 12 months after the second dose

Booster dose: All children who have received the 3 dose primary series in infancy and early childhood should receive a booster dose of 0.5 mL before entering school. However, if the third dose of the primary series is administered on or after the fourth birthday, a fourth (booster) dose is not required at school entry.

Nursing/Pharmacy Information Do not administer I.V.

Dosage Forms Injection, Suspension: Three types of poliovirus (Types 1, 2, and 3) grown in monkey kidney cell cultures (0.5 mL)

poliovirus vaccine, live, trivalent, oral

(POE lee oh VYE rus vak SEEN, live, try VAY lent, OR al)

Synonyms OPV; Sabin vaccine; TOPV

U.S. Brand Names Orimune®

Generic Available No

Therapeutic Category Vaccine, Live Virus

Use Poliovirus immunization

Usual Dosage Oral:

Infants: 0.5 mL dose at age 2 months, 4 months, and 18 months; optional dose may be administered at 6 months in areas where poliomyelitis is endemic

Older Children, Adolescents and Adults: Two 0.5 mL doses 8 weeks apart; third dose of 0.5 mL 6-12 months after second dose; a reinforcing dose of 0.5

(Continued)

poliovirus vaccine, live, trivalent, oral *(Continued)*

mL should be administered before entry to school, in children who received the third primary dose before their fourth birthday

Nursing/Pharmacy Information

Do not administer parenterally; administer directly or dilute with distilled water, simple syrup USP, or milk; may be administered on bread or sugar cubes

Stability: Keep in freezer; vaccine must remain frozen to retain potency

Dosage Forms Solution, oral: Mixture of type 1, 2, and 3 viruses in monkey kidney tissue (0.5 mL)

♦ **Polocaine®** *see* mepivacaine *on page 394*

♦ **Polycillin-N®** **Injection** *(Discontinued) see page 743*

♦ **Polycillin®** **Oral** *(Discontinued) see page 743*

♦ **Polycillin-PRB®** *(Discontinued) see page 743*

♦ **Polycitra®** *see* sodium citrate and potassium citrate mixture *on page 572*

♦ **Polycitra®-K** *see* potassium citrate and citric acid *on page 508*

♦ **Polycose®** **[OTC]** *see* glucose polymers *on page 293*

♦ **Polydine®** **[OTC]** *see* povidone-iodine *on page 510*

polyestradiol *(pol i es tra DYE ole)*

Generic Available No

Therapeutic Category Estrogen Derivative

Use Palliative treatment of advanced, inoperable carcinoma of the prostate

Usual Dosage Adults: I.M.: 40 mg every 2-4 weeks or less frequently

Nursing/Pharmacy Information

Women should inform their physicians if signs or symptoms of any of the following occur: thromboembolic or thrombotic disorders including sudden severe headache or vomiting, disturbance of vision or speech, loss of vision, numbness or weakness in an extremity, sharp or crushing chest pain, calf pain, shortness of breath, severe abdominal pain or mass, mental depression or unusual bleeding; women should discontinue taking the medication if they suspect they are pregnant or become pregnant

Stability: After reconstitution, solution is stable for 10 days at room temperature and protected from direct light

Dosage Forms Powder for injection, as phosphate: 40 mg

polyethylene glycol-electrolyte solution

(pol i ETH i leen GLY kol ee LEK troe lite soe LOO shun)

Synonyms electrolyte lavage solution; PEG-ES

U.S. Brand Names Co-Lav®; Colovage®; CoLyte®; CoLyte®-Flavored; Go-Evac®; GoLYTELY®; NuLYTELY®; OCL®

Canadian Brand Names Klean-Prep®; Peglyte™

Generic Available No

Therapeutic Category Laxative

Use For bowel cleansing prior to GI examination

Usual Dosage The recommended dose for adults is 4 L of solution prior to gastrointestinal examination, as ingestion of this dose produces a satisfactory preparation in >95% of patients. The solution is usually administered orally, but may be administered via nasogastric tube to patients who are unwilling or unable to drink the solution.

Children: Oral: 25-40 mL/kg/hour for 4-10 hours

Adults:

Oral: At a rate of 240 mL (8 oz) every 10 minutes, until 4 liters are consumed or the rectal effluent is clear; rapid drinking of each portion is preferred to drinking small amounts continuously

Nasogastric tube: At the rate of 20-30 mL/minute (1.2-1.8 L/hour); the first bowel movement should occur approximately one hour after the start of administration

Dietary Considerations Ideally the patient should fast for approximately 3-4 hours prior to administration, but in no case should solid food be given for at least 2 hours before the solution is given

Nursing/Pharmacy Information

Rapid drinking of each portion is preferred over small amounts continuously; first bowel movement should occur in one hour

Monitor electrolytes, serum glucose, BUN, urine osmolality

Stability: Use within 48 hours of preparation; refrigerate reconstituted solution; tap water may be used for preparation of the solution; shake container vigorously several times to ensure dissolution of powder

Dosage Forms Powder, for oral solution: PEG 3350 236 g, sodium sulfate 22.74 g, sodium bicarbonate 6.74 g, sodium chloride 5.86 g and potassium chloride 2.97 g (2000 mL, 4000 mL, 4800 mL, 6000 mL)

- ♦ **Polyflex® Tablet** *(Discontinued) see page 743*
- ♦ **Polygam® Injection** *(Discontinued) see page 743*
- ♦ **Polygam® S/D** *see immune globulin, intravenous on page 336*
- ♦ **Poly-Histine CS®** *see brompheniramine, phenylpropanolamine, and codeine on page 95*
- ♦ **Poly-Histine-D® Capsule** *see phenyltoloxamine, phenylpropanolamine, pyrilamine, and pheniramine on page 490*
- ♦ **Polymox®** *(Discontinued) see page 743*
- ♦ **polymyxin B and bacitracin** *see bacitracin and polymyxin B on page 71*

polymyxin B and hydrocortisone
(pol i MIKS in bee & hye droe KOR ti sone)
Synonyms hydrocortisone and polymyxin B
U.S. Brand Names Otobiotic® Otic
Generic Available No
Therapeutic Category Antibiotic/Corticosteroid, Otic
Use Treatment of superficial bacterial infections of external ear canal
Usual Dosage Otic: Instill 4 drops 3-4 times/day
Dosage Forms Solution, otic: Polymyxin B sulfate 10,000 units and hydrocortisone 0.5% [5 mg/mL] per mL (10 mL, 15 mL)

- ♦ **polymyxin B and neomycin** *see neomycin and polymyxin B on page 436*
- ♦ **polymyxin B and oxytetracycline** *see oxytetracycline and polymyxin B on page 465*
- ♦ **polymyxin B and trimethoprim** *see trimethoprim and polymyxin B on page 630*
- ♦ **polymyxin B, bacitracin, and neomycin** *see bacitracin, neomycin, and polymyxin B on page 71*
- ♦ **polymyxin B, bacitracin, neomycin, and hydrocortisone** *see bacitracin, neomycin, polymyxin B, and hydrocortisone on page 72*
- ♦ **polymyxin B, neomycin, and dexamethasone** *see neomycin, polymyxin B, and dexamethasone on page 436*
- ♦ **polymyxin B, neomycin, and gramicidin** *see neomycin, polymyxin B, and gramicidin on page 437*
- ♦ **polymyxin B, neomycin, and hydrocortisone** *see neomycin, polymyxin B, and hydrocortisone on page 437*
- ♦ **polymyxin B, neomycin, and prednisolone** *see neomycin, polymyxin B, and prednisolone on page 438*
- ♦ **Poly-Pred® Ophthalmic Suspension** *see neomycin, polymyxin B, and prednisolone on page 438*

polysaccharide-iron complex
(pol i SAK a ride-EYE ern KOM pleks)
U.S. Brand Names Hytinic® [OTC]; Niferex® [OTC]; Nu-Iron® [OTC]
Generic Available Yes
Therapeutic Category Electrolyte Supplement, Oral
Use Prevention and treatment of iron deficiency anemias
Usual Dosage Oral:
Children: 3 mg/kg 3 times/day
Adults: 200 mg 3-4 times/day
Nursing/Pharmacy Information 100% elemental iron
Dosage Forms
Capsule: Elemental iron 150 mg
Elixir: Elemental iron 100 mg/5 mL (240 mL)
Tablet: Elemental iron 50 mg

- ♦ **Polysporin® Ophthalmic** *see bacitracin and polymyxin B on page 71*
- ♦ **Polysporin® Topical** *see bacitracin and polymyxin B on page 71*
- ♦ **Polytar® [OTC]** *see coal tar on page 162*

polythiazide (pol i THYE a zide)
U.S. Brand Names Renese®
Generic Available No
Therapeutic Category Diuretic, Thiazide
Use Adjunctive therapy in treatment of edema and hypertension
Usual Dosage Adults: Oral: 1-4 mg/day
(Continued)

polythiazide *(Continued)*

Nursing/Pharmacy Information Monitor blood pressure, fluids, weight loss, serum potassium

Dosage Forms Tablet: 1 mg, 2 mg, 4 mg

- ♦ **polythiazide and prazosin** *see* prazosin and polythiazide *on page 513*
- ♦ **Polytopic®** *see* bacitracin and polymyxin B *on page 71*
- ♦ **Polytracin®** *see* bacitracin and polymyxin B *on page 71*
- ♦ **Polytrim® Ophthalmic** *see* trimethoprim and polymyxin B *on page 630*
- ♦ **Poly-Vi-Flor®** *see* vitamin, multiple (pediatric) *on page 654*
- ♦ **polyvinyl alcohol** *see* artificial tears *on page 59*
- ♦ **Poly-Vi-Sol® [OTC]** *see* vitamin, multiple (pediatric) *on page 654*
- ♦ **Pondimin® *(Discontinued)*** *see page 743*
- ♦ **Pondocillin®** *see* pivampicillin *(Canada only) on page 498*
- ♦ **Ponstan®** *see* mefenamic acid *on page 389*
- ♦ **Ponstel®** *see* mefenamic acid *on page 389*
- ♦ **Pontocaine®** *see* tetracaine *on page 600*
- ♦ **Pontocaine® With Dextrose** *see* tetracaine and dextrose *on page 601*
- ♦ **Porcelana® [OTC]** *see* hydroquinone *on page 325*
- ♦ **Porcelana® Sunscreen [OTC]** *see* hydroquinone *on page 325*

porfimer *(POR fi mer)*

U.S. Brand Names Photofrin®

Generic Available No

Therapeutic Category Antineoplastic Agent

Use Esophageal cancer: Photodynamic therapy (PDT) with porfimer for palliation of patients with completely obstructing esophageal cancer, or of patients with partially obstructing esophageal cancer who cannot be satisfactorily treated with Nd:YAG laser therapy; early-stage lung cancer (endobronchial microinvasive nonsmall cell)

Usual Dosage I.V. (refer to individual protocols):

Children: Safety and efficacy have not been established

Adults: I.V.: 2 mg/kg over 3-5 minutes

Photodynamic therapy is a two-stage process requiring administration of both drug and light. The first stage of PDT is the I.V. injection of porfimer. Illumination with laser light 40-50 hours following the injection with porfimer constitutes the second stage of therapy. A second laser light application may be administered 90-120 hours after injection, preceded by gentle debridement of residual tumor.

Patients may receive a second course of PDT a minimum of 30 days after the initial therapy; up to three courses of PDT (each separated by a minimum of 30 days) can be given. Before each course of treatment, evaluate patients for the presence of a tracheoesophageal or bronchoesophageal fistula.

Dosage Forms Powder for injection, as sodium: 75 mg

- ♦ **Pork NPH** *see* insulin preparations *on page 339*
- ♦ **Pork Regular Iletin® II** *see* insulin preparations *on page 339*
- ♦ **Portagen® [OTC]** *see* enteral nutritional products *on page 233*
- ♦ **Posicor® *(Discontinued)*** *see page 743*
- ♦ **Posipen** *see* dicloxacillin *on page 199*
- ♦ **Posture® [OTC]** *see* calcium phosphate, dibasic *on page 107*
- ♦ **Potasalan®** *see* potassium chloride *on page 506*

potassium acetate *(poe TASS ee um AS e tate)*

Generic Available Yes

Therapeutic Category Electrolyte Supplement, Oral

Use Potassium deficiency, treatment of hypokalemia, correction of metabolic acidosis through conversion of acetate to bicarbonate

Usual Dosage I.V. infusion:

Children: Not to exceed 3 mEq/kg/day

Adults: Up to 150 mEq/day administered at a rate up to 20 mEq/hour; maximum concentration: 40 mEq/L

Nursing/Pharmacy Information

Parenteral: Potassium must be diluted prior to parenteral administration; maximum recommended concentration (peripheral line): 80 mEq/L; maximum recommended concentration (central line): 150 mEq/L or 15 mEq/100 mL; in severely fluid-restricted patients (with central lines): 200 mEq/L or 20 mEq/100 mL has been used; maximum rate of infusion

Monitor serum potassium, glucose, bicarbonate, pH, urine output (if indicated), cardiac monitor (if intermittent infusion or potassium infusion rates of >0.25 mEq/kg/hour)

Dosage Forms Injection: 2 mEq/mL (20 mL, 50 mL, 100 mL); 4 mEq/mL (50 mL)

potassium acetate, potassium bicarbonate, and potassium citrate

(poe TASS ee um AS e tate, poe TASS ee um bye KAR bun ate, & poe TASS ee um SIT rate)

U.S. Brand Names Tri-K®

Generic Available Yes

Therapeutic Category Electrolyte Supplement, Oral

Use Treatment or prevention of hypokalemia

Usual Dosage Oral:

Children: 1-4 mEq/kg/24 hours in divided doses as required to maintain normal serum potassium

Adults:

Prevention: 16-24 mEq/day in 2-4 divided doses

Treatment: 40-100 mEq/day in 2-4 divided doses

Dosage Forms Solution, oral: 45 mEq/15 mL from potassium acetate 1500 mg, potassium bicarbonate 1500 mg, and potassium citrate 1500 mg per 15 mL

potassium acid phosphate (poe TASS ee um AS id FOS fate)

U.S. Brand Names K-Phos® Original

Generic Available No

Therapeutic Category Urinary Acidifying Agent

Use Acidify the urine and lower urinary calcium concentration; reduces odor and rash caused by ammoniacal urine

Usual Dosage Adults: Oral: 1000 mg dissolved in 6-8 oz of water 4 times/day with meals and at bedtime

Dietary Considerations May be administered with meals

Nursing/Pharmacy Information Monitor renal function, electrolytes, calcium, phosphorus, serum potassium

Dosage Forms Tablet, sodium free: 500 mg [potassium 3.67 mEq]

potassium bicarbonate (poe TASS ee um bye KAR bun ate)

U.S. Brand Names K+ Care® Effervescent; K-Electrolyte® Effervescent; K-Gen® Effervescent; K-Lyte® Effervescent

Generic Available No

Therapeutic Category Electrolyte Supplement, Oral

Use Potassium deficiency, hypokalemia

Usual Dosage Oral:

Normal daily requirements:

Children: 2-3 mEq/kg/day

Adults: 40-80 mEq/day

Prevention during diuretic therapy:

Children: 1-2 mEq/kg/day in 1-2 divided doses

Adults: 20-40 mEq/day in 1-2 divided doses

Treatment of hypokalemia: Children: 1-2 mEq/kg initially, then as needed based on frequently obtained lab values. If deficits are severe or ongoing losses are great, I.V. route should be considered.

Treatment of hypokalemia: Adults:

Potassium >2.5 mEq/L: 60-80 mEq/day plus additional amounts if needed

Potassium <2.5 mEq/L: Up to 40-60 mEq initial dose, followed by further doses based on lab values; deficits at a plasma level of 2 mEq/L may be as high as 400-800 mEq of potassium

Dosage Forms

Tablet for oral solution, effervescent: 6.5 mEq, 25 mEq

K+ Care® Effervescent; K-Electrolyte® Effervescent; K-Gen® Effervescent; K-Ide®; Klor-Con®/EF; K-Lyte® Effervescent: 25 mEq

potassium bicarbonate and potassium chloride, effervescent

(poe TASS ee um bye KAR bun ate & poe TASS ee um KLOR ide, ef er VES ent)

U.S. Brand Names Klorvess® Effervescent; K/Lyte/CL®

Generic Available Yes

Therapeutic Category Electrolyte Supplement, Oral

Use Treatment or prevention of hypokalemia

(Continued)

potassium bicarbonate and potassium chloride, effervescent *(Continued)*

Usual Dosage Oral:
Children: 1-4 mEq/kg/24 hours in divided doses as required to maintain normal serum potassium
Adults:
Prevention: 16-24 mEq/day in 2-4 divided doses
Treatment: 40-100 mEq/day in 2-4 divided doses
Nursing/Pharmacy Information Dissolve completely in 3-8 oz cold water, juice, or other suitable beverage and drink slowly
Dosage Forms
Granules for oral solution, effervescent (Klorvess®): 20 mEq per packet
Tablet for oral solution, effervescent
Klorvess®: 20 mEq per packet
K/Lyte/Cl®: 25 mEq, 50 mEq per packet

potassium bicarbonate and potassium citrate, effervescent

(poe TASS ee um bye KAR bun ate & poe TASS ee um SIT rate, ef er VES ent)
Synonyms potassium citrate and potassium bicarbonate, effervescent
U.S. Brand Names Effer-K™; K-Ide®; Klor-Con®/EF; K-Lyte®; K-Vescent®
Generic Available No
Therapeutic Category Electrolyte Supplement, Oral
Use Treatment or prevention of hypokalemia
Usual Dosage Oral:
Children: 1-4 mEq/kg/24 hours as required to maintain normal serum potassium
Adults:
Prevention: 16-24 mEq/day in 2-4 divided doses
Treatment: 40-100 mEq/day in 2-4 divided doses
Nursing/Pharmacy Information Monitor serum potassium
Dosage Forms
Capsule, extended release: 8 mEq, 10 mEq
Powder for oral solution: 15 mEq/packet; 20 mEq/packet; 25 mEq/packet
Tablet, effervescent: 25 mEq, 50 mEq

potassium bicarbonate, potassium chloride, and potassium citrate

(poe TASS ee um bye KAR bun ate, poe TASS ee um KLOR ide & poe TASS ee um SIT rate)
U.S. Brand Names Kaochlor-Eff®
Generic Available Yes
Therapeutic Category Electrolyte Supplement, Oral
Use Treatment or prevention of hypokalemia
Usual Dosage Oral:
Children: 1-4 mEq/kg/24 hours in divided doses as required to maintain normal serum potassium
Adults:
Prevention: 16-24 mEq/day in 2-4 divided doses
Treatment: 40-100 mEq/day in 2-4 divided doses
Dosage Forms Tablet for oral solution: 20 mEq from potassium bicarbonate 1 g, potassium chloride 600 mg, and potassium citrate 220 mg

potassium chloride (poe TASS ee um KLOR ide)

Synonyms KCl
U.S. Brand Names Cena-K®; Gen-K®; K+ 10®; Kaochlor®; Kaochlor® SF; Kaon-Cl®; Kaon-Cl-10®; Kay Ciel®; K+ Care®; K-Dur® 10; K-Dur® 20; K-Lease®; K-Lor™; Klor-Con®; Klor-Con® 8; Klor-Con® 10; Klor-Con®/25; Klorvess®; Klotrix®; K-Lyte®/Cl; K-Norm®; K-Tab®; Micro-K® 10; Micro-K® 10 Extencaps®; Micro-K® LS; Potasalan®; Rum-K®; Slow-K®; Ten-K®
Generic Available Yes
Therapeutic Category Electrolyte Supplement, Oral
Use Potassium deficiency, treatment or prevention of hypokalemia
Usual Dosage I.V. doses should be incorporated into the patient's maintenance I.V. fluids, intermittent I.V. potassium administration should be reserved for severe depletion situations in patients undergoing EKG monitoring.

Normal daily requirement: Oral, I.V.:
  Newborns: 2-6 mEq/kg/day
  Children: 2-3 mEq/kg/day
  Adults: 40-80 mEq/day
Prevention during diuretic therapy: Oral:
  Children: 1-2 mEq/kg/day in 1-2 divided doses
  Adults: 20-40 mEq/day in 1-2 divided doses
Treatment: Oral, I.V.:
  Children: 2-3 mEq/kg/day
  Adults: 40-100 mEq/day
I.V. intermittent infusion:
  Children: Dose should not exceed 0.5 mEq/kg/hour, not to exceed 20 mEq/hour
  Adults: 10-20 mEq/hour, not to exceed 40 mEq/hour and 150 mEq/day

Dietary Considerations Administer with plenty of fluid and/or food because of stomach irritation and discomfort

Nursing/Pharmacy Information

Oral liquid potassium supplements should be diluted with water or fruit juice during administration; wax matrix tablets must be swallowed and not allowed to dissolve in mouth; must be diluted prior to parenteral administration; maximum recommended concentration (peripheral line): 80 mEq/L; maximum recommended concentration (central line): 150 mEq/L or 15 mEq/100 mL; in severely fluid-restricted patients (with central lines): 200 mEq/L or 20 mEq/100 mL has been used; maximum rate of infusion

Monitor serum potassium, EKG

Stability: Store at room temperature, protect from freezing; use only clear solutions; use admixtures within 24 hours

Dosage Forms

Capsule, controlled release (microcapsulated): 600 mg [8 mEq]; 750 mg [10 mEq]
  Micro-K® Extencaps®: 600 mg [8 mEq]
  K-Lease®, K-Norm®, Micro-K® 10: 750 mg [10 mEq]
Crystals for oral suspension, extended release (Micro-K® LS®): 20 mEq per packet
Infusion, concentrate: 0.1 mEq/mL, 0.2 mEq/mL, 0.3 mEq/mL, 0.4 mEq/mL
Injection, concentrate: 1.5 mEq/mL, 2 mEq/mL, 3 mEq/mL
Liquid: 10% [20 mEq/15 mL] (480 mL, 4000 mL); 20% [40 mEq/15 mL] (480 mL, 4000 mL)
  Cena-K®, Kaochlor®, Kaochlor® SF, Kay Ciel®, Klorvess®, Potasalan®: 10% [20 mEq/15 mL] (480 mL, 4000 mL)
  Rum-K®: 15% [30 mEq/15 mL] (480 mL, 4000 mL)
  Cena-K®, Kaon-Cl® 20%: 20% [40 mEq/15 mL]
Powder: 20 mEq per packet (30s, 100s)
  K+ Care®, K-Lor™: 15 mEq per packet (30s, 100s)
  Gen-K®, Kay Ciel®, K+ Care®, K-Lor™, Klor-Con®: 20 mEq per packet (30s, 100s)
  K+ Care®, Klor-Con/25®: 25 mEq per packet (30s, 100s)
  K-Lyte/Cl®: 25 mEq per dose (30s)
Tablet, controlled release (microencapsulated)
  K-Dur® 10, Ten-K®: 750 mg [10 mEq]
  K-Dur® 20: 1500 mg [20 mEq]
Tablet, controlled release (wax matrix): 600 mg [8 mEq]; 750 mg [10 mEq]
  Kaon-Cl®: 500 mg [6.7 mEq]
  Klor-Con® 8, Slow-K®: 600 mg [8 mEq]
  K+ 10®, Kaon-Cl-10®, Klor-Con® 10, Klotrix®, K-Tab®: 750 mg [10 mEq]

potassium chloride and potassium gluconate
(poe TASS ee um KLOR ide & poe TASS ee um GLOO coe nate)
Generic Available Yes
Therapeutic Category Electrolyte Supplement, Oral
Use Treatment or prevention of hypokalemia
Usual Dosage Oral:
  Children: 1-4 mEq/kg/24 hours in divided doses as required to maintain normal serum potassium
  Adults:
    Prevention: 16-24 mEq/day in 2-4 divided doses
    Treatment: 40-100 mEq/day in 2-4 divided doses
Dosage Forms Solution, oral: Potassium 20 mEq/15 mL

potassium citrate (poe TASS ee um SIT rate)
U.S. Brand Names Urocit®-K
Generic Available Yes
Therapeutic Category Alkalinizing Agent
Use Prevention of uric acid nephrolithiasis; prevention of calcium renal stones in patients with hypocitraturia; urinary alkalinizer when sodium citrate is contraindicated
Usual Dosage Adults: Oral: 10-20 mEq 3 times/day with meals, up to 100 mEq/day
Dietary Considerations May be administered with meals
Nursing/Pharmacy Information Swallow tablets whole with a full glass of water; intact wax matrix may appear in the feces
Dosage Forms Tablet: 540 mg [5 mEq], 1080 mg [10 mEq]

potassium citrate and citric acid
(poe TASS ee um SIT rate & SI trik AS id)
Synonyms citric acid and potassium citrate
U.S. Brand Names Polycitra®-K
Generic Available No
Therapeutic Category Alkalinizing Agent
Use Treatment of metabolic acidosis; alkalinizing agent in conditions where long-term maintenance of an alkaline urine is desirable
Usual Dosage Oral:
Mild to moderate hypocitraturia: 10 mEq 3 times/day with meals
Severe hypocitraturia: Initial: 20 mEq 3 times/day or 15 mEq 4 times/day with meals or within 30 minutes after meals; do not exceed 100 mEq/day
Nursing/Pharmacy Information Potassium citrate 3.4 mmol/5 mL and citric acid 1.6 mmol/5 mL = total of 5.0 mmol/5 mL citrate content
Dosage Forms
Crystals for reconstitution: Potassium citrate 3300 mg and citric acid 1002 mg per packet
Solution, oral: Potassium citrate 1100 mg and citric acid 334 mg per 5 mL

♦ **potassium citrate and potassium bicarbonate, effervescent** *see* potassium bicarbonate and potassium citrate, effervescent *on page 506*

potassium citrate and potassium gluconate
(poe TASS ee um SIT rate & poe TASS ee um GLOO coe nate)
U.S. Brand Names Twin-K®
Generic Available Yes
Therapeutic Category Electrolyte Supplement, Oral
Use Treatment or prevention of hypokalemia
Usual Dosage Oral:
Children: 1-4 mEq/kg/24 hours in divided doses as required to maintain normal serum potassium
Adults:
Prevention: 16-24 mEq/day in 2-4 divided doses
Treatment: 40-100 mEq/day in 2-4 divided doses
Dosage Forms Solution, oral: 20 mEq/5 mL from potassium citrate 170 mg and potassium gluconate 170 mg per 5 mL

potassium gluconate (poe TASS ee um GLOO coe nate)
U.S. Brand Names Kaon®; K-G®
Generic Available Yes
Therapeutic Category Electrolyte Supplement, Oral
Use Treatment or prevention of hypokalemia
Usual Dosage Oral:
Normal daily requirement:
Children: 2-3 mEq/kg/day
Adults: 40-80 mEq/day
Prevention during diuretic therapy:
Children: 1-2 mEq/kg/day in 1-2 divided doses
Adults: 20-40 mEq/day in 1-2 divided doses
Treatment of hypokalemia:
Children: 2-3 mEq/kg/day in 2-4 divided doses
Adults: 40-100 mEq/day in 2-4 divided doses
Nursing/Pharmacy Information
Do not administer liquid full strength, must be diluted in 2-6 parts of water or juice
Monitor serum potassium, EKG

Stability: Store at room temperature, protect from freezing; use only clear solutions

Dosage Forms
Elixir: 20 mEq/15 mL
K-G®, Kaon®, Kaylixir®: 20 mEq/15 mL
Tablet:
Glu-K®: 2 mEq
Kaon®: 5 mEq

potassium iodide (poe TASS ee um EYE oh dide)

Synonyms KI; Lugol's solution; strong iodine solution
U.S. Brand Names Pima®; SSKI®; Thyro-Block®
Generic Available Yes
Therapeutic Category Antithyroid Agent; Expectorant
Use Facilitate bronchial drainage and cough; to reduce thyroid vascularity prior to thyroidectomy and management of thyrotoxic crisis; block thyroidal uptake of radioactive isotopes of iodine in a radiation emergency
Usual Dosage Oral:
Adults RDA: 130 mcg
Expectorant:
Children: 60-250 mg every 6-8 hours; maximum single dose: 500 mg
Adults: 300-1000 mg 2-3 times/day, may increase to 1-1.5 g 3 times/day
Preoperative thyroidectomy: Children and Adults: 50-250 mg 3 times/day (2-6 drops strong iodine solution); administer for 10 days before surgery
Thyrotoxic crisis:
Infants <1 year: ½ adult dosage
Children and Adults: 300 mg = 6 drops SSKI® every 8 hours
Graves' disease in neonates: 1 drop of Lugol's solution every 8 hours
Sporotrichosis:
Initial:
Preschool: 50 mg/dose 3 times/day
Children: 250 mg/dose 3 times/day
Adults: 500 mg/dose 3 times/day
Oral increase 50 mg/dose daily
Maximum dose:
Preschool: 500 mg/dose 3 times/day
Children and Adults: 1-2 g/dose 3 times/day
Continue treatment for 4-6 weeks after lesions have completely healed
Nursing/Pharmacy Information
Monitor thyroid function tests
Stability: Store in tight, light-resistant containers at temperature <40°C; freezing should be avoided
Dosage Forms
Solution, oral:
SSKI®: 1 g/mL (30 mL, 240 mL, 473 mL)
Lugol's solution, strong iodine: 100 mg/mL with iodine 50 mg/mL (120 mL)
Syrup: 325 mg/5 mL
Tablet: 130 mg

potassium phosphate (poe TASS ee um FOS fate)

U.S. Brand Names Neutra-Phos®-K
Generic Available Yes
Therapeutic Category Electrolyte Supplement, Oral
Use Treatment and prevention of hypophosphatemia
Usual Dosage I.V. doses should be incorporated into the patient's maintenance I.V. fluids; intermittent I.V. infusion should be reserved for severe depletion situations and requires continuous cardiac monitoring. It is difficult to determine total body phosphorus deficit, the following dosages are empiric guidelines: **Note:** Doses listed as mmol of **phosphate:**

Replacement intermittent infusion: I.V.:
Children:
Low dose: 0.08 mmol/kg over 6 hours; use if recent losses and uncomplicated
Intermediate dose: 0.16-0.24 mmol/kg over 4-6 hours; use if serum phosphorus level 0.5-1 mg/dL
High dose: 0.36 mmol/kg over 6 hours; use if serum phosphorus <0.5 mg/dL
Adults: Varying dosages: 0.15-0.3 mmol/kg/dose over 12 hours; may repeat as needed to achieve desired serum level **or**
15 mmol/dose over 2 hours; use if serum phosphorus <2 mg/dL **or**
(Continued)

509

potassium phosphate *(Continued)*

Low dose: 0.16 mmol/kg over 4-6 hours; use if serum phosphorus level 2.3-3 mg/dL

Intermediate dose: 0.32 mmol/kg over 4-6 hours; use if serum phosphorus level 1.6-2.2 mg/dL

High dose: 0.64 mmol/kg over 8-12 hours; use if serum phosphorus <1.5 mg/dL

Maintenance:

Children: 0.5-1.5 mmol/kg/24 hours I.V. or 2-3 mmol/kg/24 hours orally in divided doses

Adults: 50-70 mmol/24 hours I.V. or 50-150 mmol/24 hours orally in divided doses

Dietary Considerations Avoid administering with oxalate (berries, nuts, chocolate, beans, celery, tomato) or phytate (bran, whole wheat) containing foods

Nursing/Pharmacy Information

Contents of one capsule should be diluted in 75 mL water before administration; for intermittent infusion, if peripheral line, dilute to a maximum concentration of 0.05 mmol/mL; if central line, dilute to a maximum concentration of 0.12 mmol/mL; maximum rate of infusion: 0.06 mmol/kg/hour; do **not** infuse with calcium containing IV. fluids (ie, TPN)

Monitor serum potassium, phosphate, EKG

Stability: Store at room temperature, protect from freezing; use only clear solutions; up to 10-15 mEq of calcium may be added per liter before precipitate may occur

Stability of parenteral admixture at room temperature (25°C): 24 hours

Dosage Forms

Capsule: Neutra-Phos®-K: Phosphorus 250 mg [8 mmol] and potassium 556 mg [14.25 mEq] per capsule

Injection: Potassium phosphate monobasic anhydrous 224 mg and potassium phosphate dibasic anhydrous 236 mg per mL; [phosphorus 3 mmol and potassium 4.4 mEq per mL] (15 mL)

Powder: Neutra-Phos®-K: Phosphorus 250 mg [8 mmol] and potassium 556 mg [14.25 mEq] per packet

potassium phosphate and sodium phosphate

(poe TASS ee um FOS fate & SOW dee um FOS fate)

Synonyms sodium phosphate and potassium phosphate

U.S. Brand Names K-Phos® Neutral; Uro-KP-Neutral®

Generic Available Yes

Therapeutic Category Electrolyte Supplement, Oral

Use Treatment of conditions associated with excessive renal phosphate loss or inadequate GI absorption of phosphate

Usual Dosage All dosage forms to be mixed in 6-8 oz of water prior to administration

Children: 2-3 mmol phosphate/kg/24 hours administered 4 times/day

Adults: 100-150 mmol phosphate/24 hours in divided doses after meals and at bedtime; 1-8 tablets or capsules/day, administered 4 times/day

Dietary Considerations Should be administered after meals

Nursing/Pharmacy Information

Tablets may be crushed and stirred vigorously to speed dissolution

Monitor renal function, serum calcium and phosphorus, electrolytes

Dosage Forms

Capsule (Neutra-Phos®): Phosphorus 8 mmol, potassium 14.25 mEq

Powder, concentrate: Phosphate 8 mmol, sodium 7.125 mEq, and potassium 7.125 mEq per 75 mL when reconstituted

Tablet: Phosphate 8 mmol, sodium 13 mEq, and potassium 1.1 mEq (114 mg of phosphorus)

povidone-iodine (POE vi done EYE oh dyne)

U.S. Brand Names ACU-dyne® [OTC]; Aerodine® [OTC]; Betadine® [OTC]; Betadine® 5% Sterile Ophthalmic Prep Solution; Betagan® [OTC]; Biodine [OTC]; Efodine® [OTC]; Iodex® [OTC]; Iodex-p® [OTC]; Mallisol® [OTC]; Massengill® Medicated Douche w/Cepticin [OTC]; Minidyne® [OTC]; Operand® [OTC]; Polydine® [OTC]; Summer's Eve® Medicated Douche [OTC]; Yeast-Gard® Medicated Douche

Generic Available Yes

Therapeutic Category Antibacterial, Topical

Use External antiseptic with broad microbicidal spectrum against bacteria, fungi, viruses, protozoa, and yeasts

Usual Dosage Apply as needed for treatment and prevention of susceptible microbial infections

Nursing/Pharmacy Information Avoid contact with eyes

Dosage Forms

Aerosol: 5% (90 mL)

Cleanser, topical: 7.5% (30 mL, 120 mL)

Concentrate:

Whirlpool: 10% (3840 mL)

Perineal wash: 10% (240 mL)

Douche: 10% [0.3% when reconstituted]

Foam, topical: 10% (250 g)

Gel, vaginal: 10% (3 oz)

Mouthwash: 0.5% (180 mL)

Ointment, topical: 10% (0.9 g foil packet, 0.94 g, 28 g, 480 g)

Pads, antiseptic gauze: 10% (3" x 9", 5" x 9")

Scrub, surgical: 7.5% (480 mL, 946 mL)

Shampoo: 7.5% (120 mL)

Solution:

Ophthalmic, sterile prep: 5% (50 mL)

Swab aid: 10% (100s)

Swabsticks, 4": 10%

Topical: 10% (240 mL, 480 mL, 946 mL)

Suppository, vaginal: 10%

♦ **PPA** see phenylpropanolamine on page 489

♦ **PPD** see tuberculin tests on page 635

♦ **PPL** see benzylpenicilloyl-polylysine on page 82

♦ **PPS** see pentosan polysulfate sodium on page 480

pralidoxime (pra li DOKS eem)

Synonyms 2-PAM; 2-pyridine aldoxime methochloride

U.S. Brand Names Protopam® Injection

Generic Available No

Therapeutic Category Antidote

Use Reverse muscle paralysis associated with toxic exposure to organophosphate anticholinesterase pesticides and chemicals; control of overdosage by anticholinesterase drugs used to treat myasthenia gravis

Usual Dosage Poisoning: I.V.:

Children: 20-50 mg/kg/dose; repeat in 1-2 hours if muscle weakness has not been relieved, then at 10- to 12-hour intervals if cholinergic signs recur

Adults: 1-2 g; repeat in 1-2 hours if muscle weakness has not been relieved, then at 10- to 12-hour intervals if cholinergic signs recur

Nursing/Pharmacy Information

Parenteral: Reconstitute with 20 mL sterile water (preservative free) resulting in 50 mg/mL solution; dilute in normal saline 20 mg/mL and infuse over 15-30 minutes; if a more rapid onset of effect is desired or in a fluid restricted situation, the maximum concentration is 50 mg/mL; the maximum rate of infusion is over 5 minutes

Monitor heart rate, respiratory rate, blood pressure, continuous EKG

Dosage Forms

Injection: 20 mL vial containing 1 g each pralidoxime chloride with one 20 mL ampul diluent, disposable syringe, needle, and alcohol swab

Pralidoxime chloride:

Injection: 300 mg/mL (2 mL)

♦ **PrameGel® [OTC]** see pramoxine on page 512

♦ **Pramet® FA** see vitamin, multiple (prenatal) on page 654

♦ **Pramidal** see loperamide on page 374

♦ **Pramilet® FA** see vitamin, multiple (prenatal) on page 654

pramipexole (pra mi PEX ole)

U.S. Brand Names Mirapex®

Generic Available No

Therapeutic Category Dopaminergic Agent (Anti-Parkinson's)

Use Treatment of the signs and symptoms of idiopathic Parkinson's Disease

Usual Dosage Adults: Oral: Initial: 0.375 mg/day given in 3 divided doses, increase gradually by 0.125 mg/dose every 5-7 days; range: 1.5-4.5 mg/day

Dosage Forms Tablet: 0.125 mg, 0.25 mg, 1 mg, 1.5 mg

♦ **Pramosone®** see pramoxine and hydrocortisone on page 512

♦ **Pramotil** see metoclopramide on page 409

pramoxine (pra MOKS een)

U.S. Brand Names Anusol® Ointment [OTC]; Fleet® Pain Relief [OTC]; Itch-X® [OTC]; Phicon® [OTC]; PrameGel® [OTC]; Prax® [OTC]; ProctoFoam® NS [OTC]; Tronolane® [OTC]

Generic Available No

Therapeutic Category Local Anesthetic

Use Temporary relief of pain and itching associated with anogenital pruritus or irritation; dermatosis, minor burns or hemorrhoids

Usual Dosage Apply as directed, usually every 3-4 hours

Nursing/Pharmacy Information Apply sparingly, use the minimal effective dose

Dosage Forms Pramoxine hydrochloride:
Aerosol foam (ProctoFoam® NS): 1% (15 g)
Cream:
    Prax®: 1% (30 g, 113.4 g, 454 g)
    Tronolane®: 1% (30 g, 60 g)
    Tronothane® HCl: 1% (28.4 g)
Gel, topical:
    Itch-X®: 1% (35.4 g)
    PrameGel®: 1% (118 g)
Lotion (Prax®): 1% (15 mL, 120 mL, 240 mL)
Ointment (Anusol®): 1% (30 g)
Pads (Fleet® Pain Relief): 1% (100s)
Spray (Itch-X®): 1% (60 mL)

pramoxine and hydrocortisone

(pra MOKS een & hye droe KOR ti sone)

Synonyms hydrocortisone and pramoxine

U.S. Brand Names Enzone®; Pramosone®; Proctofoam®-HC; Zone-A Forte®

Generic Available No

Therapeutic Category Anesthetic/Corticosteroid

Use Treatment of severe anorectal or perianal inflammation

Usual Dosage Apply to affected areas 3-4 times/day

Nursing/Pharmacy Information When using rectally, the special applicator should be used, the aerosol container should not be placed in the rectum; for local application the foam can be placed on a tissue first

Dosage Forms
Cream, topical: Pramoxine hydrochloride 1% and hydrocortisone acetate 0.5% (30 g); pramoxine hydrochloride 1% and hydrocortisone acetate 1%
Foam, rectal: Pramoxine hydrochloride 1% and hydrocortisone acetate 1% (10 g)
Lotion, topical: Pramoxine hydrochloride 1% and hydrocortisone 0.25%; pramoxine hydrochloride 1% and hydrocortisone 2.5%; pramoxine hydrochloride 2.5% and hydrocortisone 1% (37.5 mL, 120 mL, 240 mL)

♦ **Prandin™** see repaglinide on page 544
♦ **Pravachol®** see pravastatin on page 512

pravastatin (PRA va stat in)

U.S. Brand Names Pravachol®

Generic Available No

Therapeutic Category HMG-CoA Reductase Inhibitor

Use Adjunct to diet for the reduction of elevated total and LDL-cholesterol levels in patients with hypercholesterolemia (Type IIa and IIb)

Usual Dosage Adults: Oral: 10-20 mg once daily at bedtime

Dietary Considerations May be taken with or without meals; avoid taking with high fiber meals

Nursing/Pharmacy Information Monitor creatinine phosphokinase due to possibility of myopathy

Dosage Forms Tablet, as sodium: 10 mg, 20 mg, 40 mg

♦ **Prax® [OTC]** see pramoxine on page 512
♦ **Prazidec** see omeprazole on page 455

praziquantel (pray zi KWON tel)

U.S. Brand Names Biltricide®

Mexican Brand Names Cisticid; Tecprazin

Generic Available No

Therapeutic Category Anthelmintic

Use Treatment of all stages of schistosomiasis caused by *Schistosoma* species pathogenic to humans; also active in the treatment of clonorchiasis, opisthorchiasis, cysticercosis, and many intestinal tapeworm infections and trematode

Usual Dosage Children and Adults: Oral:

Schistosomiasis: 20 mg/kg/dose 2-3 times/day for 1 day at 4- to 6-hour intervals

Flukes: 25 mg/kg/dose every 8 hours for 1-2 days

Cysticercosis: 50 mg/kg/day divided every 8 hours for 14 days

Tapeworms: 10-20 mg/kg as a single dose (25 mg/kg for *H. nana*)

Nursing/Pharmacy Information Tablets can be halved or quartered

Dosage Forms Tablet, tri-scored: 600 mg

prazosin (PRA zoe sin)

Synonyms furazosin

U.S. Brand Names Minipress®

Canadian Brand Names Apo®-Prazo; Novo-Prazin®; Nu-Prazo®

Generic Available Yes

Therapeutic Category Alpha-Adrenergic Blocking Agent

Use Hypertension, severe congestive heart failure (in conjunction with diuretics and cardiac glycosides)

Unlabeled use: Symptoms of benign prostatic hyperplasia

Usual Dosage Oral:

Children: Initial: 5 mcg/kg/dose (to assess hypotensive effects); usual dosing interval every 6 hours; increase dosage gradually up to maintenance of 25-150 mcg/kg/day divided every 6 hours

Adults: Initial: 1 mg/dose 2-3 times/day; usual maintenance dose: 3-15 mg/day in divided doses 2-4 times/day; maximum daily dose: 20 mg

Dietary Considerations Avoid natural licorice (causes sodium and water retention and increases potassium loss); food has variable effects on absorption

Nursing/Pharmacy Information

Syncope may occur usually within 90 minutes of the initial dose; administer initial dose at bedtime

Monitor blood pressure, standing and sitting/supine

Dosage Forms Capsule, as hydrochloride: 1 mg, 2 mg, 5 mg

prazosin and polythiazide (PRA zoe sin & pol i THYE a zide)

Synonyms polythiazide and prazosin

U.S. Brand Names Minizide®

Generic Available No

Therapeutic Category Antihypertensive Agent, Combination

Use Management of mild to moderate hypertension

Usual Dosage Adults: Oral: 1 capsule 2-3 times/day

Dosage Forms Capsule:

1: Prazosin 1 mg and polythiazide 0.5 mg

2: Prazosin 2 mg and polythiazide 0.5 mg

5: Prazosin 5 mg and polythiazide 0.5 mg

♦ **Precaptil** *see* captopril *on page 110*

♦ **Precose®** *see* acarbose *on page 12*

♦ **Predaject-50®** *(Discontinued) see page 743*

♦ **Predalone®** *(Discontinued) see page 743*

♦ **Pred Forte® Ophthalmic** *see* prednisolone (ophthalmic) *on page 514*

♦ **Pred-G® Ophthalmic** *see* prednisolone and gentamicin *on page 514*

♦ **Predicort-50®** *(Discontinued) see page 743*

♦ **Pred Mild® Ophthalmic** *see* prednisolone (ophthalmic) *on page 514*

prednicarbate (PRED ni kar bate)

U.S. Brand Names Dermatop®

Generic Available No

Therapeutic Category Corticosteroid, Topical

Use Relief of the inflammatory and pruritic manifestations of corticosteroid-responsive dermatoses

Usual Dosage Adults: Topical: Apply a thin film to affected area twice daily

Nursing/Pharmacy Information Use sparingly

Dosage Forms Cream: 0.1% (15 g, 60 g)

♦ **Prednicen-M®** *see* prednisone *on page 515*

♦ **prednisolone and chloramphenicol** *see* chloramphenicol and prednisolone *on page 133*

prednisolone and gentamicin
(pred NIS oh lone & jen ta MYE sin)

Synonyms gentamicin and prednisolone

U.S. Brand Names Pred-G® Ophthalmic

Generic Available Yes

Therapeutic Category Antibiotic/Corticosteroid, Ophthalmic

Use Treatment of steroid responsive inflammatory conditions and superficial ocular infections due to strains of microorganisms susceptible to gentamicin such as *Staphylococcus*, *E. coli*, *H. influenzae*, *Klebsiella*, *Neisseria*, *Pseudomonas*, *Proteus*, and *Serratia* species

Usual Dosage Children and Adults: Ophthalmic: 1 drop 2-4 times/day; during the initial 24-48 hours, the dosing frequency may be increased if necessary

Nursing/Pharmacy Information
Shake well before using
Monitor intraocular pressure with use >10 days

Dosage Forms
Ointment, ophthalmic: Prednisolone acetate 0.6% and gentamicin sulfate 0.3% (3.5 g)
Suspension, ophthalmic: Prednisolone acetate 1% and gentamicin sulfate 0.3% (2 mL, 5 mL, 10 mL)

♦ **prednisolone and sulfacetamide** *see* sulfacetamide and prednisolone *on page 585*

♦ **prednisolone, neomycin, and polymyxin B** *see* neomycin, polymyxin B, and prednisolone *on page 438*

prednisolone (ophthalmic) (pred NIS oh lone)

U.S. Brand Names AK-Pred® Ophthalmic; Econopred® Ophthalmic; Econopred® Plus Ophthalmic; Inflamase® Forte Ophthalmic; Inflamase® Mild Ophthalmic; Metreton® Ophthalmic; Pred Forte® Ophthalmic; Pred Mild® Ophthalmic

Canadian Brand Names Ophtho-tate®

Mexican Brand Names Fisopred®; Sophipren Ofteno

Generic Available Yes

Therapeutic Category Adrenal Corticosteroid

Use Treatment of palpebral and bulbar conjunctivitis; corneal injury from chemical, radiation, thermal burns, or foreign body penetration

Usual Dosage Adults: Ophthalmic: 1-2 drops into conjunctival sac every hour during day, every 2 hours at night until favorable response is obtained, then use 1 drop every 4 hours

Dietary Considerations Should be administered after meals or with food or milk to decrease GI effects; limit caffeine; increase dietary intake of pyridoxine, vitamin C, vitamin D, folate, calcium, and phosphorus

Nursing/Pharmacy Information
Do not administer acetate or tebutate salts I.V.
Monitor blood pressure, blood glucose, electrolytes

Dosage Forms
Solution, ophthalmic, as sodium phosphate: 0.125% (5 mL, 10 mL, 15 mL); 1% (5 mL, 10 mL, 15 mL)
Suspension, ophthalmic, as acetate: 0.12% (5 mL, 10 mL); 0.125% (5 mL, 10 mL, 15 mL); 1% (1 mL, 5 mL, 10 mL, 15 mL)

prednisolone (systemic) (pred NIS oh lone)

Synonyms deltahydrocortisone; metacortandralone

U.S. Brand Names Delta-Cortef® Oral; Key-Pred® Injection; Key-Pred-SP® Injection; Pediapred® Oral; Prednisol® TBA Injection; Prelone® Oral

Canadian Brand Names Novo-Prednisolone®

Generic Available Yes

Therapeutic Category Adrenal Corticosteroid

Use Treatment of endocrine disorders, rheumatic disorders, collagen diseases, dermatologic diseases, allergic states, ophthalmic diseases, respiratory diseases, hematologic disorders, neoplastic diseases, edematous states, and gastrointestinal diseases

Usual Dosage Dose depends upon condition being treated and response of patient; dosage for infants and children should be based on severity of the disease and response of the patient rather than on strict adherence to dosage indicated by age, weight, or body surface area. Consider alternate day therapy for long-term therapy. Discontinuation of long-term therapy requires gradual withdrawal by tapering the dose.

Children:
Acute asthma:
Oral: 1-2 mg/kg/day in divided doses 1-2 times/day for 3-5 days
I.V.: 2-4 mg/kg/day divided 3-4 times/day
Anti-inflammatory or immunosuppressive dose: Oral, I.V.: 0.1-2 mg/kg/day in divided doses 1-4 times/day
Nephrotic syndrome: Oral: Initial: 2 mg/kg/day (maximum: 80 mg/day) in divided doses 3-4 times/day until urine is protein free for 5 days (maximum: 28 days); if proteinuria persists, use 4 mg/kg/dose every other day for an additional 28 days (maximum: 120 mg/day); maintenance: 2 mg/kg/dose every other day for 28 days (maximum: 80 mg/dose); then taper over 4-6 weeks

Adults:
Oral, I.V.: 5-60 mg/day

Dietary Considerations Should be administered after meals or with food or milk to decrease GI effects; limit caffeine; increase dietary intake of pyridoxine, vitamin C, vitamin D, folate, calcium, and phosphorus

Nursing/Pharmacy Information
Do not administer acetate or tebutate salts I.V.
Monitor blood pressure, blood glucose, electrolytes

Dosage Forms
Injection, as acetate (for I.M., intralesional, intra-articular, or soft tissue administration only): 25 mg/mL (10 mL, 30 mL); 50 mg/mL (30 mL)
Injection, as sodium phosphate (for I.M., I.V., intra-articular, intralesional, or soft tissue administration): 20 mg/mL (2 mL, 5 mL, 10 mL)
Injection, as tebutate (for intra-articular, intralesional, soft tissue administration only): 20 mg/mL (1 mL, 5 mL, 10 mL)
Liquid, oral, as sodium phosphate: 5 mg/5 mL (120 mL)
Syrup: 15 mg/5 mL (240 mL)
Tablet: 5 mg

♦ **Prednisol® TBA Injection** *see* prednisolone (systemic) *on page 514*

prednisone (PRED ni sone)

Synonyms deltacortisone; deltadehydrocortisone

U.S. Brand Names Deltasone®; Liquid Pred®; Meticorten®; Orasone®; Prednicen-M®

Canadian Brand Names Apo®-Prednisone; Jaa-Prednisone®; Novo-Prednisone®; Winpred

Generic Available Yes

Therapeutic Category Adrenal Corticosteroid

Use Management of adrenocortical insufficiency; used for its anti-inflammatory or immunosuppressant effects

Usual Dosage Dose depends upon condition being treated and response of patient; dosage for infants and children should be based on severity of the disease and response of the patient rather than on strict adherence to dosage indicated by age, weight, or body surface area. Consider alternate day therapy for long-term therapy. Discontinuation of long-term therapy requires gradual withdrawal by tapering the dose.

Children: Oral: 0.05-2 mg/kg/day (anti-inflammatory or immunosuppressive dose) divided 1-4 times/day
Acute asthma: Oral: 1-2 mg/kg/day in divided doses 1-2 times/day for 3-5 days
Nephrotic syndrome: Oral: Initial: 2 mg/kg/day (maximum: of 80 mg/day) in divided doses 3-4 times/day until urine is protein free for 5 days (maximum: 28 days); if proteinuria persists, use 4 mg/kg/dose every other day (maximum: 120 mg/day) for an additional 28 days; maintenance: 2 mg/kg/dose every other day for 28 days (maximum: 80 mg/day); then taper over 4-6 weeks
Children and Adults: Physiologic replacement: 4-5 mg/m²/day
Adults: Oral: 5-60 mg/day in divided doses 1-4 times/day

Dietary Considerations Should be administered after meals or with food or milk; limit caffeine; increase dietary intake of pyridoxine, vitamin C, vitamin D, folate, calcium, and phosphorus

Nursing/Pharmacy Information Monitor blood pressure, blood glucose, electrolytes

Dosage Forms
Solution:
Concentrate: 5 mg/mL (5 mL, 30 mL)
Oral: 5 mg/5 mL (10 mL, 20 mL, 500 mL)
Syrup: 5 mg/5 mL (120 mL, 240 mL)
(Continued)

prednisone *(Continued)*
Tablet: 1 mg, 2.5 mg, 5 mg, 10 mg, 20 mg, 50 mg

- **Prefrin™ Liquifilm®** *see* phenylephrine *on page 487*
- **Prefrin™ Prefrin™ Ophthalmic Solution** *see* phenylephrine *on page 487*
- **Pregestimil® [OTC]** *see* enteral nutritional products *on page 233*
- **pregnenedione** *see* progesterone *on page 520*
- **Pregnyl®** *see* chorionic gonadotropin *on page 149*
- **Prelone® Oral** *see* prednisolone (systemic) *on page 514*
- **Prelu-2®** *see* phendimetrazine *on page 484*
- **Preludin® *(Discontinued)*** *see page 743*
- **Premarin®** *see* estrogens, conjugated (equine) *on page 245*
- **Premarin® Vaginal Cream *(Discontinued)*** *see page 743*
- **Premarin® With Methyltestosterone** *see* estrogens and methyltestosterone *on page 244*
- **Premphase™** *see* estrogens and medroxyprogesterone *on page 244*
- **Prempro™** *see* estrogens and medroxyprogesterone *on page 244*
- **prenatal vitamins** *see* vitamin, multiple (prenatal) *on page 654*
- **Prenavite® [OTC]** *see* vitamin, multiple (prenatal) *on page 654*
- **Prenavite® Forte** *see* vitamin, multiple (oral) *on page 654*
- **Prepcat®** *see* radiological/contrast media (ionic) *on page 539*
- **Pre-Pen®** *see* benzylpenicilloyl-polylysine *on page 82*
- **Prepidil® Vaginal Gel** *see* dinoprostone *on page 207*
- **Prepulsid®** *see* cisapride *on page 152*
- **Prescription Strength Desenex® [OTC]** *see* miconazole *on page 413*
- **Presoken** *see* diltiazem *on page 205*
- **Presoquim** *see* diltiazem *on page 205*
- **Pressyn®** *see* vasopressin *on page 645*
- **PreSun® 29 [OTC]** *see* methoxycinnamate and oxybenzone *on page 404*
- **Pretz® [OTC]** *see* sodium chloride *on page 571*
- **Pretz-D® [OTC]** *see* ephedrine *on page 233*
- **Prevacid®** *see* lansoprazole *on page 360*
- **Prevalite®** *see* cholestyramine resin *on page 147*
- **Preven™** *see* ethinyl estradiol and levonorgestrel *on page 250*
- **Preveon®** *see* adefovir *New Drug on page 22*
- **Prevex™ Baby Diaper Rash** *see* zinc oxide *on page 660*
- **Prevex™ HC** *see* hydrocortisone (topical) *on page 324*
- **Prevident®** *see* fluoride *on page 274*
- **Priftin®** *see* rifapentine *on page 550*

prilocaine *(PRIL oh kane)*
U.S. Brand Names Citanest® Forte; Citanest® Plain
Generic Available No
Therapeutic Category Local Anesthetic
Use In dentistry for infiltration anesthesia and for nerve block anesthesia
Usual Dosage Dose varies with procedure, desired depth, and duration of anesthesia, desired muscle relaxation, vascularity of tissues, physical condition, and age of patient
Dosage Forms Injection:
Citanest® Plain: 4% (1.8 mL)
Citanest® Forte: 4% with epinephrine bitartrate 1:200,000 (1.8 mL)

- **prilocaine and lidocaine** *see* lidocaine and prilocaine *on page 369*
- **Prilosec™** *see* omeprazole *on page 455*
- **primaclone** *see* primidone *on page 517*
- **Primacor®** *see* milrinone *on page 416*

primaquine *(PRIM a kween FOS fate)*
Synonyms prymaccone
Generic Available Yes
Therapeutic Category Aminoquinoline (Antimalarial)
Use In conjunction with a blood schizonticidal agent to provide radical cure of *P. vivax* or *P. ovale* malaria after a clinical attack has been confirmed by blood smear or serologic titer; prevention of relapse of *P. ovale* or *P. vivax* malaria; malaria postexposure prophylaxis

Usual Dosage Oral:

Children: 0.3 mg base/kg/day once daily for 14 days not to exceed 15 mg/day or 0.9 mg base/kg once weekly for 8 weeks not to exceed 45 mg base/week

Adults: 15 mg/day (base) once daily for 14 days or 45 mg base once weekly for 8 weeks

Nursing/Pharmacy Information Monitor periodic CBC, visual color check of urine

Dosage Forms Tablet, as phosphate: 26.3 mg [15 mg base]

♦ **primaquine and chloroquine** *see* chloroquine and primaquine *on page 136*

♦ **Primatene® Mist [OTC]** *see* epinephrine *on page 234*

♦ **Primaxin®** *see* imipenem and cilastatin *on page 334*

primidone (PRI mi done)

Synonyms desoxyphenobarbital; primaclone

U.S. Brand Names Mysoline®

Canadian Brand Names Apo®-Primidone; Sertan®

Generic Available Yes: Tablet

Therapeutic Category Anticonvulsant; Barbiturate

Use Management of generalized tonic-clonic (grand mal), complex partial and simple partial (focal) seizures

Usual Dosage Oral:

Children <8 years: Initial: 50-125 mg/day given at bedtime; increase by 50-125 mg/day increments every 3-7 days; usual dose: 10-25 mg/kg/day in divided doses 3-4 times/day

Children >8 years and Adults: Initial: 125-250 mg/day at bedtime; increase by 125-250 mg/day every 3-7 days; usual dose: 750-1500 mg/day in divided doses 3-4 times/day with maximum dosage of 2 g/day

Dietary Considerations Should be administered with food; encourage food high in vitamin K, vitamin D, and vitamin B_{12}

Food:

Folic acid: Low erythrocyte and CSF folate concentrations; megaloblastic anemia has been reported; to avoid folic acid deficiency and megaloblastic anemia, some clinicians recommend giving patients on anticonvulsants prophylactic doses of folic acid and cyanocobalamin

Protein-deficient diets: Increases duration of action of primidone should not restrict or delete protein from diet unless discussed with physician; be consistent with protein intake during primidone therapy

Fresh fruits containing vitamin C: Displaces drug from binding sites, resulting in increased urinary excretion of primidone; educate patients regarding the potential for decreased primidone effect with consumption of foods high in Vitamin C

Nursing/Pharmacy Information

Monitor serum primidone and phenobarbital concentration, CBC, SMA-12

Stability: Protect from light

Dosage Forms

Suspension, oral: 250 mg/5 mL (240 mL)

Tablet: 50 mg, 250 mg

♦ **Primolut® Depot** *see* hydroxyprogesterone caproate *on page 327*

♦ **Principen®** *see* ampicillin *on page 46*

♦ **Prinivil®** *see* lisinopril *on page 372*

♦ **Prinzide®** *see* lisinopril and hydrochlorothiazide *on page 372*

♦ **Priscoline®** *see* tolazoline *on page 617*

♦ **pristinamycin** *see* quinupristin and dalfopristin *New Drug on page 538*

♦ **Privine® Nasal [OTC]** *see* naphazoline *on page 431*

♦ **ProAmatine** *see* midodrine *on page 415*

♦ **Pro-Amox®** *see* amoxicillin *on page 43*

♦ **Proampacin®** *(Discontinued) see page 743*

♦ **Pro-Ampi®** *see* ampicillin *on page 46*

♦ **Proartinal** *see* ibuprofen *on page 332*

♦ **Pro-Banthine®** *see* propantheline *on page 524*

probenecid (proe BEN e sid)

Canadian Brand Names Benemid®; Benuryl™

Mexican Brand Names Benecid Probenecida Valdecasas

Generic Available Yes

Therapeutic Category Uricosuric Agent

Use Prevention of gouty arthritis; hyperuricemia; prolong serum levels of penicillin/cephalosporin

(Continued)

probenecid *(Continued)*

Usual Dosage Oral:

Children:

<2 years: Not recommended

2-14 years: Prolong penicillin serum levels: 25 mg/kg starting dose, then 40 mg/kg/day administered 4 times/day

Gonorrhea: <45 kg: 25 mg/kg x 1 (maximum: 1 g/dose) 30 minutes before penicillin, ampicillin or amoxicillin

Adults:

Hyperuricemia with gout: 250 mg twice daily for one week; increase to 500 mg 2 times/day; may increase by 500 mg/month, if needed, to maximum of 2-3 g/day (dosages may be decreased by 500 mg every 6 months if serum urate concentrations are controlled)

Prolong penicillin serum levels: 500 mg 4 times/day

Gonorrhea: 1 g 30 minutes before penicillin, ampicillin or amoxicillin

Dietary Considerations Should be administered with food or antacids; encourage alkaline ash foods (milk products, nuts, beets, spinach, turnip greens); may cause GI upset; drink plenty of fluids

Nursing/Pharmacy Information Monitor uric acid, renal function

Dosage Forms Tablet: 500 mg

♦ **probenecid and colchicine** *see* colchicine and probenecid *on page 165*

procainamide *(proe kane A mide)*

Synonyms procaine amide hydrochloride

U.S. Brand Names Procanbid™; Pronestyl®; Pronestyl-SR®

Canadian Brand Names Apo®-Procainamide; Procan™ SR

Generic Available Yes

Therapeutic Category Antiarrhythmic Agent, Class I-A

Use Ventricular tachycardia, premature ventricular contractions, paroxysmal atrial tachycardia, and atrial fibrillation; to prevent recurrence of ventricular tachycardia, paroxysmal supraventricular tachycardia, atrial fibrillation or flutter

Usual Dosage Must be titrated to patient's response

Children:

Oral: 15-50 mg/kg/24 hours divided every 3-6 hours; maximum 4 g/24 hours

I.M.: 20-30 mg/kg/24 hours divided every 4-6 hours in divided doses; maximum 4 g/24 hours

I.V.: Load: 3-6 mg/kg/dose over 5 minutes not to exceed 100 mg/dose; may repeat every 5-10 minutes to maximum of 15 mg/kg/load; maintenance as continuous I.V. infusion: 20-80 mcg/kg/minute; maximum: 2 g/24 hours

Adults:

Oral: 250-500 mg/dose every 3-6 hours or 500 mg to 1 g every 6 hours sustained release; usual dose: 50 mg/kg/24 hours or 2-4 g/24 hours

I.V.: Load: 50-100 mg/dose, repeated every 5-10 minutes until patient controlled; or load with 15-18 mg/kg, maximum loading dose: 1-1.5 g; maintenance: 2-6 mg/minute continuous I.V. infusion, usual maintenance: 3-4 mg/minute

Dietary Considerations Should be administered with water on an empty stomach

Nursing/Pharmacy Information

Do not administer faster than 20-30 mg/minute; severe hypotension can occur with rapid I.V. administration; administer I.V. push over at least 5 minutes; administer I.V. loading dose over 25-30 minutes, use concentration of 20-30 mg/mL for loading dose and 2-4 mg/mL for maintenance infusing

Monitor EKG, blood pressure, CBC with differential, platelet count

Stability: Parenteral admixture at room temperature and refrigeration temperature (4°C): 24 hours; use only clear or slightly yellow solutions

Dosage Forms Procainamide hydrochloride:

Capsule: 250 mg, 375 mg, 500 mg

Injection: 100 mg/mL (10 mL); 500 mg/mL (2 mL)

Tablet: 250 mg, 375 mg, 500 mg

Sustained release: 250 mg, 500 mg, 750 mg, 1000 mg

Sustained release (Procanbid™): 500 mg, 1000 mg

procaine *(PROE kane)*

U.S. Brand Names Novocain®

Generic Available Yes

Therapeutic Category Local Anesthetic

Use Produce spinal anesthesia and epidural and peripheral nerve block by injection and infiltration methods

Usual Dosage Dose varies with procedure, desired depth and duration of anesthesia, desired muscle relaxation, vascularity of tissues, physical condition, and age of patient

Nursing/Pharmacy Information Prior to instillation of anesthetic agent, withdraw plunger to ensure needle is not in artery or vein; resuscitative equipment should be available when local anesthetics are administered

Dosage Forms Injection, as hydrochloride: 1% [10 mg/mL] (2 mL, 6 mL, 30 mL, 100 mL); 2% [20 mg/mL] (30 mL, 100 mL); 10% (2 mL)

- ♦ **procaine amide hydrochloride** see procainamide on page 518
- ♦ **procaine benzylpenicillin** see penicillin G procaine on page 476
- ♦ **procaine penicillin G** see penicillin G procaine on page 476
- ♦ **Pro-Cal-Sof® [OTC]** see docusate on page 214
- ♦ **Procanbid™** see procainamide on page 518
- ♦ **Procan™ SR** see procainamide on page 518
- ♦ **Procan SR®** *(Discontinued)* see page 743

procarbazine (proe KAR ba zeen)

Synonyms ibenzmethyzin; MIH; n-methylhydrazine
U.S. Brand Names Matulane®
Canadian Brand Names Natulan®
Mexican Brand Names Natulan
Generic Available No
Therapeutic Category Antineoplastic Agent
Use Treatment of Hodgkin's disease, non-Hodgkin's lymphoma, brain tumor, bronchogenic carcinoma
Usual Dosage Refer to individual protocols. Oral:
Children: 50-100 mg/m^2/day in a single dose; doses as high as 100-200 mg/m^2/day once daily have been used for neuroblastoma and medulloblastoma
Adults: Initial: 2-4 mg/kg/day in single or divided doses for 7 days then increase dose to 4-6 mg/kg/day until response is obtained or leukocyte count decreased <4000/mm^3 or the platelet count decreased <100,000/mm^3; maintenance: 1-2 mg/kg/day
Dietary Considerations Avoid food with high tyramine content (cheese, tea, coffee, cola drinks, wine, bananas); alcohol will cause "disulfiram"-type reaction consisting of flushing, headache, nausea, and in some patients, vomiting and chest and/or abdominal pain; administer with food to decrease GI distress
Nursing/Pharmacy Information
Monitor CBC with differential, platelet and reticulocyte count, urinalysis, liver function test, renal function test
Stability: Protect from light
Dosage Forms Capsule, as hydrochloride: 50 mg

- ♦ **Procardia®** see nifedipine on page 442
- ♦ **Procardia XL®** see nifedipine on page 442
- ♦ **procetofene** see fenofibrate on page 261

prochlorperazine (proe klor PER a zeen)

U.S. Brand Names Compazine®
Canadian Brand Names Nu-Prochlor®; PMS-Prochlorperazine; Prorazin®; Stemetil®
Generic Available Yes
Therapeutic Category Phenothiazine Derivative
Use Management of nausea and vomiting; acute and chronic psychoses
Usual Dosage
Children: Oral, rectal:
>10 kg: 0.4 mg/kg/24 hours in 3-4 divided doses; **or**
9-14 kg: 2.5 mg every 12-24 hours as needed; maximum: 7.5 mg/day
14-18 kg: 2.5 mg every 8-12 hours as needed; maximum: 10 mg/day
18-39 kg: 2.5 mg every 8 hours or 5 mg every 12 hours as needed; maximum: 15 mg/day
I.M.: 0.1-0.15 mg/kg/dose; usual: 0.13 mg/kg/dose; change to oral as soon as possible
I.V.: Not recommended
Adults:
Oral: 5-10 mg 3-4 times/day; usual maximum: 40 mg/day; doses up to 150 mg/day may be required in some patients
I.M.: 5-10 mg every 3-4 hours; usual maximum: 40 mg/day; doses up to 10-20 mg every 4-6 hours may be required in some patients
I.V.: 2.5-10 mg; maximum 10 mg/dose or 40 mg/day; may repeat dose every 3-4 hours as needed
(Continued)

prochlorperazine *(Continued)*

Rectal: 25 mg twice daily

Dietary Considerations Limit caffeine; increase dietary intake of riboflavin; should be administered with food or water

Nursing/Pharmacy Information

Avoid skin contact with oral solution or injection, contact dermatitis has occurred; do not administer by S.C. route (tissue damage may occur); avoid I.V. administration; if necessary, may be administered by direct I.V. injection at a maximum rate of 5 mg/minute

Monitor CBC with differential and periodic ophthalmic exams (if chronically used)

Stability: Protect from light; clear or slightly yellow solutions may be used; **incompatible** when mixed with aminophylline, amphotericin B, ampicillin, calcium salts, cephalothin, foscarnet (Y-site), furosemide, hydrocortisone, hydromorphone, methohexital, midazolam, penicillin G, pentobarbital, phenobarbital, thiopental

Dosage Forms

Suppository, rectal: 2.5 mg, 5 mg, 25 mg (12/box)

Prochlorperazine edisylate:

Injection: 5 mg/mL (2 mL, 10 mL)

Syrup: 5 mg/5 mL (120 mL)

Prochlorperazine maleate:

Capsule, sustained action: 10 mg, 15 mg, 30 mg

Tablet: 5 mg, 10 mg, 25 mg

- ♦ **Procrit®** *see* epoetin alfa *on page 236*
- ♦ **Proctocort™ Rectal** *see* hydrocortisone (rectal) *on page 322*
- ♦ **proctofene** *see* fenofibrate *on page 261*
- ♦ **Proctofoam®-HC** *see* pramoxine and hydrocortisone *on page 512*
- ♦ **ProctoFoam® NS [OTC]** *see* pramoxine *on page 512*
- ♦ **Procyclid®** *see* procyclidine *on page 520*

procyclidine *(proe SYE kli deen)*

U.S. Brand Names Kemadrin®

Canadian Brand Names PMS-Procyclidine; Procyclid®

Generic Available No

Therapeutic Category Anticholinergic Agent; Anti-Parkinson's Agent

Use Relief of symptoms of Parkinsonian syndrome and drug-induced extrapyramidal symptoms

Usual Dosage Adults: Oral: 2-2.5 mg 3 times/day after meals; if tolerated, gradually increase dose to 4-5 mg 3 times/day

Dietary Considerations Should be administered after meals

Nursing/Pharmacy Information Do not discontinue drug abruptly

Dosage Forms Tablet, as hydrochloride: 5 mg

- ♦ **Procytox®** *see* cyclophosphamide *on page 175*
- ♦ **Prodiem® Plain** *see* psyllium *on page 531*
- ♦ **Prodium® [OTC]** *see* phenazopyridine *on page 483*
- ♦ **Profasi® HP** *see* chorionic gonadotropin *on page 149*
- ♦ **Profenal® Ophthalmic** *see* suprofen *on page 590*
- ♦ **Profenid®** *see* ketoprofen *on page 355*
- ♦ **Profenid® 200** *see* ketoprofen *on page 355*
- ♦ **Profenid®-IM** *see* ketoprofen *on page 355*
- ♦ **Profen II®** *see* guaifenesin and phenylpropanolamine *on page 301*
- ♦ **Profen II DM®** *see* guaifenesin, phenylpropanolamine, and dextromethorphan *on page 303*
- ♦ **Profen LA®** *see* guaifenesin and phenylpropanolamine *on page 301*
- ♦ **Profilate-HP®** *(Discontinued) see page 743*
- ♦ **Profilnine® SD** *see* factor IX complex (human) *on page 257*
- ♦ **Progestaject® Injection** *(Discontinued) see page 743*
- ♦ **Progestasert®** *see* progesterone *on page 520*

progesterone *(proe JES ter one)*

Synonyms pregnenedione; progestin

U.S. Brand Names Crinone™; Progestasert®; Prometrium®

Canadian Brand Names PMS-Progesterone; Progesterone Oil

Mexican Brand Names Crinone® V; Utrogestan

Generic Available Yes

Therapeutic Category Progestin

Use

Gel: Progesterone supplementation or replacement as part of an assisted reproductive technology treatment for infertile women with progesterone deficiency

Oral: Prevention of endometrial hyperplasia in nonhysterectomized postmenopausal women who are receiving conjugated estrogen tablets; secondary amenorrhea

Reservoir: Endometrial carcinoma or renal carcinoma as well as secondary amenorrhea or abnormal uterine bleeding due to hormonal imbalance

Usual Dosage Adults:

Amenorrhea: I.M.: 5-10 mg/day for 6-8 consecutive days

Functional uterine bleeding: I.M.: 5-10 mg/day for 6 doses

Contraception: Female: Intrauterine device: Insert a single system into the uterine cavity; contraceptive effectiveness is retained for 1 year and system must be replaced 1 year after insertion

Dietary Considerations Food increases oral bioavailability

Nursing/Pharmacy Information

Patients should receive a copy of the patient labeling for the drug; administer deep I.M. only

Before starting therapy, a physical exam including the breasts and pelvis are recommended, also a PAP smear; signs or symptoms of depression, glucose in diabetics

Stability: Refrigerate suppositories

Dosage Forms

Capsule: 100 mg

Gel, single use: 8% (90 mg applicator)

Intrauterine system, reservoir: 38 mg in silicone fluid

- **Progesterone Oil** *see progesterone on page 520*
- **progestin** *see progesterone on page 520*
- **Proglycem® Oral** *see diazoxide on page 197*
- **Prograf®** *see tacrolimus on page 592*
- **ProHIBiT®** *see Haemophilus B conjugate vaccine on page 306*
- **Pro-Indo®** *see indomethacin on page 337*
- **Proken M** *see metoprolol on page 410*
- **Prokine® Injection (Discontinued)** *see page 743*
- **Prolaken** *see metoprolol on page 410*
- **Prolamine® (Discontinued)** *see page 743*
- **Prolastin®** *see alpha₁-proteinase inhibitor on page 30*
- **Proleukin®** *see aldesleukin on page 26*
- **Prolixin Decanoate® Injection** *see fluphenazine on page 277*
- **Prolixin Enanthate® Injection** *see fluphenazine on page 277*
- **Prolixin® Injection** *see fluphenazine on page 277*
- **Prolixin® Oral** *see fluphenazine on page 277*
- **Proloid® (Discontinued)** *see page 743*
- **Prolopa®** *see benserazide and levodopa (Canada only) on page 77*
- **Proloprim®** *see trimethoprim on page 630*
- **Pro-Lorazepam®** *see lorazepam on page 375*

promazine (PROE ma zeen)

U.S. Brand Names Sparine®

Generic Available Yes: Injection only

Therapeutic Category Phenothiazine Derivative

Use Treatment of psychoses

Usual Dosage Oral, I.M.:

Children >12 years: Antipsychotic: 10-25 mg every 4-6 hours

Adults:

Psychosis: 10-200 mg every 4-6 hours not to exceed 1000 mg/day

Antiemetic: 25-50 mg every 4-6 hours as needed

Nursing/Pharmacy Information

I.M. injections should be deep injections; if administering I.V., dilute to at least 25 mg/mL and administer slowly; watch for hypotension; protect injection from light

Monitor orthostatic blood pressures 3-5 days after initiation of therapy or a dose increase; observe for tremor and abnormal movement or posturing (extrapyramidal symptoms)

Stability: **Incompatible** when mixed with aminophylline, dimenhydrinate, methohexital, nafcillin, penicillin G, pentobarbital, phenobarbital, sodium bicarbonate, thiopental

(Continued)

promazine (Continued)

Dosage Forms Promazine hydrochloride:
Injection: 25 mg/mL (10 mL); 50 mg/mL (1 mL, 2 mL, 10 mL)
Tablet: 25 mg, 50 mg, 100 mg

♦ **Prometa®** see metaproterenol on page 397

promethazine (proe METH a zeen)

U.S. Brand Names Phenazine® Injection; Phenergan® Injection; Phenergan®
Oral; Phenergan® Rectal; Prorex® Injection
Canadian Brand Names Histantil
Generic Available Yes
Therapeutic Category Antiemetic; Phenothiazine Derivative
Use Symptomatic treatment of various allergic conditions and motion sickness;
sedative and an antiemetic
Usual Dosage
Children:
Antihistamine: Oral: 0.1 mg/kg/dose every 6 hours during the day and 0.5
mg/kg/dose at bedtime as needed
Antiemetic: Oral, I.M., I.V., rectal: 0.25-1 mg/kg 4-6 times/day as needed
Motion sickness: Oral: 0.5 mg/kg 30 minutes to 1 hour before departure, then
every 12 hours as needed
Sedation: Oral, I.M., I.V., rectal: 0.5-1 mg/kg/dose every 6 hours as needed
Adults:
Antihistamine:
Oral: 25 mg at bedtime or 12.5 mg 3 times/day
I.M., I.V., rectal: 25 mg, may repeat in 2 hours
Antiemetic: Oral, I.M., I.V., rectal: 12.5-25 mg every 4 hours as needed
Motion sickness: Oral: 25 mg 30 minutes to 1 hour before departure, then
every 12 hours as needed
Sedation: Oral, I.M., I.V., rectal: 25-50 mg/dose
Dietary Considerations Increase dietary intake of riboflavin; should be admin-
istered with food or water
Nursing/Pharmacy Information
Avoid S.C. administration, promethazine is a chemical irritation which may
produce necrosis; avoid I.V. use; if necessary, may dilute to a maximum
concentration of 25 mg/mL and infuse at a maximum rate of 25 mg/minute
Stability: Protect from light and from freezing; promethazine is **incompatible**
when mixed with aminophylline, cefoperazone (Y-site), chloramphenicol,
dimenhydrinate (same syringe), foscarnet (Y-site), furosemide, heparin,
hydrocortisone, methohexital, penicillin G, pentobarbital, phenobarbital, thiopental
Dosage Forms Promethazine hydrochloride:
Injection: 25 mg/mL (1 mL, 10 mL); 50 mg/mL (1 mL, 10 mL)
Suppository, rectal: 12.5 mg, 25 mg, 50 mg
Syrup: 6.25 mg/5 mL (5 mL, 120 mL, 240 mL, 480 mL, 4000 mL); 25 mg/5 mL
(120 mL, 480 mL, 4000 mL)
Tablet: 12.5 mg, 25 mg, 50 mg

promethazine and codeine (proe METH a zeen & KOE deen)

Synonyms codeine and promethazine
U.S. Brand Names Phenergan® With Codeine; Pherazine® With Codeine;
Prothazine-DC®
Generic Available Yes
Therapeutic Category Antihistamine/Antitussive
Controlled Substance C-V
Use Temporary relief of coughs and upper respiratory symptoms associated
with allergy or the common cold
Usual Dosage Oral (in terms of codeine):
Children: 1-1.5 mg/kg/day every 4 hours as needed; maximum: 30 mg/day **or**
2-6 years: 1.25-2.5 mL every 4-6 hours or 2.5-5 mg/dose every 4-6 hours as
needed; maximum: 30 mg codeine/day
6-12 years: 2.5-5 mL every 4-6 hours as needed or 5-10 mg/dose every 4-6
hours as needed; maximum: 60 mg codeine/day
Adults: 10-20 mg/dose every 4-6 hours as needed; maximum: 120 mg
codeine/day; or 5-10 mL every 4-6 hours as needed
Dietary Considerations Increase fluids, fiber intake, and riboflavin in diet
Nursing/Pharmacy Information May cause sedation and drowsiness
Dosage Forms Syrup: Promethazine hydrochloride 6.25 mg and codeine phosphate 10 mg per 5 mL (120 mL, 180 mL, 473 mL)

promethazine and dextromethorphan
(proe METH a zeen & deks troe meth OR fan)

Synonyms dextromethorphan and promethazine

U.S. Brand Names Phenameth® DM; Phenergan® With Dextromethorphan; Pherazine® w/DM

Generic Available Yes

Therapeutic Category Antihistamine/Antitussive

Use Temporary relief of coughs and upper respiratory symptoms associated with allergy or the common cold

Usual Dosage Oral:

Children:

2-6 years: 1.25-2.5 mL every 4-6 hours up to 10 mL in 24 hours

6-12 years: 2.5-5 mL every 4-6 hours up to 20 mL in 24 hours

Adults: 5 mL every 4-6 hours up to 30 mL in 24 hours

Dosage Forms Syrup: Promethazine hydrochloride 6.25 mg and dextromethorphan hydrobromide 15 mg per 5 mL with alcohol 7% (120 mL, 480 mL, 4000 mL)

♦ **promethazine and meperidine** *see* meperidine and promethazine *on page 392*

promethazine and phenylephrine
(proe METH a zeen & fen il EF rin)

Synonyms phenylephrine and promethazine

U.S. Brand Names Phenergan® VC Syrup; Promethazine VC Plain Syrup; Promethazine VC Syrup; Prometh VC Plain Liquid

Generic Available Yes

Therapeutic Category Antihistamine/Decongestant Combination

Use Temporary relief of upper respiratory symptoms associated with allergy or the common cold

Usual Dosage Oral:

Children:

2-6 years: 1.25 mL every 4-6 hours, not to exceed 7.5 mL in 24 hours

6-12 years: 2.5 mL every 4-6 hours, not to exceed 15 mL in 24 hours

Children >12 years and Adults: 5 mL every 4-6 hours, not to exceed 30 mL in 24 hours

Dietary Considerations Increase dietary intake of riboflavin

Nursing/Pharmacy Information May cause drowsiness

Dosage Forms Liquid: Promethazine hydrochloride 6.25 mg and phenylephrine hydrochloride 5 mg per 5 mL (120 mL, 240 mL, 473 mL)

promethazine, phenylephrine, and codeine
(proe METH a zeen, fen il EF rin, & KOE deen)

Synonyms codeine, promethazine, and phenylephrine; phenylephrine, promethazine, and codeine

U.S. Brand Names Phenergan® VC With Codeine; Pherazine® VC w/ Codeine; Promethist® With Codeine; Prometh® VC With Codeine

Generic Available Yes

Therapeutic Category Antihistamine/Decongestant/Antitussive

Controlled Substance C-V

Use Temporary relief of coughs and upper respiratory symptoms including nasal congestion

Usual Dosage Oral:

Children (expressed in terms of codeine dosage): 1-1.5 mg/kg/day every 4 hours, maximum: 30 mg/day **or**

<2 years: Not recommended

2 to 6 years:

Weight 25 lb: 1.25-2.5 mL every 4-6 hours, not to exceed 6 mL/24 hours

Weight 30 lb: 1.25-2.5 mL every 4-6 hours, not to exceed 7 mL/24 hours

Weight 35 lb: 1.25-2.5 mL every 4-6 hours, not to exceed 8 mL/24 hours

Weight 40 lb: 1.25-2.5 mL every 4-6 hours, not to exceed 9 mL/24 hours

6 to <12 years: 2.5-5 mL every 4-6 hours, not to exceed 15 mL/24 hours

Adults: 5 mL every 4-6 hours, not to exceed 30 mL/24 hours

Dietary Considerations May be administered with food or water to decrease GI upset; avoid alcohol; increase fiber intake and riboflavin in diet

Dosage Forms Liquid: Promethazine hydrochloride 6.25 mg, phenylephrine hydrochloride 5 mg, and codeine phosphate 10 mg per 5 mL with alcohol 7% (120 mL, 240 mL, 480 mL, 4000 mL)

♦ **Promethazine VC Plain Syrup** *see* promethazine and phenylephrine *on page 523*

- **Promethazine VC Syrup** *see promethazine and phenylephrine on page 523*
- **Prometh® *(Discontinued)*** *see page 743*
- **Promethist® With Codeine** *see promethazine, phenylephrine, and codeine on page 523*
- **Prometh VC Plain Liquid** *see promethazine and phenylephrine on page 523*
- **Prometh® VC With Codeine** *see promethazine, phenylephrine, and codeine on page 523*
- **Prometrium®** *see progesterone on page 520*
- **Promit®** *see dextran 1 on page 192*
- **Pronaxil** *see naproxen on page 432*
- **Pronestyl®** *see procainamide on page 518*
- **Pronestyl-SR®** *see procainamide on page 518*
- **Pronto® Shampoo [OTC]** *see pyrethrins and piperonyl butoxide on page 533*
- **Propac™ [OTC]** *see enteral nutritional products on page 233*
- **Propacet®** *see propoxyphene and acetaminophen on page 526*
- **Propaderm®** *see beclomethasone on page 75*

propafenone (proe pa FEEN one)

U.S. Brand Names Rythmol®
Mexican Brand Names Nistaken; Norfenon®
Generic Available No
Therapeutic Category Antiarrhythmic Agent, Class I-C
Use Life-threatening ventricular arrhythmias; an oral sodium channel blocker similar to encainide and flecainide; in clinical trials was used effectively to treat atrial flutter, atrial fibrillation and other arrhythmias, but are not labeled indications; can worsen or even cause new ventricular arrhythmias (proarrhythmic effect)
Usual Dosage Adults: Oral: 150 mg every 8 hours, up to 300 mg every 8 hours
Dietary Considerations Administer at the same time in relation to meals each day, either always with meals or always between meals
Nursing/Pharmacy Information Monitor for signs of infection; monitor heart sounds and pulses for rate, rhythm and quality
Dosage Forms Tablet, as hydrochloride: 150 mg, 225 mg, 300 mg

- **Propagest® [OTC]** *see phenylpropanolamine on page 489*
- **Propanthel™** *see propantheline on page 524*

propantheline (proe PAN the leen)

U.S. Brand Names Pro-Banthine®
Canadian Brand Names Propanthel™
Generic Available Yes: 15 mg tablet
Therapeutic Category Anticholinergic Agent
Use Adjunctive treatment of peptic ulcer, irritable bowel syndrome, pancreatitis, ureteral and urinary bladder spasm; to reduce duodenal motility during diagnostic radiologic procedures
Usual Dosage Oral:
Antisecretory:
Children: 1-2 mg/kg/day in 3-4 divided doses
Elderly patients: 7.5 mg 3 times/day before meals and at bedtime
Antispasmodic:
Children: 2-3 mg/kg/day in divided doses every 4-6 hours and at bedtime
Adults: 15 mg 3 times/day before meals or food and 30 mg at bedtime
Dietary Considerations Should be administered 30 minutes before meals so that the drug's peak effect occurs at the proper time
Nursing/Pharmacy Information Monitor anticholinergic effects, orthostatic changes
Dosage Forms Tablet, as bromide: 7.5 mg, 15 mg

proparacaine (proe PAR a kane)

Synonyms proxymetacaine
U.S. Brand Names AK-Taine®; Alcaine®; I-Paracaine®; Ophthetic®
Canadian Brand Names Diocaine
Generic Available Yes
Therapeutic Category Local Anesthetic
Use Local anesthesia for tonometry, gonioscopy; suture removal from cornea; removal of corneal foreign body; cataract extraction, glaucoma surgery; short operative procedure involving the cornea and conjunctiva

Usual Dosage Children and Adults:
Ophthalmic surgery: Instill 1 drop of 0.5% solution in eye every 5-10 minutes for 5-7 doses
Tonometry, gonioscopy, suture removal: Instill 1-2 drops 0.5% solution in eye just prior to procedure

Nursing/Pharmacy Information
Do not use if discolored; protect eye from irritating chemicals, foreign bodies, and blink reflex; use eye patch if necessary
Stability: Store in tight, light-resistant containers

Dosage Forms Ophthalmic, solution, as hydrochloride: 0.5% (2 mL, 15 mL)

proparacaine and fluorescein
(proe PAR a kane & FLURE e seen)

U.S. Brand Names Fluoracaine® Ophthalmic

Generic Available Yes

Therapeutic Category Diagnostic Agent; Local Anesthetic

Use Anesthesia for tonometry, gonioscopy; suture removal from cornea; removal of corneal foreign body; cataract extraction, glaucoma surgery

Usual Dosage
Tonometry, gonioscopy, suture removal: Adults: Instill 1-2 drops 0.5% solution in eye just prior to procedure
Ophthalmic surgery: Children and Adults: Instill 1 drop of 0.5% solution in eye every 5-10 minutes for 5-7 doses

Nursing/Pharmacy Information
Do not use if discolored; protect eye from irritating chemicals, foreign bodies, and blink reflex; use eye patch if necessary
Stability: Store in tight, light-resistant containers

Dosage Forms Solution: Proparacaine hydrochloride 0.5% and fluorescein sodium 0.25% (2 mL, 5 mL)

♦ **Propine®** *see* dipivefrin *on page 211*

propiomazine (proe pee OH ma zeen)

Generic Available No

Therapeutic Category Phenothiazine Derivative

Use Relief of restlessness, nausea and apprehension before and during surgery or during labor

Usual Dosage I.M., I.V.:
Children: 0.55-1.1 mg/kg
Adults: 10-40 mg prior to procedure, additional may be repeated at 3-hour intervals

Dosage Forms Injection, as hydrochloride: 20 mg/mL (1 mL)

♦ **Pro-Piroxicam®** *see* piroxicam *on page 497*
♦ **Proplex® SX-T Injection** *(Discontinued) see page 743*
♦ **Proplex® T** *see* factor IX complex (human) *on page 257*

propofol (PROE po fole)

U.S. Brand Names Diprivan®

Generic Available No

Therapeutic Category General Anesthetic

Use Induction or maintenance of anesthesia; sedation

Usual Dosage Dosage must be individualized and titrated to the desired clinical effect; however, as a general guideline:
No pediatric dose has been established
Induction: I.V.:
Adults ≤55 years, and/or ASA I or II patients: 2-2.5 mg/kg of body weight (approximately 40 mg every 10 seconds until onset of induction)
Elderly, debilitated, hypovolemic, and/or ASA III or IV patients: 1-1.5 mg/kg of body weight (approximately 20 mg every 10 seconds until onset of induction)
Maintenance: I.V. infusion:
Adults ≤55 years, and/or ASA I or II patients: 0.1-0.2 mg/kg of body weight/minute (6-12 mg/kg of body weight/hour)
Elderly, debilitated, hypovolemic, and/or ASA III or IV patients: 0.05-0.1 mg/kg of body weight/minute (3-6 mg/kg of body weight/hour)

I.V. intermittent: 25-50 mg increments, as needed

Nursing/Pharmacy Information
Changes urine color to green
Cardiorespiratory functions (eg, oxygen saturation, hypotension, apnea, airway obstruction, bradycardia) should be monitored in all patients. Patients
(Continued)

propofol *(Continued)*

receiving propofol by intermittent bolus injection should be closely monitored for respiratory depression, transient increase in sedation depth, and prolongation of recovery. Daily monitoring of serum lipids is recommended, especially in patients receiving high doses for long periods.

Stability: Do not use if there is evidence of separation of phases of emulsion; discard any unused portions at end of the surgical procedure

Dosage Forms Injection: 10 mg/mL (20 mL, 50 mL, 100 mL)

propoxyphene (proe POKS i feen)

Synonyms dextropropoxyphene

U.S. Brand Names Darvon®; Darvon-N®; Dolene®

Canadian Brand Names 642®; Novo-Propoxyn®

Generic Available Yes: Capsule

Therapeutic Category Analgesic, Narcotic

Controlled Substance C-IV

Use Management of mild to moderate pain

Usual Dosage Adults: Oral:

Hydrochloride: 65 mg every 3-4 hours as needed for pain; maximum: 390 mg/day

Napsylate: 100 mg every 4 hours as needed for pain; maximum: 600 mg/day

Dietary Considerations

Alcohol: Additive CNS effects; avoid or limit alcohol; watch for sedation

Food: May decrease rate of absorption, but may slightly increase bioavailability; should be administered with glass of water on empty stomach;

Glucose: May cause hyperglycemia; monitor blood glucose concentrations

Nursing/Pharmacy Information Monitor pain relief, respiratory and mental status, blood pressure, excessive sedation

Dosage Forms

Capsule, as hydrochloride: 65 mg

Tablet, as napsylate: 100 mg

propoxyphene and acetaminophen

(proe POKS i feen & a seet a MIN oh fen)

Synonyms acetaminophen and propoxyphene

U.S. Brand Names Darvocet-N®; Darvocet-N® 100; Propacet®; Wygesic®

Generic Available Yes

Therapeutic Category Analgesic, Narcotic

Controlled Substance C-IV

Use Management of mild to moderate pain

Usual Dosage Adults: Oral:

Darvocet-N®: 1-2 tablets every 4 hours as needed; maximum: 600 mg propoxyphene napsylate/day

Darvocet-N® 100: 1 tablet every 4 hours as needed; maximum: 600 mg propoxyphene napsylate/day

Dietary Considerations Should be administered with water on an empty stomach; food may decrease rate of absorption of propoxyphene, but may slightly increase bioavailability; the rate of absorption of acetaminophen may be decreased when administered with food high in carbohydrates

Nursing/Pharmacy Information Monitor pain relief, respiratory and mental status, blood pressure, excessive sedation

Dosage Forms Tablet:

Darvocet-N®: Propoxyphene napsylate 50 mg and acetaminophen 325 mg

Darvocet-N® 100: Propoxyphene napsylate 100 mg and acetaminophen 650 mg

Genagesic®, Wygesic®: Propoxyphene hydrochloride 65 mg and acetaminophen 650 mg

propoxyphene and aspirin (proe POKS i feen & AS pir in)

Synonyms aspirin and propoxyphene

U.S. Brand Names Bexophene®; Darvon® Compound-65 Pulvules®

Generic Available Yes

Therapeutic Category Analgesic, Narcotic

Controlled Substance C-IV

Use Management of mild to moderate pain

Usual Dosage Oral: 1-2 capsules every 4 hours as needed

Nursing/Pharmacy Information Monitor pain relief, respiratory and mental status, blood pressure

Dosage Forms
Capsule: Propoxyphene hydrochloride 65 mg and aspirin 389 mg with caffeine 32.4 mg

Tablet (Darvon-N® with A.S.A.): Propoxyphene napsylate 100 mg and aspirin 325 mg

propranolol (proe PRAN oh lole)
U.S. Brand Names Betachron®; Inderal®; Inderal® LA
Canadian Brand Names Apo®-Propranolol; Detensol®; Nu-Propranolol®
Mexican Brand Names Inderalici; PMS-Propranolol®
Generic Available Yes
Therapeutic Category Antiarrhythmic Agent, Class II; Beta-Adrenergic Blocker
Use Management of hypertension, angina pectoris, pheochromocytoma, essential tremor, tetralogy of Fallot cyanotic spells, and arrhythmias (such as atrial fibrillation and flutter, A-V nodal re-entrant tachycardias, and catecholamine-induced arrhythmias); prevention of myocardial infarction, migraine headache; symptomatic treatment of hypertrophic subaortic stenosis; short-term adjunctive therapy of thyrotoxicosis

Usual Dosage
Tachyarrhythmias:
Oral:
Children: Initial: 0.5-1 mg/kg/day in divided doses every 6-8 hours; titrate dosage upward every 3-7 days; usual dose: 2-4 mg/kg/day; higher doses may be needed; do not exceed 16 mg/kg/day or 60 mg/day
Adults: 10-80 mg/dose every 6-8 hours
I.V.:
Children: 0.01-0.1 mg/kg slow IVP over 10 minutes; maximum dose: 1 mg
Adults: 1 mg/dose slow IVP; repeat every 5 minutes up to a total of 5 mg
Hypertension: Oral:
Children: Initial: 0.5-1 mg/kg/day in divided doses every 6-12 hours; increase gradually every 3-7 days; maximum: 2 mg/kg/24 hours
Adults: Initial: 40 mg twice daily or 60-80 mg once daily as sustained release capsules; increase dosage every 3-7 days; usual dose: ≤320 mg divided in 2-3 doses/day or once daily as sustained release; maximum daily dose: 640 mg
Migraine headache prophylaxis: Oral:
Children: 0.6-1.5 mg/kg/day **or**
≤35 kg: 10-20 mg 3 times/day
>35 kg: 20-40 mg 3 times/day
Adults: Initial: 80 mg/day divided every 6-8 hours; increase by 20-40 mg/dose every 3-4 weeks to a maximum of 160-240 mg/day administered in divided doses every 6-8 hours; if satisfactory response not achieved within 6 weeks of starting therapy, drug should be withdrawn gradually over several weeks
Tetralogy spells: Children: Oral: 1-2 mg/kg/day every 6 hours as needed, may increase by 1 mg/kg/day to a maximum of 5 mg/kg/day, or if refractory may increase slowly to a maximum of 10-15 mg/kg/day
Thyrotoxicosis:
Adolescents and Adults: Oral: 10-40 mg/dose every 6 hours
Adults: I.V.: 1-3 mg/dose slow IVP as a single dose
Adults: Oral:
Angina: 80-320 mg/day in doses divided 2-4 times/day or 80-160 mg of sustained release once daily
Pheochromocytoma: 30-60 mg/day in divided doses
Myocardial infarction prophylaxis: 180-240 mg/day in 3-4divided doses
Hypertrophic subaortic stenosis: 20-40 mg 3-4 times/day
Essential tremor: 40 mg twice daily initially; maintenance doses: usually 120-320 mg/day

Dietary Considerations Avoid natural licorice (causes sodium and water retention and increases potassium loss); protein-rich foods may increase bioavailability; a change in diet from high carbohydrate/low protein to low carbohydrate/high protein may result in increased oral clearance

Nursing/Pharmacy Information
I.V. dose much smaller than oral dose; propranolol may block hypoglycemia induced tachycardia and blood pressure changes; I.V. administration should not exceed 1 mg/minute for adults; administer slow I.V. over 10 minutes in children

Monitor blood pressure, EKG

Stability: **Compatible** in saline, **incompatible** with HCO_3^-; protect injection from light

(Continued)

propranolol *(Continued)*

Dosage Forms Propranolol hydrochloride:
Capsule, sustained action: 60 mg, 80 mg, 120 mg, 160 mg
Injection: 1 mg/mL (1 mL)
Solution, oral (strawberry-mint flavor): 4 mg/mL (5 mL, 500 mL); 8 mg/mL (5 mL, 500 mL)
Solution, oral, concentrate: 80 mg/mL (30 mL)
Tablet: 10 mg, 20 mg, 40 mg, 60 mg, 80 mg, 90 mg

propranolol and hydrochlorothiazide
(proe PRAN oh lole & hye droe klor oh THYE a zide)

Synonyms hydrochlorothiazide and propranolol
U.S. Brand Names Inderide®
Generic Available Immediate release: Yes
Therapeutic Category Antihypertensive Agent, Combination
Use Management of hypertension
Usual Dosage Dose is individualized
Dosage Forms
Capsule, long-acting (Inderide® LA):
80/50 Propranolol hydrochloride 80 mg and hydrochlorothiazide 50 mg
120/50 Propranolol hydrochloride 120 mg and hydrochlorothiazide 50 mg
160/50 Propranolol hydrochloride 160 mg and hydrochlorothiazide 50 mg
Tablet (Inderide®):
40/25 Propranolol hydrochloride 40 mg and hydrochlorothiazide 25 mg
80/25 Propranolol hydrochloride 80 mg and hydrochlorothiazide 25 mg

♦ **Propress** *see* dinoprostone *on page 207*
♦ **Propulsid®** *see* cisapride *on page 152*
♦ **propylene glycol and salicylic acid** *see* salicylic acid and propylene glycol *on page 558*

propylhexedrine (proe pil HEKS e dreen)

U.S. Brand Names Benzedrex® [OTC]
Generic Available No
Therapeutic Category Adrenergic Agonist Agent
Use Topical nasal decongestant
Usual Dosage Inhale through each nostril while blocking the other
Nursing/Pharmacy Information Drug has been extracted from inhaler and injected I.V. as an amphetamine substitute
Dosage Forms Inhaler: 250 mg

♦ **2-propylpentanoic acid** *see* valproic acid and derivatives *on page 641*

propylthiouracil (proe pil thye oh YOOR a sil)

Synonyms PTU
Canadian Brand Names Propyl-Thyracil®
Generic Available Yes
Therapeutic Category Antithyroid Agent
Use Palliative treatment of hyperthyroidism, adjunct to ameliorate hyperthyroidism in preparation for surgical treatment or radioactive iodine therapy, management of thyrotoxic crisis
Usual Dosage Oral:
Children: Initial: 5-7 mg/kg/day in divided doses every 8 hours or
6-10 years: 50-150 mg/day
>10 years: 150-300 mg/day
Maintenance: $1/3$ to $2/3$ of the initial dose in divided doses every 8-12 hours
Adults: Initial: 300-450 mg/day in divided doses every 8 hours; maintenance: 100-150 mg/day in divided doses every 8-12 hours
Dietary Considerations Administer at the same time in relation to meals each day, either always with meals or always between meals
Nursing/Pharmacy Information Monitor CBC with differential, prothrombin time, liver function tests, thyroid function tests (T_4, T_3, TSH); periodic blood counts are recommended chronic therapy
Dosage Forms Tablet: 50 mg

♦ **Propyl-Thyracil®** *see* propylthiouracil *on page 528*
♦ **2-propylvaleric acid** *see* valproic acid and derivatives *on page 641*
♦ **Prorazin®** *see* prochlorperazine *on page 519*
♦ **Prorex® Injection** *see* promethazine *on page 522*
♦ **Proscar®** *see* finasteride *on page 268*
♦ **Pro-Sof®** *(Discontinued)* *see page 743*

- ◆ **Pro-Sof® Plus [OTC]** *see docusate and casanthranol on page 215*
- ◆ **ProSom™** *see estazolam on page 242*
- ◆ **prostaglandin E₁** *see alprostadil on page 30*
- ◆ **prostaglandin E₂** *see dinoprostone on page 207*
- ◆ **prostaglandin F₂ alpha** *see dinoprost tromethamine on page 207*
- ◆ **Prostaphlin®** *(Discontinued) see page 743*
- ◆ **ProStep® Patch** *see nicotine on page 441*
- ◆ **Prostigmin®** *see neostigmine on page 438*
- ◆ **Prostin E₂® Vaginal Suppository** *see dinoprostone on page 207*
- ◆ **Prostin F₂ Alpha®** *see dinoprost tromethamine on page 207*
- ◆ **Prostin VR Pediatric® Injection** *see alprostadil on page 30*

protamine sulfate (PROE ta meen SUL fate)

Generic Available Yes

Therapeutic Category Antidote

Use Treatment of heparin overdosage; neutralize heparin during surgery or dialysis procedures

Usual Dosage Children and Adults: I.V.: 1 mg of protamine neutralizes 90 USP units of heparin (lung) and 115 USP units of heparin (intestinal); heparin neutralization occurs within 5 minutes following I.V. injection; administer 1 mg for each 100 units of heparin administered in preceding 3-4 hours up to a maximum dose of 50 mg

Nursing/Pharmacy Information

Parenteral: Reconstitute vial with 5 mL sterile water; if using protamine in neonates, reconstitute with preservative-free sterile water for injection; resulting solution equals 10 mg/mL; inject without further dilution over 1-3 minutes; maximum of 50 mg in any 10-minute period

Monitor coagulation test

Stability: Refrigerate, avoid freezing; remains stable for at least 2 weeks at room temperature; **incompatible** with cephalosporins and penicillins

Dosage Forms Injection: 10 mg/mL (5 mL, 10 mL, 25 mL)

- ◆ **Protenate®** *see plasma protein fraction on page 498*
- ◆ **Prothazine-DC®** *see promethazine and codeine on page 522*
- ◆ **Protilase®** *see pancrelipase on page 467*

protirelin (proe TYE re lin)

Synonyms lopremone

U.S. Brand Names Relefact® TRH; Thypinone®; Thyrel® TRH

Canadian Brand Names Combantrin®

Generic Available No

Therapeutic Category Diagnostic Agent

Use Adjunct in the diagnostic assessment of thyroid function, and an adjunct to other diagnostic procedures in assessment of patients with pituitary or hypothalamic dysfunction; also causes release of prolactin from the pituitary and is used to detect defective control of prolactin secretion.

Usual Dosage I.V.:

Children: 7 mcg/kg to a maximum dose of 500 mcg

Adults: 500 mcg (range: 200-500 mcg)

Nursing/Pharmacy Information

Keep patient supine during drug administration; administer undiluted direct I.V. over 15-30 seconds with the patient remaining supine for an additional 15 minutes

Monitor blood pressure, prolactin, TSH, T_4 and T_3

Dosage Forms Injection: 500 mcg/mL (1 mL)

- ◆ **Protopam® Injection** *see pralidoxime on page 511*
- ◆ **Protopam® Tablet** *(Discontinued) see page 743*
- ◆ **Protostat® Oral** *see metronidazole on page 411*
- ◆ **Pro-Trin®** *see co-trimoxazole on page 170*

protriptyline (proe TRIP ti leen)

U.S. Brand Names Vivactil®

Canadian Brand Names Triptil®

Generic Available No

Therapeutic Category Antidepressant, Tricyclic (Secondary Amine)

Use Treatment of various forms of depression, often in conjunction with psychotherapy

Usual Dosage Oral:

Adolescents: 15-20 mg/day

(Continued)

protriptyline (Continued)

Adults: 15-60 mg in 3-4 divided doses
Elderly: 15-20 mg/day

Dietary Considerations May be administered with food to decrease GI distress

Nursing/Pharmacy Information
Offer patient sugarless hard candy for dry mouth
Monitor sitting and standing blood pressure and pulse

Dosage Forms Tablet, as hydrochloride: 5 mg, 10 mg

- **Protropin®** *see* human growth hormone *on page 315*
- **Provatene®** *(Discontinued) see page 743*
- **Proventil®** *see* albuterol *on page 25*
- **Proventil® HFA** *see* albuterol *on page 25*
- **Provera® Oral** *see* medroxyprogesterone acetate *on page 389*
- **Provigil®** *see* modafinil *on page 419*
- **Provocholine®** *see* methacholine *on page 399*
- **Proxigel® Oral [OTC]** *see* carbamide peroxide *on page 112*
- **proxymetacaine** *see* proparacaine *on page 524*
- **Prozac®** *see* fluoxetine *on page 276*
- **Prozoladex** *see* goserelin *on page 297*
- **PRP-D** *see* Haemophilus B conjugate vaccine *on page 306*
- **prymaccone** *see* primaquine *on page 516*
- **Pseudo-Car® DM** *see* carbinoxamine, pseudoephedrine, and dextromethorphan *on page 114*

pseudoephedrine (soo doe e FED rin)

Synonyms d-isoephedrine

U.S. Brand Names Actifed® Allergy Tablet (Day) [OTC]; Afrinol® [OTC]; Cenafed® [OTC]; Children's Silfedrine® [OTC]; Decofed® Syrup [OTC]; Drixoral® Non-Drowsy [OTC]; Efidac/24® [OTC]; Neofed® [OTC]; PediaCare® Oral; Sudafed® [OTC]; Sudafed® 12 Hour [OTC]; Sufedrin® [OTC]; Triaminic® AM Decongestant Formula [OTC]

Canadian Brand Names Balminil® Decongestant; Eltor®; PMS-Pseudoephedrine; Robidrine®

Generic Available Yes

Therapeutic Category Adrenergic Agonist Agent

Use Temporary symptomatic relief of nasal congestion due to common cold, upper respiratory allergies, and sinusitis; also promotes nasal or sinus drainage

Usual Dosage Oral:
Children:
<2 years: 4 mg/kg/day in divided doses every 6 hours
2-5 years: 15 mg every 6 hours; maximum: 60 mg/24 hours
6-12 years: 30 mg every 6 hours; maximum: 120 mg/24 hours
Adults: 60 mg every 6 hours; maximum: 240 mg/24 hours

Dietary Considerations Should be administered with water or milk to decrease GI distress

Dosage Forms
Pseudoephedrine hydrochloride:
Capsule: 60 mg
Capsule, timed release: 120 mg
Drops, oral: 7.5 mg/0.8 mL (15 mL)
Liquid: 15 mg/5 mL (120 mL); 30 mg/5 mL (120 mL, 240 mL, 473 mL)
Syrup: 15 mg/5 mL (118 mL)
Tablet: 30 mg, 60 mg
Tablet, timed release: 120 mg
Pseudoephedrine sulfate:
Extended release: 120 mg, 240 mg

- **pseudoephedrine, acetaminophen, and dextromethorphan** *see* acetaminophen, dextromethorphan, and pseudoephedrine *on page 16*
- **pseudoephedrine and acetaminophen** *see* acetaminophen and pseudoephedrine *on page 15*
- **pseudoephedrine and acrivastine** *see* acrivastine and pseudoephedrine *on page 20*
- **pseudoephedrine and azatadine** *see* azatadine and pseudoephedrine *on page 67*
- **pseudoephedrine and carbinoxamine** *see* carbinoxamine and pseudoephedrine *on page 113*

♦ **pseudoephedrine and chlorpheniramine** *see* chlorpheniramine and pseudoephedrine *on page 140*

♦ **pseudoephedrine and dexbrompheniramine** *see* dexbrompheniramine and pseudoephedrine *on page 191*

pseudoephedrine and dextromethorphan
(soo doe e FED rin & deks troe meth OR fan)

U.S. Brand Names Drixoral® Cough & Congestion Liquid Caps [OTC]; Vicks® 44D Cough & Head Congestion; Vicks® 44 Non-Drowsy Cold & Cough Liqui-Caps [OTC]

Generic Available Yes

Therapeutic Category Antitussive/Decongestant

Use Temporary symptomatic relief of nasal congestion due to common cold, upper respiratory allergies, and sinusitis; also promotes nasal or sinus drainage; symptomatic relief of coughs caused by minor viral upper respiratory tract infections or inhaled irritants; most effective for a chronic nonproductive cough

Usual Dosage Adults: Oral: 1 capsule every 6 hours

Dosage Forms

Capsule: Pseudoephedrine hydrochloride 60 mg and dextromethorphan hydrobromide 30 mg

Liquid: Pseudoephedrine hydrochloride 20 mg and dextromethorphan hydrobromide 10 mg per 5 mL

♦ **pseudoephedrine and guaifenesin** *see* guaifenesin and pseudoephedrine *on page 302*

pseudoephedrine and ibuprofen
(soo doe e FED rin & eye byoo PROE fen)

U.S. Brand Names Advil® Cold & Sinus Caplets [OTC]; Dimetapp® Sinus Caplets [OTC]; Dristan® Sinus Caplets [OTC]; Motrin® IB Sinus [OTC]; Sine-Aid® IB [OTC]

Generic Available Yes

Therapeutic Category Decongestant/Analgesic

Use Temporary symptomatic relief of nasal congestion due to common cold, upper respiratory allergies, and sinusitis; also promotes nasal or sinus drainage; sinus headaches and pains

Usual Dosage Adults: Oral: 1-2 caplets every 4-6 hours

Dosage Forms Caplet: Pseudoephedrine hydrochloride 30 mg and ibuprofen 200 mg

♦ **pseudoephedrine and loratadine** *see* loratadine and pseudoephedrine *on page 375*

♦ **pseudoephedrine and triprolidine** *see* triprolidine and pseudoephedrine *on page 632*

♦ **pseudoephedrine, dextromethorphan, and acetaminophen** *see* acetaminophen, dextromethorphan, and pseudoephedrine *on page 16*

♦ **pseudoephedrine, dextromethorphan, and guaifenesin** *see* guaifenesin, pseudoephedrine, and dextromethorphan *on page 304*

♦ **pseudoephedrine, guaifenesin, and codeine** *see* guaifenesin, pseudoephedrine, and codeine *on page 304*

♦ **pseudoephedrine, hydrocodone, and guaifenesin** *see* hydrocodone, pseudoephedrine, and guaifenesin *on page 322*

♦ **Pseudo-Gest Plus® Tablet [OTC]** *see* chlorpheniramine and pseudoephedrine *on page 140*

♦ **pseudomonic acid A** *see* mupirocin *on page 424*

♦ **Psorcon™** *see* diflorasone *on page 202*

♦ **psoriGel® [OTC]** *see* coal tar *on page 162*

♦ **Psorion® Topical** *see* betamethasone (topical) *on page 85*

♦ **PSP** *see* phenolsulfonphthalein *on page 486*

♦ **P&S® Shampoo [OTC]** *see* salicylic acid *on page 557*

psyllium (SIL i yum)

Synonyms plantago seed; plantain seed

U.S. Brand Names Effer-Syllium® [OTC]; Fiberall® [OTC]; Fiberall® Powder [OTC]; Fiberall® Wafer [OTC]; Hydrocil® [OTC]; Konsyl® [OTC]; Konsyl-D® [OTC]; Metamucil® [OTC]; Metamucil® Instant Mix [OTC]; Modane® Bulk [OTC]; Perdiem® Plain [OTC]; Reguloid® [OTC]; Serutan® [OTC]; Syllact® [OTC]; V-Lax® [OTC]

Canadian Brand Names Fibrepur®; Novo-Mucilax®; Prodiem® Plain

Generic Available Yes

Therapeutic Category Laxative

(Continued)

psyllium *(Continued)*

Use Treatment of chronic atonic or spastic constipation and in constipation associated with rectal disorders; management of irritable bowel syndrome

Usual Dosage Oral:

Children 6-11 years: $1/2$ to 1 rounded teaspoonful 1-3 times/day

Adults: 1-2 rounded teaspoonfuls or 1-2 packets 1-4 times/day

Dietary Considerations Should be administered with large amount of fluids

Nursing/Pharmacy Information Inhalation of psyllium dust may cause sensitivity to psyllium (runny nose, watery eyes, wheezing)

Dosage Forms

Granules: 4.03 g per rounded teaspoon (100 g, 250 g); 2.5 g per rounded teaspoon

Powder: Psyllium 50% and dextrose 50% (6.5 g, 325 g, 420 g, 480 g, 500 g)

Powder:

Effervescent: 3 g/dose (270 g, 480 g); 3.4 g/dose (single-dose packets)

Psyllium hydrophilic: 3.4 g per rounded teaspoon (210 g, 300 g, 420 g, 630 g)

Squares, chewable: 1.7 g, 3.4 g

Wafers: 3.4 g

♦ **P.T.E.-4®** *see* trace metals *on page 620*
♦ **P.T.E.-5®** *see* trace metals *on page 620*
♦ **pteroylglutamic acid** *see* folic acid *on page 281*
♦ **PTU** *see* propylthiouracil *on page 528*
♦ **Pulmicort® Turbuhaler®** *see* budesonide *on page 96*
♦ **Pulmozyme®** *see* dornase alfa *on page 218*
♦ **Puralube® Tears Solution [OTC]** *see* artificial tears *on page 59*
♦ **Purge® [OTC]** *see* castor oil *on page 118*
♦ **Puri-Clens™ [OTC]** *see* methylbenzethonium chloride *on page 405*
♦ **purified protein derivative** *see* tuberculin tests *on page 635*
♦ **Purinethol®** *see* mercaptopurine *on page 394*
♦ **Purinol®** *see* allopurinol *on page 29*
♦ **PVF® K** *see* penicillin V potassium *on page 476*
♦ **P-V-Tussin®** *see* hydrocodone, phenylephrine, pyrilamine, phenindamine, chlorpheniramine, and ammonium chloride *on page 322*
♦ **P_xE_x® Ophthalmic** *see* pilocarpine and epinephrine *on page 494*

pyrantel pamoate *(pi RAN tel PAM oh ate)*

U.S. Brand Names Antiminth® [OTC]; Pin-Rid® [OTC]; Pin-X® [OTC]; Reese's® Pinworm Medicine [OTC]

Generic Available No

Therapeutic Category Anthelmintic

Use Roundworm (*Ascaris lumbricoides*), pinworm (*Enterobius vermicularis*), and hookworm (*Ancylostoma duodenale* and *Necator americanus*) infestations, and trichostrongyliasis

Usual Dosage Children and Adults: Oral:

Roundworm, pinworm, or trichostrongyliasis: 11 mg/kg administered as a single dose; maximum dose is 1 g; dosage should be repeated in 2 weeks for pinworm infection

Hookworm: 11 mg/kg/day once daily for 3 days

Nursing/Pharmacy Information

Shake well before pouring to assure accurate dosage

Monitor stool for presence of eggs, worms, and occult blood, serum AST AND ALT

Stability: Protect from light

Dosage Forms

Capsule: 180 mg

Liquid: 50 mg/mL (30 mL); 144 mg/mL (30 mL)

Suspension, oral (caramel-currant flavor): 50 mg/mL (60 mL)

pyrazinamide *(peer a ZIN a mide)*

Synonyms pyrazinoic acid amide

Canadian Brand Names PMS-Pyrazinamide; Tebrazid

Mexican Brand Names Braccoprial®

Generic Available Yes

Therapeutic Category Antitubercular Agent

Use In combination with other antituberculosis agents in the treatment of *Mycobacterium* tuberculosis infection (especially useful in disseminated and meningeal tuberculosis); CDC currently recommends a 3 or 4 multidrug regimen

which includes pyrazinamide, rifampin, INH, and at times ethambutol or streptomycin for the treatment of tuberculosis

Usual Dosage Oral:

Children: 15-30 mg/kg/day in divided doses every 12-24 hours; daily dose not
to exceed 2 g

Adults: 15-30 mg/kg/day in 3-4 divided doses; maximum daily dose: 2 g/day

Nursing/Pharmacy Information Monitor periodic liver function tests, serum
uric acid

Dosage Forms Tablet: 500 mg

♦ **pyrazinamide, rifampin, and isoniazid** *see* rifampin, isoniazid, and pyrazinamide *on page 550*

♦ **pyrazinoic acid amide** *see* pyrazinamide *on page 532*

pyrethrins and piperonyl butoxide (pye RE thrins)

Synonyms piperonyl butoxide and pyrethrins

U.S. Brand Names A-200™ Shampoo [OTC]; Barc™ Liquid [OTC]; End Lice®
Liquid [OTC]; Lice-Enz® Shampoo [OTC]; Pronto® Shampoo [OTC]; Pyrinex®
Pediculicide Shampoo [OTC]; Pyrinyl II® Liquid [OTC]; Pyrinyl Plus® Shampoo
[OTC]; R & C® Shampoo [OTC]; RID® Shampoo [OTC]; Tisit® Blue Gel [OTC];
Tisit® Liquid [OTC]; Tisit® Shampoo [OTC]; Triple X® Liquid [OTC]

Generic Available Yes

Therapeutic Category Scabicides/Pediculicides

Use Treatment of *Pediculus humanus* infestations

Usual Dosage Application of pyrethrins: Topical:

Apply enough solution to completely wet infested area, including hair

Allow to remain on area for 10 minutes

Wash and rinse with large amounts of warm water

Use fine-toothed comb to remove lice and eggs from hair

Shampoo hair to restore body and luster

Treatment may be repeated if necessary once in a 24-hours period

Repeat treatment in 7-10 days to kill newly hatched lice

Nursing/Pharmacy Information For external use only; avoid touching eyes,
mouth, or other mucous membranes; contact physician if irritation occurs or if
condition does not improve in 2-3 days

Dosage Forms

Gel, topical: Pyrethrins 0.3% and piperonyl butoxide 3% with petroleum distillate 1.2% (30 g, 480 g)

Liquid, topical: Pyrethrins 0.18% and piperonyl butoxide 2.2% with petroleum
distillate 5.52% (60 mL); pyrethrins 0.2% and piperonyl butoxide 2% with
deodorized kerosene 0.8% (60 mL, 120 mL); pyrethrins 0.3% and piperonyl
butoxide 2% (60 mL, 118 mL); pyrethrins 0.3% and piperonyl butoxide 3%
(60 mL, 120 mL, 240 mL)

Shampoo: Pyrethrins 0.2% and 2% piperonyl butoxide with deodorized kerosene 0.8% (118 mL); pyrethrins 0.3% and piperonyl butoxide 3% (60 mL,
118 mL); pyrethrins 0.33% and piperonyl butoxide 4% (60 mL, 120 mL)

♦ **Pyridiate®** *see* phenazopyridine *on page 483*

♦ **2-pyridine aldoxime methochloride** *see* pralidoxime *on page 511*

♦ **Pyridium®** *see* phenazopyridine *on page 483*

♦ **Pyridium Plus®** *(Discontinued) see page 743*

pyridostigmine (peer id oh STIG meen)

U.S. Brand Names Mestinon® Injection; Mestinon® Oral; Regonol® Injection

Generic Available No

Therapeutic Category Cholinergic Agent

Use Symptomatic treatment of myasthenia gravis by improving muscle strength;
reversal of effects of nondepolarizing neuromuscular blocking agents

Usual Dosage Normally, sustained release dosage form is used at bedtime for
patients who complain of morning weakness

Myasthenia gravis:

Oral:

Children: 7 mg/kg/day in 5-6 divided doses

Adults: Initial: 60 mg 3 times/day with maintenance dose ranging from 60
mg to 1.5 g/day; sustained release formulation should be dosed at least
every 6 hours (usually 12-24 hours)

I.M., I.V.:

Children: 0.05-0.15 mg/kg/dose (maximum single dose: 10 mg)

Adults: 2 mg every 2-3 hours or 1/30th of oral dose

Reversal of nondepolarizing neuromuscular blocker: I.M., I.V.:

Children: 0.1-0.25 mg/kg/dose preceded by atropine

(Continued)

pyridostigmine *(Continued)*

Adults: 10-20 mg preceded by atropine

Nursing/Pharmacy Information

Do not crush sustained release drug product; observe patient closely for cholinergic symptoms especially if I.V. dose is used; administer direct I.V. slowly over 2-4 minutes; patients receiving large parenteral doses should be pretreated with atropine

Monitor muscle strength, heart rate, vital capacity

Stability: Protect from light

Dosage Forms Pyridostigmine bromide:

Injection: 5 mg/mL (2 mL, 5 mL)

Syrup (raspberry flavor): 60 mg/5 mL (480 mL)

Tablet: 60 mg

Tablet, sustained release: 180 mg

pyridoxine (peer i DOKS een)

Synonyms vitamin B_6

U.S. Brand Names Nestrex®

Mexican Brand Names Benadon

Generic Available Yes

Therapeutic Category Vitamin, Water Soluble

Use Prevent and treat vitamin B_6 deficiency, pyridoxine-dependent seizures in infants, treatment of drug-induced deficiency (eg, isoniazid or hydralazine)

Usual Dosage

Pyridoxine-dependent Infants:

Oral: 2-100 mg/day

I.M., I.V.: 10-100 mg

Dietary deficiency: Oral:

Children: 5-10 mg/24 hours for 3 weeks

Adults: 10-20 mg/day for 3 weeks

Drug-induced neuritis (eg, isoniazid, hydralazine, penicillamine, cycloserine): Oral treatment:

Children: 10-50 mg/24 hours; prophylaxis: 1-2 mg/kg/24 hours

Adults: 100-200 mg/24 hours; prophylaxis: 10-100 mg/24 hours

For the treatment of seizures and/or coma from acute isoniazid toxicity, a dose of pyridoxine hydrochloride equal to the amount of INH ingested can be administered I.M./I.V. in divided doses together with other anticonvulsants

Nursing/Pharmacy Information

Parenteral: Administer slow I.V.

When administering large I.V. doses, monitor respiratory rate, heart rate, and blood pressure

Stability: Protect from light

Dosage Forms Pyridoxine hydrochloride:

Injection: 100 mg/mL (10 mL, 30 mL)

Tablet: 25 mg, 50 mg, 100 mg

Tablet, extended release: 100 mg

pyrimethamine (peer i METH a meen)

U.S. Brand Names Daraprim®

Mexican Brand Names Daraprim®

Generic Available No

Therapeutic Category Folic Acid Antagonist (Antimalarial)

Use Prophylaxis of malaria due to susceptible strains of plasmodia; used in conjunction with quinine and sulfadoxine for the treatment of uncomplicated attacks of chloroquine-resistant *P. falciparum* malaria; used in conjunction with fast-acting schizonticide to initiate transmission control and suppression cure; synergistic combination with sulfadiazine in treatment of toxoplasmosis

Usual Dosage Oral:

Malaria chemoprophylaxis:

Children: 0.5 mg/kg once weekly; not to exceed 25 mg/dose **or**

Children:

<4 years: 6.25 mg once weekly

4-10 years: 12.5 mg once weekly

Children >10 years and Adults: 25 mg once weekly

Dosage should be continued for all age groups for at least 6-10 weeks after leaving endemic areas

Chloroquine-resistant *P. falciparum* malaria (when used in conjunction with quinine and sulfadiazine):

Children:

<10 kg: 6.25 mg/day once daily for 3 days

10-20 kg: 12.5 mg/day once daily for 3 days
20-40 kg: 25 mg/day once daily for 3 days
Adults: 25 mg twice daily for 3 days
Toxoplasmosis (with sulfadiazine or trisulfapyrimidines):
Children: 1 mg/kg/day divided into 2 equal daily doses; decrease dose after 2-4 days by 50%, continue for about 1 month; used with 100 mg sulfadiazine/kg/day divided every 6 hours; or 2 mg/kg/day divided every 12 hours for 3 days followed by 1 mg/kg/day once daily for 4 weeks
Adults: 50-75 mg/day together with 1-4 g of a sulfonamide for 1-3 weeks depending on patient's tolerance and response

Nursing/Pharmacy Information
Leucovorin may be administered in a dosage of 3-9 mg/day for 3 days or 5 mg every 3 days or as required to reverse symptoms or to prevent hematologic problems due to folic acid deficiency
Monitor CBC, including platelet counts twice weekly
Stability: Pyrimethamine tablets may be crushed to prepare oral suspensions of the drug in water, cherry syrup, or sucrose-containing solutions at a concentration of 1 mg/mL; stable at room temperature for 5-7 days

Dosage Forms Tablet: 25 mg

♦ **Pyrinex® Pediculicide Shampoo [OTC]** *see* pyrethrins and piperonyl butoxide *on page 533*

♦ **Pyrinyl II® Liquid [OTC]** *see* pyrethrins and piperonyl butoxide *on page 533*

♦ **Pyrinyl Plus® Shampoo [OTC]** *see* pyrethrins and piperonyl butoxide *on page 533*

pyrithione zinc (peer i THYE one zingk)
U.S. Brand Names DHS Zinc® [OTC]; Head & Shoulders® [OTC]; Theraplex Z® [OTC]; Zincon® Shampoo [OTC]; ZNP® Bar [OTC]
Generic Available No
Therapeutic Category Antiseborrheic Agent, Topical
Use Relieves the itching, irritation and scalp flaking associated with dandruff and/or seborrheal dermatitis of the scalp
Usual Dosage Topical: Shampoo hair twice weekly, wet hair, apply to scalp and massage vigorously, rinse and repeat
Dosage Forms
Bar: 2% (119 g)
Shampoo: 1% (120 mL); 2% (120 mL, 180 mL, 240 mL, 360 mL)

♦ **Pyronium®** *see* phenazopyridine *on page 483*

♦ **Quadrax** *see* ibuprofen *on page 332*

quazepam (KWAY ze pam)
U.S. Brand Names Doral®
Generic Available No
Therapeutic Category Benzodiazepine
Controlled Substance C-IV
Use Short-term treatment of insomnia
Usual Dosage Adults: Oral: Initial: 15 mg at bedtime; in some patients the dose may be reduced to 7.5 mg after a few nights
Nursing/Pharmacy Information
Provide safety measures (ie, side rails, night light, call button); remove smoking materials from area; supervise ambulation
Monitor respiratory and cardiovascular status
Dosage Forms Tablet: 7.5 mg, 15 mg

♦ **Quelicin®** *see* succinylcholine *on page 582*

♦ **Quemicetina** *see* chloramphenicol *on page 133*

♦ **Questran®** *see* cholestyramine resin *on page 147*

♦ **Questran® Light** *see* cholestyramine resin *on page 147*

♦ **Questran® Tablet** *(Discontinued) see page 743*

quetiapine (kwe TYE a peen)
U.S. Brand Names Seroquel®
Generic Available No
Therapeutic Category Antipsychotic Agent
Use Management of psychotic disorders; this antipsychotic drug belongs to a new chemical class, the dibenzothiazepine derivatives
Usual Dosage Adults: Oral: 25-100 mg 2-3 times/day
Nursing/Pharmacy Information Seroquel® has a very low incidence of extrapyramidal symptoms such as restlessness and abnormal movement; is at least as effective as conventional antipsychotics, ie Haldol®
(Continued)

quetiapine (Continued)

Dosage Forms Tablet, as fumarate: 25 mg, 100 mg, 200 mg

- ◆ **Quibron®** see theophylline and guaifenesin on page 604
- ◆ **Quibron®-T** see theophylline on page 603
- ◆ **Quibron®-T/SR** see theophylline on page 603
- ◆ **Quiess® Injection** see hydroxyzine on page 328
- ◆ **Quilagen** see gentamicin on page 290
- ◆ **Quimocyclar** see tetracycline on page 601
- ◆ **Quinaglute® Dura-Tabs®** see quinidine on page 536
- ◆ **Quinalan®** see quinidine on page 536
- ◆ **quinalbarbitone** see secobarbital on page 561
- ◆ **Quinamm® (Discontinued)** see page 743

quinapril (KWIN a pril)

U.S. Brand Names Accupril®
Mexican Brand Names Acupril
Generic Available No
Therapeutic Category Angiotensin-Converting Enzyme (ACE) Inhibitor
Use Treatment of hypertension, either alone or in combination with other antihypertensive agents
Usual Dosage Adults: Oral: Initial: 10 mg once daily, adjust according to blood pressure response at peak and trough blood levels; in general, the normal dosage range is 40-80 mg/day
Nursing/Pharmacy Information
May cause depression in some patients; discontinue if angioedema of the face, extremities, lips, tongue, or glottis occurs; watch for hypotensive effects within 1-3 hours of first dose or new higher dose
Monitor BUN, serum creatinine, renal function; nausea, headache, diarrhea, change in taste, cough
Stability: Store at room temperature
Dosage Forms Tablet, as hydrochloride: 5 mg, 10 mg, 20 mg, 40 mg

quinapril and hydrochlorothiazide (Canada only)

(KWIN a pril & hye droe klor oh THYE a zide)
Canadian Brand Names Accuretic®
Generic Available No
Therapeutic Category Angiotensin-Converting Enzyme (ACE) Inhibitor; Diuretic, Thiazide
Use Treatment of essential hypertension when combination therapy is appropriate
Usual Dosage Dosage must be individualized; the fixed combination is not for initial therapy; the dose should be determined by titration of the individual components
Dosage Forms Tablet: Quinapril hydrochloride 10 mg and hydrochlorothiazide 12.5 mg; quinapril hydrochloride 20 mg and hydrochlorothiazide 12.5 mg

quinethazone (kwin ETH a zone)

U.S. Brand Names Hydromox®
Generic Available No
Therapeutic Category Diuretic, Thiazide
Use Adjunctive therapy in treatment of edema and hypertension
Usual Dosage Adults: Oral: 50-100 mg once daily up to a maximum of 200 mg/day
Dietary Considerations May be administered with food or milk
Nursing/Pharmacy Information Administer early in day to avoid nocturia; administer the last dose of multiple doses no later than 6 PM unless instructed otherwise. A few people who take this medication become more sensitive to sunlight and may experience skin rash, redness, itching, or severe sunburn, especially if sun block SPF 15 or higher is not used on exposed skin areas.
Dosage Forms Tablet: 50 mg

- ◆ **Quinidex® Extentabs®** see quinidine on page 536

quinidine (KWIN i deen)

U.S. Brand Names Cardioquin®; Quinaglute® Dura-Tabs®; Quinalan®; Quinidex® Extentabs®; Quinora®
Canadian Brand Names Biquin® Durules®
Mexican Brand Names Quini Durules®
Generic Available Yes

Therapeutic Category Antiarrhythmic Agent, Class I-A

Use Prophylaxis after cardioversion of atrial fibrillation and/or flutter to maintain normal sinus rhythm; also used to prevent reoccurrence of paroxysmal supraventricular tachycardia, paroxysmal A-V junctional rhythm, paroxysmal ventricular tachycardia, paroxysmal atrial fibrillation, and atrial or ventricular premature contractions; also has activity against *Plasmodium falciparum* malaria

Usual Dosage Note: Dosage expressed in terms of the salt: 267 mg of quinidine gluconate = 275 mg of quinidine polygalacturonate = 200 mg of quinidine sulfate

Children: Test dose for idiosyncratic reaction (sulfate, oral or gluconate, I.M.): 2 mg/kg or 60 mg/m^2

    Oral (quinidine sulfate): 15-60 mg/kg/day in 4-5 divided doses or 6 mg/kg every 4-6 hours (AMA 1991); usual 30 mg/kg/day or 900 mg/m^2/day administered in 5 daily doses

    I.V. **not** recommended (quinidine gluconate): 2-10 mg/kg/dose every 3-6 hours as needed

Adults: Test dose: 200 mg administered several hours before full dosage (to determine possibility of idiosyncratic reaction)

    Oral (sulfate): 100-600 mg/dose every 4-6 hours; begin at 200 mg/dose and titrate to desired effect

    Oral (gluconate): 324-972 mg every 8-12 hours

    Oral (polygalacturonate): 275 mg every 8-12 hours

    I.M.: 400 mg/dose every 4-6 hours

    I.V.: 200-400 mg/dose diluted and administered at a rate ≤10 mg/minute

Dietary Considerations Excessive intake of fruit juices or vitamin C may decrease urine pH and result in increased clearance of quinidine with decreased serum concentration; alkaline foods may result in increased quinidine serum concentrations; food has a variable effect on absorption of sustained release formulation

Nursing/Pharmacy Information

Do not crush sustained release product; patients should notify their physician if fever, rash, unusual bruising or bleeding, visual disturbances, or ringing in the ears occur; maximum I.V. rate of infusion: 10 mg/minute

Monitor complete blood counts, liver and renal function tests, should be routinely performed during long-term administration

Stability: Do not use discolored parenteral solution

Dosage Forms

Quinidine gluconate:
    Injection: 80 mg/mL (10 mL)
    Tablet, sustained release: 324 mg

Quinidine polygalacturonate:
    Tablet: 275 mg

Quinidine sulfate:
    Tablet: 200 mg, 300 mg
    Tablet, sustained action: 300 mg

♦ **Quini Durules®** *see* quinidine *on page 536* *see* quinidine *on page 536*

quinine (KWYE nine)

U.S. Brand Names Formula Q®

Generic Available Yes

Therapeutic Category Antimalarial Agent

Use Suppression or treatment of chloroquine-resistant *P. falciparum* malaria (inactive against sporozoites, pre-erythrocytic or exoerythrocytic forms of plasmodia); treatment of *Babesia microti* infection

Usual Dosage Oral (parenteral dosage form may be obtained from Centers for Disease Control if needed):

Children: Chloroquine-resistant malaria and babesiosis: 25 mg/kg/day in divided doses every 8 hours for 7 days; maximum: 650 mg/dose

Adults:
    Chloroquine-resistant malaria: 650 mg every 8 hours for 7 days in conjunction with another agent
    Babesiosis: 650 mg every 6-8 hours for 7 days

Dietary Considerations May be administered with food

Nursing/Pharmacy Information

Do not crush tablets or capsule to avoid bitter taste

Monitor CBC with platelet count, liver function tests, blood glucose, ophthalmologic examination

Stability: Protect from light

(Continued)

quinine *(Continued)*

Dosage Forms Quinine sulfate:
Capsule: 64.8 mg, 65 mg, 200 mg, 300 mg, 325 mg
Tablet: 162.5 mg, 260 mg

- ♦ **quinol** *see* hydroquinone *on page 325*
- ♦ **Quinora®** *see* quinidine *on page 536*

quinupristin and dalfopristin *New Drug*

(kwi NYOO pris tin & dal FOE pris tin)
Synonyms pristinamycin; RP59500
U.S. Brand Names Synercid®
Generic Available No
Therapeutic Category Antibiotic, Streptogramin
Use Treatment of serious or life-threatening infections associated with vanco-mycin-resistant *Enterococcus faecium* bacteremia; treatment of complicated skin and skin structure infections caused by methcillin-susceptible *Staphylococcus aureus* or *Streptococcus pyogenes*

Investigational use: Has been studied in the treatment of a variety of infections caused by *Enterococcus faecium* (not *E. fecalis*) including vancomycin-resistant strains. May also be effective in the treatment of serious infections caused by *Staphylococcus* species including those resistant to methicillin.

Usual Dosage Adults: I.V.:
Vancomycin-resistant *Enterococcus faecium*: 7.5 mg/kg every 8 hours
Complicated skin and skin structure infection: 7.5 mg/kg every 12 hours
Dosage adjustment in renal impairment: No adjustment required in renal failure, hemodialysis or peritoneal dialysis
Dosage adjustment in hepatic impairment: Pharmacokinetic data suggest dosage adjustment may be necessary, however, specific recommendations have not been proposed
Elderly: No dosage adjustment is required
Dosage Forms Powder for injection: 500 mg (350 mg dalfopristin and 150 mg quinupristin)

- ♦ **Quiphile®** *(Discontinued) see page 743*
- ♦ **Q-vel®** *(Discontinued) see page 743*

rabeprazole *New Drug* (ra BE pray zole)

Synonyms pariprazole
U.S. Brand Names Aciphex™
Generic Available No
Therapeutic Category Gastric Acid Secretion Inhibitor
Use Short-term (4-8 weeks) treatment of erosive or ulcerative gastroesophageal reflux disease (GERD); maintenance therapy in erosive or ulcerative GERD; short-term (up to 4 weeks) treatment of duodenal ulcers; long-term treatment of pathological hypersecretory conditions, including Zollinger-Ellison syndrome
Usual Dosage Adults and Elderly:
GERD: 20 mg once daily for 4-8 weeks; maintenance: 20 mg once daily
Duodenal ulcer: 20 mg/day after breakfast for 4 weeks
Hypersecretory conditions: 60 mg once daily; dose may need to be adjusted as necessary. Doses as high as 100 mg and 60 mg twice daily have been used.
Dosage Forms Tablet, delayed release: 20 mg

rabies immune globulin (human)

(RAY beez i MYUN GLOB yoo lin, HYU man)
Synonyms RIG
U.S. Brand Names Bayrab®; Hyperab®; Imogam®
Generic Available No
Therapeutic Category Immune Globulin
Use Passive immunity to rabies for postexposure prophylaxis of individuals exposed to the virus
Usual Dosage Children and Adults: I.M.: 20 units/kg in a single dose (RIG should always be administered in conjunction with rabies vaccine (HDCV)) (infiltrate ½ of the dose locally around the wound; administer the remainder I.M.)
Nursing/Pharmacy Information
Severe adverse reactions can occur if patient receives RIG I.V.
Stability: Refrigerate
Dosage Forms Injection: 150 units/mL (2 mL, 10 mL)

rabies virus vaccine (RAY beez VYE rus vak SEEN)

Synonyms HDCV; HDRS

U.S. Brand Names Imovax® Rabies I.D. Vaccine; Imovax® Rabies Vaccine

Generic Available No

Therapeutic Category Vaccine, Inactivated Virus

Use Pre-exposure rabies immunization for high risk persons; postexposure anti-rabies immunization along with local treatment and immune globulin

Usual Dosage

Pre-exposure prophylaxis: Two 1 mL doses I.M. or I.D. one week apart, third dose 3 weeks after second dose. If exposure continues, booster doses can be administered every 2 years, or an antibody titer determined and a booster dose administered if the titer is inadequate.

Postexposure prophylaxis: All postexposure treatment should begin with immediate cleansing of the wound with soap and water. Persons not previously immunized as above: Rabies immune globulin 20 units/kg body weight, half infiltrated at bite site if possible, remainder I.M.; and 5 doses of rabies vaccine, 1 mL I.M., one each on days 0, 3, 7, 14, 28.

Persons who have previously received postexposure prophylaxis with rabies vaccine, received a recommended I.M. or I.D. pre-exposure series of rabies vaccine or have a previously documented rabies antibody titer considered adequate: Two doses of rabies vaccine, 1 mL I.M., one each on days 0 and 3

Nursing/Pharmacy Information

For intramuscular injection only; this rabies vaccine product must not be administered intradermally; in older children and adults it should be given in deltoid area for best response

Stability: Refrigerate; reconstituted vaccine should be used immediately

Dosage Forms Injection:

I.M. (HDCV): Rabies antigen 2.5 units/mL (1 mL)

Intradermal: Rabies antigen 0.25 units/mL (1 mL)

♦ **Racovel** see levodopa and carbidopa on page 365

radiological/contrast media (ionic)

U.S. Brand Names Anatrast®; Angio Conray®; Angiovist®; Baricon®; Barobag®; Baro-CAT®; Baroflave®; Barosperse®; Bar-Test®; Bilopaque®; Cholebrine®; Cholografin® Meglumine; Conray®; Cystografin®; Dionosil Oily®; Enecat®; Entrobar®; Epi-C®; Ethiodol®; Flo-Coat®; Gastrografin®; HD 85®; HD 200 Plus®; Hexabrix™; Hypaque-Cysto®; Hypaque® Meglumine; Hypaque® Sodium; Liquid Barosperse®; Liquipake®; Lymphazurin®; Magnevist®; MD-Gastroview®; Oragrafin® Calcium; Oragrafin® Sodium; Perchloracap®; Prepcat®; Reno-M-30®; Reno-M-60®; Reno-M-Dip®; Renovue®-65; Renovue®-DIP; Sinografin®; Telepaque®; Tomocat®; Tonopaque®; Urovist Cysto®; Urovist® Meglumine; Urovist® Sodium 300; Vascoray®

Generic Available Yes

Therapeutic Category Radiopaque Agents

Dosage Forms

Oral cholecystographic agents:

Iocetamic acid: Tablet (Cholebrine®): 750 mg

Iopanoic acid: Tablet (Telepaque®): 500 mg

Ipodate calcium: Granules for oral suspension (Oragrafin® Calcium): 3 g

Ipodate sodium: Capsule (Bilivist®, Oragrafin® Sodium): 500 mg

Tyropanoate sodium: Capsule (Bilopaque®): 750 mg

GI contrast agents: Barium sulfate:

Paste (Anatrast®): 100% (500 g)

Powder:

Baroflave®: 100%

Baricon®, HD 200 Plus®: 98%

Barosperse®, Tonopaque®: 95%

Suspension:

Baro-CAT®, Prepcat®: 1.5%

Enecat®, Tomocat®: 5%

Entrobar®: 50%

Liquid Barasperse®: 60%

HD 85®: 85%

Barobag®: 97%

Flo-Coat®, Liquipake®: 100%

Epi-C®: 150%

Tablet (Bar-Test®): 650 mg

(Continued)

radiological/contrast media (ionic) *(Continued)*

Parenteral agents: Injection:
Diatrizoate meglumine:
 Hypaque® Meglumine
 Reno-M-DIP®
 Urovist® Meglumine
 Angiovist® 282
 Hypaque® Meglumine
 Reno-M-60®
Diatrizoate sodium:
 Hypaque® Sodium
 Hypaque® Sodium
 Urovist® Sodium 300
Gadopentetate dimeglumine: Magnevist®
Iodamide meglumine:
 Renovue®-DIP
 Renovue®-65
Iodipamide meglumine: Cholografin® meglumine
Iothalamate meglumine:
 Conray® 30
 Conray® 43
 Conray®
Iothalamate sodium:
 Angio Conray®
 Conray® 325
 Conray® 400
Diatrizoate meglumine and diatrizoate sodium:
 Angiovist® 292
 Angiovist® 370
 Hypaque-76®
 Hypaque-M®, 75%
 Hypaque-M®, 90%
 MD-60®
 MD-76®
 Renografin-60®
 Renografin-76®
 Renovist® II
 Renovist®
Iothalamate meglumine and iothalamate sodium:
 Vascoray®
 Hexabrix™

Miscellaneous agents: (**NOT** for intravascular use, for instillation into various cavities)
Diatrizoate meglumine: Urogenital solution, sterile:
 Crystografin®
 Crystografin® Dilute
 Hypaque-Cysto®
 Reno-M-30®
 Urovist Cysto®
Diatrizoate meglumine and diatrizoate sodium: Solution, oral or rectal:
 Gastrografin®
 MD-Gastroview®
Diatrizoate sodium:
 Solution, oral or rectal (Hypaque® sodium oral)
 Solution, urogenital (Hypaque® sodium 20%)
Iothalamate meglumine: Solution, urogenital:
 Cysto-Conray®
 Cysto-Conray® II

Diatrizoate meglumine and iodipamide meglumine:
 Injection, urogenital for intrauterine instillation (Sinografin®)
Ethiodized oil: Injection (Ethiodol®)
Propyliodone: Suspension (Dionosil Oily®)
Isosulfan blue: Injection (Lymphazurin® 1%)
Potassium perchlorate: Capsule (Perchloracap®): 200 mg

radiological/contrast media (non-ionic)
U.S. Brand Names Amipaque®; Isovue®; Omnipaque®; Optiray®
Generic Available Yes
Therapeutic Category Radiopaque Agents

Dosage Forms Parenteral agents: Injection:
 Iohexol: Omnipaque®: 140 mg/mL; 180 mg/mL; 210 mg/mL; 240 mg/mL; 300 mg/mL; 350 mg/mL
 Iopamidol:
  Isovue-128®
  Isovue-200®
  Isovue-M 200®
  Isovue-300®
  Isovue-M 300®
  Isovue-370®
 Ioversol:
  Optiray® 160
  Optiray® 240
  Optiray® 320
 Metrizamide: Amipaque®

♦ **Radiostol®** *see* ergocalciferol *on page 237*
♦ **R-albuterol** *see* levalbuterol *New Drug on page 363*

raloxifene (ral OX i feen)
U.S. Brand Names Evista®
Generic Available No
Therapeutic Category Selective Estrogen Receptor Modulator (SERM)
Use Prevention and treatment of osteoporosis in postmenopausal women
Usual Dosage Adults: Oral: 1 tablet daily, may be administered any time of the day without regard to meals
Dosage Forms Tablet, as hydrochloride: 60 mg

♦ **Ramace** *see* ramipril *on page 541*

ramipril (ra MI pril)
U.S. Brand Names Altace™
Mexican Brand Names Ramace; Tritace
Generic Available No
Therapeutic Category Angiotensin-Converting Enzyme (ACE) Inhibitor
Use Treatment of hypertension, alone or in combination with thiazide diuretics; congestive heart failure immediately after myocardial infarction
Usual Dosage Adults: Oral: 2.5-5 mg once daily
Nursing/Pharmacy Information
 May cause depression in some patients; discontinue if angioedema of the face, extremities, lips, tongue, or glottis occurs; watch for hypotensive effects within 1-3 hours of first dose or new higher dose
 Monitor BUN, serum creatinine, renal function; nausea, headache, diarrhea, change in taste, cough
Dosage Forms Capsule: 1.25 mg, 2.5 mg, 5 mg, 10 mg

♦ **Ramses® [OTC]** *see* nonoxynol 9 *on page 446*
♦ **Randikan** *see* kanamycin *on page 352*
♦ **Ranifur** *see* ranitidine hydrochloride *on page 541*
♦ **Ranisen** *see* ranitidine hydrochloride *on page 541*

ranitidine bismuth citrate (ra NI ti deen BIZ muth SIT rate)
Synonyms RBC
U.S. Brand Names Tritec®
Generic Available No
Therapeutic Category Gastrointestinal Agent, Gastric or Duodenal Ulcer Treatment
Use In combination with clarithromycin for the treatment of active duodenal ulcer associated with *H. pylori* infection; not to be used alone for the treatment of active duodenal ulcer
Usual Dosage Adults: Oral: 400 mg twice daily for 4 weeks (28 days) in conjunction with clarithromycin 500 mg 3 times/day for first 2 weeks
Dosage Forms Tablet: 400 mg (ranitidine 162 mg, trivalent bismuth 128 mg, and citrate 110 mg)

ranitidine hydrochloride (ra NI ti deen hye droe KLOR ide)
U.S. Brand Names Zantac®; Zantac® 75 [OTC]
Canadian Brand Names Apo®-Ranitidine; Novo-Ranidine®; Nu-Ranit®
Mexican Brand Names Acloral®; Alter-H₂®; Alvidina; Anistal; Azantac; Cauteridol®; Credaxol; Galidrin; Gastrec; Microtid; Neugal; Ranifur; Ranisen
Generic Available Yes
Therapeutic Category Histamine H₂ Antagonist
 (Continued)

541

ranitidine hydrochloride *(Continued)*

Use Short-term treatment of active duodenal ulcers and benign gastric ulcers; long-term prophylaxis of duodenal ulcer and gastric hypersecretory states; gastroesophageal reflux (GER)

Usual Dosage

Children:

Oral: 1.5-2 mg/kg/dose every 12 hours

I.M., I.V.: 0.75-1.5 mg/kg/dose every 6-8 hours, maximum daily dose: 400 mg

Continuous infusion: 0.1-0.25 mg/kg/hour (preferred for stress ulcer prophylaxis in patients with concurrent maintenance I.V.s or TPNs)

Adults:

Short-term treatment of ulceration: 150 mg/dose twice daily or 300 mg at bedtime

Prophylaxis of recurrent duodenal ulcer: 150 mg at bedtime

Gastric hypersecretory conditions: Oral: 150 mg twice daily, up to 600 mg / day

I.M., I.V.: 50 mg/dose every 6-8 hours (dose not to exceed 400 mg/day)

Nursing/Pharmacy Information

I.M. solution does not need to be diluted before use; monitor creatinine clearance for renal impairment; administering dose at 6 PM may be better than 10 PM bedtime, the highest acid production usually starts at approximately 7 PM, thus administering at 6 PM controls acid secretion better; observe caution in patients with renal function impairment and hepatic function impairment; intermittent infusion preferred over direct injection to decrease risk of bradycardia; for intermittent infusion, infuse over 15-30 minutes, at a usual concentration of 0.5 mg/mL; for direct I.V. injection, administer over a period not less than 5 minutes at a final concentration not to exceed 2.5 mg/ mL

Monitor AST, ALT, serum creatinine; when used to prevent stress-related GI bleeding, measure the intragastric pH and try to maintain pH >4

Stability: Solution for I.V. infusion in normal saline or D_5W is stable for 48 hours at room temperature or 30 days when frozen; is stable for 24 hours in TPN solutions; is stable only for 12 hours in total nutrient admixtures (TPN) when lipids are added. I.V. form is **incompatible** with amphotericin B, clindamycin, diazepam (same syringe), hetastarch (Y-line), hydroxyzine (same syringe), midazolam (same syringe), pentobarbital (same syringe), phenobarbital (same syringe)

Dosage Forms Ranitidine hydrochloride:

Capsule (GELdose™): 150 mg, 300 mg

Granules, effervescent (EFFERdose™): 150 mg

Infusion, preservative free, in NaCl 0.45%: 1 mg/mL (50 mL)

Injection: 25 mg/mL (2 mL, 10 mL, 40 mL)

Syrup (peppermint flavor): 15 mg/mL (473 mL)

Tablet: 75 mg [OTC]; 150 mg, 300 mg

Tablet, effervescent (EFFERdose™): 150 mg

rapacuronium *New Drug* (ra pa kyoo ROE nee um)

U.S. Brand Names Raplon™

Generic Available No

Therapeutic Category Neuromuscular Blocker Agent, Nondepolarizing

Use Adjunct to general anesthesia to facilitate tracheal intubation; to provide skeletal muscle relaxation during surgical procedures; does not relieve pain

Usual Dosage I.V. (do not administer I.M.):

Children 1 month to 12 years: Initial: 2 mg/kg. Repeat dosing is not recommended in pediatric patients.

Children 13-17 years: Clinicians should consider the physical maturity, height and weight of the patient in determining the dose. Adults (1.5 mg/kg), pediatric (2 mg/kg) and Cesarean section (2.5 mg/kg) dosing recommendations may serve as a general guideline in determining an intubating dose in this age group.

Adults: Tracheal Intubation:

Initial: Short surgical procedures: 1.5 mg/kg; Cesarean section: 2.5 mg/kg

Repeat dosing: Up to three maintenance doses of 0.5 mg/kg, administered at 25% recovery of control T1 may be administered. **Note:** The duration of neuromuscular blockade increases with each additional dose.

Elderly: No dosing adjustment is recommended in geriatric patients

Dosage Forms Powder for injection: 100 mg (5 mL); 200 mg (10 mL)

♦ **Rapamune®** see sirolimus *New Drug* on page 568
♦ **Raplon™** see rapacuronium *New Drug* on page 542

♦ **Rastinon** see tolbutamide on page 617
♦ **Raudixin**® see Rauwolfia serpentina on page 543
♦ **Rauverid**® see Rauwolfia serpentina on page 543

Rauwolfia serpentina (rah WOOL fee a ser pen TEEN ah)

Synonyms whole root rauwolfia
U.S. Brand Names Raudixin®; Rauverid®; Wolfina®
Generic Available Yes
Therapeutic Category Rauwolfia Alkaloid
Use Mild essential hypertension; relief of agitated psychotic states
Usual Dosage Adults: Oral: 200-400 mg/day in 2 divided doses
Dietary Considerations May be administered with food or milk to decrease GI distress
Nursing/Pharmacy Information Monitor blood pressure (standing and sitting/supine); diarrhea, weakness, mental changes
Dosage Forms Tablet: 50 mg, 100 mg

♦ **Raxar**® see grepafloxacin Withdrawn from U.S. market 10/27/99 on page 298
♦ **Raxedin** see loperamide on page 374
♦ **RBC** see ranitidine bismuth citrate on page 541
♦ **R & C**® **Shampoo [OTC]** see pyrethrins and piperonyl butoxide on page 533
♦ **Reactine**™ see cetirizine on page 130
♦ **Rea-Lo**® **[OTC]** see urea on page 638
♦ **Rebetron**™ see interferon alfa-2b and ribavirin combination pack on page 342
♦ **recombinant human deoxyribonuclease** see dornase alfa on page 218
♦ **recombinant human interleukin-11** see oprelvekin on page 457
♦ **recombinant interleukin-11** see oprelvekin on page 457
♦ **recombinant plasminogen activator** see reteplase on page 545
♦ **Recombinate**® see antihemophilic factor (recombinant) on page 52
♦ **Recombivax HB**® see hepatitis B vaccine on page 312
♦ **Rectacort**® **Suppository** *(Discontinued)* see page 743
♦ **Rectocort** see hydrocortisone (rectal) on page 322
♦ **Red Away**® see naphazoline on page 431
♦ **Redisol**® see cyanocobalamin on page 173
♦ **Redoxon**® see ascorbic acid on page 60
♦ **Redoxon**® **Forte** see ascorbic acid on page 60
♦ **Redutemp**® **[OTC]** see acetaminophen on page 13
♦ **Redux**® *(Discontinued)* see page 743
♦ **Reese's**® **Pinworm Medicine [OTC]** see pyrantel pamoate on page 532
♦ **Refludan**® see lepirudin on page 362
♦ **Refresh**® **Ophthalmic Solution [OTC]** see artificial tears on page 59
♦ **Refresh**® **Plus Ophthalmic Solution [OTC]** see artificial tears on page 59
♦ **Regitine**® see phentolamine on page 487
♦ **Reglan**® see metoclopramide on page 409
♦ **Regonol**® **Injection** see pyridostigmine on page 533
♦ **Regranex**® see becaplermin on page 75
♦ **Regulace**® **[OTC]** see docusate and casanthranol on page 215
♦ **Regular Iletin**® **I** see insulin preparations on page 339
♦ **Regular [Concentrated] Iletin**® **II U-500** see insulin preparations on page 339
♦ **Regular Insulin** see insulin preparations on page 339
♦ **Regular Purified Pork Insulin** see insulin preparations on page 339
♦ **Regulax SS**® **[OTC]** see docusate on page 214
♦ **Regulex**® see docusate on page 214
♦ **Reguloid**® **[OTC]** see psyllium on page 531
♦ **Regutol**® *(Discontinued)* see page 743
♦ **Relafen**® see nabumetone on page 427
♦ **Relefact**® **TRH** see protirelin on page 529
♦ **Relenza**® see zanamivir New Drug on page 658
♦ **Relief**® **Ophthalmic Solution** see phenylephrine on page 487
♦ **Remeron**® see mirtazapine on page 417
♦ **Remicade**® see infliximab on page 338

remifentanil (rem i FEN ta nil)
U.S. Brand Names Ultiva™
Generic Available No
Therapeutic Category Analgesic, Narcotic
Use Analgesic for use during general anesthesia for continued analgesia
Usual Dosage Adults: I.V. continuous infusion:
During induction: 0.5-1 mcg/kg/minute
During maintenance:
With nitrous oxide (66%): 0.4 mcg/kg/minute (range: 0.1-2 mcg/kg/min)
With isoflurane: 0.25 mcg/kg/minute (range: 0.05-2 mcg/kg/min)
With propofol: 0.25 mcg/kg/minute (range: 0.05-2 mcg/kg/min)
Continuation as an analgesic in immediate postoperative period: 0.1 mcg/kg/
minute (range: 0.025-0.2 mcg/kg/min)
Dosage Forms Powder for injection, lyophilized: 1 mg/3 mL vial, 2 mg/5 mL
vial, 5 mg/10 mL vial

- **Renacidin®** see citric acid bladder mixture on page 154
- **Renagel®** see sevelamer on page 564
- **Renese®** see polythiazide on page 503
- **Renitec** see enalapril on page 230
- **Reno-M-30®** see radiological/contrast media (ionic) on page 539
- **Reno-M-60®** see radiological/contrast media (ionic) on page 539
- **Reno-M-Dip®** see radiological/contrast media (ionic) on page 539
- **Renoquid®** see sulfacytine on page 586
- **Renormax®** see spirapril on page 578
- **Renovue®-65** see radiological/contrast media (ionic) on page 539
- **Renovue®-DIP** see radiological/contrast media (ionic) on page 539
- **Rentamine®** see chlorpheniramine, ephedrine, phenylephrine, and carbetapentane
  on page 141
- **ReoPro®** see abciximab on page 12

repaglinide (re PAG li nide)
U.S. Brand Names Prandin™
Generic Available No
Therapeutic Category Hypoglycemic Agent, Oral
Use As an adjunct to diet and exercise to lower blood glucose on noninsulin-
dependent (Type II) diabetes patients
Usual Dosage Oral: Adults: 0.5-4 mg before each meal
Oral hypoglycemic-naive individuals or those with HbA1c levels <8%: Initial:
0.5 mg before each meal; for other patients, the starting dose is 1-2 mg
before each meal
Dose can be adjusted (by prescribers) up to 4 mg before each meal. If a meal
is skipped, the patient should also skip the repaglinide dose.
Dosage Forms Tablet: 0.5 mg, 1 mg, 2 mg

- **Repan®** see butalbital compound and acetaminophen on page 99
- **Replasyn®** see sodium hyaluronate on page 572
- **Reposans-10® Oral** see chlordiazepoxide on page 134
- **Rep-Pred®** *(Discontinued)* see page 743
- **Repronex™** see menotropins on page 391
- **Requip™** see ropinirole on page 554
- **Resaid®** see chlorpheniramine and phenylpropanolamine on page 139
- **Rescaps-D® S.R. Capsule** see caramiphen and phenylpropanolamine on
  page 111
- **Rescon Liquid [OTC]** see chlorpheniramine and phenylpropanolamine on
  page 139
- **Rescriptor®** see delavirdine on page 185
- **Resectisol® Irrigation Solution** see mannitol on page 383

reserpine (re SER peen)
U.S. Brand Names Serpalan®
Canadian Brand Names Novo-Reserpine®
Generic Available Yes
Therapeutic Category Rauwolfia Alkaloid
Use Management of mild to moderate hypertension
Usual Dosage Adults: Oral: 0.1-0.5 mg/day in 1-2 doses
Nursing/Pharmacy Information
Alert family members to report any symptoms

Monitor blood pressure, standing and sitting/supine; observe for mental depression

Stability: Protect oral dosage forms from light

Dosage Forms Tablet: 0.1 mg, 0.25 mg

- ♦ **reserpine and chlorothiazide** *see* chlorothiazide and reserpine *on page 137*
- ♦ **reserpine and hydrochlorothiazide** *see* hydrochlorothiazide and reserpine *on page 318*
- ♦ **reserpine and hydroflumethiazide** *see* hydroflumethiazide and reserpine *on page 324*
- ♦ **reserpine, hydralazine, and hydrochlorothiazide** *see* hydralazine, hydrochlorothiazide, and reserpine *on page 317*
- ♦ **Resource®** *see* enteral nutritional products *on page 233*
- ♦ **Respa-1st®** *see* guaifenesin and pseudoephedrine *on page 302*
- ♦ **Respa-DM®** *see* guaifenesin and dextromethorphan *on page 300*
- ♦ **Respa-GF®** *see* guaifenesin *on page 299*
- ♦ **Respaire®-60 SR** *see* guaifenesin and pseudoephedrine *on page 302*
- ♦ **Respaire®-120 SR** *see* guaifenesin and pseudoephedrine *on page 302*
- ♦ **Respbid®** *see* theophylline *on page 603*
- ♦ **RespiGam™** *see* respiratory syncytial virus immune globulin (intravenous) *on page 545*

respiratory syncytial virus immune globulin (intravenous)

(RES peer rah tor ee sin SISH al VYE rus i MYUN GLOB yoo lin in tra VEE nus)

Synonyms RSV-IGIV

U.S. Brand Names RespiGam™

Generic Available No

Therapeutic Category Immune Globulin

Use Prevention of serious lower respiratory infection caused by respiratory syncytial virus (RSV) in children <24 months of age with bronchopulmonary dysplasia (BPD) or a history of premature birth (≤35 weeks gestation)

Usual Dosage I.V.: 750 mg/kg/month according to the following infusion schedule: 1.5 mL/kg/hour for 15 minutes, then at 3 mL/kg/hour for the next 15 minutes if the clinical condition does not contraindicate a higher rate, and finally, administer at 6 mL/kg/hour until completion of dose

Nursing/Pharmacy Information Observe for signs of intolerance during and after infusion; administer through an I.V. line using a constant infusion pump and through a separate I.V. line, if possible; begin infusion within 6 hours and complete within 12 hours after entering the vial; if needed, RSV-IGIV may be "piggy-backed" into dextrose with or without saline solutions, avoiding dilutions >2:1 with such line configurations

Dosage Forms Injection: 2500 mg RSV immunoglobulin/50 mL vial

- ♦ **Restoril®** *see* temazepam *on page 594*
- ♦ **Retavase™** *see* reteplase *on page 545*

reteplase (RE ta plase)

Synonyms recombinant plasminogen activator; r-PA

U.S. Brand Names Retavase™

Generic Available No

Therapeutic Category Thrombolytic Agent

Use Management of acute myocardial infarction

Usual Dosage Adults: I.V.: Given as two (2) bolus doses of 10 units each over a period of 2 minutes (second dose given 30 minutes after the initiation of the first dose)

Dosage Forms Powder for injection, lyophilized: 10.8 units [reteplase 18.8 mg]

- ♦ **Retin-A™** *see* tretinoin (topical) *on page 622*
- ♦ **retinoic acid** *see* tretinoin (topical) *on page 622*
- ♦ **Retinova™** *see* tretinoin (topical) *on page 622*
- ♦ **Retisol-A®** *see* tretinoin (topical) *on page 622*
- ♦ **Retrovir®** *see* zidovudine *on page 658*
- ♦ **Retrovir-AZT** *see* zidovudine *on page 658*
- ♦ **Revapol** *see* mebendazole *on page 387*
- ♦ **Reversol®** *see* edrophonium *on page 228*
- ♦ **Revex®** *see* nalmefene *on page 429*
- ♦ **Rēv-Eyes™** *see* dapiprazole *on page 182*

- **ReVia®** *see* naltrexone *on page 430*
- **Revitalose C-1000®** *see* ascorbic acid *on page 60*
- **Rexigen Forte®** *see* phendimetrazine *on page 484*
- **Rezulin®** *see* troglitazone *on page 633*
- **rFVIIa** *see* factor VIIa, recombinant *New Drug on page 258*
- **R-Gel® [OTC]** *see* capsaicin *on page 110*
- **R-Gen®** *(Discontinued) see page 743*
- **R-Gene®** *see* arginine *on page 58*
- **RGM-CSF** *see* sargramostim *on page 559*
- **Rheaban® [OTC]** *see* attapulgite *on page 66*
- **Rheomacrodex®** *see* dextran *on page 192*
- **Rhesonativ® Injection** *(Discontinued) see page 743*
- **Rheumatrex®** *see* methotrexate *on page 402*
- **rhIL-11** *see* oprelvekin *on page 457*
- **Rhinalar®** *see* flunisolide *on page 272*
- **Rhinall® Nasal Solution [OTC]** *see* phenylephrine *on page 487*
- **Rhinaris-F®** *see* flunisolide *on page 272*
- **Rhinatate® Tablet** *see* chlorpheniramine, pyrilamine, and phenylephrine *on page 144*
- **Rhindecon®** *(Discontinued) see page 743*
- **Rhinocort®** *see* budesonide *on page 96*
- **Rhinocort® Turbuhaler®** *see* budesonide *on page 96*
- **Rhinolar®** *(Discontinued) see page 743*
- **Rhinosyn-DMX® [OTC]** *see* guaifenesin and dextromethorphan *on page 300*
- **Rhinosyn® Liquid [OTC]** *see* chlorpheniramine and pseudoephedrine *on page 140*
- **Rhinosyn-PD® Liquid [OTC]** *see* chlorpheniramine and pseudoephedrine *on page 140*
- **Rhinosyn-X® Liquid [OTC]** *see* guaifenesin, pseudoephedrine, and dextromethorphan *on page 304*

Rh$_o$(D) immune globulin (intramuscular)

(ar aych oh (dee) i MYUN GLOB yoo lin)

U.S. Brand Names Gamulin® Rh; HypRho®-D; HypRho®-D Mini-Dose; MICRhoGAM™; Mini-Gamulin® Rh; RhoGAM™

Generic Available No

Therapeutic Category Immune Globulin

Use Prevent isoimmunization in Rh-negative individuals exposed to Rh-positive blood during delivery of an Rh-positive infant, as a result of an abortion, following amniocentesis or abdominal trauma, or following a transfusion accident; to prevent hemolytic disease of the newborn if there is a subsequent pregnancy with an Rh-positive fetus

Usual Dosage Adults: I.M.:

Obstetrical usage: 1 vial (300 mcg) prevents maternal sensitization if fetal packed red blood cell volume that has entered the circulation is <15 mL; if it is more, administer additional vials. The number of vials = RBC volume of the calculated fetomaternal hemorrhage divided by 15 mL

Postpartum prophylaxis: 300 mcg within 72 hours of delivery

Antepartum prophylaxis: 300 mcg at approximately 26-28 weeks gestation; followed by 300 mcg within 72 hours of delivery if infant is Rh-positive

Following miscarriage, abortion, or termination of ectopic pregnancy at up to 13 weeks of gestation: 50 mcg ideally within 3 hours, but may be administered up to 72 hours after; if pregnancy has been terminated at 13 or more weeks of gestation, administer 300 mcg

Nursing/Pharmacy Information

Administer I.M. preferably in the anterolateral aspects of the upper thigh or the deltoid muscle of the upper arm. The total volume can be administered in divided doses at different sites at one time or may be divided and administered at intervals, provided the total dosage is administered within 72 hours of the fetomaternal hemorrhage or transfusion.

Stability: Reconstituted solution should be refrigerated and remains stable for 30 days; solutions that have been frozen should be discarded

Dosage Forms

Injection: Each package contains one single dose 300 mcg of Rh$_o$ (D) immune globulin

Injection, microdose: Each package contains one single dose of microdose, 50 mcg of Rh$_o$ (D) immune globulin

rh₀(D) immune globulin (intravenous-human)

(ar aych oh (dee) i MYUN GLOB yoo lin in tra VEE nus HYU man)

Synonyms RhoIGIV

U.S. Brand Names WinRho SD®; WinRho SDF®

Generic Available No

Therapeutic Category Immune Globulin

Use

Prevention of Rh isoimmunization in nonsensitized Rho(D) antigen-negative women within 7 hours after spontaneous or induced abortion, amniocentesis, chorionic villus sampling, ruptured tubal pregnancy, abdominal trauma, transplacental hemorrhage, or in the normal course of pregnancy unless the blood type of the fetus or father is known to be Rho(D) antigen-negative

Suppression of Rh isoimmunization in Rho(D) antigen-negative female children and female adults in their childbearing years transfused with Rho(D) antigen-positive RBCs or blood components containing Rho(D) antigen-positive RBCs

Treatment of idiopathic thrombocytopenic purpura (ITP) in nonsplenectomized Rho(D) antigen-positive patients

Usual Dosage

Prevention of Rh isoimmunization:

I.V.: 1500 units (300 mcg) at 28 weeks gestation or immediately after amniocentesis if <34 weeks gestation or after chorionic villus sampling; repeat this dose every 12 weeks during the pregnancy, 600 units (120 mcg) at delivery (within 72 hours) and after invasive intrauterine procedures such as abortion, amniocentesis, or any other manipulation if at >34 weeks gestation. **Note:** If the Rh status of the baby is not known at 72 hours, administer Rho(D) immune globulin to the mother at 72 hours after delivery. If >72 hours have elapsed, do not withhold Rho(D) immune globulin, but administer as soon as possible, up to 28 days after delivery.

I.M.: Reconstitute vial with 1.25 mL and administer as above

Transfusion: Administer within 72 hours after exposure for treatment of incompatible blood transfusions or massive fetal hemorrhage as follows:

I.V.: 3000 units (600 mcg) every 8 hours until the total dose is administered (45 units [9 mcg] of Rh+ blood/mL blood; 90 units [18 mcg] Rh+ red cells/mL cells)

I.M.: 6000 units [1200 mcg] every 12 hours until the total dose is administered (60 units [12 mcg] of Rh+ blood/mL blood; 120 units [24 mcg] Rh+ red cells/mL cells)

Treatment of ITP: I.V.: Initial: 25-50 mcg/kg depending on the patient's Hg concentration; maintenance: 25-60 mcg/kg depending on the clinical response

Nursing/Pharmacy Information Increasing the time of infusion from 1-3 minutes to 15-20 minutes may also help; pretreatment with acetaminophen, diphenhydramine, or prednisone can prevent the fever/chill reaction; Rho(D) is IgA-depleted and is unlikely to cause an anaphylactic reaction in women with IgA deficiency and anti-IgA antibodies. Although immune globulins for I.M. use, manufactured in the U.S., have never been found to transmit any viral infection, Rho(D) is the only Rho(D) preparation treated with highly effective solvent detergent method of viral inactivation for hepatitis C, HIV, and hepatitis B; treatment of ITP in Rh+ patients with an intact spleen appears to be about as effective as IVIG.

Dosage Forms Injection: 600 units [120 mcg], 1500 units [300 mcg]

♦ **Rhodis®** *see* ketoprofen *on page 355*

♦ **Rhodis-EC®** *see* ketoprofen *on page 355*

♦ **RhoGAM™** *see* Rh₀(D) immune globulin (intramuscular) *on page 546*

♦ **RhoIGIV** *see* rh₀(D) immune globulin (intravenous-human) *on page 547*

♦ **Rhoprolene®** *see* betamethasone (topical) *on page 85*

♦ **Rhoprosone®** *see* betamethasone (topical) *on page 85*

♦ **Rhotral®** *see* acebutolol *on page 13*

♦ **Rhotrimine®** *see* trimipramine *on page 630*

♦ **RHUEPO-α** *see* epoetin alfa *on page 236*

♦ **Rhulicaine® [OTC]** *see* benzocaine *on page 79*

♦ **Rhuli® Cream *(Discontinued)*** *see page 743*

ribavirin (rye ba VYE rin)

Synonyms RTCA; tribavirin

U.S. Brand Names Virazole® Aerosol

Mexican Brand Names Vilona; Vilona Pediatrica; Virazide

Generic Available No

(Continued)

ribavirin *(Continued)*

Therapeutic Category Antiviral Agent

Use Treatment of patients with respiratory syncytial virus (RSV) infections; specially indicated for treatment of severe lower respiratory tract RSV infections in patients with an underlying compromising condition (prematurity, bronchopulmonary dysplasia and other chronic lung conditions, congenital heart disease, immunodeficiency, immunosuppression), and recent transplant recipients; may also be used in other viral infections including influenza A and B and adenovirus

Usual Dosage Infants, Children, and Adults:

Aerosol inhalation: Use with Viratek® small particle aerosol generator (SPAG-2) at a concentration of 20 mg/mL (6 g reconstituted with 300 mL of sterile water without preservatives)

Aerosol only: 12-18 hours/day for 3 days, up to 7 days in length

Nursing/Pharmacy Information

Healthcare workers who are pregnant or who may become pregnant should be advised of the potential risks of exposure and counseled about risk reduction strategies including alternate job responsibilities; ribavirin may adsorb to contact lenses; should be administered in well-ventilated rooms (at least 6 air changes/hour); can potentially be deposited in the ventilator delivery system depending on temperature, humidity, and electrostatic forces; this deposition can lead to malfunction or obstruction of the expiratory valve, resulting in inadvertently high positive end-expiratory pressures. The use of one-way valves in the spiratory lines, a breathing circuit filter in the expiratory line, and frequent monitoring and filter replacement have been effective in preventing these problems.

Monitor respiratory function

Stability: Do not use any water containing an antimicrobial agent to reconstitute drug; reconstituted solution is stable for 24 hours at room temperature

Dosage Forms Powder for aerosol: 6 g (100 mL)

riboflavin (RYE boe flay vin)

Synonyms lactoflavin; vitamin B_2; vitamin G

U.S. Brand Names Riobin®

Generic Available Yes

Therapeutic Category Vitamin, Water Soluble

Use Prevent riboflavin deficiency and treat ariboflavinosis

Usual Dosage Oral:

Riboflavin deficiency:

Children: 2.5-10 mg/day in divided doses

Adults: 5-30 mg/day in divided doses

Required daily allowance: Adults:

Male: 1.4-4.8 mg

Female: 1.2-1.3 mg

Nursing/Pharmacy Information Monitor CBC and reticulocyte counts (if anemic when treating deficiency)

Dosage Forms Tablet: 25 mg, 50 mg, 100 mg

♦ **Rid-A-Pain® [OTC]** *see benzocaine on page 79*

♦ **Ridaura®** *see auranofin on page 66*

♦ **Ridene** *see nicardipine on page 440*

♦ **Ridenol® [OTC]** *see acetaminophen on page 13*

♦ **RID® Shampoo [OTC]** *see pyrethrins and piperonyl butoxide on page 533*

rifabutin (rif a BYOO tin)

Synonyms ansamycin

U.S. Brand Names Mycobutin®

Generic Available No

Therapeutic Category Antibiotic, Miscellaneous

Use Prevention of disseminated *Mycobacterium avium* complex (MAC) in patients with advanced HIV infection; utilized in multiple drug regimens for treatment of MAC

Usual Dosage Oral:

Children: Efficacy and safety of rifabutin have not been established in children; a limited number of HIV-positive children with MAC (n=22) have been given rifabutin for MAC prophylaxis; doses of 5 mg/kg/day have been useful

Adults: 300 mg once daily; for patients who experience gastrointestinal upset, rifabutin can be administered 150 mg twice daily with food

Dietary Considerations May be administered with meals or without food or mix with applesauce; high-fat meal may decrease the rate but not the extent of absorption

Nursing/Pharmacy Information Monitor periodic liver function tests, CBC with differential, platelet count, hemoglobin, hematocrit

Dosage Forms Capsule: 150 mg

- ◆ **Rifadin® Injection** *see* rifampin *on page 549*
- ◆ **Rifadin® Oral** *see* rifampin *on page 549*
- ◆ **Rifamate®** *see* rifampin and isoniazid *on page 549*
- ◆ **rifampicin** *see* rifampin *on page 549*

rifampin (RIF am pin)

Synonyms rifampicin
U.S. Brand Names Rifadin® Injection; Rifadin® Oral; Rimactane® Oral
Canadian Brand Names Rofact™
Generic Available No
Therapeutic Category Antibiotic, Miscellaneous
Use In combination with other antitubercular drugs for the treatment of active tuberculosis; eliminate meningococci from asymptomatic carriers; prophylaxis in contacts of patients with *Haemophilus influenzae* type B infection; used in combination with other anti-infectives in the treatment of staphylococcal infections

Usual Dosage Oral (I.V. infusion dose is the same as for the oral route):
Tuberculosis:
Children: 10-20 mg/kg/day in divided doses every 12-24 hours
Adults: 10 mg/kg/day; maximum: 600 mg/day
American Thoracic Society and CDC currently recommend twice weekly therapy as part of a short-course regimen which follows 1-2 months of daily treatment of uncomplicated pulmonary tuberculosis in the compliant patient
Children: 10-20 mg/kg/dose (up to 600 mg) twice weekly under supervision to ensure compliance
Adults: 10 mg/kg (up to 600 mg) twice weekly
H. influenzae prophylaxis:
Infants and Children: 20 mg/kg/day every 24 hours for 4 days
Adults: 600 mg every 24 hours for 4 days
Meningococcal prophylaxis:
<1 month: 10 mg/kg/day in divided doses every 12 hours
Infants and Children: 20 mg/kg/day in divided doses every 12 hours for 2 days
Adults: 600 mg every 12 hours for 2 days
Nasal carriers of *Staphylococcus aureus*: Adults: 600 mg/day for 5-10 days in combination with other antibiotics

Dietary Considerations Should be administered 1 hour before or 2 hours after a meal on an empty stomach with a glass of water; food may delay and reduce the amount of rifampin absorbed

Nursing/Pharmacy Information
The compounded oral suspension must be shaken well before using; may mix contents of capsule with applesauce or jelly; administer I.V. preparation once daily by slow I.V. infusion over 30 minutes to 3 hours at a final concentration not to exceed 6 mg/mL
Monitor periodic monitoring of liver function (AST, ALT), CBC; hepatic status and mental status
Stability: Reconstituted I.V. solution is stable for 24 hours at room temperature; rifampin oral suspension can be compounded with simple syrup or wild cherry syrup at a concentration of 10 mg/mL; the suspension is stable for 4 weeks at room temperature or in a refrigerator when stored in a glass amber prescription bottle

Dosage Forms
Capsule: 150 mg, 300 mg
Powder for injection: 600 mg (contains a sulfite)

rifampin and isoniazid (RIF am pin & eye soe NYE a zid)

Synonyms isoniazid and rifampin
U.S. Brand Names Rifamate®
Generic Available No
Therapeutic Category Antibiotic, Miscellaneous
Use Management of active tuberculosis; see individual monographs for additional information
Usual Dosage Oral: 2 capsules/day
Dosage Forms Capsule: Rifampin 300 mg and isoniazid 150 mg

rifampin, isoniazid, and pyrazinamide
(RIF am pin , eye soe NYE a zid, & peer a ZIN a mide)

Synonyms isoniazid, rifampin, and pyrazinamide; pyrazinamide, rifampin, and isoniazid

U.S. Brand Names Rifater®

Generic Available No

Therapeutic Category Antibiotic, Miscellaneous

Use Management of active tuberculosis

Usual Dosage Adults: Oral: Patients weighing:
≤44 kg: 4 tablets
45-54 kg: 5 tablets
≥55 kg: 6 tablets
Doses should be administered in a single daily dose

Dietary Considerations Administer dose either 1 hour before or 2 hours after a meal with a full glass of water

Dosage Forms Tablet: Rifampin 120 mg, isoniazid 50 mg, and pyrazinamide 300 mg

rifapentine (RIF a pen teen)

U.S. Brand Names Priftin®

Generic Available No

Therapeutic Category Antitubercular Agent

Use Treatment of pulmonary tuberculosis (indication is based on the 6-month follow-up treatment outcome observed in controlled clinical trial). Rifapentine must always be used in conjunction with at least one other antituberculosis drug to which the isolate is susceptible; it may also be necessary to add a third agent (either streptomycin or ethambutol) until susceptibility is known.

Usual Dosage
Children: No dosing information available
Adults: **Rifapentine should not be used alone**; initial phase should include a 3- to 4-drug regimen
Intensive phase of short-term therapy: 600 mg (four 150 mg tablets) given weekly (every 72 hours); following the intensive phase, treatment should continue with rifapentine 600 mg once weekly for 4 months in combination with INH or appropriate agent for susceptible organisms

Dietary Considerations Food increases AUC and maximum serum concentration by 43% and 44% respectively as compared to fasting conditions

Dosage Forms Tablet, film-coated: 150 mg

- ♦ **Rifater®** see rifampin, isoniazid, and pyrazinamide on page 550
- ♦ **rIFN-A** see interferon alfa-2a on page 341
- ♦ **RIG** see rabies immune globulin (human) on page 538
- ♦ **rIL-11** see oprelvekin on page 457
- ♦ **Rilutek®** see riluzole on page 550

riluzole (RIL yoo zole)

Synonyms 2-amino-6-trifluoromethoxy-benzothiazole; RP54274

U.S. Brand Names Rilutek®

Generic Available No

Therapeutic Category Miscellaneous Product

Use Treatment of amyotrophic lateral sclerosis (ALS), also known as Lou Gehrig's disease

Usual Dosage Adults: Oral: 50 mg twice daily

Dosage Forms Tablet: 50 mg

- ♦ **Rimactane® Oral** see rifampin on page 549

rimantadine (ri MAN ta deen)

U.S. Brand Names Flumadine®

Generic Available No

Therapeutic Category Antiviral Agent

Use Prophylaxis (adults and children) and treatment (adults) of influenza A viral infection

Usual Dosage Oral:
Prophylaxis:
Children <10 years: 5 mg/kg administered once daily
Children >10 years and Adults: 100 mg twice daily
Treatment: Adults: 100 mg twice daily

Dietary Considerations Food does not affect rate or extent of absorption

Nursing/Pharmacy Information Avoid use in pregnant or breast-feeding women

Dosage Forms Rimantadine hydrochloride:
Syrup: 50 mg/5 mL (60 mL, 240 mL, 480 mL)
Tablet: 100 mg

rimexolone (ri MEKS oh lone)

U.S. Brand Names Vexol® Ophthalmic Suspension
Generic Available No
Therapeutic Category Adrenal Corticosteroid
Use Treatment of inflammation after ocular surgery and the treatment of anterior uveitis
Usual Dosage Children >2 years and Adults: Ophthalmic: Instill 1-2 drops into conjunctival sac every hour during day, every 2 hours at night until favorable response is obtained, then use 1 drop every 4 hours; for mild to moderate inflammation, instill 1-2 drops into conjunctival sac 2-4 times/day
Dosage Forms Suspension, ophthalmic: 1% (5 mL, 10 mL)

♦ **Rimso®-50** see dimethyl sulfoxide on page 207
♦ **Riobin®** see riboflavin on page 548
♦ **Riopan® [OTC]** see magaldrate on page 380
♦ **Riopan Plus® [OTC]** see magaldrate and simethicone on page 380

risedronate (ris ED roe nate)

U.S. Brand Names Actonel®
Generic Available No
Therapeutic Category Bisphosphonate Derivative
Use Treatment of hypercalcemia associated with malignancy, osteolytic bone lesions of multiple myeloma; also used in postmenopausal osteoporosis; primary hyperparathyroidism and Paget's disease (moderate to severe)
Usual Dosage Adults: Oral: 30 mg once daily for 2 months
Dosage Forms Tablet: 30 mg

♦ **Risperdal®** see risperidone on page 551

risperidone (ris PER i done)

U.S. Brand Names Risperdal®
Generic Available No
Therapeutic Category Antipsychotic Agent, Benzisoxazole
Use Management of psychotic disorders (eg, schizophrenia)
Usual Dosage Oral: Recommended starting dose: 1 mg twice daily; slowly increase to the optimum range of 4-8 mg/day; daily dosages >10 mg does not appear to confer any additional benefit, and the incidence of extrapyramidal reactions is higher than with lower doses
Nursing/Pharmacy Information Monitor for extrapyramidal effects, orthostatic blood pressure changes for 3-5 days after starting or increasing dose
Dosage Forms
Solution, oral: 1 mg/mL (30 mL, 100 mL)
Tablet: 0.25 mg, 0.5 mg, 1 mg, 2 mg, 3 mg, 4 mg

♦ **Ritalin®** see methylphenidate on page 407
♦ **Ritalin-SR®** see methylphenidate on page 407
♦ **Ritmolol** see metoprolol on page 410

ritodrine (RI toe dreen)

U.S. Brand Names Yutopar®
Generic Available No
Therapeutic Category Adrenergic Agonist Agent
Use Inhibit uterine contraction in preterm labor
Usual Dosage Adults:
Oral: Start 30 minutes before stopping I.V. infusion; 10 mg every 2 hours for 24 hours, then 10-20 mg every 4-6 hours up to 120 mg/day. Continue treatment as long as it is desirable to prolong pregnancy.
I.V.: 50-100 mcg/minute; increase by 50 mcg/minute every 10 minutes; continue for 12 hours after contractions have stopped
Nursing/Pharmacy Information
Monitor hematocrit, serum potassium, glucose, colloidal osmotic pressure, heart rate, and uterine contractions
Stability: 48 hours at room temperature after dilution in 500 mL of normal saline, D_5W, or lactated Ringer's I.V. solutions
Dosage Forms Ritodrine hydrochloride:
Injection: 10 mg/mL (5 mL); 15 mg/mL (10 mL)
(Continued)

ritodrine *(Continued)*
Tablet: 10 mg

ritonavir *(rye TON a veer)*
U.S. Brand Names Norvir®
Generic Available No
Therapeutic Category Antiviral Agent
Use Treatment of HIV, especially advanced cases; usually is used as part of triple or double therapy with other nucleoside and protease inhibitors
Usual Dosage Adults: Oral: 600 mg twice daily with meals
Dosage Forms
Capsule: 100 mg
Solution: 80 mg/mL (240 mL)

♦ **Rituxan®** *see* rituximab *on page 552*

rituximab *(ri TUK si mab)*
Synonyms anti-CD20 monoclonal antibodies; C2B8 monoclonal antibody; Pan-B antibodies
U.S. Brand Names Rituxan®
Generic Available No
Therapeutic Category Antineoplastic Agent
Use Treatment of patients with relapsed or refractory low-grade or follicular, CD20 positive, B-cell non-Hodgkin's lymphoma
Usual Dosage Adults: I.V.: 375 mg/m² given as an I.V. infusion once weekly for 4 doses (days 1, 8, 15, and 22); may be administered in an outpatient setting; **do not administer as an intravenous push or bolus**
Dosage Forms Injection: 10 mg/mL (10 mL, 50 mL)

♦ **Rivotril®** *see* clonazepam *on page 159*

rizatriptan *(rye za TRIP tan)*
U.S. Brand Names Maxalt®; Maxalt-MLT™
Generic Available No
Therapeutic Category Antimigraine Agent; Serotonin Agonist
Use Acute treatment of migraine with or without aura
Usual Dosage Oral: 10-20 mg, repeat after 2 hours if significant relief is not attained
Dosage Forms Tablet, as benzoate:
Maxalt®: 5 mg, 10 mg
Maxalt-MLT™ (orally disintegrating): 5 mg, 10 mg

♦ **rLFN-α2** *see* interferon alfa-2b *on page 341*

♦ **RMS® Rectal** *see* morphine sulfate *on page 422*

♦ **Robafen® AC** *see* guaifenesin and codeine *on page 300*

♦ **Robafen® CF [OTC]** *see* guaifenesin, phenylpropanolamine, and dextromethorphan *on page 303*

♦ **Robafen DM® [OTC]** *see* guaifenesin and dextromethorphan *on page 300*

♦ **Robaxin®** *see* methocarbamol *on page 401*

♦ **Robaxisal®** *see* methocarbamol and aspirin *on page 402*

♦ **Robicillin® Tablet *(Discontinued)*** *see page 743*

♦ **Robidrine®** *see* pseudoephedrine *on page 530*

♦ **Robinul®** *see* glycopyrrolate *on page 295*

♦ **Robinul® Forte** *see* glycopyrrolate *on page 295*

♦ **Robitet® *(Discontinued)*** *see page 743*

♦ **Robitet® Oral** *see* tetracycline *on page 601*

♦ **Robitussin® [OTC]** *see* guaifenesin *on page 299*

♦ **Robitussin® A-C** *see* guaifenesin and codeine *on page 300*

♦ **Robitussin-CF® [OTC]** *see* guaifenesin, phenylpropanolamine, and dextromethorphan *on page 303*

♦ **Robitussin® Cough Calmers [OTC]** *see* dextromethorphan *on page 194*

♦ **Robitussin®-DAC** *see* guaifenesin, pseudoephedrine, and codeine *on page 304*

♦ **Robitussin®-DM [OTC]** *see* guaifenesin and dextromethorphan *on page 300*

♦ **Robitussin-PE® [OTC]** *see* guaifenesin and pseudoephedrine *on page 302*

♦ **Robitussin® Pediatric [OTC]** *see* dextromethorphan *on page 194*

♦ **Robitussin® Severe Congestion Liqui-Gels® [OTC]** *see* guaifenesin and pseudoephedrine *on page 302*

♦ **Rocaltrol®** *see* calcitriol *on page 103*

♦ **Rocephin**® *see* ceftriaxone *on page 126*

rocuronium (roe kyoor OH nee um)
U.S. Brand Names Zemuron™
Generic Available No
Therapeutic Category Skeletal Muscle Relaxant
Use Produces skeletal muscle relaxation during surgery after induction of general anesthesia, increases pulmonary compliance during assisted mechanical respiration, facilitates endotracheal intubation
Usual Dosage I.V.:
Children:
Initial: 0.6 mg/kg under halothane anesthesia produce excellent to good intubating conditions within 1 minute and will provide a median time of 41 minutes of clinical relaxation in children 3 months to 1 year of age, and 27 minutes in children 1-12 years
Maintenance: 0.075-0.125 mg/kg administered upon return of T_1 to 25% of control provides clinical relaxation for 7-10 minutes
Adults:
Tracheal intubation:
Initial: 0.6 mg/kg is expected to provide approximately 31 minutes of clinical relaxation under opioid/nitrous oxide/oxygen anesthesia with neuromuscular block sufficient for intubation attained in 1-2 minutes; lower doses (0.45 mg/kg) may be used to provide 22 minutes of clinical relaxation with median time to neuromuscular block of 1-3 minutes; maximum blockade is achieved in <4 minutes
Maximum: 0.9-1.2 mg/kg may be administered during surgery under opioid/nitrous oxide/oxygen anesthesia without adverse cardiovascular effects and is expected to provide 58-67 minutes of clinical relaxation; neuromuscular blockade sufficient for intubation is achieved in <2 minutes with maximum blockade in <3 minutes
Maintenance: 0.1, 0.15, and 0.2 mg/kg administered at 25% recovery of control T_1 (defined as 3 twitches of train-of-four) provides a median of 12, 17, and 24 minutes of clinical duration under anesthesia
Rapid sequence intubation: 0.6-1.2 mg/kg in appropriately premedicated and anesthetized patients with excellent or good intubating conditions within 2 minutes
Continuous infusion: Initial: 0.01-0.012 mg/kg/minute only after early evidence of spontaneous recovery of neuromuscular function is evident
Nursing/Pharmacy Information
Administer I.V. only
Stability: Refrigerate
Dosage Forms Injection, as bromide: 10 mg/mL

♦ **Rofact**™ *see* rifampin *on page 549*

rofecoxib *New Drug* (roe fe COX ib)
U.S. Brand Names Vioxx®
Generic Available No
Therapeutic Category Nonsteroidal Anti-inflammatory Drug (NSAID), COX-2 Selective
Use Relief of the signs and symptoms of osteoarthritis; management of acute pain in adults; treatment of primary dysmenorrhea
Usual Dosage Adult: Oral:
Osteoarthritis: 12.5 mg once daily; may be increased to a maximum of 25 mg once daily
Acute pain and management of dysmenorrhea: 50 mg once daily as needed (use for longer than 5 days is not recommended)
Dosage Forms
Suspension, oral: 12.5 mg/5 mL (150 mL); 25 mg/5 mL (150 mL)
Tablets: 12.5 mg, 25 mg

♦ **Roferon-A**® *see* interferon alfa-2a *on page 341*
♦ **Rogaine**® **Topical** *see* minoxidil *on page 417*
♦ **Rogal** *see* piroxicam *on page 497*
♦ **Rogitine**® *see* phentolamine *on page 487*
♦ **Rolaids**® **[OTC]** *see* dihydroxyaluminum sodium carbonate *on page 205*
♦ **Rolaids**® **Calcium Rich [OTC]** *see* calcium carbonate *on page 103*
♦ **Rolatuss**® **Plain Liquid** *see* chlorpheniramine and phenylephrine *on page 139*
♦ **Romazicon**® *see* flumazenil *on page 272*
♦ **Romir** *see* captopril *on page 110*

- **Romycin® Solution** *(Discontinued)* see page 743
- **Rondamine-DM® Drops** *see* carbinoxamine, pseudoephedrine, and dextromethorphan *on page 114*
- **Rondec®-DM** *see* carbinoxamine, pseudoephedrine, and dextromethorphan *on page 114*
- **Rondec® Drops** *see* carbinoxamine and pseudoephedrine *on page 113*
- **Rondec® Filmtab®** *see* carbinoxamine and pseudoephedrine *on page 113*
- **Rondec® Syrup** *see* carbinoxamine and pseudoephedrine *on page 113*
- **Rondec-TR®** *see* carbinoxamine and pseudoephedrine *on page 113*
- **Rondomycin® Capsule** *(Discontinued)* see page 743

ropinirole (roe PIN i role)
U.S. Brand Names Requip™
Generic Available No
Therapeutic Category Anti-Parkinson's Agent
Use Treatment of idiopathic Parkinson's disease; in patients with early Parkinson's disease who were not receiving concomitant levodopa therapy as well as in patients with advanced disease on concomitant levodopa
Usual Dosage Adults: Oral: Dosage should be increased to achieve a maximum therapeutic effect, balanced against the principal side effects of nausea, dizziness, somnolence, and dyskinesia

Recommended starting dose: 0.25 mg 3 times/day; based on individual patient response, the dosage should be titrated with weekly increments
Week 1: 0.25 mg 3 times/day; total daily dose: 0.75 mg
Week 2: 0.5 mg 3 times/day; total daily dose: 1.5 mg
Week 3: 0.75 mg 3 times/day; total daily dose: 2.25 mg
Week 4: 1 mg 3 times/day; total daily dose: 3 mg
After week 4, if necessary, daily dosage may be increased by 1.5 mg/day on a weekly basis up to a dose of 9 mg/day, and then by up to 3 mg/day weekly to a total of 24 mg/day
Dietary Considerations Ropinirole can be taken with or without food.
Nursing/Pharmacy Information Hallucinations can occur and elderly are at a higher risk than younger patients with Parkinson's disease. Postural hypotension may develop with or without symptoms such as dizziness, nausea, syncope, and sometimes sweating. Hypotension and/or orthostatic symptoms may occur more frequently during initial therapy or with an increase in dose at any time. Use caution when rising rapidly after sitting or lying down, especially after having done so for prolonged periods and especially at the initiation of treatment with ropinirole. Because of additive sedative effects, caution should be used when taking CNS depressants (eg, benzodiazepines, antipsychotics, antidepressants) in combination with ropinirole.
Dosage Forms Tablet, as hydrochloride: 0.25 mg, 0.5 mg, 1 mg, 2 mg, 5 mg

ropivacaine (roe PIV a kane)
U.S. Brand Names Naropin™
Generic Available No
Therapeutic Category Local Anesthetic
Use Production of local or regional anesthesia for surgery, postoperative pain management and obstetrical procedures by infiltration anesthesia and nerve block anesthesia
Usual Dosage Administer the smallest dose and concentration required to produce the desired result
Dosage Forms Ropivacaine hydrochloride:
Infusion: 2 mg/mL (100 mL, 200 mL)
Injection: (single dose): 2 mg/mL (20 mL); 5 mg/mL (30 mL); 7.5 mg/mL (10 mL, 20 mL); 10 mg/mL (10 mL, 20 mL)

rosiglitazone *New Drug* (roe si GLI ta zone)
U.S. Brand Names Avandia®
Generic Available No
Therapeutic Category Hypoglycemic Agent, Oral; Thiazolidinedione Derivative
Use
Type II diabetes, monotherapy: Improve glycemic control as an adjunct to diet and exercise
Type II diabetes, combination therapy: In combination with metformin when diet, exercise and metformin alone or diet, exercise and rosiglitazone alone do not result in adequate glycemic control.

Usual Dosage Adults: Oral: Initial: 4 mg daily as a single daily dose or in divided doses twice daily. If response is inadequate after 12 weeks of treatment, the dosage may be increased to 8 mg daily as a single daily dose or in divided doses twice daily.

Dosage Forms Tablet: 2 mg, 4 mg

♦ **RotaShield®** see rotavirus vaccine *Withdrawn from U.S. market on page 555*

rotavirus vaccine *Withdrawn from U.S. market*
(RO ta vye rus vak SEEN)

U.S. Brand Names RotaShield®

Generic Available No

Therapeutic Category Vaccine

Use Prevention of gastroenteritis caused by the rotavirus serotypes responsible for the majority of disease in infants and children in the U.S. (serotypes G 1,2,3 and 4)

Usual Dosage For oral administration only

Children: Three 2.5 mL doses are administered. The recommended schedule for immunization is at 2, 4, and 6 months of age. The first dose may be administered as early as 6 weeks of age, with subsequent doses at least 3 weeks apart. The third dose has been administered to infants up to 33 weeks of age with no increase in adverse reactions. Initiation of vaccination after the age of 6 months is not currently recommended due to an increased risk of fever. RotaShield® does not diminish the efficacy of OPV, DTP, or Hib when administered concurrently. Repeat dosing of vaccine is not recommended if an infant should regurgitate a dose.

Adults: Not approved for administration to adults

Dosage Forms Powder, lyophilized, for oral solution: 2.5 mL diluent (Dispette®); specialized diluent contains citric acid and sodium bicarbonate

♦ **Roubac®** see co-trimoxazole *on page 170*

♦ **Rovamycine®** see spiramycin *(Canada only) on page 578*

♦ **Rowasa® Rectal** see mesalamine *on page 395*

♦ **Roxanol™ Oral** see morphine sulfate *on page 422*

♦ **Roxanol SR™ Oral** see morphine sulfate *on page 422*

♦ **Roxicet® 5/500** see oxycodone and acetaminophen *on page 462*

♦ **Roxicodone™** see oxycodone *on page 462*

♦ **Roxilox®** see oxycodone and acetaminophen *on page 462*

♦ **Roxiprin®** see oxycodone and aspirin *on page 463*

♦ **RP54274** see riluzole *on page 550*

♦ **RP59500** see quinupristin and dalfopristin *New Drug on page 538*

♦ **r-PA** see reteplase *on page 545*

♦ **RSV-IGIV** see respiratory syncytial virus immune globulin (intravenous) *on page 545*

♦ **R-Tannamine® Tablet** see chlorpheniramine, pyrilamine, and phenylephrine *on page 144*

♦ **R-Tannate® Tablet** see chlorpheniramine, pyrilamine, and phenylephrine *on page 144*

♦ **RTCA** see ribavirin *on page 547*

♦ **rubella and measles vaccines, combined** see measles and rubella vaccines, combined *on page 386*

rubella and mumps vaccines, combined
(rue BEL a & mumpz vak SEENS, kom BINED)

U.S. Brand Names Biavax® II

Generic Available No

Therapeutic Category Vaccine, Live Virus

Use Promote active immunity to rubella and mumps by inducing production of antibodies

Usual Dosage Children >12 months and Adults: 1 vial in outer aspect of the upper arm

Nursing/Pharmacy Information

Federal law requires that the date of administration, the vaccine manufacturer, lot number of vaccine, and the administering person's name, title and address be entered into the patient's permanent medical record

Stability: Refrigerate, discard unused portion within 8 hours, protect from light

Dosage Forms Injection (mixture of 2 viruses):

1. Wistar RA 27/3 strain of rubella virus
2. Jeryl Lynn (B level) mumps strain grown cell cultures of chick embryo

rubella virus vaccine, live (rue BEL a VYE rus vak SEEN, live)
Synonyms german measles vaccine
U.S. Brand Names Meruvax® II
Generic Available No
Therapeutic Category Vaccine, Live Virus
Use Provide vaccine-induced immunity to rubella
Usual Dosage S.C.: 1000 $TCID_{50}$ of rubella
Nursing/Pharmacy Information
  Reconstituted vaccine should be used within 8 hours; S.C. injection only; federal law requires that the date of administration, the vaccine manufacturer, lot number of vaccine, and the administering person's name, title, and address be entered into the patient's permanent record
  Stability: Refrigerate, discard reconstituted vaccine after 8 hours
Dosage Forms Injection, single dose: 1000 $TCID_{50}$ (Wistar RA 27/3 Strain)

♦ **rubeola vaccine** see measles virus vaccine, live on page 386
♦ **Rubex®** see doxorubicin on page 220
♦ **rubidomycin** see daunorubicin hydrochloride on page 183
♦ **Rubilem** see daunorubicin hydrochloride on page 183
♦ **Rubramin®** see cyanocobalamin on page 173
♦ **Rubramin-PC®** see cyanocobalamin on page 173
♦ **Rufen®** *(Discontinued)* see page 743
♦ **Rum-K®** see potassium chloride on page 506
♦ **Ru-Tuss®** see chlorpheniramine, phenylephrine, phenylpropanolamine, and belladonna alkaloids on page 142
♦ **Ru-Tuss® DE** see guaifenesin and pseudoephedrine on page 302
♦ **Ru-Tuss® Expectorant [OTC]** see guaifenesin, pseudoephedrine, and dextromethorphan on page 304
♦ **Ru-Tuss® Liquid** see chlorpheniramine and phenylephrine on page 139
♦ **Ru-Vert-M®** see meclizine on page 387
♦ **Rymed®** see guaifenesin and pseudoephedrine on page 302
♦ **Rymed-TR®** see guaifenesin and phenylpropanolamine on page 301
♦ **Ryna-C® Liquid** see chlorpheniramine, pseudoephedrine, and codeine on page 143
♦ **Rynacrom®** see cromolyn sodium on page 171
♦ **Ryna-CX®** see guaifenesin, pseudoephedrine, and codeine on page 304
♦ **Ryna® Liquid [OTC]** see chlorpheniramine and pseudoephedrine on page 140
♦ **Rynatan®** see azatadine and pseudoephedrine on page 67
♦ **Rynatan® Pediatric Suspension** see chlorpheniramine, pyrilamine, and phenylephrine on page 144
♦ **Rynatan® Tablet** see chlorpheniramine, pyrilamine, and phenylephrine on page 144
♦ **Rynatuss® Pediatric Suspension** see chlorpheniramine, ephedrine, phenylephrine, and carbetapentane on page 141
♦ **Rythmodan®, -LA** see disopyramide on page 213
♦ **Rythmol®** see propafenone on page 524
♦ **Sabin vaccine** see poliovirus vaccine, live, trivalent, oral on page 501
♦ **Sabulin®** see albuterol on page 25

sacrosidase *New Drug* (sak RO se dase)
U.S. Brand Names Sucraid™
Generic Available No
Therapeutic Category Enzyme
Use An enzyme replacement therapy for the treatment of the genetically determined sucrase deficiency, which is part of congenital sucrase-isomaltase deficiency (CSID)
Usual Dosage Oral:
  <15 kg: 1 mL [8500 int. units] (one full measuring scoop or 22 drops) per meal or snack
  >15 kg: 2 mL [17,000 int. units] (two full measuring scoops or 44 drops) per meal or snack
  It is recommended that approximately half of the dosage be taken at the beginning of each meal or snack, and the remainder be taken at the end of each meal or snack.
  The beverage or infant formula should be served cold or at room temperature; the beverage or infant formula should not be warmed or heated before or after addition of sacrosidase

Dosage Forms Solution, oral: 8500 int. units/mL (118 mL)

♦ **Safe Tussin® 30 [OTC]** *see* guaifenesin and dextromethorphan *on page 300*
♦ **Saizen®** *see* human growth hormone *on page 315*
♦ **Salac™** *see* salicylic acid *on page 557*
♦ **Salacid® Ointment** *see* salicylic acid *on page 557*
♦ **Sal-Acid® Plaster** *see* salicylic acid *on page 557*
♦ **Salagen® Oral** *see* pilocarpine *on page 493*
♦ **Salazopyrin®** *see* sulfasalazine *on page 587*
♦ **Salazopyrin EN-Tabs®** *see* sulfasalazine *on page 587*
♦ **Salbulin** *see* albuterol *on page 25*
♦ **Salbutalan** *see* albuterol *on page 25*
♦ **salbutamol** *see* albuterol *on page 25*
♦ **Saleto-200® [OTC]** *see* ibuprofen *on page 332*
♦ **Saleto-400®** *see* ibuprofen *on page 332*
♦ **Salflex®** *see* salsalate *on page 559*
♦ **Salgesic®** *see* salsalate *on page 559*
♦ **salicylazosulfapyridine** *see* sulfasalazine *on page 587*

salicylic acid (sal i SIL ik AS id)

U.S. Brand Names Clear Away® Disc [OTC]; Freezone® Solution [OTC]; Gordofilm® Liquid; Mediplast® Plaster [OTC]; Occlusal®-HP Liquid; Panscol® Lotion [OTC]; Panscol® Ointment [OTC]; PediaPatch Transdermal Patch [OTC]; P&S® Shampoo [OTC]; Salacid® Ointment; Sal-Acid® Plaster; Trans-Plantar® Transdermal Patch [OTC]; Trans-Ver-Sal® Transdermal Patch [OTC]; Vergogel® Gel [OTC]; Verukan® Solution

Canadian Brand Names Acnex®; Acnomel®; Duoforte® 27; Salac™; Sebcur®; Soluver®; Trans-Plantar®; X-Seb™

Generic Available Yes

Therapeutic Category Keratolytic Agent

Use Topically for its keratolytic effect in controlling seborrheic dermatitis or psoriasis of body and scalp, dandruff, and other scaling dermatoses; to remove warts, corns, calluses; also used in the treatment of acne

Usual Dosage
Shampoo: Apply to scalp and allow to remain for a few minutes, then rinse, initially use every day or every other day; 2 treatments/week are usually sufficient to maintain control
Topical: Apply to affected area and place under occlusion at night; hydrate skin for at least 5 minutes before use

Nursing/Pharmacy Information
For warts: Before applying product, soak area in warm water for 5 minutes; dry area thoroughly, then apply medication
Monitor for signs and symptoms of salicylate toxicity: nausea, vomiting, dizziness, tinnitus, loss of hearing, lethargy, diarrhea, psychic disturbances

Dosage Forms
Cream: 2% (30 g)
Disk: 40%
Gel: 5% (60 g); 6% (30 g); 17% (7.5 g)
Liquid: 13.6% (9.3 mL); 17% (9.3 mL, 13.5 mL, 15 mL); 16.7% (15 mL)
Lotion: 3% (120 mL)
Ointment: 3% (90 g)
Patch, transdermal: 15% (20 mm); 40% (20 mm)
Plaster: 40%
Soap: 2% (97.5 g)
Strip: 40%

♦ **salicylic acid and benzoic acid** *see* benzoic acid and salicylic acid *on page 80*

salicylic acid and lactic acid (sal i SIL ik AS id & LAK tik AS id)

Synonyms lactic acid and salicylic acid
U.S. Brand Names Duofilm® Solution
Generic Available Yes
Therapeutic Category Keratolytic Agent
Use Treatment of benign epithelial tumors such as warts
Usual Dosage Topical: Apply a thin layer directly to wart once daily (may be useful to apply at bedtime and wash off in morning)
Nursing/Pharmacy Information Protect normal skin tissue with a ring of petrolatum surrounding the affected area; prior to application, soak affected area in hot water for at least 5 minutes; dry thoroughly with a clean towel
(Continued)

salicylic acid and lactic acid *(Continued)*

Dosage Forms Solution, topical: Salicylic acid 16.7% and lactic acid 16.7% in flexible collodion (15 mL)

♦ **salicylic acid and podophyllin** *see* podophyllin and salicylic acid *on page 500*

salicylic acid and propylene glycol
(sal i SIL ik AS id & PROE pi leen GLYE cole)

Synonyms propylene glycol and salicylic acid
U.S. Brand Names Keralyt® Gel
Generic Available No
Therapeutic Category Keratolytic Agent
Use Removal of excessive keratin in hyperkeratotic skin disorders, including various ichthyosis, keratosis palmaris and plantaris and psoriasis; may be used to remove excessive keratin in dorsal and plantar hyperkeratotic lesions
Usual Dosage Topical: Apply to area at night after soaking region for at least 5 minutes to hydrate area, and place under occlusion; medication is washed off in morning
Dosage Forms Gel, topical: Salicylic acid 6% and propylene glycol 60% in ethyl alcohol 19.4% with hydroxypropyl methylcellulose and water (30 g)

♦ **salicylic acid and sulfur** *see* sulfur and salicylic acid *on page 589*
♦ **Saline from Otrivin®** *see* sodium chloride *on page 571*
♦ **SalineX® [OTC]** *see* sodium chloride *on page 571*
♦ **Salivart® Solution [OTC]** *see* saliva substitute *on page 558*

saliva substitute (sa LYE va SUB stee tute)

U.S. Brand Names Entertainer's Secret® Spray [OTC]; Moi-Stir® Solution [OTC]; Moi-Stir® Swabsticks [OTC]; Mouthkote® Solution [OTC]; Optimoist® Solution [OTC]; Salivart® Solution [OTC]; Salix® Lozenge [OTC]
Generic Available Yes
Therapeutic Category Gastrointestinal Agent, Miscellaneous
Use Relief of dry mouth and throat in xerostomia
Usual Dosage Use as needed
Dosage Forms
Lozenge: 100s
Solution: 60 mL, 75 mL, 120 mL, 180 mL, 240 mL
Swabstix: 3§

♦ **Salix® Lozenge [OTC]** *see* saliva substitute *on page 558*
♦ **Salk vaccine** *see* poliovirus vaccine, inactivated *on page 501*

salmeterol (sal ME te role)

U.S. Brand Names Serevent®; Serevent® Diskus®
Mexican Brand Names Zamtirel
Generic Available No
Therapeutic Category Adrenergic Agonist Agent
Use Maintenance treatment of asthma; prevention of bronchospasm in patients >12 years of age with reversible obstructive airway disease, including patients with symptoms of nocturnal asthma who require regular treatment with inhaled, short-acting beta$_2$ agonists; prevention of exercise-induced bronchospasm
Usual Dosage
Inhalation: 42 mcg (2 puffs) twice daily (12 hours apart) for maintenance and prevention of symptoms of asthma
Prevention of exercise-induced asthma: 42 mcg (2 puffs) 30-60 minutes prior to exercise; additional doses should not be used for 12 hours
Nursing/Pharmacy Information Residents requiring frequent treatment (4 inhalations/day on regular basis) with short-acting B_2 agonist for breakthrough or acute episodes while on salmeterol should be brought to the physician's attention for re-evaluation; safety in children <12 years not established. The therapeutic effect may decrease when the cannister is cold, therefore, the cannister should remain at room temperature. Do not store at temperatures >120°F.
Dosage Forms Aerosol, oral, as xinafoate: 21 mcg/spray [60 inhalations] (6.5 g), [120 inhalations] (13 g)

♦ **Salmonine®** *see* calcitonin *on page 102*
♦ **Salofalk** *see* aminosalicylate sodium *on page 39*

salsalate (SAL sa late)

Synonyms disalicylic acid

U.S. Brand Names Argesic®-SA; Artha-G®; Disalcid®; Marthritic®; Mono-Gesic®; Salflex®; Salgesic®; Salsitab®

Generic Available Yes

Therapeutic Category Analgesic, Non-narcotic; Antipyretic; Nonsteroidal Anti-inflammatory Drug (NSAID)

Use Treatment of minor pain or fever; rheumatoid arthritis, osteoarthritis, and related inflammatory conditions

Usual Dosage Adults: Oral: 1 g 2-4 times/day

Dietary Considerations May be administered with food to decrease GI distress

Nursing/Pharmacy Information Does not appear to inhibit platelet aggregation

Dosage Forms
Capsule: 500 mg
Tablet: 500 mg, 750 mg

saquinavir (sa KWIN a veer)

U.S. Brand Names Fortovase®; Invirase®

Generic Available No

Therapeutic Category Antiviral Agent

Use Treatment of advanced HIV infection, used in combination with older nucleoside analog medications

Usual Dosage Adults: Oral:
Fortovase®: Six 200 mg (1200 mg) capsules 3 times/day within 2 hours after a meal
Invirase®: Three 200 mg (600 mg) capsules 3 times/day within 2 hours after a full meal

Dosage Forms
Capsule (hard) as mesylate (Invirase®): 200 mg
Capsule (soft) (Fortovase®): 200 mg

sargramostim (sar GRAM oh stim)

Synonyms GM-CSF; granulocyte-macrophage colony-stimulating factor; RGM-CSF

U.S. Brand Names Leukine™

Mexican Brand Names Leucomax®

Generic Available No

Therapeutic Category Colony-Stimulating Factor

Use Myeloid reconstitution after autologous bone marrow transplantation; to accelerate myeloid recovery in patients with non-Hodgkin's lymphoma, Hodgkin's lymphoma, and acute lymphoblastic leukemia undergoing autologous BMT; following induction chemotherapy in patients with acute myelogenous leukemia to shorten time to neutrophil recovery

Usual Dosage
Children and Adults (may also administer S.C.):
Bone marrow transplant: I.V.: 250 mcg/m^2/day over at least 2 hours to begin 2-4 hours after the marrow infusion on day 0 of autologous bone marrow transplant or not <24 hours after chemotherapy or 12 hours after last dose
(Continued)

sargramostim *(Continued)*

of radiotherapy. If significant adverse effects or "first dose" reaction is seen at this dose, discontinue the drug until toxicity resolves, then restart at a reduced dose of 125 mcg/m^2/day

Cancer chemotherapy recovery: I.V.: 3-15 mcg/kg/day over at least 2 hours for 14-21 days; maximum daily dose is 15 mcg/kg/day due to dose-related adverse effects

Discontinue therapy if the ANC count is >20,000/mm^3.

Excessive blood counts return to normal or baseline levels within 3-7 days following cessation of therapy.

Length of therapy: Bone marrow transplant patients: GM-CSF should be administered daily for up to 30 days or until the ANC has reached 1000/mm^3 for 3 consecutive days following the expected chemotherapy-induced neutrophil-nadir.

Nursing/Pharmacy Information

Can premedicate with analgesics and antipyretics; control bone pain with non-narcotic analgesics; do not shake solution to avoid foaming. When administering GM-CSF subcutaneously, rotate injection sites. Administer as a 2-hour I.V. infusion, 6-hour I.V. infusion, or by continuous I.V. infusion. Use normal saline for dilution of the drug. If the final concentration of GM-CSF in normal saline is ≤10 mcg/mL, then add 1 mg albumin per mL of I.V. fluid. Albumin acts as a carrier molecule to prevent drug adsorption to the I.V. tubing. Albumin should be added to the saline prior to addition of GM-CSF.

Monitor vital signs, weight, CBC with differential, platelets, renal/liver function tests, especially with previous dysfunction, WBC with differential, pulmonary function

Stability: Sargramostim is available as a sterile, white, preservative-free, lyophilized powder. Sargramostim should be stored at 2°C to 8°C (36°F to 46°F). Vials should not be frozen or shaken. Sargramostim is stable after dilution in 1 mL of bacteriostatic or nonbacteriostatic sterile water for injection for 30 days at 2°C to 8°C or 25°C. Sargramostim may also be further diluted in 50 mL 0.9% sodium chloride to a concentration of ≥10 mcg/mL for I.V. infusion administration. This diluted solution is stable for 48 hours at room temperature and refrigeration. If the final concentration of sargramostim is <10 mcg/mL, human albumin should be added to the saline prior to the addition of sargramostim to prevent absorption of the components to the delivery system. It is recommended that 1 mg of human albumin per 1 mL of 0.9% sodium chloride (eg, 1 mL of 5% human albumin per 50 mL of 0.9% sodium chloride) be added.

Dosage Forms Injection: 250 mcg, 500 mcg

♦ **Sarna [OTC]** *see* camphor, menthol, and phenol *on page 108*

♦ **S.A.S™** *see* sulfasalazine *on page 587*

♦ **SAStid® Plain Therapeutic Shampoo and Acne Wash [OTC]** *see* sulfur and salicylic acid *on page 589*

♦ **Scabene® *(Discontinued)*** *see page 743*

♦ **Scabisan Shampoo** *see* lindane *on page 370*

♦ **Scalpicin® Topical** *see* hydrocortisone (topical) *on page 324*

♦ **Sclavo - PPD® Solution *(Discontinued)*** *see page 743*

♦ **Sclavo Test - PPD® *(Discontinued)*** *see page 743*

♦ **Scleromate™** *see* morrhuate sodium *on page 423*

♦ **Scopace® Tablet** *see* scopolamine *on page 560*

scopolamine *(skoe POL a meen)*

Synonyms hyoscine

U.S. Brand Names Isopto® Hyoscine; Scopace® Tablet; Transderm Scop®

Canadian Brand Names Transdermal-V®

Generic Available Yes

Therapeutic Category Anticholinergic Agent

Use Preoperative medication to produce amnesia and decrease salivary and respiratory secretions; to produce cycloplegia and mydriasis; treatment of iridocyclitis; prevention of motion sickness; prevention of nausea/vomiting associated with anesthesia or opiate analgesia (patch)

Usual Dosage

Preoperatively:

Children: I.M., S.C.: 6 mcg/kg/dose (maximum: 0.3 mg/dose) or 0.2 mg/m^2 may be repeated every 6-8 hours **or** alternatively:

4-7 months: 0.1 mg

7 months to 3 years: 0.15 mg

3-8 years: 0.2 mg

8-12 years: 0.3 mg
Adults: I.M., I.V., S.C.: 0.3-0.65 mg; may be repeated every 4-6 hours
Motion sickness: Transdermal: Children >12 years and Adults: Apply 1 disc behind the ear at least 4 hours prior to exposure and every 3 days as needed
Ophthalmic:
Refraction:
Children: Instill 1 drop of 0.25% to eye(s) twice daily for 2 days before procedure
Adults: Instill 1-2 drops of 0.25% to eye(s) 1 hour before procedure
Iridocyclitis:
Children: Instill 1 drop of 0.25% to eye(s) up to 3 times/day
Adults: Instill 1-2 drops of 0.25% to eye(s) up to 4 times/day

Nursing/Pharmacy Information
Disc is programmed to deliver *in vivo* 0.5 mg over 3 days; wash hands before and after applying the disc to avoid drug contact with eyes; after instilling ophthalmic preparation, apply pressure to the side of the nose near the eye to minimize systemic absorption
I.V.: Dilute with an equal volume of sterile water and administer by direct I.V. injection over 2-3 minutes
Stability: Avoid acid solutions, because hydrolysis occurs at pH <3

Dosage Forms
Disc, transdermal: 1.5 mg/disc (4's)
Injection, as hydrobromide: 0.3 mg/mL (1 mL); 0.4 mg/mL (0.5 mL, 1 mL); 0.86 mg/mL (0.5 mL); 1 mg/mL (1 mL)
Solution, ophthalmic, as hydrobromide: 0.25% (5 mL, 15 mL)
Tablet: 0.4 mg

♦ **scopolamine and phenylephrine** *see* phenylephrine and scopolamine *on page 489*

♦ **scopolamine, hyoscyamine, atropine, and phenobarbital** *see* hyoscyamine, atropine, scopolamine, and phenobarbital *on page 330*

♦ **Scot-Tussin® [OTC]** *see* guaifenesin *on page 299*

♦ **Scot-Tussin DM® Cough Chasers [OTC]** *see* dextromethorphan *on page 194*

♦ **Scot-Tussin® Senior Clear [OTC]** *see* guaifenesin and dextromethorphan *on page 300*

♦ **SeaMist® [OTC]** *see* sodium chloride *on page 571*

♦ **Sebcur®** *see* salicylic acid *on page 557*

♦ **Sebulex®** *(Discontinued) see page 743*

♦ **Sebulon®** *(Discontinued) see page 743*

secobarbital (see koe BAR bi tal)

Synonyms quinalbarbitone
U.S. Brand Names Seconal™ Injection
Canadian Brand Names Novo-Secobarb®
Generic Available Yes
Therapeutic Category Barbiturate
Controlled Substance C-II
Use Short-term treatment of insomnia and as preanesthetic agent
Usual Dosage Hypnotic:
Children: I.M.: 3-5 mg/kg/dose; maximum: 100 mg/dose
Adults:
I.M.: 100-200 mg/dose
I.V.: 50-250 mg/dose

Nursing/Pharmacy Information
I.V.: Administer undiluted or diluted with sterile water for injection, normal saline, or Ringer's injection; maximum infusion rate: 50 mg/15 seconds
Stability: Do not shake vial during reconstitution, rotate ampul; aqueous solutions are not stable, reconstitute with aqueous polyethylene glycol; aqueous (sterile water) solutions should be used within 30 minutes; do not use bacteriostatic water for injection or lactated Ringer's. I.V. form is **incompatible** when mixed with benzquinamide (in syringe), cimetidine (same syringe), codeine, erythromycin, glycopyrrolate (same syringe), hydrocortisone, insulin, levorphanol, methadone, norepinephrine, pentazocine, phenytoin, sodium bicarbonate, tetracycline, vancomycin

Dosage Forms Injection, as sodium: 50 mg/mL (2 mL)

♦ **secobarbital and amobarbital** *see* amobarbital and secobarbital *on page 42*

♦ **Seconal™ Injection** *see* secobarbital *on page 561*

♦ **Seconal™ Oral** *(Discontinued) see page 743*

♦ **Secran®** *see* vitamin, multiple (oral) *on page 654*

secretin (SEE kre tin)
U.S. Brand Names Secretin-Ferring Powder
Generic Available No
Therapeutic Category Diagnostic Agent
Use Diagnosis of Zollinger-Ellison syndrome, chronic pancreatic dysfunction, and some hepatobiliary diseases such as obstructive jaundice resulting from cancer or stones in the biliary tract
Usual Dosage I.V.:
Pancreatic function: 1 CU/kg slow I.V. injection over 1 minute
Zollinger-Ellison: 2 CU/kg slow I.V. injection over 1 minute
Nursing/Pharmacy Information
Patients should fast 12-15 hours before test; reconstitute with 7.5 mL of normal saline; **do not shake**; use immediately by direct I.V. injection slowly over 1 minute
Monitor duodenal fluid volume and bicarbonate content; serum gastrin (Zollinger-Ellison syndrome)
Stability: Unstable; should be used immediately after reconstitution, store in freezer (-20°C) or store at 25°C for up to 3 weeks
Dosage Forms Powder for injection: 75 units (10 mL)

♦ **Secretin-Ferring Powder** *see* secretin *on page 562*
♦ **Sectral®** *see* acebutolol *on page 13*
♦ **Sedapap-10®** *see* butalbital compound and acetaminophen *on page 99*
♦ **Sefulken** *see* diazoxide *on page 197*
♦ **Selax®** *see* docusate *on page 214*
♦ **Seldane®** *(Canada) see* terfenadine *on page 597*
♦ **Seldane-D®** *(Discontinued) see page 743*
♦ **Seldane®** *(Discontinued in U.S.) see page 743*
♦ **Selecor®** *(Discontinued) see page 743*

selegiline (seh LEDGE ah leen)
Synonyms deprenyl; *l*-deprenyl
U.S. Brand Names Eldepryl®
Canadian Brand Names Novo-Selegiline
Generic Available Yes
Therapeutic Category Anti-Parkinson's Agent; Dopaminergic Agent (Anti-Parkinson's)
Use Adjunct in the management of Parkinsonian patients in which levodopa/carbidopa therapy is deteriorating
Unlabeled uses: Early Parkinson's disease, Alzheimer's disease
Usual Dosage Adults: Oral: 5 mg twice daily
Dietary Considerations This medication may cause sudden and severe high blood pressure when taken with food high in tyramine (cheeses, sour cream, yogurt, pickled herring, chicken liver, canned figs, raisins, bananas, avocados, soy sauce, broad bean pods, yeast extracts, meats prepared with tenderizers, and many foods aged to improve flavor; wine (Chianti and hearty red) and beer); small amounts of caffeine may produce irregular heartbeat or high blood pressure and can interact with this medication for up to 2 weeks after stopping its use
Nursing/Pharmacy Information
Selegiline is a monoamine oxidase inhibitor type "B"; there should **not** be a problem with tyramine-containing products as long as the typical doses are employed
Monitor blood pressure, symptoms of parkinsonism
Dosage Forms
Capsule, as hydrochloride (Eldepryl®): 5 mg
Tablet: 5 mg

selenium sulfide (se LEE nee um SUL fide)
U.S. Brand Names Exsel® Shampoo; Selsun Blue® Shampoo [OTC]; Selsun® Shampoo
Canadian Brand Names Versel™
Generic Available Yes
Therapeutic Category Antiseborrheic Agent, Topical
Use Treat itching and flaking of the scalp associated with dandruff; to control scalp seborrheic dermatitis; treatment of tinea versicolor

Usual Dosage Topical:

Dandruff, seborrhea: Massage 5-10 mL into wet scalp, leave on scalp 2-3 minutes, rinse thoroughly and repeat application; shampoo twice weekly for 2 weeks initially, then use once every 1-4 weeks as indicated depending upon control

Tinea versicolor: Apply the 2.5% lotion to affected area and lather with small amounts of water; leave on skin for 10 minutes, then rinse thoroughly; apply every day for 7 days

Nursing/Pharmacy Information Notify physician if condition persists or worsens

Dosage Forms Shampoo: 1% (120 mL, 210 mL, 240 mL, 330 mL); 2.5% (120 mL)

- **Sele-Pak®** *see* trace metals *on page 620*
- **Selepen®** *see* trace metals *on page 620*
- **Selestoject®** *see* betamethasone (systemic) *on page 84*
- **Selestoject®** *(Discontinued) see page 743*
- **Seloken** *see* metoprolol *on page 410*
- **Selopres** *see* metoprolol *on page 410*
- **Selsun Blue® Shampoo [OTC]** *see* selenium sulfide *on page 562*
- **Selsun® Shampoo** *see* selenium sulfide *on page 562*
- **Semicid® [OTC]** *see* nonoxynol 9 *on page 446*
- **Semprex®-D** *see* acrivastine and pseudoephedrine *on page 20*

senna (SEN na)

U.S. Brand Names Black Draught® [OTC]; Senna-Gen® [OTC]; Senokot® [OTC]; X-Prep® Liquid [OTC]

Canadian Brand Names Glysennid®

Generic Available Yes

Therapeutic Category Laxative

Use Short-term treatment of constipation; evacuate the colon for bowel or rectal examinations

Usual Dosage

Children:

Oral:

>6 years: 10-20 mg/kg/dose at bedtime; maximum daily dose: 872 mg

6-12 years, >27 kg: 1 tablet at bedtime, up to 4 tablets/day **or** 1/2 teaspoonful of granules (326 mg/tsp) at bedtime (up to 2 teaspoonfuls/day)

Liquid:

2-5 years: 5-10 mL at bedtime

6-15 years: 10-15 mL at bedtime

Suppository: 1/2 at bedtime

Syrup:

1 month to 1 year: 1.25-2.5 mL at bedtime up to 5 mL/day

1-5 years: 2.5-5 mL at bedtime up to 10 mL/day

5-10 years: 5-10 mL at bedtime up to 20 mL/day

Adults:

Granules (326 mg/teaspoon): 1 teaspoonful at bedtime, not to exceed 2 teaspoonfuls twice daily

Liquid: 15-30 mL with meals and at bedtime

Suppository: 1 at bedtime, may repeat once in 2 hours

Syrup: 2-3 teaspoonfuls at bedtime, not to exceed 30 mL/day

Tablet: 187 mg: 2 tablets at bedtime, not to exceed 8 tablets/day

Tablet: 374 mg: 1 at bedtime, up to 4/day; 600 mg: 2 tablets at bedtime, up to 3 tablets/day

Dietary Considerations Liquid may be administered with fruit juice or milk to mask taste

Nursing/Pharmacy Information

May discolor urine or feces; liquid syrups contain 7% alcohol; liquids 3.5% to 4.9% alcohol

Monitor I & O

Dosage Forms

Granules: 326 mg/teaspoonful

Liquid: 7% [70 mg/mL] (130 mL, 360 mL); 6.5% [65 mg/mL] (75 mL, 150 mL)

Suppository, rectal: 652 mg

Syrup: 218 mg/5 mL (60 mL, 240 mL)

Tablet: 187 mg, 217 mg, 600 mg

- **Senna-Gen® [OTC]** *see* senna *on page 563*
- **Senokot® [OTC]** *see* senna *on page 563*

- **Senolax®** *(Discontinued) see page 743*
- **Sensibit** *see* loratadine *on page 375*
- **Sensorcaine®** *see* bupivacaine *on page 97*
- **Sensorcaine®-MPF** *see* bupivacaine *on page 97*
- **Septa® Topical Ointment [OTC]** *see* bacitracin, neomycin, and polymyxin B *on page 71*
- **Septisol®** *see* hexachlorophene *on page 312*
- **Septra®** *see* co-trimoxazole *on page 170*
- **Septra® DS** *see* co-trimoxazole *on page 170*
- **Ser-Ap-Es®** *see* hydralazine, hydrochlorothiazide, and reserpine *on page 317*
- **Serax®** *see* oxazepam *on page 460*
- **Serc®** *see* betahistine *(Canada only) on page 84*
- **Serentil®** *see* mesoridazine *on page 396*
- **Serevent®** *see* salmeterol *on page 558*
- **Serevent® Diskus®** *see* salmeterol *on page 558*

sermorelin acetate (ser moe REL in AS e tate)
U.S. Brand Names Geref®
Generic Available No
Therapeutic Category Diagnostic Agent
Use Evaluate ability of the somatotroph of the pituitary gland to secrete growth hormone
Usual Dosage I.V. (in a single dose in the morning following an overnight fast):
Children or subjects <50 kg: Draw venous blood samples for GH determinations 15 minutes before and immediately prior to administration, then administer 1 mcg/kg followed by a 3 mL normal saline flush, draw blood samples again for GH determinations
Adults or subjects >50 kg: Determine the number of ampules needed based on a dose of 1 mcg/kg, draw venous blood samples for GH determinations 15 minutes before and immediately prior to administration, then administer 1 mcg/kg followed by a 3 mL normal saline flush, draw blood samples again for GH determinations
Dosage Forms Powder for injection, lyophilized: 50 mcg

- **Serocryptin®** *see* bromocriptine *on page 93*
- **Seromycin® Pulvules®** *see* cycloserine *on page 176*
- **Serophene®** *see* clomiphene *on page 158*
- **Seroquel®** *see* quetiapine *on page 535*
- **Serostim®** *see* human growth hormone *on page 315*
- **Serozide®** *see* etoposide *on page 255*
- **Serpalan®** *see* reserpine *on page 544*
- **Serpasil®** *(Discontinued) see page 743*
- **Sertan®** *see* primidone *on page 517*

sertraline (SER tra leen)
U.S. Brand Names Zoloft®
Generic Available No
Therapeutic Category Antidepressant, Selective Serotonin Reuptake Inhibitor
Use Treatment of major depression; pediatric obsessive-compulsive disorder; also being studied for use in obesity
Usual Dosage Oral: Initial: 50 mg/day as a single dose, dosage may be increased at intervals of at least 1 week to a maximum recommended dosage of 200 mg/day
Nursing/Pharmacy Information
If patient becomes anxious or overstimulated, notify physician; if somnolent, administer dose at bedtime; offer hard, sugarless candy or ice chips for dry mouth.
Monitor nutritional intake and weight
Dosage Forms Tablet, as hydrochloride: 25 mg, 50 mg, 100 mg

- **Serutan® [OTC]** *see* psyllium *on page 531*
- **Servigenta** *see* gentamicin *on page 290*
- **Serzone®** *see* nefazodone *on page 434*

sevelamer (se VEL a mer)
U.S. Brand Names Renagel®
Generic Available No
Therapeutic Category Phosphate Binder

Use Reduction of serum phosphorous in patients with end-stage renal disease

Usual Dosage Adults: Oral: 2-4 capsules 3 times/day with meals; the initial dose may be based on serum phosphorous:

(Phosphorous: Initial dose)

>6.0 and <7.5: 2 capsules 3 times/day

>7.5 and <9.0: 3 capsules 3 times/day

≥9.0: 4 capsules 3 times/day

Dosage should be adjusted based on serum phosphorous concentration, with a goal of lowering to <6.0 mg/dL; maximum daily dose studied was 30 capsules/day

Dosage Forms Capsule: 403 mg

sevoflurane (see voe FLOO rane)
U.S. Brand Names Ultane®
Generic Available No
Therapeutic Category General Anesthetic
Use General induction and maintenance of anesthesia (inhalation)
Usual Dosage Surgical levels of anesthesia can usually be obtained with concentrations of 0.5% to 3%
Dosage Forms Liquid for inhalation: 250 mL

♦ **Shur-Seal® [OTC]** *see* nonoxynol 9 *on page 446*
♦ **Siblin® (Discontinued)** *see page 743*

sibutramine (si BYOO tra meen)
U.S. Brand Names Meridia™
Generic Available No
Therapeutic Category Anorexiant
Use Management of obesity, including weight loss and maintenance of weight loss, and should be used in conjunction with a reduced calorie diet
Usual Dosage Adults ≥16 years: Initial: 10 mg once daily; after 4 weeks may titrate up to 15 mg once daily as needed and tolerated
Dosage Forms Capsule, as hydrochloride monohydrate: 5 mg, 10 mg, 15 mg

♦ **Sigafam** *see* famotidine *on page 259*
♦ **Silace-C® [OTC]** *see* docusate and casanthranol *on page 215*
♦ **Siladryl® Oral [OTC]** *see* diphenhydramine *on page 208*
♦ **Silafed® Syrup [OTC]** *see* triprolidine and pseudoephedrine *on page 632*
♦ **Silain® [OTC]** *see* simethicone *on page 566*
♦ **Silaminic® Cold Syrup [OTC]** *see* chlorpheniramine and phenylpropanolamine *on page 139*
♦ **Silaminic® Expectorant [OTC]** *see* guaifenesin and phenylpropanolamine *on page 301*
♦ **Silapap® [OTC]** *see* acetaminophen *on page 13*

sildenafil (sil DEN a fil)
Synonyms UK 92480
U.S. Brand Names Viagra®
Generic Available No
Therapeutic Category Phosphodiesterase Enzyme Inhibitor
Use Effective in most men with erectile dysfunction (ED), the medical term for impotence, which is associated with a broad range of physical or psychological medical conditions.
Usual Dosage Oral: Adults: 50 mg taken one hour before sexual activity; individuals may need more (100 mg) or less (25 mg) and dosing should be determined by a physician depending on effectiveness and side effects. The drug should not be used more than once daily.
Dosage Forms Tablet, as citrate: 25 mg, 50 mg, 100 mg

♦ **Sildicon-E® [OTC]** *see* guaifenesin and phenylpropanolamine *on page 301*
♦ **Silphen® Cough [OTC]** *see* diphenhydramine *on page 208*
♦ **Silphen DM® [OTC]** *see* dextromethorphan *on page 194*
♦ **Siltussin® [OTC]** *see* guaifenesin *on page 299*
♦ **Siltussin-CF® [OTC]** *see* guaifenesin, phenylpropanolamine, and dextromethorphan *on page 303*
♦ **Siltussin DM® [OTC]** *see* guaifenesin and dextromethorphan *on page 300*
♦ **Silvadene®** *see* silver sulfadiazine *on page 566*

silver nitrate (SIL ver NYE trate)
Synonyms AgNO$_3$
U.S. Brand Names Dey-Drop® Ophthalmic Solution
(Continued)

silver nitrate *(Continued)*
Generic Available Yes
Therapeutic Category Topical Skin Product
Use Prevention of gonococcal ophthalmia neonatorum; cauterization of wounds and sluggish ulcers, removal of granulation tissue and warts
Usual Dosage
Neonates: Ophthalmic: Instill 2 drops immediately after birth into conjunctival sac of each eye as a single dose; do not irrigate eyes following instillation of eye drops
Children and Adults:
Sticks: Apply to mucous membranes and other moist skin surfaces only on area to be treated 2-3 times/week for 2-3 weeks
Topical solution: Apply a cotton applicator dipped in solution on the affected area 2-3 times/week for 2-3 weeks
Nursing/Pharmacy Information
Silver nitrate solutions stain skin and utensils
Monitor methemoglobin levels with prolonged use
Stability: Must be stored in a dry place; exposure to light causes silver to oxidize and turn brown, dipping in water causes oxidized film to readily dissolve
Dosage Forms
Applicator, topical: 75% with potassium nitrate 25% (6")
Ointment, topical: 10% (30 g)
Solution:
Ophthalmic: 1% (wax ampuls)
Topical: 10% (30 mL); 25% (30 mL); 50% (30 mL)

silver protein, mild (SIL ver PRO teen mild)
Generic Available No
Therapeutic Category Antibiotic, Topical
Use Stain and coagulate mucus in eye surgery which is then removed by irrigation; eye infections
Usual Dosage
Preop in eye surgery: Place 2-3 drops into eye(s), then rinse out with sterile irrigating solution
Eye infections: 1-3 drops into the affected eye(s) every 3-4 hours for several days
Dosage Forms Solution, ophthalmic: 20% (15 mL, 30 mL)

silver sulfadiazine (SIL ver sul fa DYE a zeen)
U.S. Brand Names Silvadene®; SSD® AF; SSD® Cream; Thermazene®
Canadian Brand Names Dermazin™; Flamazine®
Generic Available Yes
Therapeutic Category Antibacterial, Topical
Use Adjunct in the prevention and treatment of infection in second and third degree burns
Usual Dosage Children and Adults: Topical: Apply once or twice daily with a sterile gloved hand; apply to a thickness of 1/16"; burned area should be covered with cream at all times
Nursing/Pharmacy Information
Evaluate the development of granulation
Monitor serum electrolytes, urinalysis, renal function tests, CBC in patients with extensive burns on long-term treatment
Stability: Discard if cream is darkened (reacts with heavy metals resulting in release of silver)
Dosage Forms Cream, topical: 1% [10 mg/g] (20 g, 50 g, 100 g, 400 g, 1000 g)

simethicone (sye METH i kone)
Synonyms activated dimethicone; activated methylpolysiloxane
U.S. Brand Names Degas® [OTC]; Flatulex® [OTC]; Gas-X® [OTC]; Maalox Anti-Gas® [OTC]; Mylanta Gas® [OTC]; Mylicon® [OTC]; Phazyme® [OTC]; Silain® [OTC]
Canadian Brand Names Ovol®
Generic Available Yes: Tablet
Therapeutic Category Antiflatulent
Use Relieve flatulence, functional gastric bloating, and postoperative gas pains
Usual Dosage Oral:
Infants: 20 mg 4 times/day
Children <12 years: 40 mg 4 times/day

Children >12 years and Adults: 40-120 mg after meals and at bedtime as needed, not to exceed 500 mg/day

Dietary Considerations Avoid carbonated beverages and gas-forming foods; should be administered after meals

Nursing/Pharmacy Information
Shake suspension before using; mix with water, infant formula or other liquids
Stability: Protect from light

Dosage Forms
Capsule: 125 mg
Drops, oral: 40 mg/0.6 mL (30 mL)
Tablet: 50 mg, 60 mg, 95 mg
Chewable: 40 mg, 80 mg, 125 mg

- ♦ **simethicone and calcium carbonate** *see* calcium carbonate and simethicone *on page 104*
- ♦ **simethicone and magaldrate** *see* magaldrate and simethicone *on page 380*
- ♦ **Simron® [OTC]** *see* ferrous gluconate *on page 265*
- ♦ **Simulect®** *see* basiliximab *on page 74*

simvastatin (SIM va stat in)

U.S. Brand Names Zocor®
Generic Available No
Therapeutic Category HMG-CoA Reductase Inhibitor
Use Adjunct to dietary therapy to decrease elevated serum total and LDL cholesterol concentrations in primary hypercholesterolemia; lowering elevated triglyceride levels
Usual Dosage Adults: Oral: Start with 5-10 mg/day as a single bedtime dose; starting dose of 5 mg/day should be considered for patients with LDL-C of ≤190 mg/dL and for the elderly; patients with LDL-C levels >190 mg/dL should be started on 10 mg/day; adjustments of dosage should be made at intervals of 4 weeks or more; maximum recommended dose: 40 mg/day
Nursing/Pharmacy Information
Monitor creatine phosphokinase levels due to possibility of myopathy
Stability: Tablets should be stored in well-closed containers at temperatures between 5°C to 30°C (41°F to 86°F)
Dosage Forms Tablet: 5 mg, 10 mg, 20 mg, 40 mg

- ♦ **Sinaplin** *see* ampicillin *on page 46*
- ♦ **Sinarest® 12 Hour Nasal Solution** *see* oxymetazoline *on page 463*
- ♦ **Sinarest® Nasal Solution [OTC]** *see* phenylephrine *on page 487*
- ♦ **Sinarest®, No Drowsiness [OTC]** *see* acetaminophen and pseudoephedrine *on page 15*

sincalide (SIN ka lide)

Synonyms C8-CCK; OP-CCK
U.S. Brand Names Kinevac®
Generic Available No
Therapeutic Category Diagnostic Agent
Use Postevacuation cholecystography; gallbladder bile sampling; stimulate pancreatic secretion for analysis
Usual Dosage Adults: I.V.:
Contraction of gallbladder: 0.02 mcg/kg over 30 seconds to 1 minute, may repeat in 15 minutes a 0.04 mcg/kg dose
Pancreatic function: 0.02 mcg/kg over 30 minutes
Nursing/Pharmacy Information Stability: Reconstituted solution may be kept at room temperature for 24 hours
Dosage Forms Injection: 5 mcg

- ♦ **Sine-Aid® IB [OTC]** *see* pseudoephedrine and ibuprofen *on page 531*
- ♦ **Sine-Aid®, Maximum Strength [OTC]** *see* acetaminophen and pseudoephedrine *on page 15*
- ♦ **Sinedol** *see* acetaminophen *on page 13*
- ♦ **Sinedol 500** *see* acetaminophen *on page 13*
- ♦ **Sinemet®** *see* levodopa and carbidopa *on page 365*
- ♦ **Sine-Off® Maximum Strength No Drowsiness Formula [OTC]** *see* acetaminophen and pseudoephedrine *on page 15*
- ♦ **Sinequan® Oral** *see* doxepin *on page 219*
- ♦ **Sinex® Long-Acting [OTC]** *see* oxymetazoline *on page 463*
- ♦ **Singulair®** *see* montelukast *on page 421*
- ♦ **Sinografin®** *see* radiological/contrast media (ionic) *on page 539*
- ♦ **Sintrom®** *see* nicoumalone *(Canada only) on page 442*

- **Sinuberase®** *see* Lactobacillus *on page 358*
- **Sinubid®** *see* phenyltoloxamine, phenylpropanolamine, and acetaminophen *on page 490*
- **Sinufed® Timecelles®** *see* guaifenesin and pseudoephedrine *on page 302*
- **Sinumist®-SR Capsulets®** *see* guaifenesin *on page 299*
- **Sinupan®** *see* guaifenesin and phenylephrine *on page 301*
- **Sinus Excedrin® Extra Strength [OTC]** *see* acetaminophen and pseudoephedrine *on page 15*
- **Sinus-Relief® [OTC]** *see* acetaminophen and pseudoephedrine *on page 15*
- **Sinutab® Tablets [OTC]** *see* acetaminophen, chlorpheniramine, and pseudoephedrine *on page 16*
- **Sinutab® Without Drowsiness [OTC]** *see* acetaminophen and pseudoephedrine *on page 15*

sirolimus *New Drug* (sir OH li mus)
U.S. Brand Names Rapamune®
Generic Available No
Therapeutic Category Immunosuppressant Agent
Use Prophylaxis of organ rejection in patients receiving renal transplants, in combination with cyclosporin and corticosteroids
> **Unlabeled use:** Prophylaxis of organ rejection in solid organ transplant patients in combination with tacrolimus and corticosteriods

Usual Dosage Oral:
> Adults ≥40 kg: Loading dose: For *de novo* transplant recipients, a loading dose of 3 times the daily maintenance dose should be administered on day 1 of dosing. Maintenance dose: 2 mg/day. Doses should be taken 4 hours after cyclosporine, and should be taken consistently either with or without food.
> Children ≥13 years or Adults <40 kg: Loading dose: 3 mg/m² (day 1); followed by a maintenance of 1 mg/m²/day.

Dosage Forms Solution, oral: 1 mg/mL (1 mL, 2 mL, 5 mL, 60 mL, 150 mL)

- **SK** *see* streptokinase *on page 580*
- **Skelaxin®** *see* metaxalone *on page 398*
- **Skelex®** *(Discontinued)* *see* page 743
- **Skelid®** *see* tiludronate *on page 613*
- **SKF 104864** *see* topotecan *on page 619*

skin test antigens, multiple (skin test AN tee gens, MUL ti pul)
U.S. Brand Names Multitest CMI®
Generic Available No
Therapeutic Category Diagnostic Agent
Use Detection of nonresponsiveness to antigens by means of delayed hypersensitivity skin testing
Usual Dosage Select only test sites that permit sufficient surface area and subcutaneous tissue to allow adequate penetration of all 8 points, avoid hairy areas

> Press loaded unit into the skin with sufficient pressure to puncture the skin and allow adequate penetration of all points, maintain firm contact for at least five seconds, during application the device should not be "rocked" back and forth and side to side without removing any of the test heads from the skin sites
> If adequate pressure is applied it will be possible to observe:
> 1. The puncture marks of the nine tines on each of the eight test heads
> 2. An imprint of the circular platform surrounding each test head
> 3. Residual antigen and glycerin at each of the eight sites
> If any of the above three criteria are not fully followed, the test results may not be reliable
> Reading should be done in good light, read the test sites at both 24 and 48 hours, the largest reaction recorded from the two readings at each test site should be used; if two readings are not possible, a single 48 hour is recommended
> A positive reaction from any of the seven delayed hypersensitivity skin test antigens is **induration of ≥2 mm** providing there is no induration at the negative control site; the size of the induration reactions with this test may be smaller than those obtained with other intradermal procedures

Nursing/Pharmacy Information Contains disposable plastic applicator consisting of eight sterile test heads preloaded with the following seven delayed hypersensitivity skin test antigens and glycerin negative control for percutaneous administration
> Test Head No. 1 = Tetanus toxoid antigen
> Test Head No. 2 = Diphtheria toxoid antigen

Test Head No. 3 = *Streptococcus* antigen
Test Head No. 4 = Tuberculin, old
Test Head No. 5 = Glycerin negative control
Test Head No. 6 = *Candida* antigen
Test Head No. 7 = *Trichophyton* antigen
Test Head No. 8 = *Proteus* antigen
Stability: Refrigerate at 2°C to 8°C (35°F to 46°F)

Dosage Forms Individual carton containing one preloaded skin test antigen for cellular hypersensitivity

- ◆ **Sleep-eze 3® Oral [OTC]** *see* diphenhydramine *on page 208*
- ◆ **Sleepinal® [OTC]** *see* diphenhydramine *on page 208*
- ◆ **Sleepwell 2-nite® [OTC]** *see* diphenhydramine *on page 208*
- ◆ **Slim-Mint® [OTC]** *see* benzocaine *on page 79*
- ◆ **Slo-bid™** *see* theophylline *on page 603*
- ◆ **Slo-Niacin® [OTC]** *see* niacin *on page 440*
- ◆ **Slo-Phyllin®** *see* theophylline *on page 603*
- ◆ **Slo-Phyllin® GG** *see* theophylline and guaifenesin *on page 604*
- ◆ **Slo-Salt® *(Discontinued)*** *see page 743*
- ◆ **Slow FE® [OTC]** *see* ferrous sulfate *on page 265*
- ◆ **Slow-K®** *see* potassium chloride *on page 506*
- ◆ **Slow-Mag® [OTC]** *see* magnesium chloride *on page 380*
- ◆ **smelling salts** *see* ammonia spirit, aromatic *on page 41*
- ◆ **SMX-TMP** *see* co-trimoxazole *on page 170*
- ◆ **snake (pit vipers) antivenin** *see* antivenin (*Crotalidae*) polyvalent *on page 54*
- ◆ **Snaplets-EX® [OTC]** *see* guaifenesin and phenylpropanolamine *on page 301*
- ◆ **Snaplets-FR® Granules [OTC]** *see* acetaminophen *on page 13*
- ◆ **sodium 2-mercaptoethane sulfonate** *see* mesna *on page 395*

sodium acetate (SOW dee um AS e tate)

Generic Available Yes
Therapeutic Category Alkalinizing Agent; Electrolyte Supplement, Oral
Use Sodium salt replacement; correction of acidosis through conversion of acetate to bicarbonate
Usual Dosage Sodium acetate is metabolized to bicarbonate on an equimolar basis outside the liver; administer in large volume I.V. fluids as a sodium source. Refer to sodium bicarbonate monograph.

Maintenance electrolyte requirements of sodium in parenteral nutrition solutions:
Daily requirements: 3-4 mEq/kg/24 hours or 25-40 mEq/1000 kcal/24 hours
Maximum: 100-150 mEq/24 hours

Nursing/Pharmacy Information
Sodium and acetate content of 1 g: 7.3 mEq
Stability: Protect from light, heat, and from freezing; **incompatible** with acids, acidic salts, alkaloid salts, calcium salts, catecholamines, atropine
Dosage Forms Injection: 2 mEq/mL (20 mL, 50 mL); 4 mEq/mL (50 mL)

- ◆ **sodium acid carbonate** *see* sodium bicarbonate *on page 570*

sodium ascorbate (SOW dee um a SKOR bate)

U.S. Brand Names Cenolate®
Generic Available Yes
Therapeutic Category Vitamin, Water Soluble
Use Prevention and treatment of scurvy and to acidify the urine; large doses may decrease the severity of "colds"
Usual Dosage Oral, I.V.:
Children:
Scurvy: 100-300 mg/day in divided doses for at least 2 weeks
Urinary acidification: 500 mg every 6-8 hours
Dietary supplement: 35-45 mg/day
Adults:
Scurvy: 100-250 mg 1-2 times/day for at least 2 weeks
Urinary acidification: 4-12 g/day in divided doses
Dietary supplement: 50-60 mg/day
Prevention and treatment of cold: 1-3 g/day
Nursing/Pharmacy Information Do not exceed recommended daily allowance
Dosage Forms
Crystals: 1020 mg per ¼ teaspoonful [ascorbic acid 900 mg]
(Continued)

sodium ascorbate *(Continued)*

Injection: 250 mg/mL [ascorbic acid 222 mg/mL] (30 mL); 562.5 mg/mL [ascorbic acid 500 mg/mL] (1 mL, 2 mL)
Tablet: 585 mg [ascorbic acid 500 mg]

♦ **sodium benzoate and caffeine** *see* caffeine and sodium benzoate *on page 101*

sodium bicarbonate (SOW dee um bye KAR bun ate)

Synonyms baking soda; $NaHCO_3$; sodium acid carbonate; sodium hydrogen carbonate

U.S. Brand Names Neut®

Generic Available Yes

Therapeutic Category Alkalinizing Agent; Antacid; Electrolyte Supplement, Oral

Use Management of metabolic acidosis; antacid; alkalinize urine; stabilization of acid base status in cardiac arrest, and treatment of life-threatening hyperkalemia

Usual Dosage

Cardiac arrest (patient should be adequately ventilated before administering $NaHCO_3$):

Infants: Use 1:1 dilution of 1 mEq/mL $NaHCO_3$ or use 0.5 mEq/mL $NaHCO_3$ at a dose of 1 mEq/kg slow IVP initially; may repeat with 0.5 mEq/kg in 10 minutes one time or as indicated by the patient's acid-base status. Rate of administration should not exceed 10 mEq/minute.

Children and Adults: IVP: 1 mEq/kg initially; may repeat with 0.5 mEq/kg in 10 minutes one time or as indicated by the patient's acid-base status

Metabolic acidosis: Dosage should be based on the following formula if blood gases and pH measurements are available:

Infants and Children: HCO_3-(mEq) = 0.3 x weight (kg) x base deficit (mEq/L) **or** HCO_3-(mEq) = 0.5 x weight (kg) x (24 - serum HCO_3-) (mEq/L)

Adults: HCO_3-(mEq) = 0.2 x weight (kg) x base deficit (mEq/L) **or** HCO_3-(mEq) = 0.5 x weight (kg) x (24 - serum HCO_3-) (mEq/L)

If acid-base status is not available: Dose for older Children and Adults: 2-5 mEq/kg I.V. infusion over 4-8 hours; subsequent doses should be based on patient's acid-base status

Chronic renal failure: Oral: Children: 1-3 mEq/kg/day

Renal tubular acidosis: Oral:

Distal:

Children: 2-3 mEq/kg/day

Adults: 1 mEq/kg/day

Proximal: Children: Initial: 5-10 mEq/kg/day; maintenance: Increase as required to maintain serum bicarbonate in the normal range

Urine alkalinization: Oral:

Children: 1-10 mEq (84-840 mg)/kg/day in divided doses; dose should be titrated to desired urinary pH .

Adults: Initial: 48 mEq (4 g), then 12-24 mEq (1-2 g) every 4 hours; dose should be titrated to desired urinary pH; doses up to 16 g/day have been used

Dietary Considerations Oral product should be administered 1-3 hours after meals; concurrent doses with iron may decrease iron absorption

Nursing/Pharmacy Information

Advise patient of milk-alkali syndrome if use is long-term; observe for extravasation when administering I.V.; for I.V. administration to infants, use the 0.5 mEq/mL solution or dilute the 1 mEq/mL solution 1:1 with **sterile water**; for direct I.V. infusion in emergencies, administer slowly (maximum rate in infants: 10 mEq/minute); for infusion, dilute to a maximum concentration of 0.5 mEq/mL in dextrose solution and infuse over 2 hours (maximum rate of administration: 1 mEq/kg/hour)

Monitor serum electrolytes including calcium, urinary pH, arterial blood gases (if indicated)

Stability: Store injection at room temperature; protect from heat and from freezing; use only clear solutions; Advise patient of milk-alkali syndrome if use is long-term; observe for extravasation when administering I.V. **incompatible** with acids, acidic salts, alkaloid salts, calcium salts, catecholamines, atropine

Dosage Forms

Injection: 4% [40 mg/mL = 2.4 mEq/5 mL] (5 mL); 4.2% [42 mg/mL = 5 mEq/10 mL] (10 mL); 7.5% [75 mg/mL = 8.92 mEq/10 mL] (10 mL, 50 mL); 8.4% [84 mg/mL = 10 mEq/10 mL] (10 mL, 50 mL)

Powder: 120 g, 480 g

Tablet: 300 mg [3.6 mEq]; 325 mg [3.8 mEq]; 520 mg [6.3 mEq]; 600 mg [7.3 mEq]; 650 mg [7.6 mEq]

♦ **sodium cellulose phosphate** *see* cellulose sodium phosphate *on page 127*

sodium chloride (SOW dee um KLOR ide)

Synonyms NaCl; normal saline; salt

U.S. Brand Names Adsorbonac® Ophthalmic [OTC]; Afrin® Saline Mist [OTC]; AK-NaCl® [OTC]; Ayr® Nasal [OTC]; Breathe Free® [OTC]; Dristan® Saline Spray [OTC]; HuMist® Nasal Mist [OTC]; Muro 128® Ophthalmic [OTC]; Muroptic-5® [OTC]; NaSal™ [OTC]; Nasal Moist® [OTC]; Ocean Nasal Mist [OTC]; Pretz® [OTC]; SalineX® [OTC]; SeaMist® [OTC]

Canadian Brand Names Saline from Otrivin®

Generic Available Yes

Therapeutic Category Electrolyte Supplement, Oral; Lubricant, Ocular

Use Prevention of muscle cramps and heat prostration; restoration of sodium ion in hyponatremia; restore moisture to nasal membranes; reduction of corneal edema

Usual Dosage

Newborn electrolyte requirement:

Premature: 2-8 mEq/kg/24 hours

Term:

0-48 hours: 0-2 mEq/kg/24 hours

>48 hours: 1-4 mEq/kg/24 hours

Children: I.V.: Hypertonic solutions (>0.9%) should only be used for the initial treatment of acute serious symptomatic hyponatremia; maintenance: 3-4 mEq/kg/day; maximum: 100-150 mEq/day; dosage varies widely depending on clinical condition

Replacement: Determined by laboratory determinations mEq

Sodium deficiency (mEq/kg) = [% dehydration (L/kg)/100 x 70 (mEq/L) = [0.6 (L/kg) x (140 - serum sodium) (mEq/L)]

Nasal: Use as often as needed

Adults:

GI irrigant: 1-3 L/day by intermittent irrigation

Heat cramps: Oral: 0.5-1 g with full glass of water, up to 4.8 g/day

Replacement I.V.: Determined by laboratory determinations mEq

Sodium deficiency (mEq/kg) = [% dehydration (L/kg)/100 x 70 (mEq/L)] + [0.6 (L/kg) x (140 - serum sodium) (mEq/L)]

To correct acute, serious hyponatremia: mEq sodium = (desired sodium (mEq/L) - actual sodium (mEq/L) x 0.6 x wt (kg)); for acute correction use 125 mEq/L as the desired serum sodium; acutely correct serum sodium in 5 mEq/L/dose increments; more gradual correction in increments of 10 mEq/L/day is indicated in the asymptomatic patient

Chloride maintenance electrolyte requirement in parenteral nutrition: 2-4 mEq/kg/24 hours or 25-40 mEq/1000 kcals/24 hours; maximum: 100-150 mEq/24 hours

Sodium maintenance electrolyte requirement in parenteral nutrition: 3-4 mEq/kg/24 hours or 25-40 mEq/1000 kcals/24 hours; maximum: 100-150 mEq/24 hours.

Nasal: Use as often as needed

Ophthalmic:

Ointment: Apply once daily or more often

Solution: Instill 1-2 drops into affected eye(s) every 3-4 hours

Abortifacient: 20% (250 mL) administered by transabdominal intra-amniotic instillation

Nursing/Pharmacy Information

Bacteriostatic NS should not be used for diluting or reconstituting drugs for administration in neonates; infuse hypertonic solutions (>NaCl 0.9%) via central line only; maximum rate of administration: 1 mEq/kg/hour

Monitor serum sodium, potassium, chloride, and bicarbonate levels.

Stability: Store injection at room temperature; protect from heat and from freezing; use only clear solutions

Dosage Forms

Drops, nasal: 0.9% with dropper

Injection: 0.2% (3 mL); 0.45% (3 mL, 5 mL, 500 mL, 1000 mL); 0.9% (1 mL, 2 mL, 3 mL, 4 mL, 5 mL, 10 mL, 20 mL, 25 mL, 30 mL, 50 mL, 100 mL, 130 mL, 150 mL, 250 mL, 500 mL, 1000 mL); 3% (500 mL); 5% (500 mL); 20% (250 mL); 23.4% (30 mL, 100 mL)

Injection:

Admixtures: 50 mEq (20 mL); 100 mEq (40 mL); 625 mEq (250 mL)

Bacteriostatic: 0.9% (30 mL)

(Continued)

sodium chloride *(Continued)*

Concentrated: 14.6% (20 mL, 40 mL, 200 mL); 23.4% (10 mL, 20 mL, 30 mL)
Irrigation: 0.45% (500 mL, 1000 mL, 1500 mL); 0.9% (250 mL, 500 mL, 1000 mL, 1500 mL, 2000 mL, 3000 mL, 4000 mL)
Ointment, ophthalmic (Muro 128®): 5% (3.5 g)
Solution:
Irrigation: 0.9% (1000 mL, 2000 mL)
Nasal: 0.4% (15 mL, 50 mL); 0.6% (15 mL); 0.65% (20 mL, 45 mL, 50 mL)
Ophthalmic (Adsorbonac®): 2% (15 mL); 5% (15 mL, 30 mL)
Tablet: 650 mg, 1 g, 2.25 g
Enteric coated: 1 g
Slow release: 600 mg

sodium citrate and potassium citrate mixture
(SOW dee um SIT rate & poe TASS ee um SIT rate MIKS chur)
U.S. Brand Names Polycitra®
Generic Available Yes
Therapeutic Category Alkalinizing Agent
Use Conditions where long-term maintenance of an alkaline urine is desirable as in control and dissolution of uric acid and cystine calculi of the urinary tract
Usual Dosage Oral:
Children: 5-15 mL diluted in water after meals and at bedtime
Adults: 15-30 mL diluted in water after meals and at bedtime
Dietary Considerations Should be administered after meals
Nursing/Pharmacy Information Dilute each dose in 30-90 mL of water prior to administration
Dosage Forms Syrup: Sodium citrate 500 mg, potassium citrate 550 mg, with citric acid 334 mg per 5 mL [sodium 1 mEq, potassium 1 mEq, bicarbonate 2 mEq]

♦ **sodium edetate** *see* edetate disodium *on page 228*
♦ **sodium ethacrynate** *see* ethacrynic acid *on page 247*
♦ **sodium etidronate** *see* etidronate disodium *on page 254*
♦ **Sodium Fusidate** *see* fusidic acid *(Canada only) on page 286*

sodium hyaluronate (SOW dee um hye al yoor ON nate)
Synonyms hyaluronic acid
U.S. Brand Names AMO Vitrax®; Amvisc®; Amvisc® Plus; Healon®; Healon® GV
Canadian Brand Names Replasyn®
Generic Available No
Therapeutic Category Ophthalmic Agent, Viscoelastic
Use Surgical aid in cataract extraction, intraocular implantation, corneal transplant, glaucoma filtration, and retinal attachment surgery
Usual Dosage Depends upon procedure (slowly introduce a sufficient quantity into eye)
Nursing/Pharmacy Information
Monitor intraocular pressure
Stability: Store in refrigerator (2°C to 8°C); do not freeze
Dosage Forms Injection, intraocular:
Healon®: 10 mg/mL (0.4 mL, 0.55 mL, 0.85 mL, 2 mL)
Amvisc®: 12 mg/mL (0.5 mL, 0.8 mL)
Healon® GV: 14 mg/mL (0.55 mL, 0.85 mL)
Amvisc® Plus: 16 mg/mL (0.5 mL, 8 mL)
AMO Vitrax®: 30 mg/mL (0.65 mL)

♦ **sodium hyaluronate-chrondroitin sulfate** *see* chondroitin sulfate-sodium hyaluronate *on page 148*
♦ **sodium hydrogen carbonate** *see* sodium bicarbonate *on page 570*

sodium hypochlorite solution
(SOW dee um hye poe KLOR ite soe LOO shun)
Synonyms Dakin's solution; modified Dakin's solution
Generic Available Yes
Therapeutic Category Disinfectant
Use Treatment of athlete's foot (0.5%); wound irrigation (0.5%); to disinfect utensils and equipment (5%)
Usual Dosage Topical irrigation
Nursing/Pharmacy Information
Monitor healing rate of lesions/ulcers
Stability: Use prepared solution within 7 days

Dosage Forms
Solution: 5% (4000 mL)
  Modified Dakin's solution:
    Full strength: 0.5% (1000 mL)
    Half strength: 0.25% (1000 mL)
    Quarter strength: 0.125% (1000 mL)

sodium lactate (SOW dee um LAK tate)
Generic Available Yes
Therapeutic Category Alkalinizing Agent
Use Source of bicarbonate for prevention and treatment of mild to moderate metabolic acidosis
Usual Dosage Dosage depends on degree of acidosis
Nursing/Pharmacy Information Monitor fluid and electrolyte status during therapy
Dosage Forms Injection:
  1.87 g/100 mL [sodium 16.7 mEq and lactate 16.7 mEq per 100 mL] (1000 mL)
  560 mg/mL [sodium 5 mEq sodium and lactate 5 mEq per mL] (10 mL)

♦ **sodium nitroferricyanide** *see* nitroprusside *on page 445*
♦ **Sodium P.A.S.® *(Discontinued)*** *see page 743*
♦ **sodium-pca and lactic acid** *see* lactic acid and sodium-PCA *on page 358*

sodium phenylacetate and sodium benzoate
(SOW dee um fen il AS e tate & SOW dee um BENZ oh ate)
U.S. Brand Names Ucephan®
Generic Available No
Therapeutic Category Ammonium Detoxicant
Use Adjunctive therapy to prevent/treat hyperammonemia in patients with urea cycle enzymopathy involving partial or complete deficiencies of carbamoyl-phosphate synthetase, ornithine transcarbamoylase or argininosuccinate synthetase
Usual Dosage Infants and Children: Oral: 2.5 mL (250 mg sodium benzoate and 250 mg sodium phenylacetate)/kg/day divided 3-6 times/day; total daily dose should not exceed 100 mL
Dietary Considerations Dilute each dose in 4-8 oz of infant formula or milk and administer with meals
Nursing/Pharmacy Information
Monitor serum electrolytes, blood ammonia
Stability: Diluting Ucephan® with an acidic solution can result in precipitation of the drug
Dosage Forms Solution: Sodium phenylacetate 100 mg and sodium benzoate 100 mg per mL (100 mL)

sodium phenylbutyrate (SOW dee um fen il BYOO ti rate)
Synonyms ammonapse
U.S. Brand Names Buphenyl®
Generic Available No
Therapeutic Category Miscellaneous Product
Use Adjunctive therapy in the chronic management of patients with urea cycle disorder involving deficiencies of carbamoylphosphate synthetase, ornithine transcarbamylase, or argininosuccinic acid synthetase
Usual Dosage
Powder: Patients weighing <20 kg: 450-600 mg/kg/day or 9.9-13 g/m²/day, administered in equally divided amounts with each meal or feeding, 4-6 times/day; safety and efficacy of doses >20 g/day have not been established
Tablet: Children >20 kg and Adults: 450-600 mg/kg/day or 9.9-13 g/m²/day, administered in equally divided amounts with each meal; safety and efficacy of doses >20 g/day have not been established
Dosage Forms
Powder: 3.2 g [sodium phenylbutyrate 3 g] per teaspoon (500 mL, 950 mL); 9.1 g [sodium phenylbutyrate 8.6 g] per **tablespoon** (500 mL, 950 mL)
Tablet: 500 mg

♦ **sodium phosphate and potassium phosphate** *see* potassium phosphate and sodium phosphate *on page 510*

sodium phosphates (SOW dee um FOS fate)
U.S. Brand Names Fleet® Enema [OTC]; Fleet® Phospho®-Soda [OTC]
Canadian Brand Names Enemol™
Generic Available Yes
(Continued)

sodium phosphates (Continued)

Therapeutic Category Electrolyte Supplement, Oral; Laxative

Use Source of phosphate in large volume I.V. fluids; short-term treatment of constipation (oral/rectal) and to evacuate the colon for rectal and bowel exams; treatment and prevention of hypophosphatemia

Usual Dosage

Normal requirements elemental phosphate: Oral:

0-6 months: 240 mg

6-12 months: 360 mg

1-10 years: 800 mg

>10 years: 1200 mg

Pregnancy lactation: Additional 400 mg/day

Treatment:

It is difficult to provide concrete guidelines for the treatment of severe hypophosphatemia because the extent of total body deficits and response to therapy are difficult to predict. Aggressive doses of phosphate may result in a transient serum elevation followed by redistribution into intracellular compartments or bone tissue. It is recommended that repletion of severe hypophosphatemia (<1 mg/dL in adults) be done I.V. because large doses of oral phosphate may cause diarrhea and intestinal absorption may be unreliable

Pediatric I.V. phosphate repletion:

Children: 0.25-0.5 mmol/kg **administer over 4-6 hours and repeat if symptomatic hypophosphatemia persists**; to assess the need for further phosphate administration: obtain serum inorganic phosphate after administration of the first dose and base further doses on serum levels and clinical status

Adult I.V. phosphate repletion:

Initial dose: 0.08 mmol/kg if recent uncomplicated hypophosphatemia

Initial dose: 0.16 mmol/kg if prolonged hypophosphatemia with presumed total body deficits; increase dose by 25% to 50% if patient symptomatic with severe hypophosphatemia

Severe hypophosphatemia:

High-dose = 0.36 mmol/kg over 6 hours; use if serum PO_4 <0.5 mg/dL

Adults: 0.15-0.3 mmol/kg/dose over 12 hours, may repeat as needed to achieve desired serum level

With orders for I.V. phosphate, there is considerable confusion associated with the use of millimoles (mmol) versus milliequivalents (mEq) to express the phosphate requirement. Because inorganic phosphate exists as monobasic and dibasic anions, with the mixture of valences is dependent on pH, ordering by mEq amounts is unreliable and may lead to large dosing errors. In addition, I.V. phosphate is available in the sodium and potassium salt; therefore, the content of these cations must be considered when ordering phosphate. The most reliable method of ordering I.V. phosphate is by millimoles, then specifying the potassium or sodium salt. For example, an order for 15 mmol of phosphate as potassium phosphate in one liter of normal saline would also provide 22 mEq of potassium.

Phosphate maintenance electrolyte requirement in parenteral nutrition: 2 mmol/kg/24 hours or 35 mmol/kcal/24 hours; Maximum: 15-30 mmol/24 hours

Maintenance:

Children: 0.5-1.5 mmol/kg/24 hours I.V. **or** 2-3 mmol/kg/24 hours orally in divided doses

Adults: 15-30 mmol/24 hours I.V. **or** 50-150 mmol/24 hours orally in divided doses

Laxative (Fleet®): Rectal:

Children 2-12 years: 67.5 mL (½ bottle) as a single dose, may repeat

Children ≥12 years and Adults: 133 mL enema as a single dose, may repeat

Laxative (Fleet® Phospho®-Soda): Oral:

Children:

5-9 years: 5 mL as a single dose

10-12 years: 10 mL as a single dose

Children ≥12 years and Adults: 20-30 mL as a single dose

Dietary Considerations Should be administered on an empty stomach with water

Nursing/Pharmacy Information

Contents of one packet should be diluted in 75 mL water before administration; maintain adequate fluid intake; for intermittent I.V. infusion, dilute at a maximum concentration of 0.12 mmol/mL and infuse over 4-6 hours; maximum, rate of infusion: 0.06 mmol/kg/hour

Monitor serum sodium and phosphorous levels

Stability: Phosphate salts may precipitate in the presence of calcium; check on the maximum concentrations at which they are compatible

Dosage Forms

Enema: Sodium phosphate 6 g and sodium biphosphate 16 g/100 mL (67.5 mL pediatric enema unit, 135 mL adult enema unit)

Injection: Phosphate 3 mmol and sodium 4 mEq per mL (5 mL, 10 mL, 15 mL, 30 mL, 50 mL)

Solution, oral: Sodium phosphate 18 g and sodium biphosphate 48 g/100 mL (45 mL, 90 mL, 273 mL)

See table.

	Phosphate (mmol)	Sodium (mEq)	Potassium (mEq)
Oral			
Whole cow's milk	0.29/mL	0.025/mL	0.035/mL
Fleet® Phospho®-Soda	4.15/mL	4.8/mL	None
Intravenous			
Sodium phosphate	3/mL	4/mL	None

sodium polystyrene sulfonate

(SOW dee um pol ee STYE reen SUL fon ate)

U.S. Brand Names Kayexalate®; Kionex®; SPS®

Generic Available Yes

Therapeutic Category Antidote

Use Treatment of hyperkalemia

Usual Dosage

Children:

Oral: 1 g/kg/dose every 6 hours

Rectal: 1 g/kg/dose every 2-6 hours (In small children and infants employ lower doses by using the practical exchange ratio of 1 mEq potassium/g of resin as the basis for calculation)

Adults:

Oral: 15 g (60 mL) 1-4 times/day

Rectal: 30-50 g every 6 hours

Dietary Considerations Do **not** mix in orange juice

Nursing/Pharmacy Information

Administer oral (or NG) as ~25% sorbitol solution; enema route is less effective than oral administration; retain enema in colon for at least 30-60 minutes and for several hours, if possible

Monitor serum electrolytes, EKG

Dosage Forms Oral or rectal:

Powder for suspension: 454 g

Suspension: 1.25 g/5 mL with sorbitol 33% and alcohol 0.3% (60 mL, 120 mL, 200 mL, 500 mL)

sodium salicylate (SOW dee um sa LIS i late)

U.S. Brand Names Uracel®

Generic Available Yes

Therapeutic Category Analgesic, Non-narcotic; Antipyretic

Use Treatment of minor pain or fever; arthritis

Usual Dosage Adults: Oral: 325-650 mg every 4 hours

Nursing/Pharmacy Information Sodium content of 1 g: 6.25 mEq; less effective than an equal dose of aspirin in reducing pain or fever; patients hypersensitive to aspirin may be able to tolerate

Dosage Forms Tablet, enteric coated: 325 mg, 650 mg

♦ **Sodium Sulamyd®** see sulfacetamide on page 584

sodium tetradecyl (SOW dee um tetra DEK il)

U.S. Brand Names Sotradecol®

Canadian Brand Names Trombovar®

Generic Available Yes

Therapeutic Category Sclerosing Agent

Use Treatment of small, uncomplicated varicose veins of the lower extremities; endoscopic sclerotherapy in the management of bleeding esophageal varices

Usual Dosage I.V.: 0.5-2 mL of 1% (5-20 mg) for small veins; 0.5-2 mL of 3% (15-60 mg) for medium or large veins

(Continued)

sodium tetradecyl *(Continued)*

Nursing/Pharmacy Information

Observe for signs and symptoms of embolism

Stability: Store at controlled room temperature in a well-closed container; protect from light

Dosage Forms Injection, as sulfate: 1% [10 mg/mL] (2 mL); 3% [30 mg/mL] (2 mL)

sodium thiosulfate (SOW dee um thye oh SUL fate)

U.S. Brand Names Tinver® [OTC]; Versiclear™

Generic Available Yes

Therapeutic Category Antidote; Antifungal Agent

Use

Parenteral: Used alone or with sodium nitrite or amyl nitrite in cyanide poisoning or arsenic poisoning; reduce the risk of nephrotoxicity associated with cisplatin therapy; local infiltration (in diluted form) of selected chemotherapy extravasation

Topical: Treatment of tinea versicolor

Usual Dosage I.V.:

Cyanide and nitroprusside antidote:

Children <25 kg: 50 mg/kg after receiving 4.5-10 mg/kg sodium nitrite; a half dose of each may be repeated if necessary

Children >25 kg and Adults: 12.5 g after 300 mg of sodium nitrite; a half dose of each may be repeated if necessary

Cyanide poisoning: Dose should be based on determination as with nitrite, at rate of 2.5-5 mL/minute to maximum of 50 mL

Nursing/Pharmacy Information

Do not apply topically to or near eyes; inject I.V. slowly, over at least 10 minutes; rapid administration may cause hypotension

Monitor for signs of thiocyanate toxicity

Dosage Forms

Injection: 100 mg/mL (10 mL); 250 mg/mL (50 mL)

Lotion: 25% with salicylic acid 1% and isopropyl alcohol 10% (120 mL, 180 mL)

sorbitol (SOR bi tole)
Generic Available Yes

Therapeutic Category Genitourinary Irrigant; Laxative

Use Humectant; sweetening agent; hyperosmotic laxative; facilitate the passage of sodium polystyrene sulfonate or a charcoal-toxin complex through the intestinal tract

Usual Dosage Hyperosmotic laxative (as single dose, at infrequent intervals):
Children 2-11 years:
Oral: 2 mL/kg (as 70% solution)
Rectal enema: 30-60 mL as 25% to 30% solution
Children >12 years and Adults:
Oral: 30-150 mL (as 70% solution)
Rectal enema: 120 mL as 25% to 30% solution
Adjunct to sodium polystyrene sulfonate: 15 mL as 70% solution orally until diarrhea occurs (10-20 mL/2 hours) or 20-100 mL as an oral vehicle for the sodium polystyrene sulfonate resin

When administered with charcoal: Oral:
Children: 4.3 mL/kg of 35% sorbitol with 1 g/kg of activated charcoal
Adults: 4.3 mL/kg of 70% sorbitol with 1 g/kg of activated charcoal

Nursing/Pharmacy Information
Do not use unless solution is clear
Monitor serum electrolytes, I & O

Dosage Forms
Solution: 70%
Solution, genitourinary irrigation: 3% (1500 mL, 3000 mL); 3.3% (2000 mL)

♦ **Sorbitrate®** *see* isosorbide dinitrate *on page 349*
♦ **Soriatane™** *see* acitretin *on page 20*
♦ **Sotacor®** *see* sotalol *on page 577*

sotalol (SOE ta lole)
U.S. Brand Names Betapace®

Canadian Brand Names Sotacor®

Generic Available No

Therapeutic Category Antiarrhythmic Agent, Class II; Antiarrhythmic Agent, Class III

Use Treatment of ventricular arrhythmias

Usual Dosage Adults: Oral: Initial: 80 mg twice daily; may be increased to 240-320 mg/day and up to 480-640 mg/day in patients with life-threatening refractory ventricular arrhythmias

Dietary Considerations Food decreases absorption; administer on an empty stomach

Nursing/Pharmacy Information
Initiation of therapy and dose escalation should be done in a hospital with cardiac monitoring; lidocaine and other resuscitative measures should be available
Monitor serum magnesium, potassium, EKG

Dosage Forms Tablet, as hydrochloride: 80 mg, 120 mg, 160 mg, 240 mg

♦ **Sotradecol®** *see* sodium tetradecyl *on page 575*
♦ **Soyacal®** *see* fat emulsion *on page 259*
♦ **Soyalac® [OTC]** *see* enteral nutritional products *on page 233*
♦ **Span-FF® [OTC]** *see* ferrous fumarate *on page 264*

sparfloxacin (spar FLOKS a sin)
U.S. Brand Names Zagam®

Generic Available No

Therapeutic Category Quinolone

Use Treatment of adult patients with community acquired pneumonia caused by susceptible strains of *Chlamydia pneumoniae*, *Haemophilus influenzae*, *Haemophilus parainfluenzae*, *Moraxella catarrhalis*, *Mycoplasma pneumoniae*, or *Streptococcus pneumoniae* and acute bacterial exacerbations of acute bronchitis caused by susceptible strains of *Chlamydia pneumoniae*, *Enterobacter cloacae*, *Haemophilus influenzae*, *Haemophilus parainfluenzae*, *Klebsiella pneumoniae*, *Moraxella catarrhalis*, *Staphylococcus aureus*, or *Streptococcus pneumoniae*

Usual Dosage Adults: Oral: 400 mg on day 1, then 200 mg/day for the next 9 days (11 tablets total). In patients with creatinine clearance <50 mL/minute, administer 400 mg on day 1, then begin 200 mg every 48 hours on day 3 for a total of 9 days (6 tablets total).
(Continued)

sparfloxacin *(Continued)*
Dosage Forms Tablet: 200 mg

- **Sparine®** *see promazine on page 521*
- **Spasmoject®** *(Discontinued) see page 743*
- **Spasmolin®** *see hyoscyamine, atropine, scopolamine, and phenobarbital on page 330*
- **Spec-T®** [OTC] *see benzocaine on page 79*
- **Spectazole™** *see econazole on page 227*

spectinomycin (spek ti noe MYE sin)
U.S. Brand Names Trobicin®
Generic Available No
Therapeutic Category Antibiotic, Miscellaneous
Use Treatment of uncomplicated gonorrhea (ineffective against syphilis)
Usual Dosage I.M.:
  Children:
    <45 kg: 40 mg/kg/dose 1 time
    ≥45 kg: See adult dose
    Children >8 years who are allergic to penicillins/cephalosporins may be treated with oral tetracycline
  Adults: 2 g deep I.M. or 4 g where antibiotic resistance is prevalent 1 time; 4 g (10 mL) dose should be administered as 2-5 mL injections
Nursing/Pharmacy Information
  For I.M. use only
  Stability: Use reconstituted solutions within 24 hours
Dosage Forms Injection, as hydrochloride: 2 g, 4 g

- **Spectrobid® Oral Suspension** *(Discontinued) see page 743*
- **Spectrobid® Tablet** *see bacampicillin on page 70*
- **Spectrum™ Forte 29** *see vitamin, multiple (oral) on page 654*
- **Spherulin®** *see coccidioidin skin test on page 163*

spiramycin *(Canada only)* (speer a MYE sin)
Canadian Brand Names Rovamycine®
Generic Available No
Therapeutic Category Antibiotic, Macrolide
Use The treatment of infections of the respiratory tract, buccal cavity, skin and soft tissues due to susceptible organisms. *N. gonorrheae*: as an alternate choice of treatment for gonorrhea in patients allergic to the penicillins. Before treatment of gonorrhea, the possibility of concomitant infection due to *T. pallidum* should be excluded.
Usual Dosage Oral:
  Children: The usual daily dosage is based on 150,000 units/kg body weight in 2 or 3 divided doses Adults: Oral: 6,000,000-9,000,000 units per 24 hours, in 2 divided doses. In severe infections, the daily dosage may be increased to 12,000,000-15,000,000 units per day
  Gonorrhea: 12,000,000-13,500000 units in a single dose.
Dosage Forms Capsule: 250 [750,000 units]; 500 [1,500,000 units]

spirapril (SPYE ra pril)
U.S. Brand Names Renormax®
Generic Available No
Therapeutic Category Angiotensin-Converting Enzyme (ACE) Inhibitor
Use Management of mild to severe hypertension
Usual Dosage Adults: Oral: 12 mg/day in 1-2 divided doses
Dosage Forms Tablet: 3 mg, 6 mg, 12 mg, 24 mg

- **Spironazide®** *see hydrochlorothiazide and spironolactone on page 318*

spironolactone (speer on oh LAK tone)
U.S. Brand Names Aldactone®
Canadian Brand Names Novo-Spiroton®
Generic Available Yes
Therapeutic Category Diuretic, Potassium Sparing
Use Management of edema associated with excessive aldosterone excretion; hypertension; primary hyperaldosteronism; hypokalemia; treatment of hirsutism
Usual Dosage Oral:
  Children: 1.5-3.5 mg/kg/day in divided doses every 6-24 hours
    Diagnosis of primary aldosteronism: 125-375 mg/m²/day in divided doses

Vaso-occlusive disease: 7.5 mg/kg/day in divided doses twice daily (non-FDA approved dose)

Adults:
Edema, hypertension, hypokalemia: 25-200 mg/day in 1-2 divided doses
Diagnosis of primary aldosteronism: 100-400 mg/day in 1-2 divided doses

Dietary Considerations This diuretic does not cause you to lose potassium; because salt substitutes and low-salt milk may contain potassium, do not use these products without checking with your physician, too much potassium can be as harmful as too little; should be administered with food, avoid natural licorice

Nursing/Pharmacy Information
Diuretic effect may be delayed 2-3 days and maximum hypertensive may be delayed 2-3 weeks
Monitor blood pressure, serum electrolytes, renal function
Stability: Protect from light

Dosage Forms Tablet: 25 mg, 50 mg, 100 mg

- ♦ **spironolactone and hydrochlorothiazide** *see* hydrochlorothiazide and spironolactone *on page 318*
- ♦ **Spirozide®** *see* hydrochlorothiazide and spironolactone *on page 318*
- ♦ **Sporanox®** *see* itraconazole *on page 351*
- ♦ **Sportscreme® [CTC]** *see* triethanolamine salicylate *on page 627*
- ♦ **SPS®** *see* sodium polystyrene sulfonate *on page 575*
- ♦ **S-P-T** *see* thyroid *on page 610*
- ♦ **SRC® Expectorant** *see* hydrocodone, pseudoephedrine, and guaifenesin *on page 322*
- ♦ **SSD® AF** *see* silver sulfadiazine *on page 566*
- ♦ **SSD® Cream** *see* silver sulfadiazine *on page 566*
- ♦ **SSKI®** *see* potassium iodide *on page 509*
- ♦ **Stadol®** *see* butorphanol *on page 100*
- ♦ **Stadol® NS** *see* butorphanol *on page 100*
- ♦ **Stagesic®** *see* hydrocodone and acetaminophen *on page 319*
- ♦ **Stahist®** *see* chlorpheniramine, phenylephrine, phenylpropanolamine, and belladonna alkaloids *on page 142*

stanozolol (stan OH zoe lole)

U.S. Brand Names Winstrol®
Generic Available No
Therapeutic Category Anabolic Steroid
Controlled Substance C-III
Use Prophylactic use against angioedema
Usual Dosage
Children: Acute attacks:
<6 years: 1 mg/day
6-12 years: 2 mg/day
Adults: Oral: Initial: 2 mg 3 times/day, may then reduce to a maintenance dose of 2 mg/day or 2 mg every other day after 1-3 months
Nursing/Pharmacy Information High protein, high caloric diet is suggested, restrict salt intake; glucose tolerance may be altered in diabetics
Dosage Forms Tablet: 2 mg

- ♦ **Staphcillin®** *(Discontinued) see page 743*
- ♦ **Statex®** *see* morphine sulfate *on page 422*
- ♦ **Staticin® Topical** *see* erythromycin (ophthalmic/topical) *on page 239*
- ♦ **Statobex®** *(Discontinued) see page 743*

stavudine (STAV yoo deen)

Synonyms d4T
U.S. Brand Names Zerit®
Generic Available No
Therapeutic Category Antiviral Agent
Use Treatment of advanced HIV infection in patients who experience intolerance, toxicity, resistance, or HIV disease progression with either zidovudine or didanosine therapy; active against most zidovudine-resistant strains; in adults, stavudine used alone in patients with 50-500 CD4 cells/mm^3 and at least 6 months previous treatment with zidovudine was more effective than continued zidovudine in preventing disease progression and more death
Usual Dosage Oral:
Children 7 months to 15 years: 1-2 mg/kg/day divided twice daily
Adults: 0.5-1 mg/kg/day **or**
(Continued)

stavudine *(Continued)*

<60 kg: 30 mg every 12 hours

≥60 kg: 40 mg every 12 hours

If peripheral neuropathy or elevations in liver enzymes occur, stavudine should be discontinued; once adverse effects resolve, reinitiate therapy at a lower dose of 20 mg every 12 hours (for ≥60 kg patients) or 15 mg every 12 hours (for <60 kg patients)

Nursing/Pharmacy Information Monitor liver function tests and signs and symptoms of peripheral neuropathy

Dosage Forms

Capsule: 15 mg, 20 mg, 30 mg, 40 mg

Powder for oral solution: 1 mg/mL (200 mL)

♦ **S-T Cort® Topical** *see* hydrocortisone (topical) *on page 324*

♦ **Stelazine®** *see* trifluoperazine *on page 627*

♦ **Stemetil®** *see* prochlorperazine *on page 519*

♦ **Stemex®** *see* paramethasone acetate *on page 470*

♦ **Stenox** *see* fluoxymesterone *on page 276*

♦ **Sterapred®** *(Discontinued) see page 743*

♦ **Stieva-A®** *see* tretinoin (topical) *on page 622*

♦ **Stieva-A® 0.025%** *see* tretinoin (topical) *on page 622*

♦ **Stieva-A® Forte** *see* tretinoin (topical) *on page 622*

♦ **stilbestrol** *see* diethylstilbestrol *on page 201*

♦ **Stilphostrol®** *see* diethylstilbestrol *on page 201*

♦ **Stimate®** *see* desmopressin acetate *on page 188*

♦ **St. Joseph® Cough Suppressant [OTC]** *see* dextromethorphan *on page 194*

♦ **St. Joseph® Measured Dose Nasal Solution [OTC]** *see* phenylephrine *on page 487*

♦ **Stop® [OTC]** *see* fluoride *on page 274*

♦ **Streptase®** *see* streptokinase *on page 580*

streptokinase *(strep toe KYE nase)*

Synonyms SK

U.S. Brand Names Kabikinase®; Streptase®

Generic Available No

Therapeutic Category Thrombolytic Agent

Use Thrombolytic agent used in treatment of recent severe or massive deep vein thrombosis, pulmonary emboli, myocardial infarction, and occluded arteriovenous cannulas

Usual Dosage I.V.:

Children: Safety and efficacy not established; limited studies have used: 3500-4000 units/kg over 30 minutes followed by 1000-1500 units/kg/hour; clotted catheter: 25,000 units, clamp for 2 hours then aspirate contents and flush with normal saline

Adults (best results are realized if used within 5-6 hours of myocardial infarction; antibodies to streptokinase remain for 3-6 months after initial dose, use another thrombolytic enzyme, ie, urokinase, if thrombolytic therapy is indicated):

Guidelines for Acute Myocardial Infarction (AMI):

1.5 million units infused over 60 minutes. Monitor for the first few hours for signs of anaphylaxis or allergic reaction. **Infusion should be slowed if lowering of 25 mm Hg in blood pressure or terminated if asthmatic symptoms appear.** Begin heparin 5000-10,000 unit bolus followed by 1000 units/hour approximately 3-4 hours after completion of streptokinase infusion or when PTT is <100 seconds.

Guidelines for Acute Pulmonary Embolism (APE):

3 million unit dose; administer 250,000 units over 30 minutes followed by 100,000 units/hour for 24 hours. Monitor for the first few hours for signs of anaphylaxis or allergic reaction. **Infusion should be slowed if blood pressure is lowered by 25 mm Hg or if asthmatic symptoms appear.** Begin heparin 1000 units/hour approximately 3-4 hours after completion of streptokinase infusion or when PTT is <100 seconds.

Thromboses: 250,000 units to start, then 100,000 units/hour for 24-72 hours depending on location

Cannula occlusion: 250,000 units into cannula, clamp for 2 hours, then aspirate contents and flush with normal saline

Nursing/Pharmacy Information

For intravenous or intracoronary use only; avoid I.M. injections

Monitor blood pressure, PT, APTT, fibrinogen, platelet count, hematocrit

Stability: Keep in refrigerator, use reconstituted solutions within 24 hours; store unopened vials at room temperature

Dosage Forms Powder for injection: 250,000 units (5 mL, 6.5 mL); 600,000 units (5 mL); 750,000 units (6 mL, 6.5 mL); 1,500,000 units (6.5 mL, 10 mL, 50 mL)

streptomycin (strep toe MYE sin)

Generic Available Yes

Therapeutic Category Antibiotic, Aminoglycoside; Antitubercular Agent

Use Combination therapy of active tuberculosis; used in combination with other agents for treatment of streptococcal or enterococcal endocarditis, mycobacterial infections, plague, tularemia, and brucellosis. Streptomycin is indicated for persons from endemic areas of drug-resistant *Mycobacterium tuberculosis* or who are HIV infected.

Usual Dosage Intramuscular (may also be given intravenous piggyback):

Tuberculosis therapy: **Note:** A four-drug regimen (isoniazid, rifampin, pyrazinamide and either streptomycin or ethambutol) is preferred for the initial, empiric treatment of TB. When the drug susceptibility results are available, the regimen should be altered as appropriate.

Patients with TB and without HIV infection:

OPTION 1:

Isoniazid resistance rate <4%: Administer daily isoniazid, rifampin, and pyrazinamide for 8 weeks followed by isoniazid and rifampin daily or directly observed therapy (DOT) 2-3 times/week for 16 weeks

If isoniazid resistance rate is not documented, ethambutol or streptomycin should also be administered until susceptibility to isoniazid or rifampin is demonstrated. Continue treatment for at least 6 months or 3 months beyond culture conversion.

OPTION 2: Administer daily isoniazid, rifampin, pyrazinamide, and either streptomycin or ethambutol for 2 weeks followed by DOT 2 times/week administration of the same drugs for 6 weeks, and subsequently, with isoniazid and rifampin DOT 2 times/week administration for 16 weeks

OPTION 3: Administer isoniazid, rifampin, pyrazinamide, and either ethambutol or streptomycin by DOT 3 times/week for 6 months

Patients with TB and with HIV infection: Administer any of the above OPTIONS 1, 2 or 3, however, treatment should be continued for a total of 9 months and at least 6 months beyond culture conversion

Note: Some experts recommend that the duration of therapy should be extended to 9 months for patients with disseminated disease, miliary disease, disease involving the bones or joints, or tuberculosis lymphadenitis

Children:

Daily therapy: 20-30 mg/kg/day (maximum: 1 g/day)

Directly observed therapy (DOT): Twice weekly: 25-30 mg/kg (maximum: 1.5 g)

DOT: 3 times/week: 25-30 mg/kg (maximum: 1 g)

Adults:

Daily therapy: 15 mg/kg/day (maximum: 1 g)

Directly observed therapy (DOT): Twice weekly: 25-30 mg/kg (maximum: 1.5 g)

DOT: 3 times/week: 25-30 mg/kg (maximum: 1 g)

Enterococcal endocarditis: 1 g every 12 hours for 2 weeks, 500 mg every 12 hours for 4 weeks in combination with penicillin

Streptococcal endocarditis: 1 g every 12 hours for 1 week, 500 mg every 12 hours for 1 week

Tularemia: 1-2 g/day in divided doses for 7-10 days or until patient is afebrile for 5-7 days

Plague: 2-4 g/day in divided doses until the patient is afebrile for at least 3 days

Elderly: 10 mg/kg/day, not to exceed 750 mg/day; dosing interval should be adjusted for renal function; some authors suggest not to give more than 5 days/week or give as 20-25 mg/kg/dose twice weekly

Dosage Forms Injection, as sulfate: 400 mg/mL (2.5 mL)

♦ **Streptomycin® *(Discontinued)*** see page 743

streptozocin (strep toe ZOE sin)

U.S. Brand Names Zanosar®

Generic Available No

Therapeutic Category Antineoplastic Agent

(Continued)

streptozocin *(Continued)*

Use Treat metastatic islet cell carcinoma of the pancreas, carcinoid tumor and syndrome, Hodgkin's disease, palliative treatment of colorectal cancer

Usual Dosage Children and Adults: I.V.: 500 mg/m^2 for 5 days every 6 weeks until optimal benefit or toxicity occurs; or may be administered in single dose 1000 mg/m^2 at weekly intervals for 2 doses, then increased to 1500 mg/m^2 weekly; the median total dose to onset of response is about 2000 mg/m^2 and the median total dose to maximum response is about 4000 mg/m^2

Nursing/Pharmacy Information

Monitor renal function closely

Stability: Refrigerate vials; solution is stable 48 hours at room temperature and 96 hours with refrigeration; may be diluted in D$_5$W or sodium chloride; protect from light

Dosage Forms Injection: 1 g

♦ **Stresstabs® 600 Advanced Formula Tablets [OTC]** *see* vitamin, multiple (oral) *on page 654*

♦ **Stromectol®** *see* ivermectin *on page 351*

♦ **strong iodine solution** *see* potassium iodide *on page 509*

strontium-89 *(STRON shee um atey nine)*

U.S. Brand Names Metastron®

Generic Available No

Therapeutic Category Radiopharmaceutical

Use Relief of bone pain in patients with skeletal metastases

Usual Dosage Adults: I.V.: 148 megabecquerel (4 millicurie) administered by slow I.V. injection over 1-2 minutes or 1.5-2.2 megabecquerel (40-60 microcurie)/kg; repeated doses are generally not recommended at intervals <90 days

Nursing/Pharmacy Information

Monitor routine blood tests

Stability: Store vial and its contents inside its transportation container at room temperature

Dosage Forms Injection, as chloride: 10.9-22.6 mg/mL [148 megabecquerel, 4 millicurie] (10 mL)

♦ **Stuartnatal® 1 + 1** *see* vitamin, multiple (prenatal) *on page 654*

♦ **Stuart Prenatal® [OTC]** *see* vitamin, multiple (prenatal) *on page 654*

♦ **Sublimaze® Injection** *see* fentanyl *on page 263*

succimer *(SUKS i mer)*

U.S. Brand Names Chemet®

Generic Available No

Therapeutic Category Chelating Agent

Use Treatment of lead poisoning in children with blood levels >45 mcg/dL. It is not indicated for prophylaxis of lead poisoning in a lead-containing environment.

Usual Dosage Children and Adults: Oral: 30 mg/kg/day in divided doses every 8 hours for an additional 5 days followed by 20 mg/kg/day for 14 days

Nursing/Pharmacy Information

Ensure adequate patient hydration; for patients who cannot swallow the capsule, sprinkle the medicated beads on a small amount of soft food or administer with a fruit juice to mask the odor

Monitor blood lead levels, serum amino transferases

Dosage Forms Capsule: 100 mg

♦ **succinate mafenide acetate** *see* mafenide *on page 379*

succinylcholine *(suks in il KOE leen)*

Synonyms suxamethonium

U.S. Brand Names Anectine® Chloride; Anectine® Flo-Pack®; Quelicin®

Generic Available Yes

Therapeutic Category Skeletal Muscle Relaxant

Use Produces skeletal muscle relaxation in procedures of short duration such as endotracheal intubation or endoscopic exams

Usual Dosage I.M., I.V.:

Children: 1-2 mg/kg

Intermittent: Initial: 1 mg/kg/dose one time; maintenance: 0.3-0.6 mg/kg every 5-10 minutes as needed

Adults: 0.6 mg/kg (range: 0.3-1.1 mg/kg) over 10-30 seconds, up to 150 mg total dose

Maintenance: 0.04-0.07 mg/kg every 5-10 minutes as needed

Continuous infusion: 2.5 mg/minute (or 0.5-10 mg/minute); dilute to concentration of 1-2 mg/mL in D_5W or NS

Note: Pretreatment with atropine may reduce occurrence of bradycardia

Nursing/Pharmacy Information

Parenteral: May be administered by rapid I.V. injection without further dilution

Monitor temperature, serum potassium and calcium

Stability: Refrigerate; however, remains stable for 14 days unrefrigerated; stability of parenteral admixture at refrigeration temperature (4°C): 24 hours; I.V. form is **incompatible** when mixed with sodium bicarbonate, pentobarbital, thiopental

Dosage Forms Succinylcholine chloride:

Injection: 20 mg/mL (10 mL); 50 mg/mL (10 mL); 100 mg/mL (5 mL, 10 mL, 20 mL)

Powder for injection: 100 mg, 500 mg, 1 g

+ **Sucostrin®** *(Discontinued) see page 743*
+ **Sucraid™** *see sacrosidase New Drug on page 556*

sucralfate (soo KRAL fate)

Synonyms aluminum sucrose sulfate, basic

U.S. Brand Names Carafate®; Sulcrate®

Canadian Brand Names Novo-Sucralate®; Sulcrate®; Sulcrate® Suspension Plus

Mexican Brand Names Antepsin

Generic Available Yes

Therapeutic Category Gastrointestinal Agent, Gastric or Duodenal Ulcer Treatment

Use Short-term management of duodenal ulcers; gastric ulcers; suspension may be used topically for treatment of stomatitis due to cancer chemotherapy or other causes of esophageal and gastric erosions

Usual Dosage

Children: Dose not established, doses of 40-80 mg/kg/day divided every 6 hours have been used

Stomatitis: Oral: 2.5-5 mL (1 g/10 mL suspension), swish and spit or swish and swallow 4 times/day

Adults:

Duodenal ulcer treatment: Oral: 1 g 4 times/day, 1 hour before meals or food and at bedtime for 4-8 weeks, or alternatively 2 g twice daily

Duodenal ulcer maintenance therapy: Oral: 1 g twice daily

Stomatitis: Oral: 1 g/10 mL suspension, swish and spit or swish and swallow 4 times/day

Dietary Considerations Should be administered before meals or on an empty stomach; interferes with absorption of vitamin A, vitamin D, vitamin E, and vitamin K

Nursing/Pharmacy Information

Tablet may be broken or dissolved in water before ingestion

Stability: Shake well and store suspension at controlled room temperature

Dosage Forms

Suspension, oral: 1 g/10 mL (420 mL)

Tablet: 1 g

+ **Sucrets® [OTC]** *see dyclonine on page 226*
+ **Sucrets® Cough Calmers [OTC]** *see dextromethorphan on page 194*
+ **Sucrets® Sore Throat [OTC]** *see hexylresorcinol on page 313*
+ **Sudafed® [OTC]** *see pseudoephedrine on page 530*
+ **Sudafed® 12 Hour [OTC]** *see pseudoephedrine on page 530*
+ **Sudafed® Children** *(Discontinued) see page 743*
+ **Sudafed® Cold & Cough Liquid Caps [OTC]** *see guaifenesin, pseudoephedrine, and dextromethorphan on page 304*
+ **Sudafed® Cough** *(Discontinued) see page 743*
+ **Sudafed Plus® Liquid** *(Discontinued) see page 743*
+ **Sudafed® Plus Tablet [OTC]** *see chlorpheniramine and pseudoephedrine on page 140*
+ **Sudafed® Severe Cold [OTC]** *see acetaminophen, dextromethorphan, and pseudoephedrine on page 16*
+ **Sufedrin® [OTC]** *see pseudoephedrine on page 530*
+ **Sufenta®** *see sufentanil on page 584*

sufentanil (soo FEN ta nil)
U.S. Brand Names Sufenta®
Generic Available No
Therapeutic Category Analgesic, Narcotic; General Anesthetic
Controlled Substance C-II
Use Analgesia; analgesia adjunct; anesthetic agent
Usual Dosage I.V.:
Children <12 years: 10-25 mcg/kg with 100% O_2, maintenance: 25-50 mcg as needed (total dose of up to 1-2 mcg/kg)
Adults: Dose should be based on body weight. **Note:** In obese patients (ie, >20% above ideal body weight), use lean body weight to determine dosage
1-2 mcg/kg with N_2O/O_2 for endotracheal intubation; maintenance: 10-25 mcg as needed
2-8 mcg/kg with N_2O/O_2 more complicated major surgical procedures; maintenance: 10-50 mcg as needed
8-30 mcg/kg with 100% O_2 and muscle relaxant produces sleep; at doses of ≥8 mcg/kg maintains a deep level of anesthesia; maintenance: 10-50 mcg as needed
Nursing/Pharmacy Information Patient may develop rebound respiratory depression postoperatively
Dosage Forms Injection, as citrate: 50 mcg/mL (1 mL, 2 mL, 5 mL)

♦ **Sufisal** see pentoxifylline on page 480
♦ **Sular®** see nisoldipine on page 443
♦ **sulbactam and ampicillin** see ampicillin and sulbactam on page 47

sulconazole (sul KON a zole)
U.S. Brand Names Exelderm® Topical
Generic Available No
Therapeutic Category Antifungal Agent
Use Treatment of superficial fungal infections of the skin, including tinea cruris, tinea corporis, tinea versicolor and possibly tinea pedis
Usual Dosage Topical: Apply once or twice daily for 4-6 weeks
Nursing/Pharmacy Information For external use only; avoid contact with eyes; if burning or irritation develops, notify physician
Dosage Forms Sulconazole nitrate:
Cream: 1% (15 g, 30 g, 60 g)
Solution, topical: 1% (30 mL)

♦ **Sulcrate®** see sucralfate on page 583
♦ **Sulcrate® Suspension Plus** see sucralfate on page 583
♦ **Sulf-10®** see sulfacetamide on page 584

sulfabenzamide, sulfacetamide, and sulfathiazole
(sul fa BENZ a mide, sul fa SEE ta mide & sul fa THYE a zole)
Synonyms sulfacetamide, sulfabenzamide, and sulfathiazole; sulfathiazole, sulfacetamide, and sulfabenzamide; triple sulfa
U.S. Brand Names Femguard®; Gyne-Sulf®; Sulfa-Gyn®; Sulfa-Trip®; Sultrin™; Trysul®; V.V.S.®
Generic Available Yes
Therapeutic Category Antibiotic, Vaginal
Use Treatment of *Haemophilus vaginalis* vaginitis
Usual Dosage Adults: Vaginal:
Cream: Insert 1 applicatorful in vagina twice daily for 4-6 days; dosage may then be decreased to 1/2 to 1/4 of an applicatorful twice daily
Tablet: Insert 1 intravaginally twice daily for 10 days
Nursing/Pharmacy Information Complete full course of therapy; notify physician if burning, irritation, or signs of a systemic allergic reaction occur
Dosage Forms
Cream, vaginal: Sulfabenzamide 3.7%, sulfacetamide 2.86%, and sulfathiazole 3.42% (78 g with applicator, 90 g, 120 g)
Tablet, vaginal: Sulfabenzamide 184 mg, sulfacetamide 143.75 mg, and sulfathiazole 172.5 mg (20 tablets/box with vaginal applicator)

sulfacetamide (sul fa SEE ta mide)
U.S. Brand Names AK-Sulf®; Bleph®-10; Cetamide®; I-Sulfacet®; Ophthacet®; Sodium Sulamyd®; Sulf-10®; Sulfair®
Canadian Brand Names Sulfex® 10%
Generic Available Yes
Therapeutic Category Antibiotic, Ophthalmic

Use Treatment and prophylaxis of conjunctivitis, corneal ulcers, and other superficial ocular infections due to susceptible organisms; adjunctive treatment with systemic sulfonamides for therapy of trachoma

Usual Dosage Children >2 months and Adults: Ophthalmic:
Ointment: Apply to lower conjunctival sac 1-4 times/day and at bedtime
Solution: 1-2 drops every 2-3 hours in the lower conjunctival sac during the waking hours and less frequently at night

Nursing/Pharmacy Information
Eye drops will burn upon instillation (especially 30% solution); wait at least 10 minutes before administering another eye preparation
Monitor response to therapy
Stability: Protect from light; discolored solution should not be used; **incompatible** with silver and zinc sulfate; sulfacetamide is inactivated by blood or purulent exudates

Dosage Forms Sulfacetamide sodium:
Lotion: 10% (85 g)
Ointment, ophthalmic: 10% (3.5 g)
Solution, ophthalmic: 10% (1 mL, 2 mL, 2.5 mL, 5 mL, 15 mL); 15% (5 mL, 15 mL); 30% (15 mL)

sulfacetamide and phenylephrine
(sul fa SEE ta mide & fen il EF rin)

Synonyms phenylephrine and sulfacetamide
U.S. Brand Names Vasosulf® Ophthalmic
Generic Available Yes
Therapeutic Category Antibiotic, Ophthalmic
Use Treatment of conjunctivitis, corneal ulcer, and other superficial ocular infections due to susceptible microorganisms; adjunctive in systemic sulfonamide therapy
Usual Dosage Ophthalmic: Instill 1-3 drops in lower conjunctival sac every 3-4 hours
Nursing/Pharmacy Information Keep tightly closed; protect from light
Dosage Forms Solution, ophthalmic: Sulfacetamide sodium 15% and phenylephrine hydrochloride 0.125% (5 mL, 15 mL)

sulfacetamide and prednisolone
(sul fa SEE ta mide & pred NIS oh lone)

Synonyms prednisolone and sulfacetamide
U.S. Brand Names AK-Cide® Ophthalmic; Blephamide® Ophthalmic; Cetapred® Ophthalmic; Isopto® Cetapred® Ophthalmic; Metimyd® Ophthalmic; Vasocidin® Ophthalmic
Generic Available Yes
Therapeutic Category Antibiotic/Corticosteroid, Ophthalmic
Use Steroid-responsive inflammatory ocular conditions where infection is present or there is a risk of infection; ophthalmic suspension may be used as an otic preparation
Usual Dosage Children >2 and Adults: Ophthalmic:
Ointment: Apply to lower conjunctival sac 1-4 times/day
Solution: Instill 1-3 drops every 2-3 hours while awake
Nursing/Pharmacy Information Shake ophthalmic suspension before using
Dosage Forms
Ointment, ophthalmic:
AK-Cide®, Metimyd®, Vasocidin®: Sulfacetamide sodium 10% and prednisolone acetate 0.5% (3.5 g)
Blephamide®: Sulfacetamide sodium 10% and prednisolone acetate 0.2% (3.5 g)
Cetapred®: Sulfacetamide sodium 10% and prednisolone acetate 0.25% (3.5 g)
Suspension, ophthalmic: Sulfacetamide sodium 10% and prednisolone sodium phosphate 0.25% (5 mL)
Suspension, ophthalmic:
AK-Cide®, Metimyd®: Sulfacetamide sodium 10% and prednisolone acetate 0.5% (5 mL)
Blephamide®: Sulfacetamide sodium 10% and prednisolone acetate 0.2% (2.5 mL, 5 mL, 10 mL)
Isopto® Cetapred®: Sulfacetamide sodium 10% and prednisolone acetate 0.25% (5 mL, 15 mL)
Vasocidin®: Sulfacetamide sodium 10% and prednisolone sodium phosphate: 0.25% (5 mL, 10 mL)

♦ **sulfacetamide and sulfur** *see* sulfur and sulfacetamide *on page 589*

sulfacetamide sodium and fluorometholone
(sul fa SEE ta mide & flure oh METH oh lone)
Synonyms fluorometholone and sulfacetamide
U.S. Brand Names FML-S® Ophthalmic Suspension
Generic Available Yes
Therapeutic Category Antibiotic/Corticosteroid, Ophthalmic
Use Steroid-responsive inflammatory ocular conditions where infection is present or there is a risk of infection
Usual Dosage Children >2 months and Adults: Ophthalmic: Instill 1-3 drops every 2-3 hours while awake
Dosage Forms Suspension, ophthalmic: Sulfacetamide sodium 10% and fluorometholone 0.1% (5 mL, 10 mL)

♦ **sulfacetamide, sulfabenzamide, and sulfathiazole** *see* sulfabenzamide, sulfacetamide, and sulfathiazole *on page 584*

♦ **Sulfacet-R® Topical** *see* sulfur and sulfacetamide *on page 589*

sulfacytine (sul fa SYE teen)
U.S. Brand Names Renoquid®
Generic Available No
Therapeutic Category Sulfonamide
Use Treatment of urinary tract infections
Usual Dosage Adults: Oral: Initial: 500 mg, then 250 mg every 4 hours for 10 days
Dietary Considerations Should be administered 1 hour before or 2 hours after a meal on an empty stomach
Dosage Forms Tablet: 250 mg

sulfadiazine (sul fa DYE a zeen)
Canadian Brand Names Coptin®
Generic Available Yes
Therapeutic Category Sulfonamide
Use Adjunctive treatment in toxoplasmosis; treatment of urinary tract infections and nocardiosis; rheumatic fever prophylaxis in penicillin-allergic patient; uncomplicated attack of malaria
Usual Dosage Oral:
Congenital toxoplasmosis:
Newborns and Children <2 months: 100 mg/kg/day divided every 6 hours in conjunction with pyrimethamine 1 mg/kg/day once daily and supplemental folinic acid 5 mg every 3 days for 6 months
Children >2 months: 25-50 mg/kg/dose 4 times/day
Toxoplasmosis:
Children: 120-150 mg/kg/day, maximum dose: 6 g/day; divided every 6 hours in conjunction with pyrimethamine 2 mg/kg/day divided every 12 hours for 3 days followed by 1 mg/kg/day once daily (maximum: 25 mg/day) with supplemental folinic acid
Adults: 2-8 g/day divided every 6 hours in conjunction with pyrimethamine 25 mg/day and with supplemental folinic acid
Dietary Considerations Supplemental folinic acid should be administered to reverse symptoms or prevent problems due to folic acid deficiency; avoid large quantities of vitamin C or acidifying agents (cranberry juice) to prevent crystalluria
Nursing/Pharmacy Information
Monitor CBC, renal function tests, urinalysis
Stability: Tablets may be crushed to prepare oral suspension of the drug in water or with a sucrose-containing solution; aqueous suspension with concentrations of 100 mg/mL should be stored in the refrigerator and used within 7 days
Dosage Forms Tablet: 500 mg

sulfadiazine, sulfamethazine, and sulfamerazine
(sul fa DYE a zeen, sul fa METH a zeen & sul fa MER a zeen)
Synonyms multiple sulfonamides; trisulfapyrimidines
Generic Available No
Therapeutic Category Sulfonamide
Use Treatment of toxoplasmosis
Usual Dosage Adults: Oral: 2-4 g to start, then 2-4 g/day in 3-6 divided doses
Dietary Considerations Should be administered 1 hour before or 2 hours after a meal on an empty stomach
Nursing/Pharmacy Information Drink plenty of fluids

Dosage Forms Tablet: Sulfadiazine 167 mg, sulfamethazine 167 mg, and sulfamerazine 167 mg

♦ **Sulfa-Gyn®** *see* sulfabenzamide, sulfacetamide, and sulfathiazole *on page 584*

♦ **Sulfair®** *see* sulfacetamide *on page 584*

♦ **Sulfalax® [OTC]** *see* docusate *on page 214*

♦ **Sulfamethoprim®** *see* co-trimoxazole *on page 170*

sulfamethoxazole (sul fa meth OKS a zole)

U.S. Brand Names Gantanol®; Urobak®
Canadian Brand Names Apo®-Sulfamethoxazole
Generic Available Yes: Tablet
Therapeutic Category Sulfonamide
Use Treatment of urinary tract infections, nocardiosis, chlamydial infections, toxoplasmosis, acute otitis media, and acute exacerbations of chronic bronchitis due to susceptible organisms
Usual Dosage Oral:
Children >2 months: 50-60 mg/kg/day divided every 12 hours; maximum: 3 g/ 24 hours or 75 mg/kg/day
Adults: 2 g stat, 1 g 2-3 times/day; maximum: 3 g/24 hours
Dietary Considerations Should be administered 1 hour before or 2 hours after a meal on an empty stomach; avoid large quantities of vitamin C or acidifying agents (cranberry juice) to prevent crystalluria; presence of food delays but does not reduce absorption
Nursing/Pharmacy Information
Shake suspension before administering
Monitor CBC, urinalysis, renal function test; watch for signs of adverse reactions
Stability: Protect from light
Dosage Forms
Suspension, oral (cherry flavor): 500 mg/5 mL (480 mL)
Tablet: 500 mg

sulfamethoxazole and phenazopyridine
(sul fa meth OKS a zole & fen az oh PEER i deen)
Synonyms phenazopyridine and sulfamethoxazole
Generic Available Yes
Therapeutic Category Sulfonamide
Use Treatment of urinary tract infections complicated with pain
Usual Dosage Oral: Initial: 4 tablets, then 2 tablets twice daily for up to 2 days, then switch to sulfamethoxazole only
Dietary Considerations Should be administered 1 hour before or 2 hours after a meal on an empty stomach
Nursing/Pharmacy Information Urine may be discolored orange-red; when possible, obtain specimens for culture and sensitivity before the first dose; review allergy history
Dosage Forms Tablet: Sulfamethoxazole 500 mg and phenazopyridine 100 mg

♦ **sulfamethoxazole and trimethoprim** *see* co-trimoxazole *on page 170*

♦ **Sulfamylon® Topical** *see* mafenide *on page 379*

sulfanilamide (sul fa NIL a mide)

U.S. Brand Names AVC™ Cream; AVC™ Suppository; Vagitrol®
Generic Available No
Therapeutic Category Antifungal Agent
Use Treatment of vulvovaginitis caused by *Candida albicans*
Usual Dosage Vaginal: 1 applicatorful once or twice daily continued through 1 complete menstrual cycle
Nursing/Pharmacy Information Avoid excessive exposure to sunlight; complete full course of therapy; notify physician if burning or irritation become severe or persist or if allergic symptoms occur
Dosage Forms
Cream, vaginal (AVC™, Vagitrol®): 15% [150 mg/g] (120 g with applicator)
Suppository, vaginal (AVC™): 1.05 g (16s)

sulfasalazine (sul fa SAL a zeen)

Synonyms salicylazosulfapyridine
U.S. Brand Names Azulfidine®; Azulfidine® EN-tabs®
(Continued)

sulfasalazine *(Continued)*

Canadian Brand Names Apo®-Sulfasalazine; PMS-Sulfasalazine; Salazo-pyrin®; Salazopyrin EN-Tabs®; S.A.S™

Generic Available Yes

Therapeutic Category 5-Aminosalicylic Acid Derivative

Use Management of ulcerative colitis; treatment of active Crohn's disease

Usual Dosage Oral:

Children >2 years:

Initial: 40-60 mg/kg/day divided every 4-6 hour

Maintenance dose: 20-30 mg/kg/day divided every 6 hours, up to a maximum of 2 g/day

Adults:

Initial: 3-4 g/day divided every 4-6 hours

Maintenance dose: 2 g/day divided every 6 hours

Dietary Considerations Dietary intake of iron should be increased; since sulfasalazine impairs folate absorption, consider providing 1 mg/day folate supplement

Nursing/Pharmacy Information

GI intolerance is common during the first few days of therapy; drug commonly imparts an orange-yellow discoloration to urine and skin, shake suspension well

Monitor stool frequency, hematocrit, reticulocyte count, CBC, urinalysis, renal function tests, liver function tests

Stability: Protect from light; shake suspension well

Dosage Forms

Tablet: 500 mg

Tablet, enteric coated: 500 mg

♦ **sulfathiazole, sulfacetamide, and sulfabenzamide** *see* sulfabenzamide, sulfa-cetamide, and sulfathiazole *on page 584*

♦ **Sulfatrim®** *see* co-trimoxazole *on page 170*

♦ **Sulfatrim® DS** *see* co-trimoxazole *on page 170*

♦ **Sulfa-Trip®** *see* sulfabenzamide, sulfacetamide, and sulfathiazole *on page 584*

♦ **Sulfex® 10%** *see* sulfacetamide *on page 584*

sulfinpyrazone *(sul fin PEER a zone)*

U.S. Brand Names Anturane®

Canadian Brand Names Antazone®; Anturan®; Apo-Sulfinpyrazone®; Novo-Pyrazone; Nu-Sulfinpyrazone

Generic Available Yes

Therapeutic Category Uricosuric Agent

Use Treatment of chronic gouty arthritis and intermittent gouty arthritis

Usual Dosage Oral: 200 mg twice daily

Dietary Considerations Should be administered with food or milk

Nursing/Pharmacy Information Monitor serum and urinary uric acid

Dosage Forms

Capsule: 200 mg

Tablet: 100 mg

sulfisoxazole *(sul fi SOKS a zole)*

Synonyms sulphafurazole

U.S. Brand Names Gantrisin®

Canadian Brand Names Novo-Soxazole®; Sulfizole®

Generic Available Yes

Therapeutic Category Sulfonamide

Use Treatment of uncomplicated urinary tract infections, otitis media, *Chla-mydia*; nocardiosis; treatment of acute pelvic inflammatory disease in prepu-bertal children

Usual Dosage

Children >2 months: Oral: 75 mg/kg stat, 120-150 mg/kg/day in divided doses every 4-6 hours; not to exceed 6 g/day

Pelvic inflammatory disease: 100 mg/kg/day in divided doses every 6 hours; used in combination with ceftriaxone

Chlamydia trachomatis: 100 mg/kg/day divided every 6 hours

Adults: Oral: 2-4 g stat, 4-8 g/day in divided doses every 4-6 hours

Dietary Considerations Should be administered with a glass of water on an empty stomach; interferes with folate absorption

Nursing/Pharmacy Information

Maintain adequate patient fluid intake

Monitor CBC, urinalysis, renal function tests
Stability: Protect from light
Dosage Forms
Suspension, oral, pediatric, as acetyl (raspberry flavor): 500 mg/5 mL (480 mL)
Tablet: 500 mg

♦ **sulfisoxazole and erythromycin** *see* erythromycin and sulfisoxazole *on page 239*

sulfisoxazole and phenazopyridine
(sul fi SOKS a zole & fen az oh PEER i deen)
Synonyms phenazopyridine and sulfisoxazole
Generic Available Yes
Therapeutic Category Sulfonamide
Use Treatment of urinary tract infections and nocardiosis
Usual Dosage Oral: 4-6 tablets to start, then 2 tablets 4 times/day for 2 days, then continue with sulfisoxazole only
Dietary Considerations Should be administered 1 hour before or 2 hours after a meal on an empty stomach
Nursing/Pharmacy Information May cause reddish-orange discoloration of urine; staining of contact lenses has also been reported; drink plenty of fluids; administer on an empty stomach; avoid prolonged exposure to sunlight or wear protective clothing and sunscreen; notify physician if rash, difficulty breathing, severe or persistent fever, or sore throat occurs
Dosage Forms Tablet: Sulfisoxazole 500 mg and phenazopyridine 50 mg

♦ **Sulfizole®** *see* sulfisoxazole *on page 588*

sulfur and salicylic acid (SUL fur & sal i SIL ik AS id)
Synonyms salicylic acid and sulfur
U.S. Brand Names Aveeno® Cleansing Bar [OTC]; Fostex® [OTC]; Pernox® [OTC]; SAStid® Plain Therapeutic Shampoo and Acne Wash [OTC]
Generic Available Yes
Therapeutic Category Antiseborrheic Agent, Topical
Use Therapeutic shampoo for dandruff and seborrheal dermatitis; acne skin cleanser
Usual Dosage Children and Adults: Topical:
Shampoo: Initial: Use daily or every other day; 1-2 treatments/week will usually maintain control
Soap: Use daily or every other day
Nursing/Pharmacy Information
Avoid contact with the eyes; contact physician if condition worsens or rash or irritation develops
Stability: Preparations containing sulfur may react with metals including silver and copper, resulting in discoloration of the metal
Dosage Forms
Cake: Sulfur 2% and salicylic acid 2% (123 g)
Cleanser: Sulfur 2% and salicylic acid 1.5% (60 mL, 120 mL)
Shampoo: Micropulverized sulfur 2% and salicylic acid 2% (120 mL, 240 mL)
Soap: Micropulverized sulfur 2% and salicylic acid 2% (113 g)
Wash: Sulfur 1.6% and salicylic acid 1.6% (75 mL)

sulfur and sulfacetamide (SUL fur & sul fa SEE ta mide)
Synonyms sulfacetamide and sulfur
U.S. Brand Names Novacet® Topical; Sulfacet-R® Topical
Generic Available Yes
Therapeutic Category Antiseborrheic Agent, Topical
Use Aid in the treatment of acne vulgaris, acne rosacea and seborrheic dermatitis
Usual Dosage Topical: Apply in a thin film 1-3 times/day
Dosage Forms Lotion, topical: Sulfur colloid 5% and sulfacetamide sodium 10% (30 mL)

sulindac (sul IN dak)
U.S. Brand Names Clinoril®
Canadian Brand Names Apo®-Sulin; Novo-Sundac®
Generic Available Yes
Therapeutic Category Analgesic, Non-narcotic; Nonsteroidal Anti-inflammatory Drug (NSAID)
Use Management of inflammatory disease, rheumatoid disorders; acute gouty arthritis
(Continued)

sulindac *(Continued)*

Usual Dosage Oral:
Children: Dose not established
Adults: 150-200 mg twice daily; not to exceed 400 mg/day

Dietary Considerations Food may decrease the rate but not the extent of oral absorption; may cause GI upset, bleeding, ulceration, perforation; administer with food or milk to minimize GI upset

Nursing/Pharmacy Information Monitor liver enzymes, BUN, serum creatinine, CBC, blood pressure

Dosage Forms Tablet: 150 mg, 200 mg

♦ **sulphafurazole** *see* sulfisoxazole *on page 588*

♦ **Sultrin**™ *see* sulfabenzamide, sulfacetamide, and sulfathiazole *on page 584*

♦ **Sumacal®** [OTC] *see* glucose polymers *on page 293*

sumatriptan succinate *(SOO ma trip tan SUKS i nate)*

U.S. Brand Names Imitrex®
Mexican Brand Names Imigran
Generic Available No
Therapeutic Category Antimigraine Agent
Use Acute treatment of migraine with or without aura
Unlabeled use: Cluster headaches

Usual Dosage Adults:
Oral: 25 mg (taken with fluids); maximum recommended dose is 100 mg. If a satisfactory response has not been obtained at 2 hours, a second dose of up to 100 mg may be given. Efficacy of this second dose has not been examined. If a headache returns, additional doses may be taken at intervals of at least 2 hours up to a daily maximum of 300 mg. There is no evidence that an initial dose of 100 mg provides substantially greater relief than 25 mg.

Intranasal: Single dose of 5, 10, or 20 mg administered in one nostril; a 10 mg dose may be achieved by administration of a single 5 mg dose in each nostril; if headache returns, the dose may be repeated once after 2 hours, not to exceed a total daily dose of 40 mg

S.C.: 6 mg; a second injection may be administered at least 1 hour after the initial dose, but not more than two injections in a 24-hour period

Nursing/Pharmacy Information
Do not administer I.V., may cause coronary vasospasm; if pain or tightness in chest occurs, notify physician; females should avoid pregnancy; pain at injection site lasts <1 hour
Stability: Store at 2°C to 20°C (36°F to 86°F); protect from light

Dosage Forms
Injection: 12 mg/mL (0.5 mL, 2 mL)
Spray, nasal: 5 mg (100 mcL); 20 mg (100 mcL)
Tablet: 25 mg, 50 mg

♦ **Summer's Eve® Medicated Douche** [OTC] *see* povidone-iodine *on page 510*

♦ **Sumycin® Oral** *see* tetracycline *on page 601*

♦ **sunscreen (paba-free)** *see* methoxycinnamate and oxybenzone *on page 404*

♦ **Superchar®** *(Discontinued) see page 743*

♦ **Superchar® With Sorbitol** *(Discontinued) see page 743*

♦ **Suplena** *see* vitamin, multiple (oral) *on page 654*

♦ **Supprelin**™ *see* histrelin *on page 313*

♦ **Suppress®** [OTC] *see* dextromethorphan *on page 194*

♦ **Supracaine®** *see* tetracaine *on page 600*

♦ **Supradol®** *see* naproxen *on page 432*

♦ **Suprane®** *see* desflurane *on page 187*

♦ **Suprax®** *see* cefixime *on page 121*

suprofen *(soo PROE fen)*

U.S. Brand Names Profenal® Ophthalmic
Generic Available No
Therapeutic Category Nonsteroidal Anti-inflammatory Drug (NSAID)
Use Inhibition of intraoperative miosis
Usual Dosage Ophthalmic: On day of surgery, instill 2 drops in conjunctival sac at 3, 2, and 1 hour prior to surgery; or 2 drops in sac every 4 hours, while awake, the day preceding surgery

Nursing/Pharmacy Information Avoid aspirin and aspirin-containing products while taking this medication; get instructions on administration of eye drops

Dosage Forms Solution, ophthalmic: 1% (2.5 mL)

- **Surbex® [OTC]** *see* vitamin B complex *on page 651*
- **Surbex-T® Filmtabs® [OTC]** *see* vitamin B complex with vitamin C *on page 651*
- **Surbex® With C Filmtabs® [OTC]** *see* vitamin B complex with vitamin C *on page 651*
- **Surfak® [OTC]** *see* docusate *on page 214*
- **Surgam®** *see* tiaprofenic acid *(Canada only) on page 611*
- **Surgam® SR** *see* tiaprofenic acid *(Canada only) on page 611*
- **Surgicel®** *see* cellulose, oxidized *on page 127*
- **Surital®** *(Discontinued) see page 743*
- **Surmontil®** *see* trimipramine *on page 630*
- **Survanta®** *see* beractant *on page 83*
- **Sus-Phrine®** *see* epinephrine *on page 234*
- **Sustaire®** *see* theophylline *on page 603*
- **Sustiva™** *see* efavirenz *on page 229*
- **suxamethonium** *see* succinylcholine *on page 582*
- **Sween Cream® [OTC]** *see* methylbenzethonium chloride *on page 405*
- **Swim-Ear® Otic [OTC]** *see* boric acid *on page 90*
- **Sydolil** *see* ergotamine *on page 238*
- **Syllact® [OTC]** *see* psyllium *on page 531*
- **Symadine®** *see* amantadine *on page 35*
- **Symmetrel® Capsule** *(Discontinued) see page 743*
- **Symmetrel® Syrup** *see* amantadine *on page 35*
- **Synacol® CF [OTC]** *see* guaifenesin and dextromethorphan *on page 300*
- **Synacort® Topical** *see* hydrocortisone (topical) *on page 324*
- **synacthen** *see* cosyntropin *on page 170*
- **Synacthen® Depot** *see* cosyntropin *on page 170*
- **Synagis®** *see* palivizumab *on page 466*
- **Synalar-HP® Topical** *see* fluocinolone *on page 273*
- **Synalar® Topical** *see* fluocinolone *on page 273*
- **Synalgos®-DC** *see* dihydrocodeine compound *on page 204*
- **Synarel®** *see* nafarelin *on page 428*
- **Syn-Captopril®** *see* captopril *on page 110*
- **Syn-Diltiazem®** *see* diltiazem *on page 205*
- **Synemol® Topical** *see* fluocinolone *on page 273*
- **Synercid®** *see* quinupristin and dalfopristin *New Drug on page 538*
- **Synflex®** *see* naproxen *on page 432*
- **Syn-Flunisolide®** *see* flunisolide *on page 272*
- **Syngestal** *see* norethindrone *on page 447*
- **Synkayvite®** *(Discontinued) see page 743*
- **Syn-Minocycline®** *see* minocycline *on page 416*
- **Syn-Nadolol®** *see* nadolol *on page 427*
- **Synphasic®** *see* ethinyl estradiol and norethindrone *on page 250*
- **Syn-Pindol®** *see* pindolol *on page 495*
- **synthetic lung surfactant** *see* colfosceril palmitate *on page 166*
- **Synthroid®** *see* levothyroxine *on page 367*
- **Syntocinon®** *see* oxytocin *on page 465*
- **Syntocinon® Nasal** *(Discontinued) see page 743*
- **Syprine®** *see* trientine *on page 627*
- **Syracol-CF® [OTC]** *see* guaifenesin and dextromethorphan *on page 300*
- **Syraprim** *see* co-trimoxazole *on page 170*
- **Syscor** *see* nisoldipine *on page 443*
- **Systen** *see* estradiol *on page 242*
- **Sytobex®** *see* cyanocobalamin *on page 173*
- **t₃/t₄ liotrix** *see* liotrix *on page 371*
- **t₃ thyronine** *see* liothyronine *on page 371*
- **t₄ thyroxine** *see* levothyroxine *on page 367*
- **Tabalon** *see* ibuprofen *on page 332*
- **Tabron®** *(Discontinued) see page 743*
- **Tac™-3 Injection** *see* triamcinolone (systemic) *on page 624*

+ **Tac™-40 Injection** *see* triamcinolone (systemic) *on page 624*
+ **Tacaryl®** *(Discontinued) see page 743*
+ **TACE®** *see* chlorotrianisene *on page 137*
+ **Tacex** *see* ceftriaxone *on page 126*
+ **Tacozin®** *see* piperacillin and tazobactam sodium *on page 496*

tacrine (TAK reen)
Synonyms tetrahydroaminoacrine; THA
U.S. Brand Names Cognex®
Generic Available No
Therapeutic Category Acetylcholinesterase Inhibitor
Use Treatment of Alzheimer's disease
Usual Dosage Adults: Oral: 40 mg/day
Nursing/Pharmacy Information Monitor ALT levels and other liver enzymes weekly for at least the first 18 weeks, then monitor once every 3 months
Dosage Forms Capsule, as hydrochloride: 10 mg, 20 mg, 30 mg, 40 mg

tacrolimus (ta KROE li mus)
Synonyms FK506
U.S. Brand Names Prograf®
Generic Available No
Therapeutic Category Immunosuppressant Agent
Use Potent immunosuppressive drug used in liver, kidney, heart, lung, or small bowel transplant recipients
Usual Dosage
Initial: I.V. continuous infusion: 0.1 mg/kg/day until the tolerance of oral intake
Oral: Usually 3-4 times the I.V. dose, or 0.3 mg/kg/day in divided doses every 12 hours
Nursing/Pharmacy Information
Monitor renal function, hepatic function, plasma drug concentrations (trough for oral dosing), and the patient's clinical status, including serum electrolytes and blood pressure
Stability: 24 hours in dextrose 5% solutions or normal saline; tacrolimus is completely available from plastic syringes, glass or polyolefin containers; polyvinyl-containing sets (eg, Venoset®, Accuset®) adsorb significant amounts of the drug, and their use may lead to a lower dose being delivered to the patient
Dosage Forms
Capsule: 1 mg, 5 mg
Injection, with alcohol and surfactant: 5 mg/mL (1 mL)

+ **Tafil** *see* alprazolam *on page 30*
+ **Tagal** *see* ceftazidime *on page 124*
+ **Tagamet®** *see* cimetidine *on page 150*
+ **Tagamet-HB® [OTC]** *see* cimetidine *on page 150*
+ **Talacen®** *see* pentazocine compound *on page 479*
+ **Taloken** *see* ceftazidime *on page 124*
+ **Talpramin** *see* imipramine *on page 334*
+ **Talwin®** *see* pentazocine *on page 478*
+ **Talwin® Compound** *see* pentazocine compound *on page 479*
+ **Talwin® NX** *see* pentazocine *on page 478*
+ **Tambocor™** *see* flecainide *on page 269*
+ **Tamiflu™** *see* oseltamivir *New Drug on page 459*
+ **Tamine® [OTC]** *see* brompheniramine and phenylpropanolamine *on page 94*
+ **Tamofen®** *see* tamoxifen *on page 592*
+ **Tamone®** *see* tamoxifen *on page 592*
+ **Tamoxan** *see* tamoxifen *on page 592*

tamoxifen (ta MOKS i fen)
U.S. Brand Names Nolvadex®
Canadian Brand Names Alpha-Tamoxifen®; Apo-Tamox®; Novo-Tamoxifen; Tamofen®; Tamone®
Mexican Brand Names Bilem; Cryoxifeno; Tamoxan; Taxus
Generic Available Yes
Therapeutic Category Antineoplastic Agent
Use Palliative or adjunctive treatment of advanced breast cancer in postmenopausal women
Usual Dosage Oral: 10-20 mg twice daily
Nursing/Pharmacy Information Monitor WBC and platelet counts, tumor

Dosage Forms Tablet, as citrate: 10 mg, 20 mg

tamsulosin (tam SOO loe sin)

U.S. Brand Names Flomax®
Generic Available No
Therapeutic Category Alpha-Adrenergic Blocking Agent
Use Treatment of signs and symptoms of benign prostatic hyperplasia (BPH)
Usual Dosage Oral: Adults: 0.4 mg once daily approximately 30 minutes after the same meal each day
Dosage Forms Capsule, as hydrochloride: 0.4 mg

- ◆ Tanac® [OTC] see benzocaine on page 79
- ◆ Tanoral® Tablet see chlorpheniramine, pyrilamine, and phenylephrine on page 144
- ◆ Tantaphen® see acetaminophen on page 13
- ◆ Tao® see troleandomycin on page 633
- ◆ Tapanol® [OTC] see acetaminophen on page 13
- ◆ Tapazole® see methimazole on page 401
- ◆ Taporin see cefotaxime on page 122
- ◆ Tarabine® PFS see cytarabine on page 178
- ◆ Taractan® (Discontinued) see page 743
- ◆ Tarka® see trandolapril and verapamil on page 620
- ◆ Taro-Ampicillin® see ampicillin on page 46
- ◆ Taro-Atenol® see atenolol on page 63
- ◆ Taro-Cloxacillin® see cloxacillin on page 161
- ◆ Taro-Sone® see betamethasone (topical) on page 85
- ◆ Tasedan see estazolam on page 242
- ◆ Tasmar® see tolcapone on page 617
- ◆ TAT see tetanus antitoxin on page 599
- ◆ Tavanic see levofloxacin on page 366
- ◆ Tavist® see clemastine on page 155
- ◆ Tavist®-1 [OTC] see clemastine on page 155
- ◆ Tavist-D® see clemastine and phenylpropanolamine on page 156
- ◆ Taxol® see paclitaxel on page 465
- ◆ Taxotere® see docetaxel on page 214
- ◆ Taxus see tamoxifen on page 592

tazarotene (taz AR oh teen)

U.S. Brand Names Tazorac®
Generic Available No
Therapeutic Category Keratolytic Agent
Use Topical treatment of facial acne vulgaris; topical treatment of stable plaque psoriasis of up to 20% body surface area involvement
Usual Dosage Children >12 years and Adults: Topical:
Acne: Cleanse the face gently. After the skin is dry, apply a thin film of tazarotene (2 mg/cm²) once daily, in the evening, to the skin where the acne lesions appear. Use enough to cover the entire affected area. Tazarotene was investigated ≤12 weeks during clinical trials for acne.
Psoriasis: Apply tazarotene once daily, in the evening, to psoriatic lesions using enough (2 mg/cm²) to cover only the lesion with a thin film to no more than 20% of body surface area. If a bath or shower is taken prior to application, dry the skin before applying the gel. Because unaffected skin may be more susceptible to irritation, avoid application of tazarotene to these areas. Tazarotene was investigated for up to 12 months during clinical trials for psoriasis.
Dosage Forms Gel: 0.05% (30 g, 100 g); 0.1% (30 g, 100 g)

- ◆ Tazicef® see ceftazidime on page 124
- ◆ Tazidime® see ceftazidime on page 124
- ◆ Taziken see terbutaline on page 596
- ◆ tazobactam and piperacillin see piperacillin and tazobactam sodium on page 496
- ◆ Tazorac® see tazarotene on page 593
- ◆ 3TC® see lamivudine on page 359
- ◆ T-Caine® Lozenge (Discontinued) see page 743
- ◆ TCN see tetracycline on page 601
- ◆ Td see diphtheria and tetanus toxoid on page 209
- ◆ Tear Drop® Solution [OTC] see artificial tears on page 59

- **TearGard® Ophthalmic Solution [OTC]** *see* artificial tears *on page 59*
- **Teargen® Ophthalmic Solution [OTC]** *see* artificial tears *on page 59*
- **Tearisol® Solution [OTC]** *see* artificial tears *on page 59*
- **Tears Naturale® Free Solution [OTC]** *see* artificial tears *on page 59*
- **Tears Naturale® II Solution [OTC]** *see* artificial tears *on page 59*
- **Tears Naturale® Solution [OTC]** *see* artificial tears *on page 59*
- **Tears Plus® Solution [OTC]** *see* artificial tears *on page 59*
- **Tears Renewed® Solution [OTC]** *see* artificial tears *on page 59*
- **Tebamide®** *see* trimethobenzamide *on page 629*
- **Tebrazid** *see* pyrazinamide *on page 532*
- **Tecprazin** *see* praziquantel *on page 512*
- **Teczem®** *see* enalapril and diltiazem *on page 231*
- **Tedral®** *see* theophylline, ephedrine, and phenobarbital *on page 605*
- **Teejel®** *see* choline salicylate *on page 148*
- **Tega-Vert® Oral** *see* dimenhydrinate *on page 206*
- **Tegison®** *see* etretinate *on page 256*
- **Tegopen® *(Discontinued)*** *see page 743*
- **Tegretol®** *see* carbamazepine *on page 112*
- **Tegretol-XR®** *see* carbamazepine *on page 112*
- **Tegrin®-HC Topical [OTC]** *see* hydrocortisone (topical) *on page 324*
- **Telachlor® Oral** *see* chlorpheniramine *on page 138*
- **Teladar® Topical** *see* betamethasone (topical) *on page 85*
- **Teldrin® Oral [OTC]** *see* chlorpheniramine *on page 138*
- **Telepaque®** *see* radiological/contrast media (ionic) *on page 539*
- **Teline® *(Discontinued)*** *see page 743*

telmisartan (tel mi SAR tan)
U.S. Brand Names Micardis®
Generic Available No
Therapeutic Category Angiotensin II Antagonist
Use Treatment of hypertension alone or in combination with other antihypertensives
Usual Dosage Adults: Oral: The usual starting dose is 40 mg once daily. Blood pressure response is dose-related over the range of 20 mg-80 mg/day; when additional antihypertensive effects are needed beyond that achieved with 80 mg/day, a diuretic may be added.
Dosage Forms Tablet: 40 mg, 80 mg

- **Temaril® *(Discontinued)*** *see page 743*

temazepam (te MAZ e pam)
U.S. Brand Names Restoril®
Generic Available Yes
Therapeutic Category Benzodiazepine
Controlled Substance C-IV
Use Treatment of anxiety and as an adjunct in the treatment of depression; also may be used in the management of panic attacks; transient insomnia and sleep latency
Usual Dosage Adults: Oral: 15-30 mg at bedtime
Nursing/Pharmacy Information
Provide safety measures (ie, side rails, night light, and call button); remove smoking materials from area; supervise ambulation
Monitor respiratory and cardiovascular status
Dosage Forms Capsule: 7.5 mg, 15 mg, 30 mg

- **Temazin® Cold Syrup [OTC]** *see* chlorpheniramine and phenylpropanolamine *on page 139*
- **Temgesic®** *see* buprenorphine *on page 97*
- **Temodar®** *see* temozolomide *New Drug on page 594*
- **Temovate®** *see* clobetasol *on page 157*

temozolomide *New Drug* (te mo ZOLE oh mide)
U.S. Brand Names Temodar®
Generic Available No
Therapeutic Category Antineoplastic Agent, Alkylating Agent
Use Treatment of adult patients with refractory (first relapse) anaplastic astrocytoma who have experienced disease progression on nitrosourea and procarbazine

Unlabeled use: Glioma, first relapse/advanced metastatic malignant melanoma

Usual Dosage The dosage is adjusted according to nadir neutrophil and platelet counts of previous cycle and counts at the time of the next cycle.

Adults: Initial dose: 150 mg/m² once daily for 5 consecutive days per 28-day treatment cycle

Measure day 22 ANC and platelets. Measure day 29 ANC and platelets. Based on lowest counts at either day 22 or day 29:

On day 22 or day 29, if ANC <1,000/µL or the platelet count is <50,000/µL, postpone therapy until ANC >1,500/µL and platelet count >100,000/µL. Reduce dose by 50 mg/m² for subsequent cycle.

If ANC 1,000-1,500/µL or platelets 50,000-100,000/µL, postpone therapy until ANC >1,500/µL and platelet count >100,000/µL; maintain initial dose.

If ANC >1,500/µL (on day 22 and day 29) and platelet count >100,000/µL, increase dose to, or maintain dose at 200 mg/m²/day for 5 for subsequent cycle.

Dosage Forms Capsule: 5 mg, 20 mg, 100 mg, 250 mg

♦ **Temperal** *see* acetaminophen *on page 13*
♦ **Tempra® [OTC]** *see* acetaminophen *on page 13*
♦ **Tenex®** *see* guanfacine *on page 305*

teniposide (ten i POE side)
Synonyms EPT; VM-26
U.S. Brand Names Vumon
Generic Available No
Therapeutic Category Antineoplastic Agent
Use Treatment of Hodgkin's and non-Hodgkin's lymphomas, acute lymphocytic leukemia, bladder carcinoma and neuroblastoma
Usual Dosage I.V.:
Children: 130 mg/m²/week, increasing to 150 mg/m² after 3 weeks and to 180 mg/m² after 6 weeks
Adults: 50-180 mg/m² once or twice weekly for 4-6 weeks
Nursing/Pharmacy Information
Do not use in-line filter during I.V. infusion; slow I.V. infusion over ≥30 minutes
Monitor blood pressure during infusion; observe for chemical phlebitis at injection site
Stability: Store ampuls in refrigerator at 2°C to 8°C (36°F to 46°F); solutions containing 0.5-2 mg/mL remain stable for 4 hours, while those containing 0.1-0.4 mg/mL are stable for 24 hours in glass containers and 8 hours in plastic containers at refrigeration and room temperature; precipitation may occur; **incompatible** with heparin
Dosage Forms Injection: 10 mg/mL (5 mL)

♦ **Ten-K®** *see* potassium chloride *on page 506*
♦ **Tenoretic®** *see* atenolol and chlorthalidone *on page 63*
♦ **Tenormin®** *see* atenolol *on page 63*
♦ **Tensilon®** *see* edrophonium *on page 228*
♦ **Tenuate®** *see* diethylpropion *on page 201*
♦ **Tenuate® Dospan®** *see* diethylpropion *on page 201*
♦ **Tepanil®** *(Discontinued) see page 743*
♦ **Tepanil® TenTabs®** *(Discontinued) see page 743*
♦ **Tequin™** *see* gatifloxacin *New Drug on page 288*
♦ **Terak® Ophthalmic Ointment** *see* oxytetracycline and polymyxin B *on page 465*
♦ **Terazol® Vaginal** *see* terconazole *on page 597*

terazosin (ter AY zoe sin)
U.S. Brand Names Hytrin®
Generic Available Yes
Therapeutic Category Alpha-Adrenergic Blocking Agent
Use Management of mild to moderate hypertension; considered a step 2 drug in stepped approach to hypertension; benign prostate hypertrophy
Usual Dosage Adults: Oral: 1 mg; slowly increase dose to achieve desired blood pressure, up to 20 mg/day
Dietary Considerations May be administered without regard to meals at the same time each day
Nursing/Pharmacy Information
Syncope may occur usually within 90 minutes of the initial dose; administer initial dose at bedtime
Monitor blood pressure, standing and sitting/supine
(Continued)

terazosin *(Continued)*

Dosage Forms
Capsule: 1 mg, 2 mg, 5 mg, 10 mg
Tablet: 1 mg, 2 mg, 5 mg, 10 mg

terbinafine, oral *(TER bin a feen, OR al)*
U.S. Brand Names Lamisil® Oral
Generic Available No
Therapeutic Category Antifungal Agent
Use Treatment of onychomycosis infections of the toenail or fingernail
Usual Dosage Adults: Oral:
Fingernail onychomycosis: 250 mg once daily for 6 weeks
Toenail onychomycosis: 250 mg once daily for 12 weeks
Dosage Forms Tablet: 250 mg

terbinafine, topical *(TER bin a feen, TOP i kal)*
U.S. Brand Names Lamisil® Cream
Generic Available No
Therapeutic Category Antifungal Agent
Use Topical antifungal for the treatment of tinea pedis (athlete's foot), tinea cruris (jock itch), and tinea corporis (ring worm); tinea versicolor (lotion)
Unlabeled use: Cutaneous candidiasis
Usual Dosage Adults: Topical:
Athlete's foot: Apply to affected area twice daily for at least 1 week, not to exceed 4 weeks
Ringworm and jock itch: Apply to affected area once or twice daily for at least 1 week, not to exceed 4 weeks
Dosage Forms
Cream: 1% (15 g, 30 g)
Lotion: 1%

terbutaline *(ter BYOO ta leen)*
U.S. Brand Names Brethaire®; Brethine®; Bricanyl®
Mexican Brand Names Taziken
Generic Available No
Therapeutic Category Adrenergic Agonist Agent
Use Bronchodilator in reversible airway obstruction and bronchial asthma
Usual Dosage
Children <6 years:
Oral: Initial: 0.05 mg/kg/dose 3 times/day, increased gradually as required; maximum: 0.15 mg/kg/dose 3-4 times/day or a total of 5 mg/24 hours
S.C.: 0.005-0.01 mg/kg/dose to a maximum of 0.3 mg/dose every 15-20 minutes for 3 doses
Inhalation nebulization dose: 0.06 mg/kg; maximum: 8 mg
Inhalation: 0.3 mg/kg/dose up to maximum of 10 mg/dose every 4-6 hours
Children >6 years and Adults:
Oral:
6-15 years: 2.5 mg every 6 hours 3 times/day; not to exceed 7.5 mg in 24 hours
>15 years: 5 mg/dose every 6 hours 3 times/day; if side effects occur, reduce dose to 2.5 mg every 6 hours; not to exceed 15 mg in 24 hours
S.C.: 0.25 mg/dose repeated in 15-30 minutes for one time only; a total dose of 0.5 mg should not be exceeded within a 4-hour period
Nebulization: 0.01-0.03 mL/kg (1 mg = 1 mL); minimum dose: 0.1 mL; maximum dose: 2.5 mL diluted with 1-2 mL normal saline
Inhalation: 2 inhalations every 4-6 hours; wait 1 minute between inhalations
Nursing/Pharmacy Information
Parenteral form is only for S.C. use. Before using, the inhaler must be shaken well; assess lung sounds, pulse, and blood pressure before administration and during peak of medication; observe patient for wheezing after administration, if this occurs, call physician
Monitor serum potassium, heart rate, blood pressure, respiratory rate
Stability: Store injection at room temperature; protect from heat, light, and from freezing; use only clear solutions
Dosage Forms Terbutaline sulfate:
Aerosol, oral: 0.2 mg/actuation (10.5 g)
Injection: 1 mg/mL (1 mL)
Tablet: 2.5 mg, 5 mg

terconazole (ter KONE a zole)
Synonyms triaconazole
U.S. Brand Names Terazol® Vaginal
Mexican Brand Names Fungistat; Fungistat Dual
Generic Available No
Therapeutic Category Antifungal Agent
Use Local treatment of vulvovaginal candidiasis
Usual Dosage Vaginal: 1 applicatorful in vagina at bedtime for 7 consecutive days
Nursing/Pharmacy Information
 Assist patient in administration, if necessary
 Monitor local irritation
 Stability: Room temperature (13°C to 30°C/59°F to 86°F)
Dosage Forms
 Cream, vaginal: 0.4% (45 g); 0.8% (20 g)
 Suppository, vaginal: 80 mg (3s)

terfenadine *(Canada only)* (ter FEN a deen)
U.S. Brand Names Seldane®
Canadian Brand Names Apo®-Terfenadine; Novo-Terfenadine®
Generic Available Yes
Therapeutic Category Antihistamine
Use Perennial and seasonal allergic rhinitis and other allergic symptoms including urticaria
Usual Dosage Oral:
 Children:
  3-6 years: 15 mg twice daily
  6-12 years: 30 mg twice daily
 Children >12 years and Adults: 60 mg twice daily
Dietary Considerations May be administered with food
Nursing/Pharmacy Information
 Monitor for relief of symptoms
 Stability: Keep away from direct sunlight
Dosage Forms Tablet: 60 mg

teriparatide (ter i PAR a tide)
U.S. Brand Names Parathar™
Generic Available No
Therapeutic Category Diagnostic Agent
Use Diagnosis of hypocalcemia in either hypoparathyroidism or pseudohypoparathyroidism
Usual Dosage I.V.:
 Children ≥3 years: 3 units/kg up to 200 units
 Adults: 200 units over 10 minutes
Dosage Forms Powder for injection: 200 units hPTH activity (10 mL)

terpin hydrate (TER pin HYE drate)
Generic Available Yes
Therapeutic Category Expectorant
Use Symptomatic relief of cough
Usual Dosage Adults: Oral: 5-10 mL every 4-6 hours as needed
Dosage Forms Elixir: 85 mg/5 mL (120 mL)

terpin hydrate and codeine (TER pin HYE drate & KOE deen)
Synonyms ETH and C
Generic Available Yes
Therapeutic Category Antitussive/Expectorant
Controlled Substance C-V
Use Symptomatic relief of cough
Usual Dosage Based on codeine content: Oral:
 Children (not recommended): 1-1.5 mg/kg/24 hours divided every 4 hours; maximum: 30 mg/24 hours
  2-6 years: 1.25-2.5 mL every 4-6 hours as needed
  6-12 years: 2.5-5 mL every 4-6 hours as needed
 Adults: 10-20 mg/dose every 4-6 hours as needed
Dosage Forms Elixir: Terpin hydrate 85 mg and codeine 10 mg per 5 mL with alcohol 42.5%

♦ **Terra-Cortril® Ophthalmic Suspension** *see* oxytetracycline and hydrocortisone *on page 465*

- **Terramicina** *see* oxytetracycline *on page 464*
- **Terramycin® I.M. Injection** *see* oxytetracycline *on page 464*
- **Terramycin® Ophthalmic Ointment** *see* oxytetracycline and polymyxin B *on page 465*
- **Terramycin® Oral** *see* oxytetracycline *on page 464*
- **Terramycin® w/Polymyxin B Ophthalmic Ointment** *see* oxytetracycline and polymyxin B *on page 465*
- **Terranumonyl** *see* tetracycline *on page 601*
- **Tesalon** *see* benzonatate *on page 80*
- **Tesamone® Injection** *see* testosterone *on page 598*
- **Teslac®** *see* testolactone *on page 598*
- **TESPA** *see* thiotepa *on page 608*
- **Tessalon® Perles** *see* benzonatate *on page 80*
- **Tes-Tape®** *(Discontinued) see page 743*
- **Testoderm® Transdermal System** *see* testosterone *on page 598*

testolactone (tes toe LAK tone)

U.S. Brand Names Teslac®
Generic Available No
Therapeutic Category Androgen
Use Palliative treatment of advanced disseminated breast carcinoma
Usual Dosage Adults: Females: Oral: 250 mg 4 times/day for at least 3 months; desired response may take as long as 3 months
Nursing/Pharmacy Information Monitor plasma calcium levels
Dosage Forms Tablet: 50 mg

- **Testopel® Pellet** *see* testosterone *on page 598*

testosterone (tes TOS ter one)

Synonyms aqueous testosterone
U.S. Brand Names Androderm® Transdermal System; Andro-L.A.® Injection; Andropository® Injection; Delatest® Injection; Delatestryl® Injection; depAndro® Injection; Depotest® Injection; Depo®-Testosterone Injection; Duratest® Injection; Durathate® Injection; Everone® Injection; Histerone® Injection; Tesamone® Injection; Testoderm® Transdermal System; Testopel® Pellet
Generic Available Yes
Therapeutic Category Androgen
Controlled Substance C-III
Use Androgen replacement therapy in the treatment of delayed male puberty; male hypogonadism
Usual Dosage I.M.:
Delayed puberty: Children: 40-50 mg/m^2/dose (cypionate or enanthate) monthly for 6 months
Male hypogonadism: 50-400 mg every 2-4 weeks
Initiation of pubertal growth: 40-50 mg/m^2/dose (cypionate or enanthate) monthly until the growth rate falls to prepubertal levels (~5 cm/year)
During terminal growth phase: 100 mg/m^2/dose (cypionate or enanthate) monthly until growth ceases
Maintenance virilizing dose: 100 mg/m^2/dose (cypionate or enanthate) twice monthly or 50-400 mg/dose every 2-4 weeks
Inoperable breast cancer: Adults: 200-400 mg every 2-4 weeks
Hypogonadism: Adults:
Testosterone or testosterone propionate: 10-25 mg 2-3 times/week
Testosterone cypionate or enanthate: 50-400 mg every 2-4 weeks
Postpubertal cryptorchism: Testosterone or testosterone propionate: 10-25 mg 2-3 times/week
Transdermal system: Males: Place the patch on clean, dry, scrotal skin; dry-shaved scrotal hair for optimal skin contact, do not use chemical depilatories; patients should start therapy with 6 mg/day system applied daily; if scrotal area is inadequate, use a 4 mg/day system; the system should be worn for 22-24 hours
Nursing/Pharmacy Information
Administer deep I.M.
Monitor periodic liver function tests, radiologic examination of wrist and hand every 6 months (when using in prepubertal children)
Dosage Forms
Injection:
Aqueous suspension: 25 mg/mL (10 mL, 30 mL); 50 mg/mL (10 mL, 30 mL); 100 mg/mL (10 mL, 30 mL)
In oil, as cypionate: 100 mg/mL (1 mL, 10 mL); 200 mg/mL (1 mL, 10 mL)

In oil, as enanthate: 100 mg/mL (5 mL, 10 mL); 200 mg/mL (5 mL, 10 mL)
In oil, as propionate: 50 mg/mL (10 mL, 30 mL); 100 mg/mL (10 mL, 30 mL)
Pellet: 75 mg (1 pellet per vial)
Transdermal system: 2.5 mg/day; 4 mg/day; 5 mg/day; 6 mg/day

♦ **Testred®** *see* methyltestosterone *on page 408*
♦ **tetanus and diphtheria toxoid** *see* diphtheria and tetanus toxoid *on page 209*

tetanus antitoxin (TET a nus an tee TOKS in)

Synonyms TAT
Generic Available No
Therapeutic Category Antitoxin
Use Tetanus prophylaxis or treatment of active tetanus only when tetanus immune globulin (TIG) is not available
Usual Dosage
Prophylaxis: I.M., S.C.:
Children <30 kg: 1500 units
Children and Adults >30 kg: 3000-5000 units
Treatment: Children and Adults: Inject 10,000-40,000 units into wound; administer 40,000-100,000 units I.V.
Nursing/Pharmacy Information
All patients should have sensitivity testing prior to starting therapy with tetanus antitoxin
Stability: Refrigerate, do not freeze
Dosage Forms Injection, equine: Not less than 400 units/mL (12.5 mL, 50 mL)

tetanus immune globulin (human)
(TET a nus i MYUN GLOB yoo lin, HYU man)
Synonyms TIG
U.S. Brand Names Hyper-Tet®
Generic Available No
Therapeutic Category Immune Globulin
Use Passive immunization against tetanus; tetanus immune globulin is preferred over tetanus antitoxin for treatment of active tetanus; part of the management of an unclean, nonminor wound in a person whose history of previous receipt of tetanus toxoid is unknown or who has received less than three doses of tetanus toxoid
Usual Dosage I.M.:
Prophylaxis of tetanus:
Children: 4 units/kg; some recommend administering 250 units to small children
Adults: 250 units
Treatment of tetanus:
Children: 500-3000 units; some should infiltrate locally around the wound
Adults: 3000-6000 units
Nursing/Pharmacy Information
Do not administer I.V.
Stability: Refrigerate
Dosage Forms Injection: 250 units/mL

tetanus toxoid (adsorbed) (TET a nus TOKS oyd, ad SORBED)
Generic Available No
Therapeutic Category Toxoid
Use Active immunization against tetanus
Usual Dosage Adults: I.M.:
Primary immunization: 0.5 mL; repeat 0.5 mL at 4-8 weeks after first dose and at 6-12 months after second dose
Routine booster doses are recommended only every 5-10 years
Nursing/Pharmacy Information
Inject intramuscularly in the area of the vastus lateralis (midthigh laterally) or deltoid
Stability: Refrigerate, do not freeze
Dosage Forms Injection, adsorbed:
Tetanus 5 Lf units per 0.5 mL dose (0.5 mL, 5 mL)
Tetanus 10 Lf units per 0.5 mL dose (0.5 mL, 5 mL)

tetanus toxoid (fluid) (TET a nus TOKS oyd FLOO id)
Synonyms tetanus toxoid plain
Generic Available No
Therapeutic Category Toxoid
(Continued)

tetanus toxoid (fluid) *(Continued)*

Use Active immunization against tetanus in adults and children

Usual Dosage Inject 3 doses of 0.5 mL I.M. or S.C. at 4- to 8-week intervals with fourth dose administered only 6-12 months after third dose

Nursing/Pharmacy Information
Must not be used I.V.
Stability: Refrigerate

Dosage Forms Injection, fluid:
Tetanus 4 Lf units per 0.5 mL dose (7.5 mL)
Tetanus 5 Lf units per 0.5 mL dose (0.5 mL, 7.5 mL)

♦ **tetanus toxoid plain** *see* tetanus toxoid (fluid) *on page 599*
♦ **Tetra-Atlantis®** *see* tetracycline *on page 601*

tetrabenazine *(Canada only)* (tet ra BENZ a zeen)

Canadian Brand Names Nitoman®

Generic Available No

Therapeutic Category Monoamine Depleting Agent

Use Treatment of hyperkinetic movement disorders such as Huntington's chorea, hemiballismus, senile chorea, tic and Gilles de la Tourette syndrome and tardive dyskinesia; not indicated for the treatment of levodopa-induced dyskinetic/choreiform movements; should only be used by (or in consultation with) physicians who are experienced in the treatment of hyperkinetic movement diso

Usual Dosage Oral:
Children: No adequately controlled clinical studies have been performed in children. Limited clinical experience suggests that treatment should be started at approximately half the adult dose, and titrated slowly and carefully according to tolerance and individual response.
Adults: An initial starting dose of 12.5 mg two to three times a day is recommended. This can be increased by 12.5 mg a day every three to five days until the maximal tolerated and effective dose is reached for the individual, and may have to be up/down titrated depending on individual tolerance. In most cases the maximal tolerated dose will be 25 mg three times/day. In very rare cases, a 200 mg dose has been reached (the maximum recommended dose in some publications). If there is no improvement at the maximal tolerated dose in seven days, it is unlikely that Nitoman® will be of benefit to the patient, either by increasing the dose or by extending the duration of treatment.
Elderly and debilitated patients: No adequately controlled clinical studies have been performed in the elderly and/or debilitated patients. Clinical experience suggests that a reduced initial and maintenance dose should be used. Parkinsonian-like adverse reactions are relatively common in these patients and may be dose-limiting.

Dosage Forms Tablet: 25 mg

tetracaine (TET ra kane)

Synonyms amethocaine

U.S. Brand Names Pontocaine®

Canadian Brand Names Supracaine®

Generic Available Yes

Therapeutic Category Local Anesthetic

Use Local anesthesia in the eye for various diagnostic and examination purposes; spinal anesthesia; topical anesthesia for local skin disorders; local anesthesia for mucous membranes

Usual Dosage
Children: Safety and efficacy have not been established
Adults:
Ophthalmic (not for prolonged use):
Ointment: Apply ½" to 1" to lower conjunctival fornix
Solution: Instill 1-2 drops
Spinal anesthesia 1% solution:
Subarachnoid injection: 5-20 mg
Saddle block: 2-5 mg; a 1% solution should be diluted with equal volume of CSF before administration
Topical mucous membranes (2% solution): Apply as needed; dose should not exceed 20 mg
Topical for skin: Apply to affected areas as needed

Nursing/Pharmacy Information
Not for prolonged use topically
Stability: Store solution in the refrigerator

Dosage Forms Tetracaine hydrochloride:
Cream: 1% (28 g)
Injection: 1% [10 mg/mL] (2 mL)
Injection, with dextrose 6%: 0.2% [2 mg/mL] (2 mL); 0.3% [3 mg/mL] (5 mL)
Ointment:
Ophthalmic: 0.5% [5 mg/mL] (3.75 g)
Topical: 0.5% [5 mg/mL] (28 g)
Powder for injection: 20 mg
Solution:
Ophthalmic: 0.5% [5 mg/mL] (1 mL, 2 mL, 15 mL, 59 mL)
Topical: 2% [20 mg/mL] (30 mL, 118 mL)

tetracaine and dextrose (TET ra kane & DEKS trose)
U.S. Brand Names Pontocaine® With Dextrose
Generic Available Yes
Therapeutic Category Local Anesthetic
Use Spinal anesthesia (saddle block)
Usual Dosage Dose varies with procedure, depth of anesthesia, duration desired, and physical condition of patient
Dosage Forms Injection: Tetracaine hydrochloride 0.2% and dextrose 6% (2 mL); tetracaine hydrochloride 0.3% and dextrose 6% (5 mL)

♦ **tetracaine hydrochloride, benzocaine, butyl aminobenzoate, and benzalkonium chloride** *see* benzocaine, butyl aminobenzoate, tetracaine, and benzalkonium chloride *on page 79*

♦ **Tetracap® Oral** *see* tetracycline *on page 601*

♦ **tetracosactide** *see* cosyntropin *on page 170*

tetracycline (tet ra SYE kleen)
Synonyms TCN
U.S. Brand Names Achromycin® Ophthalmic; Achromycin® Topical; Nor-tet® Oral; Panmycin® Oral; Robitet® Oral; Sumycin® Oral; Tetracap® Oral; Topicycline® Topical
Canadian Brand Names Apo®-Tetra; Novo-Tetra®; Nu-Tetra®; Tetracyn®
Mexican Brand Names Acromicina; Ambotetra; Quimocyclar; Terranumonyl; Tetra-Atlantis®; Zorbenal-G
Generic Available Yes
Therapeutic Category Antibiotic, Ophthalmic; Antibiotic, Topical; Tetracycline Derivative
Use
Children, Adolescents, and Adults: Treatment of Rocky mountain spotted fever caused by susceptible Rickettsia or brucellosis
Adolescents and Adults: Presumptive treatment of chlamydial infection in patients with gonorrhea
Older Children, Adolescents, and Adults: Treatment of Lyme disease, mycoplasmal disease or *Legionella*
Usual Dosage
Children >8 years:
Oral: 25-50 mg/kg/day in divided doses every 6 hours; not to exceed 3 g/day
Ophthalmic:
Suspension: Instill 1-2 drops 2-4 times/day or more often as needed
Ointment: Instill every 2-12 hours
Adults:
Oral: 250-500 mg/dose every 6 hours
Ophthalmic:
Suspension: Instill 1-2 drops 2-4 times/day or more often as needed
Ointment: Instill every 2-12 hours
Topical: Apply to affected areas 1-4 times/day
Dietary Considerations Should be administered 2 hours before or after meals with adequate amounts of fluid; avoid taking antacids, iron, dairy products, or milk formulas within 2 hours of tetracyclines; decreased absorption of magnesium, zinc, calcium, iron, and amino acids
Nursing/Pharmacy Information
Do not administer I.M. injection I.V., or I.V. injection I.M. (specific products available for each). I.V. should be infused over at least 2 hours
Monitor renal, hepatic, and hematologic function test
Stability: Outdated tetracyclines have caused a Fanconi-like syndrome
Dosage Forms Tetracycline hydrochloride:
Capsule: 100 mg, 250 mg, 500 mg
Ointment:
Ophthalmic: 1% [10 mg/mL] (3.5 g)
(Continued)

tetracycline *(Continued)*
Topical: 3% [30 mg/mL] (14.2 g, 30 g)
Solution, topical: 2.2 mg/mL (70 mL)
Suspension:
Ophthalmic: 1% [10 mg/mL] (0.5 mL, 1 mL, 4 mL)
Oral: 125 mg/5 mL (60 mL, 480 mL)
Tablet: 250 mg, 500 mg

♦ **Tetracyn®** *see* tetracycline *on page 601*
♦ **tetrahydroaminoacrine** *see* tacrine *on page 592*
♦ **tetrahydrocannabinol** *see* dronabinol *on page 223*

tetrahydrozoline (tet ra hye DROZ a leen)
Synonyms tetryzoline
U.S. Brand Names Collyrium Fresh® Ophthalmic [OTC]; Eyesine® Ophthalmic [OTC]; Geneye® Ophthalmic [OTC]; Mallazine® Eye Drops [OTC]; Murine® Plus Ophthalmic [OTC]; Optigene® Ophthalmic [OTC]; Tetrasine® Extra Ophthalmic [OTC]; Tetrasine® Ophthalmic [OTC]; Tyzine® Nasal; Visine® Extra Ophthalmic [OTC]
Generic Available Yes
Therapeutic Category Adrenergic Agonist Agent
Use Symptomatic relief of nasal congestion and conjunctival congestion
Usual Dosage
Nasal congestion:
Children 2-6 years: Instill 2-3 drops of 0.05% solution every 4-6 hours as needed
Children >6 years and Adults: Instill 2-4 drops or 0.1% spray nasal mucosa every 4-6 hours as needed
Conjunctival congestion: Adults: Instill 1-2 drops in each eye 2-3 times/day
Nursing/Pharmacy Information
Do not use for >3-4 days without direct physician supervision
Monitor blood pressure, heart rate, symptom response
Stability: Do not use if solution changes color or becomes cloudy
Dosage Forms Solution, as hydrochloride:
Nasal: 0.05% (15 mL), 0.1% (30 mL, 473 mL)
Ophthalmic: 0.05% (15 mL)

♦ **Tetralan®** *(Discontinued) see page 743*
♦ **Tetram®** *(Discontinued) see page 743*
♦ **Tetramune®** *see* diphtheria, tetanus toxoids, whole-cell pertussis, and *Haemophilus* B conjugate vaccine *on page 211*
♦ **Tetrasine® Extra Ophthalmic [OTC]** *see* tetrahydrozoline *on page 602*
♦ **Tetrasine® Ophthalmic [OTC]** *see* tetrahydrozoline *on page 602*
♦ **tetryzoline** *see* tetrahydrozoline *on page 602*
♦ **Texacort® Topical** *see* hydrocortisone (topical) *on page 324*
♦ **TG** *see* thioguanine *on page 607*
♦ **6-TG** *see* thioguanine *on page 607*
♦ **T/Gel® [OTC]** *see* coal tar *on page 162*
♦ **T-Gen®** *see* trimethobenzamide *on page 629*
♦ **T-Gesic®** *see* hydrocodone and acetaminophen *on page 319*
♦ **THA** *see* tacrine *on page 592*

thalidomide (tha LI doe mide)
U.S. Brand Names Contergan®; Distaval®; Kevadon®; Thalomid®
Generic Available No
Therapeutic Category Immunosuppressant Agent
Use Treatment or prevention of graft-versus-host reactions after bone marrow transplantation; in aphthous ulceration in HIV-positive patients; reactional lepromatous or erythema nodosum leprosy; Langerhans cell histiocytosis, Behçet's syndrome; hypnotic agent; also may be effective in rheumatoid arthritis, discoid lupus, and erythema multiforme; useful in type 2 lepra reactions, but not type 1; can assist in healing mouth ulcers in AIDS patients
Usual Dosage
Leprosy: Up to 400 mg/day; usual maintenance dose: 50-100 mg/day
Behçet's syndrome: 100-400 mg/day
Graft-vs-host reactions:
Children: 3 mg/kg 4 times/day
Adults: 100-1600 mg/day; usual initial dose: 200 mg 4 times/day for use up to 700 days

AIDS-related aphthous stomatitis: 200 mg twice daily for 5 days, then 200 mg/day for up to 8 weeks

Discoid lupus erythematosus: 100-400 mg/day; maintenance dose: 25-50 mg

Dosage Forms Capsule: 50 mg

- ◆ **Thalitone®** *see* chlorthalidone *on page 146*
- ◆ **Thalomid®** *see* thalidomide *on page 602*
- ◆ **THAM®** *see* tromethamine *on page 633*
- ◆ **THAM-E®** *see* tromethamine *on page 633*
- ◆ **THC** *see* dronabinol *on page 223*
- ◆ **Theelin® Aqueous Injection** *(Discontinued) see page 743*
- ◆ **Theo-24®** *see* theophylline *on page 603*
- ◆ **Theobid®** *see* theophylline *on page 603*
- ◆ **Theobid® Jr Duracaps®** *(Discontinued) see page 743*
- ◆ **Theochron®** *see* theophylline *on page 603*
- ◆ **Theoclear-80®** *see* theophylline *on page 603*
- ◆ **Theoclear® L.A.** *see* theophylline *on page 603*
- ◆ **Theo-Dur®** *see* theophylline *on page 603*
- ◆ **Theo-Dur® Sprinkle®** *(Discontinued) see page 743*
- ◆ **Theolair™** *see* theophylline *on page 603*
- ◆ **Theo-Organidin®** *(Discontinued) see page 743*

theophylline (thee OF i lin)

U.S. Brand Names Aerolate III®; Aerolate JR®; Aerolate SR®; Aquaphyllin®; Asmalix®; Elixomin®; Elixophyllin®; Quibron®-T; Quibron®-T/SR; Respbid®; Slo-bid™; Slo-Phyllin®; Sustaire®; Theo-24®; Theobid®; Theochron®; Theoclear-80®; Theoclear® L.A.; Theo-Dur®; Theolair™; Theo-Sav®; Theospan®-SR; Theostat-80®; Theovent®; Theo-X®; T-Phyl®; Uni-Dur®; Uniphyl®

Generic Available Yes

Therapeutic Category Theophylline Derivative

Use Treatment of symptoms and reversible airway obstruction due to chronic asthma, chronic bronchitis, or COPD; for treatment of idiopathic apnea of prematurity in neonates

Usual Dosage

Apnea: Dosage should be determined by plasma level monitoring; each 0.5 mg/kg of theophylline administered as a loading dose will result in a 1 mcg/mL increase in serum theophylline concentration

Loading dose: 5 mg/kg; dilute dose in 1-hour I.V. fluid via syringe pump over 1 hour

Maintenance: 2 mg/kg every 8-12 hours or 1-3 mg/kg/dose every 8-12 hours; administer I.V. push 1 mL/minute (2 mg/minute)

Treatment of acute bronchospasm in older patients: (>6 months of age): Loading dose (in patients not currently receiving theophylline): 6 mg/kg (based on aminophylline) administered I.V. over 20-30 minutes; 4.7 mg/kg (based on theophylline) administered I.V. over 20-30 minutes; administration rate should not exceed 20 mg (1 mL)/minute (theophylline) or 25 mg (1 mL)/minute (aminophylline)

Approximate maintenance dosage for treatment of acute bronchospasm:

Children:

6 months to 9 years: 1.2 mg/kg/hour (aminophylline); 0.95 mg/kg/hour (theophylline)

9-16 years and young adult smokers: 1 mg/kg/hour (aminophylline); 0.79 mg/kg/hour (theophylline)

Adults (healthy, nonsmoking): 0.7 mg/kg/hour (aminophylline); 0.55 mg/kg/hour (theophylline)

Older patients and patients with cor pulmonale: 0.6 mg/kg/hour (aminophylline); 0.47 mg/kg/hour (theophylline)

Patients with CHF or liver failure: 0.5 mg/kg/hour (aminophylline); 0.39 mg/kg/hour (theophylline)

Chronic therapy: Slow clinical titration is generally preferred

Initial dose: 16 mg/kg/24 hours or 400 mg/24 hours, whichever is less

Increasing dose: The above dosage may be increased in ~25% increments at 2- to 3-day intervals so long as the drug is tolerated or until the maximum dose is reached; monitor serum levels

Exercise caution in younger children who cannot complain of minor side effects, older adults, and those with cor pulmonale; CHF or liver disease may have unusually low dosage requirements

(Continued)

theophylline *(Continued)*

Dietary Considerations Avoid drinking or eating large quantities of caffeine-containing beverages or food; avoid extremes of dietary protein and carbohydrate intake; limit charcoal-broiled foods; should be administered with water 1 hour before or 2 hours after meals

Nursing/Pharmacy Information

Do not crush Theo-Dur® tablets; tablets may only be cut in half

Monitor heart rate, CNS effects (insomnia, irritability); respiratory rate (COPD patients often have resting controlled respiratory rates in low 20s), serum theophylline level, arterial or capillary blood gases (if applicable)

Stability: Store injection at room temperature; protect from heat and from freezing; use only clear solutions; stability of parenteral admixture at room temperature (25°C): 30 days

Dosage Forms

Capsule:

Immediate release (Bronkodyl®, Elixophyllin®): 100 mg, 200 mg

Timed release:

8-12 hours (Aerolate®): 65 mg [III]; 130 mg [JR], 260 mg [SR]

8-12 hours (Slo-bid™): 50 mg, 75 mg, 100 mg, 125 mg, 200 mg, 300 mg

8-12 hours (Slo-Phyllin® Gyrocaps®): 60 mg, 125 mg, 250 mg

12 hours (Theobid® Duracaps®): 260 mg

12 hours (Theoclear® L.A.): 130 mg, 260 mg

12 hours (Theospan®-SR): 130 mg, 260 mg

12 hours (Theovent®): 125 mg, 250 mg

24 hours (Theo-24®): 100 mg, 200 mg, 300 mg

Elixir (Asmalix®, Elixomin®, Elixophyllin®, Lanophyllin®): 80 mg/15 mL (15 mL, 30 mL, 480 mL, 4000 mL)

Infusion, in D₅W: 0.4 mg/mL (1000 mL); 0.8 mg/mL (500 mL, 1000 mL); 1.6 mg/mL (250 mL, 500 mL); 2 mg/mL (100 mL); 3.2 mg/mL (250 mL); 4 mg/mL (50 mL, 100 mL);

Solution, oral:

Theolair™: 80 mg/15 mL (15 mL, 18.75 mL, 30 mL, 480 mL)

Syrup:

Aquaphyllin®, Slo-Phyllin®, Theoclear-80®, Theostat-80®: 80 mg/15 mL (15 mL, 30 mL, 500 mL)

Accurbron®: 150 mg/15 mL (480 mL)

Tablet: Immediate release:

Slo-Phyllin®: 100 mg, 200 mg

Theolair™: 125 mg, 250 mg

Quibron®-T: 300 mg

Tablet:

Controlled release (Theo-X®): 100 mg, 200 mg, 300 mg

Timed release:

12-24 hours: 100 mg, 200 mg, 300 mg, 450 mg

8-12 hours (Quibron®-T/SR): 300 mg

8-12 hours (Respbid®): 250 mg, 500 mg

8-12 hours (Sustaire®): 100 mg, 300 mg

8-12 hours (T-Phyl®): 200 mg

12-24 hours (Theochron®): 100 mg, 200 mg, 300 mg

8-24 hours (Theo-Dur®): 100 mg, 200 mg, 300 mg, 450 mg

8-24 hours (Theo-Sav®): 100 mg, 200 mg, 300 mg

24 hours (Theolair™-SR): 200 mg, 250 mg, 300 mg, 500 mg

24 hours (Uni-Dur®, Uniphyl®): 400 mg, 600 mg

theophylline and guaifenesin *(thee OF i lin & gwye FEN e sin)*

Synonyms guaifenesin and theophylline

U.S. Brand Names Bronchial®; Glycerol-T®; Quibron®; Slo-Phyllin® GG

Generic Available Yes

Therapeutic Category Theophylline Derivative

Use Symptomatic treatment of bronchospasm associated with bronchial asthma, chronic bronchitis and pulmonary emphysema

Usual Dosage Adults: Oral: 1-2 capsules every 6-8 hours

Dietary Considerations Should be administered with water 1 hour before or 2 hours after meals

Dosage Forms

Capsule: Theophylline 150 mg and guaifenesin 90 mg; theophylline 300 mg and guaifenesin 180 mg

Elixir: Theophylline 150 mg and guaifenesin 90 mg per 15 mL (480 mL)

theophylline, ephedrine, and hydroxyzine
(thee OF i lin, e FED rin, & hye DROKS i zeen)

Synonyms ephedrine, theophylline, and hydroxyzine; hydroxyzine, theophylline, and ephedrine

U.S. Brand Names Hydrophed®; Marax®

Generic Available Yes

Therapeutic Category Theophylline Derivative

Use Possibly effective for controlling bronchospastic disorders

Usual Dosage Oral:
Children:
2-5 years: $^1/_2$ tablet 2-4 times/day or 2.5 mL 3-4 times/day
>5 years: $^1/_2$ tablet 2-4 times/day or 5 mL 3-4 times/day
Adults: 1 tablet 2-4 times/day

Dietary Considerations Should be administered with water 1 hour before or 2 hours after meals

Dosage Forms
Syrup, dye free: Theophylline 32.5 mg, ephedrine 6.25 mg, and hydroxyzine 2.5 mg per 5 mL
Tablet: Theophylline 130 mg, ephedrine 25 mg, and hydroxyzine 10 mg

theophylline, ephedrine, and phenobarbital
(thee OF i lin, e FED rin, & fee noe BAR bi tal)

Synonyms ephedrine, theophylline, and phenobarbital; phenobarbital, theophylline, and ephedrine

U.S. Brand Names Tedral®

Generic Available Yes

Therapeutic Category Theophylline Derivative

Use Prevention and symptomatic treatment of bronchial asthma; relief of asthmatic bronchitis and other bronchospastic disorders

Usual Dosage Oral:
Children >60 lb: 1 tablet or 5 mL every 4 hours
Adults: 1-2 tablets or 10-20 mL every 4 hours

Dietary Considerations Should be administered with water 1 hour before or 2 hours after meals

Dosage Forms
Suspension: Theophylline 65 mg, ephedrine sulfate 12 mg, and phenobarbital 4 mg per 5 mL
Tablet: Theophylline 118 mg, ephedrine sulfate 25 mg, and phenobarbital 11 mg; theophylline 130 mg, ephedrine sulfate 24 mg, and phenobarbital 8 mg

♦ **theophylline ethylenediamine** *see* aminophylline *on page 38*

♦ **Theo-Sav®** *see* theophylline *on page 603*

♦ **Theospan®-SR** *see* theophylline *on page 603*

♦ **Theostat-80®** *see* theophylline *on page 603*

♦ **Theovent®** *see* theophylline *on page 603*

♦ **Theo-X®** *see* theophylline *on page 603*

♦ **Therabid® [OTC]** *see* vitamin, multiple (oral) *on page 654*

♦ **Thera-Combex® H-P Kapseals® [OTC]** *see* vitamin B complex with vitamin C *on page 651*

♦ **TheraCys®** *see* BCG vaccine *on page 74*

♦ **Theraflu® Non-Drowsy Formula Maximum Strength [OTC]** *see* acetaminophen, dextromethorphan, and pseudoephedrine *on page 16*

♦ **Thera-Flur®** *see* fluoride *on page 274*

♦ **Thera-Flur-N®** *see* fluoride *on page 274*

♦ **Theragran® [OTC]** *see* vitamin, multiple (oral) *on page 654*

♦ **Theragran® Hematinic®** *see* vitamin, multiple (oral) *on page 654*

♦ **Theragran® Liquid [OTC]** *see* vitamin, multiple (oral) *on page 654*

♦ **Theragran-M® [OTC]** *see* vitamin, multiple (oral) *on page 654*

♦ **Thera-Hist® Syrup [OTC]** *see* chlorpheniramine and phenylpropanolamine *on page 139*

♦ **Theramine® Expectorant *(Discontinued)*** *see page 743*

♦ **Theraplex Z® [OTC]** *see* pyrithione zinc *on page 535*

♦ **Thermazene®** *see* silver sulfadiazine *on page 566*

♦ **Theroxide® Wash [OTC]** *see* benzoyl peroxide *on page 81*

thiabendazole (thye a BEN da zole)

Synonyms tiabendazole

U.S. Brand Names Mintezol®

Generic Available No

(Continued)

thiabendazole *(Continued)*

Therapeutic Category Anthelmintic

Use Treatment of strongyloidiasis, cutaneous larva migrans, visceral larva migrans, dracunculosis, trichinosis, and mixed helminthic infections

Usual Dosage Children and Adults: Oral: 50 mg/kg/day divided every 12 hours (maximum dose: 3 g/day)

Strongyloidiasis: For 2 consecutive days

Cutaneous larva migrans: For 2-5 consecutive days

Visceral larva migrans: For 5-7 consecutive days

Trichinosis: For 2-4 consecutive days

Dracunculosis: 50-75 mg/kg/day divided every 12 hours for 3 days

Nursing/Pharmacy Information

Purgation is not required prior to use

Monitor periodic renal and hepatic function tests

Dosage Forms

Suspension, oral: 500 mg/5 mL (120 mL)

Tablet, chewable (orange flavor): 500 mg

♦ **Thiacide®** *(Discontinued)* see page 743

♦ **thiamazole** *see* methimazole *on page 401*

thiamine (THYE a min)

Synonyms aneurine; thiaminium; vitamin B$_1$

U.S. Brand Names Betalin®S

Canadian Brand Names Betaxin®; Bewon®

Generic Available Yes

Therapeutic Category Vitamin, Water Soluble

Use Treatment of thiamine deficiency including beriberi, Wernicke's encephalopathy syndrome, and peripheral neuritis associated with pellagra; alcoholic patients with altered sensorium; various genetic metabolic disorders

Usual Dosage Dietary supplement (depends on caloric or carbohydrate content of the diet):

Infants: 0.3-0.5 mg/day

Children: 0.5-1 mg/day

Adults: 1-2 mg/day

Note: The above doses can be found as a combination in multivitamin preparations

Children:

Noncritically ill thiamine deficiency: Oral: 10-50 mg/day in divided doses every day for 2 weeks followed by 5-10 mg/day for one month

Beriberi: I.M.: 10-25 mg/day for 2 weeks, then 5-10 mg orally every day for one month (oral as therapeutic multivitamin)

Adults:

Wernicke's encephalopathy: I.M., I.V.: 50 mg as a single dose, then 50 mg I.M. every day until normal diet resumed

Noncritically ill thiamine deficiency: Oral: 10-50 mg/day in divided doses

Beriberi: I.M., I.V.: 10-30 mg 3 times/day for 2 weeks, then switch to 5-10 mg orally every day for one month (oral as therapeutic multivitamin)

Dietary Considerations High carbohydrate diets may increase thiamine requirement

Nursing/Pharmacy Information

Parenteral: Administer by slow I.V. injection

Stability: Protect oral dosage forms from light; **incompatible** with alkaline or neutral solutions and with oxidizing or reducing agents

Dosage Forms Thiamine hydrochloride:

Injection: 100 mg/mL (1 mL, 2 mL, 10 mL, 30 mL); 200 mg/mL (30 mL)

Tablet: 50 mg, 100 mg, 250 mg, 500 mg

Tablet, enteric coated: 20 mg

♦ **thiaminium** *see* thiamine *on page 606*

thiethylperazine (thye eth il PER a zeen)

Generic Available No

Therapeutic Category Phenothiazine Derivative

Use Relief of nausea and vomiting

Usual Dosage Children >12 years and Adults:

Oral, I.M., rectal: 10 mg 1-3 times/day as needed

I.V. and S.C. routes of administration are not recommended

Nursing/Pharmacy Information Inject I.M. deeply into large muscle mass, patient should be lying down and remain so for at least 1 hour after administration; help with ambulation

Dosage Forms Thiethylperazine maleate:
Injection: 5 mg/mL (2 mL)
Tablet: 10 mg

thimerosal (thye MER oh sal)

U.S. Brand Names Aeroaid® [OTC]; Mersol® [OTC]; Merthiolate® [OTC]
Generic Available Yes
Therapeutic Category Antibacterial, Topical
Use Organomercurial antiseptic with sustained bacteriostatic and fungistatic activity
Usual Dosage Apply 1-3 times/day
Dosage Forms
Ointment, ophthalmic: 0.02% [0.2 mg/mL] (3.5 g)
Solution, topical: 0.1% [1 mg/mL = 1:1000] (120 mL, 480 mL, 4000 mL)
Spray, antiseptic: 0.1% [1 mg/mL = 1:1000] with alcohol 2% (90 mL)
Tincture: 0.1% [1 mg/mL = 1:1000] with alcohol 50% (120 mL, 480 mL, 4000 mL)

thioguanine (thye oh GWAH neen)

Synonyms 2-amino-6-mercaptopurine; TG; 6-TG; 6-thioguanine; tioguanine
Canadian Brand Names Lanvis®
Generic Available No
Therapeutic Category Antineoplastic Agent
Use Remission induction in acute myelogenous (nonlymphocytic) leukemia; treatment of chronic myelogenous leukemia and acute lymphocytic leukemia
Usual Dosage Refer to individual protocols. Oral:
Infants <3 years: Combination drug therapy for acute nonlymphocytic leukemia: 3.3 mg/kg/day in divided doses twice daily for 4 days
Children and Adults: 2-3 mg/kg/day calculated to nearest 20 mg or 75-200 mg/m^2/day in 1-2 divided doses for 5-7 days or until remission is attained
Dietary Considerations Enhanced absorption if administered between meals
Nursing/Pharmacy Information Monitor CBC with differential and platelet count, liver function tests, hemoglobin, hematocrit, serum uric acid
Dosage Forms Tablet, scored: 40 mg

♦ **6-thioguanine** see thioguanine on page 607
♦ **Thiola™** see tiopronin on page 614

thiopental (thye oh PEN tal)

U.S. Brand Names Pentothal® Sodium
Generic Available Yes
Therapeutic Category Barbiturate
Controlled Substance C-III
Use Induction of anesthesia; adjunct for intubation in head injury patients; control of convulsive states; treatment of elevated intracranial pressure
Usual Dosage I.V.:
Induction anesthesia:
Infants: 5-8 mg/kg
Children 1-12 years: 5-6 mg/kg
Adults: 3-5 mg/kg
Maintenance anesthesia:
Children: 1 mg/kg as needed
Adults: 25-100 mg as needed
Increased intracranial pressure: Children and Adults: 1.5-5 mg/kg/dose; repeat as needed to control intracranial pressure
Seizures:
Children: 2-3 mg/kg/dose, repeat as needed
Adults: 75-250 mg/dose, repeat as needed
Rectal administration: (Patient should be NPO for no less than 3 hours prior to administration)
Suggested initial doses of thiopental rectal suspension are:
<3 months: 15 mg/kg/dose
>3 months: 25 mg/kg/dose
Note: The age of a premature infant should be adjusted to reflect the age that the infant would have been if full-term (eg, an infant, now age 4 months, who was 2 months premature should be considered to be a 2-month old infant).
Doses should be rounded downward to the nearest 50 mg increment to allow for accurate measurement of the dose
(Continued)

thiopental *(Continued)*

Inactive or debilitated patients and patients recently medicated with other sedatives, (eg, chloral hydrate, meperidine, chlorpromazine, and promethazine), may require smaller doses than usual

If the patient is not sedated within 15-20 minutes, a single repeat dose of thiopental can be administered; the single repeat doses are:
<3 months of age: <7.5 mg/kg/dose
>3 months of age: 15 mg/kg/dose
Adults weighing >90 kg should not receive >3 g as a total dose (initial plus repeat doses)
Children weighing >34 kg should not receive >1 g as a total dose (initial plus repeat doses)
Neither adults nor children should receive more than one course of thiopental rectal suspension (initial dose plus repeat dose) per 24-hour period

Nursing/Pharmacy Information
Parenteral: Rapid I.V. injection may cause hypotension or decreased cardiac output
Monitor respiratory rate, heart rate, blood pressure
Stability: Reconstituted solutions remain stable for 3 days at room temperature and 7 days when refrigerated; solutions are alkaline and **incompatible** with drugs with acidic pH, such as succinylcholine, atropine sulfate, etc. I.V. form is **incompatible** when mixed with amikacin, codeine, dimenhydrinate, diphenhydramine, hydromorphone, insulin, levorphanol, meperidine, metaraminol, morphine, norepinephrine, penicillin G, prochlorperazine, succinylcholine, tetracycline, benzquinamide, chlorpromazine, glycopyrrolate

Dosage Forms Thiopental sodium:
Injection: 250 mg, 400 mg, 500 mg, 1 g, 2.5 g, 5 g
Suspension, rectal: 400 mg/g (2 g)

♦ **Thioplex®** *see* thiotepa *on page 608*

thioridazine *(thye oh RID a zeen)*

U.S. Brand Names Mellaril®; Mellaril-S®
Canadian Brand Names Apo®-Thioridazine; Novo-Ridazine®; PMS-Thioridazine
Generic Available Yes
Therapeutic Category Phenothiazine Derivative
Use Management of psychotic disorders; depressive neurosis; dementia in elderly; severe behavioral problems in children
Usual Dosage Oral:
Children >2 years: Range: 0.5-3 mg/kg/day in 2-3 divided doses; usual: 1 mg/kg/day; maximum: 3 mg/kg/day
Behavior problems: Initial: 10 mg 2-3 times/day, increase gradually
Severe psychoses: Initial: 25 mg 2-3 times/day, increase gradually
Adults:
Psychoses: Initial: 50-100 mg. 3 times/day with gradual increments as needed and tolerated; maximum daily dose: 800 mg/day in 2-4 divided doses
Depressive disorders, dementia: Initial: 25 mg 3 times/day; maintenance dose: 20-200 mg/day
Dietary Considerations Increase dietary intake of riboflavin; liquid formulation is **incompatible** with enteral formulas; should be administered with food
Nursing/Pharmacy Information
Dilute the oral concentrate with water or juice before administration; avoid skin contact with oral suspension or solution, may cause contact dermatitis
Monitor patients on prolonged therapy; CBC, ophthalmologic exam, blood pressure, liver function tests
Stability: Protect all dosage forms from light
Dosage Forms Thioridazine hydrochloride:
Concentrate, oral, as hydrochloride: 30 mg/mL (120 mL); 100 mg/mL (3.4 mL, 120 mL)
Suspension, oral, as hydrochloride: 25 mg/5 mL (480 mL); 100 mg/5 mL (480 mL)
Tablet, as hydrochloride: 10 mg, 15 mg, 25 mg, 50 mg, 100 mg, 150 mg, 200 mg

thiotepa *(thye oh TEP a)*

Synonyms TESPA; triethylenethiophosphoramide; TSPA
U.S. Brand Names Thioplex®
Generic Available No
Therapeutic Category Antineoplastic Agent

Use Treatment of superficial tumors of the bladder; palliative treatment of adenocarcinoma of breast or ovary; lymphomas and sarcomas; meningeal neoplasms; control pleural, pericardial or peritoneal effusions caused by metastatic tumors; high-dose regimens with autologous bone marrow transplantation

Usual Dosage Refer to individual protocols

Children: Sarcomas: I.V.: 25-65 mg/m² as a single dose every 21 days

Adults:

I.M., I.V., S.C.: 8 mg/m² daily for 5 days or 30-60 mg/m² once per week

High-dose therapy for bone marrow transplant: I.V.: 500 mg/m²

Intracavitary: 0.6-0.8 mg/kg or 60 mg in 60 mL SWI instilled into the bladder at 1- to 4-week intervals

Intrathecal: Doses of 1-10 mg/m² administered 1-2 times/week

Nursing/Pharmacy Information

Parenteral: Can be administered slow IVP over 5 minutes at a concentration not to exceed 10 mg/mL or I.V. infusion at a final concentration for administration of 1 mg/mL

Monitor CBC with differential and platelet count, uric acid, urinalysis

Stability: Refrigerate, protect from light; the reconstituted solution is stable for 5 days when refrigerated, **compatible** with D_5W, 0.9% sodium chloride, D_5NS, or lactated Ringer's

Dosage Forms Powder for injection: 15 mg

thiothixene (thye oh THIKS een)

Synonyms tiotixene

U.S. Brand Names Navane® Capsule

Generic Available Yes

Therapeutic Category Thioxanthene Derivative

Use Management of psychotic disorders

Usual Dosage

Children <12 years: Oral: Not well established; 0.25 mg/kg/24 hours in divided doses

Children >12 years and Adults:

Oral: Initial: 2 mg 3 times/day, up to 20-30 mg/day; maximum: 60 mg/day

I.M. (administer undiluted injection): 4 mg 2-4 times/day, increase dose gradually; usual: 16-20 mg/day; maximum: 30 mg/day; change to oral dose as soon as able

Dietary Considerations May be administered with food; may cause increase in dietary riboflavin requirements

Nursing/Pharmacy Information

Store injection in the refrigerator; injection for intramuscular use only; dilute the oral concentrate with water or juice before administration; avoid skin contact with oral suspension or solution; may cause contact dermatitis; monitor orthostatic blood pressures 3-5 days after initiation of therapy or a dose increase

Monitor orthostatic blood pressures; tremors, gait changes, abnormal movement in trunk, neck, buccal area or extremities; monitor target behaviors for which the agent is given; monitor hepatic function (especially if fever with flu-like symptoms)

Stability: Refrigerate

Dosage Forms

Capsule: 1 mg, 2 mg, 5 mg, 10 mg, 20 mg

Concentrate, as hydrochloride: 5 mg/mL

- **Thorazine®** see chlorpromazine on page 144
- **Thrombate III™** see antithrombin III on page 53
- **Thrombinar®** see thrombin, topical on page 609

thrombin, topical (THROM bin, TOP i kal)

U.S. Brand Names Thrombinar®; Thrombogen®; Thrombostat®

Generic Available No

Therapeutic Category Hemostatic Agent

Use Hemostasis whenever minor bleeding from capillaries and small venules is accessible

Usual Dosage Use 1000-2000 units/mL of solution where bleeding is profuse; apply powder directly to the site of bleeding or on oozing surfaces; use 100 units/mL for bleeding from skin or mucosal surfaces

Nursing/Pharmacy Information

Parenteral: May be applied directly as a powder or as reconstituted solution; use sterile water or 0.9% sodium chloride to reconstitute powder to desired concentration; sponge surface free of blood prior to application, if possible

(Continued)

thrombin, topical *(Continued)*

Stability: Refrigerate

Dosage Forms Powder: 1000 units, 5000 units, 10,000 units, 20,000 units, 50,000 units

♦ **Thrombogen®** *see* thrombin, topical *on page 609*

♦ **Thrombostat®** *see* thrombin, topical *on page 609*

♦ **Thypinone®** *see* protirelin *on page 529*

♦ **Thyrar®** *see* thyroid *on page 610*

♦ **Thyrel® TRH** *see* protirelin *on page 529*

♦ **Thyro-Block®** *see* potassium iodide *on page 509*

♦ **Thyrogen®** *see* thyrotropin alpha *New Drug on page 610*

thyroid (THYE royd)

Synonyms desiccated thyroid; thyroid extract

U.S. Brand Names Armour® Thyroid; S-P-T; Thyrar®; Thyroid Strong®

Generic Available Yes

Therapeutic Category Thyroid Product

Use Replacement or supplemental therapy in hypothyroidism

Usual Dosage Adults: Oral: Start at 30 mg/day and titrate by 30 mg/day in increments of 2- to 3-week intervals; usual maintenance dose: 60-120 mg/day

Dietary Considerations Should be administered on an empty stomach

Nursing/Pharmacy Information Monitor T_4, TSH, heart rate, blood pressure, clinical signs of hypo- and hyperthyroidism; in cases where T_4 remains low and TSH is within normal limits, an evaluation of "free" (unbound) T_4 is needed to evaluate further increase in dosage. Thyroid replacement requires periodic assessment of thyroid status; TSH is the most reliable guide for evaluating adequacy of thyroid replacement dosage. TSH may be elevated during the first few months of thyroid replacement despite patients being clinically euthyroid.

Dosage Forms

Capsule, pork source in soybean oil (S-P-T): 60 mg, 120 mg, 180 mg, 300 mg
Tablet:
Armour® Thyroid: 15 mg, 30 mg, 60 mg, 90 mg, 120 mg, 180 mg, 240 mg, 300 mg
Thyrar® (bovine source): 30 mg, 60 mg, 120 mg
Thyroid Strong® (60 mg is equivalent to 90 mg thyroid USP):
Regular: 30 mg, 60 mg, 120 mg
Sugar coated: 30 mg, 60 mg, 120 mg, 180 mg
Thyroid USP: 15 mg, 30 mg, 60 mg, 120 mg, 180 mg, 300 mg

♦ **thyroid extract** *see* thyroid *on page 610*

♦ **thyroid-stimulating hormone** *see* thyrotropin *on page 610*

♦ **Thyroid Strong®** *see* thyroid *on page 610*

♦ **Thyrolar®** *see* liotrix *on page 371*

thyrotropin (thye roe TROE pin)

Synonyms thyroid-stimulating hormone; TSH

U.S. Brand Names Thytropar®

Generic Available No

Therapeutic Category Diagnostic Agent

Use Diagnostic aid to determine subclinical hypothyroidism or decreased thyroid reserve, to differentiate between primary and secondary hypothyroidism and between primary hypothyroidism and euthyroidism in patients receiving thyroid replacement

Usual Dosage I.M., S.C.: 10 units/day for 1-3 days; follow by a radioiodine study 24 hours past last injection, no response in thyroid failure, substantial response in pituitary failure

Nursing/Pharmacy Information Stability: After reconstitution, store in refrigerator at 2°C to 8°C (36°F to 46°F); use within 2 weeks

Dosage Forms Injection: 10 units

thyrotropin alpha *New Drug* (thye roe TROE pin AL fa)

Synonyms human thyroid-stimulating hormone; TSH

U.S. Brand Names Thyrogen®

Generic Available No

Therapeutic Category Diagnostic Agent

Use As an adjunctive diagnostic tool for serum thyroglobulin (Tg) testing with or without radioiodine imaging in the follow-up of patients with well-differentiated thyroid cancer

Potential clinical uses:

1. Patients with an undetectable Tg on thyroid hormone suppressive therapy to exclude the diagnosis of residual or recurrent thyroid cancer
2. Patients requiring serum Tg testing and radioiodine imaging who are unwilling to undergo thyroid hormone withdrawal testing and whose treating physician believes that use of a less sensitive test is justified
3. Patients who are either unable to mount an adequate endogenous TSH response to thyroid hormone withdrawal or in whom withdrawal is medically contraindicated

Usual Dosage Children >16 years and Adults: I.M.: 0.9 mg every 24 hours for 2 doses or every 72 hours for 3 doses. For radioiodine imaging, radioiodine administration should be given 24 hours following the final Thyrogen® injection. Scanning should be performed 48 hours after radioiodine administration (72 hours after the final injection of Thyrogen®).

Dosage Forms Kits containing two 1.1 mg vials (>4 int. units) of thyrogen® and two 10 mL vials of sterile water for injection

♦ **Thytropar®** *see* thyrotropin *on page 610*

♦ **tlabendazole** *see* thiabendazole *on page 605*

tiagabine (tye AG a bene)
U.S. Brand Names Gabitril®
Generic Available No
Therapeutic Category Anticonvulsant
Use Adjunctive therapy in adults and children 12 years and older in the treatment of partial seizures
Usual Dosage Children >12 years and Adults: Oral: Initial: 4 mg, once daily; the total daily dose may be increased in 4 mg increments beginning the second week of therapy; thereafter, the daily dose may be increased by 4-8 mg/day until clinical response is achieved, up to a maximum of 32 mg/day; the total daily dose at higher levels should be given in divided doses, 2-4 times/day
Dosage Forms Tablet, as hydrochloride: 4 mg, 12 mg, 16 mg, 20 mg

♦ **Tiamate®** *see* diltiazem *on page 205*

♦ **Tiamol®** *see* fluocinonide *on page 273*

tiaprofenic acid *(Canada only)* (tye ah PRO fen ik AS id)
Canadian Brand Names Surgam®; Surgam® SR
Generic Available No
Therapeutic Category Nonsteroidal Anti-Inflammatory Agent (NSAID)
Use Relief of signs and symptoms of rheumatoid arthritis and osteoarthritis (degenerative joint disease)
Usual Dosage Adults: Oral:
Tablet:
Rheumatoid arthritis: Usual initial and maintenance dose: 600 mg/day in 3 divided doses; some patients may do well on 300 mg twice daily; maximum daily dose: 600 mg.
Osteoarthritis: Usual initial and maintenance dose: 600 mg/day in 2 or 3 divided doses; in rare instances patients may be maintained on 300 mg daily in divided doses; maximum daily dose: 600 mg
Extended release capsule:
Rheumatoid arthritis or osteoarthritis: Initial and maintenance dose: 2 sustained release capsules of 300 mg once daily. Surgam® SR capsules should be swallowed whole
Dosage Forms
Capsule, sustained release: 300 mg
Tablet: 200 mg, 300 mg

♦ **Tiazac®** *see* diltiazem *on page 205*

♦ **Ticar®** *see* ticarcillin *on page 611*

ticarcillin (tye kar SIL in)
U.S. Brand Names Ticar®
Generic Available No
Therapeutic Category Penicillin
Use Treatment of infections such as septicemia, acute and chronic respiratory tract infections, skin and soft tissue infections, and urinary tract infections due to susceptible strains of *Pseudomonas*, *Proteus*, *Escherichia coli*, and *Enterobacter*
Usual Dosage I.V. (ticarcillin is generally administered I.M. only for the treatment of uncomplicated urinary tract infections):
(Continued)

ticarcillin (Continued)

Infants and Children: 200-300 mg/kg/day in divided doses every 4-6 hours; maximum dose: 24 g/day

Adults: 1-4 g every 4-6 hours

Nursing/Pharmacy Information

Administer 1 hour apart from aminoglycosides; dosage modification required in patients with impaired renal function; do not administer I.M.; can be administered I.V. push over 10-20 minutes or by I.V. intermittent infusion over 30-120 minutes at a final concentration not to exceed 100 mg/mL; concentrations of ≤50 mg/mL are preferred for peripheral intermittent infusions to avoid vein irritation

Monitor serum electrolytes, bleeding time, and periodic tests of renal, hepatic, and hematologic function

Stability: Reconstituted solution is stable for 72 hours at room temperature and 14 days when refrigerated; for I.V. infusion in normal saline or D_5W, solution is stable for 72 hours at room temperature, 14 days when refrigerated, or 30 days when frozen; after freezing, thawed solution is stable for 72 hours at room temperature or 14 days when refrigerated; **incompatible** with aminoglycosides

Dosage Forms Powder for injection, as disodium: 1 g, 3 g, 6 g, 20 g, 30 g

ticarcillin and clavulanate potassium

(tye kar SIL in & klav yoo LAN ate poe TASS ee um)

Synonyms clavulanic acid and ticarcillin; ticarcillin and clavulanic acid

U.S. Brand Names Timentin®

Generic Available No

Therapeutic Category Penicillin

Use Treatment of infections caused by susceptible organisms involving the lower respiratory tract, urinary tract, skin and skin structures, bone and joint, and septicemia. Clavulanate expands activity of ticarcillin to include beta-lactamase producing strains of *S. aureus*, *H. influenzae*, *Moraxella catarrhalis*, *B. fragilis*, *Klebsiella*, and *Proteus* species

Usual Dosage I.V.:

Children: 200-300 mg of ticarcillin/kg/day in divided doses every 4-6 hours

Adults: 3.1 g (ticarcillin 3 g plus clavulanic acid 0.1 g) every 4-6 hours; maximum: 18-24 g/day; for urinary tract infections: 3.1 g every 6-8 hours

Nursing/Pharmacy Information

Do not administer I.M.; administer by I.V. intermittent infusion over 30 minutes; final concentration for administration should not exceed 100 mg/mL of ticarcillin; however, concentrations ≤50 mg/mL are preferred

Monitor serum electrolytes, periodic renal, hepatic and hematologic function tests

Stability: Reconstituted solution is stable for 6 hours at room temperature and 72 hours when refrigerated; for I.V. infusion in >normal saline is stable for 24 hours at room temperature, 7 days when refrigerated, or 30 days when frozen; after freezing, thawed solution is stable for 8 hours at room temperature; for I.V. infusion in D_5W, solution is stable for 24 hours at room temperature, 3 days when refrigerated, or 7 days when frozen; after freezing, thawed solution is stable for 8 hours at room temperature; darkening of drug indicates loss of potency of clavulanate potassium; **incompatible** with sodium bicarbonate, aminoglycosides

Dosage Forms

Infusion, premixed (frozen): Ticarcillin disodium 3 g and clavulanate potassium 0.1 g (100 mL)

Powder for injection: Ticarcillin disodium 3 g and clavulanate potassium 0.1 g (3.1 g, 31 g)

♦ **ticarcillin and clavulanic acid** *see* ticarcillin and clavulanate potassium *on page 612*

♦ **TICE® BCG** *see* BCG vaccine *on page 74*

♦ **Ticlid®** *see* ticlopidine *on page 612*

ticlopidine (tye KLOE pi deen)

U.S. Brand Names Ticlid®

Generic Available Yes

Therapeutic Category Antiplatelet Agent

Use Platelet aggregation inhibitor that reduces the risk of thrombotic stroke in patients who have had a stroke or stroke precursors

Usual Dosage Adults: Oral: 1 tablet twice daily with food

Dietary Considerations Should be administered with food to reduce stomach upset; high fat meals increase absorption, antacids decrease absorption

Nursing/Pharmacy Information Monitor bleeding times, platelets, CBC, hemoglobin and hematocrit

Dosage Forms Tablet, as hydrochloride: 250 mg

♦ **Ticon®** *see* trimethobenzamide *on page 629*
♦ **Tienam®** *see* imipenem and cilastatin *on page 334*
♦ **TIG** *see* tetanus immune globulin (human) *on page 599*
♦ **Tigan®** *see* trimethobenzamide *on page 629*
♦ **Tiject-20®** *(Discontinued) see page 743*
♦ **Tikosyn™** *see* dofetilide *New Drug on page 215*
♦ **Tilade® Inhalation Aerosol** *see* nedocromil (inhalation) *on page 434*
♦ **Tilazem** *see* diltiazem *on page 205*

tiludronate (tye LOO droe nate)

Synonyms tiludronic acid
U.S. Brand Names Skelid®
Generic Available No
Therapeutic Category Bisphosphonate Derivative
Use Paget's disease of the bone
Usual Dosage Adults: Oral: 400 mg/day (2 tablets) [tiludronic acid]
Dosage Forms Tablet, as disodium: 240 mg [tiludronic acid 200 mg]; dosage is expressed in terms of tiludronic acid.

♦ **tiludronic acid** *see* tiludronate *on page 613*
♦ **Tim-AK** *see* timolol *on page 613*
♦ **Timecelles® [OTC]** *see* ascorbic acid *on page 60*
♦ **Timentin®** *see* ticarcillin and clavulanate potassium *on page 612*

timolol (TYE moe lole)

U.S. Brand Names Blocadren® Oral; Timoptic® Ophthalmic; Timoptic-XE® Ophthalmic
Canadian Brand Names Apo®-Timol; Apo®-Timop; Beta-Tim®; Gen-Timolol®; Novo-Timol®; Nu-Timolol®; Tim-AK
Mexican Brand Names Imot Ofteno; Timoptol®; Timoptol® XE
Generic Available Yes
Therapeutic Category Beta-Adrenergic Blocker
Use Ophthalmic dosage form used to treat elevated intraocular pressure such as glaucoma or ocular hypertension; orally for treatment of hypertension and angina and for prevention of myocardial infarction and migraine headaches
Usual Dosage
Children and Adults: Ophthalmic: Initial: 0.25% solution, instill 1 drop twice daily; increase to 0.5% solution if response not adequate; decrease to 1 drop/day if controlled; do not exceed 1 drop twice daily of 0.5% solution
Adults: Oral:
Hypertension: Initial: 10 mg twice daily, increase gradually every 7 days, usual dosage: 20-40 mg/day in 2 divided doses; maximum: 60 mg/day
Prevention of myocardial infarction: 10 mg twice daily initiated within 1-4 weeks after infarction
Migraine headache: Initial: 10 mg twice daily, increase to maximum of 30 mg/day
Dietary Considerations Oral product should be administered with food at the same time each day
Nursing/Pharmacy Information
Use cautiously in diabetics receiving hypoglycemic agents; teach proper instillation of eye drops
Monitor signs of congestive heart failure, hypotension, respiratory difficulty (bronchospasm); monitor blood pressure and heart rate
Dosage Forms
Timolol hemihydrate:
Solution, ophthalmic (Betimol®): 0.25% (2.5 mL, 5 mL, 10 mL, 15 mL); 0.5% (2.5 mL, 5 mL, 10 mL, 15 mL)
Timolol maleate:
Gel, ophthalmic (Timoptic-XE®): 0.25% (2.5 mL, 5 mL); 0.5% (2.5 mL, 5 mL)
Solution, ophthalmic (Timoptic®): 0.25% (2.5 mL, 5 mL, 10 mL, 15 mL); 0.5% (2.5 mL, 5 mL, 10 mL, 15 mL)
Solution, ophthalmic, preservative free, single use (Timoptic® OcuDose®): 0.25%, 0.5%
Tablet (Blocadren®): 5 mg, 10 mg, 20 mg

♦ **Timoptic® Ophthalmic** *see* timolol *on page 613*
♦ **Timoptic-XE® Ophthalmic** *see* timolol *on page 613*

- **Timoptol®** *see* timolol *on page 613*
- **Timoptol® XE** *see* timolol *on page 613*
- **Tinactin® [OTC]** *see* tolnaftate *on page 618*
- **TinBen® [OTC]** *see* benzoin *on page 80*
- **TinCoBen® [OTC]** *see* benzoin *on page 80*
- **Tindal® *(Discontinued)* see page 743**
- **Tine Test PPD** *see* tuberculin tests *on page 635*
- **Tiniazol** *see* ketoconazole *on page 354*
- **Tinver® [OTC]** *see* sodium thiosulfate *on page 576*

tinzaparin *(Canada only)* (tin ZA pa rin)
Canadian Brand Names Innohep®
Generic Available No
Therapeutic Category Anticoagulant
Use Prevention of postoperative venous thromboembolism in patients undergoing orthopedic surgery; may be used in the management of the prevention of postoperative venous thromboembolism in patients undergoing general surgery who are at high risk of developing postoperative venous thromboembolism; postoperative administration does not preclude other prophylactic modalities including physical and mechanical methods of adjunct therapy
Usual Dosage Adults: S.C.: Postoperative venous thromboembolism in general surgery patients: 3500 anti-Xa int. units 2 hours before surgery followed by 3500 anti-Xa int. units once daily for 7 to 10 days
Dosage Forms Injection, as sodium:
Syringe: 10,000 anti-Xa int. units/mL (0.35 mL, 0.45 mL); 20,000 anti-Xa int. units/mL (0.5 mL, 0.7 mL, 0.9 mL)
Vial: 10,000 anti-Xa int. units/mL (2 mL); 20,000 anti-Xa int. units/mL (2 mL)

tioconazole (tye oh KONE a zole)
U.S. Brand Names Vagistat®-1 Vaginal [OTC]
Generic Available No
Therapeutic Category Antifungal Agent
Use Local treatment of vulvovaginal candidiasis
Usual Dosage Vaginal: Insert 1 applicatorful in vagina, just prior to bedtime, as a single dose
Nursing/Pharmacy Information Insert high into vagina; contact physician if itching or burning continues
Dosage Forms Cream, vaginal: 6.5% with applicator (4.6 g)

- **tioguanine** *see* thioguanine *on page 607*

tiopronin (tye oh PROE nin)
U.S. Brand Names Thiola™
Generic Available No
Therapeutic Category Urinary Tract Product
Use Prevention of kidney stone (cystine) formation in patients with severe homozygous cystinuric who have urinary cystine >500 mg/day who are resistant to treatment with high fluid intake, alkali, and diet modification, or who have had adverse reactions to penicillamine
Usual Dosage Adults: Initial: 800 mg/day; average dose: 1000 mg/day
Dosage Forms Tablet: 100 mg

- **tiotixene** *see* thiothixene *on page 609*

tirofiban (tye roe FYE ban)
U.S. Brand Names Aggrastat®
Generic Available No
Therapeutic Category Antiplatelet Agent
Use In combination with heparin, is indicated for the treatment of acute coronary syndrome, including patients who are to be managed medically and those undergoing PTCA or atherectomy. In this setting, it has been shown to decrease the rate of a combined endpoint of death, new myocardial infarction or refractory ischemia/repeat cardiac procedure.
Usual Dosage Adults: I.V.: Initial rate of 0.4 mcg/kg/minute for 30 minutes and then continued at 0.1 mcg/kg/minute
Dosage Forms Injection: 50 mcg/mL (500 mL); 250 mcg/mL (50 mL)

- **Tiroidine** *see* levothyroxine *on page 367*
- **Ti-Screen® [OTC]** *see* methoxycinnamate and oxybenzone *on page 404*
- **Tisit® Blue Gel [OTC]** *see* pyrethrins and piperonyl butoxide *on page 533*
- **Tisit® Liquid [OTC]** *see* pyrethrins and piperonyl butoxide *on page 533*

- **Tisit® Shampoo [OTC]** *see* pyrethrins and piperonyl butoxide *on page 533*
- **tissue plasminogen activator, recombinant** *see* alteplase *on page 31*
- **Titralac® Plus Liquid [OTC]** *see* calcium carbonate and simethicone *on page 104*

tizanidine (tye ZAN i deen)

U.S. Brand Names Zanaflex®
Generic Available No
Therapeutic Category Alpha₂-Adrenergic Agonist Agent
Use Intermittent management of increased muscle tone associated with spasticity (eg, multiple sclerosis, spinal cord injury)
Usual Dosage Adults: Oral: Initial: 4 mg every 6-8 hours, not to exceed 3 doses/day or 36 mg in a 24-hour period; doses may be increased at 2 mg or 4 mg increments with single doses not exceeding 12 mg
Dosage Forms Tablet, as hydrochloride: 4 mg

- **TMP** *see* trimethoprim *on page 630*
- **TMP-SMX** *see* co-trimoxazole *on page 170*
- **TOBI™ Inhalation Solution** *see* tobramycin *on page 615*
- **Tobra** *see* tobramycin *on page 615*
- **TobraDex® Ophthalmic** *see* tobramycin and dexamethasone *on page 616*

tobramycin (toe bra MYE sin)

U.S. Brand Names AKTob® Ophthalmic; Nebcin® Injection; TOBI™ Inhalation Solution; Tobrex® Ophthalmic
Mexican Brand Names Tobra; Trazil Ofteno/Ungena
Generic Available Yes
Therapeutic Category Aminoglycoside (Antibiotic); Antibiotic, Ophthalmic
Use Treatment of documented or suspected infections caused by susceptible gram-negative bacilli including *Pseudomonas aeruginosa*; infection with a nonpseudomonal enteric bacillus which is more sensitive to tobramycin than gentamicin based on susceptibility tests; susceptible organisms in lower respiratory tract infections, septicemia; intra-abdominal, skin, bone, and urinary tract infections; empiric therapy in cystic fibrosis and immunocompromised patients; used topically to treat superficial ophthalmic infections caused by susceptible bacteria
Usual Dosage Dosage should be based on an estimate of ideal body weight
Infants and Children: I.M., I.V.: 2.5 mg/kg/dose every 8 hours
  Note: Some patients may require larger or more frequent doses if serum levels document the need (ie, cystic fibrosis or febrile granulocytopenic patients)
Adults: I.M., I.V.: 3-5 mg/kg/day in 3 divided doses

Children and Adults:
  Renal dysfunction: 2.5 mg/kg (2-3 serum level measurements should be obtained after the initial dose to measure the half-life in order to determine the frequency of subsequent doses)
  Ophthalmic: 1-2 drops every 4 hours; apply ointment 2-3 times/day; for severe infections apply ointment every 3-4 hours, or 2 drops every 30-60 minutes initially, then reduce to less frequent intervals
Dietary Considerations Calcium, magnesium, potassium: Renal wasting may cause hypocalcemia, hypomagnesemia and/or hypokalemia
Nursing/Pharmacy Information
  Obtain serum concentration after the third dose except in neonates and patients with rapidly changing renal function in whom levels need to be measured sooner; peak levels are drawn 30 minutes after the end of a 30-minute infusion; the trough is drawn just before the next dose; administer other antibiotics such as penicillins and cephalosporins at least one hour before or after tobramycin; provide optimal patient hydration and perfusion; final concentration for administration should not exceed 10 mg/mL
  Monitor urinalysis, urine output, BUN, serum creatinine, peak and trough plasma tobramycin levels; be alert to ototoxicity; hearing should be tested before and during treatment
  Stability: Reconstituted solution is stable for 24 hours at room temperature and 96 hours when refrigerated; **incompatible** with penicillins
Dosage Forms Tobramycin sulfate:
  Injection, (Nebcin®): 10 mg/mL (2 mL); 40 mg/mL (1.5 mL, 2 mL)
  Ointment, ophthalmic (Tobrex®): 0.3% (3.5 g)
  Powder for injection (Nebcin®): 40 mg/mL (1.2 g vials)
  Solution, ophthalmic: 0.3% (5 mL)
    AKTob®, Tobrex®: 0.3% (5 mL)

tobramycin and dexamethasone
(toe bra MYE sin & deks a METH a sone)

Synonyms dexamethasone and tobramycin

U.S. Brand Names TobraDex® Ophthalmic

Generic Available No

Therapeutic Category Antibiotic/Corticosteroid, Ophthalmic

Use Treatment of external ocular infection caused by susceptible gram-negative bacteria and steroid responsive inflammatory conditions of the palpebral and bulbar conjunctiva, lid, cornea, and anterior segment of the globe

Usual Dosage Ophthalmic: Adults:

Ointment: Apply 1.25 cm (1/2") every 3-4 hours to 2-3 times/day

Suspension: Instill 1-2 drops every 4-6 hours (first 24-48 hours may increase frequency to every 2 hours until signs of clinical improvement are seen); apply every 30-60 minutes for severe infections

Nursing/Pharmacy Information Shake well before using, do not touch dropper to eye, apply light finger pressure on lacrimal sac for 1 minute following instillation; notify physician if condition fails to improve or worsens

Dosage Forms

Ointment, ophthalmic: Tobramycin 0.3% and dexamethasone 0.1% (3.5 g)

Suspension, ophthalmic: Tobramycin 0.3% and dexamethasone 0.1% (2.5 mL, 5 mL)

♦ **Tobrex® Ophthalmic** see tobramycin on page 615

tocainide (toe KAY nide)

U.S. Brand Names Tonocard®

Generic Available No

Therapeutic Category Antiarrhythmic Agent, Class I-B

Use Suppress and prevent symptomatic ventricular arrhythmias

Usual Dosage Adults: Oral: 1200-1800 mg/day in 3 divided doses

Dietary Considerations Should be administered with food

Nursing/Pharmacy Information Monitor for tremors; titration of dosing and initiation of therapy require cardiac monitoring

Dosage Forms Tablet, as hydrochloride: 400 mg, 600 mg

tocophersolan (toe kof er SOE lan)

Synonyms TPGS

U.S. Brand Names Liqui-E®

Generic Available No

Therapeutic Category Vitamin, Fat Soluble

Use Treatment of vitamin E deficiency resulting from malabsorption due to prolonged cholestatic hepatobiliary disease

Usual Dosage Dietary supplement: Oral: 15 mg (400 units) every day

Nursing/Pharmacy Information Studies indicate that TPGS is absorbed better than fat soluble forms of vitamin E in patients with impaired digestion and absorption and when coadministered with cyclosporin to transplant recipients it improves cyclosporin absorption. Due to these findings, this product has a valuable role in the liver transplant patient population.

Dosage Forms Liquid: 26.6 units/mL

♦ **Toesen®** see oxytocin on page 465

♦ **Tofranil®** see imipramine on page 334

♦ **Tofranil-PM®** see imipramine on page 334

tolazamide (tole AZ a mide)

U.S. Brand Names Tolinase®

Generic Available Yes

Therapeutic Category Antidiabetic Agent, Oral

Use Adjunct to diet for the management of mild to moderately severe, stable, noninsulin-dependent (type II) diabetes mellitus

Usual Dosage Adults: Oral: 100-1000 mg/day

Nursing/Pharmacy Information

Patients who are anorexic or NPO may need to have their dose held to avoid hypoglycemia

Monitor for signs and symptoms of hypoglycemia, (fatigue, sweating, numbness of extremities); urine for glucose and ketones; fasting blood glucose; hemoglobin A, C, or fructosamine

Dosage Forms Tablet: 100 mg, 250 mg, 500 mg

tolazoline (tole AZ oh leen)
Synonyms benzazoline
U.S. Brand Names Priscoline®
Generic Available No
Therapeutic Category Alpha-Adrenergic Blocking Agent
Use Persistent pulmonary hypertension of the newborn (PPHN), also known as persistent fetal circulation (PFC); peripheral vasospastic disorders
Usual Dosage
Neonates: Initial: I.V.: 1-2 mg/kg over 10-15 minutes via scalp vein or upper extremity; maintenance: 1-2 mg/kg/hour; use lower maintenance doses in patients with decreased renal function. Also used in neonates for acute vasospasm "cath toes" at 0.25 mg/kg/hour (no load)
Adults: Peripheral vasospastic disorder: I.M., I.V., S.C.: 10-50 mg 4 times/day
Dietary Considerations Alcohol will cause "disulfiram"-type reaction consisting of flushing, headache, nausea, and in some patients, vomiting and chest and/or abdominal pain
Nursing/Pharmacy Information
Parenteral: I.V.: Usual maximum concentration: 0.1 mg/mL
Monitor vital signs, blood gases
Stability: **Compatible** in D_5W, $D_{10}W$, and saline solutions
Dosage Forms Injection, as hydrochloride: 25 mg/mL (4 mL)

tolbutamide (tole BYOO ta mide)
U.S. Brand Names Orinase® Diagnostic Injection; Orinase® Oral
Canadian Brand Names Apo-Tolbutamide®; Mobenol®; Novo-Butamide®
Mexican Brand Names Artosin; Diaval; Rastinon
Generic Available Yes
Therapeutic Category Antidiabetic Agent, Oral
Use Adjunct to diet for the management of mild to moderately severe, stable, noninsulin-dependent (type II) diabetes mellitus
Usual Dosage Adults:
Oral: 250-2000 mg/day
I.V. bolus: 20 mg/kg
Dietary Considerations Drug takes 30 minutes to be absorbed and become effective
Nursing/Pharmacy Information
Patients who are anorexic or NPO may need to have their dose held to avoid hypoglycemia
Monitor fasting blood glucose, hemoglobin A_{1c} or fructosamine
Stability: Use parenteral formulation within 1 hour following reconstitution
Dosage Forms Tolbutamide sodium:
Injection, diagnostic: 1 g (20 mL)
Tablet: 250 mg, 500 mg

tolcapone (TOLE ka pone)
U.S. Brand Names Tasmar®
Generic Available No
Therapeutic Category Anti-Parkinson's Agent
Use Adjunct to levodopa and carbidopa for the treatment of signs and symptoms of idiopathic Parkinson's disease
Usual Dosage Adults: Oral: Initial: 100 mg 3 times/day, may increase to 200 mg 3 times/day
Dosage Forms Tablet: 100 mg, 200 mg

♦ **Tolectin®** see tolmetin on page 617
♦ **Tolectin® DS** see tolmetin on page 617
♦ **Tolerex®** see enteral nutritional products on page 233
♦ **Tolinase®** see tolazamide on page 616

tolmetin (TOLE met in)
U.S. Brand Names Tolectin®; Tolectin® DS
Canadian Brand Names Novo-Tolmetin®
Generic Available Yes
Therapeutic Category Analgesic, Non-narcotic; Nonsteroidal Anti-inflammatory Drug (NSAID)
Use Treatment of inflammatory and rheumatoid disorders, including juvenile rheumatoid arthritis
Usual Dosage Oral:
Children ≥2 years: Anti-inflammatory: Initial: 20 mg/kg/day in 3 divided doses, then 15-30 mg/kg/day in 3 divided doses; maximum dose: 30 mg/kg/day
(Continued)

tolmetin *(Continued)*

Adults: 400 mg 3 times/day; usual dose: 600 mg to 1.8 g/day; maximum: 2 g/day

Dietary Considerations Should be administered with food, milk, or antacids to decrease GI adverse effects; food or milk may decrease the extent of oral absorption

Nursing/Pharmacy Information Monitor occult blood loss, CBC, liver enzymes, BUN, serum creatinine, periodic liver function test

Dosage Forms Tolmetin sodium:
Capsule (Tolectin® DS): 400 mg
Tablet (Tolectin®): 200 mg, 600 mg

tolnaftate *(tole NAF tate)*

U.S. Brand Names Absorbine® Antifungal [OTC]; Absorbine® Jock Itch [OTC]; Absorbine Jr.® Antifungal [OTC]; Aftate® [OTC]; Desenex® [OTC]; Genaspor® [OTC]; NP-27® [OTC]; Tinactin® [OTC]; Zeasorb-AF® [OTC]

Canadian Brand Names Pitrex®

Generic Available Yes

Therapeutic Category Antifungal Agent

Use Treatment of tinea pedis, tinea cruris, tinea corporis, tinea manuum caused by *Trichophyton rubrum*, *T. mentagrophytes*, *T. tonsurans*, *M. canis*, *M. audouinii*, and *E. floccosum*; also effective in the treatment of tinea versicolor infections due to *Malassezia furfur*

Usual Dosage Children and Adults: Topical: Wash and dry affected area; apply 1-2 drops of solution or a small amount of cream or powder and rub into the affected areas twice daily for 2-4 weeks

Nursing/Pharmacy Information
Itching, burning, and soreness are usually relieved within 24-72 hours
Monitor resolution of skin infection

Dosage Forms
Aerosol, topical:
Liquid: 1% (59.2 mL, 90 mL, 120 mL)
Powder: 1% (56.7 g, 100 g, 105 g, 150 g)
Cream: 1% (15 g, 30 g)
Gel, topical: 1% (15 g)
Powder, topical: 1% (45 g, 90 g)
Solution, topical: 1% (10 mL)

tolterodine *(tole TER oh dine)*

U.S. Brand Names Detrol™

Generic Available No

Therapeutic Category Anticholinergic Agent

Use Treatment of patients with an overactive bladder with symptoms of urinary frequency, urgency, or urge incontinence

Usual Dosage Adults: Oral: 2 mg twice daily, dose may be reduced to 1 mg twice daily

Dosage Forms Tablet, as tartrate: 1 mg, 2 mg

♦ **Tolu-Sed® DM [OTC]** *see* guaifenesin and dextromethorphan *on page 300*
♦ **Tomocat®** *see* radiological/contrast media (ionic) *on page 539*
♦ **Tonocard®** *see* tocainide *on page 616*
♦ **Tonopaque®** *see* radiological/contrast media (ionic) *on page 539*
♦ **Topactin®** *see* fluocinonide *on page 273*
♦ **Topamax®** *see* topiramate *on page 618*
♦ **Topicort®** *see* desoximetasone *on page 189*
♦ **Topicort®-LP** *see* desoximetasone *on page 189*
♦ **Topicycline® Topical** *see* tetracycline *on page 601*
♦ **Topilene®** *see* betamethasone (topical) *on page 85*

topiramate *(toe PYE ra mate)*

U.S. Brand Names Topamax®

Generic Available No

Therapeutic Category Anticonvulsant

Use Adjunctive therapy for partial onset seizures in adults

Usual Dosage Adults: Oral: 200 mg twice daily (400 mg/day)

Dosage Forms Tablet: 25 mg, 100 mg, 200 mg

♦ **Topisone®** *see* betamethasone (topical) *on page 85*
♦ **Toposar® Injection** *see* etoposide *on page 255*

topotecan (toe poe TEE kan)
Synonyms hycamptamine; SKF 104864
U.S. Brand Names Hycamtin™
Generic Available No
Therapeutic Category Antineoplastic Agent
Use Metastatic carcinoma of the ovary after failure of initial or subsequent chemotherapy; experimentally in childhood solid tumors and leukemia resistant to standard therapies; treatment of small cell lung cancer sensitive disease after failure of first-line chemotherapy (sensitive disease is defined as disease responding to chemotherapy but subsequently progressing at least 60 days or at least 90 days after chemotherapy)
Usual Dosage
Children: A phase I study in pediatric patients by CCSG determined the recommended phase II dose to be 5.5 mg/m^2 as a 24-hour continuous infusion
Adults: Most phase II studies currently utilize topotecan at 1.5-2.0 mg/m^2/day for 5 days, repeated every 21-28 days. Alternative dosing regimens evaluated in phase I studies have included 21-day continuous infusion (recommended phase II dose: 0.53-0.7 mg/m^2/day) and weekly 24-hour infusions (recommended phase II dose: 1.5 mg/m^2/week).
Dose modifications: Dosage modification may be required for toxicity
Dosage Forms Powder for injection, as hydrochloride, lyophilized: 4 mg (base)

- ◆ **Toprol XL**® *see metoprolol on page 410*
- ◆ **Topsyn**® *see fluocinonide on page 273*
- ◆ **TOPV** *see poliovirus vaccine, live, trivalent, oral on page 501*
- ◆ **Toradol**® *see ketorolac tromethamine on page 355*
- ◆ **Torecan**® **Suppository** *(Discontinued) see page 743*

toremifene (TORE em i feen)
Synonyms FC1157a
U.S. Brand Names Fareston®
Generic Available No
Therapeutic Category Antineoplastic Agent
Use Treatment of advanced breast cancer; management of desmoid tumors and endometrial carcinoma
Usual Dosage Refer to individual protocols
Adults: Oral: 60 mg once daily, generally continued until disease progression is observed
Dosage Forms Tablet, as citrate: 60 mg

- ◆ **Tornalate**® *see bitolterol on page 89*

torsemide (TOR se mide)
U.S. Brand Names Demadex®
Generic Available No
Therapeutic Category Diuretic, Loop
Use Management of edema associated with congestive heart failure and hepatic or renal disease; used alone or in combination with antihypertensives in treatment of hypertension
Usual Dosage Adults:
Oral: 5-10 mg once daily; if ineffective, may double dose until desired effect is achieved
I.V.: 10-20 mg/dose repeated in 2 hours as needed with a doubling of the dose with each succeeding dose until desired diuresis is achieved
Continues to be effective in patients with cirrhosis, no apparent change in dose is necessary
Nursing/Pharmacy Information
Administer the I.V. dose slowly over 2 minutes
Monitor renal function, electrolytes, and fluid states closely including weight and I & O
Dosage Forms
Injection: 10 mg/mL (2 mL, 5 mL)
Tablet: 5 mg, 10 mg, 20 mg, 100 mg

- ◆ **Totacillin**® *see ampicillin on page 46*
- ◆ **Totacillin-N**® *(Discontinued) see page 743*
- ◆ **Touro Ex**® *see guaifenesin on page 299*
- ◆ **Touro LA**® *see guaifenesin and pseudoephedrine on page 302*
- ◆ **t-PA** *see alteplase on page 31*
- ◆ **TPGS** *see tocophersolan on page 616*
- ◆ **T-Phyl**® *see theophylline on page 603*

♦ **Trace-4®** *see* trace metals *on page 620*

trace metals (trase MET als)

Synonyms chromium injection; copper injection; manganese injection; molybdenum injection; neonatal trace metals; zinc injection

U.S. Brand Names Chroma-Pak®; Iodopen®; Molypen®; M.T.E.-4®; M.T.E.-5®; M.T.E.-6®; MulTE-PAK-4®; MulTE-PAK-5®; Neotrace-4®; PedTE-PAK-4®; Pedtrace-4®; P.T.E.-4®; P.T.E.-5®; Sele-Pak®; Selepen®; Trace-4®; Zinca-Pak®

Generic Available Yes

Therapeutic Category Trace Element

Use Prevent and correct trace metal deficiencies

Dietary Considerations Decreased absorption of oral zinc when administered with bran products, protein, and phytates

Nursing/Pharmacy Information Persistent diarrhea or excessive gastrointestinal fluid losses from ostomy sites may grossly increase zinc losses

Dosage Forms
Chromium: Injection: 4 mcg/mL, 20 mcg/mL
Copper: Injection: 0.4 mg/mL, 2 mg/mL
Manganese: Injection: 0.1 mg/mL (as chloride or sulfate salt)
Molybdenum: Injection: 25 mcg/mL
Selenium: Injection: 40 mcg/mL
Zinc: Injection: 1 mg/mL (sulfate); 1 mg/mL (chloride); 5 mg/mL (sulfate)

♦ **Tracrium®** *see* atracurium *on page 64*
♦ **Tradol** *see* tramadol *on page 620*
♦ **Tral® (Discontinued)** *see page 743*

tramadol (TRA ma dole)

U.S. Brand Names Ultram®
Mexican Brand Names Tradol
Generic Available No
Therapeutic Category Analgesic, Non-narcotic
Use Relief of moderate to moderately severe pain
Usual Dosage Adults: Oral: 50-100 mg every 4-6 hours, not to exceed 400 mg/day
Nursing/Pharmacy Information Avoid driving or operating machinery until the effect of drug wears off; tramadol has not been fully evaluated for its abuse potential, report cravings to your physician immediately
Dosage Forms Tablet, as hydrochloride: 50 mg

♦ **Trandate®** *see* labetalol *on page 357*

trandolapril (tran DOE la pril)

U.S. Brand Names Mavik®
Generic Available No
Therapeutic Category Angiotensin-Converting Enzyme (ACE) Inhibitor
Use Management of hypertension alone or in combination with other antihypertensive agents
Unlabeled use: As a class, ACE inhibitors are recommended in the treatment of systolic congestive heart failure
Usual Dosage Adults:
Non-Black patients: 0.5-1 mg for those not receiving diuretics; increase dose at 0.5-1 mg increments at 1- to 2-week intervals; maximum dose: 4 mg/day
Black patients: Initiate doses of 1-2 mg; maximum dose: 4 mg/day
Nursing/Pharmacy Information May cause depression in some patients; discontinue if angioedema of the face, extremities, lips, tongue, or glottis occurs; watch for hypotensive effects within 1-3 hours of first dose or new higher dose; patients taking diuretics are at risk for developing hypotension on initial dosing; to prevent this, discontinue diuretics 2-3 days prior to initiating trandolapril; may restart diuretics if blood pressure is not controlled by trandolapril alone
Dosage Forms Tablet: 1 mg, 2 mg, 4 mg

trandolapril and verapamil (tran DOE la pril & ver AP a mil)

U.S. Brand Names Tarka®
Generic Available No
Therapeutic Category Antihypertensive Agent, Combination
Use Combination drug for the treatment of hypertension
Usual Dosage Dose is individualized
Dosage Forms Tablet:
Trandolapril 1 mg and verapamil hydrochloride 240 mg

Trandolapril 2 mg and verapamil hydrochloride 180 mg
Trandolapril 2 mg and verapamil hydrochloride 240 mg
Trandolapril 4 mg and verapamil hydrochloride 240 mg

tranexamic acid (tran eks AM ik AS id)
U.S. Brand Names Cyklokapron®
Generic Available No
Therapeutic Category Antihemophilic Agent
Use Short-term use (2-8 days) in hemophilia patients during and following tooth extraction to reduce or prevent hemorrhage
Usual Dosage Children and Adults: I.V.: 10 mg/kg immediately before surgery, then 25 mg/kg/dose orally 3-4 times/day for 2-8 days
Alternatively:
   Oral: 25 mg/kg 3-4 times/day beginning 1 day prior to surgery
   I.V.: 10 mg/kg 3-4 times/day in patients who are unable to take oral
Nursing/Pharmacy Information
Parenteral: May be administered by direct I.V. injection at a maximum rate of 100 mg/minute; **compatible** with dextrose, saline, and electrolyte solutions
Monitor ophthalmologic exams (baseline and at regular intervals) of chronic therapy
Stability: **Incompatible** with solutions containing penicillin
Dosage Forms
Injection: 100 mg/mL (10 mL)
Tablet: 500 mg

♦ **transamine** see tranylcypromine on page 621
♦ **Transdermal-NTG® Patch** see nitroglycerin on page 444
♦ **Transdermal-V®** see scopolamine on page 560
♦ **Transderm-Nitro® Patch** see nitroglycerin on page 444
♦ **Transderm Scop®** see scopolamine on page 560
♦ **Trans-Plantar®** see salicylic acid on page 557
♦ **Trans-Plantar® Transdermal Patch [OTC]** see salicylic acid on page 557
♦ **Trans-Ver-Sal® Transdermal Patch [OTC]** see salicylic acid on page 557
♦ **Tranxene®** see clorazepate on page 160

tranylcypromine (tran il SIP roe meen)
Synonyms transamine
U.S. Brand Names Parnate®
Generic Available No
Therapeutic Category Antidepressant, Monoamine Oxidase Inhibitor
Use Symptomatic treatment of depressed patients refractory to or intolerant to tricyclic antidepressants or electroconvulsive therapy; has a more rapid onset of therapeutic effect than other MAO inhibitors, but causes more severe hypertensive reactions
Usual Dosage Adults: Oral: 10 mg twice daily, increase by 10 mg increments at 1- to 3-week intervals; maximum: 60 mg/day
Dietary Considerations This medication may cause sudden and severe high blood pressure when administered with food high in tyramine (cheeses, sour cream, yogurt, pickled herring, chicken liver, canned figs, raisins, bananas, avocados, soy sauce, broad bean pods, yeast extracts, meats prepared with tenderizers, and many foods aged to improve flavor, wine (Chianti and hearty red) and beer); small amounts of caffeine may produce irregular heartbeat or high blood pressure and can interact with this medication for up to 2 weeks after stopping its use
Nursing/Pharmacy Information
Assist with ambulation during initiation of therapy; administer second dose before 4 PM to avoid insomnia
Monitor blood pressure, blood glucose
Dosage Forms Tablet, as sulfate: 10 mg

♦ **Trasicor®** see oxprenolol (Canada only) on page 461

trastuzumab (tras TU zoo mab)
U.S. Brand Names Herceptin®
Generic Available No
Therapeutic Category Antineoplastic Agent
Use Treatment of patients with metastatic breast cancer whose tumors overexpress the HER2 protein
Usual Dosage Adults: I.V.:
Loading dose: 4 mg/kg over 90 minutes; do not administer as an I.V. bolus or I.V. push
(Continued)

trastuzumab *(Continued)*

Maintenance dose: 2 mg/kg once weekly (may be infused over 30 minutes if prior infusions are well tolerated)

Dosage Forms Powder for injection: 440 mg

- ◆ **Trasylol®** *see* aprotinin *on page 57*
- ◆ **Travase®** *(Discontinued) see page 743*
- ◆ **Travasol®** *see* enteral nutritional products *on page 233*
- ◆ **Travel Aid®** *see* dimenhydrinate *on page 206*
- ◆ **Travel Tabs** *see* dimenhydrinate *on page 206*
- ◆ **Trazil Ofteno/Ungena** *see* tobramycin *on page 615*

trazodone (TRAZ oh done)

U.S. Brand Names Desyrel®
Generic Available Yes
Therapeutic Category Antidepressant, Triazolopyridine
Use Treatment of depression
Usual Dosage Oral:
   Adolescents: Initial: 25-50 mg/day; increase to 100-150 mg/day in divided doses
   Adults: Initial: 150 mg/day in 3 divided doses (may increase by 50 mg/day every 3-7 days); maximum: 600 mg/day
Dietary Considerations Dosing after meals may decrease lightheadedness and postural hypotension; should be administered with food
Dosage Forms Tablet, as hydrochloride: 50 mg, 100 mg, 150 mg, 300 mg

- ◆ **Trecator®-SC** *see* ethionamide *on page 253*
- ◆ **Tremytoine®** *see* phenytoin *on page 490*
- ◆ **Trendar®** [OTC] *see* ibuprofen *on page 332*
- ◆ **Trental®** *see* pentoxifylline *on page 480*

tretinoin (oral) (TRET i noyn, oral)

Synonyms all-*trans*-retinoic acid
U.S. Brand Names Vesanoid®
Generic Available No
Therapeutic Category Antineoplastic Agent
Use Acute promyelocytic leukemia (APL): Induction of remission in patients with APL, French American British (FAB) classification M3 (including the M3 variant), characterized by the presence of the t(15;17) translocation or the presence of the PML/RARα gene who are refractory to or who have relapsed from anthracycline chemotherapy, or for whom anthracycline-based chemotherapy is contraindicated. Tretinoin is for the induction of remission only. All patients should receive an accepted form of remission consolidation or maintenance therapy for APL after completion of induction therapy with tretinoin.
Usual Dosage Oral:
   Children: There are limited clinical data on the pediatric use of tretinoin. Of 15 pediatric patients (age range: 1-16 years) treated with tretinoin, the incidence of complete remission was 67%. Safety and efficacy in pediatric patients <1 year of age have not been established. Some pediatric patients experience severe headache and pseudotumor cerebri, requiring analgesic treatment and lumbar puncture for relief. Increased caution is recommended. Consider dose reduction in children experiencing serious or intolerable toxicity; however, the efficacy and safety of tretinoin at doses <45 mg/m²/day have not been evaluated.
   Adults: 45 mg/m²/day administered as two evenly divided doses until complete remission is documented. Discontinue therapy 30 days after achievement of complete remission or after 90 days of treatment, whichever occurs first. If after initiation of treatment the presence of the t(15;17) translocation is not confirmed by cytogenetics or by polymerase chain reaction studies and the patient has not responded to tretinoin, consider alternative therapy.

   Note: Tretinoin is for the induction of remission only. Optimal consolidation or maintenance regimens have not been determined. All patients should, therefore, receive a standard consolidation or maintenance chemotherapy regimen for APL after induction therapy with tretinoin unless otherwise contraindicated.
Dosage Forms Capsule: 10 mg

tretinoin (topical) (TRET i noyn, TOP i kal)

Synonyms retinoic acid; vitamin A acid
U.S. Brand Names Retin-A™

Canadian Brand Names Retinova™; Retisol-A®; Stieva-A®; Stieva-A® Forte; Vitinoin™

Mexican Brand Names Stieva-A®; Stieva-A® 0.025%

Generic Available Yes

Therapeutic Category Retinoic Acid Derivative

Use Treatment of acne vulgaris, photodamaged skin, and some skin cancers

Usual Dosage Children >12 years and Adults: Topical: Apply once daily before retiring; if stinging or irritation develop, decrease frequency of application

Dietary Considerations Avoid excessive intake of vitamin A

Nursing/Pharmacy Information Therapeutic effects seen after 2-3 weeks; optimum results may require 3-5 months of continuous therapy

Dosage Forms
Cream:
Retin-A™: 0.025% (20 g, 45 g); 0.05% (20 g, 45 g); 0.1% (20 g, 45 g)
Avita®: 0.025% (20 g, 45 g)
Gel, topical:
Retin-A™: 0.01% (15 g, 45 g); 0.025% (15 g, 45 g)
Retin-A™ Micro: 0.1% (20 g, 45 g)
Liquid, topical (Retin-A™): 0.05% (28 mL)

triacetin (trye a SEE tin)

Synonyms glycerol triacetate

U.S. Brand Names Ony-Clear® Nail

Generic Available No

Therapeutic Category Antifungal Agent

Use Fungistat for athlete's foot and other superficial fungal infections

Usual Dosage Topical: Apply twice daily, cleanse areas with dilute alcohol or mild soap and water before application; continue treatment for 7 days after symptoms have disappeared

Nursing/Pharmacy Information Cover treated area with clean cloth or bandage, avoid contact with rayon fabrics

Dosage Forms
Cream: With cetylpyridinium chloride and chloroxylenol (30 g)
Liquid: With cetylpyridinium chloride and chloroxylenol (30 mL)
Solution: With cetylpyridinium chloride, chloroxylenol, and benzalkonium chloride in an oil base (15 mL)
Spray, aerosol: With cetylpyridinium chloride, chloroxylenol, and benzalkonium chloride (45 mL, 60 mL)

♦ **Triacet™ Topical** see triamcinolone (topical) on page 624
♦ **triacetyloleandomycin** see troleandomycin on page 633
♦ **Triacin-C®** see triprolidine, pseudoephedrine, and codeine on page 632
♦ **triaconazole** see terconazole on page 597
♦ **Triadapin®** see doxepin on page 219
♦ **Triaken** see ceftriaxone on page 126
♦ **Triam-A® Injection** see triamcinolone (systemic) on page 624
♦ **triamcinolone and nystatin** see nystatin and triamcinolone on page 452

triamcinolone (inhalation, nasal) (trye am SIN oh lone)

U.S. Brand Names Nasacort®; Nasacort® AQ

Generic Available Yes

Therapeutic Category Corticosteroid, Topical

Use Symptoms of seasonal and perennial allergic rhinitis

Usual Dosage Children >12 years and Adults: Intranasal: 2 sprays in each nostril once daily; may increase after 4-7 days up to 4 sprays once daily or 1 spray 4 times/day in each nostril

Dosage Forms
Aerosol: Nasal: 55 mcg per actuation (15 mL)
Spray, nasal: 55 mcg per actuation in aqueous base (16.5 g)

triamcinolone (inhalation, oral) (trye am SIN oh lone)

U.S. Brand Names Azmacort™ Oral Inhaler

Generic Available Yes

Therapeutic Category Adrenal Corticosteroid

Use Asthma

Usual Dosage
Children 6-12 years:
Inhalation: 1-2 inhalations 3-4 times/day, not to exceed 12 inhalations/day
Children >12 years and Adults:
Oral inhalation: 2 inhalations 3-4 times/day, not to exceed 16 inhalations/day
(Continued)

triamcinolone (inhalation, oral) *(Continued)*

Nursing/Pharmacy Information Rinse mouth and throat after oral inhalation use to prevent candidiasis

Dosage Forms Aerosol: Oral inhalation: 100 mcg/metered spray (2 oz)

triamcinolone (systemic) (trye am SIN oh lone)

U.S. Brand Names Amcort® Injection; Aristocort® Forte Injection; Aristocort® Intralesional Injection; Aristocort® Oral; Aristospan® Intra-articular Injection; Aristospan® Intralesional Injection; Atolone® Oral; Kenacort® Oral; Kenaject® Injection; Kenalog® Injection; Tac™-3 Injection; Tac™-40 Injection; Triam-A® Injection; Triam Forte® Injection; Triamonide® Injection; Tri-Kort® Injection; Trilog® Injection; Trilone® Injection; Trisoject® Injection

Mexican Brand Names Kenacort®; Ledercort; Zamacort®

Generic Available Yes

Therapeutic Category Adrenal Corticosteroid

Use Severe inflammation or immunosuppression

Usual Dosage In general, single I.M. dose of 4-7 times oral dose will control patient from 4-7 days up to 3-4 weeks

Children 6-12 years:
  I.M.: Acetonide or hexacetonide: 0.03-0.2 mg/kg at 1- to 7-day intervals
Children >12 years and Adults:
  Oral: 4-100 mg/day
  I.M.: Acetonide or hexacetonide: 60 mg (of 40 mg/mL), additional 20-100 mg doses (usual: 40-80 mg) may be administered when signs and symptoms recur, best at 6-week intervals to minimize HPA suppression
  Intra-articularly, intrasynovially, intralesionally: 2.5-40 mg as diacetate salt or acetonide salt, dose may be repeated when signs and symptoms recur
  Intra-articularly: Hexacetonide: 2-20 mg every 3-4 weeks as hexacetonide salt
  Intralesional (use 10 mg/mL): Diacetate or acetonide: 1 mg/injection site, may be repeated one or more times/week depending upon patients response; maximum; 30 mg at any one time; may use multiple injections if they are more than 1 cm apart
  Intra-articular, intrasynovial, and soft-tissue injection (use 10 mg/mL or 40 mg/mL): Diacetate or acetonide: 2.5-40 mg depending upon location, size of joints, and degree of inflammation; repeat when signs and symptoms recur
  Sublesionally (as acetonide): Up to 1 mg per injection site and may be repeated one or more times weekly; multiple sites may be injected if they are 1 cm or more apart, not to exceed 30 mg

Dietary Considerations May be administered with food to decrease GI distress

Nursing/Pharmacy Information Avoid S.C. use

Dosage Forms
Syrup: 2 mg/5 mL (120 mL); 4 mg/5 mL (120 mL)
Tablet: 1 mg, 2 mg, 4 mg, 8 mg

Triamcinolone acetonide:
  Injection: 10 mg/mL (5 mL); 40 mg/mL (1 mL, 5 mL, 10 mL)

Triamcinolone diacetate: Injection: 25 mg/mL (5 mL); 40 mg/mL (1 mL, 5 mL, 10 mL)

Triamcinolone hexacetonide: Injection: 5 mg/mL (5 mL); 20 mg/mL (1 mL, 5 mL)

triamcinolone (topical) (trye am SIN oh lone)

U.S. Brand Names Aristocort® A Topical; Aristocort® Topical; Delta-Tritex® Topical; Flutex® Topical; Kenalog® in Orabase®; Kenalog® Topical; Kenonel® Topical; Triacet™ Topical

Generic Available Yes

Therapeutic Category Corticosteroid, Topical

Use Severe inflammation or immunosuppression; nasal spray for symptoms of seasonal and perennial allergic rhinitis

Usual Dosage Children >12 years and Adults: Topical: Apply a thin film 2-3 times/day

Dietary Considerations May be administered with food to decrease GI distress

Nursing/Pharmacy Information Avoid topical application on face; for topical use do not occlude area unless directed

Dosage Forms
Ointment, oral: 0.1% (5 g)

Aerosol, topical: 0.2 mg/2 second spray (23 g, 63 g)
Cream: 0.025% (15 g, 60 g, 80 g, 240 g, 454 g); 0.1% (15 g, 30 g, 60 g, 80 g, 90 g, 120 g, 240 g); 0.5% (15 g, 20 g, 30 g, 240 g)
Lotion: 0.025% (60 mL); 0.1% (15 mL, 60 mL)
Ointment, topical: 0.025% (15 g, 30 g, 60 g, 80 g, 120 g, 454 g); 0.1% (15 g, 30 g, 60 g, 80 g, 120 g, 240 g, 454 g); 0.5% (15 g, 20 g, 30 g, 240 g)

- ♦ **Triam Forte® Injection** *see* triamcinolone (systemic) *on page 624*
- ♦ **Triaminic® Allergy Tablet [OTC]** *see* chlorpheniramine and phenylpropanolamine *on page 139*
- ♦ **Triaminic® AM Decongestant Formula [OTC]** *see* pseudoephedrine *on page 530*
- ♦ **Triaminic® Cold Tablet [OTC]** *see* chlorpheniramine and phenylpropanolamine *on page 139*
- ♦ **Triaminic DM** *see* dextromethorphan *on page 194*
- ♦ **Triaminic® Expectorant [OTC]** *see* guaifenesin and phenylpropanolamine *on page 301*
- ♦ **Triaminicol® Multi-Symptom Cold Syrup [OTC]** *see* chlorpheniramine, phenylpropanolamine, and dextromethorphan *on page 143*
- ♦ **Triaminic® Oral Infant Drops** *see* pheniramine, phenylpropanolamine, and pyrilamine *on page 485*
- ♦ **Triaminic® Syrup [OTC]** *see* chlorpheniramine and phenylpropanolamine *on page 139*
- ♦ **Triamonide® Injection** *see* triamcinolone (systemic) *on page 624*

triamterene (trye AM ter een)
U.S. Brand Names Dyrenium®
Generic Available No
Therapeutic Category Diuretic, Potassium Sparing
Use Alone or in combination with other diuretics to treat edema and hypertension; decreases potassium excretion caused by kaliuretic diuretics
Usual Dosage Oral:
Children: 2-4 mg/kg/day in 1-2 divided doses; maximum: 300 mg/day
Adults: 100-300 mg/day in 1-2 divided doses; maximum: 300 mg/day
Dietary Considerations This diuretic does not cause you to lose potassium; because salt substitutes and low-salt milk may contain potassium, do not use these products without checking with your physician, too much potassium can be as harmful as too little; may be administered with food
Nursing/Pharmacy Information Monitor serum electrolytes, liver function tests; observe for hyperkalemia in elderly patients and in patients with renal insufficiency; assess weight and I & O daily to determine weight loss
Dosage Forms Capsule: 50 mg, 100 mg

- ♦ **triamterene and hydrochlorothiazide** *see* hydrochlorothiazide and triamterene *on page 318*
- ♦ **Triapin®** *see* butalbital compound and acetaminophen *on page 99*
- ♦ **Triavil®** *see* amitriptyline and perphenazine *on page 40*

triazolam (trye AY zoe lam)
U.S. Brand Names Halcion®
Canadian Brand Names Apo®-Triazo; Gen-Triazolam®; Novo-Triolam®; Nu-Triazo®
Generic Available Yes
Therapeutic Category Benzodiazepine
Controlled Substance C-IV
Use Short-term treatment of insomnia
Usual Dosage Oral (onset of action is rapid, patient should be in bed when taking medication):
Children <18 years: Dosage not established
Adults: 0.125-0.25 mg at bedtime
Dietary Considerations Food may decrease the rate of absorption
Nursing/Pharmacy Information
Provide safety measures (ie, side rails, night light, call button); remove smoking materials from area; supervise ambulation
Monitor respiratory and cardiovascular status
Dosage Forms Tablet: 0.125 mg, 0.25 mg

- ♦ **Tribakin** *see* co-trimoxazole *on page 170*
- ♦ **Triban®** *see* trimethobenzamide *on page 629*
- ♦ **tribavirin** *see* ribavirin *on page 547*
- ♦ **Tri-Chlor®** *see* trichloroacetic acid *on page 626*

trichlormethiazide (trye klor meth EYE a zide)
U.S. Brand Names Metahydrin®; Naqua®
Generic Available Yes
Therapeutic Category Diuretic, Thiazide
Use Management of mild to moderate hypertension; treatment of edema in congestive heart failure and nephrotic syndrome
Usual Dosage Oral:
Children >6 months: 0.07 mg/kg/24 hours or 2 mg/m^2/24 hours
Adults: 1-4 mg/day
Dietary Considerations May be administered with food or milk
Nursing/Pharmacy Information Administer early in day to avoid nocturia; administer the last dose of multiple doses no later than 6 PM unless instructed otherwise. A few people who take this medication become more sensitive to sunlight and may experience skin rash, redness, itching, or severe sunburn, especially if sun block ≥SPF 15 is not used on exposed skin areas.
Dosage Forms Tablet: 2 mg, 4 mg

♦ **trichloroacetaldehyde monohydrate** see chloral hydrate on page 132

trichloroacetic acid (trye klor oh a SEE tik AS id)
U.S. Brand Names Tri-Chlor®
Generic Available Yes
Therapeutic Category Keratolytic Agent
Use Debride callous tissue
Usual Dosage Apply to verruca, cover with bandage for 5-6 days, remove verruca, reapply as needed
Dosage Forms Liquid: 80% (15 mL)

Trichophyton skin test (trye koe FYE ton skin test)
U.S. Brand Names Dermatophytin®
Generic Available No
Therapeutic Category Diagnostic Agent
Use Assess cell-mediated immunity
Usual Dosage 0.1 mL intradermally, examine reaction site in 24-48 hours; induration of ≥5 mm in diameter is a positive reaction
Nursing/Pharmacy Information
Administer by intradermal injection into flexor surface of forearm using a tuberculin syringe with a $^3/_8$" to $^1/_2$" 26- or 27-gauge needle; do not administer I.V.
Stability: Refrigerate at 2°C to 8°C (36°F to 46°F)
Dosage Forms Injection:
Diluted: 1:30 V/V (5 mL)
Undiluted: 5 mL

♦ **Tri-Clear® Expectorant [OTC]** see guaifenesin and phenylpropanolamine on page 301
♦ **TriCor™** see fenofibrate on page 261
♦ **Tridesilon® Topical** see desonide on page 188

tridihexethyl (trye dye heks ETH il)
U.S. Brand Names Pathilon®
Generic Available No
Therapeutic Category Anticholinergic Agent
Use Adjunctive therapy in peptic ulcer treatment
Usual Dosage Adults: Oral: 1-2 tablets 3-4 times/day before meals and 2 tablets at bedtime
Dietary Considerations Should be administered 30 minutes before meals and at bedtime
Nursing/Pharmacy Information Maintain good oral hygiene habits, because lack of saliva may increase chance of cavities; observe caution while driving or performing other tasks requiring alertness, as drug may cause drowsiness, dizziness, or blurred vision; notify physician if skin rash, flushing or eye pain occurs; or if difficulty in urinating, constipation, or sensitivity to light becomes severe or persists
Dosage Forms Tablet, as chloride: 25 mg

♦ **Tridil® Injection** see nitroglycerin on page 444
♦ **Tridione® Oral** see trimethadione on page 629
♦ **Tridione® Suppository (Discontinued)** see page 743

trientine (TRYE en teen)

U.S. Brand Names Syprine®
Generic Available No
Therapeutic Category Chelating Agent
Use Treatment of Wilson's disease in patients intolerant to penicillamine
Usual Dosage Oral (administer on an empty stomach):
Children <12 years: 500-750 mg/day in divided doses 2-4 times/day; maximum: 1.5 g/day
Adults: 750-1250 mg/day in divided doses 2-4 times/day; maximum daily dose: 2 g
Dietary Considerations Should be administered 1 hour before or 2 hours after meals and at least 1 hour apart from any drug, food, or milk
Nursing/Pharmacy Information Do not chew capsule, swallow whole followed by a full glass of water; notify physician of any fever or skin changes; any skin exposed to the contents of a capsule should be promptly washed with water
Dosage Forms Capsule, as hydrochloride: 250 mg

triethanolamine polypeptide oleate-condensate
(trye eth a NOLE a meen pol i PEP tide OH lee ate-KON den sate)
U.S. Brand Names Cerumenex® Otic
Generic Available No
Therapeutic Category Otic Agent, Cerumenolytic
Use Removal of ear wax (cerumen)
Usual Dosage Children and Adults: Otic: Fill ear canal, insert cotton plug; allow to remain 15-30 minutes; flush ear with lukewarm water
Nursing/Pharmacy Information
Avoid undue exposure of the drug to the periaural skin
Monitor hearing before and after instillation of medication
Dosage Forms Solution, otic: 6 mL, 12 mL

triethanolamine salicylate (trye eth a NOLE a meen sa LIS i late)
U.S. Brand Names Myoflex® [OTC]; Sportscreme® [OTC]
Generic Available No
Therapeutic Category Analgesic, Topical
Use Relief of pain of muscular aches, rheumatism, neuralgia, sprains, arthritis on intact skin
Usual Dosage Topical: Apply to area as needed
Dosage Forms Cream: 10% in a nongreasy base

♦ **triethylenethiophosphoramide** *see* thiotepa *on page 608*

♦ **Trifed-C®** *see* triprolidine, pseudoephedrine, and codeine *on page 632*

trifluoperazine (trye floo oh PER a zeen)

U.S. Brand Names Stelazine®
Mexican Brand Names Flupazine
Generic Available Yes
Therapeutic Category Phenothiazine Derivative
Use Treatment of psychoses and management of anxiety
Usual Dosage
Children 6-12 years: Psychoses:
Oral: Hospitalized or well supervised patients: Initial dose: 1 mg 1-2 times/day, gradually increase until symptoms are controlled or adverse effects become troublesome; maximum: 15 mg/day
I.M.: 1 mg twice daily
Adults:
Psychoses:
Outpatients: Oral: 1-2 mg twice daily
Hospitalized or well supervised patients: Initial dose: 2-5 mg twice daily with optimum response in the 15-20 mg/day range; do not exceed 40 mg/day
I.M.: 1-2 mg every 4-6 hours as needed up to 10 mg/24 hours maximum
Nonpsychotic anxiety: Oral: 1-2 mg twice daily; maximum: 6 mg/day; therapy for anxiety should not exceed 12 weeks; do not exceed 6 mg/day for longer than 12 weeks when treating anxiety; agitation, jitteriness or insomnia may be confused with original neurotic or psychotic symptoms
Dietary Considerations May be administered with food to decrease GI distress
(Continued)

trifluoperazine *(Continued)*

Nursing/Pharmacy Information

Administer I.M. injection deep in upper outer quadrant of buttock; watch for hypotension when administering I.M. or I.V.; dilute the oral concentrate with water or juice before administration; avoid skin contact with oral suspension or solution; may cause contact dermatitis; administer the I.V. dose slowly over 2 minutes

Monitor orthostatic blood pressures 3-5 days after initiation of therapy or a dose increase; observe for tremor and abnormal movement or posturing (extrapyramidal symptoms)

Stability: Store injection at room temperature; protect from heat and from freezing; use only clear or slightly yellow solutions

Dosage Forms Trifluoperazine hydrochloride:

Concentrate, oral: 10 mg/mL (60 mL)
Injection: 2 mg/mL (10 mL)
Tablet: 1 mg, 2 mg, 5 mg, 10 mg

♦ **trifluorothymidine** *see* trifluridine *on page 628*

triflupromazine *(trye floo PROE ma zeen)*

U.S. Brand Names Vesprin®
Generic Available No
Therapeutic Category Phenothiazine Derivative
Use Treatment of psychoses, nausea, vomiting, and intractable hiccups
Usual Dosage
Children: I.M.: 0.2-0.25 mg/kg
Adults:
I.M.: 5-15 mg every 4 hours
I.V.: 1 mg
Dietary Considerations Should be administered with food, milk, or water
Dosage Forms Injection, as hydrochloride: 20 mg/mL (1 mL)

trifluridine *(trye FLURE i deen)*

Synonyms f_3t; trifluorothymidine
U.S. Brand Names Viroptic® Ophthalmic
Generic Available No
Therapeutic Category Antiviral Agent
Use Treatment of primary keratoconjunctivitis and recurrent epithelial keratitis caused by herpes simplex virus types I and II
Usual Dosage Adults: Ophthalmic: Instill 1 drop into affected eye every 2 hours while awake, to a maximum of 9 drops/day, until re-epithelialization of corneal ulcer occurs; then use 1 drop every 4 hours for another 7 days; do **not** exceed 21 days of treatment

Nursing/Pharmacy Information

Monitor ophthalmologic exam (test for corneal staining with fluorescein or rose bengal)

Stability: Refrigerate at 2°C to 8°C (36°F to 46°F); storage at room temperature may result in a solution altered pH which could result in ocular discomfort upon administration and/or decreased potency

Dosage Forms Solution, ophthalmic: 1% (7.5 mL)

♦ **triglycerides, medium chain** *see* medium chain triglycerides *on page 388*
♦ **Trihexy®** *see* trihexyphenidyl *on page 628*
♦ **Trihexyphen®** *see* trihexyphenidyl *on page 628*

trihexyphenidyl *(trye heks ee FEN i dil)*

Synonyms benzhexol
U.S. Brand Names Artane®; Trihexy®
Canadian Brand Names Apo®-Trihex; Novo-Hexidyl®; PMS-Trihexyphenidyl; Trihexyphen®
Mexican Brand Names Hipokinon
Generic Available Yes: Tablet
Therapeutic Category Anticholinergic Agent; Anti-Parkinson's Agent
Use Adjunctive treatment of Parkinson's disease; also used in treatment of drug-induced extrapyramidal effects and acute dystonic reactions
Usual Dosage Oral:
Parkinsonism: Initial: Administer 1-2 mg the first day; increase by 2 mg increments at intervals of 3-5 days, until a total of 6-10 mg is administered daily. Many patients derive maximum benefit from a total daily dose of 6-10 mg; however, postencephalitic patients may require a total daily dose of 12-15 mg in 3-4 divided doses

Concomitant use with levodopa: 3-6 mg/day in divided doses is usually adequate

Drug-induced extrapyramidal disorders: Start with a single 1 mg dose; daily dosage usually ranges between 5-15 mg in 3-4 divided doses

Dietary Considerations Tolerated best if administered in 3 daily doses and with food; high doses may be divided into 4 doses, at meal times and at bedtime

Nursing/Pharmacy Information Monitor IOP and gonioscopic evaluations should be performed periodically

Dosage Forms Trihexyphenidyl hydrochloride:
Capsule, sustained release: 5 mg
Elixir: 2 mg/5 mL (480 mL)
Tablet: 2 mg, 5 mg

♦ **Tri-Immunol®** *see* diphtheria, tetanus toxoids, and whole-cell pertussis vaccine *on page 211*

♦ **Tri-K®** *see* potassium acetate, potassium bicarbonate, and potassium citrate *on page 505*

♦ **TriKacide®** *see* metronidazole *on page 411*

♦ **Tri-Kort® Injection** *see* triamcinolone (systemic) *on page 624*

♦ **Trilafon®** *see* perphenazine *on page 482*

♦ **Tri-Levlen®** *see* ethinyl estradiol and levonorgestrel *on page 250*

♦ **Trilisate®** *see* choline magnesium trisalicylate *on page 147*

♦ **Trilog® Injection** *see* triamcinolone (systemic) *on page 624*

♦ **Trilone® Injection** *see* triamcinolone (systemic) *on page 624*

♦ **Trimazide®** *see* trimethobenzamide *on page 629*

trimebutine *(Canada only)* (trye me BYOO teen)

Canadian Brand Names Modulon®
Generic Available No
Therapeutic Category Antispasmodic Agent, Gastrointestinal
Use For the treatment and relief of symptoms associated with the irritable bowel syndrome (spastic colon). In postoperative paralytic ileus in order to accelerate the resumption of the intestinal transit following abdominal surgery.
Usual Dosage Adults:
Parenteral: Dosage should be individually tailored according to response, but the total parenteral daily dose should not exceed 300 mg. The usual adult dose is 50-100 mg 3 times daily, administered as an I.M. injection, as a 3 minute I.V. injection, or as a 60 minute I.V. infusion (in D_5W or NS), until resumption of intestinal motility.
Tablets: Up to 600 mg daily in divided doses. It may be administered as two 100 mg tablets 3 times daily before meals or one 200 mg tablet 3 times daily before meals.
Dosage Forms
Injection, as maleate: 10 mg/mL (5 mL)
Tablet, as maleate: 100 mg, 200 mg

♦ **Trimesuxol** *see* co-trimoxazole *on page 170*

trimethadione (trye meth a DYE one)

Synonyms troxidone
U.S. Brand Names Tridione® Oral
Generic Available No
Therapeutic Category Anticonvulsant
Use Control absence (petit mal) seizures refractory to other drugs
Usual Dosage Oral:
Children: Initial: 25-50 mg/kg/24 hours in 3-4 equally divided doses every 6-8 hours
Adults: Initial: 900 mg/day in 3-4 equally divided doses, increase by 300 mg/day at weekly intervals until therapeutic results or toxic symptoms appear
Nursing/Pharmacy Information Caution patient that even minor skin rash and signs of infection or bleeding must be reported to the physician
Dosage Forms
Capsule: 300 mg
Tablet, chewable: 150 mg

trimethobenzamide (trye meth oh BEN za mide)

U.S. Brand Names Arrestin®; Pediatric Triban®; Tebamide®; T-Gen®; Ticon®; Tigan®; Triban®; Trimazide®
Generic Available No
Therapeutic Category Anticholinergic Agent; Antiemetic
(Continued)

trimethobenzamide *(Continued)*

Use Control of nausea and vomiting (especially for long term antiemetic therapy)

Usual Dosage Rectal use: Contraindicated in neonates and premature infants

Children:

Oral, rectal: 15-20 mg/kg/day or 400-500 mg/m^2/day divided into 3-4 doses

I.M.: Not recommended

Adults:

Oral: 250 mg 3-4 times/day

I.M., rectal: 200 mg 3-4 times/day

Nursing/Pharmacy Information Stability: Store injection at room temperature; protect from heat and from freezing; use only clear solutions

Dosage Forms Trimethobenzamide hydrochloride:

Capsule: 100 mg, 250 mg

Injection: 100 mg/mL (2 mL, 20 mL)

Suppository, rectal: 100 mg, 200 mg

trimethoprim *(trye METH oh prim)*

Synonyms TMP

U.S. Brand Names Proloprim®; Trimpex®

Generic Available Yes

Therapeutic Category Antibiotic, Miscellaneous

Use Treatment and prophylaxis of urinary tract infections; in combination with other agents for treatment of *Pneumocystis carinii* pneumonia

Usual Dosage Adults: Oral: 100 mg every 12 hours or 200 mg every 24 hours

Dietary Considerations May be administered with food; may cause folic acid deficiency, supplements may be needed

Nursing/Pharmacy Information Monitor for signs of bone marrow suppression such as fever, sore throat, or bleeding; tablets can be crushed

Dosage Forms Tablet: 100 mg, 200 mg

trimethoprim and polymyxin B

(trye METH oh prim & pol i MIKS in bee)

Synonyms polymyxin B and trimethoprim

U.S. Brand Names Polytrim® Ophthalmic

Generic Available No

Therapeutic Category Antibiotic, Ophthalmic

Use Treatment of surface ocular bacterial conjunctivitis and blepharoconjunctivitis

Usual Dosage Ophthalmic: Instill 1-2 drops in eye(s) every 4-6 hours

Nursing/Pharmacy Information Avoid contamination of the applicator tip; if redness, swelling, pain, or irritation persists, contact your physician

Dosage Forms Solution, ophthalmic: Trimethoprim sulfate 1 mg and polymyxin B sulfate 10,000 units per mL (10 mL)

♦ **trimethoprim and sulfamethoxazole** *see* co-trimoxazole *on page 170*

♦ **trimethylpsoralen** *see* trioxsalen *on page 631*

♦ **Trimetoger** *see* co-trimoxazole *on page 170*

♦ **Trimetox** *see* co-trimoxazole *on page 170*

trimetrexate glucuronate *(tri me TREKS ate gloo KYOOR oh nate)*

U.S. Brand Names Neutrexin®

Generic Available No

Therapeutic Category Antibiotic, Miscellaneous

Use Alternative therapy for the treatment of moderate-to-severe *Pneumocystis carinii* pneumonia (PCP) in immunocompromised patients, including patients with acquired immunodeficiency syndrome (AIDS), who are intolerant of, or are refractory to, co-trimoxazole therapy or for whom co-trimoxazole is contraindicated

Usual Dosage Adults: I.V.: 45 mg/m^2 once daily over 60 minutes for 21 days; it is necessary to reduce the dose in patients with liver dysfunction, although no specific recommendations exist

Dosage Forms Powder for injection: 25 mg

trimipramine *(trye MI pra meen)*

U.S. Brand Names Surmontil®

Canadian Brand Names Apo-Trimip®; Novo-Tripramine; Nu-Trimipramine®; Rhotrimine®

Generic Available Yes

Therapeutic Category Antidepressant, Tricyclic (Tertiary Amine)

Use Treatment of various forms of depression, often in conjunction with psycho-therapy

Usual Dosage Oral: 50-150 mg/day as a single bedtime dose

Nursing/Pharmacy Information Monitor blood pressure and pulse rate prior to and during initial therapy; evaluate mental status; monitor weight

Dosage Forms Capsule, as maleate: 25 mg, 50 mg, 100 mg

♦ **Trimox®** see amoxicillin on page 43

♦ **Trimox® 500 mg (Discontinued)** see page 743

♦ **Trimpex®** see trimethoprim on page 630

♦ **Trimzol** see co-trimoxazole on page 170

♦ **Trinalin®** see azatadine and pseudoephedrine on page 67

♦ **Tri-Nefrin® Extra Strength Tablet [OTC]** see chlorpheniramine and phenylpropanolamine on page 139

♦ **Tri-Norinyl®** see ethinyl estradiol and norethindrone on page 250

♦ **Triofed® Syrup [OTC]** see triprolidine and pseudoephedrine on page 632

♦ **Triostat™ Injection** see liothyronine on page 371

♦ **Triotann® Tablet** see chlorpheniramine, pyrilamine, and phenylephrine on page 144

trioxsalen (trye OKS a len)

Synonyms trimethylpsoralen

U.S. Brand Names Trisoralen®

Generic Available No

Therapeutic Category Psoralen

Use In conjunction with controlled exposure to ultraviolet light or sunlight for repigmentation of idiopathic vitiligo; increasing tolerance to sunlight with albinism; enhance pigmentation

Usual Dosage Children >12 years and Adults: Oral: 10 mg/day as a single dose, 2-4 hours before controlled exposure to UVA or sunlight

Nursing/Pharmacy Information To minimize gastric discomfort, tablets may be administered with milk or after a meal; wear sunglasses during exposure and a light-screening lipstick; do not exceed dose or exposure duration

Dosage Forms Tablet: 5 mg

♦ **Tripedia®** see diphtheria, tetanus toxoids, and acellular pertussis vaccine on page 210

tripelennamine (tri pel EN a meen)

U.S. Brand Names PBZ®; PBZ-SR®

Generic Available Yes

Therapeutic Category Antihistamine

Use Perennial and seasonal allergic rhinitis and other allergic symptoms including urticaria

Usual Dosage Oral:

Infants and Children: 5 mg/kg/day in 4-6 divided doses, up to 300 mg/day maximum

Adults: 25-50 mg every 4-6 hours, extended release tablets 100 mg morning and evening up to 100 mg every 8 hours

Nursing/Pharmacy Information Raise bed rails, institute safety measures, assist with ambulation

Dosage Forms Tripelennamine hydrochloride:

Tablet: 25 mg, 50 mg

Tablet, extended release: 100 mg

♦ **Triphasil®** see ethinyl estradiol and levonorgestrel on page 250

♦ **Tri-Phen-Chlor®** see chlorpheniramine, phenyltoloxamine, phenylpropanolamine, and phenylephrine on page 143

♦ **Triphenyl® Expectorant [OTC]** see guaifenesin and phenylpropanolamine on page 301

♦ **Triphenyl® Syrup [OTC]** see chlorpheniramine and phenylpropanolamine on page 139

♦ **Triple Antibiotic® Topical** see bacitracin, neomycin, and polymyxin B on page 71

♦ **triple sulfa** see sulfabenzamide, sulfacetamide, and sulfathiazole on page 584

♦ **Triple X® Liquid [OTC]** see pyrethrins and piperonyl butoxide on page 533

♦ **Triposed® Syrup [OTC]** see triprolidine and pseudoephedrine on page 632

♦ **Triposed® Tablet [OTC]** see triprolidine and pseudoephedrine on page 632

triprolidine and pseudoephedrine
(trye PROE li deen & soo doe e FED rin)

Synonyms pseudoephedrine and triprolidine

U.S. Brand Names Actagen® Syrup [OTC]; Actagen® Tablet [OTC]; Allercon® Tablet [OTC]; Allerfrin® Syrup [OTC]; Allerfrin® Tablet [OTC]; Allerphed® Syrup [OTC]; Aprodine® Syrup [OTC]; Aprodine® Tablet [OTC]; Cenafed® Plus Tablet [OTC]; Genac® Tablet [OTC]; Silafed® Syrup [OTC]; Triofed® Syrup [OTC]; Triposed® Syrup [OTC]; Triposed® Tablet [OTC]

Generic Available Yes

Therapeutic Category Antihistamine/Decongestant Combination

Use Temporary relief of nasal congestion, running nose, sneezing, itching of nose or throat and itchy, watery eyes due to common cold, hay fever or other upper respiratory allergies

Usual Dosage May dose according to **pseudoephedrine** component (4 mg/kg/day in divided doses 3-4 times/day) Oral:

Children:
4 months to 2 years: 1.25 mL 3-4 times/day
2-4 years: 2.5 mL 3-4 times/day
4-6 years: 3.75 mL 3-4 times/day
6-12 years: 5 mL or $\frac{1}{2}$ tablet 3-4 times/day, not to exceed 2 tablets/day
Children >12 years and Adults: 10 mL or 1 tablet 3-4 times/day, not to exceed 4 tablets/day

Dietary Considerations Should be administered with food or milk

Nursing/Pharmacy Information Do not crush extended release capsule

Dosage Forms
Capsule: Triprolidine hydrochloride 2.5 mg and pseudoephedrine hydrochloride 60 mg
Extended release: Triprolidine hydrochloride 5 mg and pseudoephedrine hydrochloride 120 mg
Syrup: Triprolidine hydrochloride 1.25 mg and pseudoephedrine hydrochloride 30 mg per 5 mL
Tablet: Triprolidine hydrochloride 2.5 mg and pseudoephedrine hydrochloride 60 mg

triprolidine, pseudoephedrine, and codeine
(trye PROE li deen, soo doe e FED rin, & KOE deen)

U.S. Brand Names Actagen-C®; Allerfrin® w/Codeine; Aprodine® w/C; Triacin-C®; Trifed-C®

Generic Available Yes

Therapeutic Category Antihistamine/Decongestant/Antitussive

Controlled Substance C-V

Use Symptomatic relief of cough

Usual Dosage Oral:
Children:
2-6 years: 2.5 mL 4 times/day
7-12 years: 5 mL 4 times/day
Children >12 years and Adults: 10 mL 4 times/day

Nursing/Pharmacy Information Contains 4.3% alcohol

Dosage Forms Syrup: Triprolidine hydrochloride 1.25 mg, pseudoephedrine hydrochloride 30 mg, and codeine phosphate 10 mg per 5 mL with alcohol 4.3%

- ♦ **Triptil®** *see* protriptyline *on page 529*
- ♦ **TripTone® Caplets® [OTC]** *see* dimenhydrinate *on page 206*
- ♦ **tris buffer** *see* tromethamine *on page 633*
- ♦ **tris(hydroxymethyl)aminomethane** *see* tromethamine *on page 633*
- ♦ **Trisoject® Injection** *see* triamcinolone (systemic) *on page 624*
- ♦ **Trisoralen®** *see* trioxsalen *on page 631*
- ♦ **Tri-Statin® II Topical** *see* nystatin and triamcinolone *on page 452*
- ♦ **Trisulfa®** *see* co-trimoxazole *on page 170*
- ♦ **trisulfapyrimidines** *see* sulfadiazine, sulfamethazine, and sulfamerazine *on page 586*
- ♦ **Trisulfa-S®** *see* co-trimoxazole *on page 170*
- ♦ **Tritace** *see* ramipril *on page 541*
- ♦ **Tri-Tannate Plus®** *see* chlorpheniramine, ephedrine, phenylephrine, and carbetapentane *on page 141*
- ♦ **Tri-Tannate® Tablet** *see* chlorpheniramine, pyrilamine, and phenylephrine *on page 144*
- ♦ **Tritec®** *see* ranitidine bismuth citrate *on page 541*

- **Tri-Vi-Flor®** *see* vitamin, multiple (pediatric) *on page 654*
- **Tri-Vi-Sol® [OTC]** *see* vitamin, multiple (pediatric) *on page 654*
- **Trixilem** *see* daunorubicin hydrochloride *on page 183*
- **Trobicin®** *see* spectinomycin *on page 578*
- **Trocaine® [OTC]** *see* benzocaine *on page 79*
- **Trocal® [OTC]** *see* dextromethorphan *on page 194*
- **Trofan®** *(Discontinued)* see page 743
- **Trofan DS®** *(Discontinued)* see page 743

troglitazone (TROE gli to zone)
U.S. Brand Names Rezulin®
Generic Available No
Therapeutic Category Thiazolidinedione Derivative
Use Troglitazone is indicated for the following:
To improve glycemic control in patients with type 2 diabetes mellitus as an adjunct to diet and exercise in combination (and not substituted for):
- sulfonylureas in patients who are not adequately controlled with a sulfonylurea alone, or
- a sulfonylurea together with metformin for patients who are not adequately controlled with the combination of a sulfonylurea and metformin or
- insulin in patients who are not adequately controlled with insulin alone
Troglitazone is not indicated as initial therapy or monotherapy in patients with type 2 diabetes
Usual Dosage Adults: Oral: 200 mg once daily with a meal; for patients on insulin therapy continue current insulin dose; dose may be increased to 400 mg/day after 2-4 weeks in those who are not responding adequately; maximum recommended dose: 600 mg/day. It is recommended that the insulin dose should be reduced by 10% to 25% when fasting plasma glucose concentrations decrease to <120 mg/dL in those patients receiving concomitant insulin. Combination therapy with metformin and sulfonylureas: 400 mg once daily.
Nursing/Pharmacy Information Patients taking this drug should be monitored more frequently for signs of injury to the liver; the increased monitoring of patients taking this drug is designed to detect those few patients in whom use of the drug can lead to liver damage; liver enzymes should be measured at the start of therapy, every month for the first 6 months of treatment, every other month for the next 6 months, and periodically thereafter; in addition, liver function tests should be performed on any patient who develops symptoms of liver dysfunction, such as nausea, vomiting, fatigue, loss of appetite, or dark urine and jaundice
Dosage Forms Tablet: 200 mg, 400 mg

troleandomycin (troe lee an doe MYE sin)
Synonyms triacetyloleandomycin
U.S. Brand Names Tao®
Generic Available No
Therapeutic Category Macrolide (Antibiotic)
Use Adjunct in the treatment of severe corticosteroid-dependent asthma due to its steroid-sparing properties; obsolete antibiotic with spectrum of activity similar to erythromycin
Usual Dosage Oral:
Children: 25-40 mg/kg/day divided every 6 hours
Adjunct in corticosteroid-dependent asthma: 14 mg/kg/day in divided doses every 6-12 hours not to exceed 250 mg every 6 hours; dose is tapered to once daily then alternate day dosing
Adults: 250-500 mg 4 times/day
Dietary Considerations May be administered with food; presence of food delays absorption, but has no effect on the extent of absorption
Nursing/Pharmacy Information Monitor hepatic function tests
Dosage Forms Capsule: 250 mg

- **Trombovar®** *see* sodium tetradecyl *on page 575*

tromethamine (troe METH a meen)
Synonyms tris buffer; tris(hydroxymethyl)aminomethane
U.S. Brand Names THAM®; THAM-E®
Generic Available No
Therapeutic Category Alkalinizing Agent
Use Correction of metabolic acidosis associated with cardiac bypass surgery or cardiac arrest; to correct excess acidity of stored blood that is preserved with
(Continued)

tromethamine *(Continued)*

acid citrate dextrose (ACD); to prime the pump-oxygenator during cardiac bypass surgery; indicated in severe metabolic acidosis in patients in whom sodium or carbon dioxide elimination is restricted [eg, infants needing alkalinization after receiving maximum sodium bicarbonate (8-10 mEq/kg/24 hours)]

Usual Dosage Dose depends on buffer base deficit; when deficit is known: tromethamine mL of 0.3 M solution = body weight (kg) x base deficit (mEq/L); when base deficit is not known: 3-6 mL/kg/dose I.V. (1-2 mEq/kg/dose)

Metabolic acidosis with cardiac arrest:
I.V.: 3.5-6 mL/kg (1-2 mEq/kg/dose) into large peripheral vein; 500-1000 mL if needed in adults
I.V. continuous drip: Infuse slowly by syringe pump over 3-6 hours
Excess acidity of ACD priming blood: 14-70 mL of 0.3 molar solution added to each 500 mL of blood

Nursing/Pharmacy Information
Parenteral: Maximum concentration: 0.3 molar; infuse slowly over at least 1 hour (Tham-E® requires the reconstitution with 1 L sterile water before use)
Monitor blood pH, CO_2 tension, bicarbonate, glucose, serum electrolytes

Dosage Forms Injection:
Tham®: 18 g [0.3 molar] (500 mL)
Tham-E®: 36 g with sodium 30 mEq, potassium 5 mEq, and chloride 35 mEq (1000 mL)

- ◆ **Tromigal** *see* erythromycin (systemic) *on page 240*
- ◆ **Trompersantin** *see* dipyridamole *on page 212*
- ◆ **Tronolane® [OTC]** *see* pramoxine *on page 512*
- ◆ **Tropicacyl®** *see* tropicamide *on page 634*

tropicamide (troe PIK a mide)

Synonyms bistropamide
U.S. Brand Names I-Picamide®; Mydriacyl®; Tropicacyl®
Canadian Brand Names Diotrope
Generic Available Yes
Therapeutic Category Anticholinergic Agent
Use Short-acting mydriatic used in diagnostic procedures; as well as preoperatively and postoperatively; treatment of some cases of acute iritis, iridocyclitis, and keratitis
Usual Dosage Children and Adults: Ophthalmic:
Cycloplegia: 1-2 drops (1%); may repeat in 5 minutes
Mydriasis: 1-2 drops (0.5%) 15-20 minutes before exam; may repeat every 30 minutes as needed
Nursing/Pharmacy Information
Monitor IOP
Stability: Store in tightly closed containers
Dosage Forms Solution, ophthalmic: 0.5% (2 mL, 15 mL); 1% (2 mL, 3 mL, 15 mL)

- ◆ **Tropyn Z** *see* atropine *on page 64*

trovafloxacin (TROE va flox a sin)

Synonyms alatrofloxacin; CP-99,219-27
U.S. Brand Names Trovan™
Generic Available No
Therapeutic Category Antibiotic, Quinolone
Use Should be used only in life- or limb-threatening infections
Treatment of nosocomial pneumonia, community-acquired pneumonia, complicated intra-abdominal infections, gynecologic/pelvic infections, complicated skin and skin structure infections
Usual Dosage Adults:
Nosocomial pneumonia: I.V.: 300 mg single dose followed by 200 mg/day orally for a total duration of 10-14 days
Community-acquired pneumonia: Oral, I.V.: 200 mg/day for 7-14 days
Complicated intra-abdominal infections, including postsurgical infections/gynecologic and pelvic infections: I.V.: 300 mg as a single dose followed by 200 mg/day orally for a total duration of 7-14 days
Skin and skin structure infections, complicated, including diabetic foot infections: Oral, I.V.: 200 mg/day for 10-14 days
Dosage Forms
Injection, as mesylate (alatrofloxacin): 5 mg/mL (40 mL, 60 mL)
Tablet, as mesylate (trovafloxacin): 100 mg, 200 mg

♦ **Trovan**™ *see* trovafloxacin *on page 634*

♦ **troxidone** *see* trimethadione *on page 629*

♦ **Truphylline**® *see* aminophylline *on page 38*

♦ **Trusopt**® *see* dorzolamide *on page 218*

trypsin, balsam Peru, and castor oil
(TRIP sin, BAL sam pe RUE , & KAS tor oyl)
U.S. Brand Names Granulex
Generic Available No
Therapeutic Category Protectant, Topical
Use Treatment of decubitus ulcers, varicose ulcers, debridement of eschar, dehiscent wounds and sunburn
Usual Dosage Topical: Apply a minimum of twice daily or as often as necessary
Nursing/Pharmacy Information Clean wound prior to application and at each redressing; shake well before spraying; hold can upright ~12" from area to be treated
Dosage Forms Aerosol, topical: Trypsin 0.1 mg, balsam Peru 72.5 mg, and castor oil 650 mg per 0.82 mL (60 g, 120 g)

♦ **Tryptacin**® *(Discontinued) see page 743*

♦ **Tryptanol**® *see* amitriptyline *on page 40*

♦ **Trysul**® *see* sulfabenzamide, sulfacetamide, and sulfathiazole *on page 584*

♦ **TSH** *see* thyrotropin *on page 610*

♦ **TSH** *see* thyrotropin alpha *New Drug on page 610*

♦ **TSPA** *see* thiotepa *on page 608*

♦ **T-Stat**® **Topical** *see* erythromycin (ophthalmic/topical) *on page 239*

♦ **Tubasal**® *see* aminosalicylate sodium *on page 39*

tuberculin tests (too BER kyoo lin tests)
Synonyms Mantoux; old tuberculin; PPD; purified protein derivative
U.S. Brand Names Aplisol®; Aplitest®; Tine Test PPD; Tubersol®
Generic Available Yes
Therapeutic Category Diagnostic Agent
Use Skin test in diagnosis of tuberculosis, to aid in assessment of cell-mediated immunity; routine tuberculin testing is recommended at 12 months of age and at every 1-2 years thereafter, before the measles vaccination
Usual Dosage Children and Adults: Intradermally: 0.1 mL approximately 4" below elbow; use ¹/₄" to ¹/₂" or 26- or 27-gauge needle; significant reactions are ≥5 mm in diameter
Nursing/Pharmacy Information
Test dose: 0.1 mL intracutaneously; store in refrigerator; examine site at 48-72 hours after administration; whenever tuberculin is administered, a record should be made of the administration technique (Mantoux method, disposable multiple-puncture device), tuberculin used (OT or PPD), manufacturer and lot number of tuberculin used, date of administration, date of test reading, and the size of the reaction in millimeters (mm)
Stability: Refrigerate
Dosage Forms Injection:
First test strength: 1 TU/0.1 mL (1 mL)
Intermediate test strength: 5 TU/0.1 mL (1 mL, 5 mL, 10 mL)
Second test strength: 250 TU/0.1 mL (1 mL)
Tine: 5 TU each test

♦ **Tubersol**® *see* tuberculin tests *on page 635*

tubocurarine (too boe kyoor AR een)
Synonyms d-tubocurarine
Generic Available Yes
Therapeutic Category Skeletal Muscle Relaxant
Use Adjunct to anesthesia to induce skeletal muscle relaxation
Usual Dosage Children and Adults: I.V.: 0.2-0.4 mg/kg as a single dose; maintenance: 0.04-0.2 mg/kg/dose as needed to maintain paralysis
Alternative adult dose: 6-9 mg once daily, then 3-4.5 mg as needed to maintain paralysis
Nursing/Pharmacy Information
Parenteral: May infuse direct I.V. without further dilution over a period of 1-1¹/₂ minutes
Monitor mean arterial pressure, heart rate, respiratory status, serum potassium
Stability: Refrigerate; **incompatible** with barbiturates
(Continued)

tubocurarine *(Continued)*

Dosage Forms Injection, as chloride: 3 mg/mL [3 units/mL] (5 mL, 10 mL, 20 mL)

- ♦ **Tucks® [OTC]** *see* witch hazel *on page 655*
- ♦ **Tucks® Cream *(Discontinued)*** *see page 743*
- ♦ **Tuinal®** *see* amobarbital and secobarbital *on page 42*
- ♦ **Tums® [OTC]** *see* calcium carbonate *on page 103*
- ♦ **Tums® E-X Extra Strength Tablet [OTC]** *see* calcium carbonate *on page 103*
- ♦ **Tums® Extra Strength Liquid [OTC]** *see* calcium carbonate *on page 103*
- ♦ **Tusal® *(Discontinued)*** *see page 743*
- ♦ **Tusibron® [OTC]** *see* guaifenesin *on page 299*
- ♦ **Tusibron-DM® [OTC]** *see* guaifenesin and dextromethorphan *on page 300*
- ♦ **Tussafed® Drops** *see* carbinoxamine, pseudoephedrine, and dextromethorphan *on page 114*
- ♦ **Tussafin® Expectorant** *see* hydrocodone, pseudoephedrine, and guaifenesin *on page 322*
- ♦ **Tuss-Allergine® Modified T.D. Capsule** *see* caramiphen and phenylpropanolamine *on page 111*
- ♦ **Tussar® SF Syrup** *see* guaifenesin, pseudoephedrine, and codeine *on page 304*
- ♦ **Tuss-DM® [OTC]** *see* guaifenesin and dextromethorphan *on page 300*
- ♦ **Tussigon®** *see* hydrocodone and homatropine *on page 320*
- ♦ **Tussionex®** *see* hydrocodone and chlorpheniramine *on page 320*
- ♦ **Tussi-Organidin® *(Discontinued)*** *see page 743*
- ♦ **Tussi-Organidin® DM *(Discontinued)*** *see page 743*
- ♦ **Tussi-Organidin® DM NR** *see* guaifenesin and dextromethorphan *on page 300*
- ♦ **Tussi-Organidin® NR** *see* guaifenesin and codeine *on page 300*
- ♦ **Tuss-LA®** *see* guaifenesin and pseudoephedrine *on page 302*
- ♦ **Tusso-DM® *(Discontinued)*** *see page 743*
- ♦ **Tussogest® Extended Release Capsule** *see* caramiphen and phenylpropanolamine *on page 111*
- ♦ **Tuss-Ornade® *(Discontinued)*** *see page 743*
- ♦ **Tusstat® Syrup** *see* diphenhydramine *on page 208*
- ♦ **Twice-A-Day® Nasal Solution [OTC]** *see* oxymetazoline *on page 463*
- ♦ **Twilite® Oral [OTC]** *see* diphenhydramine *on page 208*
- ♦ **Twin-K®** *see* potassium citrate and potassium gluconate *on page 508*
- ♦ **Two-Dyne®** *see* butalbital compound and acetaminophen *on page 99*
- ♦ **Tylenol® [OTC]** *see* acetaminophen *on page 13*
- ♦ **Tylenol® Cold Effervescent Medication Tablet [OTC]** *see* chlorpheniramine, phenylpropanolamine, and acetaminophen *on page 142*
- ♦ **Tylenol® Cold No Drowsiness [OTC]** *see* acetaminophen, dextromethorphan, and pseudoephedrine *on page 16*
- ♦ **Tylenol® Flu Maximum Strength [OTC]** *see* acetaminophen, dextromethorphan, and pseudoephedrine *on page 16*
- ♦ **Tylenol® Sinus, Maximum Strength [OTC]** *see* acetaminophen and pseudoephedrine *on page 15*
- ♦ **Tylenol® With Codeine** *see* acetaminophen and codeine *on page 14*
- ♦ **Tylex 750** *see* acetaminophen *on page 13*
- ♦ **Tylex CD** *see* acetaminophen and codeine *on page 14*
- ♦ **Tylox®** *see* oxycodone and acetaminophen *on page 462*
- ♦ **Ty-Pap [OTC]** *see* acetaminophen *on page 13*
- ♦ **Typhim Vi®** *see* typhoid vaccine *on page 636*

typhoid vaccine (TYE foid vak SEEN)

Synonyms typhoid vaccine live oral Ty21a

U.S. Brand Names Typhim Vi®; Vivotif Berna™ Oral

Generic Available Yes: Injection only

Therapeutic Category Vaccine, Inactivated Bacteria

Use Promotes active immunity to typhoid fever for patients exposed to typhoid carrier or foreign travel to typhoid fever endemic area

Usual Dosage

Oral: Adults:

Primary immunization: 1 capsule on alternate days (day 1, 3, 5, and 7)

Booster immunization: Repeat full course of primary immunization every 5 years

S.C.:

Children 6 months to 10 years: 0.25 mL; repeat in ≥4 weeks (total immunization is 2 doses)

Children >10 years and Adults: 0.5 mL; repeat dose in ≥4 weeks (total immunization is 2 doses)

Booster: 0.25 mL every 3 years for children 6 months to 10 years and 0.5 mL every 3 years for adults and children >10 years

Nursing/Pharmacy Information

Doses of vaccine are different between S.C. and intradermal; S.C. injection only should be used

Stability: Refrigerate, do not freeze

Dosage Forms

Capsule, enteric coated (Vivotif Berna™): Viable *S. typhi* Ty21a Colony-forming units 2-6 x 10^9 and nonviable *S. typhi* Ty21a Colony-forming units 50 x 10^9 with sucrose, ascorbic acid, amino acid mixture, lactose and magnesium stearate

Injection, suspension (H-P): Heat- and phenol-inactivated, killed Ty-2 strain of *S. typhi* organisms; provides 8 units/mL, ≤1 billion/mL and ≤35 mcg nitrogen/mL (5 mL, 10 mL)

Injection (Typhim Vi®): Purified Vi capsular polysaccharide 25 mcg/0.5 mL (0.5 mL)

Powder for suspension (AKD): 8 units/mL ≤1 billion/mL, acetone inactivated dried (50 doses)

♦ **typhoid vaccine live oral Ty21a** *see* typhoid vaccine *on page 636*
♦ **Tyrodone® Liquid** *see* hydrocodone and pseudoephedrine *on page 321*
♦ **Tyzine® Nasal** *see* tetrahydrozoline *on page 602*
♦ **U-90152S** *see* delavirdine *on page 185*
♦ **UAD Otic®** *see* neomycin, polymyxin B, and hydrocortisone *on page 437*
♦ **UCB-P071** *see* cetirizine *on page 130*
♦ **Ucephan®** *see* sodium phenylacetate and sodium benzoate *on page 573*
♦ **U-Cort™ Topical** *see* hydrocortisone (topical) *on page 324*
♦ **UK** *see* urokinase *on page 639*
♦ **UK-68-798** *see* dofetilide *New Drug on page 215*
♦ **UK 92480** *see* sildenafil *on page 565*
♦ **Ukidan®** *see* urokinase *on page 639*
♦ **Ulcedine** *see* cimetidine *on page 150*
♦ **Ulcerease® [OTC]** *see* phenol *on page 486*
♦ **ULR-LA®** *see* guaifenesin and phenylpropanolamine *on page 301*
♦ **Ulsen** *see* omeprazole *on page 455*
♦ **Ultane®** *see* sevoflurane *on page 565*
♦ **Ultiva™** *see* remifentanil *on page 544*
♦ **Ultracef®** *see* ceftizoxime *on page 125*
♦ **Ultralente® U** *(Discontinued) see page 743*
♦ **Ultram®** *see* tramadol *on page 620*
♦ **Ultra Mide® Topical** *see* urea *on page 638*
♦ **Ultramop™** *see* methoxsalen *on page 403*
♦ **Ultraquin™** *see* hydroquinone *on page 325*
♦ **Ultrase® MT** *see* pancrelipase *on page 467*
♦ **Ultrase® MT24** *(Discontinued) see page 743*
♦ **Ultra Tears® Solution [OTC]** *see* artificial tears *on page 59*
♦ **Ultravate™** *see* halobetasol *on page 307*
♦ **Unamol** *see* cisapride *on page 152*
♦ **Unasyn®** *see* ampicillin and sulbactam *on page 47*
♦ **Unasyna** *see* ampicillin and sulbactam *on page 47*
♦ **Unasyna Oral** *see* ampicillin and sulbactam *on page 47*

undecylenic acid and derivatives
(un de sil EN ik AS id & dah RIV ah tivs)

Synonyms zinc undecylenate

U.S. Brand Names Caldesene® Topical [OTC]; Fungoid® AF Topical Solution [OTC]; Pedi-Pro Topical [OTC]

Generic Available Yes

Therapeutic Category Antifungal Agent

(Continued)

undecylenic acid and derivatives *(Continued)*

Use Treatment of athlete's foot (tinea pedis), ringworm (except nails and scalp), prickly heat, jock itch (tinea cruris), diaper rash and other minor skin irritations due to superficial dermatophytes

Usual Dosage Children and Adults: Topical: Apply as needed twice daily after cleansing the affected area for 2-4 weeks

Nursing/Pharmacy Information
Clean and dry the affected area before topical application
Monitor resolution of skin infection

Dosage Forms
Cream: Total undecylenate 20% (15 g, 82.5 g)
Foam, topical: Undecylenic acid 10% (42.5 g)
Liquid, topical: Undecylenic acid 10% (42.5 g)
Ointment, topical: Total undecylenate 22% (30 g, 60 g, 454 g); total undecylenate 25% (60 g, 454 g)
Powder, topical: Calcium undecylenate 10% (45 g, 60 g, 120 g); total undecylenate 22% (45 g, 54 g, 81 g, 90 g, 105 g, 165 g, 454 g)
Solution, topical: Undecylenic acid 25% (29.57 mL)

♦ **Unguentine®** [OTC] *see* benzocaine *on page 79*

♦ **Uni-Ace®** [OTC] *see* acetaminophen *on page 13*

♦ **Uni-Bent® Cough Syrup** *see* diphenhydramine *on page 208*

♦ **Unicap®** [OTC] *see* vitamin, multiple (oral) *on page 654*

♦ **Uni-Decon®** *see* chlorpheniramine, phenyltoloxamine, phenylpropanolamine, and phenylephrine *on page 143*

♦ **Uni-Dur®** *see* theophylline *on page 603*

♦ **Unipen®** *(Discontinued) see page 743*

♦ **Uniphyl®** *see* theophylline *on page 603*

♦ **Unipres®** *(Discontinued) see page 743*

♦ **Uni-Pro®** [OTC] *see* ibuprofen *on page 332*

♦ **Uniretic™** *see* moexipril and hydrochlorothiazide *on page 420*

♦ **Unitrol®** [OTC] *see* phenylpropanolamine *on page 489*

♦ **Uni-tussin®** [OTC] *see* guaifenesin *on page 299*

♦ **Uni-tussin® DM** [OTC] *see* guaifenesin and dextromethorphan *on page 300*

♦ **Univasc®** *see* moexipril *on page 420*

♦ **Unizuric 300** *see* allopurinol *on page 29*

♦ **Unna's boot** *see* zinc gelatin *on page 660*

♦ **Unna's paste** *see* zinc gelatin *on page 660*

♦ **Urabeth®** *see* bethanechol *on page 86*

♦ **Uracel®** *see* sodium salicylate *on page 575*

uracil mustard *(YOOR a sil MUS tard)*

Canadian Brand Names Ursofalk®
Generic Available No
Therapeutic Category Antineoplastic Agent
Use Palliative treatment in symptomatic chronic lymphocytic leukemia; non-Hodgkin's lymphomas
Usual Dosage Oral:
Children: 0.3 mg/kg in a single weekly dose for 4 weeks
Adults: 0.15 mg/kg in a single weekly dose for 4 weeks
Thrombocytosis: 1-2 mg/day for 14 days
Nursing/Pharmacy Information Notify physician of persistent or severe nausea, diarrhea, fever, sore throat, chills, bleeding, or bruising
Dosage Forms Capsule: 1 mg

♦ **Urasal®** *see* methenamine *on page 400*

urea *(yoor EE a)*

Synonyms carbamide
U.S. Brand Names Amino-Cerv™ Vaginal Cream; Aquacare® Topical [OTC]; Carmol® Topical [OTC]; Gormel® Creme [OTC]; Lanaphilic® Topical [OTC]; Nutraplus® Topical [OTC]; Rea-Lo® [OTC]; Ultra Mide® Topical; Ureacin®-20 Topical [OTC]; Ureaphil® Injection
Canadian Brand Names Onyvul®; Uremol®; Urisec®; Velvelan®
Generic Available Yes
Therapeutic Category Diuretic, Osmotic; Topical Skin Product
Use Reduce intracranial pressure and intraocular pressure (30%); promotes hydration and removal of excess keratin in hyperkeratotic conditions and dry skin; mild cervicitis

Usual Dosage
Children: I.V. slow infusion:
<2 years: 0.1-0.5 g/kg
>2 years: 0.5-1.5 g/kg
Adults:
I.V. infusion: 1-1.5 g/kg by slow infusion (1-2½ hours); maximum: 120 g/24 hours
Topical: Apply 1-3 times/day
Vaginal: 1 applicatorful in vagina at bedtime for 2-4 weeks
Nursing/Pharmacy Information Do not infuse into leg veins; injection dosage form may be used orally by mixing with carbonated beverages, jelly or jam, to mask unpleasant flavor
Dosage Forms
Cream:
Topical: 2% [20 mg/mL] (75 g); 10% [100 mg/mL] (75 g, 90 g, 454 g); 20% [200 mg/mL] (45 g, 75 g, 90 g, 454 g); 30% [300 mg/mL] (60 g, 454 g); 40% (30 g)
Vaginal: 8.34% [83.4 mg/g] (82.5 g)
Injection: 40 g/150 mL
Lotion: 2% (240 mL); 10% (180 mL, 240 mL, 480 mL); 15% (120 mL, 480 mL); 25% (180 mL)

urea and hydrocortisone (yoor EE a & hye droe KOR ti sone)
Synonyms hydrocortisone and urea
U.S. Brand Names Carmol-HC® Topical
Generic Available No
Therapeutic Category Corticosteroid, Topical
Use Inflammation of corticosteroid-responsive dermatoses
Usual Dosage Topical: Apply thin film and rub in well 1-4 times/day
Dosage Forms Cream, topical: Urea 10% and hydrocortisone acetate 1% in a water-washable vanishing cream base (30 g)

♦ **Ureacin®-20 Topical [OTC]** see urea on page 638
♦ **Ureacin®-40 Topical** *(Discontinued)* see page 743
♦ **urea peroxide** see carbamide peroxide on page 112
♦ **Ureaphil® Injection** see urea on page 638
♦ **Urecholine®** see bethanechol on page 86
♦ **Uremol®** see urea on page 638
♦ **Urex®** see methenamine on page 400
♦ **Uridon®** see chlorthalidone on page 146
♦ **Urisec®** see urea on page 638
♦ **Urispas®** see flavoxate on page 268
♦ **Uri-Tet®** *(Discontinued)* see page 743
♦ **Uritol®** see furosemide on page 285
♦ **Urobak®** see sulfamethoxazole on page 587
♦ **Urobiotic-25®** *(Discontinued)* see page 743
♦ **Urocit®-K** see potassium citrate on page 508
♦ **Urodine®** see phenazopyridine on page 483

urofollitropin (yoor oh fol li TROE pin)
U.S. Brand Names Fertinex®; Metrodin®
Mexican Brand Names Fertinorm® H.P.
Generic Available No
Therapeutic Category Ovulation Stimulator
Use Induction of ovulation in patients with polycystic ovarian disease and to stimulate the development of multiple oocytes
Usual Dosage Adults: Female: S.C.: 75 units/day for 7-12 days, used with hCG may repeat course of treatment 2 more times
Nursing/Pharmacy Information Stability: Protect from light; refrigerate at 3°C to 25°C (37°F to 77°F)
Dosage Forms Injection: 0.83 mg [75 units FSH activity] (2 mL); 1.66 mg [150 units FSH activity]

♦ **Urogesic®** see phenazopyridine on page 483

urokinase (yoor oh KIN ase)
Synonyms UK
U.S. Brand Names Abbokinase®
Mexican Brand Names Ukidan®
Generic Available No
(Continued)

urokinase *(Continued)*

Therapeutic Category Thrombolytic Agent

Use Treatment of recent severe or massive deep vein or arterial thrombosis, pulmonary emboli, and occluded arteriovenous cannulas

Usual Dosage

Children and Adults: Deep vein thrombosis: I.V.: Loading: 4400 units/kg over 10 minutes, then 4400 units/kg/hour for 12 hours

Adults:

Myocardial infarction: Intracoronary: 750,000 units over 2 hours (6000 units/minute over up to 2 hours)

Occluded I.V. catheters:

5000 units (use only Abbokinase® Open Cath) in each lumen over 1-2 minutes, leave in lumen for 1-4 hours, then aspirate; may repeat with 10,000 units in each lumen if 5000 units fails to clear the catheter; **do not infuse into the patient**; volume to instill into catheter is equal to the volume of the catheter

I.V. infusion: 200 units/kg/hour in each lumen for 12-48 hours at a rate of at least 20 mL/hour

Dialysis patients: 5000 units is administered in each lumen over 1-2 minutes; leave urokinase in lumen for 1-2 days, then aspirate

Clot lysis (large vessel thrombi): Loading: I.V.: 4400 units/kg over 10 minutes, increase to 6000 units/kg/hour; maintenance: 4400-6000 units/kg/hour adjusted to achieve clot lysis or patency of affected vessel; doses up to 50,000 units/kg/hour have been used. **Note:** Therapy should be initiated as soon as possible after diagnosis of thrombi and continued until clot is dissolved (usually 24-72 hours).

Acute pulmonary embolism: Three treatment alternatives: 3 million unit dosage

Alternative 1: 12-hour infusion: 4400 units/kg (2000 units/lb) bolus over 10 minutes followed by 4400 units/kg/hour (2000 units/lb); begin heparin 1000 units/hour approximately 3-4 hours after completion of urokinase infusion or when PTT is <100 seconds

Alternative 2: 2-hour infusion: 1 million unit bolus over 10 minutes followed by 2 million units over 110 minutes; begin heparin 1000 units/hour approximately 3-4 hours after completion of urokinase infusion or when PTT is <100 seconds

Alternative 3: Bolus dose only: 15,000 units/kg over 10 minutes; begin heparin 1000 units/hour approximately 3-4 hours after completion of urokinase infusion or when PTT is <100 seconds

Nursing/Pharmacy Information

Use 0.22 or 0.45 micron filter during I.V. systemic therapy; I.V. infusion: Usual concentration: 1250-1500 units/mL; maximum concentration not yet defined

Monitor CBC, reticulocyte, platelet count, DIC panel (fibrinogen, plasminogen, FDP, D Dimers, PT, PTT), thrombosis panel (AT-III, protein C), urinalysis, ACT

Stability: Store in refrigerator; reconstitute by gently rolling and tilting; do not shake; contains no preservatives, should not be reconstituted until immediately before using, discard unused portion; stable at room temperature for 24 hours after reconstitution

Dosage Forms

Powder for injection: 250,000 units (5 mL)

Powder for injection, catheter clear: 5000 units (1 mL)

♦ **Uro-KP-Neutral®** *see* potassium phosphate and sodium phosphate *on page 510*

♦ **Urolene Blue®** *see* methylene blue *on page 406*

♦ **Uro-Mag® [OTC]** *see* magnesium oxide *on page 382*

♦ **Uroplus® DS** *see* co-trimoxazole *on page 170*

♦ **Uroplus® SS** *see* co-trimoxazole *on page 170*

♦ **Urovalidin** *see* phenazopyridine *on page 483*

♦ **Urovist Cysto®** *see* radiological/contrast media (ionic) *on page 539*

♦ **Urovist® Meglumine** *see* radiological/contrast media (ionic) *on page 539*

♦ **Urovist® Sodium 300** *see* radiological/contrast media (ionic) *on page 539*

♦ **Urozide®** *see* hydrochlorothiazide *on page 317*

♦ **Urso®** *see* ursodiol *on page 640*

♦ **ursodeoxycholic acid** *see* ursodiol *on page 640*

ursodiol *(ER soe dye ole)*

Synonyms ursodeoxycholic acid

U.S. Brand Names Actigall™; Urso®

Mexican Brand Names Ursofalk

Generic Available No
Therapeutic Category Gallstone Dissolution Agent
Use Gallbladder stone dissolution
Usual Dosage Oral: 8-10 mg/kg/day in 2-3 divided doses
Nursing/Pharmacy Information
   Monitor ALT, AST, sonogram
   Stability: Do not store >30°C (86°F)
Dosage Forms Capsule: 300 mg

- **Ursofalk®** *see* uracil mustard *on page 638*
- **Ursofalk** *see* ursodiol *on page 640*
- **Uticort®** *(Discontinued) see page 743*
- **Utrogestan** *see* progesterone *on page 520*
- **Vagifem®** *see* estradiol *on page 242*
- **Vagistat®-1 Vaginal [OTC]** *see* tioconazole *on page 614*
- **Vagitrol®** *see* sulfanilamide *on page 587*

valacyclovir (val ay SYE kloe veer)

U.S. Brand Names Valtrex®
Generic Available No
Therapeutic Category Antiviral Agent
Use Treatment of herpes zoster (shingles) in immunocompetent patients; once daily therapy for the suppression of genital herpes
Usual Dosage Adults: Oral: 1000 mg 3 times/day for 7 days
Dosage Forms Tablet: 500 mg, 1000 mg

- **Valadol®** *(Discontinued) see page 743*
- **Valergen® Injection** *(Discontinued) see page 743*
- **Valertest No.1®** *see* estradiol and testosterone *on page 243*
- **Valisone® Topical** *see* betamethasone (topical) *on page 85*
- **Valium® Injection** *see* diazepam *on page 196*
- **Valium® Oral** *see* diazepam *on page 196*
- **Valmid® Capsule** *(Discontinued) see page 743*
- **Valpin® 50** *(Discontinued) see page 743*

valproic acid and derivatives

(val PROE ik AS id & dah RIV ah tives)
Synonyms dipropylacetic acid; DPA; 2-propylpentanoic acid; 2-propylvaleric acid
U.S. Brand Names Depacon®; Depakene®; Depakote®
Mexican Brand Names Atemperator-S®; Cryoval; Epival®; Leptilan®; Valprosid®
Generic Available Yes
Therapeutic Category Anticonvulsant
Use Management of simple and complex absence seizures; mixed seizure types; myoclonic and generalized tonic-clonic (grand mal) seizures; prevent migraine headaches in adults (Depakote®); mania associated with bipolar disorder; may be effective in partial seizures and infantile spasms; Depakote® can be used for the treatment of complex partial seizures; Depacon® is indicated as a temporary intravenous alternative when oral administration is not possible
Usual Dosage Children and Adults:
   Oral: Initial: 10-15 mg/kg/day in 1-3 divided doses; increase by 5-10 mg/kg/day at weekly intervals until therapeutic levels are achieved; maintenance: 30-60 mg/kg/day in 2-3 divided doses
      Children receiving more than one anticonvulsant (ie, polytherapy) may require doses up to 100 mg/kg/day in 3-4 divided doses
   I.V.: Administer as a 60 minute infusion (≤20 mg/min) with the same frequency as oral products; switch patient to oral products as soon as possible
   Rectal: Dilute syrup 1:1 with water for use as a retention enema; loading dose: 17-20 mg/kg one time; maintenance: 10-15 mg/kg/dose every 8 hours
Dietary Considerations
   Alcohol: Additive CNS depression; avoid or limit alcohol
   Food:
      Valproic acid may cause GI upset; administer with large amount of water or food to decrease GI upset; may need to split doses to avoid GI upset
      Food may delay but does not affect the extent of absorption
         Coated particles of divalproex sodium may be mixed with semisolid food (eg, applesauce or pudding) in patients having difficulty swallowing; particles should be swallowed and not chewed
(Continued)

valproic acid and derivatives *(Continued)*

Valproate sodium oral solution will generate valproic acid in carbonated beverages and may cause mouth and throat irritation; do not mix valproate sodium oral solution with carbonated beverages

Milk: No effect on absorption; may administer with milk

Sodium: SIADH and water intoxication; monitor fluid status; may need to restrict fluid

Nursing/Pharmacy Information

Instruct patients/parents to report signs or symptoms of hepatotoxicity; do not chew, break or crush the tablet or capsule; GI side effects of divalproex may be less than valproic acid

Monitor liver enzymes, CBC with platelets

Dosage Forms

Divalproex sodium:

Capsule, sprinkle (Depakote® Sprinkle®): 125 mg

Tablet, delayed release, as divalproex sodium (Depakote®): 125 mg, 250 mg, 500 mg

Valproic acid: Capsule (Depakene®): 250 mg

Valproate sodium:

Injection (Depacon®): 100 mg/mL (5 mL)

Syrup (Depakene®): 250 mg/5 mL (5 mL, 50 mL, 480 mL)

♦ **Valprosid®** *see* valproic acid and derivatives *on page 641*

♦ **Valrelease®** *(Discontinued) see page 743*

valrubicin (val ru BYE cin)

U.S. Brand Names Valstar™

Generic Available No

Therapeutic Category Antineoplastic Agent

Use Intravesical therapy of BCG-refractory carcinoma *in situ* of the urinary bladder

Usual Dosage Adults: Intravesical: 800 mg once weekly for 6 weeks

Dosage Forms Injection: 40 mg/mL (5 mL)

valsartan (val SAR tan)

U.S. Brand Names Diovan™

Generic Available No

Therapeutic Category Angiotensin II Antagonist

Use Treatment of hypertension alone or in combination with other antihypertensives

Usual Dosage Adults: Oral: 80 mg/day; may be increased to 160 mg if needed (maximal effects observed in 4-6 weeks)

Dosage Forms Capsule: 80 mg, 160 mg

valsartan and hydrochlorothiazide

(val SAR tan & hye droe klor oh THYE a zide)

U.S. Brand Names Diovan HCT™

Generic Available No

Therapeutic Category Angiotensin II Antagonist; Diuretic, Thiazide

Use Treatment of hypertension

Usual Dosage Adults: Oral: Dose is individualized

Dosage Forms Tablet: Valsartan 80 mg and hydrochlorothiazide 12.5 mg; valsartan 160 mg and hydrochlorothiazide 12.5 mg

♦ **Valstar™** *see* valrubicin *on page 642*

♦ **Valtrex®** *see* valacyclovir *on page 641*

♦ **Vamate® Oral** *see* hydroxyzine *on page 328*

♦ **Vancenase® AQ 84 mcg** *see* beclomethasone *on page 75*

♦ **Vancenase® AQ Inhaler** *see* beclomethasone *on page 75*

♦ **Vancenase® Nasal Inhaler** *see* beclomethasone *on page 75*

♦ **Vanceril® 84 mcg Double Strength** *see* beclomethasone *on page 75*

♦ **Vanceril® Oral Inhaler** *see* beclomethasone *on page 75*

♦ **Vancocin® CP** *see* vancomycin *on page 642*

♦ **Vancocin® Injection** *see* vancomycin *on page 642*

♦ **Vancocin® Oral** *see* vancomycin *on page 642*

♦ **Vancoled® Injection** *see* vancomycin *on page 642*

vancomycin (van koe MYE sin)

U.S. Brand Names Lyphocin® Injection; Vancocin® Injection; Vancocin® Oral; Vancoled® Injection

Canadian Brand Names Vancocin® CP
Mexican Brand Names Balcoran; Vanmicina®
Generic Available Yes
Therapeutic Category Antibiotic, Miscellaneous
Use Treatment of patients with the following infections or conditions: treatment of infections due to documented or suspected methicillin-resistant *S. aureus* or beta-lactam resistant coagulase negative *Staphylococcus*; treatment of serious or life-threatening infections (ie, endocarditis, meningitis, osteomyelitis) due to documented or suspected staphylococcal or streptococcal infections in patients who are allergic to penicillins and/or cephalosporins; empiric therapy of infections associated with central lines, VP shunts, hemodialysis shunts, vascular grafts, prosthetic heart valves; used orally for staphylococcal enterocolitis or for antibiotic-associated pseudomembranous colitis produced by *C. difficile*

Usual Dosage I.V. (initial dosage recommendation):
Infants >1 month and Children: 40 mg/kg/day in divided doses every 6 hours
Infants >1 month and Children with staphylococcal central nervous system infection: 60 mg/kg/day in divided doses every 6 hours
Adults: With normal renal function: 0.5 g every 6 hours or 1 g every 12 hours

Intrathecal:
Children: 5-20 mg/day
Adults: 20 mg/day

Oral:
Children: 10-50 mg/kg/day in divided doses every 6-8 hours; not to exceed 2 g/day
Adults: 0.5-2 g/day in divided doses every 6-8 hours

Pseudomembranous colitis produced by *C. difficile*:
Children: 40 mg/kg/day in divided doses, added to fluids
Adults: 500 mg to 2 g/day administered in 3 or 4 divided doses for 7-10 days

Dietary Considerations May be administered with food
Nursing/Pharmacy Information
Do not administer I.M.; peak levels are drawn 1 hour after the completion of a 1-hour infusion; troughs are obtained just before the next dose; if a maculopapular rash appears on face, neck, trunk, and upper extremities, slow the infusion rate to over 1½ to 2 hours and increase the dilution volume; administration of antihistamines just before the infusion may also prevent or minimize this reaction; administer vancomycin by I.V. intermittent infusion over 60 minutes at a final concentration not to exceed 5 mg/mL

Monitor periodic renal function tests, urinalysis, serum vancomycin concentrations, WBC

Stability: After the oral or parenteral solution is reconstituted, refrigerate and discard after 14 days; after further dilution, the parenteral solution is stable, at room temperature, for 24 hours

Dosage Forms Vancomycin hydrochloride:
Capsule: 125 mg, 250 mg
Powder for oral solution: 1 g, 10 g
Powder for injection: 500 mg, 1 g, 2 g, 5 g, 10 g

♦ **Vanex-LA®** *(Discontinued) see page 743*
♦ **Vanmicina®** *see vancomycin on page 642*
♦ **Vanoxide® [OTC]** *see benzoyl peroxide on page 81*
♦ **Vanoxide-HC®** *see benzoyl peroxide and hydrocortisone on page 81*
♦ **Vanseb-T® Shampoo** *(Discontinued) see page 743*
♦ **Vansil™** *see oxamniquine on page 460*
♦ **Vantin®** *see cefpodoxime on page 124*
♦ **Vapocet®** *see hydrocodone and acetaminophen on page 319*
♦ **Vaponefrin® [OTC]** *see epinephrine on page 234*

varicella virus vaccine (var i SEL a VYE rus vak SEEN)

Synonyms chicken pox vaccine; varicella-zoster virus (VZV) vaccine
U.S. Brand Names Varivax®
Generic Available No
Therapeutic Category Vaccine, Live Virus
Use The American Association of Pediatrics recommends that the chickenpox vaccine should be given to all healthy children between 12 months and 18 years; children between 12 months and 13 years who have not been immunized or who have not had chickenpox should receive 1 vaccination while children 13-18 years of age require 2 vaccinations 4-8 weeks apart; the vaccine has been added to the childhood immunization schedule for infants 12-28 months of age and children 11-12 years of age who have not been (Continued)

varicella virus vaccine *(Continued)*

vaccinated previously or who have not had the disease; it is recommended to be given with the measles, mumps, and rubella (MMR) vaccine

Usual Dosage S.C.:

Children 12 months to 12 years: 0.5 mL

Children 12 years to Adults: 2 doses of 0.5 mL separated by 4-8 weeks

Nursing/Pharmacy Information

Obtain the previous immunization history (including allergic reactions) to previous vaccines; do not inject into a blood vessel; use the supplied diluent only for reconstitution; inject immediately after reconstitution

Store in freezer (-15°C), store diluent separately at room temperature or in refrigerator; discard if reconstituted vaccine is not used within 30 minutes

Dosage Forms Powder for injection, lyophilized powder, preservative free: 1350 plaque forming units (PFU)/0.5 mL (0.5 mL single-dose vials)

varicella-zoster immune globulin (human)

(var i SEL a- ZOS ter i MYUN GLOB yoo lin HYU man)

Synonyms VZIG

Generic Available No

Therapeutic Category Immune Globulin

Use Passive immunization of susceptible immunodeficient patients after exposure to varicella; most effective if begun within 96 hours of exposure

VZIG supplies are limited, restrict administration to those meeting the following criteria:

One of the following underlying illnesses or conditions:

Neoplastic disease (eg, leukemia or lymphoma)

Congenital or acquired immunodeficiency

Immunosuppressive therapy with steroids, antimetabolites or other immunosuppressive treatment regimens

Newborn of mother who had onset of chickenpox within 5 days before delivery or within 48 hours after delivery

Premature (≥28 weeks gestation) whose mother has no history of chickenpox

Premature (<28 weeks gestation or ≤1000 g VZIG) regardless of maternal history

One of the following types of exposure to chickenpox or zoster patient(s):

Continuous household contact

Playmate contact (>1 hour play indoors)

Hospital contact (in same 2-4 bedroom or adjacent beds in a large ward or prolonged face-to-face contact with an infectious staff member or patient)

Susceptible to varicella-zoster

Age of <15 years; administer to immunocompromised adolescents and adults and to other older patients on an individual basis

An acceptable alternative to VZIG prophylaxis is to treat varicella, if it occurs, with high-dose I.V. acyclovir

Usual Dosage High-risk susceptible patients who are exposed again more than 3 weeks after a prior dose of VZIG should receive another full dose; there is no evidence VZIG modifies established varicella-zoster infections.

I.M.: Administer by deep injection in the gluteal muscle or in another large muscle mass. Inject 125 units/10 kg (22 lb); maximum dose: 625 units (5 vials); minimum dose: 125 units; do not administer fractional doses. Do not inject I.V.

Nursing/Pharmacy Information

Administer as soon as possible after presumed exposure; do not inject I.V.; administer by deep I.M. injection into gluteal muscle or other large muscle; administer entire contents of each vial

Stability: Refrigerate

Dosage Forms Injection: 125 units of antibody in single dose vials

♦ **varicella-zoster virus (VZV) vaccine** *see* varicella virus vaccine *on page 643*

♦ **Varivax®** *see* varicella virus vaccine *on page 643*

♦ **Vascor®** *see* bepridil *on page 83*

♦ **Vascoray®** *see* radiological/contrast media (ionic) *on page 539*

♦ **Vaseretic® 10-25** *see* enalapril and hydrochlorothiazide *on page 231*

♦ **Vasocidin® Ophthalmic** *see* sulfacetamide and prednisolone *on page 585*

♦ **VasoClear® Ophthalmic [OTC]** *see* naphazoline *on page 431*

- **Vasocon-A® [OTC] Ophthalmic** *see* naphazoline and antazoline *on page 431*
- **Vasocon Regular® Ophthalmic** *see* naphazoline *on page 431*
- **Vasodilan®** *see* isoxsuprine *on page 350*

vasopressin (vay soe PRES in)
Synonyms antidiuretic hormone (ADH); 8-arginine vasopressin
U.S. Brand Names Pitressin®
Canadian Brand Names Pressyn®
Generic Available Yes
Therapeutic Category Hormone, Posterior Pituitary
Use Treatment of diabetes insipidus; prevention and treatment of postoperative abdominal distention; differential diagnosis of diabetes insipidus; adjunct in the treatment of acute massive hemorrhage of GI tract or esophageal varices
Usual Dosage
Diabetes insipidus:
I.M., S.C.:
Children: 2.5-5 units 2-4 times/day as needed
Adults: 5-10 units 2-4 times/day as needed (dosage range 5-60 units/day)
Intranasal: Administer on cotton pledget or nasal spray
Abdominal distention Adults: I.M.: 5 mg stat, 10 mg every 3-4 hours
GI hemorrhage: I.V.: Administer in a peripheral vein; dilute aqueous in NS or D_5W to 0.1-1 unit/mL and infuse at 0.2-0.4 unit/minute and progressively increase to 0.9 unit/minute if necessary; I.V. infusion administration requires the use of an infusion pump and should be administered in a peripheral line to minimize adverse reactions on coronary arteries
Nursing/Pharmacy Information
Before withdrawing a dose, vasopressin tannate in oil should be shaken thoroughly to obtain a uniform suspension; vasopressin tannate in oil must not be administered I.V.; monitor fluid I & O; watch for signs of I.V. infiltration and gangrene; dilute in normal saline or 5% dextrose to a final concentration of 0.1-1 unit/mL
Monitor serum and urine sodium, urine output, fluid I & O, urine specific gravity, urine and serum osmolality
Stability: Store injection at room temperature; protect from heat and from freezing; use only clear solutions
Dosage Forms Injection, aqueous: 20 pressor units/mL (0.5 mL, 1 mL)

- **Vasosulf® Ophthalmic** *see* sulfacetamide and phenylephrine *on page 585*
- **Vasotec® I.V.** *see* enalapril *on page 230*
- **Vasotec® Oral** *see* enalapril *on page 230*
- **Vasoxyl®** *see* methoxamine *on page 403*
- **Vatrix-S** *see* metronidazole *on page 411*
- **V-Cillin K® (Discontinued)** *see page 743*
- **VCR** *see* vincristine *on page 648*
- **V-Dec-M®** *see* guaifenesin and pseudoephedrine *on page 302*
- **Vectrin®** *see* minocycline *on page 416*

vecuronium (ve KYOO roe nee um)
Synonyms ORG NC 45
U.S. Brand Names Norcuron®
Generic Available No
Therapeutic Category Skeletal Muscle Relaxant
Use Adjunct to anesthesia, to facilitate endotracheal intubation, and provide skeletal muscle relaxation during surgery or mechanical ventilation
Usual Dosage I.V.:
Infants >7 weeks to 1 year: Initial: 0.08-0.1 mg/kg/dose; maintenance: 0.05-0.1 mg/kg/every hour as needed
Children >1 year and Adults: Initial: 0.08-0.1 mg/kg/dose; maintenance: 0.05-0.1 mg/kg/every hour as needed; may be administered as a continuous infusion at 0.1 mg/kg/hour
Note: Children may require slightly higher initial doses and slightly more frequent supplementation
Nursing/Pharmacy Information
Does not alter the patient's state of consciousness; addition of sedation and analgesia are recommended; dilute vial to a maximum concentration of 2 mg/mL and administer by rapid direct injection; for continuous infusion, dilute to a maximum concentration of 1 mg/mL
Monitor blood pressure, heart rate
(Continued)

vecuronium *(Continued)*

Stability: 5 days at room temperature when reconstituted with bacteriostatic water; 24 hours at room temperature when reconstituted with preservative-free sterile water (avoid preservatives in neonates); do not mix with alkaline drugs

Dosage Forms Powder for injection:
With diluent: 10 mg (10 mL)
Without diluent: 10 mg (10 mL); 20 mg (20 mL)

- ◆ **Veetids®** *see* penicillin V potassium *on page 476*
- ◆ **Velban®** *see* vinblastine *on page 648*
- ◆ **Velbe®** *see* vinblastine *on page 648*
- ◆ **Velosef®** *see* cephradine *on page 129*
- ◆ **Velosulin®** *see* insulin preparations *on page 339*
- ◆ **Velosulin® BR Human (Buffered)** *see* insulin preparations *on page 339*
- ◆ **Velsar® Injection *(Discontinued)*** *see page 743*
- ◆ **Velsay** *see* naproxen *on page 432*
- ◆ **Velvelan®** *see* urea *on page 638*

venlafaxine *(VEN la faks een)*

U.S. Brand Names Effexor®; Effexor-XR®
Generic Available No
Therapeutic Category Antidepressant, Phenethylamine
Use Treatment of depression
Usual Dosage Adults: Oral:
Capsule: One capsule daily
Tablet: 75 mg/day, administered in 2 or 3 divided doses, taken with food; dose may be increased in 75 mg/day increments at intervals of at least 4 days, up to 225-375 mg/day
Dietary Considerations Should be administered with food
Nursing/Pharmacy Information Avoid use of alcohol; use caution when operating hazardous machinery
Dosage Forms
Capsule, extended release: 37.5 mg, 75 mg, 150 mg
Tablet: 25 mg, 37.5 mg, 50 mg, 75 mg, 100 mg, 150 mg

- ◆ **Venoglobulin®-I** *see* immune globulin, intravenous *on page 336*
- ◆ **Venoglobulin®-S** *see* immune globulin, intravenous *on page 336*
- ◆ **Ventolin®** *see* albuterol *on page 25*
- ◆ **Ventolin® Rotocaps®** *see* albuterol *on page 25*
- ◆ **VePesid®** *see* etoposide *on page 255*
- ◆ **Veracef** *see* cephradine *on page 129*
- ◆ **Veraken** *see* verapamil *on page 646*

verapamil *(ver AP a mil)*

Synonyms iproveratril
U.S. Brand Names Calan®; Calan® SR; Covera-HS®; Isoptin®; Isoptin® SR; Verelan®
Canadian Brand Names Apo®-Verap; Novo-Veramil®; Nu-Verap®
Mexican Brand Names Dilacoran; Dilacoran HTA; Dilacoran Retard; Veraken; Verdilac
Generic Available Yes
Therapeutic Category Antiarrhythmic Agent, Class IV; Calcium Channel Blocker
Use Angina, hypertension; I.V. for supraventricular tachyarrhythmias (PSVT, atrial fibrillation, atrial flutter)
Usual Dosage
Children: I.V.:
0-1 year: 0.1-0.2 mg/kg/dose, repeated after 30 minutes as needed
1-16 years: 0.1-0.3 mg/kg over 2-3 minutes; maximum: 5 mg/dose, may repeat dose once in 30 minutes if adequate response not achieved; maximum for second dose: 10 mg/dose
Children: Oral (dose not well established):
4-8 mg/kg/day in 3 divided doses **or** 1-5 years: 40-80 mg every 8 hours
>5 years: 80 mg every 6-8 hours
Adults:
Oral: 240-480 mg/24 hours divided 3-4 times/day
I.V.: 5-10 mg (0.075-0.15 mg/kg); may repeat 10 mg (0.15 mg/kg) 15-30 minutes after the initial dose if needed and if patient tolerated initial dose

Dietary Considerations Sustained release product should be administered with food or milk, other formulations may be administered without regard to meals; sprinkling contents of capsule onto food does not affect oral absorption

Nursing/Pharmacy Information

Do not crush sustained release products; infuse I.V. dose over 2-3 minutes; infuse I.V. over 3-4 minutes if blood pressure is in the lower range of normal; I.V. push: Maximum concentration: 2.5 mg/mL

Monitor EKG, blood pressure, heart rate

Stability: Store injection at room temperature; protect from heat and from freezing; use only clear solutions; **compatible** in solutions of pH of 3-6, but may precipitate in solutions having a pH of ≥6

Dosage Forms Verapamil hydrochloride:

Capsule, sustained release (Verelan®): 120 mg, 180 mg, 240 mg, 360 mg

Injection: 2.5 mg/mL (2 mL, 4 mL)

Isoptin®: 2.5 mg/mL (2 mL, 4 mL)

Tablet: 40 mg, 80 mg, 120 mg

Calan®, Isoptin®: 40 mg, 80 mg, 120 mg

Tablet sustained release: 180 mg, 240 mg

Calan® SR, Isoptin® SR: 120 mg, 180 mg, 240 mg

Covera-HS®: 180 mg, 240 mg

- ♦ **Verazinc® Oral [OTC]** *see* zinc sulfate *on page 660*
- ♦ **Vercyte®** *(Discontinued) see page 743*
- ♦ **Verdilac** *see* verapamil *on page 646*
- ♦ **Verelan®** *see* verapamil *on page 646*
- ♦ **Vergogel® Gel [OTC]** *see* salicylic acid *on page 557*
- ♦ **Vergon® [OTC]** *see* meclizine *on page 387*
- ♦ **Vermicol** *see* mebendazole *on page 387*
- ♦ **Vermox®** *see* mebendazole *on page 387*
- ♦ **Verr-Canth®** *(Discontinued) see page 743*
- ♦ **Verrex-C&M®** *see* podophyllin and salicylic acid *on page 500*
- ♦ **Verrex®** *(Discontinued) see page 743*
- ♦ **Verrusol®** *(Discontinued) see page 743*
- ♦ **Versacaps®** *see* guaifenesin and pseudoephedrine *on page 302*
- ♦ **Versed®** *see* midazolam *on page 415*
- ♦ **Versel™** *see* selenium sulfide *on page 562*
- ♦ **Versiclear™** *see* sodium thiosulfate *on page 576*
- ♦ **Vertisal** *see* metronidazole *on page 411*
- ♦ **Verukan® Solution** *see* salicylic acid *on page 557*
- ♦ **Vesanoid®** *see* tretinoin (oral) *on page 622*
- ♦ **Vesprin®** *see* triflupromazine *on page 628*
- ♦ **Vexol® Ophthalmic Suspension** *see* rimexolone *on page 551*
- ♦ **V-Gan® Injection** *(Discontinued) see page 743*
- ♦ **Viagra®** *see* sildenafil *on page 565*
- ♦ **Vibramicina®** *see* doxycycline *on page 222*
- ♦ **Vibramycin®** *see* doxycycline *on page 222*
- ♦ **Vibra-Tabs®** *see* doxycycline *on page 222*
- ♦ **Vicks® 44D Cough & Head Congestion** *see* pseudoephedrine and dextromethorphan *on page 531*
- ♦ **Vicks® 44E [OTC]** *see* guaifenesin and dextromethorphan *on page 300*
- ♦ **Vicks® 44 Non-Drowsy Cold & Cough Liqui-Caps [OTC]** *see* pseudoephedrine and dextromethorphan *on page 531*
- ♦ **Vicks Children's Chloraseptic® [OTC]** *see* benzocaine *on page 79*
- ♦ **Vicks Chloraseptic® Sore Throat [OTC]** *see* benzocaine *on page 79*
- ♦ **Vicks® DayQuil® Allergy Relief 4 Hour Tablet [OTC]** *see* brompheniramine and phenylpropanolamine *on page 94*
- ♦ **Vicks® DayQuil® Sinus Pressure & Congestion Relief [OTC]** *see* guaifenesin and phenylpropanolamine *on page 301*
- ♦ **Vicks Formula 44® [OTC]** *see* dextromethorphan *on page 194*
- ♦ **Vicks Formula 44® Pediatric Formula [OTC]** *see* dextromethorphan *on page 194*
- ♦ **Vicks® Pediatric Formula 44E [OTC]** *see* guaifenesin and dextromethorphan *on page 300*
- ♦ **Vicks® Sinex® Nasal Solution [OTC]** *see* phenylephrine *on page 487*
- ♦ **Vicks® Vatronol®** *(Discontinued) see page 743*
- ♦ **Vicodin®** *see* hydrocodone and acetaminophen *on page 319*
- ♦ **Vicodin® ES** *see* hydrocodone and acetaminophen *on page 319*
- ♦ **Vicon-C® [OTC]** *see* vitamin B complex with vitamin C *on page 651*

- **Vicon Forte®** *see* vitamin, multiple (oral) *on page 654*
- **Vicon® Plus [OTC]** *see* vitamin, multiple (oral) *on page 654*
- **Vicoprofen®** *see* hydrocodone and ibuprofen *on page 321*

vidarabine (vye DARE a been)
Synonyms adenine arabinoside; ARA-A; arabinofuranosyladenine
U.S. Brand Names Vira-A® Ophthalmic
Mexican Brand Names Adena a Ungena
Generic Available No
Therapeutic Category Antiviral Agent
Use Treatment of acute keratoconjunctivitis and epithelial keratitis due to herpes simplex virus; herpes simplex encephalitis; neonatal herpes simplex virus infections; disseminated varicella-zoster in immunosuppressed patients
Usual Dosage Children and Adults: Ophthalmic: Keratoconjunctivitis: $\frac{1}{2}$" of ointment in lower conjunctival sac 5 times/day every 3 hours while awake until complete re-epithelialization has occurred, then twice daily for an additional 7 days
Dosage Forms Ointment, ophthalmic, as monohydrate: 3% [30 mg/mL = 28 mg/mL base] (3.5 g)

- **Vi-Daylin® [OTC]** *see* vitamin, multiple (pediatric) *on page 654*
- **Vi-Daylin/F®** *see* vitamin, multiple (pediatric) *on page 654*
- **Videx®** *see* didanosine *on page 200*
- **Viken** *see* cefotaxime *on page 122*
- **Vilona** *see* ribavirin *on page 547*
- **Vilona Pediatrica** *see* ribavirin *on page 547*

vinblastine (vin BLAS teen)
Synonyms vincaleukoblastine; VLB
U.S. Brand Names Alkaban-AQ®; Velban®
Canadian Brand Names Velbe®
Mexican Brand Names Lemblastine
Generic Available Yes
Therapeutic Category Antineoplastic Agent
Use Palliative treatment of Hodgkin's disease; advanced testicular germinal-cell cancers; non-Hodgkin's lymphoma, histiocytosis, and choriocarcinoma
Usual Dosage Refer to individual protocol. Varies depending upon clinical and hematological response. Administer at intervals of at least 7 days and only after leukocyte count has returned to at least 4000/mm^3; maintenance therapy should be titrated according to leukocyte count. Dosage should be reduced in patients with recent exposure to radiation therapy or chemotherapy; single doses in these patients should not exceed 5.5 mg/m^2.

Children and Adults: I.V.: 4-12 mg/m^2 every 7-10 days **or** 5-day continuous infusion of 1.4-1.8 mg/m^2/day **or** 0.1-0.5 mg/kg/week
Nursing/Pharmacy Information
Maintain adequate hydration. Allopurinol may be given to prevent uric acid nephropathy; vinblastine is a tissue irritant and can cause sloughing upon extravasation; care should be taken to avoid extravasation. If extravasation occurs, hyaluronidase and a warm pack can be used for treatment. May be administered IVP or into a free flowing I.V. over a 1-minute period at a concentration for administration of 1 mg/mL.
Monitor CBC with differential and platelet count, serum uric acid, hepatic function tests
Stability: Refrigerate; however, is stable for up to 1-3 months (depending on manufacturer) at room temperature; constituted solutions remain stable for 30 days when refrigerated; protect from light, must be dispersed in amber bag. **Compatible** with doxorubicin, metoclopramide, dacarbazine, bleomycin.
Dosage Forms Vinblastine sulfate:
Injection: 1 mg/mL (10 mL)
Powder for reconstitution: 10 mg

- **vincaleukoblastine** *see* vinblastine *on page 648*
- **Vincasar® PFS™** *see* vincristine *on page 648*

vincristine (vin KRIS teen)
Synonyms LCR; leurocristine; VCR
U.S. Brand Names Oncovin®; Vincasar® PFS™
Mexican Brand Names Citomid
Generic Available Yes

Therapeutic Category Antineoplastic Agent

Use Treatment of leukemias, Hodgkin's disease, neuroblastoma, malignant lymphomas, Wilms' tumor, and rhabdomyosarcoma

Usual Dosage Refer to individual protocol as dosages vary with protocol used. Adjustments are made depending upon clinical and hematological response and upon adverse reactions.

Children: I.V.:
≤10 kg or BSA <1 m²: 0.05 mg/kg once weekly
2 mg/m²; may repeat every week
Adults: I.V.: 0.4-1.4 mg/m², up to 2 mg maximum; may repeat every week

Nursing/Pharmacy Information

Maintain adequate hydration. Allopurinol may be given to prevent uric acid nephropathy; vincristine is a tissue irritant; care should be taken to avoid extravasation. If extravasation occurs, hyaluronidase and a warm pack can be used for treatment. Avoid contact with the eye since vincristine is very irritating. Vincristine is administered IVP or into a free flowing I.V. over a period of 1 minute at a concentration for administration of 1 mg/mL

Monitor Serum electrolytes (sodium), hepatic function tests, neurologic examination, CBC, serum uric acid

Stability: Refrigerate; however, is stable for up to 1 month at room temperature; drug may be administered IVP or IVPB and is **compatible** with D₅W; should be protected from light; **compatible** with doxorubicin, bleomycin, cytarabine, fluorouracil, methotrexate, and metoclopramide

Dosage Forms Injection, as sulfate: 1 mg/mL (1 mL, 2 mL, 5 mL)

vinorelbine (vi NOR el been)

Synonyms vinorelbine tartrate hydrochloride

U.S. Brand Names Navelbine®

Generic Available No

Therapeutic Category Antineoplastic Agent

Use Treatment of nonsmall cell lung cancer (as a single agent or in combination with cisplatin)

Unlabeled use: Breast cancer, ovarian carcinoma (cisplatin-resistant), Hodgkin's disease

Usual Dosage Varies depending upon clinical and hematological response (refer to individual protocols)

Adults: I.V.: 30 mg/m² every 7 days

Dosage adjustment in hematological toxicity (based on granulocyte counts):
Granulocytes ≥1500 cells/mm³ on day of treatment: Administer 30 mg/m²
Granulocytes 1000-1499 cells/mm³ on day of treatment: Administer 15 mg/m²
Granulocytes <1000 cells/mm³ on day of treatment: Do not administer. Repeat granulocyte count in one week; if 3 consecutive doses are held because granulocyte count is <1000 cells/mm³, discontinue vinorelbine

For patients who, during treatment, have experienced fever or sepsis while granulocytopenic or had 2 consecutive weekly doses held due to granulocytopenia, subsequent doses of vinorelbine should be:
22.5 mg/m² for granulocytes ≥1,500 cells/mm³
11.25 mg/m² for granulocytes 1000-1499 cells/mm³

Nursing/Pharmacy Information

Administer I.V. over 6-10 minutes; vesicant with extravasation; maintain adequate hydration; allopurinol may be given to prevent uric acid nephropathy; may cause sloughing upon extravasation

Extravasation treatment: Inject 3-5 mL of hyaluronidase (10 units/mL) S.C. clockwise into the infiltrated area using a 25-gauge needle; change the needle with each injection; apply heat immediately for 1 hour, repeat 4 times/day for 3-5 days (application of cold and injection of hydrocortisone is contraindicated). Hair may be lost during treatment but will regrow to its pretreatment extent even with continued treatment; report any bleeding; examine mouth daily and report soreness to a physician; jaw pain or pain in the organs containing tumor tissue; avoid constipation. Any signs of infection, easy bruising or bleeding, shortness of breath, or painful or burning urination should be brought to physician's attention. Nausea, vomiting or hair loss sometimes occur. The drug may cause permanent sterility and may cause birth defects. The drug may be excreted in breast milk, therefore, an alternative form of feeding your baby should be used.

Dosage Forms Injection, as tartrate: 10 mg/mL (1 mL, 5 mL)

♦ **vinorelbine tartrate hydrochloride** *see* vinorelbine *on page 649*

- **Vioform®** [OTC] *see* clioquinol *on page 157*
- **Vioform®-Hydrocortisone Topical** *(Discontinued)* *see page 743*
- **Viokase®** *see* pancrelipase *on page 467*
- **viosterol** *see* ergocalciferol *on page 237*
- **Vioxx®** *see* rofecoxib *New Drug on page 553*
- **Viprinex®** *see* ancrod *on page 49*
- **Vira-A® Ophthalmic** *see* vidarabine *on page 648*
- **Viracept®** *see* nelfinavir *on page 434*
- **Viramune®** *see* nevirapine *on page 440*
- **Virazide** *see* ribavirin *on page 547*
- **Virazole® Aerosol** *see* ribavirin *on page 547*
- **Virilon®** *see* methyltestosterone *on page 408*
- **Viroptic® Ophthalmic** *see* trifluridine *on page 628*
- **Viscoat®** *see* chondroitin sulfate-sodium hyaluronate *on page 148*
- **Visine®** *(Discontinued)* *see page 743*
- **Visine® Extra Ophthalmic** [OTC] *see* tetrahydrozoline *on page 602*
- **Visine® L.R. Ophthalmic** [OTC] *see* oxymetazoline *on page 463*
- **Visken®** *see* pindolol *on page 495*
- **Vistacon-50® Injection** *see* hydroxyzine *on page 328*
- **Vistaject-25®** *(Discontinued)* *see page 743*
- **Vistaject-50®** *(Discontinued)* *see page 743*
- **Vistaquel® Injection** *see* hydroxyzine *on page 328*
- **Vistaril® Injection** *see* hydroxyzine *on page 328*
- **Vistaril® Oral** *see* hydroxyzine *on page 328*
- **Vistazine® Injection** *see* hydroxyzine *on page 328*
- **Vistide®** *see* cidofovir *on page 149*
- **Vi-Syneral** *see* vitamin, multiple (oral) *on page 654*
- **Vita-C®** [OTC] *see* ascorbic acid *on page 60*
- **VitaCarn® Oral** *see* levocarnitine *on page 365*
- **Vital HN®** [OTC] *see* enteral nutritional products *on page 233*

vitamin A (VYE ta min aye)

Synonyms oleovitamin A
U.S. Brand Names Aquasol A®; Del-Vi-A®; Palmitate-A® 5000 [OTC]
Mexican Brand Names Arovit; A-Vicon; A-Vitex
Generic Available Yes
Therapeutic Category Vitamin, Fat Soluble
Use Treatment and prevention of vitamin A deficiency; supplementation in patients with measles
Usual Dosage
RDA:
0-3 years: 400 mcg*
4-6 years: 500 mcg*
7-10 years: 700 mcg*
>10 years: 800-1000 mcg*
*mcg retinol equivalent (0.3 mcg retinol = 1 unit vitamin A)

Supplementation in measles: Children: Oral:
<1 year: 100,000 units/day for 2 days
>1 year: 200,000 units/day for 2 days
Severe deficiency with xerophthalmia:
Children 1-8 years:
Oral: 5000-10,000 units/kg/day for 5 days or until recovery occurs
I.M.: 5000-15,000 units/day for 10 days
Children >8 years and Adults:
Oral: 500,000 units/day for 3 days, then 50,000 units/day for 14 days, then 10,000-20,000 units/day for 2 months
I.M.: 50,000-100,000 units/day for 3 days, 50,000 units/day for 14 days
Deficiency (without corneal changes): Oral:
Infants <1 year: 10,000 units/kg/day for 5 days, then 7500-15,000 units/day for 10 days
Children 1-8 years: 5000-10,000 units/kg/day for 5 days, then 17,000-35,000 units/day for 10 days
Children >8 years and Adults: 100,000 units/day for 3 days then 50,000 units/day for 14 days
Malabsorption syndrome (prophylaxis): Children >8 years and Adults: Oral: 10,000-50,000 units/day of water miscible product

Dietary supplement: Oral:
Infants up to 6 months: 1500 units/day
Children:
6 months to 3 years: 1500-2000 units/day
4-6 years: 2500 units/day
7-10 years: 3300-3500 units/day
Children >10 years and Adults: 4000-5000 units/day

Nursing/Pharmacy Information
1 mg equals 3333 units
Stability: Protect from light

Dosage Forms
Capsule: 10,000 units [OTC], 25,000 units, 50,000 units
Drops, oral (water miscible) [OTC]: 5000 units/0.1 mL (30 mL)
Injection: 50,000 units/mL (2 mL)
Tablet [OTC]: 5000 units

♦ **vitamin A acid** *see* tretinoin (topical) *on page 622*

vitamin A and vitamin D (VYE ta min aye & VYE ta min dee)

Synonyms cod liver oil
U.S. Brand Names A and D™ Ointment [OTC]
Generic Available Yes
Therapeutic Category Protectant, Topical
Use Temporary relief of discomfort due to chapped skin, diaper rash, minor burns, abrasions, as well as irritations associated with ostomy skin care
Usual Dosage
Oral, oil: Dietary supplement: 2.5 mL/day
Topical: Apply locally with gentle massage as needed
Nursing/Pharmacy Information Discontinue use if irritation develops and consult physician; for external use only
Dosage Forms Ointment, topical: In a lanolin-petrolatum base (60 g)

♦ **vitamin B₁** *see* thiamine *on page 606*
♦ **vitamin B₂** *see* riboflavin *on page 548*
♦ **vitamin B₃** *see* niacin *on page 440*
♦ **vitamin B₅** *see* pantothenic acid *on page 469*
♦ **vitamin B₆** *see* pyridoxine *on page 534*
♦ **vitamin B₁₂** *see* cyanocobalamin *on page 173*
♦ **vitamin B₁₂ₐ** *see* hydroxocobalamin *on page 326*

vitamin B complex (VYE ta min bee KOM pleks)

U.S. Brand Names Apatate® [OTC]; Gevrabon® [OTC]; Lederplex® [OTC]; Lipovite® [OTC]; Mega B® [OTC]; Megaton™ [OTC]; Mucoplex® [OTC]; NeoVadrin® B Complex [OTC]; Orexin® [OTC]; Surbex® [OTC]
Generic Available Yes
Therapeutic Category Vitamin, Water Soluble
Usual Dosage Dosage is usually 1 tablet or capsule/day; please refer to package insert
Dosage Forms
Capsule
Solution: 5 mL, 360 mL

vitamin B complex with vitamin C
(VYE ta min bee KOM pleks with VYE ta min see)
U.S. Brand Names Allbee® With C [OTC]; Surbex-T® Filmtabs® [OTC]; Surbex® With C Filmtabs® [OTC]; Thera-Combex® H-P Kapseals® [OTC]; Vicon-C® [OTC]
Generic Available Yes
Therapeutic Category Vitamin, Water Soluble
Use Supportive nutritional supplementation in conditions in which water-soluble vitamins are required like GI disorders, chronic alcoholism, pregnancy, severe burns, and recovery from surgery
Usual Dosage Adults: Oral: 1 tablet/capsule daily
Dosage Forms Actual vitamin content may vary slightly depending on product used
Tablet/capsule: Vitamin B₁ 10-15 mg, vitamin B₂ 10 mg, vitamin B₃ 100 mg, vitamin B₅ 20 mg, vitamin B₆ 2-5 mg, vitamin B₁₂ 6-10 mg, vitamin C 300-500 mg

vitamin B complex with vitamin C and folic acid
(VYE ta min bee KOM pleks with VYE ta min see & FOE lik AS id)
U.S. Brand Names Berocca®; Nephrocaps®
Generic Available Yes
Therapeutic Category Vitamin, Water Soluble
Use Supportive nutritional supplementation in conditions in which water-soluble vitamins are required like GI disorders, chronic alcoholism, pregnancy, severe burns, and recovery from surgery
Usual Dosage Adults: Oral: 1 capsule/day
Dosage Forms Capsule

♦ **vitamin C** *see* ascorbic acid *on page 60*
♦ **Vitamin C Drops [OTC]** *see* ascorbic acid *on page 60*
♦ **vitamin D$_2$** *see* ergocalciferol *on page 237*

vitamin E (VYE ta min ee)
Synonyms *d*-alpha tocopherol; *dl*-alpha tocopherol
U.S. Brand Names Amino-Opti-E® [OTC]; Aquasol E® [OTC]; E-Complex-600® [OTC]; E-Vitamin® [OTC]; Vita-Plus® E Softgels® [OTC]; Vitec® [OTC]; Vite E® Creme [OTC]
Generic Available Yes
Therapeutic Category Vitamin, Fat Soluble; Vitamin, Topical
Use Prevention and treatment of vitamin E deficiency
Usual Dosage
RDA: Oral:
Premature Infants ≤3 months: 25 units/day
Infants:
≤6 months: 4.5 units/day
6-12 months: 6 units/day
Children:
1-3 years: 9 units/day
4-10 years: 10.5 units/day
Adults >11 years:
Female: 12 units/day
Male: 15 units/day
Prevention of vitamin E deficiency: Neonates, premature, low birthweight (results in normal levels within 1 week): Oral: 25-50 units/24 hours until 6-10 weeks of age or 125-150 units/kg total in 4 doses on days 1, 2, 7, and 8 of life
Vitamin E deficiency treatment: Adults: Oral: 50-200 units/24 hours for 2 weeks
Topical: Apply a thin layer over affected areas as needed
Nursing/Pharmacy Information
Monitor plasma tocopherol concentrations (normal range: 6-14 mcg/mL)
Stability: Protect from light
Dosage Forms
Capsule: 100 units, 200 units, 330 mg, 400 units, 500 units, 600 units, 1000 units
Capsule, water miscible: 73.5 mg, 147 mg, 165 mg, 330 mg, 400 units
Cream: 50 mg/g (15 g, 30 g, 60 g, 75 g, 120 g, 454 g)
Drops, oral: 50 mg/mL (12 mL, 30 mL)
Liquid, topical: 10 mL, 15 mL, 30 mL, 60 mL
Lotion: 120 mL
Oil: 15 mL, 30 mL, 60 mL
Ointment, topical: 30 mg/g (45 g, 60 g)
Tablet: 200 units, 400 units

♦ **vitamin G** *see* riboflavin *on page 548*
♦ **vitamin K$_1$** *see* phytonadione *on page 493*

vitamin, multiple (injectable)
U.S. Brand Names M.V.C.® 9 + 3; M.V.I.®-12; M.V.I.® Concentrate; M.V.I.® Pediatric
Generic Available Yes
Therapeutic Category Vitamin
Usual Dosage I.V.:
Children:
≤5 kg: 10 mL/1000 mL TPN (M.V.I.® Pediatric)
5.1 kg to 11 years: 5 mL/one TPN bag/day (M.V.I.® Pediatric)
Children >11 years and Adults: 5 mL of vials 1 and 2 (M.V.I.®-12)/one TPN bag/day
Dosage Forms See Multivitamins table.

Multivitamin Products Available

Product	Content Given Per	A IU	D IU	E IU	C mg	FA mg	B₁ mg	B₂ mg	B₃ mg	B₆ mg	B₁₂ mcg	Other
Theragran®	5 mL liquid	10,000	400		200		10	10	100	4.1	5	B₅ 21.4 mg
Vi-Daylin®	1 mL drops	1500	400	4.1	35		0.5	0.6	8	0.4	1.5	Alcohol <0.5%
Vi-Daylin® Iron	1 mL	1500	400	4.1	35		0.5	0.6	8	0.4		Fe 10 mg
Albee® with C	tablet				300		15	10.2		5		Niacinamide 50 mg, pantothenic acid 10 mg
Vitamin B Complex	tablet					400 mcg	1.5	1.7		2	6	Niacinamide 20 mg
Hexavitamin	cap/tab	5000	400		75		2	3	20			
Iberet®-Folic - 500	tablet				500	0.8	6	6	30	5	25	B₅ 10 mg, Fe 105 mg
Stuartnatal 1+1	tablet	4000	400	11	120	1	1.5	3	20	10	12	Cu, Zn 25 mg, Fe 65 mg, Ca 200 mg
Theragran® M	tablet	5000	400	30	90	0.4	3	3.4	30	3	9	Cl, Cr, I, K, B₅ 10 mg, Mg, Mn, Mo, P, Se, Zn 15 mg, Fe 27 mg, biotin 30 mcg, beta-carotene 1250 IU
Vi-Daylin®	tablet	2500	400	15	60	0.3	1.05	1.2	13.5	1.05	4.5	
M.V.I.-12 injection	5 mL	3300	200	10	100	0.4	3	3.6	40	4	5	B₅ 15 mg, biotin 60 mcg
M.V.I.-12 unit vial	20 mL											
M.V.I. pediatric powder	5 mL	2300	400	7	80	0.14	1.2	1.4	17	1	1	B₅ 5 mg, biotin 20 mcg, vitamin K 200 mcg

vitamin, multiple (oral) (VYE ta mins, MUL ti pul)

U.S. Brand Names Becotin® Pulvules®; Cefol® Filmtab®; Eldercaps® [OTC]; NeoVadrin® [OTC]; Niferex®-PN; Secran®; Stresstabs® 600 Advanced Formula Tablets [OTC]; Therabid® [OTC]; Theragran® [OTC]; Theragran® Hematinic®; Theragran® Liquid [OTC]; Theragran-M® [OTC]; Unicap® [OTC]; Vicon Forte®; Vicon® Plus [OTC]

Canadian Brand Names Icaps®; Infantol®; Maltlevol®; Materna®; Ocuvite™; Orifer® F; Penta/3B® Plus; Prenavite® Forte; Sopalamine/3B Plus C; Spectrum™ Forte 29

Mexican Brand Names Clanda®; Complan; Suplena; Vi-Syneral

Generic Available Yes

Therapeutic Category Vitamin

Use Dietary supplement

Usual Dosage Adults: Oral: 1 tablet/day or 5 mL/day liquid

Nursing/Pharmacy Information Doses may be higher for burn or cystic fibrosis patients

Dosage Forms See Multivitamins table.

vitamin, multiple (pediatric)

Synonyms children's vitamins; multivitamins/fluoride

U.S. Brand Names Adeflor®; ADEKs® Pediatric Drops; LKV-Drops® [OTC]; Multi Vit® Drops [OTC]; Poly-Vi-Flor®; Poly-Vi-Sol® [OTC]; Tri-Vi-Flor®; Tri-Vi-Sol® [OTC]; Vi-Daylin® [OTC]; Vi-Daylin/F®

Generic Available Yes

Therapeutic Category Vitamin

Use Nutritional supplement, vitamin deficiency

Usual Dosage Oral: 0.6 mL or 1 mL/day; please refer to package insert

Dosage Forms See Multivitamins table.

vitamin, multiple (prenatal)

Synonyms prenatal vitamins

U.S. Brand Names Chromagen® OB [OTC]; Natabec® [OTC]; Natabec® FA [OTC]; Natabec® Rx; Natalins® [OTC]; Natalins® Rx; Pramet® FA; Pramilet® FA; Prenavite® [OTC]; Stuartnatal® 1 + 1; Stuart Prenatal® [OTC]

Generic Available Yes

Therapeutic Category Vitamin

Use Nutritional supplement, vitamin deficiency

Usual Dosage Oral: 1 tablet or capsule daily; please refer to package insert

♦ **Vitaneed™ [OTC]** *see* enteral nutritional products *on page 233*

♦ **Vita-Plus® E Softgels® [OTC]** *see* vitamin E *on page 652*

♦ **Vitec® [OTC]** *see* vitamin E *on page 652*

♦ **Vite E® Creme [OTC]** *see* vitamin E *on page 652*

♦ **Vitinoin™** *see* tretinoin (topical) *on page 622*

♦ **Vito Reins®** *see* phenazopyridine *on page 483*

♦ **Vitrasert®** *see* ganciclovir *on page 287*

♦ **Vitravene™** *see* fomivirsen *New Drug on page 282*

♦ **Vivactil®** *see* protriptyline *on page 529*

♦ **Viva-Drops® Solution [OTC]** *see* artificial tears *on page 59*

♦ **Vivelle™ Transdermal** *see* estradiol *on page 242*

♦ **Vivol®** *see* diazepam *on page 196*

♦ **Vivonex® [OTC]** *see* enteral nutritional products *on page 233*

♦ **Vivonex® Plus** *see* enteral nutritional products *on page 233*

♦ **Vivonex® T.E.N. [OTC]** *see* enteral nutritional products *on page 233*

♦ **Vivotif Berna™ Oral** *see* typhoid vaccine *on page 636*

♦ **V-Lax® [OTC]** *see* psyllium *on page 531*

♦ **VLB** *see* vinblastine *on page 648*

♦ **VM-26** *see* teniposide *on page 595*

♦ **Volmax®** *see* albuterol *on page 25*

♦ **Voltaren® Ophthalmic** *see* diclofenac *on page 198*

♦ **Voltaren® Oral** *see* diclofenac *on page 198*

♦ **Voltaren®-XR Oral** *see* diclofenac *on page 198*

♦ **Vontrol®** *(Discontinued) see page 743*

♦ **VōSol® HC Otic** *see* acetic acid, propylene glycol diacetate, and hydrocortisone *on page 18*

♦ **VōSol® Otic** *see* acetic acid *on page 17*

♦ **VP-16** *see* etoposide *on page 255*

♦ **Vumon** *see* teniposide *on page 595*

- **V.V.S.®** *see* sulfabenzamide, sulfacetamide, and sulfathiazole *on page 584*
- **Vytone® Topical** *see* iodoquinol and hydrocortisone *on page 344*
- **VZIG** *see* varicella-zoster immune globulin (human) *on page 644*

warfarin (WAR far in)

U.S. Brand Names Coumadin®
Canadian Brand Names Warfilone®
Mexican Brand Names Dimantil
Generic Available Yes: Tablet
Therapeutic Category Anticoagulant
Use Prophylaxis and treatment of venous thromboembolic disorders; prevention of arterial thromboembolism in patients with prosthetic heart valves or atrial fibrillation; prevention of death, venous thromboembolism, and recurrent MI after acute MI

Usual Dosage
Oral:
Infants and Children: 0.05-0.34 mg/kg/day; infants <12 months of age may require doses at or near the high end of this range; consistent anticoagulation may be difficult to maintain in children <5 years of age
Adults: 5-15 mg/day for 2-5 days, then adjust dose according to results of prothrombin time; usual maintenance dose ranges from 2-10 mg/day
I.V. (administer as a slow bolus injection): 2-5 mg/day

Dietary Considerations Vitamin K can reverse the anticoagulation effects of warfarin; large amounts of food high in vitamin K (such as green leafy vegetables) may reverse warfarin, decrease prothrombin time, and lead to therapeutic failure; a balanced diet with a consistent intake of vitamin K is essential; avoid large amounts of alfalfa, asparagus, broccoli, Brussel sprouts, cabbage, cauliflower, green teas, kale, lettuce, spinach, turnip greens, watercress

High doses of vitamin A, E, or C may alter PT; use caution with fish oils or omega 3 fatty acids; avoid fried or boiled onions as they may increase drug effect by increasing fibrinolytic activity; avoid herbal teas and remedies such as tonka beans, melilot and woodruff as they contain natural coumarins and will increase effect of warfarin; avoid enteral feeds high in vitamin K, large amounts of liver, avocado, soy protein, soybean oil, papain

Nursing/Pharmacy Information
Be aware of drug interactions and foods that contain vitamin K which can alter anticoagulant effects
Monitor prothrombin time, hematocrit, INR
Stability: Protect from light

Dosage Forms Warfarin sodium:
Powder for injection, lyophilized: 2 mg, 5 mg
Tablet: 1 mg, 2 mg, 2.5 mg, 3 mg, 4 mg, 5 mg, 6 mg, 7.5 mg, 10 mg

- **Warfilone®** *see* warfarin *on page 655*
- **4-Way® Long Acting Nasal Solution [OTC]** *see* oxymetazoline *on page 463*
- **Waytrax** *see* ceftazidime *on page 124*
- **Wehamine® Injection *(Discontinued)*** *see page 743*
- **Wehdryl® *(Discontinued)*** *see page 743*
- **Wellbutrin®** *see* bupropion *on page 97*
- **Wellbutrin® SR** *see* bupropion *on page 97*
- **Wellcovorin®** *see* leucovorin *on page 362*
- **Wesprin® Buffered *(Discontinued)*** *see page 743*
- **Westcort® Topical** *see* hydrocortisone (topical) *on page 324*
- **Whitfield's Ointment [OTC]** *see* benzoic acid and salicylic acid *on page 80*
- **whole root rauwolfia** *see* Rauwolfia serpentina *on page 543*
- **Wigraine®** *see* ergotamine *on page 238*
- **Winasorb** *see* acetaminophen *on page 13*
- **Winks® [OTC]** *see* diphenhydramine *on page 208*
- **Winpred** *see* prednisone *on page 515*
- **WinRho SD®** *see* rh₀(D) immune globulin (intravenous-human) *on page 547*
- **WinRho SDF®** *see* rh₀(D) immune globulin (intravenous-human) *on page 547*
- **Winstrol®** *see* stanozolol *on page 579*

witch hazel (witch HAY zel)

Synonyms hamamelis water
U.S. Brand Names Tucks® [OTC]
Generic Available Yes
(Continued)

witch hazel *(Continued)*

Therapeutic Category Astringent

Use After-stool wipe to remove most causes of local irritation; temporary management of vulvitis, pruritus ani and vulva; help relieve the discomfort of simple hemorrhoids, anorectal surgical wounds, and episiotomies

Usual Dosage Apply to anorectal area as needed

Nursing/Pharmacy Information Consult physician if anorectal symptoms do not improve in 7 days, or if bleeding, protrusion or seepage occurs

Dosage Forms
Gel: 50% with glycerin (19.8 g)
Pads: 50% with glycerin, water and methylparaben (40/jar)

- ◆ **Wolfina®** *see Rauwolfia serpentina on page 543*
- ◆ **wood sugar** *see d-xylose on page 225*
- ◆ **Wyamine® Sulfate** *see mephentermine on page 393*
- ◆ **Wyamycin® S** *see erythromycin (systemic) on page 240*
- ◆ **Wyamycin S® *(Discontinued)*** *see page 743*
- ◆ **Wycillin®** *see penicillin G procaine on page 476*
- ◆ **Wydase®** *see hyaluronidase on page 315*
- ◆ **Wygesic®** *see propoxyphene and acetaminophen on page 526*
- ◆ **Wymox®** *see amoxicillin on page 43*
- ◆ **Wytensin®** *see guanabenz on page 305*
- ◆ **Xalatan®** *see latanoprost on page 361*
- ◆ **Xanax®** *see alprazolam on page 30*
- ◆ **Xeloda™** *see capecitabine on page 109*
- ◆ **Xenical®** *see orlistat New Drug on page 458*
- ◆ **Xitocin** *see oxytocin on page 465*
- ◆ **Xopenex™** *see levalbuterol New Drug on page 363*
- ◆ **X-Prep® Liquid [OTC]** *see senna on page 563*
- ◆ **X-Seb™** *see salicylic acid on page 557*
- ◆ **X-seb® T [OTC]** *see coal tar and salicylic acid on page 163*
- ◆ **Xylocaina** *see lidocaine on page 368*
- ◆ **Xylocaine® HCl I.V. Injection for Cardiac Arrhythmias** *see lidocaine on page 368*
- ◆ **Xylocaine® Oral** *see lidocaine on page 368*
- ◆ **Xylocaine® Topical Ointment** *see lidocaine on page 368*
- ◆ **Xylocaine® Topical Solution** *see lidocaine on page 368*
- ◆ **Xylocaine® Topical Spray** *see lidocaine on page 368*
- ◆ **Xylocaine® With Epinephrine** *see lidocaine and epinephrine on page 369*
- ◆ **Xylocard®** *see lidocaine on page 368*

xylometazoline *(zye loe met AZ oh leen)*

U.S. Brand Names Otrivin® Nasal [OTC]

Generic Available Yes

Therapeutic Category Adrenergic Agonist Agent

Use Symptomatic relief of nasal and nasopharyngeal mucosal congestion

Usual Dosage
Children <12 years: 2-3 drops (0.05%) in each nostril every 8-10 hours
Children >12 years and Adults: 2-3 drops or sprays (0.1%) in each nostril every 8-10 hours

Nursing/Pharmacy Information Do not exceed recommended dosage; do not use for more than 4 consecutive days

Dosage Forms Solution, nasal, as hydrochloride: 0.05% [0.5 mg/mL] (20 mL); 0.1% [1 mg/mL] (15 mL, 20 mL)

- ◆ **Xylo-Pfan® [OTC]** *see d-xylose on page 225*
- ◆ **Yeast-Gard® Medicated Douche** *see povidone-iodine on page 510*
- ◆ **Yectamicina** *see gentamicin on page 290*
- ◆ **Yectamid** *see amikacin on page 36*

yellow fever vaccine *(YEL oh FEE ver vak SEEN)*

U.S. Brand Names YF-VAX®

Generic Available No

Therapeutic Category Vaccine, Live Virus

Use Active immunization against yellow fever

Usual Dosage Single-dose S.C.: 0.5 mL

Nursing/Pharmacy Information
Federal law requires that the date of administration, the vaccine manufacturer, lot number of vaccine, and the administering person's name, title and address be entered into the patient's permanent medical record
Stability: Yellow fever vaccine is shipped with dry ice; do not use vaccine unless shipping case contains some dry ice on arrival; maintain vaccine continuously at a temperature between 0°C to 5°C (32°F to 41°F)
Dosage Forms Injection: Not less than 5.04 Log_{10} Plaque Forming Units (PFU) per 0.5 mL

♦ **yellow mercuric oxide** see mercuric oxide on page 395
♦ **YF-VAX®** see yellow fever vaccine on page 656
♦ **Yocon®** see yohimbine on page 657
♦ **Yodoxin®** see iodoquinol on page 344

yohimbine (yo HIM bine)
U.S. Brand Names Aphrodyne™; Dayto Himbin®; Yocon®; Yohimex™
Generic Available Yes
Therapeutic Category Miscellaneous Product
Use No FDA sanctioned indications
Usual Dosage Adults: Oral: 1 tablet 3 times/day
Dosage Forms Tablet, as hydrochloride: 5.4 mg

♦ **Yohimex™** see yohimbine on page 657
♦ **Yutopar®** see ritodrine on page 551
♦ **Zaditor™** see ketotifen New Drug on page 356

zafirlukast (za FIR loo kast)
Synonyms ICI 204, 219
U.S. Brand Names Accolate®
Generic Available No
Therapeutic Category Leukotriene Receptor Antagonist
Use Prophylaxis and chronic treatment of asthma in adults and children ≥7 years of age
Usual Dosage
Children <7 years: Safety and effectiveness has not been established
Children 7-11 years: 10 mg twice daily
Adults: Oral: 20 mg twice daily; administer 1 hour before food or 2 hours after food
Dosage Forms Tablet: 10 mg, 20 mg

♦ **Zagam®** see sparfloxacin on page 577

zalcitabine (zal SITE a been)
Synonyms ddC; dideoxycytidine
U.S. Brand Names Hivid®
Generic Available No
Therapeutic Category Antiviral Agent
Use Treatment of HIV infections as monotherapy (in patients intolerant to zidovudine or with disease progression while on zidovudine) or in combination with zidovudine in patients with advanced HIV disease (adult CD4 cell count of 150-300 cells/mm³)
Usual Dosage Oral:
Safety and efficacy in children <13 years of age have not been established
Adults (dosed in combination with zidovudine): Daily dose: 0.750 mg every 8 hours, administered together with 200 mg of zidovudine (ie, total daily dose: 2.25 mg of zalcitabine and 600 mg of zidovudine)
Dietary Considerations Should be administered on an empty stomach; food decreases oral absorption by 14%
Nursing/Pharmacy Information
Monitor renal function, CD4 counts, CBC, serum amylase, triglyceride
Stability: Tablets should be stored in tightly closed bottles at 59°F to 86°F
Dosage Forms Tablet: 0.375 mg, 0.75 mg

zaleplon *New Drug* (ZAL e plon)
U.S. Brand Names Sonata®
Generic Available No
Therapeutic Category Hypnotic, Nonbenzodiazepine (Pyrazolopyrimidine)
Use Short-term treatment of insomnia
Usual Dosage
Adults: Oral: 10 mg at bedtime (range: 5-20 mg)
(Continued)

zaleplon *New Drug* (Continued)

Elderly: 5 mg at bedtime
Dosage Forms Capsule: 5 mg, 10 mg

♦ **Zamacort®** see triamcinolone (systemic) on page 624
♦ **Zamtirel** see salmeterol on page 558
♦ **Zanaflex®** see tizanidine on page 615

zanamivir *New Drug* (za NA mi veer)

U.S. Brand Names Relenza®
Generic Available No
Therapeutic Category Antiviral Agent, Inhalation Therapy
Use Treatment of uncomplicated acute illness due to influenza virus in adults and adolescents 12 years of age or older. Treatment should only be initiated in patients who have been symptomatic for no more than 2 days.
Usual Dosage Adolescents ≥12 years and Adults: 2 Inhalations: (10 mg total) twice daily for 5 days. Two doses should be taken on the first day of dosing, regardless of interval, while doses should be spaced by approximately 12 hours on subsequent days.
Dosage Forms Powder, for inhalation: 5 mg per blister

♦ **Zanosar®** see streptozocin on page 581
♦ **Zantac®** see ranitidine hydrochloride on page 541
♦ **Zantac® 75 [OTC]** see ranitidine hydrochloride on page 541
♦ **Zapex®** see oxazepam on page 460
♦ **Zarontin®** see ethosuximide on page 253
♦ **Zaroxolyn®** see metolazone on page 410
♦ **Zartan®** see cephalexin on page 128
♦ **Z-Chlopenthixol** see zuclopenthixol (Canada only) on page 661
♦ **Zeasorb-AF® [OTC]** see tolnaftate on page 618
♦ **Zeasorb-AF® Powder [OTC]** see miconazole on page 413
♦ **Zebeta®** see bisoprolol on page 89
♦ **Zebrax®** *(Discontinued)* see page 743
♦ **Zefazone®** see cefmetazole on page 121
♦ **Zemplar™** see paricalcitol on page 470
♦ **Zemuron™** see rocuronium on page 553
♦ **Zenapax®** see daclizumab on page 179
♦ **Zephiran® [OTC]** see benzalkonium chloride on page 78
♦ **Zephrex®** see guaifenesin and pseudoephedrine on page 302
♦ **Zephrex LA®** see guaifenesin and pseudoephedrine on page 302
♦ **Zerit®** see stavudine on page 579
♦ **Zestoretic®** see lisinopril and hydrochlorothiazide on page 372
♦ **Zestril®** see lisinopril on page 372
♦ **Zetar® [OTC]** see coal tar on page 162
♦ **Zetran®** *(Discontinued)* see page 743
♦ **Ziac™** see bisoprolol and hydrochlorothiazide on page 89
♦ **Ziagen™** see abacavir New Drug on page 12

zidovudine (zye DOE vyoo deen)

Synonyms azidothymidine; AZT; compound S
U.S. Brand Names Retrovir®
Canadian Brand Names Apo®-Zidovudine; Novo-AZT®
Mexican Brand Names Dipedyne; Kenamil; Retrovir-AZT
Generic Available No
Therapeutic Category Antiviral Agent
Use Management of patients with HIV infections who have had at least one episode of *Pneumocystis carinii* pneumonia or who have CD4 cell counts (cells/mm^3) of ≤500 in children >6 years and adults, <750 in children 2-6 years, <1000 in children 1-2 years, and <1750 for children <1 year; patients who have HIV-related symptoms or who are asymptomatic with abnormal laboratory values indicating HIV-related immunosuppression; prevention of maternal-fetal HIV transmission
Usual Dosage
Children 3 months to 12 years:
Oral: 90-180 mg/m^2/dose every 6 hours; maximum: 200 mg every 6 hours
I.V. continuous infusion: 0.5-1.8 mg/kg/hour
I.V. intermittent infusion: 100 mg/m^2/dose every 6 hours

Adults:
  Oral:
    Asymptomatic infection: 100 mg every 4 hours while awake (500 mg/day)
    Symptomatic HIV infection: Initial: 200 mg every 4 hours (1200 mg/day),
      then after 1 month, 100 mg every 4 hours (600 mg/day)
  I.V.: 1-2 mg/kg/dose every 4 hours

Dietary Considerations Oral zidovudine should be administered 1 hour before or 2 hours after a meal with a glass of water; folate or vitamin B_{12} deficiency increases zidovudine-associated myelosuppression

Nursing/Pharmacy Information
Do not administer I.M.; do not administer I.V. push or by rapid infusion; infuse I.V. zidovudine over 1 hour at a final concentration not to exceed 4 mg/mL in D_5W

Monitor CBC, hemoglobin, MCV, serum creatinine kinase

Stability: Storage of capsules, syrup, undiluted vials need to be protected from light

Dosage Forms
Capsule: 100 mg
Injection: 10 mg/mL (20 mL)
Syrup (strawberry flavor): 50 mg/5 mL (240 mL)
Tablet: 300 mg

zidovudine and lamivudine
(zye DOE vyoo deen & la MI vyoo deen)
Synonyms AZT + 3TC
U.S. Brand Names Combivir®
Generic Available No
Therapeutic Category Antiviral Agent
Use Combivir® given twice a day, provides an alternative regimen to lamivudine 150 mg twice a day plus zidovudine 600 mg per day in divided doses; this drug form reduces capsule/tablet intake for these two drugs to two per day instead of up to eight
Usual Dosage Children >12 years and Adults: Oral: One tablet twice daily
Dosage Forms Tablet: Zidovudine 300 mg and lamivudine 150 mg

♦ **Zilactin-B® Medicated [OTC]** see benzocaine on page 79

zileuton (zye LOO ton)
U.S. Brand Names Zyflo™
Generic Available No
Therapeutic Category 5-Lipoxygenase Inhibitor
Use Prophylaxis and chronic treatment of asthma in adults and children ≥12 years of age
Usual Dosage Children ≥12 years and Adults: Oral: 1 tablet 4 times/day, may be taken with meals and at bedtime
Dosage Forms Tablet: 600 mg

♦ **Zinacef® Injection** see cefuroxime on page 126

♦ **Zinaderm** see zinc oxide on page 660

♦ **Zinca-Pak®** see trace metals on page 620

♦ **Zincate® Oral** see zinc sulfate on page 660

zinc chloride (zingk KLOR ide)
Generic Available Yes
Therapeutic Category Trace Element
Use Cofactor for replacement therapy to different enzymes helps maintain normal growth rates, normal skin hydration and senses of taste and smell
Usual Dosage Clinical response may not occur for up to 6-8 weeks
Supplemental to I.V. solutions:
  Premature Infants <1500 g, up to 3 kg: 300 mcg/kg/day
  Full-term Infants and Children ≤5 years: 100 mcg/kg/day
  Adults:
    Stable with fluid loss from small bowel: 12.2 mg zinc/liter TPN or 17.1 mg zinc/kg (added to 1000 mL I.V. fluids) of stool or ileostomy output
    Metabolically stable: 2.5-4 mg/day, add 2 mg/day for acute catabolic states
Nursing/Pharmacy Information Patients on TPN therapy should have periodic serum copper and serum zinc levels
Dosage Forms Injection: 1 mg/mL (10 mL)

♦ **Zincfrin® Ophthalmic [OTC]** see phenylephrine and zinc sulfate on page 489

zinc gelatin (zingk JEL ah tin)
Synonyms Unna's boot; Unna's paste
U.S. Brand Names Gelucast®
Generic Available Yes
Therapeutic Category Protectant, Topical
Use Protectant and to support varicosities and similar lesions of the lower limbs
Usual Dosage Apply externally as an occlusive boot
Nursing/Pharmacy Information After a period of ~2 weeks, the dressing is removed by soaking in warm water
Dosage Forms Bandage: 3" x 10 yards, 4" x 10 yards

- **zinc injection** *see* trace metals *on page 620*
- **Zincofax®** *see* zinc oxide *on page 660*
- **Zincon® Shampoo [OTC]** *see* pyrithione zinc *on page 535*

zinc oxide (zingk OKS ide)
Synonyms Lassar's zinc paste
Canadian Brand Names Prevex™ Baby Diaper Rash; Zinaderm; Zincofax®
Generic Available Yes
Therapeutic Category Topical Skin Product
Use Protective coating for mild skin irritations and abrasions; soothing and protective ointment to promote healing of chapped skin, diaper rash
Usual Dosage Infants, Children, and Adults: Topical: Apply several times daily to affected area
Nursing/Pharmacy Information
If irritation develops, discontinue use and consult a physician; paste is easily removed with mineral oil; for external use only; do not use in the eyes
Stability: Avoid prolonged storage at temperatures >30°C
Dosage Forms
Ointment, topical: 20% in white ointment (480 g)
Paste, topical: 25% in white petrolatum (480 g)

zinc oxide, cod liver oil, and talc
(zingk OKS ide, kod LIV er oyl, & talk)
U.S. Brand Names Desitin® [OTC]
Generic Available Yes
Therapeutic Category Protectant, Topical
Use Relief of diaper rash, superficial wounds and burns, and other minor skin irritations
Usual Dosage Topical: Apply thin layer as needed
Nursing/Pharmacy Information If condition persists, or if rash, irritation or sensitivity develops, discontinue and contact physician; for external use only
Dosage Forms Ointment, topical: Zinc oxide, cod liver oil and talc in a petrolatum and lanolin base (30 g, 60 g, 120 g, 240 g, 270 g)

zinc sulfate (zingk SUL fate)
U.S. Brand Names Eye-Sed® Ophthalmic [OTC]; Orazinc® Oral [OTC]; Verazinc® Oral [OTC]; Zincate® Oral
Generic Available Yes
Therapeutic Category Electrolyte Supplement, Oral
Use Zinc supplement (oral and parenteral); may improve wound healing in those who are deficient
Usual Dosage
RDA: Oral:
Birth to 6 months: 3 mg elemental zinc/day
6-12 months: 5 mg elemental zinc/day
1-10 years: 10 mg elemental zinc/day
≥11 years: 15 mg elemental zinc/day

Zinc deficiency: Oral:
Infants and Children: 0.5-1 mg elemental zinc/kg/day divided 1-3 times/day; somewhat larger quantities may be needed if there is impaired intestinal absorption or an excessive loss of zinc
Adults: 110-220 mg zinc sulfate (25-50 mg elemental zinc)/dose 3 times/day
Dietary Considerations May be administered with food if GI upset occurs; avoid foods high in calcium or phosphorus
Nursing/Pharmacy Information
Injection must be diluted before use; refrigerate suspension
Monitor patients on TPN therapy should have periodic serum copper and serum zinc levels
Stability: Store oral liquid (injectable used orally) in refrigerator

Dosage Forms
Capsule: 110 mg [elemental zinc 25 mg]; 220 mg [elemental zinc 50 mg]
Injection: 1 mg/mL (10 mL, 30 mL); 4 mg/mL (10 mL); 5 mg/mL (5 mL, 10 mL, 50 mL)
Tablet: 66 mg [elemental zinc 15 mg]; 200 mg [elemental zinc 46 mg]

- **zinc undecylenate** *see* undecylenic acid and derivatives *on page 637*
- **Zinecard®** *see* dexrazoxane *on page 192*
- **Zinnat** *see* cefuroxime *on page 126*
- **Zithromax™** *see* azithromycin *on page 68*
- **ZNP® Bar [OTC]** *see* pyrithione zinc *on page 535*
- **Zocor®** *see* simvastatin *on page 567*
- **Zofran®** *see* ondansetron *on page 455*
- **Zofran® ODT** *see* ondansetron *on page 455*
- **Zoladex® Implant** *see* goserelin *on page 297*
- **Zoldan-A** *see* danazol *on page 181*
- **Zolicef®** *see* cefazolin *on page 120*

zolmitriptan (zohl mi TRIP tan)

Synonyms 311C90
U.S. Brand Names Zomig®
Generic Available No
Therapeutic Category Antimigraine Agent; Serotonin Agonist
Use Acute treatment of adult migraine, with or without auras.
Usual Dosage Adults: Oral: Single doses of 1, 2.5, or 5 mg are effective in reducing symptoms of a migraine attack. Patients should be started at a dose of 2.5 mg or lower since the incidence of side effects increases somewhat with dose. If the headache returns, the dose may be repeated after 2 hours but **not to exceed** 10 mg within a 24-hour period.
Dosage Forms Tablet: 2.5 mg, 5 mg

- **Zoloft®** *see* sertraline *on page 564*

zolpidem (zole PI dem)

U.S. Brand Names Ambien™
Generic Available No
Therapeutic Category Hypnotic, Nonbarbiturate
Use Short-term treatment of insomnia
Usual Dosage Adults: Oral: 10 mg immediately before bedtime
Nursing/Pharmacy Information
Patients may require assistance with ambulation; lower doses in the elderly are usually effective; institute safety measures; administer on an empty stomach
Monitor daytime alertness; respiratory and cardiac status
Dosage Forms Tablet, as tartrate: 5 mg, 10 mg

- **Zolyse® (Discontinued)** *see page 743*
- **Zomig®** *see* zolmitriptan *on page 661*
- **Zonal** *see* fluconazole *on page 270*
- **Zonalon® Topical Cream** *see* doxepin *on page 219*
- **Zone-A Forte®** *see* pramoxine and hydrocortisone *on page 512*
- **Zorbenal-G** *see* tetracycline *on page 601*
- **ZORprin®** *see* aspirin *on page 61*
- **Zostrix® [OTC]** *see* capsaicin *on page 110*
- **Zostrix®-HP [OTC]** *see* capsaicin *on page 110*
- **Zosyn™** *see* piperacillin and tazobactam sodium *on page 496*
- **Zovia®** *see* ethinyl estradiol and ethynodiol diacetate *on page 249*
- **Zovirax®** *see* acyclovir *on page 21*

zuclopenthixol (Canada only) (zoo kloe pen THIX ol)

Synonyms Z-Chlopenthixol
Canadian Brand Names Clopixol®; Clopixol-Acuphase®; Clopixol® Depot
Generic Available No
Therapeutic Category Antipsychotic Agent
Use Schizophrenia, bipolar disorder, psychoses; usually useful in agitated states
Usual Dosage
Oral: Zuclopenthixol hydrochloride: Initial: 20-30 mg/day in divided doses; usual maintenance dose: 20-75 mg/day; maximum daily dose: 150 mg
(Continued)

zuclopenthixol *(Canada only)* *(Continued)*

I.M.:

Zuclopenthixol acetate: 50-150 mg; may be repeated in 2-3 days; no more than 4 injections should be given in the course of treatment; maximum dose during course of treatment: 400 mg

Zuclopenthixol decanoate: 100 mg by deep I.M. injection; additional doses of 100-200 mg (I.M.) may be given over the following 1-4 weeks; maximum weekly dose: 600 mg

Dosage Forms

Injection:

Acuphase, as acetate: 50 mg/mL [zuclopenthixol 42.5 mg/mL] (1 mL, 2 mL)

Depot, as decanoate: 200 mg/mL [zuclopenthixol 144.4 mg/mL] (10 mL)

Tablet, as dihydrochloride: 10 mg, 25 mg, 40 mg

- ◆ **Zyban™** *see* bupropion *on page 97*
- ◆ **Zyban 100 mg** *(Discontinued)* *see page 743*
- ◆ **Zydone®** *see* hydrocodone and acetaminophen *on page 319*
- ◆ **Zyflo™** *see* zileuton *on page 659*
- ◆ **Zyloprim®** *see* allopurinol *on page 29*
- ◆ **Zymase®** *see* pancrelipase *on page 467*
- ◆ **Zymerol** *see* cimetidine *on page 150*
- ◆ **Zyprexa™** *see* olanzapine *on page 454*
- ◆ **Zyrtec®** *see* cetirizine *on page 130*

APPENDIX TABLE OF CONTENTS

ABBREVIATIONS & SYMBOLS COMMONLY USED IN MEDICAL ORDERS

Abbreviation	From	Meaning
μg		microgram
μmol		micromole
°C		degrees Celsius (Centigrade)
<		less than
>		greater than
≤		less than or equal to
≥		greater than or equal to
a͞a, aa	ana	of each
ABG		arterial blood gas
ac	ante cibum	before meals or food
ACE		angiotensin-converting enzyme
ACLS		adult cardiac life support
ad	ad	to, up to
a.d.	aurio dextra	right ear
ADH		antidiuretic hormone
ad lib	ad libitum	at pleasure
AED		antiepileptic drug
a.l.	aurio laeva	left ear
ALL		acute lymphoblastic leukemia
ALT		alanine aminotransferase (was SGPT)
AM	ante meridiem	morning
AML		acute myeloblastic leukemia
amp		ampul
amt		amount
ANA		antinuclear antibodies
ANC		absolute neutrophil count
ANL		acute nonlymphoblastic leukemia
aq	aqua	water
aq. dest.	aqua destillata	distilled water
APTT		activated partial thromboplastin time
a.s.	aurio sinister	left ear
ASA (class I-IV)		classification of surgical patients according to their baseline health (eg, healthy ASA I and II or increased severity of illness ASA III or IV)
ASAP		as soon as possible
AST		aspartate aminotransferase (was SGOT)
a.u.	aures utrae	each ear
A-V		atrial-ventricular
bid	bis in die	twice daily
bm		bowel movement
BMT		bone marrow transplant
bp		blood pressure
BSA		body surface area
BUN		blood urea nitrogen
c	cong	a gallon
c̄	cum	with
cal		calorie
cAMP		cyclic adenosine monophosphate
cap	capsula	capsule
CBC		complete blood count
cc		cubic centimeter
CHF		congestive heart failure
CI		cardiac index
Cl$_{cr}$		creatinine clearance
cm		centimeter

Abbreviation	From	Meaning
CNS		central nervous system
comp	compositus	compound
cont		continue
COPD		chronic obstructive pulmonary disease
CSF		cerebral spinal fluid
CT		computed tomography
CVA		cerebral vascular accident
CVP		central venous pressure
d	dies	day
D_5W		dextrose 5% in water
$D_{5/0.45}$ NaCl		dextrose 5% in sodium chloride 0.45%
$D_{10}W$		dextrose 10% in water
d/c		discontinue
DIC		disseminated intravascular coagulation
dil	dilue	dilute
disp	dispensa	dispense
div	divide	divide
DNA		deoxyribonucleic acid
dtd	dentur tales doses	give of such a dose
DVT		deep vein thrombosis
EEG		electroencephalogram
EKG		electrocardiogram
elix, el	elixir	elixir
emp		as directed
ESR		erythrocyte sedimentation rate
E.T.		endotracheal
et	et	and
ex aq		in water
f, ft	fac, fiat, fiant	make, let be made
FDA		Food and Drug Administration
FEV_1		forced expiratory volume
FVC		forced vital capacity
g	gramma	gram
G-6-PD		glucose-6-phosphate dehydrogenase
GA		gestational age
GABA		gamma-aminobutyric acid
GE		gastroesophageal
GI		gastrointestinal
gr	granum	grain
gtt	gutta	a drop
GU		genitourinary
h	hora	hour
HIV		human immunodeficiency virus
HPLC		high performance liquid chromatography
hs	hora somni	at bedtime
IBW		ideal body weight
ICP		intracranial pressure
IgG		immune globulin G
I.M.		intramuscular
INR		international normalized ratio
I.O.		intraosseous
I & O		input and output
IOP		intraocular pressure
I.T.		intrathecal
I.V.		intravenous
IVH		intraventricular hemorrhage
IVP		intravenous push
JRA		juvenile rheumatoid arthritis

ABBREVIATIONS & SYMBOLS COMMONLY USED IN MEDICAL ORDERS *(Continued)*

Abbreviation	From	Meaning
kcal		kilocalorie
kg		kilogram
L		liter
LDH		lactate dehydrogenase
LE		lupus erythematosus
liq	liquor	a liquor, solution
LP		lumbar puncture
M.	misce	mix
MAO		monoamine oxidase
MAP		mean arterial pressure
mcg		microgram
m. dict	more dictor	as directed
mEq		milliequivalent
mg		milligram
MI		myocardial infarction
min		minute
mixt	mixtura	a mixture
mL		milliliter
mm		millimeter
mo		month
mOsm		milliosmols
MRI		magnetic resonance image
ND		nasoduodenal
NF		National Formulary
ng		nanogram
NG		nasogastric
NMDA		n-methyl-d-aspartate
nmol		nanomole
no.	numerus	number
noc	nocturnal	in the night
non rep	non repetatur	do not repeat, no refills
NPO		nothing by mouth
NSAID		nonsteroidal anti-inflammatory drug
O, Oct	octarius	a pint
o.d.	oculus dexter	right eye
o.l.	oculus laevus	left eye
O.R.		operating room
o.s.	oculus sinister	left eye
OTC		over-the-counter (nonprescription)
o.u.	oculo uterque	each eye
PALS		pediatric advanced life support
pc, post cib	post cibos	after meals
PCA		postconceptional age
PCP		*Pneumocystis carinii* pneumonia
PCWP		pulmonary capillary wedge pressure
PDA		patent ductus arteriosus
per		through or by
PM	post meridiem	afternoon or evening
PNA		postnatal age
P.O.	per os	by mouth
P.R.	per rectum	rectally
prn	pro re nata	as needed
PSVT		paroxysmal supraventricular tachycardia
PT		prothrombin time
PTT		partial thromboplastin time
PUD		peptic ulcer disease
pulv	pulvis	a powder
PVC		premature ventricular contraction

Abbreviation	From	Meaning
q		every
qad	quoque alternis die	every other day
qd		every day
qh	quiaque hora	every hour
qid	quater in die	four times a day
qod		every other day
qs	quantum sufficiat	a sufficient quantity
qs ad		a sufficient quantity to make
qty		quantity
qv	quam volueris	as much as you wish
Rx	recipe	take, a recipe
RAP		right atrial pressure
rep	repetatur	let it be repeated
$\bar{s}$	sine	without
S-A		sino-atrial
sa	secundum artem	according to art
sat	sataratus	saturated
S.C.		subcutaneous
S_{cr}		serum creatinine
SIADH		syndrome of inappropriate antidiuretic hormone
sig	signa	label, or let it be printed
S.L.		sublingual
SLE		systemic lupus erythematosus
sol	solutio	solution
solv		dissolve
$\overline{ss}$, ss	semis	one-half
sos	si opus sit	if there is need
stat	statim	at once, immediately
supp	suppositorium	suppository
SVR		systemic vascular resistance
SVT		supraventricular tachycardia
SWI		sterile water for injection
syr	syrupus	syrup
tab	tabella	tablet
tal		such
tid	ter in die	three times a day
tr, tinct	tincture	tincture
trit		triturate
tsp		teaspoonful
TT		thrombin time
u.d., ut dict	ut dictum	as directed
ung	unguentum	ointment
USAN		United States Adopted Names
USP		United States Pharmacopeia
UTI		urinary tract infection
V_d		volume of distribution
V_{dss}		volume of distribution at steady-state
v.o.		verbal order
w.a.		while awake
x3		3 times
x4		4 times
y		year

BODY SURFACE AREA OF ADULTS AND CHILDREN

Calculating Body Surface Area in Children

In a child of average size, find weight and corresponding surface area on the boxed scale to the left; or, use the nomogram to the right. Lay a straightedge on the correct height and weight points for the child, then read the intersecting point on the surface area scale.

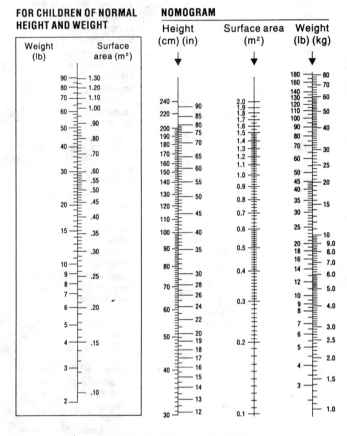

FOR CHILDREN OF NORMAL HEIGHT AND WEIGHT

NOMOGRAM

BODY SURFACE AREA FORMULA
(Adult and Pediatric)

$$\text{BSA (m}^2) = \sqrt{\frac{\text{Ht (in) x Wt (lb)}}{3131}} \quad \text{or, in metric: BSA (m}^2) = \sqrt{\frac{\text{Ht (cm) x Wt (kg)}}{3600}}$$

References

Lam TK and Leung DT, "More on Simplified Calculation of Body Surface Area," *N Engl J Med,* 1988, 318(17):1130 (Letter).

Mosteller RD, "Simplified Calculation of Body Surface Area", *N Engl J Med,* 1987, 317(17):1098 (Letter).

AVERAGE WEIGHTS AND SURFACE AREAS

Average Weight and Surface Area of Preterm Infants, Term Infants, and Children

Age	Average Weight (kg)*	Approximate Surface Area (m²)
Weeks Gestation		
26	0.9-1	0.1
30	1.3-1.5	0.12
32	1.6-2	0.15
38	2.9-3	0.2
40 (term infant at birth)	3.1-4	0.25
Months		
3	5	0.29
6	7	0.38
9	8	0.42
Year		
1	10	0.49
2	12	0.55
3	15	0.64
4	17	0.74
5	18	0.76
6	20	0.82
7	23	0.90
8	25	0.95
9	28	1.06
10	33	1.18
11	35	1.23
12	40	1.34
Adult	70	1.73

*Weights from age 3 months and older are rounded off to the nearest kilogram.

IDEAL BODY WEIGHT CALCULATION

Adults (18 years and older) (IBW is in kg)

IBW (male)	=	50 + (2.3 x height in inches over 5 feet)
IBW (female)	=	45.5 + (2.3 x height in inches over 5 feet)

*IBW is in kg.

Children (IBW is in kg; height is in cm)

a. 1-18 years

$$IBW = \frac{(height^2 \times 1.65)}{1000}$$

b. 5 feet and taller

IBW (male) = 39 + (2.27 x height in inches over 5 feet)

IBW (female) = 42.2 + (2.27 x height in inches over 5 feet)

IDEAL BODY WEIGHTS IN KILOGRAMS TABLE*

Height	Male	Female
5′0″	50.0	45.0
5′1″	52.3	47.3
5′2″	54.6	49.6
5′3″	56.9	51.9
5′4″	59.2	54.2
5′5″	61.5	56.5
5′6″	63.8	58.8
5′7″	66.1	61.1
5′8″	68.4	63.4
5′9″	70.7	65.7
5′10″	73.0	68.0
5′11″	75.3	70.3
6′0″	77.6	72.6
6′1″	79.9	
6′2″	82.2	
6′3″	84.5	
6′4″	86.8	

*Calculated from:

IBW (kg)	male	=	50 kg + 2.3 kg/inch over 5′0″
	female	=	45 kg + 2.3 kg/inch over 5′0″

APOTHECARY/METRIC EQUIVALENTS

Approximate Liquid Measures
Basic equivalent: 1 fluid ounce = 30 mL

Examples:

1 gallon .... 3800 mL	1 gallon ... 128 fluid ounces
1 quart .... 960 mL	1 quart ..... 32 fluid ounces
1 pint .... 480 mL	1 pint ...... 16 fluid ounces
8 fluid oz .... 240 mL	15 minims .... 1 mL
4 fluid oz .... 120 mL	10 minims .... 0.6 mL

Approximate Household Equivalents

1 teaspoonful ...... 5 mL	1 tablespoonful ...... 15 mL

Weights
Basic equivalents:

1 oz .... 30 g	15 gr .... 1 g

Examples:

4 oz .... 120 g	1 gr .... 60 mg
2 oz .... 60 g	1/100 gr .... 600 mcg
10 gr .... 600 mg	1/150 gr .... 400 mcg
7½ gr .... 500 mg	1/200 gr .... 300 mcg
16 oz .... 1 lb	

Metric Conversions
Basic equivalents:

1 g .... 1000 mg	1 mg .... 1000 mcg

Examples:

5 g .... 5000 mg	5 mg .... 5000 mcg
0.5 g .... 500 mg	0.5 g .... 500 mcg
0.05 g .... 50 mg	0.05 mg .... 50 mcg

Exact Equivalents

1 g	=	15.43 gr	0.1 mg	=	1/600 gr
1 mL	=	16.23 minims	0.12 mg	=	1/500 gr
1 minim	=	0.06 mL	0.15 mg	=	1/400 gr
1 gr	=	64.8 mg	0.2 mg	=	1/300 gr
1 pint (pt)	=	473.2 mL	0.3 mg	=	1/200 gr
1 oz	=	28.35 g	0.4 mg	=	1/150 gr
1 lb	=	453.6 g	0.5 mg	=	1/120 gr
1 kg	=	2.2 lbs	0.6 mg	=	1/100 gr
1 qt	=	946.4 mL	0.8 mg	=	1/80 gr
			1 mg	=	1/65 gr

Solids*

¼ grain	=	15 mg
½ grain	=	30 mg
1 grain	=	60 mg
1½ grains	=	100 mg
5 grains	=	300 mg
10 grains	=	600 mg

*Use exact equivalents for compounding and calculations requiring a high degree of accuracy.

POUNDS-KILOGRAMS CONVERSION

1 pound = 0.45359 kilograms
1 kilogram = 2.2 pounds

lb	=	kg	lb	=	kg	lb	=	kg
1		0.45	70		31.75	140		63.50
5		2.27	75		34.02	145		65.77
10		4.54	80		36.29	150		68.04
15		6.80	85		38.56	155		70.31
20		9.07	90		40.82	160		72.58
25		11.34	95		43.09	165		74.84
30		13.61	100		45.36	170		77.11
35		15.88	105		47.63	175		79.38
40		18.14	110		49.90	180		81.65
45		20.41	115		52.16	185		83.92
50		22.68	120		54.43	190		86.18
55		24.95	125		56.70	195		88.45
60		27.22	130		58.91	200		90.72
65		29.48	135		61.24			

TEMPERATURE CONVERSION

Celsius to Fahrenheit = (°C x 9/5) + 32 = °F
Fahrenheit to Celsius = (°F -32) x 5/9 = °C

°C	=	°F	°C	=	°F	°C	=	°F
100.0		212.0	39.0		102.2	36.8		98.2
50.0		122.0	38.8		101.8	36.6		97.9
41.0		105.8	38.6		101.5	36.4		97.5
40.8		105.4	38.4		101.1	36.2		97.2
40.6		105.1	38.2		100.8	36.0		96.8
40.4		104.7	38.0		100.4	35.8		96.4
40.2		104.4	37.8		100.1	35.6		96.1
40.0		104.0	37.6		99.7	35.4		95.7
39.8		103.6	37.4		99.3	35.2		95.4
39.6		103.3	37.2		99.0	35.0		95.0
39.4		102.9	37.0		98.6	0		32.0
39.2		102.6						

CANCER CHEMOTHERAPY REGIMENS

ADULT REGIMENS

Adenocarcinoma – Unknown Primary

Carbo-Tax

Paclitaxel, I.V., 135 mg/m^2 over 24 hours, day 1, followed by
Carboplatin dose targeted by Calvert equation to AUC 7.5 I.V.

Repeat cycle every 21 days

EP

Cisplatin, I.V., 60-100 mg/m^2, day 1
Etoposide, I.V., 80-100 mg/m^2, days 1-3

Repeat cycle every 21 days

FAM

Fluorouracil, I.V., 600 mg/m^2, days 1, 8, 29, 36
Doxorubicin, I.V., 30 mg/m^2, days 1, 29
Mitomycin, I.V., 10 mg/m^2, day 1

Repeat cycle every 8 weeks

Paclitaxel/Carboplatin/Etoposide

Paclitaxel, I.V., 200 mg/m^2 over 1 hour, day 1, followed by
Carboplatin dose targeted by Calvert equation to AUC 6 I.V.
Etoposide, P.O., 50 mg/day alternated with 100 mg/day, days 1-10

Repeat cycle every 21 days

Breast Cancer

Standard adjuvant chemotherapy includes 4 cycles of AC or
6 cycles of CMF (d$_1$/d$_8$ variety)

AC

Doxorubicin, I.V., 60 mg/m^2, day 1
Cyclophosphamide, I.V., 400-600 mg/m^2, day 1

Repeat cycle every 21 days

ACe

Doxorubicin, I.V., 40 mg/m^2, day 1
Cyclophosphamide, P.O., 200 mg/m^2/day, days 1-3 or 3-6

Repeat cycle every 21-28 days

CAF

Cyclophosphamide, P.O., 100 mg/m^2, days 1-14 or 600 mg/m^2 I.V.,
  day 1
Doxorubicin, I.V., 25 mg/m^2, days 1, 8 or 60 mg/m^2 I.V., day 1
Fluorouracil, I.V., 500-600 mg/m^2, days 1, 8

Repeat cycle every 28 days

or

Cyclophosphamide, I.V., 500 mg/m^2, day 1
Doxorubicin, I.V., 50 mg/m^2, day 1
Fluorouracil, I.V., 500 mg/m^2, day 1

Repeat cycle every 21 days

CFM

Cyclophosphamide, I.V., 500-600 mg/m^2, day 1
Fluorouracil, I.V., 500-600 mg/m^2, day 1
Mitoxantrone, I.V., 10-12 mg/m^2, day 1

Repeat cycle every 21 days

CFPT

Cyclophosphamide, I.V., 150 mg/m^2, days 1-5
Fluorouracil, I.V., 300 mg/m^2, days 1-5
Prednisone, P.O., 10 mg tid, days 1-7
Tamoxifen, P.O., 10 mg bid, days 1-42

Repeat cycle every 42 days

CANCER CHEMOTHERAPY REGIMENS *(Continued)*

CMF

Cyclophosphamide, P.O., 100 mg/m^2, days 1-14 or 600 mg/m^2 I.V., days 1, 8
Methotrexate, I.V., 40 mg/m^2, days 1, 8
Fluorouracil, I.V., 600 mg/m^2, days 1, 8

Repeat cycle every 28 days

or

Cyclophosphamide, I.V., 600 mg/m^2, day 1
Methotrexate, I.V., 40 mg/m^2, day 1
Fluorouracil, I.V., 400-600 mg/m^2, day 1

Repeat cycle every 21 days

CMFP

Cyclophosphamide, P.O., 100 mg/m^2, days 1-14
Methotrexate, I.V., 40-60 mg/m^2, days 1, 8
Fluorouracil, I.V., 600-700 mg/m^2, days 1, 8
Prednisone, P.O., 40 mg (first 3 cycles only), days 1-14

Repeat cycle every 28 days

FAC

Fluorouracil, I.V., 500 mg/m^2, days 1, 8
Doxorubicin, I.V., 50 mg/m^2, day 1
Cyclophosphamide, I.V., 500 mg/m^2, day 1

Repeat cycle every 21 days

IMF

Ifosfamide, I.V., 1.5 g/m^2, days 1, 8
Mesna, I.V., 20% of ifosfamide dose, give immediately before and 4 and 8 hours after ifosfamide infusion, days 1, 8
Methotrexate, I.V., 40 mg/m^2, days 1, 8
Fluorouracil, I.V., 600 mg/m^2, days 1, 8

Repeat cycle every 28 days

NFL

Mitoxantrone, I.V., 12 mg/m^2, day 1
Fluorouracil, I.V., 350 mg/m^2, days 1-3, given after leucovorin calcium
Leucovorin calcium, I.V., 300 mg/m^2, days 1-3

or

Mitoxantrone, I.V., 10 mg/m^2, day 1
Fluorouracil, I.V., 1000 mg/m^2 continuous infusion, given after leucovorin calcium, days 1-3
Leucovorin calcium, I.V., 100 mg/m^2, days 1-3

Repeat cycle every 21 days

Sequential Dox-CMF

Doxorubicin, I.V., 75 mg/m^2, every 21 days for 4 cycles followed by 21- or 28-day CMF for 8 cycles

Vinorelbine/Doxorubicin

Vinorelbine, I.V., 25 mg/m^2, days 1, 8
Doxorubicin, I.V., 50 mg/m^2, day 1

Repeat cycle every 21 days

VATH

Vinblastine, I.V., 4.5 mg/m^2, day 1
Doxorubicin, I.V., 45 mg/m^2, day 1
Thiotepa, I.V., 12 mg/m^2, day 1
Fluoxymesterone, P.O., 10 mg tid, days 1-21

Repeat cycle every 21 days

Single-Agent Regimens

Anastrozole, P.O., 1 mg qd

Capecitabine, P.O., 2500 mg/m^2/day, bid regimen, days 1-14, repeat cycle every 21 days

Docetaxel, I.V., 60-100 mg/m^2 over 1 hour; patient must be premedicated with dexamethasone 8 mg bid P.O. for 5 days, start 1 day before docetaxel; repeat cycle every 3 weeks

Gemcitabine, I.V., 725 mg/m^2 over 30 minutes, weekly for 3 weeks, followed by 1-week rest, repeat cycle every 28 days

Letrozole, P.O., 2.5 mg qd

Megestrol, P.O., 40 mg qid

Paclitaxel, I.V., 175 mg/m^2 over 3 hours, every 21 days or 250 mg/m^2
over 3-24 hours, every 21 days
Patient must be premedicated with:
Dexamethasone 20 mg P.O., 12 and 6 hours prior
Diphenhydramine 50 mg I.V., 30 minutes prior
Cimetidine 300 mg I.V., or ranitidine 50 mg I.V., 30 minutes prior

Tamoxifen, P.O., 20 mg qd

Toremifene citrate, P.O., 60 mg qd

Vinorelbine, I.V., 30 mg/m^2, every 7 days

Cervical Cancer

CLD-BOMP

Bleomycin, I.V., 5 mg continuous infusion, days 1-7
Cisplatin, I.V., 10 mg/m^2, day 1, 22
Vincristine, I.V., 0.7 mg/m^2, day 7
Mitomycin-C. I.V., 7 mg/m^2, day 7

Repeat cycle every 21 days

MOBP

Bleomycin, I.V., 30 units/day continuous infusion, days 1, 4
Vincristine, I.V., 0.5 mg/m^2, days 1, 4
Mitomycin-C. I.V., 10 mg/m^2, day 1
Cisplatin, I.V., 50 mg/m^2, days 1, 22

Repeat cycle every 28 days

Single-Agent Regimen

Cisplatin, I.V., 50-100 mg/m^2, every 21 days

Colon Cancer

F-CL

Fluorouracil, I.V., 375 mg/m^2, days 1-5
Leucovorin calcium, I.V., 200 mg/m^2, days 1-5

Repeat cycle every 28 days

or

Fluorouracil, I.V., 500 mg/m^2/week 1 hour after initiating the calcium
leucovorin infusion for 6 weeks
Leucovorin calcium, I.V., 500 mg/m^2, over 2 hours, weekly for 6 weeks
2-week break, then repeat cycle

FLe

Fluorouracil, I.V., 450 mg/m^2 for 5 days, then, after a pause of 4
weeks, 450 mg/m^2/week for 48 weeks
Levamisole, P.O., 50 mg tid for 3 days, repeated every 2 weeks for 1
year

FMV

Fluorouracil, I.V., 10 mg/kg/day, days 1-5
Methyl-CCNU, P.O., 175 mg/m^2, day 1
Vincristine, I.V., 1 mg/m^2 (max: 2 mg), day 1

Repeat cycle every 35 days

FU/LV

Fluorouracil, I.V., 370-400 mg/m^2/day, days 1-5
Leucovorin calcium, I.V., 200 mg/m^2/day, commence infusion 15
minutes prior to fluorouracil infusion, days 1-5

Repeat cycle every 21 days

or

Fluorouracil, I.V., 1000 mg/m^2/day by continuous infusion, days 1-4
Leucovorin calcium, I.V., 200 mg/m^2/day, days 1-4

Repeat cycle every 28 days

Weekly 5FU/LV

Fluorouracil, I.V., 600 mg/m^2 over 1 hour given after leucovorin, repeat
weekly x 6 then 2-week rest period = 1 cycle, days 1, 8, 15, 22,
29, 36
Leucovorin calcium, I.V., 500 mg/m^2 over 2 hours, days 1, 8, 15, 22,
29, 36

Repeat cycle every 56 days

CANCER CHEMOTHERAPY REGIMENS *(Continued)*

5FU/LDLF

Fluorouracil, I.V., 425 mg/m^2/day, days 1-5
Leucovorin calcium, I.V., 20-25 mg/m^2/day, days 1-5
Repeat cycle every 28 days

Single-Agent Regimens

5-FU, I.V., 1000 mg/m^2/day, continuous infusion, days 1-5
Repeat cycle every 21-28 days

Irinotecan, I.V., 125 mg/m^2 over 90 minutes every 7 days for 4 cycles
or 350 mg/m^2 over 30 minutes
Repeat cycle every 21 days

Endometrial Cancer

AP

Doxorubicin, I.V., 60 mg/m^2, day 1
Cisplatin, I.V., 60 mg/m^2, day 1
Repeat cycle every 21 days

Single-Agent Regimens

Doxorubicin, I.V., 40-60 mg/m^2, day 1
Repeat cycle every 21-28 days

Medroxyprogesterone, P.O., 200 mg/day

Gastric Cancer

EAP

Etoposide, I.V., 120 mg/m^2, days 4, 5, 6
Doxorubicin, I.V., 20 mg/m^2, days 1, 7
Cisplatin, I.V., 40 mg/m^2, days 2, 8
Repeat cycle every 28 days

ELF

Leucovorin calcium, I.V., 300 mg/m^2, days 1-3 followed by
Etoposide, I.V., 120 mg/m^2, days 1-3 followed by
Fluorouracil, I.V., 500 mg/m^2, days 1-3
Repeat cycle every 21-28 days

FAM

Fluorouracil, I.V., 600 mg/m^2, days 1, 8, 29, 36
Doxorubicin, I.V., 30 mg/m^2, days 1, 29
Mitomycin C, I.V., 10 mg/m^2, day 1
Repeat cycle every 8 weeks

FAME

Fluorouracil, I.V., 350 mg/m^2, days 1-5, 36-40
Doxorubicin, I.V., 40 mg/m^2, days 1, 36
Methyl-CCNU, P.O., 150 mg/m^2, day 1
Repeat cycle every 70 days

FAMTX

Methotrexate, IVPB, 1500 mg/m^2, day 1
Fluorouracil, IVPB, 1500 mg/m^2 1 hour after methotrexate, day 1
Leucovorin calcium, P.O., 15 mg/m^{2}q6h x 48 hours, 24 hours after
methotrexate, day 2
Doxorubicin, IVPB, 30 mg/m^2, day 15
Repeat cycle every 28 days

FCE

Fluorouracil, I.V., 900 mg/m^2/day continuous infusion, days 1-5
Cisplatin, I.V., 20 mg/m^2, days 1-5
Etoposide, I.V., 90 mg/m^2, days 1, 3, 5
Repeat cycle every 21 days

PFL

Cisplatin, I.V., 25 mg/m^2 continuous infusion, days 1-5
Fluorouracil, I.V., 800 mg/m^{2}continuous infusion, days 2-5
Leucovorin calcium, I.V., 500 mg/m^{2}continuous infusion, days 1-5
Repeat cycle every 28 days

Single-Agent Regimens

Irinotecan, I.V., over 90 minutes: 125 mg/m^2/week; repeat weekly for 4 weeks, then 2-week rest period

or

Irinotecan, I.V. over 30-90 minutes: 350 mg/m^2; repeat every 21 days

Genitourinary Cancer

Bladder

CAP

Cyclophosphamide, I.V., 400 mg/m^2, day 1
Doxorubicin, I.V., 40 mg/m^2, day 1
Cisplatin, I.V., 60 mg/m^2, day 1

Repeat cycle every 21 days

CISCA

Cisplatin, I.V., 70-100 mg/m^2, day 2
Cyclophosphamide, I.V., 650 mg/m^2, day 1
Doxorubicin, I.V., 50 mg/m^2, day 1

Repeat cycle every 21-28 days

CMV

Cisplatin, I.V., 100 mg/m^2 over 4 hours, start 12 hours after MTX, day 2
Methotrexate, I.V., 30 mg/m^2, days 1, 8
Vinblastine, I.V., 4 mg/m^2, days 1, 8

Repeat cycle every 21 days

m-PFL

Methotrexate, I.V., 60 mg/m^2, day 1
Cisplatin, I.V., 25 mg/m^2 continuous infusion, days 2-6
Fluorouracil, I.V., 800 mg/m^2 continuous infusion, days 2-6
Leucovorin calcium, I.V., 500 mg/m^2 continuous infusion, days 2-6

Repeat cycle every 28 days for 4 cycles

MVAC

Methotrexate, I.V., 30 mg/m^2, days 1, 15, 22
Vinblastine, I.V., 3 mg/m^2, days 2, 15, 22
Doxorubicin, I.V., 30 mg/m^2, day 2
Cisplatin, I.V., 70 mg/m^2, day 2

Repeat cycle every 28 days

PC

Paclitaxel, I.V., 200 mg/m^2 or 225 mg/m^2 over 3 hours, day 1
Carboplatin, I.V., dose targeted by Calvert equation to AUC 5 or 6 after paclitaxel, day 1

Repeat cycle every 21 days

Single-Agent Regimens

Gemcitabine, I.V., 1200 mg/m^2, days 1, 8, 15

Repeat cycle every 28 days

Paclitaxel, I.V., 250 mg/m^2 over 24 hours, day 1

Repeat cycle every 21 days

Ovarian, Epithelial

Carbo-Tax

Paclitaxel, I.V., 135 mg/m^2 over 24 hours, day 1

or

175 mg/m^2 over 3 hours, day 1, followed by
Carboplatin dose targeted by Calvert equation to AUC 7.5 I.V.

Repeat cycle every 21 days

CC

Carboplatin, I.V., dose targeted by Calvert equation to AUC 6-7
Cyclophosphamide, I.V., 600 mg/m^2, day 1

Repeat cycle every 28 days

CP

Cyclophosphamide, I.V., 750 mg/m^2, day 1
Cisplatin, I.V., 75 mg/m^2, day 1

Repeat cycle every 21 days

CANCER CHEMOTHERAPY REGIMENS *(Continued)*

CT

Paclitaxel, I.V., 135 mg/m² over 24 hours, day 1

or

175 mg/m² over 3 hours, day 1, followed by
Cisplatin, I.V., 75 mg/m²

Repeat cycle every 21 days

PAC (CAP)

Cisplatin, I.V., 50 mg/m², day 1
Doxorubicin, I.V., 50 mg/m², day 1
Cyclophosphamide, I.V., 750 mg/m², day 1

Repeat cycle every 21 days x 8 cycles

Single-Agent Regimens

Altretamine, P.O., 260 mg/m²/day, qid for 14-21 days

Repeat cycle every 28 days

Etoposide, I.V., 50-60 mg/m²/day, days 1-21

Repeat cycle every 28 days

Liposomal doxorubicin, I.V., 50 mg/m², 1-hour infusion, day 1

Repeat cycle every 21 days

Paclitaxel, I.V., 135 mg/m², over 3 or 24 hours, day 1

Repeat cycle every 21 days

Topotecan, I.V., 1.5 mg/m², over 30 minutes, days 1-5

Repeat cycle every 21 days

Ovarian, Germ Cell

BEP

Bleomycin, I.V., 30 units, days 2, 9, 16
Etoposide, I.V., 100 mg/m², days 1-5
Cisplatin, I.V., 20 mg/m², days 1-5

VAC

Vincristine, I.V., 1.2-1.5 mg/m² (max: 2 mg) weekly for 10-12 weeks, or
every 2 weeks for 12 doses
Dactinomycin, I.V., 0.3-0.4 mg/m², days 1-5
Cyclophosphamide, I.V., 150 mg/m², days 1-5

Repeat every 28 days

Prostate

EV

Estramustine, P.O., 200 mg tid, days 1-42
Vinblastine, I.V., 4 mg/m²/week, begin day 1

Repeat cycle every 6 weeks

FL

Flutamide, P.O., 250 mg tid, days 1-28
Leuprolide acetate, S.C., 1 mg qd, days 1-28

Repeat cycle every 28 days

or

Flutamide, P.O., 250 mg tid, days 1-28
Leuprolide acetate depot, I.M., 7.5 mg, day 1

Repeat cycle every 28 days

FZ

Flutamide, P.O., 250 mg tid
Goserelin acetate, S.C., 3.6 mg implant, every 28 days or goserelin
S.C., 10.8 mg depot every 12 weeks

L-VAM

Leuprolide acetate, S.C., 1 mg qd, days 1-28
Vinblastine, I.V., 1.5 mg/m²/day continuous infusion, days 2-7
Doxorubicin, I.V., 50 mg/m² continuous infusion, day 1
Mitomycin C, I.V., 10 mg/m², day 2

Repeat cycle every 28 days

Mitoxantrone/Prednisone

Mitoxantrone, I.V., 12 mg/m², day 1
Prednisone, P.O., 5 mg bid

Repeat cycle every 21 days

No Known Acronym

Bicalutamide, P.O., 50 mg/day
Leuprolide acetate depot, I.M., 7.5 mg or goserelin S.C. 3.6 mg implant every 28 days

PE

Paclitaxel, I.V., 120 mg/m^2, days 1-4
Estramustine, P.O., 600 mg qd, 24 hours before paclitaxel
Repeat cycle every 21 days

Single-Agent Regimens

Estramustine, P.O., 14 mg/kg/day, tid or qid

Goserelin acetate implant, S.C., 3.6 mg every 28 days or 10.8 mg every 12 weeks

Nilutamide, P.O., 300 mg qd, days 1-30, then 150 mg qd in combination with surgical castration; begin on same day or day after castration

Prednisone, P.O., 5 mg bid

Renal

Interleukin-2 (rIL-2), S.C.
20 million units/m^2, days 3-5, weeks 1, 4
5 million units/m^2, days 1, 3, 5, weeks 2, 3, 5, 6
or
Interferon alfa (rIFNα2), S.C.
6 million units/m^2, day 1, weeks 1, 4;
6 million units/m^2, days 1, 3, 5, weeks 2, 3, 5, 6
Repeat cycle every 8 weeks

Single-Agent Regimen

Interleukin-2:
High dose: I.V. bolus over 15 minutes, 600,000-720,000 units/kg q8h until toxicity or 14 days; administer 2 courses separated by 7-10 days
Low dose: S.C., 18 million units/day for 5 days, then 9 million units/day for 2 days, then 18 million units/day 3 days/week for 6 weeks
or
3 million units/m^2/day for 5 days/week, every 2 weeks for 1 month, then every 4 weeks

Testicular

EP

Etoposide, I.V., 100 mg/m^2, days 1-5
Cisplatin, I.V., 20 mg/m^2, days 1-5
Repeat cycle every 21 days

Testicular, Induction, Good Risk

BEP

Bleomycin, I.V., 30 units, days 2, 9, 16
Etoposide, I.V., 100 mg/m^2, days 1-5
Cisplatin, I.V., 20 mg/m^2, days 1-5
Repeat cycle every 21 days

PVB

Cisplatin, I.V., 20 mg/m^2, days 1-5
Vinblastine, I.V., 0.15 mg/kg, days 1, 2
Bleomycin, I.V., 30 units, days 2, 9, 16
Repeat cycle every 21 days

Testicular, Induction, Poor Risk

VIP

Etoposide, I.V., 75 mg/m^2, days 1-5
Ifosfamide, I.V., 1.2 g/m^2, days 1-5
Cisplatin, I.V., 20 mg/m^2, days 1-5
Mesna, I.V., 400 mg/m^2, then 1200 mg/m^2/day continuous infusion, days 1-5
Repeat cycle every 21 days

CANCER CHEMOTHERAPY REGIMENS *(Continued)*

VIP (Einhorn)

Vinblastine, I.V., 0.11 mg/kg, days 1-2
Ifosfamide, I.V., 1200 mg/m², days 1-5
Cisplatin, I.V., 20 mg/m², days 1-5
Mesna, I.V., 400 mg/m², then 1200 mg/m²/day continuous infusion, days 1-5

Repeat cycle every 21 days

Testicular, Induction, Salvage

VAB VI

Vinblastine, I.V., 4 mg/m², day 1
Dactinomycin, I.V., 1 mg/m², day 1
Bleomycin, I.V., 30 units push day 1, then 20 units/m²/day continuous infusion, days 1-3
Cisplatin, I.V., 120 mg/m², day 4
Cyclophosphamide, I.V., 600 mg/m², day 1

Repeat cycle every 21 days

VBP (PVB)

Vinblastine, I.V., 6 mg/m², days 1, 2
Bleomycin, I.V., 30 units, days 1, 8, 15, (22)
Cisplatin, I.V., 20 mg/m², days 1-5

Repeat cycle every 21-28 days

Gestational Trophoblastic Cancer

DMC

Dactinomycin, I.V., 0.37 mg/m², days 1-5
Methotrexate, I.V., 11 mg/m², days 1-5
Cyclophosphamide, I.V., 110 mg/m², days 1-5

Repeat cycle every 21 days

Head and Neck Cancer

CAP

Cyclophosphamide, I.V., 500 mg/m², day 1
Doxorubicin, I.V., 50 mg/m², day 1
Cisplatin, I.V., 50 mg/m², day 1

Repeat cycle every 28 days

CF

Cisplatin, I.V., 100 mg/m², day 1
Fluorouracil, I.V., 1000 mg/m²/day continuous infusion, days 1-5

Repeat cycle every 21-28 days

CF

Carboplatin, I.V., 400 mg/m², day 1
Fluorouracil, I.V., 1000 mg/m²/day continuous infusion, days 1-5

Repeat cycle every 21-28 days

COB

Cisplatin, I.V., 100 mg/m², day 1
Vincristine, I.V., 1 mg/m², days 2, 5
Bleomycin, I.V., 30 units/day continuous infusion, days 2-5

Repeat cycle every 21 days

5-FU HURT

Hydroxyurea, P.O., 1000 mg q12h x 11 doses; start PM of admission, give 2 hours prior to radiation therapy, days 0-5
Fluorouracil, I.V., 800 mg/m²/day continuous infusion, start AM after admission, days 1-5
Paclitaxel, I.V., 5-25 mg/m²/day continuous infusion, start AM after admission; dose escalation study – refer to protocol, days 1-5
G-CSF, S.C., 5 mcg/kg/day, days 6-12, start ≥12 hours after completion of 5-FU infusion

5-7 cycles may be administered

PFL

Cisplatin, I.V., 100 mg/m², day 1
Fluorouracil, I.V., 600-800 mg/m²/day continuous infusion, days 1-5
Leucovorin calcium, I.V., 200-300 mg/m²/day, days 1-5

Repeat cycle every 21 days

PFL+IFN

Cisplatin, I.V., 100 mg/m², day 1
Fluorouracil, I.V., 640 mg/m²/day continuous infusion, days 1-5
Leucovorin calcium, P.O., 100 mg q4h, days 1-5
Interferon alfa-2b, S.C., 2 x 10⁶units/m², days 1-6

TIP

Paclitaxel, I.V., 175 mg/m² 3-hour infusion, day 1
Ifosfamide, I.V., 1000 mg/m² 2-hour infusion, days 1-3
Mesna, I.V., 400 mg/m² before ifosfamide and 200 mg/m² I.V., 4 hours
after ifosfamide
Cisplatin, I.V., 60 mg/m², day 1

Repeat cycle every 21-28 days

Single-Agent Regimens

Carboplatin, I.V., 300-400 mg/m², over 2 hours every 21-28 days

Methotrexate, I.V., 40 mg/m², every week, escalating day 14 by
5 mg/m²/week as tolerated

Cisplatin I.V., 100 mg/m², every 28 days divided into 1, 2, or 4 equal
doses per month

Vinorelbine, I.V., 25-30 mg/m², repeat weekly

Leukemia

Acute Lymphoblastic, Induction

VAD

Vincristine, I.V., 0.4 mg continuous infusion, days 1-4
Doxorubicin, I.V., 12 mg/m² continuous infusion, days 1-4
Dexamethasone, P.O., 40 mg, days 1-4, 9-12, 17-20

VP

Vincristine, I.V., 2 mg/m²/week for 4-6 weeks (max: 2 mg)
Prednisone, P.O., 60 mg/m²/day in divided doses for 4 weeks, taper
weeks 5-7

VP-L-Asparaginase

Vincristine, I.V., 2 mg/m²/week for 4-6 weeks (max: 2 mg)
Prednisone, P.O., 60 mg/m²/day for 4-6 weeks, then taper
L-asparaginase, I.V., 10,000 units/m²/day

No Known Acronym

Cyclophosphamide, I.V., 1200 mg/m², day 1
Daunorubicin, I.V., 45 mg/m², days 1-3
Prednisone, P.O., 60 mg/m², days 1-21
Vincristine, I.V., 2 mg/m²/week
L-asparaginase, I.V., 6000 units/m², 3 times/week

or

Pegaspargase, I.M./I.V., 2500 units/m², every 14 days if patient
develops hypersensitivity to native L-asparaginase

Acute Lymphoblastic, Maintenance

MM

Mercaptopurine, P.O., 50-75 mg/m², days 1-7
Methotrexate, P.O./I.V., 20 mg/m², day 1

Repeat cycle every 7 days

MMC (MTX + MP + CTX)*

Methotrexate, I.V., 20 mg/m²/week
Mercaptopurine, P.O., 50 mg/m²/day
Cyclophosphamide, I.V., 200 mg/m²/week

*Continue all 3 drugs until relapse of disease or after 3 years of remission.

CANCER CHEMOTHERAPY REGIMENS *(Continued)*

Acute Lymphoblastic, Relapse

AVDP

Asparaginase, I.V., 15,000 units/m^2, days 1-5, 8-12, 15-19, 22-26
Vincristine, I.V., 2 mg/m^2 (max: 2 mg), days 8, 15, 22
Daunorubicin, I.V., 30-60 mg/m^2, days 8, 15, 22
Prednisone, P.O., 40 mg/m^2, days 8-12, 15-19, 22-26

Acute Myeloid Leukemia, Induction

7+3

Cytarabine, I.V., 100-200 mg/m^2/day continuous infusion, days 1-7
with
Daunorubicin, I.V., 45 mg/m^2, days 1-3
or
Idarubicin, I.V., 12 mg/m^2, days 1-3
or
Mitoxantrone, I.V., 12 mg/m^2, days 1-3

5+2*

Cytarabine, I.V., 100-200 mg/m^2/day continuous infusion, days 1-5
with
Daunorubicin, I.V., 45 mg/m^2, days 1-2
or
Mitoxantrone, I.V., 12 mg/m^2, days 1-2

*For reinduction

D-3+7

Daunorubicin, I.V., 45 mg/m^2, days 1-3
Cytarabine, I.V., 100-200 mg/m^2 continuous infusion, days 1-7

DAT/DCT

Daunorubicin, I.V., 60 mg/m^2/day, days 1-3
Cytarabine, I.V., 200 mg/m^2/day continuous infusion, days 1-5
Thioguanine, P.O., 100 mg/m^2 q12h, days 1-5

Modified DAT (considerations in elderly patients)
Daunorubicin, I.V., 50 mg/m^2, day 1
Cytarabine, S.C., 100 mg/m^2/day q12h, days 1-5
Thioguanine, P.O., 100 mg/m^2 q12h, days 1-5

EMA-86

Etoposide, I.V., 200 mg/m^2/day continuous infusion, days 8-10
Mitoxantrone, I.V., 12 mg/m^2, days 1-3
Cytarabine, I.V., 500 mg/m^2/day continuous infusion, days 1-3, 8-10

I-3+7

Idarubicin, I.V., 12 mg/m^2, days 1-3
Cytarabine, I.V., 100 mg/m^2 continuous infusion, days 1-7

IC

Idarubicin, I.V., 12 mg/m^2/day, days 1-3
Cytarabine, I.V., 100-200 mg/m^2/day continuous infusion, days 1-7

LDAC

Considerations in Elderly Patients
Cytarabine, S.C., 10 mg/m^2 bid, days 10-21

MC

Mitoxantrone, I.V., 12 mg/m^2/day, days 1-3
Cytarabine, I.V., 100-200 mg/m^2/day continuous infusion, days 1-7

Consolidation
Mitoxantrone, I.V., 12 mg/m^2, days 1-2
Cytarabine, I.V., 100 mg/m^2 continuous infusion, days 1-5
Repeat cycle every 28 days

MV

Mitoxantrone, I.V., 10 mg/m^2/day, days 1-5
Etoposide, I.V., 100 mg/m^2/day, days 1-3

Single-Agent Regimen

All transrelincic acid (ATRA), P.O., 45 mg/m^2/day (1 or 2 divided
doses) with or without 7+3 induction regimen

Acute Myeloid Leukemia, Postremission

Single-Agent Regimens

Cytarabine, I.V., 100 mg/m^2/day continuous infusion, days 1-5*; repeat cycle every 28 days

*For patients >60 years of age

Cytarabine (HiDAC), I.V. 3000 mg/m^2 over 1-3 hours, every 12 hours, days 1-6

or

3000 mg/m^2 over 1-3 hours, every 12 hours, days 1, 3, 5. Administer with saline, methylcellulose, or steroid eyedrops OU, every 2-4 hours, beginning with cytarabine and continuing 48-72 hours after last cytarabine dose

Repeat cycle every 28 days

Acute Nonlymphoblastic, Consolidation

CD

Cytarabine, I.V., 3000 mg/m^2 q12h, days 1-6
Daunorubicin, I.V., 30 mg/m^2/day, days 7-9

Chronic Lymphocytic Leukemia

CHL + PRED

Chlorambucil, P.O., 0.4 mg/kg/day for 1 day every other week
Prednisone, P.O., 100 mg/day for 2 days every other week; adjust dosage according to blood counts every 2 weeks prior to therapy; increase initial dose of 0.4 mg/kg by 0.1 mg/kg every 2 weeks until toxicity or disease control is achieved

CVP

Cyclophosphamide, P.O., 400 mg/m^2/day, days 1-5
Vincristine, I.V., 1.4 mg/m^2 (max: 2 mg), day 1
Prednisone, P.O., 100 mg/m^2, days 1-5

Repeat cycle every 21 days

Single-Agent Regimens

Chlorambucil, P.O., 0.1-0.2 mg/kg/day for 3-6 weeks

or

Chlorambucil, P.O., 20-30 mg/m^2, day 1

Repeat cycle every 14-28 days

Cladribine, I.V., 0.1 mg/kg/day continuous infusion, days 1-5 or 1-7

Repeat cycle every 28-35 days

Cyclophosphamide, P.O., 2-4 mg/kg, days 1-10

Repeat cycle every 21-28 days

Fludarabine, I.V., 25-30 mg/m^2, days 1-5

Repeat cycle every 28 days

Prednisone,* P.O., 30-60 mg/m^2, days 1-5 or 1-7

*Use if patient symptomatic with autoimmune thrombocytopenia or hemolytic anemia.

Chronic Myelogenous Leukemia

Single-Agent Regimens

Busulfan, P.O., 4-8 mg/day
Hydroxyurea, P.O., 2-5 g/day
Interferon alfa-2a, S.C., 3-5 million units/day

Hairy-Cell Leukemia

Single-Agent Regimens

Cladribine, I.V., 0.1 mg/kg/day continuous infusion, days 1-7

Administer one cycle

Interferon alfa-2a, S.C., 3 million units, 3 times/week

Pentostatin, I.V., 4 mg/m^2, day 1

Repeat cycle every 14 days

CANCER CHEMOTHERAPY REGIMENS *(Continued)*

Lung Cancer
Small Cell

CAV/VAC

Cyclophosphamide, I.V., 750-1000 mg/m^2, day 1
Doxorubicin, I.V., 50 mg/m^2, day 1
Vincristine, I.V., 1.4 mg/m^2 (max: 2 mg), day 1
Repeat cycle every 3 weeks

CAVE

Cyclophosphamide, I.V., 750 mg/m^2, day 1
Doxorubicin, I.V., 50 mg/m^2, day 1
Vincristine, I.V., 1.4 mg/m^2 (max: 2 mg), day 1
Etoposide, I.V., 60-100 mg/m^2, days 1-3
Repeat cycle every 21 days

EC

Etoposide, I.V., 100-120 mg/m^2, days 1-3
Carboplatin, I.V., 325-400 mg/m^2, day 1
Repeat cycle every 28 days

EP/PE

Etoposide, I.V., 120 mg/m^2, days 1-3
Cisplatin, I.V., 60-120 mg/m^2, day 1
Repeat cycle every 21-28 days

Single-Agent Regimen

Etoposide, P.O., 50 mg/m^2, days 1-21
Repeat cycle every 28 days

Topotecan, I.V., 1.5 mg/m^2/day, over 30 minutes, days 1-5
Repeat cycle every 21 days

Nonsmall Cell

Carbo-Tax

Paclitaxel, I.V., 135 mg/m^2 over 24 hours, day 1 **or**
175 mg/m^{2}over 3 hours, day 1, followed by
Carboplatin dose targeted by Calvert equation to AUC 7.5 I.V.
Repeat cycle every 21 days

EC

Etoposide, I.V., 100-120 mg/m^2, days 1-3
with
Carboplatin, I.V., 300-325 mg/m^2, day 1
Repeat cycle every 21-28 days

EP

Etoposide, I.V., 80 mg/m^2, days 1-3
Cisplatin, I.V., 60-100 mg/m^2, day 1
Repeat cycle every 21-28 days

Gemcitabine-Cis

Gemcitabine, I.V., 1000 mg/m^2, days 1, 8, 15
Cisplatin, I.V., 100 mg/m^2, day 2 or 15
Repeat cycle every 28 days

PC

Paclitaxel, I.V., 175 mg/m^2, 3-hour infusion, day 1
Cisplatin, I.V., 80 mg/m^2, day 1
Repeat cycle every 21 days

Vinorelbine-Cis

Vinorelbine, I.V., 30 mg/m^2, every 7 days
Cisplatin, I.V., 120 mg/m^2, day 1, 29, then every 6 weeks

Single-Agent Regimens

Topotecan, I.V., 1.5 mg/m^2/day, over 30 minutes, days 1-5
Repeat cycle every 21 days

Vinorelbine, I.V., 30 mg/m^2, every 7 days

Lymphoma
Hodgkin's

ABVD

Doxorubicin, I.V., 25 mg/m^2, days 1, 15
Bleomycin, I.V., 10 units/m^2, days 1, 15
Vinblastine, I.V., 6 mg/m^2, days 1, 15
Dacarbazine, I.V., 150 mg/m^2, days 1-5

or

Dacarbazine, I.V., 350-375 mg/m^2, days 1, 15

Repeat cycle every 28 days

ChlVPP

Chlorambucil, P.O., 6 mg/m^2 (max: 10 mg/day), days 1-14
Vinblastine, I.V., 6 mg/m^2 (max: 10 mg dose), days 1, 8
Procarbazine, P.O., 100 mg/m^2 (max: 150 mg/day), days 1-14
Prednisone, P.O., 40 mg/day, days 1-14

Repeat cycle every 28 days

CVPP

Lomustine, P.O., 75 mg/m^2, day 1
Vinblastine, I.V., 4 mg/m^2, days 1, 8
Procarbazine, P.O., 100 mg/m^2, days 1-14
Prednisone, P.O., 30 mg/m^2, days 1-14 (cycles 1 and 4 only)

Repeat cycle every 28 days

DHAP

Dexamethasone, P.O./I.V., 40 mg, days 1-4
Cytarabine, I.V., 2 g/m^2, q12h for 2 doses, day 2
Cisplatin, I.V., 100 mg/m^2 continuous infusion, day 1

Repeat cycle every 3-4 weeks

EVA

Etoposide, I.V., 100 mg/m^2, days 1-3
Vinblastine, I.V., 6 mg/m^2, day 1
Doxorubicin, I.V., 50 mg/m^2, day 1

Repeat cycle every 28 days

MOPP

Mechlorethamine, I.V., 6 mg/m^2, days 1, 8
Vincristine, I.V., 1.4 mg/m^2 (max: 2.5 mg), days 1, 8
Procarbazine, P.O., 100 mg/m^2, days 1-14
Prednisone, P.O., 40 mg/m^2 (cycles 1 and 4 only), days 1-14

Repeat cycle every 28 days

MOPP/ABV Hybrid

Mechlorethamine, I.V., 6 mg/m^2, day 1
Vincristine, I.V., 1.4 mg/m^2 (max: 2 mg), day 1
Procarbazine, P.O., 100 mg/m^2, days 1-7
Prednisone, P.O., 40 mg/m^2, days 1-14
Doxorubicin, I.V., 35 mg/m^2, day 8
Bleomycin, I.V., 10 units/m^2, day 8
Vinblastine, I.V., 6 mg/m^2, day 8

Repeat cycle every 28 days

MVPP

Mechlorethamine, I.V., 6 mg/m^2, days 1, 8
Vinblastine, I.V., 6 mg/m^2, days 1, 8
Procarbazine, P.O., 100 mg/m^2, days 1-14
Prednisone, P.O., 40 mg/m^2, days 1-14

Repeat cycle every 42 days

NOVP

Mitoxantrone, I.V., 10 mg/m^2, day 1
Vincristine, I.V., 2 mg, day 8
Vinblastine, I.V., 6 mg/m^2, day 1
Prednisone, P.O., 100 mg/m^2, days 1-5

Repeat cycle every 21 days

CANCER CHEMOTHERAPY REGIMENS *(Continued)*

Stanford V*

Mechlorethamine, I.V., 6 mg/m^2, day 1

        Doxorubicin, I.V., 25 mg/m^2, days 1, 15

        Vinblastine, I.V., 6 mg/m^2, days 1, 15

        Vincristine, I.V., 1.4 mg/m^2, days 8, 22

        Bleomycin, I.V., 5 units/m^2, days 8, 22

        Etoposide, I.V., 60 mg/m^2, days 15, 16

        Prednisone, P.O., 40 mg/m^2/day, dose tapered over the last 15 days

                        Repeat cycle every 28 days

*In patients >50 years of age, vinblastine dose decreased to 4 mg/m^2 and vincristine dose decreased to 1 mg/m^2 on weeks 9-12. Concomitant trimethoprim/sulfamethoxazole DS P.O. bid; acyclovir 200 mg P.O. tid; ketoconazole 200 mg P.O. qd and stool softeners used.

Non-Hodgkin's

BACOP

        Bleomycin, I.V., 5 units/m^2, days 15, 22

        Doxorubicin, I.V., 25 mg/m^2, days 1, 8

        Cyclophosphamide, I.V., 650 mg/m^2, days 1, 8

        Vincristine, I.V., 1.4 mg/m^2 (max: 2 mg), days 1, 8

        Prednisone, P.O., 60 mg/m^2, days 15-28

                        Repeat cycle every 28 days

CHOP

        Cyclophosphamide, I.V., 750 mg/m^2, day 1

        Doxorubicin, I.V., 50 mg/m^2, day 1

        Vincristine, I.V., 1.4 mg/m^2 (max: 2 mg), day 1

        Prednisone, P.O., 100 mg/m^2, days 1-5

                        Repeat cycle every 21 days

CHOP-Bleo

        Cyclophosphamide, I.V., 750 mg/m^2, day 1

        Doxorubicin, I.V., 50 mg/m^2, day 1

        Vincristine, I.V., 2 mg, days 1, 5

        Prednisone, P.O., 100 mg, days 1-5

        Bleomycin, I.V., 15 units, days 1, 5

                    Repeat cycle every 21-28 days

CNOP

        Cyclophosphamide, I.V., 750 mg/m^2, day 1

        Mitoxantrone, I.V., 10 mg/m^2, day 1

        Vincristine, I.V., 1.4 mg/m^2, day 1

        Prednisone, P.O., 50 mg/m^2, days 1-5

                        Repeat cycle every 21 days

COMLA

        Cyclophosphamide, I.V., 1500 mg/m^2, day 1

        Vincristine, I.V., 1.4 mg/m^2 (max: 2.5 mg), days 1, 8, 15

        Methotrexate, I.V., 120 mg/m^2, days 22, 29, 36, 43, 50, 57, 64, 71

        Leucovorin calcium rescue, P.O., 25 mg/m^2, q6h for 4 doses, beginning 24 hours after each methotrexate dose

        Cytarabine, I.V., 300 mg/m^2, days 22, 29, 36, 43, 50, 57, 64, 71

                    Repeat cycle every 21 days

COP

        Cyclophosphamide, I.V., 800 mg/m^2, day 1

        Vincristine, I.V., 1.4 mg/m^2 (max: 2 mg), day 1

        Prednisone, P.O., 60 mg/m^2, days 1-5

                        Repeat cycle every 21 days

COP-BLAM

        Cyclophosphamide, I.V., 400 mg/m^2, day 1

        Vincristine, I.V., 1 mg/m^2, day 1

        Prednisone, P.O., 40 mg/m^2, days 1-10

        Bleomycin, I.V., 15 mg, day 14

        Doxorubicin, I.V., 40 mg/m^2, day 1

        Procarbazine, P.O., 100 mg/m^2, days 1-10

COPP (or "C" MOPP)

Cyclophosphamide, I.V., 400-650 mg/m^2, days 1, 8
Vincristine, I.V., 1.4-1.5 mg/m^2(max: 2 mg), days 1, 8
Procarbazine, P.O., 100 mg/m^2, days 1-14
Prednisone, P.O., 40 mg/m^2, days 1-14

Repeat cycle every 28 days

CVP

Cyclophosphamide, P.O., 400 mg/m^2, days 1-5
Vincristine, I.V., 1.4 mg/m^2 (max: 2 mg), day 1
Prednisone, P.O., 100 mg/m^2, days 1-5

Repeat cycle every 21 days

DHAP*

Dexamethasone, I.V., 10 mg q6h, days 1-4
Cytarabine, I.V., 2 g/m^2 q12h x 2 doses, day 2
Cisplatin, I.V., 100 mg/m^{2}continuous infusion, day 1

Repeat cycle every 21-28 days

*Administer with saline, methylcellulose, or steroid eyedrops OU, every 2-4 hours, beginning with cytarabine and continuing 48-72 hours after last cytarabine dose.

ESHAP*

Etoposide, I.V., 60 mg/m^2, days 1-4
Cisplatin, I.V., 25 mg/m^2 continuous infusion, days 1-4
Cytarabine, I.V., 2 g/m^2, immediately following completion of etoposide and cisplatin therapy
Methylprednisolone, I.V., 500 mg/day, days 1-4

Repeat cycle every 21-28 days

*Administer with saline, methylcellulose, or steroid eyedrops OU, every 2-4 hours, beginning with cytarabine and continuing 48-72 hours after last cytarabine dose.

IMVP-16

Ifosfamide, I.V., 4 g/m^2 continuous infusion over 24 hours, day 1
Mesna, I.V., 800 mg/m^2 bolus prior to ifosfamide, then 4 g/m^2 continuous infusion over 12 hours concurrent w/ifosfamide; then 2.4 g/m^2 continuous infusion over 12 hours after ifosfamide infusion, day 1
Methotrexate, I.V., 30 mg/m^2, days 3, 10
Etoposide, I.V., 100 mg/m^2, days 1-3

Repeat cycle every 21-28 days

MACOP-B

Methotrexate, I.V., 400 mg/m^2, weeks 2, 6, 10
Doxorubicin, I.V., 50 mg/m^2, weeks 1, 3, 5, 7, 9, 11
Cyclophosphamide, I.V., 350 mg/m^2, weeks 1, 3, 5, 7, 9, 11
Vincristine, I.V., 1.4 mg/m^2 (max: 2 mg), weeks 2, 4, 8, 10, 12
Bleomycin, I.V., 10 units/m^2, weeks 4, 8, 12
Prednisone, P.O., 75 mg/day tapered over 15 d, days 1-15
Leucovorin calcium, P.O., 15 mg/m^2, q6h x 6 doses 24 hours after methotrexate, weeks 2, 6, 10
Trimethoprim/sulfamethoxazole DS, P.O., tablet, bid, for 12 weeks
Ketoconazole, P.O., 200 mg/day

Administer one cycle

m-BACOD

Methotrexate, I.V., 200 mg/m^2, days 8, 15
Leucovorin calcium, P.O., 10 mg/m^{2}q6h x 8 doses beginning 24 hours after each methotrexate dose, days 8, 15
Bleomycin, I.V., 4 units/m^2, day 1
Doxorubicin, I.V., 45 mg/m^2, day 1
Cyclophosphamide, I.V., 600 mg/m^2, day 1
Vincristine, I.V., 1 mg/m^2, day 1
Dexamethasone, P.O., 6 mg/m^2, days 1-5

Repeat cycle every 21 days

CANCER CHEMOTHERAPY REGIMENS *(Continued)*

m-BACOS

Methotrexate, I.V., 1 g/m^2, day 2
Bleomycin, I.V., 10 units/m^2, day 1
Doxorubicin, I.V., 50 mg/m^{2}continuous infusion, day 1
Cyclophosphamide, I.V., 750 mg/m^2, day 1
Vincristine, I.V., 1.4 mg/m^2 (max: 2 mg), day 1
Leucovorin calcium rescue, P.O., 15 mg q6h for 8 doses, starting 24 hours after methotrexate
Methylprednisolone, I.V., 500 mg, days 1-3

Repeat cycle every 21-25 days

MINE

Mesna, I.V., 1.33 g/m^2/day concurrent with ifosfamide dose, then 500 mg P.O. 4 hours after each ifosfamide infusion, days 1-3
Ifosfamide, I.V., 1.33 g/m^2/day, days 1-3
Mitoxantrone, I.V., 8 mg/m^2, day 1
Etoposide, I.V., 65 mg/m^2/day, days 1-3

Repeat cycle every 28 days

MINE-ESHAP

Mesna, I.V., 1.33 g/m^2, administered at same time as ifosfamide, then 500 mg P.O., 4 hours after ifosfamide, days 1-3
Ifosfamide, I.V., 1.33 g/m^2, over 1 hour, days 1-3
Mitoxantrone, I.V., 8 mg/m^2, day 1
Etoposide, I.V., 65 mg/m^2, days 1-3

Repeat cycle every 21 days for 6 cycles, followed by 3-6 cycles of ESHAP

NOVP

Mitoxantrone, I.V., 10 mg/m^2, day 1
Vinblastine, I.V., 6 mg/m^2, day 1
Prednisone, P.O., 100 mg, days 1-5
Vincristine, I.V., 2 mg, day 8

Repeat cycle every 21 days

Pro-MACE

Prednisone, P.O., 60 mg/m^2, days 1-14
Methotrexate, I.V., 1.5 g/m^2, day 14
Leucovorin calcium, I.V., 50 mg/m^{2}q6h x 5 doses beginning 24 hours after methotrexate dose, day 14
Doxorubicin, I.V., 25 mg/m^2, days 1, 8
Cyclophosphamide, I.V., 650 mg/m^2, days 1, 8
Etoposide, I.V., 120 mg/m^2, days 1, 8

Repeat cycle every 28 days

Pro-MACE-CytaBOM

Prednisone, P.O., 60 mg/m^2, days 1-14
Doxorubicin, I.V., 25 mg/m^2, day 1
Cyclophosphamide, I.V., 650 mg/m^2, day 1
Etoposide, I.V., 120 mg/m^2, day 1
Cytarabine, I.V., 300 mg/m^2, day 8
Bleomycin, I.V., 5 units/m^2, day 8
Vincristine, I.V., 1.4 mg/m^2 (max: 2 mg), day 8
Methotrexate, I.V., 120 mg/m^2, day 8
Leucovorin calcium, P.O., 25 mg/m^{2}q6h x 4 doses, day 9
Concomitant trimethoprim/sulfamethoxazole DS, P.O., bid

Repeat cycle every 21-28 days

Single-Agent Regimens

CDA cladribine, S.C., 0.1 mg/kg/day for 5 days or 0.1 mg/kg/day I.V., for 7 days

Repeat cycle every 28 days

Rituximab, I.V., 375 mg/m^2, days 1, 8, 15, 22

Malignant Melanoma

CVD

Cisplatin, I.V., 20 mg/m^2, days 1-5
Vinblastine, I.V., 1.6 mg/m^2, days 1-5
Dacarbazine, I.V., 800 mg/m^2, day 1

Repeat cycle every 21 days

CVD + IL-21

Cisplatin, I.V., 20 mg/m^2/day, days 1-4
Vinblastine, I.V., 1.6 mg/m^2/day, days 1-4
Dacarbazine, I.V., 800 mg/m^2, day 1
IL-2, I.V., 9 million units/m^{2}continuous infusion, days 1-4
Interferon alfa, S.C., 5 million units/m^2, every day, days 1-5, 7, 9, 11, 13

Repeat cycle every 21 days

Dacarbazine/Tamoxifen

Dacarbazine, I.V., 250 mg/m^2, days 1-5, every 21 days
Tamoxifen,* P.O., 20 mg/day

No Known Acronym

Dacarbazine, I.V., 220 mg/m^2, days 1-3, every 21-28 days
Carmustine, I.V., 150 mg/m^2, day 1, every 42-56 days
Cisplatin, I.V., 25 mg/m^2, days 1-3, every 21-28 days
Tamoxifen,* P.O., 20 mg/day

*Use of tamoxifen is optional.

Single-Agent Regimens

Interferon alfa-2b adjuvant therapy, I.M., 20 million units/m^2, days 1-30, **then**

10 million units/m^2 S.C., 3 times/week for 48 weeks

Interferon alfa-2a, I.M., 20 million units/m^{2}3 times/week for 12 weeks

Multiple Myeloma

EDAP

Etoposide, I.V., 100-200 mg/m^2, days 1-4
Dexamethasone, P.O./I.V., 40 mg/m^2, days 1-5
Cytarabine, 1000 mg, day 5
Cisplatin, I.V., 20 mg continuous infusion, days 1-4

MP

Melphalan, P.O., 8-10 mg/m^2, days 1-4
Prednisone, P.O., 40-60 mg/m^2/day, days 1-4

Repeat cycle every 28-42 days

M-2

Vincristine, I.V., 0.03 mg/kg (max: 2 mg), day 1
Carmustine, I.V., 0.5-1 mg/kg, day 1
Cyclophosphamide, I.V., 10 mg/kg, day 1
Melphalan, P.O., 0.25 mg/kg, days 1-4 or 0.1 mg/kg, days 1-7 or 1-10
Prednisone, P.O., 1 mg/kg/day, days 1-7

Repeat cycle every 35-42 days

VAD

Vincristine, I.V., 0.4 mg/day continuous infusion, days 1-4
Doxorubicin, I.V., 9 mg/m^2/day continuous infusion, days 1-4
Dexamethasone, P.O., 40 mg, days 1-4, 9-12, 17-20

Repeat cycle every 28-35 days

VAD induction therapy followed by maintenance
Interferon alfa, S.C., 3 million units/m^2, 3 times/week
Prednisone, P.O., 50 mg, 3 times/week, after interferon

VBAP

Vincristine, I.V., 1 mg, day 1
Carmustine, I.V., 30 mg/m^2, day 1
Doxorubicin, I.V., 30 mg/m^2, day 1
Prednisone, P.O., 100 mg, days 1-4

Repeat cycle every 21 days

VBMCP

Vincristine, I.V., 1.2 mg/m^2, day 1
Carmustine, I.V., 20 mg/m^2, day 1
Melphalan, P.O., 8 mg/m^2, days 1-4
Cyclophosphamide, I.V., 400 mg/m^2, day 1
Prednisone, P.O., 40 mg/m^2, days 1-7 all cycles, and 20 mg/m^2, days 8-14 first 3 cycles only

Repeat cycle every 35 days

CANCER CHEMOTHERAPY REGIMENS *(Continued)*

VCAP

Vincristine, I.V., 1 mg, day 1
Cyclophosphamide, P.O., 100 mg/m^2, days 1-4
Doxorubicin, I.V., 25 mg/m^2, day 2
Prednisone, P.O., 60 mg/m^2, days 1-4

Repeat cycle every 28 days

Single-Agent Regimens

Aldesleukin, 600,000-700,000 int. units/kg every 8 hours x 14 doses

Repeat cycle every 14 days

Dexamethasone, P.O., 20 mg/m^2 for 4 days beginning on days 1-4, 9-12, and 17-20

Repeat cycle every 35 days

Interferon alfa-2b, S.C., 2 million units/m^2, 3 times/week for maintenance therapy in selected patients with significant response to initial chemotherapy treatment

Melphalan, I.V., 90-140 mg/m^2

Administer one cycle

Pancreatic Cancer

FAM

Fluorouracil, I.V., 600 mg/m^2, days 1, 8, 29, 36
Doxorubicin, I.V., 30 mg/m^2, days 1, 29
Mitomycin, I.V., 10 mg/m^2, day 1

Repeat cycle every 72 days

SMF

Streptozocin, I.V., 1000 mg/m^2, days 1, 8, 29, 36
Mitomycin, I.V., 10 mg/m^2, day 1
Fluorouracil, I.V., 600 mg/m^2, days 1, 8, 29, 36

Repeat cycle every 72 days

Single-Agent Regimens

Gemcitabine, I.V., 1000 mg/m^2 over 30 minutes once weekly for 7 weeks, followed by a 1-week rest period; subsequent cycles once weekly for 3 consecutive weeks out of every 4 weeks

Sarcoma

AC

Doxorubicin, I.V., 75-90 mg/m^2 96-hour continuous infusion
Cisplatin, I.A./I.V., 90-120 mg/m^2, 6 days

Repeat cycle every 28 days

AD

Doxorubicin, I.V., 22.5 mg/m^2/day continuous infusion, days 1-4
Dacarbazine, I.V., 225 mg/m^2/day continuous infusion, days 1-4

Repeat cycle every 21 days

CYVADIC

Cyclophosphamide, I.V., 500 mg/m^2, day 1
Vincristine, I.V., 1.4 mg/m^2, days 1, 5
Doxorubicin, I.V., 50 mg/m^2, day 1
Dacarbazine, I.V., 250 mg/m^2, days 1-5

Repeat cycle every 21 days

DI

Doxorubicin, I.V., 50 mg/m^2 bolus, day 1
Ifosfamide, I.V., 5000 mg/m^2/day continuous infusion, following doxorubicin, day 1
Mesna, I.V., 600 mg/m^2, bolus before ifosfamide, followed by 2500 mg/m^2/day, continuous infusion, for 36 hours

Repeat cycle every 21 days

HDMTX

Methotrexate, I.V., 8-12 g/m^2
Leucovorin calcium, P.O./I.V., 15-25 mg q6h for at least 10 doses beginning 24 hours after methotrexate dose; courses repeated weekly for 2-4 weeks, alternating with various cancer chemotherapy combination regimens

IE

Etoposide, I.V., 100 mg/m^2, days 1-5
Ifosfamide, I.V., 1800 mg/m^2, days 1-5
Mesna, I.V., at 20% of ifosfamide dose prior to and 4 and 8 hours
    after ifosfamide administration

Repeat cycle every 21-28 days

MAID

Mesna, I.V., 2500 mg/m^2/day continuous infusion, days 1-4
Doxorubicin, I.V., 15 mg/m^2/day continuous infusion, days 1-4
Ifosfamide, I.V., 2500 mg/m^2/day continuous infusion, days 1-3
Dacarbazine, I.V., 250 mg/m^2/day continuous infusion, days 1-4

Repeat cycle every 21-28 days

VAC

Vincristine, I.V., 2 mg/m^2/week (max: 2 mg), during weeks 1-12
Dactinomycin, I.V., 0.015 mg/kg (max: 0.5 mg) every 3 months for 5-6
    courses, days 1-5
Cyclophosphamide, P.O., 2.5 mg/kg/day for 2 years

Single-Agent Regimens

Doxorubicin, I.V., 75 mg/m^2, day 1

Repeat cycle every 21 days

ANTACID DRUG INTERACTIONS

Drug	Antacid			
	Aluminum Salts	Calcium Salts	Magnesium Salts	Magnesium Aluminum Combinations
Allopurinol	↓			
Benzodiazepines	↑		↓	↓
Calcitriol			x*	x*
Captopril				↓
Cimetidine				↓
Corticosteroids	↓		↓	↓
Dicumarol			↑	
Diflunisal	↓			
Digoxin	↓		↓	
Iron	↓	↓	↓	↓
Isoniazid	↓			
Ketoconazole				↓
Levodopa				↑
Nitrofurantoin			↓	
Penicillamine	↓		↓	↓
Phenothiazines	↓		↓	↓
Phenytoin		↓		↓
Quinidine		↑	↑	↑
Quinolones				↓
Ranitidine	↓			↓
Salicylates		↓		↓
Sodium polystyrene sulfonate	x†		x†	x†
Tetracyclines	↓	↓	↓	↓
Valproic acid				↑

Pharmacologic effect increased (↑) or decreased (↓) by antacids.

*Concomitant use in patients on chronic renal dialysis may lead to hypermagnesemia.

†Concomitant use may cause metabolic alkalosis in patients with renal failure.

CORTICOSTEROIDS, TOPICAL COMPARISON

	Steroid	Vehicle
Lowest Potency (may be ineffective for some indications)		
0.1%	Betamethasone	Cream
0.2%	Betamethasone (Celestone®)	Cream
0.05%	Desonide	Cream
0.04%	Dexamethasone (Hexadrol®)*	Cream
0.1%	Dexamethasone (Decadron® Phosphate, Decaderm®)*	Cream, gel
1%	Hydrocortisone	Cream, ointment, lotion
2.5%	Hydrocortisone	Cream, ointment
0.25%	Methylprednisolone acetate (Medrol®)	Ointment
1%	Methylprednisolone acetate (Medrol®)	Ointment
0.5%	Prednisolone (Meti-Derm®)	Cream
Low Potency		
0.01%	Betamethasone valerate (Valisone®, reduced strength)	Cream
0.1%	Clocortolone (Cloderm®)	Cream
0.03%	Flumethasone pivalate (Locorten®)	Cream
0.01%	Fluocinolone acetonide (Synalar®)*	Cream, solution
0.025%	Fluorometholone (Oxylone®)	Cream
0.025%	Flurandrenolide (Cordran®, Cordran® SP)*	Cream, ointment
0.2%	Hydrocortisone valerate (Westcort®)	Cream
0.025%	Triamcinolone acetonide (Kenalog®)*	Cream, ointment
Intermediate Potency		
0.025%	Betamethasone benzoate	Cream, gel, lotion
0.1%	Betamethasone valerate (Valisone®)*	Cream, ointment, lotion
0.05%	Desonide (Tridesilon®)	Cream, ointment
0.05%	Desoximetasone (Topicort® LP)	Cream
0.025%	Fluocinolone acetonide*	Cream, ointment
0.05%	Flurandrenolide (Cordran®, Cordran® SP)*	Cream, ointment, lotion
0.025%	Halcinonide (Halog®)	Cream, ointment
0.1%	Triamcinolone acetonide (Kenalog®)*	Cream, ointment
High Potency		
0.1%	Amcinonide (Cyclocort®)	Cream, ointment
0.05%	Betamethasone dipropionate (Diprosone®)	Cream, ointment, lotion
0.05%	Clobetasol dipropionate	Cream, ointment
0.25%	Desoximetasone (Topicort®)	Cream
0.05%	Diflorasone diacetate (Florone®, Maxiflor®)	Cream, ointment
0.2%	Fluocinolone (Synalar-HP®)	Cream
0.05%	Fluocinonide (Lidex®)*	Cream, ointment
0.1%	Halcinonide (Halog®)	Cream, ointment, solution
0.5%	Triamcinolone acetonide*	Cream, ointment

*Fluorinated.

NORMAL LABORATORY VALUES FOR CHILDREN

CHEMISTRY		Normal Values
Albumin	0-1 year	2-4 g/dL
	1 year-adult	3.5-5.5 g/dL
Ammonia	Newborn	90-150 µg/dL
	Child	40-120 µg/dL
	Adult	18-54 µg/dL
Amylase	Newborn	0-60 units/L
	Adult	30-110 units/L
Bilirubin, conjugated, direct	Newborn	<1.5 mg/dL
	1 month-adult	0-0.5 mg/dL
Bilirubin, total	0-3 days	2-10 mg/dL
	1 month-adult	0-1.5 mg/dL
Bilirubin, unconjugated, indirect		0.6-10.5 mg/dL
Calcium	Newborn	7-12 mg/dL
	0-2 years	8.8-11.2 mg/dL
	2 years-adult	9-11 mg/dL
Calcium, ionized, whole blood		4.4-5.4 mg/dL
Carbon dioxide, total		23-33 mEq/L
Chloride		95-105 mEq/L
Cholesterol	Newborn	45-170 mg/dL
	0-1 year	65-175 mg/dL
	1-20 years	120-230 mg/dL
Creatinine	0-1 year	≤0.6 mg/dL
	1 year-adult	0.5-1.5 mg/dL
Glucose	Newborn	30-90 mg/dL
	0-2 years	60-105 mg/dL
	Child-adult	70-110 mg/dL
Iron	Newborn	110-270 µg/dL
	Infant	30-70 µg/dL
	Child	55-120 µg/dL
	Adult	70-180 µg/dL
Iron binding	Newborn	59-175 µg/dL
	Infant	100-400 µg/dL
	Adult	250-400 µg/dL
Lactic acid, lactate		2-20 mg/dL
Lead, whole blood		<30 µg/dL
Lipase	Child	20-140 units/L
	Adult	0-190 units/L
Magnesium		1.5-2.5 mEq/L
Osmolality, serum		275-296 mOsm/kg
Osmolality, urine		50-1400 mOsm/kg
Phosphorus	Newborn	4.2-9 mg/dL
	6 weeks-18 months	3.8-6.7 mg/dL
	18 months-3 years	2.9-5.9 mg/dL
	3-15 years	3.6-5.6 mg/dL
	>15 years	2.5-5 mg/dL
Potassium, plasma	Newborn	4.5-7.2 mEq/L
	2 days-3 months	4-6.2 mEq/L
	3 months-1 year	3.7-5.6 mEq/L
	1-16 years	3.5-5 mEq/L
Protein, total	0-2 years	4.2-7.4 g/dL
	>2 years	6-8 g/dL
Sodium		136-145 mEq/L
Triglycerides	Infant	0-171 mg/dL
	Child	20-130 mg/dL
	Adult	30-200 mg/dL
Urea nitrogen, blood	0-2 years	4-15 mg/dL
	2 years - Adult	5-20 mg/dL
Uric acid	Male	3-7 mg/dL

CHEMISTRY

		Normal Values
	Female	2-6 mg/dL

ENZYMES

Alanine aminotransferase (ALT) (SGPT)	0-2 months	8-78 units/L
	>2 months	8-36 units/L
Alkaline phosphatase (ALKP)	Newborn	60-130 units/L
	0-16 years	85-400 units/L
	>16 years	30-115 units/L
Aspartate aminotransferase (AST) (SGOT)	Infant	18-74 units/L
	Child	15-46 units/L
	Adult	5-35 units/L
Creatine kinase (CK)	Infant	20-200 units/L
	Child	10-90 units/L
	Adult male	0-206 units/L
	Adult female	0-175 units/L
Lactate dehydrogenase (LDH)	Newborn	290-501 units/L
	1 month-2 years	110-144 units/L
	>16 years	60-170 units/L

BLOOD GASES

	Arterial	Capillary	Venous
pH	7.35-7.45	7.35-7.45	7.32-7.42
pCO_2 (mm Hg)	35-45	35-45	38-52
pO_2 (mm Hg)	70-100	60-80	24-48
HCO_3 (mEq/L)	19-25	19-25	19-25
TCO_2 (mEq/L)	19-29	19-29	23-33
O_2 saturation (%)	90-95	90-95	40-70
Base excess (mEq/L)	-5 to +5	-5 to +5	-5 to +5

THYROID FUNCTION TESTS

		Normal Values
T_4 (thyroxine)	1-7 d	10.1-20.9 µg/dL
	8-14 d	9.8-16.6 µg/dL
	1 mo to 1 y	5.5-16.0 µg/dL
	>1 y	4.0-12.0 µg/dL
FTI	1-3 d	9.3-26.6
	1-4 wk	7.6-20.8
	1-4 mo	7.4-17.9
	4-12 mo	5.1-14.5
	1-6 y	5.7-13.3
	>6 y	4.8-14.0
T_3	Newborns	100-470 ng/dL
	1-5 y	100-260 ng/dL
	5-10 y	90-240 ng/dL
	10 y to adult	70-210 ng/dL
T_3 uptake		35%-45%
TSH	Cord	3-22 µIU/mL
	1-3 d	<40 µIU/mL
	3-7 d	<25 µIU/mL
	>7 d	0-10 µIU/mL

NORMAL LABORATORY VALUES FOR CHILDREN
(Continued)

HEMATOLOGY
Complete Blood Count

Age	Hgb (g/dL)	Hct (%)	RBC (mill/mm³)	RDW
0-3 d	15.0-20.0	45-61	4.0-5.9	<18
1-2 wk	12.5-18.5	39-57	3.6-5.5	<17
1-6 mo	10.0-13.0	29-42	3.1-4.3	<16.5
7 mo to 2 y	10.5-13.0	33-38	3.7-4.9	<16
2-5 y	11.5-13.0	34-39	3.9-5.0	<15
5-8 y	11.5-14.5	35-42	4.0-4.9	<15
13-18 y	12.0-15.2	36-47	4.5-5.1	<14.5
Adult male	13.5-16.5	41-50	4.5-5.5	<14.5
Adult female	12.0-15.0	36-44	4.0-4.9	<14.5

Age	MCV (fL)	MCH (pg)	MCHC (%)	PLTS (x 10³/mm³)
0-3 d	95-115	31-37	29-37	250-450
1-2 wk	86-110	28-36	28-38	250-450
1-6 mo	74-96	25-35	30-36	300-700
7 mo to 2 y	70-84	23-30	31-37	250-600
2-5 y	75-87	24-30	31-37	250-550
5-8 y	77-95	25-33	31-37	250-550
13-18 y	78-96	25-35	31-37	150-450
Adult male	80-100	26-34	31-37	150-450
Adult female	80-100	26-34	31-37	150-450

WBC and Diff

Age	WBC (x 10³/mm³)	Segs	Bands	Lymphs	Monos
0-3 d	9.0-35.0	32-62	10-18	19-29	5-7
1-2 wk	5.0-20.0	14-34	6-14	36-45	6-10
1-6 mo	6.0-17.5	13-33	4-12	41-71	4-7
7 mo to 2 y	6.0-17.0	15-35	5-11	45-76	3-6
2-5 y	5.5-15.5	23-45	5-11	35-65	3-6
5-8 y	5.0-14.5	32-54	5-11	28-48	3-6
13-18 y	4.5-13.0	34-64	5-11	25-45	3-6
Adults	4.5-11.0	35-66	5-11	24-44	3-6

Age	Eosinophils	Basophils	Atypical Lymphs	No. of NRBCs
0-3 d	0-2	0-1	0-8	0-2
1-2 wk	0-2	0-1	0-8	0
1-6 mo	0-3	0-1	0-8	0
7 mo to 2 y	0-3	0-1	0-8	0
2-5 y	0-3	0-1	0-8	0
5-8 y	0-3	0-1	0-8	0
13-18 y	0-3	0-1	0-8	0
Adults	0-3	0-1	0-8	0

Segs = segmented neutrophils   Lymphs = lymphocytes
Bands = band neutrophils   Monos = monocytes

Erythrocyte Sedimentation Rates and Reticulocyte Counts

Sedimentation rate, Westergren	Children	0-20 mm/hour
	Adult male	0-15 mm/hour
	Adult female	0-20 mm/hour
Sedimentation rate, Wintrobe	Children	0-13 mm/hour
	Adult male	0-10 mm/hour
	Adult female	0-15 mm/hour
Reticulocyte count	Newborns	2%-6%
	1-6 mo	0%-2.8%
	Adults	0.5%-1.5%

NORMAL LABORATORY VALUES FOR ADULTS

Automated Chemistry (CHEMISTRY A)

Test	Values	Remarks
SERUM PLASMA		
Acetone	Negative	
Albumin	3.2-5 g/dL	
Alcohol, ethyl	Negative	
Aldolase	1.2-7.6 IU/L	
Ammonia	20-70 mcg/dL	Specimen to be placed on ice as soon as collected
Amylase	30-110 units/L	
Bilirubin, direct	0-0.3 mg/dL	
Bilirubin, total	0.1-1.2 mg/dL	
Calcium	8.6-10.3 mg/dL	
Calcium, ionized	2.24-2.46 mEq/L	
Chloride	95-108 mEq/L	
Cholesterol, total	≤220 mg/dL	Fasted blood required – normal value affected by dietary habits. This reference range is for a general adult population
HDL cholesterol	40-60 mg/dL	Fasted blood required – normal value affected by dietary habits
LDL cholesterol	65-170 mg/dL	LDLC calculated by Friewald formula... which has certain inaccuracies and is invalid at trig levels >300 mg/dL
CO_2	23-30 mEq/L	
Creatine kinase (CK) isoenzymes		
CK-BB	0%	
CK-MB	0%-3.9%	
CK-MM	96%-100%	
CK-MB levels must be both ≥4% and 10 IU/L to meet diagnostic criteria for CK-MB positive result consistent with myocardial injury.		
Creatine phosphokinase (CPK)	8-150 IU/L	
Creatinine	0.5-1.4 mg/dL	
Ferritin	13-300 ng/mL	
Folate	3.6-20 ng/dL	
GGT (gamma-glutamyltranspeptidase)		
male	11-63 IU/L	
female	8-35 IU/L	
GLDH	To be determined	
Glucose (2-h postprandial)	Up to 140 mg/dL	
Glucose, fasting	60-110 mg/dL	
Glucose, nonfasting (2-h postprandial)	60-140 mg/dL	
Hemoglobin A_{1c}	8	
Hemoglobin, plasma free	<2.5 mg/100 mL	
Hemoglobin, total glycosolated (Hb A_1)	4%-8%	
Iron	65-150 mcg/dL	
Iron binding capacity, total (TIBC)	250-420 mcg/dL	
Lactic acid	0.7-2.1 mEq/L	Specimen to be kept on ice and sent to lab as soon as possible
Lactate dehydrogenase (LDH)	56-194 IU/L	
Lactate dehydrogenase (LDH) isoenzymes		
LD_1	20%-34%	
LD_2	29%-41%	
LD_3	15%-25%	

697

NORMAL LABORATORY VALUES FOR ADULTS *(Continued)*

Automated Chemistry (CHEMISTRY A) *(continued)*

Test	Values	Remarks
LD$_4$	1%-12%	
LD$_5$	1%-15%	
Flipped LD$_1$/LD$_2$ ratios (>1 may be consistent with myocardial injury) particularly when considered in combination with a recent CK-MB positive result		
Lipase	23-208 units/L	
Magnesium	1.6-2.5 mg/dL	Increased by slight hemolysis
Osmolality	289-308 mOsm/kg	
Phosphatase, alkaline		
adults 25-60 y	33-131 IU/L	
adults 61 y or older	51-153 IU/L	
infancy-adolescence	Values range up to 3-5 times higher than adults	
Phosphate, inorganic	2.8-4.2 mg/dL	
Potassium	3.5-5.2 mEq/L	Increased by slight hemolysis
Prealbumin	>15 mg/dL	
Protein, total	6.5-7.9 g/dL	
SGOT (AST)	<35 IU/L	
SGPT (ALT)	<35 IU/L	
Sodium	134-149 mEq/L	
Transferrin	>200 mg/dL	
Triglycerides	45-155 mg/dL	Fasted blood required
Urea nitrogen (BUN)	7-20 mg/dL	
Uric acid		
male	2.0-8.0 mg/dL	
female	2.0-7.5 mg/dL	

CEREBROSPINAL FLUID

Glucose	50-70 mg/dL	
Protein		
adults and children	15-45 mg/dL	CSF obtained by lumbar puncture
newborn infants	60-90 mg/dL	
On CSF obtained by cisternal puncture: About 25 mg/dL		
On CSF obtained by ventricular puncture: About 10 mg/dL		

Note: Bloody specimen gives erroneously high value due to contamination with blood proteins

URINE

(24-hour specimen is required for all these tests unless specified)

Amylase	32-641 units/L	The value is in units/L and **not** calculated for total volume
Amylase, fluid (random samples)		Interpretation of value left for physician, depends on the nature of fluid
Calcium	Depends upon dietary intake	
Creatine		
male	150 mg/24 h	Higher value on children and during pregnancy
female	250 mg/24 h	
Creatinine	1000-2000 mg/24 h	
Creatinine clearance (endogenous)		
male	85-125 mL/min	A blood sample must accompany urine specimen
female	75-115 mL/min	
Glucose	1 g/24 h	
5-hydroxyindoleacetic acid	2-8 mg/24 h	
Iron	0.15 mg/24 h	Acid washed container required
Magnesium	146-209 mg/24 h	

Automated Chemistry (CHEMISTRY A) *(continued)*

Test	Values	Remarks
Osmolality	500-800 mOsm/kg	With normal fluid intake
Oxalate	10-40 mg/24 h	
Phosphate	400-1300 mg/24 h	
Potassium	25-120 mEq/24 h	Varies with diet; the interpretation of urine electrolytes and osmolality should be left for the physician
Sodium	40-220 mEq/24 h	
Porphobilinogen, qualitative	Negative	
Porphyrins, qualitative	Negative	
Proteins	0.05-0.1 g/24 h	
Salicylate	Negative	
Urea clearance	60-95 mL/min	A blood sample must accompany specimen
Urea N	10-40 g/24 h	Dependent on protein intake
Uric acid	250-750 mg/24 h	Dependent on diet and therapy
Urobilinogen	0.5-3.5 mg/24 h	For qualitative determination on random urine, send sample to urinalysis section in Hematology Lab
Xylose absorption test		
children	16%-33% of ingested xylose	
adults	>4 g in 5 h	

FECES

Fat, 3-day collection	<5 g/d	Value depends on fat intake of 100 g/d for 3 days preceding and during collection

GASTRIC ACIDITY

Acidity, total, 12 h	10-60 mEq/L	Titrated at pH 7

BLOOD GASES

	Arterial	Capillary	Venous
pH	7.35-7.45	7.35-7.45	7.32-7.42
pCO_2 (mm Hg)	35-45	35-45	38-52
pO_2 (mm Hg)	70-100	60-80	24-48
HCO_3 (mEq/L)	19-25	19-25	19-25
TCO_2 (mEq/L)	19-29	19-29	23-33
O_2 saturation (%)	90-95	90-95	40-70
Base excess (mEq/L)	-5 to +5	-5 to +5	-5 to +5

BLOOD LEVEL SAMPLING TIME GUIDELINES

Drug	Infusion Time	Therapeutic Range	When to Draw Levels
Amikacin sulfate			
I.V.	30 min	Peak: 20-30 mcg/mL	Peak: 30 min after end of 30 min infusion
		Trough: <10 mcg/mL	Trough: Within 30 min before next dose
I.M.			Peak: 1 h after I.M. injection
			Trough: Within 30 min before next dose
Carbamazepine		4-12 mcg/mL	Just before next dose
Chloramphenicol			
I.V.	30 min	Peak: 15-25 mcg/mL	Peak: 90 min after end of 30 min infusion
			Trough: Just before next dose
P.O.			Peak: 2 h post P.O. dose
Cyclosporine			
I.V./P.O.		BMT 100-200 ng/mL	Just before next dose
		Liver transplant 200-300 ng/mL	
		Renal transplant 100-200 ng/mL	
Digoxin			
I.V./P.O.		Age and disease related: 0.8-2 ng/mL	6 h post dose to just before next dose
Ethosuximide			
P.O.		40-100 mcg/mL	Just before next dose
Flucytosine			
P.O.		25-100 mcg/mL	Peak: 2 h post dose after at least 4 d of therapy
Gentamicin			
I.V.	30 min	Peak: 4-10 mcg/mL	Peak: 30 min after end of 30 min infusion
		Trough: 0.5-2 mcg/mL	Trough: Within 30 min before next dose
I.M.			Peak: 1 h after I.M. injection
			Trough: Within 30 min before next dose
Phenobarbital		15-40 mcg/mL	Trough: Just before next dose
Phenytoin			
P.O.		10-20 mcg/mL	Trough: Just before next dose
Theophylline			
I.V. bolus	30 min	10-20 mcg/mL	Peak: 30 min after end of 30 min infusion
Continuous infusion			16-24 h after the start or change in a constant I.V. infusion
P.O. liquid, fast-release tablet			Peak: 1 h post dose
(Somophyllin®, Slo-Phyllin® liquid & tablet)			Trough: Just before next dose
P.O. slow-release			Peak: 4 h post dose
(Theo-Dur®, Slo-Phyllin® GC, Slo-bid®)			Trough: Just before next dose

Drug	Infusion Time	Therapeutic Range	When to Draw Levels
Tobramycin			
I.V.	30 min	Peak: 4-10 mcg/ mL	Peak: 30 min after end of 30 min infusion
		Trough: 0.5-2 mcg/mL	Trough: Within 30 min before next dose
I.M.			Peak: 1 h post I.M. injection
			Trough: Within 30 min before next dose
Trimethoprim			
I.V., dose 20 mg/kg	60 min	Peak: 5-10 mcg/ mL	Peak: 30 min after end of 60 min infusion
I.V., dose 8-10 mg/kg		Peak 1-3 mcg/ mL	
P.O.			Peak: 1 h post dose
Valproic acid			
P.O.		50-100 mcg/mL	Trough: Just before next dose
Vancomycin	60 min	Peak: 25-40 mcg/mL	Peak: 20-30 min after end of 60 min infusion*
		Trough: 5-15 mcg/mL	Trough: Within 30 min before next dose

*Some institutions may draw vancomycin peak 1 h after 1 h infusion and accept the lower range of therapeutic.

COMPATIBILITY OF MEDICATIONS MIXED IN A SYRINGE

	Atropine	Chlorpromazine	Codeine	Diphenhydramine	Droperidol	Fentanyl	Glycopyrrolate	Hydroxyzine	Meperidine	Metoclopramide	Midazolam	Morphine	Pentazocine	Pentobarbital†	Prochlorperazine	Promazine	Promethazine	Trimethobenzamide
Atropine		C	•	C	C	C	C	C	C	C	C	C	C	C	C	C	C	•
Chlorpromazine	C		•	C	C	C	C	C	C	C	C	C	C	X	C	C	C	•
Codeine	•	•		•	•	•	C	C	•	•	•	•	•	X	•	•	•	•
Diphenhydramine	C	C	•		C	C	C	C	C	C	C	C	C	X	C	C	C	•
Droperidol	C	C	•	C		C	C	C	C	C	C	C	C	X	C	C	C	•
Fentanyl	C	C	•	C	C		C	C	C	C	C	C	C	X	C	C	C	•
Glycopyrrolate	C	C	C	C	C	C		C	C	•	C	C	X	X	C	C	C	C
Hydroxyzine	C	C	C	C	C	C	C		C	C	C	C	C	X	C	C	C	•
Meperidine	C	C	•	C	C	C	C	C		C	C	X	C	X	C	C	C	•
Metoclopramide	C	C	•	C	C	C	•	C	C		C	C	C	•	C	C	C	•
Midazolam	C	C	•	C	C	C	C	C	C	C		C	•	X	X	C	C	C
Morphine	C	C	•	C	C	C	C	C	C	C	C		C	X	C*	C	C	•
Pentazocine	C	C	•	C	C	C	C	C	C	C	•	C		X	C	C	C	C
Pentobarbital†	C	X	X	X	X	X	X	X	X	•	X	X	X		X	X	X	•
Prochlorperazine	C	C	•	C	C	C	C	C	C	C	X	C*	C	X		C	C	•
Promazine	C	C	•	C	C	C	C	C	C	C	C	C	C	X	C		C	•
Promethazine	C	C	•	C	C	C	C	C	C	C	C	C	C	X	C	C		•
Trimethobenzamide	•	•	•	•	•	•	C	•	•	•	C	•	C	•	•	•	•	

C = Physically compatible if used within 15 minutes after mixing in a syringe
X = Incompatible
• = No documented information
C* = Potential incompatibility produced by certain manufacturers
† = Compatibility profile is characteristic of most barbiturate salts, such as phenobarbital and secobarbital

The following combinations have been found to be compatible:
atropine / meperidine / promethazine
atropine / meperidine / hydroxyzine
meperidine / promethazine / chlorpromazine

The following drugs should **_not_** be mixed with any other drugs in the same syringe:
diazepam, chlordiazepoxide

CONTROLLED SUBSTANCES

Schedule I = C-I

The drugs and other substances in this schedule have no legal medical uses except research. They have a **high** potential for abuse. They include selected opiates such as heroin, opium derivatives, and hallucinogens.

Schedule II = C-II

The drugs and other substances in this schedule have legal medical uses and a **high** abuse potential which may lead to severe dependence. They include former "Class A" narcotics, amphetamines, barbiturates, and other drugs.

Schedule III = C-III

The drugs and other substances in this schedule have legal medical uses and a **lesser** degree of abuse potential which may lead to **moderate** dependence. They include former "Class B" narcotics and other drugs.

Schedule IV = C-IV

The drugs and other substances in this schedule have legal medial uses and **low** abuse potential which may lead to **moderate** dependence. They include barbiturates, benzodiazepines, propoxyphenes, and other drugs.

Schedule V = C-V

The drugs and other substances in this schedule have legal medical uses and **low** abuse potential which may lead to **moderate** dependence. They include narcotic cough preparations, diarrhea preparations, and other drugs.

Note: These are federal classifications. Your individual state may place a substance into a more restricted category. When this occurs, the more restricted category applies. Consult your state law.

FOOD-DRUG INTERACTIONS, KEY SUMMARY

Drug	Food	Interaction
Aspirin Captopril Isoniazid Mercaptopurine Methotrexate Methyldopa Penicillin G and V Phenobarbital Propantheline Rifampin Tetracycline	Any food	Decreased absorption
Carbamazepine Hydralazine Lithium Metoprolol Propranolol	Any food	Increased absorption
Cefuroxime	Any food	Increased absorption
Chlorpropamide Disulfiram Griseofulvin Metronidazole Procarbazine Quinacrine Tolazoline	Alcohol	Antabuse reaction consisting of flushing, headache, nausea, and in some patients, vomiting, and chest and/or abdominal pain
Cyclosporine	Many foods Fatty foods	Decreased absorption Increased absorption
Cyclosporine Felodipine	Grapefruit juice	Increased absorption
Erythromycin stearate	Any food	Increased or decreased absorption
Furosemide	Any food	Decreased rate of absorption, potentially decreasing effect
Levodopa	High-protein diet	Decreased absorption
Lithium	Sodium	Enhanced elimination requiring higher doses
MAO inhibitors: Isocarboxazid Phenelzine Procarbazine Tranylcypromine	High-protein foods that have undergone aging, fermentation, pickling, or smoking; aged cheeses, red wines, pods of broad beans and fava beans; bananas, raisins, avocados; caffeine-containing beverages, beer, ale, and chocolate	Elevated blood pressure
Phenobarbital Phenytoin	High doses of vitamin B_6 (pyridoxine) and folic acid	Decreased absorption
Phenobarbital Phenytoin Theophylline Warfarin	Charcoal-broiled foods	Increased metabolism requiring higher doses
Phenytoin	Most foods Pudding	Absorption increased by 25% Absorption decreased by 50%
Quinolones (eg, ciprofloxacin) Tetracycline	Iron, calcium, aluminum, zinc, magnesium (eg, dairy products)	Decreased absorption
Warfarin	Diets rich in vitamin K such as cauliflower, spinach, broccoli, turnip greens, liver, beans, rice, pork, fish, and some cheeses	Antagonism of effect

Reprinted with permission from Saltiel E, "Food-Drug Interactions," *New Developments in Medicine & Drug Therapy*, Glenview, IL: Physicians & Scientists Publishing Co, Inc, 1994, 3(4):61.

HERBS AND COMMON NATURAL AGENTS

The authors have chosen to include this list of natural products and proposed medical claims. However, due to limited scientific investigation to support these claims, this list is not intended to imply that these claims have been scientifically proven.

Proposed Medicinal Claims

Herb	Medicinal Claim
Agrimony	Digestive disorders
Alfalfa	Source of carotene (vitamin A); contains natural fluoride
Allspice	General health
Aloe	Healing agent
Anise seed	Prevent gas
Astragalus	Enhance energy reserves; immune system modulation; adaptogen
Barberry bark	Treat halitosis
Bayberry bark	Relieve and prevent varicose veins
Bay leaf	Relieves cramps
Bee pollen	Renewal of enzymes, hormones, vitamins, amino acids, and others
Bergamot herb	Calming effect
Bilberry leaf	Increases night vision; reduces eye fatigue; antioxidant; circulation
Birch bark	Treat urinary problems; used for rheumatism
Blackberry leaf	Treat diarrhea
Black cohosh	Relieves menstrual cramps; phytoestrogen
Blueberry leaf	Diarrhea
Blue Cohosh	Regulate menstrual flow
Blue flag	Treatment of skin diseases and constipation
Boldo leaf	Stimulates digestion; treatment of gallstones
Boneset	Treatment of colds and flu
Bromelain	Digestive enzyme
Buchu leaf	Diuretic
Buckthorn bark	Expels worms; laxative
Burdock leaf and root	Treatment of severe skin problems; cases of arthritis
Butternut bark	Works well for constipation
Calendula flower	Mending and healing of cuts or wounds topically
Capsicum (Cayenne)	Normalizes blood pressure; circulation
Caraway seed	Aids digestion
Cascara sagrada bark	Remedies for chronic constipation
Catnip	Calming effect in children
Celery leaf and seed	Blood pressure; diuretic
Centaury	Stimulates the salivary gland
Chamomile flower	Excellent for a nervous stomach; relieves cramping associated with the menstrual cycle
Chickweed	Rich in vitamin C and minerals (calcium, magnesium, and potassium); diuretic; thyroid stimulant
Chicory root	Effective in disorders of the kidneys, liver, and urinary canal
Cinnamon bark	Prevents infection and indigestion; helps break down fats during digestion
Cleavers	Treatment of kidney and bladder disorders; useful in obstructions of the urinary organ

HERBS AND COMMON NATURAL AGENTS *(Continued)*

Proposed Medicinal Claims *(continued)*

Herb	Medicinal Claim
Cloves	General medicinal
Coriander seed	Stomach tonic
Cornsilk	Diuretic
Cranberry	Urinary tract health
Cubeb berry	Chronic bladder trouble; increases flow of urine
Damiana leaf	Sexual impotency
Dandelion leaf	Diuretic
Dandelion root	Detoxify poisons in the liver; beneficial in lowering blood pressure
Dill weed	Digestive health
Dong Quai root	Female troubles; menopause and PMS symptoms; anemia; blood pressure
Echinacea root	Treat strep throat, lymph glands; immune modulating
Eucalyptus leaf	Mucolytic
Elder	Antiviral
Elecampane root	Cough with mucus
Eyebright herb	Eyesight
Fennel seed	Remedies for gas and acid stomach
Fenugreek seed	Allergies, coughs, digestion, emphysema, headaches, migraines, intestinal inflammation, ulcers, lungs, mucous membranes, and sore throat
Feverfew herb	Migraines; helps reduce inflammation in arthritis joints
Garlic capsules	Lowers blood cholesterol; anti-infective
Gentian	Digestive health
Ginger root	Antiemetic
Ginkgo biloba	Improves blood circulation to the brain; asthma; vertigo; tinnitus; impotence
Ginseng root, Siberian	Resistance against stress; slows the aging process; adaptogen
Goldenseal	Treatment of bladder infections, cankers, mouth sores, mucous membranes, and ulcers
Gota kola	"Memory herb"; nerve tonic; wound healing
Gravelroot (Queen of the Meadow)	Remedy for stones in the kidney and bladder
Green barley	Antioxidant
Hawthorn	Antioxidant; cardiotonic
Henna	External use only
Hibiscus flower	Diuretic
Hops flower	Insomnia; used to decrease the desire for alcohol
Horehound	Acute or chronic sore throat and coughs
Horsetail (Shavegrass)	Rich in minerals, especially silica; used to develop strong fingernails and hair, good for split ends; diuretic
Ho shou wu	Rejuvenator
Hydrangea root	Backaches
Juniper berry	Diuretic
Kava kava root	Calm nervousness; anxiety; pain
Kelp	High contents of natural plant iodine, for proper function of the thyroid; high levels of natural calcium, potassium, and magnesium
Lavender oil	Wound healing; decrease scarring (topical)
Lecithin	Break up cholesterol; prevent arteriosclerosis

Proposed Medicinal Claims *(continued)*

Herb	Medicinal Claim
Licorice root	Expectorant; used in peptic ulceration; adrenal exhaustion
Malva flower	Soothes inflammation in the mouth and throat; helpful for earaches
Marjoram	Beneficial for a sour stomach or loss of appetite
Marshmallow leaf	Demulcent
Milk thistle herb	Liver detoxifier; antioxidant
Motherwort	Nervousness
Mugwort	Used for rheumatism and gout
Mullein leaf	High in iron, magnesium, and potassium; sinuses; relieves swollen joints; soothing bronchial tissue
Mustard seed	General medicinal
Myrrh gum	Removes bad breath; sinus problems
Nettle leaf	Remedy for dandruff; antihistiminic qualities
Nettle root	Used in benign prostatic hyperplasia (BPH)
Nutmeg	Gas
Oregano leaf	Settles the stomach after meals; helps treat colds
Oregon grape root	Gallbladder problems
Papaya leaf	Digestive stimulant; contains the enzyme papain
Paprika (sweet)	Stimulates the appetite and gastric secretions
Passion flower	Mild sedative
Pau d'arco	Protects immune system; antifungal
Peppermint leaf	Excellent for headaches; digestive stimulation
Pleurisy root	Mucolytic
Poppy seed blue	Excellent in the making of breads and desserts
Prickly ash bark	Increases circulation
Psyllium seed	Lubricant to the intestinal tract
Red clover	Phytoestrogenic properties
Red raspberry leaf	Decreases menstrual bleeding
Rhubarb root	Powerful laxative
Rose hips	High content of vitamin C
Saw palmetto berry	Used in benign prostatic hyperplasia (BPH)
Scullcap	Nerve sedative
Seawrack (Bladderwrack)	Combat obesity; contains iodine
Senna leaf	Laxative
Shepherd's purse	Female reproductive health
Sheep sorrel	Diuretic
Slippery elm bark	Normalize bowel movement; beneficial for hemorrhoids and constipation
Solomon's seal root	Poultice for bruises
Spikenard	Skin ailments such as acne, pimples, blackheads, rashes, and general skin problems
Star anise	Promotes appetite and relieves flatulence
St John's wort	Mild to moderate depression
Summer savory leaf	Treats diarrhea, upset stomach, and sore throat
Thyme leaf	Ulcers (peptic)
Uva-ursi leaf	Diuretic; used in urinary tract health
Valerian root	Promotes sleep
Vervain	Remedy for fevers
White oak bark	Strong astringent
White willow bark	Used for minor aches and pains in the body; aspirin content

HERBS AND COMMON NATURAL AGENTS *(Continued)*

Proposed Medicinal Claims *(continued)*

Herb	Medicinal Claim
Wild alum root	Powerful astringent; used as rinse for sores in mouth and bleeding gums
Wild cherry	Cough suppressant
Wild Oregon grape root	Chronic skin disease
Wild yam root	Used in female reproductive health
Wintergreen leaf	Valuable for colic and gas in the bowels
Witch hazel bark and leaf	Hemorrhoids
Wormwood	Antiparasitic
Yarrow root	Fevers
Yellow dock root	Good in all skin problems
Yerba santa	Bronchial congestion
Yohimbe	Natural aphrodisiac
Yucca root	Reduces inflammation of the joints

POTASSIUM CONTENT OF FOODS*

BEVERAGES (8 fluid ounces)	mg	mEq
Apple juice, canned	250	6.4
Apricot juice	372	9.5
Coffee, instant, 2 g	238	6.1
Grape juice, canned, sweetened	285	7.3
Grapefruit juice, canned	360	9.2
Milk, whole (high in sodium)	352	9
Milk, nonfat (high in sodium)	408	10.4
Orange juice, fresh or canned	496	12.7
Pineapple juice, canned	379	9.7
Prune juice, canned	563	14.4
Tea	66	1.7
Tomato juice, canned (high in sodium)	544	13.9

FOODS		
Apricots, raw, 2-3 medium	281	7.2
Banana, fresh, 1 medium	550	14.1
Bouillon, 1 meat extract cube (high in sodium)	108	2.8
Bouillon, 1 vegetable extract cube (high in sodium)	138	3.3
Cantaloupe, 1/2, 5" diameter	251	6.4
Cauliflower, raw, 1 1/4 cup (10 oz)	500	12.8
Dates, dried, 10 medium	648	16.6
Figs, dried, 5 medium	640	16.4
Fruit cocktail, canned sweet, 1 cup	330	8.4
Molasses, 1 tablespoonful	269	6.9
Peaches, dried, 1/2 cup (4 oz) uncooked	1100	28.2
Pears, raw, 1, 2 1/2 x 2"	180	4.6
Prunes, dried, 5 large, raw	349	8.9
Raisins, dried, 2 tablespoonfuls	152	3.9
Strawberries, raw, 8 oz	246	6.3
Watermelon, 1/2 slice, 3/4 x 10"	380	9.7
Wheat germ, 100 g	737	18.9

SALT SUBSTITUTES		
Adolph's, 1 packet	430	11
Co-Salt, 1 g	450	11.5
Diasal, 1 g	442	11.3
Lite-Salt, 1 g (high in sodium)	260	6.6
Neocurtasal, 1 g	470	12.1
Nu-Salt, 1 g	404	10.4
Salfree, 1 g	548	14.1

*Pearson RE and Fish KH Jr, "Potassium Content of Selected Medicines, Foods and Salt Substitutes," *Hosp Pharm*, 1971, 6(9):6-9.

SOUND-ALIKE COMPARISON LIST

The following list contains over 1031 pairs of sound-alike drugs accompanied by a subjective pronunciation of each drug name. Any such list can only suggest possible pronunciation or enunciation miscues and is by no means meant to be exhaustive.

New or rarely used drugs are likely to cause the most problems related to interpretation. Healthcare workers should be made aware of the existence of both drugs in a sound-alike pair in order to avoid (or minimize) the potential for error. Drug companies attempt to avoid naming different drugs with similar-sounding names; however, mix-ups do occur. Reading current drug advertisements, professional literature, and drug handbooks is a good way to avert or surely lessen such sound-alike drug errors at all levels of the healthcare industry.

Drug Name	Pronunciation	Drug Name	Pronunciation
Accolate®	(ak' cue late)	Adapin®	(ad' da pin)
Accutane®	(ak' yu tane)	Adalat®	(ad' da lat)
Accolate®	(ak' cue late)	Adapin®	(ad' a pin)
Accupril®	(ak' yu pril)	adapalene	(a dap' a lene)
Accubron®	(ak' cue bron)	Adapin®	(ad' da pin)
Accutane®	(ak' yu tane)	Adipex-P®	(ad' di pex pea)
Accupril®	(ak' cue pril)	Adapin®	(ad' da pin)
Accolate®	(ak' cue late)	Ativan®	(at' tee van)
Accupril®	(ak' cue pril)	Adderall®	(ad' der all)
Accutane®	(ak' yu tane)	Inderal®	(in' der al)
Accutane®	(ak' yu tane)	Adipex-P®	(ad' di pex pea)
Accubron®	(ak' cue bron)	Adapin®	(ad' da pin)
Accutane®	(ak' yu tane)	Adriamycin™	(ade rya mye' sin)
Accolate®	(ak' cue late)	Achromycin®	(ak roe mye' sin)
Accutane®	(ak' yu tane)	Adriamycin™	(ade rya mye' sin)
Accupril®	(ak' cue pril)	Idamycin®	(eye da mye' sin)
Accutane®	(ak' yu tane)	Aerolone®	(air' o lone)
Acutrim®	(ak' yu trim)	Aralen®	(air' a len)
Acephen®	(a' ce fen)	Afrin®	(aye' frin or af' rin)
Aciphex™	(a' si fecks)	aspirin	(as' pir in)
acetazolamide	(a set a zole' a mide)	Afrinol®	(af' ree nol)
acetohexamide	(a set o heks' a mide)	Arfonad®	(arr' foe nad)
acetohexamide	(a set o heks' a mide)	Agoral®	(ag' a ral)
acetazolamide	(a set a zole' a mide)	Argyrol®	(ar' gee roll)
Achromycin®	(ak roe mye' sin)	AK-Mycin®	(aye kay mye' sin)
Adriamycin™	(ade rya mye' sin)	Akne-Mycin®	(ak nee mye' sin)
Achromycin®	(ak roe mye' sin)	Akne-Mycin®	(ak nee mye' sin)
actinomycin	(ak ti noe mye' sin)	AK-Mycin®	(aye kay mye' sin)
Aciphex™	(a' si fecks)	AKTob®	(ak' tobe)
Acephen®	(a' ce fen)	AK-Trol®	(aye' kay trol)
Acthar®	(ac' thar)	AK-Trol®	(aye' kay trol)
Acular®	(ac' yu lar)	AKTob®	(ak' tobe)
Actidil®	(ak' tee dill)	Alazide®	(al' a zide)
Actifed®	(ak' tee fed)	Alazine®	(al' a zine)
Actidose®	(ac' ti dose)	Alazine®	(al' a zine)
Actos®	(ac' tose)	Alazide®	(al' a zide)
Actifed®	(ak' tee fed)	albuterol	(al byoo' ter ole)
Actidil®	(ak' tee dil)	atenolol	(a ten' oh lole)
actinomycin	(ak ti noe mye' sin)	Aldactazide®	(al dak' ta zide)
Achromycin®	(ak roe mye' sin)	Aldactone®	(al' dak tone)
Actos®	(ac' tose)	Aldactone®	(al' dak tone)
Actidose®	(ac' ti dose)	Aldactazide®	(al dak' ta zide)
Actron®	(ak' tron)	Aldomet®	(al' doe met)
Acutrim®	(ak' yu trim)	Aldoril®	(al' doe ril)
Acular®	(ac' yu lar)	Aldomet®	(al' doe met)
Acthar®	(ac' thar)	Anzemet®	(an' ze met)
Acutrim®	(ak' yu trim)	Aldoril®	(al' doe ril)
Accutane®	(ak' yu tane)	Aldomet®	(al' doe met)
Acutrim®	(ak' yu trim)	Aldoril®	(al' doe ril)
Actron®	(ak' tron)	Elavil®	(el' a vil)
Adalat®	(ad' da lat)	Alesse®	(a less')
Adapin®	(ad' da pin)	Aleve®	(a leve')
adapalene	(a dap' a lene)	Aleve®	(a leve')
Adapin®	(ad' a pin)	Alesse®	(a less')

Drug Name	Pronunciation	Drug Name	Pronunciation
Alfenta®	(al fen' tah)	amlodipine	(am lo' di pine)
Sufenta®	(sue fen' tah)	amiloride	(a mil' o ride)
alfentanil	(al fen' ta nill)	Amipaque®	(am' ne pak)
Anafranil®	(a naf' ra nil)	Omnipaque®	(om' ne pak)
alfentanil	(al fen' ta nil)	amoxapine	(a moks' a peen)
remifentanil	(rem i fen' ta nil)	amoxicillin	(a moks a sil' in)
alfentanil	(al fen' ta nil)	amoxicillin	(a moks a sil' in)
sufentanil	(sue fen' ta nil)	amoxapine	(a moks' a peen)
Alferon®	(al' fer on)	ampicillin	(am pi sil' in)
Alkeran®	(al' ker an)	bacampicillin	(ba kam pi sil' in)
Allegra®	(al leg' ra)	hydrochloride	
Viagra®	(vye ag' ra)	amrinone	(am' ri none)
Alkeran®	(al' ker an)	amiodarone	(a mee' oh da rone)
Alferon®	(al' fer on)	Anafranil®	(a naf' ra nil)
Allerfrin®	(al' er frin)	alfentanil	(al fen' ta nil)
Allergan®	(al' er gan)	Anafranil®	(a naf' ra nil)
Allergan®	(al' er gan)	enalapril	(e nal' a pril)
Allerfrin®	(al' er frin)	Anaprox®	(an' a prox)
Allergan®	(al' er gan)	Anaspaz®	(an' a spaz)
Auralate®	(ahl' a late)	Anaspaz®	(an' a spaz)
alprazolam	(al pray' zoe lam)	Anaprox®	(an' a prox)
alprostadil	(al pros' ta dil)	Anaspaz®	(an' a spaz)
alprazolam	(al pray' zoe lam)	Antispas®	(an' te spaz)
triazolam	(trye ay' zoe lam)	Anatrast®	(an' a trast)
alprostadil	(al pros' ta dil)	Anatuss®	(an' a tuss)
alprazolam	(al pray' zoe lam)	Anatuss®	(an' a tuss)
Altace™	(al' tase)	Anatrast®	(an' a trast)
alteplase	(al' te place)	Ancobon®	(an' coe bon)
alteplase	(al' te place)	Oncovin®	(on' coe vin)
Altace™	(al' tase)	anistreplase	(a nis' tre place)
alteplase	(al' te place)	alteplase	(al' te place)
anistreplase	(a nis' tre place)	Ansaid®	(an' said)
Alupent®	(al' yu pent)	Axid®	(aks' id)
Atrovent®	(at' troe vent)	Antagon™	(an' ta gon)
amantadine	(a man' ta deen)	Auralgon®	(a ral' gon)
rimantadine	(ri man' to deen)	Antispas®	(an' te spaz)
Amaryl®	(am' ah ril)	Anaspaz®	(an' a spaz)
Ambenyl®	(am' ba nil)	Anturane®	(ann' chu rane)
Amaryl®	(am' ah ril)	Artane®	(ar' tane)
Amerge®	(a merge')	Anusol®	(an' yu sol)
Ambenyl®	(am' ba nil)	Aquasol®	(ah' kwa sol)
Amaryl®	(am' ah ril)	Anzemet®	(an' ze met)
Ambenyl®	(am' ba nil)	Aldomet®	(al' doe met)
Aventyl®	(a ven' til)	Aplisol®	(ap' lee sol)
Ambi 10®	(am' bee ten')	A.P.L.®	(aye pee el')
Ambien™	(am' bee en)	A.P.L.®	(aye pee el')
Ambien™	(am' bee en)	Aplisol®	(ap' lee sol)
Ambi 10®	(am' bee ten')	Apresoline®	(aye press' sow leen)
Amerge®	(a merge')	Priscoline®	(pris' coe leen)
Amaryl®	(am' ah ril)	Aquasol®	(ah' kwa sol)
Amicar®	(am' i car)	Anusol®	(an' yu sol)
Amikin®	(am' i kin)	AquaTar®	(ah' kwa tar)
Amikin®	(am' i kin)	Aquatag®	(ah' kwa tag)
Amicar®	(am' i car)	Aquatag®	(ah' kwa tag)
amiloride	(a mil' o ride)	AquaTar®	(ah' kwa tar)
amiodarone	(a mee' oh da rone)	ara-C	(a ra cee')
amiloride	(a mil' o ride)	Arasine®	(a ra seen')
amlodipine	(am lo' di pine)	Aralen®	(air' a len)
aminophylline	(am in off' l lin)	Aerolone®	(air' o lone)
amitriptyline	(a mee' trip ti leen)	Aralen®	(air' a len)
amiodarone	(a mee' oh da rone)	Arlidin®	(ar' le din)
amiloride	(a mil' o ride)	Aramine®	(air' a meen)
amiodarone	((a mee' oh da rone)	Artane®	(ar' tane)
amrinone	(am' ri none)	Arasine®	(a ra seen')
amitriptyline	(a mee' trip ti leen)	ara-C	(a ra cee')
aminophylline	(am in off' l lin)	Arfonad®	(arr' foe nad)
amitriptyline	(a mee trip' ti leen)	Afrinol®	(af' ree nol)
imipramine	(im ip' ra meen)	Argyrol®	(ar' gee roll)
		Agoral®	(ag' a ral)

SOUND-ALIKE COMPARISON LIST *(Continued)*

Drug Name	Pronunciation	Drug Name	Pronunciation
Aricept®	(ar' e cept)	Aygestin®	(aye ges' tin)
Ascriptin®	(a crip' tin)	Arrestin®	(aye res' tin)
Arlidin®	(ar' le din)	Azulfidine®	(ay zul' fi deen)
Aralen®	(air' a len)	Augmentin®	(aug men' tin)
Arrestin®	(aye res' tin)	bacampicillin	(ba kam pi sil' in)
Aygestin®	(aye ges' tin)	hydrochloride	
Artane®	(ar' tane)	ampicillin	(am pi sil' in)
Anturane®	(an' chu rane)	bacitracin	(bas i tray' sin)
Artane®	(ar' tane)	Bactrim®	(bac' trim)
Aramine®	(air' a meen)	baclofen	(bak' loe fen)
Asacol®	(as' a col)	Bactroban®	(bak' troe ban)
Os-Cal®	(os' cal)	baclofen	(bak' loe fen)
Asbron®	(as' bron)	Beclovent®	(bec' lo vent)
aspirin	(as' pir in)	Bactocill®	(bak' tow sill)
Ascriptin®	(a crip' tin)	Pathocil®	(path' o sill)
Aricept®	(ar' e cept)	Bactrim®	(bac' trim)
aspirin	(as' pir in)	bacitracin	(bas i tray' sin)
Afrin®	(aye' frin or af' rin)	Bactroban®	(bak' troe ban)
aspirin	(as' pir in)	baclofen	(bak' loe fen)
Asbron®	(as' bron)	Banophen®	(ban' o fen)
Atarax®	(at' a raks)	Barophen®	(bear' o fen)
Ativan®	(at' tee van)	Banthine®	(ban' theen)
Atarax®	(at' a raks)	Brethine®	(breath' een)
Marax®	(may' raks)	Banthine®	(ban' theen)
atenolol	(a ten' oh lole)	Pro-Banthine®	(pro ban' theen)
albuterol	(al byoo' ter ole)	Barophen®	(bear' o fen)
atenolol	(a ten' oh lole)	Banophen®	(ban' o fen)
Tylenol®	(tye' le nole)	Beclovent®	(bec' lo vent)
Atgam®	(at' gam)	baclofen	(bak' loe fen)
Ativan®	(at' tee van)	Beconase®	(beck' o nase)
Ativan®	(at' tee van)	Bexophene®	(beks' o feen)
Adapin®	(add' da pin)	Beminal®	(bem' eh nall)
Ativan®	(at' tee van)	Benemid®	(ben' a mid)
Atarax®	(at' a raks)	Benadryl®	(ben' a drill)
Ativan®	(at' tee van)	benazepril	(ban ay' ze pril)
Atgam®	(at' gam)	Benadryl®	(ben' a drill)
Ativan®	(at' tee van)	Bentyl®	(ben' till)
ATnativ®	(aye tee nay' tif)	benazepril	(ban ay' ze pril)
Ativan®	(at' tee van)	Benadryl®	(ben' a drill)
Avitene®	(aye' va teen)	Benemid®	(ben' a mid)
ATnativ®	(aye tee nay' tif)	Beminal®	(bem' eh nall)
Ativan®	(at' tee van)	Benoxyl®	(ben ox' ill)
Atrovent®	(at' troe vent)	Brevoxyl®	(brev ox' il)
Alupent®	(al' yu pent)	Bentyl®	(ben' till)
Augmentin®	(aug men' tin)	Aventyl®	(a ven' til)
Azulfidine®	(ay zul' fi deen)	Bentyl®	(ben' till)
Auralate®	(ahl' a late)	Benadryl®	(ben' a drill)
Allergan®	(al' er gan)	Bentyl®	(ben' till)
Auralgon®	(a ral' gon)	Cantil®	(can' til)
Antagon™	(an' ta gon)	Bentyl®	(ben' til)
Auralgan®	(a ral' gan)	Trental®	(tren' tal)
Larylgan®	(la ril' gan)	Benylin®	(ben' eh lin)
Auralgan®	(a ral' gan)	Ventolin®	(ven' tow lin)
Ophthalgan®	(opp thal' gan)	Benza®	(ben' zah)
Avalide®	(av' a lide)	Benzac®	(ben' zak)
Avandia®	(a van' de a)	Benzac®	(ben' zak)
Avandia®	(a van' de a)	Benza®	(ben' zah)
Avalide®	(av' a lide)	Bepridil®	(be' pri dil)
Aventyl®	(a ven' til)	Prepidil®	(pre' pi dil)
Ambenyl®	(am' ba nil)	Betadine®	(bay' ta deen)
Aventyl®	(a ven' til)	Betagan®	(bay' ta gan)
Bentyl®	(ben' till)	Betagan®	(bay' ta gan)
Avitene®	(aye' va teen)	Betadine®	(bay' ta deen)
Ativan®	(at' tee van)	Betapace®	(bay' ta pace)
Axid®	(aks' id)	Betapen®	(bay' ta pen)
Ansaid®	(an' said)	Betapen®	(bay' ta pen)
		Betapace®	(bay' ta pace)

Drug Name	Pronunciation	Drug Name	Pronunciation
Bexophene®	(beks' o feen)	Capitrol®	(kap' i trol)
Beconase®	(beck' o nase)	Capital®	(kap' i tal)
Bicillin®	(bye sil' lin)	Capitrol®	(kap' i trol)
V-Cillin K®	(vee sil' lin kay)	captopril	(kap' toe pril)
Bicillin®	(bye sil' lin)	captopril	(kap' toe pril)
Wycillin®	(wye sil' lin)	Capitrol®	(kap' i trol)
bleomycin	(blee o mye' sin)	carboplatin	(kar' boe pla tin)
Cleocin®	(klee' o sin)	cisplatin	(sis' pla tin)
Bleph®-10	(blef ten')	Cardio-Green®	(kar' dee yo green')
Blephamide®	(blef' a mide)	Cardioquin®	(kar' dee yo kwin)
Blephamide®	(blef' a mide)	Cardioquin®	(kar' dee yo kwin)
Bleph®-10	(blef ten')	Cardio-Green®	(kar' dee yo green')
Borofax®	(boroe' faks)	Cardura®	(kar dur' ah)
Boropak®	(boroe' pak)	Cordarone®	(kor da rone')
Boropak®	(boroe' pak)	Cardura®	(kar dur' ah)
Borofax®	(boroe' faks)	Cordran®	(kor' dran)
Brethine®	(breath' een)	Catapres®	(kat' a pres)
Banthine®	(ban' theen)	Catarase®	(kat' a race)
Bretylol®	(brett' tee loll)	Catapres®	(kat' a pres)
Brevital®	(brev' i tall)	Combipres®	(kom' bee pres)
Brevital®	(brev' i tall)	Catapres®	(kat' a pres)
Bretylol®	(brett' tee loll)	Ser-Ap-Es®	(ser ap' ess)
Brevoxyl®	(brev ox' il)	Catarase®	(kat' a race)
Benoxyl®	(ben ox' ill)	Catapres®	(kat' a pres)
brimonidine	(bri moe' ni deen)	cefazolin	(sef a' zoe lin)
bromocriptine	(broe moe krip' teen)	cephalexin	(sef a leks' in)
Bromfed®	(brom' fed)	cefazolin	(sef a' zoe lin)
Bromphen®	(brom' fen)	cephalothin	(sef a' loe thin)
bromocriptine	(broe moe krip' teen)	cefotaxime	(sef o taks' eem)
brimonidine	(bri moe' ni deen)	cefoxitin	(se fox' i tin)
Bromphen®	(brom' fen)	cefoxitin	(se fox' i tin)
Bromfed®	(brom' fed)	cefotaxime	(sef o taks' eem)
bumetanide	(byoo met' a nide)	ceftizoxime	(sef ti zoks' eem)
Buminate®	(byoo' mi nate)	cefuroxime	(se fyoor ox' eem)
Bumex®	(byoo' mex)	cefuroxime	(se fyoor ox' eem)
Buprenex®	(byoo' pre nex)	ceftizoxime	(sef ti zoks' eem)
Buprenex®	(byoo' pre nex)	Cefzil®	(sef' zil)
Bumex®	(byoo' mex)	Kefzol®	(kef' zol)
Buminate®	(byoo' mi nate)	Celebrex®	(sel' a brex)
bumetanide	(byoo met' a nide)	Cerebyx®	(ser' e bix)
bupivacaine	(byoo piv' a kane)	Celexa®	(se lex' a)
mepivacaine	(me piv' a kane)	Zyprexa®	(zye preks' a)
busalfan	(byoo sul' fan)	Cenestin®	(se nes' tin)
Butalan®	(byoo' ta lan)	Senexon®	(sen' e son)
butabarbital	(byoo ta bar' bi tal)	cephalexin	(sef a leks' in)
butalbital	(byoo tal' bi tal)	cefazolin	(sef a' zoe lin)
Butalan®	(byoo' ta lan)	cephalothin	(sef a' loe thin)
busalfan	(byoo sul' fan)	cefazolin	(sef a' zoe lin)
butalbital	(byoo tal' bi tal)	cephapirin	(sef a pye' rin)
butabarbital	(byoo ta bar' bi tal)	cephradine	(sef' ra deen)
Byclomine®	(bye' clo meen)	cephradine	(sef' ra deen)
Bydramine®	(bye' dra meen)	cephapirin	(sef a pye' rin)
Byclomine®	(bye' clo meen)	Cerebyx®	(ser' e bix)
Hycomine®	(hye' coe meen)	Celebrex®	(sel' a brex)
Bydramine®	(bye' dra meen)	Cerebyx®	(ser' e bix)
Byclomine®	(bye' clo meen)	Cerezyme®	(ser' e zime)
Bydramine®	(bye' dra meen)	Cerezyme®	(ser' e zime)
Hydramyn®	(hye' dra min)	Cerebyx®	(ser' e bix)
Cepastat®	(sea' pa stat)	chlorambucil	(klor am' byoo sil)
Capastat®	(kap' a stat)	Chloromycetin®	(klor oh my see' tin)
Cankaid®	(kan' kaid)	Chloromycetin®	(klor oh my see' tin)
Enkaid®	(enn' kaid)	chlorambucil	(klor am' byoo sil)
Cantil®	(can' til)	chloroxine	(klor ox' een)
Bentyl®	(ben' till)	Choloxin®	(koe lox' in)
Capastat®	(kap' a stat)	Choloxin®	(koe lox' in)
Cepastat®	(sea' pa stat)	chloroxine	(klor ox' een)
Capital®	(kap' i tal)	chlorpropamide	(klor proe' pa mide)
Capitrol®	(kap' i trol)	chlorpromazine	(klor proe' ma zeen)

SOUND-ALIKE COMPARISON LIST *(Continued)*

Drug Name	Pronunciation	Drug Name	Pronunciation
chlorpromazine	(klor proe' ma zeen)	CodAphen®	(kod' a fen)
chlorpropamide	(klor proe' pa mide)	Codafed®	(kode' a fed)
Chorex®	(ko' reks)	Codafed®	(kode' a fed)
Chymex®	(kye' meks)	CodAphen®	(kod' a fen)
Chymex®	(kye' meks)	codeine	(koe' deen)
Chorex®	(ko' reks)	Cophene®	(koe' feen)
Cidex®	(sy' tecks)	codeine	(koe' deen)
Lidex®	(ly' decks)	Cordran®	(kor' dran)
Ciloxan®	(sy loks' an)	codeine	(koe' deen)
cinoxacin	(sin oks' a sin)	Lodine®	(low' deen)
Ciloxan®	(sy loks' an)	Colax®	(koe' laks)
Cytoxan®	(sy toks' an)	Co-Lav®	(koe' lav)
cinoxacin	(sin oks' a sin)	Colestid®	(koe les' tid)
Ciloxan®	(sy loks' an)	colistin	(koe lis' tin)
cisplatin	(sis' pla tin)	colistin	(koe lis' tin)
carboplatin	(kar' boe pla tin)	Colestid®	(koe les' tid)
Citracal®	(sit' tra cal)	Combipres®	(kom' bee pres)
Citrucel®	(sit' tru cel)	Catapres®	(kat' a pres)
Citrucel®	(sit' tru cel)	Combivent®	(kom' bi vent)
Citracal®	(sit' tra cal)	Combivir®	(kom' bi veer)
clarithromycin	(kla rith' roe mye sin)	Combivir®	(kom' bi veer)
erythromycin	(er ith roe mye' sin)	Combivent®	(kom® bi vent)
Cleocin®	(klee' o sin)	Congestac®	(kon ges' tin)
bleomycin	(blee o mye' sin)	Congestant®	(kon ges' tant)
Cleocin®	(klee' o sin)	Congestant®	(kon ges' tant)
Lincocin®	(link' o sin)	Congestac®	(kon ges' tin)
Clinoxide®	(klin ox' ide)	Cophene®	(koe' feen)
Clipoxide®	(kleh pox' ide)	codeine	(koe' deen)
Clipoxide®	(kleh pox' ide)	Cordarone®	(kor da rone')
Clinoxide®	(klin ox' ide)	Cardura®	(kar dur' ah)
Clocort®	(klo' kort)	Cordarone®	(kor da rone')
Cloderm®	(klo' derm)	Cordran®	(kor' dran)
Cloderm®	(klo' derm)	Cordran®	(kor' dran)
Clocort®	(klo' kort)	Cardura®	(kar dur' ah)
clofibrate	(kloe fye' brate)	Cordran®	(kor' dran)
clorazepate	(klor az' a pate)	codeine	(koe' deen)
clomiphene	(kloe' mi feen)	Cordran®	(kor' dran)
clomipramine	(kloe mi' pra meen)	Cordarone®	(kor da rone')
clomiphene	(kloe' mi feen)	Cort-Dome®	(kort' dome)
clonidine	(kloe' ni deen)	Cortone®	(kor' tone)
clomipramine	(kloe mi' pra meen)	cortisone	(kor' ti sone)
clomiphene	(kloe' mi feen)	Cortizone®	(kor' ti sone)
clonidine	(kloe' ni deen)	Cortizone®	(kor' ti sone)
clomiphene	(kloe' mi feen)	cortisone	(kor' ti sone)
clonidine	(kloe' ni deen)	Cortone®	(kor' tone)
clozapine	(kloe' za peen)	Cort-Dome®	(kort' dome)
clonidine	(kloe' ni deen)	Coumadin®	(ku' ma din)
Klonopin™	(klon' o pin)	Kemadrin®	(kem' a drin)
clonidine	(kloe' ni deen)	Cozaar®	(koe' zar)
Loniten®	(lon' eh ten)	Zocor®	(zoe' cor)
clonidine	(kloe' ni deen)	Crysticillin®	(kris ta sil' lin)
quinidine	(kwin' i deen)	Crystodigin®	(kris toe dig' in)
clorazepate	(klor az' a pate)	Crystodigin®	(kris toe dig' in)
clofibrate	(kloe fye' brate)	Crysticillin®	(kris ta sil' lin)
clotrimazole	(kloe trim' a zole)	cycloserine	(sye kloe ser' een)
co-trimoxazole	(koe-trye moks' a zole)	cyclosporine	(sye' kloe spor een)
Cloxapen®	(klox' a pen)	Cyclospasmol®	(sye kloe spas' mol)
clozapine	(kloe' za peen)	cyclosporine	(sye' kloe spor een)
clozapine	(kloe' za peen)	cyclosporine	(sye' kloe spor een)
clonidine	(kloe' ni deen)	Cyclospasmol®	(sye kloe spas' mol)
clozapine	(kloe' za peen)	cyclosporine	(sye' kloe spor een)
Cloxapen®	(klox' a pen)	Cyklokapron®	(sye kloe kay' pron)
Co-Lav®	(koe' lav)	cyclosporine	(sye' kloe spor een)
Colax®	(koe' laks)	cycloserine	(sye kloe ser' een)
co-trimoxazole	(koe-trye moks' a zole)	Cyklokapron®	(sye kloe kay' pron)
clotrimazole	(kloe trim' a zole)	cyclosporine	(sye' kloe spor een)

Drug Name	Pronunciation	Drug Name	Pronunciation
cytarabine	(sye tare' a been)	Demerol®	(dem' eh rol)
vidarabine	(vye dare' a been)	Dymelor®	(dye' meh lo)
Cytogam®	(sy' to gam)	Demerol®	(dem' eh rol)
Cytoxan®	(sy toks' an)	Temaril®	(tem' a ril)
Cytotec®	(sye' toe tek)	Demulen®	(dem' yu len)
Cytoxan®	(sye tox' an)	Dalmane®	(dal' mane)
Cytotec®	(sye' toe tek)	Demulen®	(dem' yu len)
Sytobex®	(sye' toe beks)	Demerol®	(dem' eh rol)
Cytoxan®	(sy toks' an)	Denorex®	(den' o reks)
Ciloxan®	(sy loks' an)	Demadex®	(dem' a deks)
Cytoxan®	(sy toks' an)	Depakene®	(dep' a keen)
Cytogam®	(sy' to gam)	Depakote®	(dep' a kote)
Cytoxan®	(sye tox' an)	Depakote®	(dep' a kote)
Cytotec®	(sye' toe tek)	Depakene®	(dep' a keen)
dacarbazine	(da kar' ba zeen)	DepoCyt®	(de' po set)
Dicarbosil®	(dye kar' bow sil)	Depoject®	(de' po ject)
dacarbazine	(da kar' ba zeen)	Depogen®	(dep' o gen)
procarbazine	(proe kar' ba zeen)	Depoject®	(dep' o ject)
dactinomycin	(dak ti noe mye' sin)	Depoject®	(de' po ject)
daunorubicin	(daw noe roo' bi sin)	DepoCyt®	(de' po set)
Dalmane®	(dal' mane)	Depoject®	(dep' o ject)
Demulen®	(dem' yu len)	Depogen®	(dep' o gen)
Dalmane®	(dal' mane)	Depo-Testadiol®	(dep o tes ta dye' ol)
Dialume®	(dy' a lume)	Depotestogen®	(dep o tes' tow gen)
dapsone	(dap' sone)	Depotestogen®	(dep o tes' tow gen)
Diprosone®	(dip' ro sone)	Depo-Testadiol®	(dep o tes ta dye' ol)
Daranide®	(dare' a nide)	Deprol®	(deh' prol)
Daraprim®	(dare' a prim)	Daypro®	(day' pro)
Daraprim®	(dare' a prim)	Dermacort®	(der' ma kort)
Daranide®	(dare' a nide)	DermiCort®	(der' meh kort)
Daricon®	(dare' eh kon)	Dermatop®	(der' ma top)
Darvon®	(dar' von)	DermiCort®	(der' meh kort)
Darvon®	(dar' von)	Dermatop®	(der' ma top)
Daricon®	(dare' eh kon)	Dimetapp®	(dime' tap)
Darvon®	(dar' von)	DermiCort®	(der' meh kort)
Devrom®	(dev' rom)	Dermacort®	(der' ma kort)
Darvon®	(dar' von)	DermiCort®	(der' meh kort)
Diovan®	(dye oh' van)	Dermatop®	(der' ma top)
daunorubicin	(daw noe roo' bi sin)	deserpidine	(de ser' pi deen)
dactinomycin	(dak ti noe mye' sin)	desipramine	(dess ip' ra meen)
daunorubicin	(daw noe roo' bi sin)	Desferal®	(des' fer al)
doxorubicin	(dox o roo' bi sin)	Disophrol®	(dye' so frol)
Daypro®	(day' pro)	Desferal®	(des' fer al)
Deprol®	(deh' prol)	desflurane	(des flu' rane)
Decadron®	(dek' a dron)	desflurane	(des flu' rane)
Decholin®	(dek' o lin)	Desferal®	(des' fer al)
Decadron®	(dek' a dron)	desipramine	(dess ip' ra meen)
Percodan®	(per' coe dan)	deserpidine	(de ser' pi deen)
Decholin®	(dek' o lin)	desoximetasone	(des ox i met' a sone)
Decadron®	(dek' a dron)	dexamethasone	(deks a meth' a sone)
Deconal®	(dek' o nal)	Desoxyn®	(de soks' in)
Deconsal®	(dek' on sal)	digoxin	(di joks' in)
Deconsal®	(dek' on sal)	Devrom®	(dev' rom)
Deconal®	(dek' o nal)	Darvon®	(dar' von)
Delacort®	(del' a kort)	dexamethasone	(deks a meth' a sone)
Delcort®	(del' kort)	desoximetasone	(des ox i met' a sone)
Delcort®	(del' kort)	Diaβeta®	(dye a bay' tah)
Delacort®	(del' a kort)	Diabinese®	(dye ab' beh neese)
Delfen®	(del' fen)	Diaβeta®	(dye a bay' tah)
Delsym®	(del' sim)	Zebeta®	(ze' bay tah)
Delsym®	(del' sim)	Diabinese®	(dye ab' beh neese)
Delfen®	(del' fen)	Diaβeta®	(dye a bay' tah)
Demadex®	(dem' a deks)	Dialume®	(dy' a lume)
Denorex®	(den' o reks)	Dalmane®	(dal' mane)
Demerol®	(dem' eh rol)	Diamox®	(dye' a moks)
dicumarol	(dye koo' ma role)	Trimox®	(trye' moks)
Demerol®	(dem' eh rol)	diazoxide	(dye a soks' ide)
Demulen®	(dem' yu len)	Dyazide®	(dye' a zide)

SOUND-ALIKE COMPARISON LIST *(Continued)*

Drug Name	Pronunciation	Drug Name	Pronunciation
Dicarbosil®	(dye kar' bow sil)	docusate	(dok' yoo sate)
dacarbazine	(da kar' ba zeen)	Doxinate®	(dox' eh nate)
diclofenac	(dye kloe' fen ak)	Dolobid®	(dol' ah bid)
Diflucan®	(dye flu' can)	Slo-Bid®	(slo' bid)
dicumarol	(dye koo' ma role)	Donnapine®	(don' a peen)
Demerol®	(dem' eh rol)	Donnazyme®	(don' a zime)
Diflucan®	(dye flu' can)	Donnazyme®	(don' a zime)
diclofenac	(dye kloe' fen ak)	Donnapine®	(don' a peen)
Diflucan®	(dye flu' can)	dopamine	(doe' pa meen)
Diprivan®	(dye' pri van)	dobutamine	(doe byoo' ta meen)
digitoxin	(di ji tox' in)	dopamine	(doe' pa meen)
digoxin	(di jox' in)	Dopram®	(doe' pram)
digoxin	(di joks' in)	Dopar®	(doe' par)
Desoxyn®	(de soks' in)	Dopram®	(doe' pram)
digoxin	(di jox' in)	Dopram®	(doe' pram)
digitoxin	(di ji tox' in)	dopamine	(doe' pa meen)
Dilantin®	(dye lan' tin)	Dopram®	(doe' pram)
Dilaudid®	(dye law' did)	Dopar®	(doe' par)
Dilantin®	(dye lan' tin)	doxepin	(dox' e pin)
diltiazem	(dil tye' a zem)	Doxidan®	(dox' e dan)
Dilantin®	(dye lan' tin)	Doxidan®	(dox' e dan)
Dipentum®	(dye pen' tum)	doxepin	(dox' e pin)
Dilaudid®	(dye law' did)	Doxil®	(doks' il)
Dilantin®	(dye lan' tin)	Paxil®	(paks' il)
diltiazem	(dil tye' a zem)	Doxinate®	(dox' eh nate)
Dilantin®	(dye lan' tin)	docusate	(dok' yoo sate)
dimenhydrinate	(dye men hye' dri nate)	doxorubicin	(dox o roo' bi sin)
diphenhydramine	(dye fen hye' dra meen)	daunorubicin	(daw noe roo' bi sin)
Dimetabs®	(dime' tabs)	Duo-Cyp®	(du' o sip)
Dimetapp®	(dime' tap)	DuoCet™	(du' o set)
Dimetapp®	(dime' tap)	DuoCet™	(du' o set)
Dermatop®	(der' ma top)	Duo-Cyp®	(du' o sep)
Dimetapp®	(dime' tap)	Dura-Gest®	(dur' a gest)
Dimetabs®	(dime' tabs)	Duragen®	(dur' a gen)
Diovan®	(dye oh' van)	Duragen®	(dur' a gen)
Darvon®	(dar' von)	Dura-Gest®	(dur' a gest)
Dipentum®	(dye pen' tum)	Dyazide®	(dye' a zide)
Dilantin®	(dye lan' tin)	diazoxide	(dye a soks' ide)
diphenhydramine	(dye fen hye' dra meen)	Dyazide®	(dye' a zide)
dimenhydrinate	(dye men hye' dri nate)	Dynacin®	(dye' na sin)
Diphenatol®	(dye fen' ah tol)	Dymelor®	(dye' meh lo)
diphenidiol	(dye fen' i dole)	Demerol®	(dem' eh rol)
diphenidiol	(dye fen' i dole)	Dymelor®	(dye' meh lor)
Diphenatol®	(dye fen' ah tol)	Pamelor®	(pam' meh lor)
Diphenylan®	(dye fen' eh lan)	Dynabac®	(dye' na bac)
dyphenylan	(dye fen' eh lan)	Dynapen®	(dye' na pen)
Diprivan®	(dye' pri van)	Dynacin®	(dye' na sin)
Diflucan®	(dye flu' can)	DynaCirc®	(dye' na sirk)
Diprivan®	(dip' riv an)	Dynacin®	(dye' na sin)
Ditropan®	(di troe' pan)	Dyazide®	(dye' a zide)
Diprosone®	(dip' ro sone)	Dynacin®	(dye' na sin)
dapsone	(dap' sone)	Dynapen®	(dye' ne pen)
dipyridamole	(dye peer id' a mole)	DynaCirc®	(dye' na sirk)
disopyramide	(dye soe peer' a mide)	Dynacin®	(dye' na sin)
Disophrol®	(dye' so frol)	Dynapen®	(dye' na pen)
Desferal®	(des' fer al)	Dynabac®	(dye' na bac)
disopyramide	(dye soe peer' a mide)	Dynapen®	(dye' ne pen)
dipyridamole	(dye peer id' a mole)	Dynacin®	(dye' na sin)
Ditropan®	(di troe' pan)	dyphenylan	(dye fen' eh lan)
Diprivan®	(dip' riv an)	Diphenylan®	(dye fen' eh lan)
Ditropan®	(di troe' pan)	Dyrenium®	(dye ren' e um)
Intropin®	(in troe' pin)	Pyridium®	(pye rid' dee um)
Diutensin®	(dye yu ten' sin)	Dwelle®	(dwell)
Salutensin®	(sal yu ten' sin)	Kwell®	(kwell)
dobutamine	(doe byoo' ta meen)	Ecotrin®	(eh' ko trin)
dopamine	(doe' pa meen)	Edecrin®	(ed' eh crin)

Drug Name	Pronunciation	Drug Name	Pronunciation
Edecrin®	(ed′ eh crin)	Esimil®	(es′ eh mil)
Ecotrin®	(eh′ ko trin)	Ismelin®	(is′ meh lin)
Edecrin®	(ed′ eh crin)	Esimil®	(es′ eh mil)
Ethaquin®	(eth′ a kwin)	F.M.L.®	(ef′ em el)
Elase®	(e′ lase)	Estinyl®	(es′ teh nil)
Ellence®	(el′ lens)	Esimil®	(es′ eh mil)
Elavil®	(el′ a vil)	Estratab®	(es′ tra tab)
Aldoril®	(al′ doe ril)	Ethatab®	(eth′ a tab)
Elavil®	(el′ a vil)	Eskalith®	(es′ ka lith)
Eldepryl®	(el′ de pril)	Estratest®	(es′ tra test)
Elavil®	(el′ a vil)	Estratest®	(es′ tra test)
Equanil®	(eh′ kwa nil)	Eskalith®	(es′ ka lith)
Elavil®	(el′ a vil)	ethanol	(eth′ e nol)
Mellaril®	(mel′ la ril)	Ethyol®	(eth′ e ole)
Elavil®	(el′ a vil)	Ethaquin®	(eth′ a kwin)
Oruvail®	(or′ yu vale)	Edecrin®	(ed′ eh crin)
Eldepryl®	(el′ de pril)	Ethatab®	(eth′ a tab)
Elavil®	(el′ a vil)	Estratab®	(es′ tra tab)
Eldepryl®	(el de pril)	ethosuximide	(eth o sux′ i mide)
enalapril	(e nal′ a pril)	methsuximide	(meth sux′ i mide)
Elixicon®	(eh lix′ i con)	Ethyol®	(eth′ e ole)
Elocon®	(ee′ lo con)	ethanol	(eth′ e nol)
Ellence®	(el′ lens)	etidocaine	(e ti′ doe kane)
Elase®	(e′ lase)	etidronate	(e ti droe′ nate)
Elocon®	(ee′ lo con)	etidronate	(e ti droe′ nate)
Elixicon®	(eh lix′ i con)	etidocaine	(e ti′ doe kane)
emetine	(em′ eh teen)	etidronate	(e ti droe′ nate)
Emetrol®	(em′ eh trol)	etretinate	(e tret′ i nate)
Emetrol®	(em′ eh trol)	etretinate	(e tret′ i nate)
emetine	(em′ eh teen)	etidronate	(e ti droe′ nate)
enalapril	(e nal′ a pril)	Eurax®	(yoor′ aks)
Anafranil®	(a naf′ ra nil)	Serax®	(sear′ aks)
enalapril	(e nal′ a pril)	Eurax®	(yoor′ aks)
Eldepryl®	(el de pril)	Urex®	(yu′ eks)
Endal®	(en′ dal)	Factrel®	(fak′ trel)
Intal®	(in′ tal)	Sectral®	(sek′ tral)
Enduron®	(en′ du ron)	Feldene®	(fel′ deen)
Imuran®	(im′ yu ran)	Seldane®	(sel′ dane)
Enduron®	(en′ du ron)	fenoprofen	(fen o proe′ fen)
Inderal®	(in′ der al)	flurbiprofen	(flure bi′ proe fen)
Enduronyl®	(en dur′ o nil)	Feosol®	(fee′ o sol)
Inderal®	(in′ der al)	Fer-In-Sol®	(fehr′ in sol)
Enduronyl® Forte	(en dur′ o nil for′ tay)	Feosol®	(fee′ o sol)
Inderal® 40	(in′ der al for′ tee)	Festal®	(fes′ tal)
enflurane	(en′ floo rane)	Feosol®	(fee′ o sol)
isoflurane	(eye soe flure′ ane)	Fluosol®	(flu′ o sol)
Enkaid®	(enn′ kaid)	Fer-In-Sol®	(fehr′ in sol)
Cankaid®	(kan′ kaid)	Feosol®	(fee′ o sol)
Entex®	(en′ teks)	Ferralet®	(fer′ a let)
Tenex®	(ten′ eks)	Ferrlecit®	(fer′ le set)
ephedrine	(e fed′ rin)	Ferrlecit®	(fer′ le set)
Epifrin®	(ep′ eh frin)	Ferralet®	(fer′ a let)
EpiPen®	(ep′ eh pen)	Festal®	(fes′ tal)
Epifrin®	(ep′ eh frin)	Feosol®	(fee′ o sol)
Epifrin®	(ep′ eh frin)	Feverall™	(fee′ ver all)
ephedrine	(e fed′ rin)	Fiberall®	(fye′ ber all)
Epifrin®	(ep′ eh frin)	Fiberall®	(fye′ ber all)
EpiPen®	(ep′ eh pen)	Feverall™	(fee′ ver all)
Epinal®	(ep′ eh nal)	Fioricet®	(fee oh′ reh set)
Epitol®	(ep′ eh tol)	Lorcet®	(lor′ set)
Epitol®	(ep′ eh tol)	Fiorinal®	(fee or′ reh nal)
Epinal®	(ep′ eh nal)	Florinef®	(flor′ eh nef)
Equanil®	(eh′ kwa nil)	Flaxedil®	(flaks′ eh dil)
Elavil®	(el′ a vil)	Flexeril®	(fleks′ eh ril)
erythromycin	(er ith roe mye′ sin)	Flexeril®	(fleks′ eh ril)
clarithromycin	(kla rith′ roe mye sin)	Flaxedil®	(flaks′ eh dil)
Esimil®	(es′ eh mil)	Flexeril®	(fleks′ eh ril)
Estinyl®	(es′ teh nil)	Hectoral™	(hek′ to ral)

SOUND-ALIKE COMPARISON LIST *(Continued)*

Drug Name	Pronunciation	Drug Name	Pronunciation
Flexon®	(fleks' on)	gonadorelin	(goe nad o rell' in)
Floxin®	(floks' in)	guanadrel	(gwahn' a drel)
Flomax™	(flo' maks)	Gonak™	(gon' ak)
Fosamax®	(fos' a maks)	Gonic®	(gon' ik)
Flomax™	(flo' maks)	Gonic®	(gon' ik)
Volmax®	(vol' maks)	Gonak™	(gon' ak)
Florinef®	(flor' eh nef)	Granulex®	(gran' u lecks)
Fiorinal®	(fee or' reh nal)	Regranex®	(re gra' neks)
Floxin®	(floks' in)	guaifenesin	(gwye fen' e sin)
Flexon®	(fleks' on)	guanfacine	(gwahn' fa seen)
flunisolide	(floo nis' o lide)	guanadrel	(gwahn' a drel)
fluocinonide	(floo o sin' o nide)	gonadorelin	(goe nad o rell' in)
fluocinolone	(floo o sin' o lone)	guanethidine	(gwahn eth' i deen)
fluocinonide	(floo o sin' o nide)	guanidine	(gwahn' i deen)
fluocinonide	(floo o sin' o nide)	guanfacine	(gwahn' fa seen)
flunisolide	(floo nis' o lide)	guaifenesin	(gwye fen' e sin)
fluocinonide	(floo o sin' o nide)	guanidine	(gwahn' i deen)
fluocinolone	(floo o sin' o lone)	guanethidine	(gwahn eth' i deen)
Fluosol®	(flu' o sol)	Haldol®	(hal' dol)
Feosol®	(fee' o sol)	Halenol®	(hal' e nol)
flurbiprofen	(flure bi' proe fen)	Haldol®	(hal' dol)
fenoprofen	(fen o proe' fen)	Halog®	(hay' log)
F.M.L.®	(ef' em el)	Halenol®	(hal' e nol)
Esimil®	(es' eh mil)	Haldol®	(hal' dol)
Fosamax®	(fos' a maks)	Halfan®	(hal' fan)
Flomax™	(flo' maks)	Halfprin®	(half' prin)
Fostex®	(fos' teks)	Halfprin®	(half' prin)
pHisoHex®	(fye' so heks)	Halfan®	(hal' fan)
Fulvicin®	(ful' vi sin)	Halfprin®	(half' prin)
Furacin®	(fur' a sin)	Haltran®	(hal' tran)
Furacin®	(fur' a sin)	Halog®	(hay' log)
Fulvicin®	(ful' vi sin)	Haldol®	(hal' dol)
Gamastan®	(gam' a stan)	Halotestin®	(hay lo tes' tin)
Garamycin®	(gar a mye' sin)	Halotex®	(hay' lo teks)
Gantanol®	(gan' ta nol)	Halotestin®	(hay lo tes' tin)
Gantrisin®	(gan' tri sin)	Halotussin®	(hay lo tus' sin)
Gantrisin®	(gan' tri sin)	Halotex®	(hay' lo teks)
Gantanol®	(gan' ta nol)	Halotestin®	(hay lo tes' tin)
Gantrisin®	(gan' tri sin)	Halotussin®	(hay lo tus' sin)
Gastrosed™	(gas' troe sed)	Halotestin®	(hay lo tes' tin)
Garamycin®	(gar a mye' sin)	Haltran®	(hal' tran)
Gamastan®	(gam' a stan)	Halfprin®	(half' prin)
Garamycin®	(gar a mye' sin)	Hectoral™	(hek' to ral)
kanamycin	(kan a mye' sin)	Flexeril®	(fleks' eh ril)
Garamycin®	(gar a mye' sin)	Herplex®	(her' pleks)
Terramycin®	(tehr a mye' sin)	Hiprex®	(hi' preks)
Gastrosed™	(gas' troe sed)	Hespan®	(hes' pan)
Gantrisin®	(gan' tri sin)	Histaspan®	(his' ta span)
Genapap®	(gen' a pap)	Hexadrol®	(heks' a drol)
Genapax®	(gen' a paks)	Hexalol®	(heks' a drol)
Genapap®	(gen' a pap)	Hexalol®	(heks' a drol)
Genatap®	(gen' a tap)	Hexadrol®	(heks' a drol)
Genapax®	(gen' a paks)	Hiprex®	(hi' preks)
Genapap®	(gen' a pap)	Herplex®	(her' pleks)
Genatap®	(gen' a tap)	Histaspan®	(his' ta span)
Genapap®	(gen' a pap)	Hespan®	(hes' pan)
gentamicin	(jen ta mye' sin)	Hycamtin®	(hye cam' tin)
kanamycin	(kan a mye' sin)	Hycomine®	(hye' co meen)
Glucophage®	(glue' co faagsch)	Hycodan®	(hye' co dan)
Glucotrol®	(glue' co trol)	Hycomine®	(hye' co meen)
Glucotrol®	(glue' co trol)	Hycodan®	(hye' co dan)
Glucophage®	(glue' co faagsch)	Vicodin®	(vye' co din)
Glycotuss®	(glye' co tuss)	Hycomine®	(hye' coe meen)
Glytuss®	(glye' tuss)	Byclomine®	(bye' clo meen)
Glytuss®	(glye' tuss)	Hycomine®	(hye' co meen)
Glycotuss®	(glye' co tuss)	Hycamtin®	(hye cam' tin)

Drug Name	Pronunciation	Drug Name	Pronunciation
Hycomine®	(hye′ co meen)	interferon	(in ter fer′ on)
Hycodan®	(hye′ co dan)	Imferon®	(im′ fer on)
Hydergine®	(hye′ der geen)	Intropin®	(in tro′ pin)
Hydramyn®	(hye′ dra min)	Isoptin®	(eye sop′ tin)
hydralazine	(hye dral′ a zeen)	Intropin®	(in troe′ pin)
hydroxyzine	(hye drox′ i zeen)	Ditropan®	(di troe′ pan)
Hydramyn®	(hye′ dra min)	Ismelin®	(is′ meh lin)
Hydergine®	(hye′ der geen)	Esimil®	(es′ eh mil)
Hydramyn®	(hye′ dra min)	Ismelin®	(is′ meh lin)
Bydramine®	(bye′ dra meen)	Ritalin®	(ri′ ta lin)
Hydrocet®	(hye′ dro set)	isoflurane	(eye soe flure′ ane)
Hydrocil®	(hye′ dro sil)	enflurane	(en′ floo rane)
Hydrocil®	(hye′ dro sil)	isoflurane	(eye soe flure′ ane)
Hydrocet®	(hye′ dro set)	isoflurophate	(eye soe flure′ o fate)
hydroxyurea	(hye drox ee yoor ee′ a)	isoflurophate	(eye soe flure′ o fate)
hydroxyzine	(hye drox′ i zeen)	Isoflurane	(eye soe flure′ ane)
hydroxyzine	(hye drox′ i zeen)	Isoptin®	(eye sop′ tin)
hydralazine	(hye dral′ a zeen)	Intropin®	(in tro′ pin)
hydroxyzine	(hye drox′ i zeen)	Isoptin®	(eye sop′ tin)
hydroxyurea	(hye drox ee yoor ee′ a)	Isopto® Tears	(eye sop′ tow tears)
Hygroton®	(hye gro′ ton)	Isopto® Tears	(eye sop′ tow tears)
Regroton®	(reg′ ro ton)	Isoptin®	(eye sop′ tin)
Hyperab®	(hye′ per ab)	Isordil®	(eye′ sor dil)
HyperHep®	(hye′ per hep)	Inderal®	(in′ der al)
Hyperstat®	(hye′ per stat)	Isordil®	(eye′ sor dil)
Hyper-Tet®	(hye′ per tet)	Isuprel®	(eye′ sue prel)
Hyperstat®	(hye′ per stat)	Isuprel®	(eye′ sue prel)
Nitrostat®	(nye′ troe stat)	Isordil®	(eye′ sor dil)
Hyper-Tet®	(hye′ per tet)	K-Lor™	(kay′ lor)
HyperHep®	(hye′ per hep)	Kaochlor®	(kay′ o klor)
Hyper-Tet®	(hye′ per tet)	kanamycin	(kan a mye′ sin)
Hyperstat®	(hye′ per stat)	Garamycin®	(gar a mye′ sin)
HyperHep®	(hye′ per hep)	kanamycin	(kan a mye′ sin)
Hyperab®	(hye′ per ab)	gentamicin	(jen ta mye′ sin)
HyperHep®	(hye′ per hep)	Kaochlor®	(kay′ o klor)
Hyper-Tet®	(hye′ per tet)	K-Lor™	(kay′ lor)
Hytone®	(hye′ tone)	kaolin	(kay′ oh lin)
Vytone®	(vye′ tone)	Kaon®	(kay′ on)
Idamycin®	(eye da mye′ sin)	Kaon®	(kay′ on)
Adriamycin™	(ade rya mye′ sin)	kaolin	(kay′ oh lin)
Imferon®	(im′ fer on)	Kaopectate®	(kay oh pek′ tate)
interferon	(in ter fer′ on)	Kayexelate®	(kay eks′ e late)
imipramine	(im ip′ ra meen)	Kayexelate®	(kay eks′ e late)
amitripyline	(a mee trip′ ti leen)	Kaopectate®	(kay oh pek′ tate)
imipramine	(im ip′ ra meen)	Keflex®	(keh′ fleks)
Norpramin®	(nor pray′ min)	Keflin®	(keh′ flin)
Imuran®	(im′ yu ran)	Keflin®	(keh′ flin)
Enduron®	(en′ du ron)	Keflex®	(keh′ fleks)
Inapsine®	(i nap′ seen)	Ketzol®	(kef′ zol)
Nebcin®	(neb′ sin)	Cefzil®	(sef′ zil)
Inderal®	(in′ der al)	Kemadrin®	(kem′ a drin)
Adderall®	(ad′ der all)	Coumadin®	(ku′ ma din)
Inderal®	(in′ der al)	Klonopin™	(klon′ o pin)
Enduron®	(en′ du ron)	clonidine	(kloe′ ni deen)
Inderal®	(in′ der al)	Komex®	(koe′ meks)
Enduronyl®	(en dur′ o nil)	Koromex®	(kor′ o meks)
Inderal®	(in′ der al)	Koromex®	(kor′ o meks)
Isordil®	(eye′ sor dil)	Komex®	(koe′ meks)
Inderal®	(in′ der al)	Kwell®	(kwell)
Medrol®	(meh′ drol)	Dwelle®	(dwell)
Inderal® 40	(in′ der al for′ tee)	lactose	(lak′ tose)
Enduronyl® Forte	(en dur′ o nil for′ tay)	lactulose	(lak′ tu lose)
Indocin®	(in′ doe sin)	lactulose	(lak′ tu lose)
Lincocin®	(lin′ coe sin)	lactose	(lak′ tose)
Indocin®	(in′ doe sin)	Lamictal®	(la mic′ tal)
Minocin®	(min′ o sin)	Lamisil®	(lam′ eh sil)
Intal®	(in′ tal)	Lamictal®	(la mic′ tal)
Endal®	(en′ dal)	Lomotil®	(lo′ mo til)

SOUND-ALIKE COMPARISON LIST *(Continued)*

Drug Name	Pronunciation	Drug Name	Pronunciation
Lamisil®	(lam' eh sil)	Lomotil®	(lo' mo til)
Lamictal®	(la mic' tal)	Lamictal®	(la mic' tal)
lamotrigine	(la moe' tri jeen)	Loniten®	(lon' eh ten)
lamivudine	(la mi' vyoo deen)	clonidine	(kloe' ni deen)
lamivudine	(la mi' vyoo deen)	Lopressor®	(lo pres' sor)
lamotrigine	(la moe' tri jeen)	Lopurin®	(lo pure' in)
Lanoxin®	(lan ox' in)	Lopurin®	(lo pure' in)
Levoxine®	(lev ox een)	Lopressor®	(lo pres' sor)
Lanoxin®	(lan ox' in)	Lopurin®	(lo pure' in)
Levsinex®	(lev' si neks)	Lupron®	(lu' pron)
Lanoxin®	(lan ox' in)	Lorcet®	(lor' set)
Mefoxin®	(me fox' in)	Fioricet®	(fee oh' reh set)
Larylgan®	(la ril' gan)	Lotrimin®	(low' tri min)
Auralgan®	(a ral' gan)	Otrivin®	(oh' tri vin)
Lasix®	(lay' siks)	Lovenox®	(lo' ve nox)
Lidex®	(lye' deks)	Lomodix®	(lo' mo dix)
Lasix®	(lay' siks)	Loxitane®	(loks' e tane)
Luvox®	(lu' voks)	Soriatane®	(sor' e ah tane)
leucovorin	(loo koe vor' in)	Luminal®	(lu' mi nal)
Leukeran®	(lu' keh ran)	Tuinal®	(tu' i nal)
Leukeran®	(lu' keh ran)	Lupron®	(lu' pron)
leucovorin	(loo koe vor' in)	Lopurin®	(lo pure' in)
levodopa	(lee voe doe' pa)	Lupron®	(lu' pron)
methyldopa	(meth ill doe' pa)	Nuprin®	(nu' prin)
levothyroxine	(lee voe thye rox' een)	Luvox®	(lu' voks)
liothyronine	(lye o thye' roe neen)	Lasix®	(lay' siks)
Levoxine®	(lev ox een)	Maalox®	(may' loks)
Lanoxin®	(lan ox' in)	Maox®	(may' oks)
Levsinex®	(lev' si neks)	Maalox®	(may' loks)
Lanoxin®	(lan ox' in)	Marax®	(mare' aks)
Lidex®	(ly' decks)	Maalox®	(may' loks)
Cidex®	(sy' tecks)	Monodox®	(mon' o doks)
Lidex®	(lye' deks)	Maltsupex®	(malt' su peks)
Lasix®	(lay' siks)	Manoplax®	(man' o laks)
Lidex®	(lye' deks)	Mandol®	(man' dole)
Lidox®	(lye' dox)	nadolol	(nay doe' lole)
Lidex®	(lye' deks)	Manoplax®	(man' o laks)
Videx®	(vye' deks)	Maltsupex®	(malt' su peks)
Lidex®	(lye' deks)	Maox®	(may' oks)
Wydase®	(wye' dase)	Maalox®	(may' loks)
Lidox®	(lye' dox)	Maox®	(may' oks)
Lidex®	(lye' deks)	Marax®	(may' raks)
Lincocin®	(link' o sin)	Marax®	(mare' aks)
Cleocin®	(klee' o sin)	Maalox®	(may' loks)
Lincocin®	(lin' coe sin)	Marax®	(may' raks)
Indocin®	(in' doe sin)	Atarax®	(at' a raks)
Lincocin®	(link' o sin)	Marax®	(may' raks)
Minocin®	(min' o sin)	Maox®	(may' oks)
Lioresal®	(lye or' reh sal)	Marcaine®	(mar' kane)
lisinopril	(lyse in' o pril)	Narcan®	(nar' kan)
liothyronine	(lye o thye' roe neen)	Marinol®	(mare' i nole)
levothyroxine	(lee voe thye rox' een)	Marnal®	(mar' nal)
lisinopril	(lyse in' o pril)	Marnal®	(mar' nal)
Lioresal®	(lye or' reh sal)	Marinol®	(mare' i nole)
Lithane®	(lith' ane)	Matulane®	(mat' chu lane)
Lithonate®	(lith' o nate)	Modane®	(moe' dane)
Lithonate®	(lith' o nate)	Maxidex®	(maks' i deks)
Lithane®	(lith' ane)	Maxzide®	(maks' zide)
Lithostat®	(lith' o stat)	Maxzide®	(maks' zide)
Lithotabs®	(lith' o tabs)	Maxidex®	(maks' i deks)
Lithotabs®	(lith' o tabs)	Mebaral®	(meb' a ral)
Lithostat®	(lith' o stat)	Medrol®	(med' role)
Lodine®	(low' deen)	Mebaral®	(meb' a ral)
codeine	(koe' deen)	Mellaril®	(mel' a ril)
Lomodix®	(lo' mo dix)	Mebaral®	(meb' a ral)
Lovenox®	(lo' ve nox)	Tegretol®	(teg' ree tol)

Drug Name	Pronunciation	Drug Name	Pronunciation
mecamylamine	(mek a mill' a meen)	methyldopa	(meth ill doe' pa)
mesalamine	(me sal' a meen)	levodopa	(lee voe doe' pa)
Meclan®	(me' klan)	metolazone	(me tole' a zone)
Meclomen®	(meh' klo men)	metaxalone	(me taks' a lone)
Meclan®	(me' klan)	metolazone	(me tole' a zone)
Mezlin®	(mes' lin)	methazolamide	(meth a zoe' la mide)
Meclomen®	(meh' klo men)	metolazone	(me tole' a zone)
Meclan®	(me' klan)	minoxidil	(mi nox' i dill)
Medrol®	(med' role)	metoprolol	(me toe' proe lole)
Mebaral®	(meb' a ral)	metaproterenol	(met a proe ter' e nol)
Medrol®	(meh' drol)	metyrapone	(me teer' a pone)
Inderal®	(in' der al)	metyrosine	(me tye' roe seen)
Mefoxin®	(me fox' in)	metyrosine	(me tye' roe seen)
Lanoxin®	(lan ox' in)	metyrapone	(me teer' a pone)
Mellaril®	(mel' la ril)	Mevacor®	(me' va cor)
Elavil®	(el' a vil)	Mivacron®	(mi' va cron)
Mellaril®	(mel' a ril)	Mexitil®	(meks' i til)
Mebaral®	(meb' a ral)	Mezlin®	(mes' lin)
melphalan	(mel' fa lan)	Mezlin®	(mes' lin)
Mephyton®	(meh fye' ton)	Meclan®	(me' klan)
mephenytoin	(me fen' i toyn)	Mezlin®	(mes' lin)
Mephyton®	(meh fye' ton)	Mexitil®	(meks' i til)
mephenytoin	(me fen' i toyn)	mezlocillin	(mez loe sill' in)
Mesantoin®	(meh san' toyn)	methicillin	(meth i sill' in)
mephenytoin	(me fen' i toyn)	miconazole	(mi kon' a zole)
phenytoin	(fen' i toyn)	Micronase®	(mye' croe nase)
mephobarbital	(me foe bar' bi tal)	Micro-K®	(mye' cro kay)
methocarbamol	(meth o kar' ba mole)	Micronase®	(mye' croe nase)
Mephyton®	(meh fye' ton)	Micronase®	(mye' croe nase)
melphalan	(mel' fa lan)	Micro-K®	(mye' cro kay)
Mephyton®	(meh fye' ton)	Micronase®	(mye' croe nase)
mephenytoin	(me fen' i toyn)	Micronor®	(mye' croe nor)
Mephyton®	(meh fye' ton)	Micronase®	(mye' croe nase)
methadone	(meth' a done)	miconazole	(mi kon' a zole)
mepivacaine	(me piv' a kane)	Micronor®	(mye' croe nor)
bupivacaine	(byoo piv' a kane)	Micronase®	(mye' croe nase)
Meprospan®	(meh' pro span)	Midrin®	(mid' rin)
Naprosyn®	(na' pro sin)	Mydfrin®	(mid' frin)
mesalamine	(me sal' a meen)	Milontin®	(mi lon' tin)
mecamylamine	(mek a mill' a meen)	Miltown®	(mil' town)
Mesantoin®	(meh san' toyn)	Milontin®	(mi lon' tin)
mephenytoin	(me fen' i toyn)	Mylanta®	(mye lan' tah)
Mesantoin®	(meh san' toyn)	Miltown®	(mil' town)
Mestinon®	(meh' sti non)	Milontin®	(mi lon' tin)
Mestinon®	(meh' sti non)	Minizide®	(min' i zide)
Mesantoin®	(meh san' toyn)	Minocin®	(min' o sin)
Metahydrin®	(me ta hye' drin)	Minocin®	(min' o sin)
Metandren®	(me tan' dren)	Indocin®	(in' doe sin)
Metandren®	(me tan' dren)	Minocin®	(min' o sin)
Metahydrin®	(me ta hye' drin)	Lincocin®	(link' o sin)
metaproterenol	(met a proe ter' e nol)	Minocin®	(min' o sin)
metoprolol	(me toe' proe lole)	Minizide®	(min' i zide)
metaxalone	(me taks' a lone)	Minocin®	(min' o sin)
metolazone	(me tole' a zone)	Mithracin®	(mith' ra sin)
methadone	(meth' a done)	Minocin®	(min' o sin)
Mephyton®	(meh fye' ton)	niacin	(nye' a sin)
methazolamide	(meth a zoe' la mide)	minoxidil	(mi nox' i dill)
metolazone	(me tole' a zone)	metolazone	(me tole' a zone)
methenamine	(meth en' a meen)	Mithracin®	(mith' ra sin)
methionine	(me thye' o neen)	Minocin®	(min' o sin)
methicillin	(meth i sill' in)	mitomycin	(mye toe mye' sin)
mezlocillin	(mez loe sill' in)	Mutamycin®	(mute a mye' sin)
methionine	(me thye' o neen)	Mivacron®	(mi' va cron)
methenamine	(meth en' a meen)	Mevacor®	(me' va cor)
methocarbamol	(meth o kar' ba mole)	Moban®	(moe' ban)
mephobarbital	(me foe bar' bi tal)	Modane®	(moe' dane)
methsuximide	(meth sux' i mide)	Modane®	(moe' dane)
ethosuximide	(eth o sux' i mide)	Matulane®	(mat' chu lane)

SOUND-ALIKE COMPARISON LIST *(Continued)*

Drug Name	Pronunciation	Drug Name	Pronunciation
Modane®	(moe' dane)	Nasalcrom®	(nay' sal crome)
Moban®	(moe' ban)	Nasacort®	(nay' sa cort)
Modicon®	(mod' i kon)	Natacyn®	(na' ta sin)
Mylicon®	(mye' li kon)	Naprosyn®	(na' pro sin)
moexipril	(mo ex' i pril)	Navane®	(nav' ane)
Monopril®	(mon' oh pril)	Norvasc®	(nor' vask)
Monodox®	(mon' o doks)	Nebcin®	(neb' sin)
Maalox®	(may' loks)	Inapsine®	(i nap' seen)
Monopril®	(mon' oh pril)	Nebcin®	(neb' sin)
moexipril	(mo ex' i pril)	Naprosyn®	(na' pro sin)
Mutamycin®	(mute a mye' sin)	nelfinavir	(nel fin' a vir)
mitomycin	(mye toe mye' sin)	nevirapine	(ne vir' a peen)
Myambutol®	(mya am' byoo tol)	Nembutal®	(nem' byoo tal)
Nembutal®	(nem' byoo tal)	Myambutol®	(mya am' byoo tol)
Mycelex®	(mye' si leks)	Neptazane®	(nep' ta zane)
Myoflex®	(mye' o fleks)	Nesacaine®	(nes' a kane)
Mycifradin®	(mye ce fray' din)	Nesacaine®	(nes' a kane)
Mycitracin®	(mye ce tray' sin)	Neptazane®	(nep' ta zane)
Mycitracin®	(mye ce tray' sin)	Neupogen®	(nu' po gen)
Mycifradin®	(mye ce fray' din)	Nutramigen®	(nu' tra gen)
Mydfrin®	(mid' frin)	nevirapine	(ne vir' a peen)
Midrin®	(mid' rin)	nelfinavir	(nel fin' a vir)
Mylanta®	(mye lan' tah)	niacin	(nye' a sin)
Milontin®	(mi lon' tin)	Minocin®	(min' o sin)
Myleran®	(mye' leh ran)	nicardipine	(nye kar' de peen)
Mylicon®	(mye' li kon)	nifedipine	(nye fed' i peen)
Mylicon®	(mye' li kon)	Nicobid®	(nye' ko bid)
Modicon®	(mod' i kon)	Nitro-Bid®	(nye' troe bid)
Mylicon®	(mye' li kon)	Nicoderm®	(nye' co derm)
Myleran®	(mye' leh ran)	Nitroderm®	(nye' tro derm)
Myochrysine®	(mye o kris' seen)	Nicorette®	(nik' o ret)
vincristine	(vin kris' teen)	Nordette®	(nor det')
Myoflex®	(mye' o fleks)	nifedipine	(nye fed' i peen)
Mycelex®	(mye' si leks)	nicardipine	(nye kar' de peen)
nadolol	(nay doe' lole)	nifedipine	(nye fed' i peen)
Mandol®	(man' dole)	nimodipine	(nye moe' di peen)
Naldecon®	(nal' dee kon)	nifedipine	(nye fed' i peen)
Nalfon®	(nal' fon)	nisoldipine	(nye' sole di peen)
Nalfon®	(nal' fon)	Nilstat®	(nil' stat)
Naldecon®	(nal' dee kon)	Nitrostat®	(nye' troe stat)
Nallpen®	(nall' pen)	Nimodipine	(nye moe' di peen)
Nalspan®	(nal' span)	nifedipine	(nye fed' i peen)
naloxone	(nal ox' one)	nisoldipine	(nye' sole di peen)
naltrexone	(nal treks' one)	nifedipine	(nye fed' i peen)
Nalspan®	(nal' span)	Nitro-Bid®	(nye' troe bid)
Nallpen®	(nall' pen)	Nicobid®	(nye' ko bid)
naltrexone	(nal treks' one)	Nitroderm®	(nye' tro derm)
naloxone	(nal ox' one)	Nicroderm®	(nye' co derm)
Naprosyn®	(na' pro sin)	Nitroglycerin	(nye troe gli' ser in)
Meprospan®	(meh' pro span)	Nitroglyn®	(nye' troe glin)
Naprosyn®	(na' pro sin)	Nitroglyn®	(nye' troe glin)
naproxen	(na prox' en)	nitroglycerin	(nye troe gli' ser in)
Naprosyn®	(na' pro sin)	Nitrostat®	(nye' troe stat)
Natacyn®	(na' ta sin)	Hyperstat®	(hye' per stat)
Naprosyn®	(na' pro sin)	Nitrostat®	(nye' troe stat)
Nebcin®	(neb' sin)	Nilstat®	(nil' stat)
naproxen	(na prox' en)	Norcuron®	(nor' ku ron)
Naprosyn®	(na' pro sin)	Narcan®	(nar' can)
Narcan®	(nar' kan)	Nordette®	(nor det')
Marcaine®	(mar' kane)	Nicorette®	(nik' o ret)
Narcan®	(nar' kan)	Norinyl®	(nor' eh nil)
Norcuron®	(nor' ku ron)	Nardil®	(nar' dil)
Nardil®	(nar' dil)	Norlutate®	(nor' lu tate)
Norinyl®	(nor' eh nil)	Norlutin®	(nor lu' tin)
Nasacort®	(nay' sa cort)	Norlutin®	(nor lu' tin)
Nasalcrom®	(nay' sal crome)	Norlutate®	(nor' lu tate)

Drug Name	Pronunciation	Drug Name	Pronunciation
Norpramin®	(nor pray' min)	Ornade®	(or' nade)
imipramine	(im ip' ra meen)	Orinase®	(or' in ase)
Norvasc®	(nor' vask)	Oruvail®	(or' yu vale)
Navane®	(nav' ane)	Elavil®	(el' a vil)
Norvasc®	(nor' vask)	Os-Cal®	(os' cal)
Norvir®	(nor' vir)	Asacol®	(as' a col)
Norvir®	(nor' vir)	Otrivin®	(oh' tri vin)
Norvasc®	(nor' vask)	Lotrimin®	(low' tri min)
Novacet®	(no' va set)	oxymetazoline	(ox i met az' o leen)
NovaSeven®	(no' va se ven)	oxymetholone	(ox i meth' o lone)
Novafed®	(nove' a fed)	oxymetholone	(ox i meth' o lone)
Nucofed®	(nu' co fed)	oxymetazoline	(ox i met az' o leen)
NovaSeven®	(no' va se ven)	oxymetholone	(ox i meth' o lone)
Novacet®	(no' va set)	oxymorphone	(ox i mor' fone)
Nucofed®	(nu' co fed)	oxymorphone	(ox i mor' fone)
Novafed®	(nove' a fed)	oxymetholone	(ox i meth' o lone)
Nuprin®	(nu' prin)	Pamelor®	(pam' meh lor)
Lupron®	(lu' pron)	Dymelor®	(dye' meh lor)
Nutramigen®	(nu' tra gen)	pancreatin	(pan kre' a tine)
Neupogen®	(nu' po gen)	Panretin®	(pan ree' tin)
olanzapine	(oh lan' za peen)	Panretin®	(pan ree' tin)
olsalazine sodium	(ole sal' a zeen)	pancreatin	(pan kre' a tine)
olsalazine sodium	(ole sal' a zeen)	Patanol®	(pa' ta nol)
olanzapine	(oh lan' za peen)	Platinol®	(pla' ti nol)
Omnipaque®	(om' ne pak)	Pathilon®	(path' i lon)
Amipaque®	(am' ne pak)	Pathocil®	(path' o sil)
Omnipaque®	(om' ni pak)	Pathocil®	(path' o sil)
Omnipen®	(om' ni pen)	Pathilon®	(path' i lon)
Omnipen®	(om' ni pen)	Pathocil®	(path' o sil)
Omnipaque®	(om' ni pak)	Placidyl®	(pla' ce dil)
Omnipen®	(om' ni pen)	Pathocil®	(path' o sill)
Unipen®	(yu' ni pen)	Bactocill®	(bak' tow sill)
Oncet®	(on' set)	Pavabid®	(pav' a bid)
Ontak®	(on' tak)	Pavased®	(pav' a sed)
Oncovin®	(on' coe vin)	Pavased®	(pav' a sed)
Ancobon®	(an' coe bon)	Pavabid®	(pav' a bid)
Ontak®	(on' tak)	Paxil®	(paks' il)
Oncet®	(on' set)	Doxil®	(doks' il)
Ophthaine®	(op' thane)	Paxil®	(paks' il)
Ophthetic®	(op thet' ik)	Taxol®	(tacks' ol)
Ophthalgan®	(opp thal' gan)	pentobarbital	(pen toe bar' bi tal)
Auralgan®	(a ral' gan)	phenobarbital	(fee noe bar' bi tal)
Ophthetic®	(op thet' ik)	Percodan®	(per' coe dan)
Ophthaine®	(op' thane)	Decadron®	(dek' a dron)
Ophthochlor®	(op' tho klor)	Perdiem®	(per dee' em)
Ophthocort®	(op' tho kort)	Pyridium®	(pye rid' dee um)
Ophthocort®	(op' tho kort)	Persantine®	(per san' teen)
Ophthochlor®	(op' tho klor)	Pertofrane®	(per' toe frane)
oprelvekin	(op rel' ve kin)	Pertofrane®	(per' toe frane)
Proleukin®	(pro lu' kin)	Persantine®	(per san' teen)
Orabase®	(or' a base)	Phazyme®	(fay' zeem)
Orinase®	(or' in ase)	Pherazine®	(fer' a zeen)
Orasol®	(or' a sol)	Phenergan®	(fen' er gan)
Orasone®	(or' a sone)	Phrenilin®	(fren' ni lin)
Orasone®	(or' a sone)	Phenergan®	(fen' er gan)
Orasol®	(or' a sol)	Theragran®	(ther' a gran)
Oretic®	(or et' ik)	phenobarbital	(fee noe bar' bi tal)
Oreton®	(or' eh ton)	pentobarbital	(pen toe bar' bi tal)
Oreton®	(or' eh ton)	phentermine	(fen' ter meen)
Oretic®	(or et' ik)	phentolamine	(fen tole' a meen)
Orex®	(or' ecks)	phentolamine	(fen tole' a meen)
Urex®	(yur' ecks)	phentermine	(fen' ter meen)
Orinase®	(or' in ase)	phentolamine	(fen tole' a meen)
Orabase®	(or' a base)	Ventolin®	(ven' to lin)
Orinase®	(or' in ase)	phenytoin	(fen' i toyn)
Ornade®	(or' nade)	mephenytoin	(me fen' i toyn)
Orinase®	(or' in ase)	Pherazine®	(fer' a zeen)
Tolinase®	(tole' i nase)	Phazyme®	(fay' zeem)

SOUND-ALIKE COMPARISON LIST *(Continued)*

Drug Name	Pronunciation	Drug Name	Pronunciation
pHisoHex®	(fye' so heks)	prednisone	(pred' ni sone)
Fostex®	(fos' teks)	prednisolone	(pred nis' o lone)
Phos-Flur®	(fos' flur)	prednisone	(pred' ni sone)
PhosLo®	(fos' lo)	primidone	(pri' mi done)
PhosLo®	(fos' lo)	Premarin®	(prem' a rin)
Phos-Flur®	(fos' flur)	Primaxin®	(pri maks' in)
PhosLo®	(fos' lo)	Prepidil®	(pre' pi dil)
ProSom™	(pro' som)	Bepridil®	(be' pri dil)
Phosphaljel®	(fos' fal gel)	prilocaine	(pril' o kane)
Phospholine®	(fos' fo leen)	Prilosec™	(pre' lo sek)
Phospholine®	(fos' fo leen)	Prilosec™	(pre' lo sek)
Phosphaljel®	(fos' fal gel)	Prozac®	(proe' zak)
Phrenilin®	(fren' ni lin)	Prilosec™	(pre' lo sek)
Phenergan®	(fen' er gan)	prilocaine	(pril' o kane)
Phrenilin®	(fren' ni lin)	Primaxin®	(pri maks' in)
Trinalin®	(tri' na lin)	Premarin®	(prem' a rin)
physostigmine	(fye zoe stig' meen)	primidone	(pri' mi done)
Prostigmin®	(pro stig' min)	prednisone	(pred' ni sone)
physostigmine	(fye zoe stig' meen)	Priscoline®	(pris' coe leen)
pyridostigmine	(peer id o stig' meen)	Apresoline®	(aye press' sow leen)
Pitocin®	(pi toe' sin)	Pro-Banthine®	(pro ban' theen)
Pitressin®	(ph tres' sin)	Banthine®	(ban' theen)
Pitressin®	(ph tres' sin)	procaine	(pro' cane)
Pitocin®	(ph toe' sin)	Prokine®	(pro' keen)
Placidyl®	(pla' ce dil)	procarbazine	(proe kar' ba zeen)
Pathocil®	(path' o sil)	dacarbazine	(da kar' ba zeen)
Plaquenil®	(pla' kwe nil)	Prokine®	(pro' keen)
Platinol®	(pla' tee nol)	procaine®	(pro' cane)
Platinol®	(pla' ti nol)	Proleukin®	(pro lu' kin)
Patanol®	(pa' ta nol)	oprelvekin	(op rel' ve kin)
Platinol®	(pla' tee nol)	promazine	(proe' ma zeen)
Plaquenil®	(pla' kwe nil)	promethazine	(proe meth' a zeen)
Plendil®	(plen' dil)	Prometh®	(proe' meth)
Isordil®	(eye' tal)	Promit®	(proe' mit)
Plendil®	(plen' dil)	promethazine	(proe meth' a zeen)
Pletal®	(ple' tal)	promazine	(proe' ma zeen)
Pletal®	(ple' tal)	Promit®	(proe' mit)
Plendil®	(plen' dil)	Prometh®	(proe' meth)
Ponstel®	(pon' stel)	Pronestyl®	(pro nes' til)
Pronestyl®	(pro nes' til)	Ponstel®	(pon' stel)
Posicor®	(pos' e cor)	Propacet®	(proe' pa set)
Proscar®	(pros' car)	Propagest®	(proe' pa gest)
pralidoxime	(pra li dox' eem)	Propagest®	(proe' pa gest)
pramoxine	(pra moks' een)	Propacet®	(proe' pa set)
pralidoxime	(pra li dox' eem)	Proscar®	(pros' car)
pyridoxine	(peer i dox' een)	Posicor®	(pos' e cor)
Pramosone®	(pra' mo sone)	Pro-Sof®	(proe' sof)
prednisone	(pred' ni sone)	ProSom™	(pro' som)
pramoxine	(pra moks' een)	ProSom™	(pro' som)
pralidoxime	(pra li dox' eem)	PhosLo®	(fos' lo)
prazepam	(pra' ze pam)	ProSom™	(pro' som)
prazosin	(pra' zoe sin)	Pro-Sof Plus	(proe' sof)
prazosin	(pra' zoe sin)	ProStep®	(proe' step)
prazepam	(pra' ze pam)	Prozac®	(proe' zak)
Precare®	(pre' kare)	Prostigmin®	(pro stig' min)
Precose®	(pre' kose)	physostigmine	(fye zoe stig' meen)
Precose®	(pre' kose)	protamine	(proe' ta meen)
Precare®	(pre' kare)	Protopam®	(proe' toe pam)
Predalone®	(pred' a lone)	Protopam®	(proe' toe pam)
prednisone	(pred' ni sone)	protamine	(proe' ta meen)
prednisolone	(pred nis' o lone)	Protopam®	(proe' toe pam)
prednisone	(pred' ni sone)	Protropin®	(proe tro' pin)
prednisone	(pred' ni sone)	Protropin®	(proe tro' pin)
Pramosone®	(pra' mo sone)	Protopam®	(proe' toe pam)
prednisone	(pred' ni sone)	Prozac®	(proe' zak)
Predalone®	(pred' a lone)	Prilosec™	(pre' lo sek)

Drug Name	Pronunciation	Drug Name	Pronunciation
Prozac®	(proe' zak)	Riopan®	(rye' o pan)
ProStep®	(proe' step)	Repan®	(ree' pan)
Pyridium®	(pye rid' dee um)	Riopan®	(rye' o pan)
Dyrenium®	(dye ren' e um)	Riobin®	(rye' o bin)
Pyridium®	(pye rid' dee um)	Ritalin®	(ri' ta lin)
Perdiem®	(per dee' em)	Ismelin®	(is' meh lin)
Pyridium®	(pye rid' dee um)	Ritalin®	(ri' ta lin)
pyridoxine	(peer i dox' een)	Rifadin®	(rif' a din)
Pyridium®	(pye rid' dee um)	Ritalin®	(ri' ta lin)
pyrithione	(peer i thye' one)	ritodrine	(ri' toe dreen)
pyridostigmine	(peer id o stig' meen)	ritodrine	(ri' toe dreen)
physostigmine	(fye zoe stig' meen)	Ritalin®	(ri' ta lin)
pyridoxine	(peer i dox' een)	ritonavir	(ri ton' o vir)
Pyridium®	(pye rid' dee um)	Retrovir®	(re' tro vir)
pyridoxine	(peer i dox' een)	Rocephin®	(roe sef' fen)
pralidoxime	(pra li dox' eem)	Roferon®	(roe fer' on)
pyrithione	(peer i thye' one)	Roferon®	(roe fer' on)
Pyridium®	(pye rid' dee um)	Rocephin®	(roe sef' fen)
quinidine	(kwin' i deen)	Rynatan®	(rye' na tan)
clonidine	(kloe' ni deen)	Rynatuss®	(rye' na tuss)
quinidine	(kwin' i deen)	Rynatuss®	(rye' na tuss)
quinine	(kwye' nine)	Rynatan®	(rye' na tan)
quinine	(kwye' nine)	Rythmol®	(rith' mol)
quinidine	(kwin' i deen)	Rhythmin®	(rith' min)
Reglan®	(reg' lan)	Salacid®	(sal as' sid)
Regonol®	(reg' o nol)	Salagen®	(sal' a gen)
Regonol®	(reg' o nol)	Salagen®	(sal' a gen)
Reglan®	(reg' lan)	Salacid®	(sal as' sid)
Regonol®	(reg' o nol)	Salutensin®	(sal yu ten' sin)
Regutol®	(reg' yu tol)	Diutensin®	(dye yu ten' sin)
Regranex®	(re gra' neks)	saquinavir	(sa kwin' a veer)
Granulex®	(gran' u lecks)	Sinequan®	(si' ne kwan)
Regroton®	(reg' ro ton)	Seconal™	(sek' o nal)
Hygroton®	(hye gro' ton)	Sectral®	(sek' tral)
Regutol®	(reg' yu tol)	Sectral®	(sek' tral)
Regonol®	(reg' o nol)	Factrel®	(fak' trel)
remifentanil	(rem i fen' ta nil)	Sectral®	(sek' tral)
alfentanil	(al fen' ta nil)	Seconal™	(sek' o nal)
Repan®	(ree' pan)	Seldane®	(sel' dane)
Riopan®	(rye' o pan)	Feldene®	(fel' deen)
Restore®	(res tore')	Senexon®	(sen' e son)
Restoril®	(res' tor ril)	Cenestin®	(se nes' tin)
Restoril®	(res' tor ril)	Septa®	(sep' tah)
Restore®	(res tore')	Septra®	(sep' trah)
Restoril®	(res' tor ril)	Septra®	(sep' trah)
Vistaril®	(vis' tar ril)	Septa®	(sep' tah)
Retrovir®	(re' tro vir)	Ser-Ap-Es®	(ser ap' ess)
ritonavir	(ri ton' o vir)	Catapres®	(kat' a pres)
Revex®	(rev' ex)	Serax®	(sear' aks)
Revia®	(rev' ve ah)	Eurax®	(yoor' aks)
Revia®	(rev' ve ah)	Serax®	(sear' aks)
Revex®	(rev' ex)	Urex®	(yu' eks)
Rhythmin®	(rith' min)	Serax®	(sear' aks)
Rythmol®	(rith' mol)	Zyrtec®	(zir' tec)
ribavirin	(rye ba vye' rin)	Serentil®	(su ren' til)
riboflavin	(rye' boe flay vin)	Surital®	(su' ri tal)
riboflavin	(rye' boe flay vin)	Seroquel®	(seer' oh kwel)
ribavirin	(rye ba vye' rin)	Sinequan®	(si' ne kwan)
Rifadin®	(rif' a din)	Silace®	(sye' lace)
Ritalin®	(ri' ta lin)	Silain®	(sye' lain)
Rimactane®	(ri mak' tane)	Silain®	(sye' lain)
rimantadine	(ri man' to deen)	Silace®	(sye' lace)
rimantadine	(ri man' to deen)	Sinequan®	(si' ne kwan)
Rimactane®	(ri mak' tane)	saquinavir	(sa kwin' a veer)
rimantadine	(ri man' to deen)	Sinequan®	(si' ne kwan)
amantadine	(a man' ta deen)	Seroquel®	(seer' oh kwel)
Riobin®	(rye' o bin)	Slo-Bid®	(slo' bid)
Riopan®	(rye' o pan)	Dolobid®	(dol' ah bid)

SOUND-ALIKE COMPARISON LIST *(Continued)*

Drug Name	Pronunciation	Drug Name	Pronunciation
Solarcaine®	(sole' ar kane)	Tegrin®	(teg' rin)
Solatene®	(sole' a teen)	Tegopen®	(teg' o pen)
Solatene®	(sole' a teen)	Teldrin®	(tel' drin)
Solarcaine®	(sole' ar kane)	Tedral®	(ted' ral)
Soriatane®	(sor' e ah tane)	Temaril®	(tem' a ril)
Loxitane®	(loks' e tane)	Demerol®	(dem' eh rol)
Staphcillin®	(staf sil' lin)	Temaril®	(tem' a ril)
Staticin®	(stat' i sin)	Tepanil®	(tep' a nil)
Staticin®	(stat' i sin)	Tenex®	(ten' eks)
Staphcillin®	(staf sil' lin)	Entex®	(en' teks)
streptomycin	(strep toe mye' sin)	Tenex®	(ten' eks)
streptozocin	(strep toe zoe' sin)	Xanax®	(zan' aks)
streptozocin	(strep toe zoe' sin)	Tepanil®	(tep' a nil)
streptomycin	(strep toe mye' sin)	Temaril®	(tem' a ril)
Sudafed®	(sue' da fed)	Tepanil®	(tep' a nil)
Sufenta®	(sue fen' tah)	Tofranil®	(toe fray' nil)
Sufenta®	(sue fen' tah)	terbinafine	(ter' bin a feen)
Alfenta®	(al fen' tah)	terfenadine	(ter fen' na deen)
Sufenta®	(sue fen' tah)	terbinafine	(ter' bin a feen)
Sudafed®	(sue' da fed)	terbutaline	(ter byoo' ta leen)
sufentanil	(sue fen' ta nil)	terbutaline	(ter byoo' ta leen)
alfentanil	(al fen' ta nil)	terbinafine	(ter' bin a feen)
sulfasalazine	(sul fa sal' a zeen)	terbutaline	(ter byoo' ta leen)
sulfisoxazole	(sul fi sox' a zole)	tolbutamide	(tole byoo' ta mide)
sulfisoxazole	(sul fi sox' a zole)	terconazole	(ter kone' a zole)
sulfasalazine	(sul fa sal' a zeen)	tioconazole	(tye o kone' a zole)
sumatriptan	(soo ma trip' tan)	terfenadine	(ter fen' na deen)
zolmitriptan	(zohl mi trip' tan)	terbinafine	(ter' bin a feen)
Suprax®	(su' prax)	Terramycin®	(tehr a mye' sin)
Surbex®	(sur' beks)	Garamycin®	(gar a mye' sin)
Surbex®	(sur' beks)	testolactone	(tess toe lak' tone)
Suprax®	(su' prax)	testosterone	(tess toss' ter one)
Surbex®	(sur' beks)	testosterone	(tess toss' ter one)
Surfak®	(sur' fak)	testolactone	(tess toe lak' tone)
Surfak®	(sur' fak)	Theelin®	(thee' lin)
Surbex®	(sur' beks)	Theolair™	(thee' o lare)
Surital®	(su' ri tal)	Theoclear®	(thee' o clear)
Serentil®	(su ren' til)	Theolair™	(thee' o lare)
Sytobex®	(sye' toe beks)	Theolair™	(thee' o lare)
Cytotec®	(sye' toe tek)	Theelin®	(thee' lin)
Tacaryl®	(tak' a ril)	Theolair™	(thee' o lare)
tacrine	(tak' reen)	Theoclear®	(thee' o clear)
tacrine	(tak' reen)	Theolair™	(thee' o lare)
Tacaryl®	(tak' a ril)	Thiola™	(thye oh' la)
Tagamet®	(tag' a met)	Theolair™	(thee' o lare)
Tegopen®	(teg' o pen)	Thyrolar®	(thye' roe lar)
Talacen®	(tal' a sen)	Theragran®	(ther' a gran)
Tegison®	(teg' i son)	Phenergan®	(fen' er gan)
Talacen®	(tal' a sen)	Theramin®	(there' a min)
Tinactin®	(tin ak' tin)	thiamine	(thye' a min)
Taxol®	(tacks' ol)	thiamine	(thye' a min)
Paxil®	(packs' ol)	Theramin®	(there' a min)
Tedral®	(ted' ral)	Thiola™	(thye oh' la)
Teldrin®	(tel' drin)	Theolair™	(thee' o lare)
Tegison®	(teg' i son)	thioridazine	(thye o rid' a zeen)
Talacen®	(tal' a sen)	thiothixene	(thye o thix' een)
Tegopen®	(teg' o pen)	thiothixene	(thye o thix' een)
Tagamet®	(tag' a met)	thioridazine	(thye o rid' a zeen)
Tegopen®	(teg' o pen)	Thyrar®	(thyer' are)
Tegretol®	(teg' ree tol)	Thyrolar®	(thye' roe lar)
Tegopen®	(teg' o pen)	Thyrar®	(thyer' are)
Tegrin®	(teg' rin)	Ticar®	(tye' kar)
Tegretol®	(teg' ree tol)	Thyrolar®	(thye' roe lar)
Mebaral®	(meb' a ral)	Theolair™	(thee' o lare)
Tegretol®	(teg' ree tol)	Thyrolar®	(thye' roe lar)
Tegopen®	(teg' o pen)	Thyrar®	(thyer' are)

Drug Name	Pronunciation	Drug Name	Pronunciation
Thyrolar⁵	(thye' roe lar)	triacetin	(trye a see' tin)
Thytropar⁵	(thye' troe par)	Triacin⁵	(trye' a sin)
Thytropar⁵	(thye' troe par)	Triacin⁵.	(trye' a sin)
Thyrolar⁵	(thye' roe lar)	triacetin	(trye a see' tin)
Ticar⁵	(tye' kar)	triamterene	(trye am' ter een)
Thyrar®	(thyer' are)	trimipramine	(trye mi' pra meen)
Ticar⁵	(tye' kar)	Triapin⁵	(trye a pin)
Tigan®	(tye' gan)	Triban⁵	(trye' ban)
Ticon®	(tye' kon)	triazolam	(trye ay' zoe lam)
Tigan®	(tye' gan)	alprazolam	(al pray' zoe lam)
Tigan®	(tye' gan)	Triban⁵	(trye' ban)
Ticar⁵	(tye' kar)	Triapin⁵	(trye a pin)
Tigan®	(tye' gan)	trientine	(trye' en teen)
Ticon®	(tye' kon)	tretinoin	(tret' i noyn)
timolol	(tye' moe lole)	Trilafon®	(tri' la fon)
Tylenol®	(tye' le nole)	Tri-Levlen®	(trye' lev len)
Timoptic®	(tim op' tik)	trimeprazine	(trye mep' ra zeen)
Viroptic®	(vir op' tik)	trimipramine	(trye mi' pra meen)
Tinactin®	(tin ak' tin)	trimethaphan	(trye meth' a fan)
Talacen®	(tal' a sen)	trimethoprim	(trye meth' o prim)
Tindal⁵	(tin' dal)	trimethoprim	(trye meth' o prim)
Trental®	(tren' tal)	trimethaphan	(trye meth' a fan)
tioconazole	(tye o kone' a zole)	trimipramine	(trye mi' pra meen)
terconazole	(ter kone' a zole)	triamterene	(trye am' ter een)
TobraDex®	(toe' bra deks)	trimipramine	(trye mi' pra meen)
Tobrex®	(toe' breks)	trimeprazine	(trye mep' ra zeen)
tobramycin	(toe bra mye' sin)	Trimox®	(trye' moks)
Trobicin®	(troe' bi sin)	Diamox®	(dye' a moks)
Tobrex®	(toe' breks)	Trimox®	(trye' moks)
TobraDex®	(toe' bra deks)	Tylox®	(tye' loks)
Tofranil®	(toe fray' nil)	Trinalin⁵	(tri' na lin)
Tepanil®	(tep' a nil)	Phrenilin®	(fren' ni lin)
tolazamide	(tole az' a mide)	Triofed®	(trye' o fed)
tolazoline	(tole az' o leen)	Triostat™	(tree' o stat)
tolazamide	(tole az' a mide)	Triostat™	(tree' o stat)
tolbutamide	(tole byoo' ta mide)	Triofed®	(trye' o fed)
tolazoline	(tole az' o leen)	Trisoralen⁵	(trye sore' a len)
tolazamide	(tole az' a mide)	Trysul⁵	(trye' sul)
tolbutamide	(tole byoo' ta mide)	Trobicin®	(troe' bi sin)
terbutaline	(ter byoo' ta leen)	tobramycin	(toe bra mye' sin)
tolbutamide	(tole byoo' ta mide)	Tronolane®	(tron' o lane)
tolazamide	(tole az' a mide)	Tronothane®	(tron' o thane)
Tolinase⁵	(tole' i nase)	Tronothane®	(tron' o thane)
Orinase®	(or' in ase)	Tronolane®	(tron' o lane)
tolnaftate	(tole naf' tate)	Trysul®	(trye' sul)
Tornalate®	(tor' na late)	Trisoralen®	(trye sore' a len)
Tonocard®	(ton' o kard)	Tuinal⁵	(tu' i nal)
Torecan®	(tor' e kan)	Luminal®	(lu' mi nal)
Torecan⁵	(tor' e kan)	Tuinal⁵	(tu' i nal)
Tonocard®	(ton' o kard)	Tylenol®	(tye' le nole)
Tornalate®	(tor' na late)	Tussafed®	(tus' a fed)
tolnaftate	(tole naf' tate)	Tussafin®	(tus' a fin)
Trandate⁵	(tran' date)	Tussafin®	(tus' a fin)
Trendar®	(tren' dar)	Tussafed®	(tus' a fed)
Trandate⁵	(tran' date)	Tylenol®	(tye' le nole)
Trental®	(tren' tal)	atenolol	(a ten' oh lole)
Trendar®	(tren' dar)	Tylenol®	(tye' le nole)
Trandate®	(tran' date)	timolol	(tye' moe lole)
Trental®	(tren' tal)	Tylenol®	(tye' le nole)
Bentyl®	(ben' til)	Tuinal®	(tu' i nal)
Trental®	(tren' tal)	Tylenol®	(tye' le nole)
Tindal®	(tin' dal)	Tylox®	(tye' loks)
Trental⁵	(tren' tal)	Tylox®	(tye' loks)
Trandate®	(tran' date)	Trimox®	(trye' moks)
tretinoin	(tret' i noyn)	Tylox⁺	(tye' loks)
trientine	(trye' en teen)	Tylenol⁵	(tye' le nole)
Tri-Levlen⁵	(trye' lev len)	Tylox®	(tye' loks)
Trilafon®	(tri' la fon)	Wymox⁺	(wye' moks)

SOUND-ALIKE COMPARISON LIST *(Continued)*

Drug Name	Pronunciation	Drug Name	Pronunciation
Uni-Bent▲	(yu′ ni bent)	Volmax‡	(vol′ maks)
Unipen▼	(yu′ ni pen)	Flomax‡	(flo′ maks)
Unipen▼	(yu′ ni pen)	Voltaren®	(vo tare′ en)
Uni-Bent®	(yu′ ni bent)	Verelan®	(ver′ e lan)
Unipen▼	(yu′ ni pen)	Voltaren▲	(vo tare′ en)
Omnipen®	(om′ ni pen)	Vontrol▲	(von′ trole)
Urex®	(yu′ eks)	Vontrol▲	(von′ trole)
Eurax®	(yoor′ aks)	Voltaren®	(vo tare′ en)
Urex®	(yur′ ecks)	Vytone®	(vye′ tone)
Orex®	(or′ ecks)	Hytone®	(hye′ tone)
Urex®	(yu′ eks)	Vytone▲	(vye′ tone)
Serax®	(sear′ aks)	Zydone®	(zye′ doan)
V-Cillin K®	(vee sil′ lin kay)	Wycillin®	(wye sil′ lin)
Bicillin®	(bye sil′ lin)	Bicillin®	(bye sil′ lin)
V-Cillin K®	(vee′ sil lin kay)	Wycillin®	(wye sil′ lin)
Wycillin®	(wye sil′ lin)	V-Cillin K®	(vee′ sil lin kay)
Vamate®	(vam′ ate)	Wydase®	(wye′ dase)
Vancenase®	(van′ sen ase)	Lidex®	(lye′ deks)
Vancenase®	(van′ sen ase)	Wymox®	(wye′ moks)
Vamate®	(vam′ ate)	Tylox®	(tye′ loks)
Vanceril®	(van′ ser il)	Xanax®	(zan′ aks)
Vansil™	(van′ sil)	Tenex®	(ten′ eks)
Vansil™	(van′ sil)	Xanax®	(zan′ aks)
Vanceril®	(van′ ser il)	Zantac®	(zan′ tak)
Vasocidin®	(vay so sye′ din)	Xalatan®	(za lan′ tan)
Vasodilan®	(vay so di′ lan)	Zarontin®	(za ron′ tin)
Vasodilan®	(vay so di′ lan)	Xylo-Pfan®	(zye′ lo fan)
Vasocidin®	(vay so sye′ din)	Zyloprim®	(zye′ lo prim)
Vasosulf®	(vay′ so sulf)	Yocon®	(yo′ con)
Velosef®	(vel′ o sef)	Zocor®	(zoe′ cor)
VePesid®	(veh′ pe sid)	Zantac®	(zan′ tak)
Versed®	(ver′ sed)	Xanax®	(zan′ aks)
Velosef®	(vel′ o sef)	Zarontin®	(za ron′ tin)
Vasosulf®	(vay′ so sulf)	Xalatan®	(za lan′ tan)
Ventolin®	(ven′ tow lin)	Zarontin®	(za ron′ tin)
Benylin®	(ben′ eh lin)	Zaroxolyn®	(za roks′ o lin)
Ventolin®	(ven′ to lin)	Zaroxolyn®	(za roks′ o lin)
phentolamine	(fen tole′ a meen)	Zarontin®	(za ron′ tin)
Verelan®	(ver′ e lan)	Zebeta®	(ze′ bay tah)
Voltaren®	(vo tare′ en)	Diaβeta®	(dye a bay′ tah)
Versed®	(ver′ sed)	Zerit®	(zer′ it)
VePesid®	(veh′ pe sid)	Ziac™	(zye′ ak)
Viagra®	(vye ag′ ra)	Ziac™	(zye′ ak)
Allegra®	(al leg′ ra)	Zerit®	(zer′ it)
Vicodin®	(vye′ co din)	Zocor®	(zoe′ cor)
Hycodan®	(hye′ co dan)	Cozaar®	(koe′ zar)
vidarabine	(vye dare′ a been)	Zocor®	(zoe′ cor)
cytarabine	(sye tare′ a been)	Yocon®	(yo′ con)
Videx®	(vye′ deks)	Zofran®	(zoe′ fran)
Lidex®	(lye′ deks)	Zosyn™	(zoe′ sin)
vinblastine	(vin blas′ teen)	zolmitriptan	(zohl mi trip′ tan)
vincristine	(vin kris′ teen)	sumatriptan	(soo ma trip′ tan)
vincristine	(vin kris′ teen)	Zosyn™	(zoe′ sin)
Myochrysine®	(mye o kris′ seen)	Zofran®	(zoe′ fran)
vincristine	(vin kris′ teen)	Zydone®	(zye′ doan)
vinblastine	(vin blas′ teen)	Vytone®	(vye′ tone)
Viroptic®	(vir op′ tik)	Zyloprim®	(zye′ lo prim)
Timoptic®	(tim op′ tik)	Xylo-Pfan®	(zye′ lo fan)
Visine®	(vye′ seen)	Zyprexa®	(zye preks′ a)
Visken®	(vis′ ken)	Celexa®	(se lex′ a)
Visken®	(vis′ ken)	Zyrtec®	(zir′ tec)
Visine®	(vye′ seen)	Serax®	(sear′ aks)
Vistaril®	(vis′ tar ril)		
Restoril®	(res′ tor ril)		

TABLETS THAT CANNOT BE CRUSHED OR ALTERED

There are a variety of reasons for crushing tablets or capsule contents prior to administering to the patient. Patients may have nasogastric tubes which do not permit the administration of tablets or capsules; an oral solution for a particular medication may not be available from the manufacturer or readily prepared by pharmacy; patients may have difficulty swallowing capsules or tablets; or mixing of powdered medication with food or drink may make the drug more palatable.

Generally, medications which should not be crushed fall into one of the following categories.

- **Extended-Release Products**. The formulation of some tablets is specialized as to allow the medication within it to be slowly released into the body. This is sometimes accomplished by centering the drug within the core of the tablet, with a subsequent shedding of multiple layers around the core. Wax melts in the GI tract. Slow-K® is an example of this. Capsules may contain beads which have multiple layers which are slowly dissolved with time.

- **Medications Which Are Irritating to the Stomach**. Tablets which are irritating to the stomach may be enteric-coated which delays release of the drug until the time when it reaches the small intestine. Enteric-coated aspirin is an example of this.

- **Foul-Tasting Medication**. Some drugs are quite unpleasant to taste so the manufacturer coats the tablet in a sugar coating to increase its palatability. By crushing the tablet, this sugar coating is lost and the patient tastes the unpleasant tasting medication.

- **Sublingual Medication**. Medication intended for use under the tongue should not be crushed. While it appears to be obvious, it is not always easy to determine if a medication is to be used sublingually. Sublingual medications should indicate on the package that they are intended for sublingual use.

- **Effervescent Tablets**. These are tablets which, when dropped into a liquid, quickly dissolve to yield a solution. Many effervescent tablets, when crushed, lose their ability to quickly dissolve.

Recommendations

1. It is not advisable to crush certain medications.

2. Consult individual monographs prior to crushing capsule or tablet.

3. If crushing a tablet or capsule is contraindicated, consult with your pharmacist to determine whether an oral solution exists or can be compounded.

Drug Product	Dosage Forms	Reasons/Comments
Accutane®	Capsule	Mucous membrane irritant
Actifed 12® Hour	Capsule	Slow release†
Acutrim®	Tablet	Slow release
Adalat® CC	Tablet	Slow release
Aerolate® SR, JR, III	Capsule	Slow release*†
Allerest® 12-Hour	Tablet	Slow release
Artane® Sequels®	Capsule	Slow release*†
Arthritis Bayer® Time Release	Capsule	Slow release
A.S.A.® Enseals®	Tablet	Enteric-coated
Atrohist® Plus	Tablet	Slow release*
Atrohist® Sprinkle	Capsule	Slow release
Azulfidine® EN-tabs®	Tablet	Enteric-coated
Baros	Tablet	Effervescent tablet¶
Bayer® Aspirin, low adult 81 mg strength	Tablet	Enteric-coated
Bayer® Aspirin, regular strength 325 mg caplet	Tablet	Enteric-coated
Bayer® Aspirin, regular strength EC caplet	Tablet	Enteric-coated
Betachron E-R®	Capsule	Slow release
Betapen®-VK	Tablet	Taste††

TABLETS THAT CANNOT BE CRUSHED OR ALTERED
(Continued)

Drug Product	Dosage Forms	Reasons/Comments
Biohist® LA	Tablet	Slow release♦
Bisacodyl	Tablet	Enteric-coated‡
Bisco-Lax®	Tablet	Enteric-coated‡
Bontril® Slow-Release	Capsule	Slow release
Breonesin®	Capsule	Liquid filled§
Brexin® L.A.	Capsule	Slow release
Bromfed®	Capsule	Slow release†
Bromfed-PD®	Capsule	Slow release†
Calan® SR	Tablet	Slow release♦
Cama® Arthritis Pain Reliever	Tablet	Multiple compressed tablet
Carbiset-TR®	Tablet	Slow release
Cardizem®	Tablet	Slow release
Cardizem® CD	Capsule	Slow release*
Cardizem® SR	Capsule	Slow release*
Carter's Little Pills®	Tablet	Enteric-coated
Ceftin®	Tablet	Taste **Note:** Use suspension for children
Charcoal Plus®	Tablet	Enteric-coated
Chloral Hydrate	Capsule	**Note:** Product is in liquid form within a special capsule†
Chlorpheniramine Maleate Time Release	Capsule	Slow release
Chlor-Trimeton® Repetab®	Tablet	Slow release†
Choledyl® SA	Tablet	Slow release†
Cipro™	Tablet	Taste††
Claritin-D®	Tablet	Slow release
Codimal-L.A.®	Capsule	Slow release
Codimal-L.A.® Half	Capsule	Slow release
Colace®	Capsule	Taste††
Comhist® LA	Capsule	Slow release*
Compazine® Spansule®	Capsule	Slow release†
Congess SR, JR	Capsule	Slow release
Contac®	Capsule	Slow release*
Cotazym-S®	Capsule	Enteric-coated*
Covera-HS™	Tablet	Slow release
Creon® 10 Minimicrospheres™	Capsule	Enteric-coated*
Creon® 20	Capsule	Enteric-coated*
Cytospaz-M®	Capsule	Slow release
Cytoxan®	Tablet	**Note:** Drug may be crushed, but maker recommends using injection
Dallergy®	Capsule	Slow release†
Dallergy-D®	Capsule	Slow release
Dallergy-JR®	Capsule	Slow release
Deconamine® SR	Capsule	Slow release†
Deconsal® II	Tablet	Slow release
Deconsal® Sprinkle®	Capsule	Slow release*
Defen L.A.®	Tablet	Slow release♦
Demazin® Repetabs®	Tablet	Slow release†
Depakene®	Capsule	Slow-release-mucous membrane irritant†
Depakote®	Capsule	Enteric-coated
Desoxyn® Gradumets®	Tablet	Slow release
Desyrel®	Tablet	Taste††
Dexatrim® Max Strength	Tablet	Slow release
Dexedrine® Spansule®	Capsule	Slow release
Diamox® Sequels®	Capsule	Slow release§
Dilatrate-SR®	Capsule	Slow release
Disobrom®	Tablet	Slow release
Disophrol® Chronotab®	Tablet	Slow release
Dital®	Capsule	Slow release
Donnatal® Extentab®	Tablet	Slow release†
Donnazyme®	Tablet	Enteric-coated

Drug Product	Dosage Forms	Reasons/Comments
Drisdol⁴	Capsule	Liquid filled§
Drixoral⁴	Tablet	Slow release†
Drixoral⁵ Sinus	Tablet	Slow release
Dulcolax⁴	Tablet	Enteric-coated‡
Dynabac⁴	Tablet	Enteric-coated
Easprin⁵	Tablet	Enteric-coated
Ecotrin⁴	Tablet	Enteric-coated
E.E.S.⁵ 400	Tablet	Enteric-coated†
Efidac/24⁴	Tablet	Slow release
Efidac⁴ 24 Chlorpheniramine	Tablet	Slow release
E-Mycin⁵	Tablet	Enteric-coated
Endafed⁴	Capsule	Slow release
Entex® LA	Tablet	Slow release†
Equanil⁵	Tablet	Taste††
Eryc®	Capsule	Enteric-coated*
Ery-Tab®	Tablet	Enteric-coated
Erythrocin Stearate	Tablet	Enteric-coated
Erythromycin Base	Tablet	Enteric-coated
Eskalith CR®	Tablet	Slow release
Exgest⁵ LA	Tablet	Slow release
Fedahist⁴ Timecaps⁵	Capsule	Slow release†
Feldene®	Capsule	Mucous membrane irritant
Feocyte	Tablet	Slow release
Feosol⁴	Tablet	Enteric-coated†
Feosol⁴ Spansule®	Capsule	Slow release*†
Feratab⁵	Tablet	Enteric-coated†
Fero-Grad 500®	Tablet	Slow release
Fero-Gradumet®	Tablet	Slow release
Ferralet S.R.®	Tablet	Slow release
Feverall™ Sprinkle Caps	Capsule	Taste* **Note:** Capsule contents intended to be placed in a teaspoonful of water or soft food.
Fumatinic®	Capsule	Slow release
Gastrocrom®	Capsule	**Note:** Contents should be dissolved in water for administration.
Geocillin®	Tablet	Taste
Glucotrol® XL	Tablet	Slow release
Gris-PEG®	Tablet	**Note:** Crushing may result in precipitation of larger particles.
Guaifed⁵	Capsule	Slow release
Guaifed⁵-PD	Capsule	Slow release
Guaifenex⁵ LA	Tablet	Slow release♦
Guaifenex® PSE	Tablet	Slow release♦
GuaiMAX-D⁵	Tablet	Slow release
Humibid⁴ DM	Tablet	Slow release
Humibid⁴ DM Sprinkle	Capsule	Slow release*
Humibid⁵ LA	Tablet	Slow release
Humibid⁵ Sprinkle	Capsule	Slow release*
Hydergine⁵ LC	Capsule	**Note:** Product is in liquid form within a special capsule††
Hydergine⁵ Sublingual	Tablet	Sublingual route†
Hytakerol⁴	Capsule	Liquid filled§†
Iberet⁴	Tablet	Slow release†
Iberet-500®	Tablet	Slow release†
ICAPS⁴ Plus	Tablet	Slow release
ICAPS⁴ Time Release	Tablet	Slow release
Ilotycin⁴	Tablet	Enteric-coated
Imdur™	Tablet	Slow release♦
Inderal⁴ LA	Capsule	Slow release
Inderide⁵ LA	Capsule	Slow release
Indocin⁴ SR	Capsule	Slow release*†
Ionamin⁴	Capsule	Slow release
Isoptin⁴ SR	Tablet	Slow release

TABLETS THAT CANNOT BE CRUSHED OR ALTERED
(Continued)

Drug Product	Dosage Forms	Reasons/Comments
Isordil® Sublingual	Tablet	Sublingual form•
Isordil® Tembid®	Tablet	Slow release
Isosorbide Dinitrate Sublingual	Tablet	Sublingual form•
Isosorbide Dinitrate SR	Tablet	Slow release
K+ 8®	Tablet	Slow release†
K+ 10®	Tablet	Slow release†
Kaon-Cl® 6.7	Tablet	Slow release†
Kaon-Cl® 10	Tablet	Slow release†
K+ Care® ET	Tablet	Effervescent tablet†¶
K-Lease®	Capsule	Slow release•†
Klor-Con®	Tablet	Slow release†
Klor-Con/EF®	Tablet	Effervescent tablet†¶
Klorvess®	Tablet	Effervescent tablet†¶
Klotrix®	Tablet	Slow release†
K-Lyte®	Tablet	Effervescent tablet¶
K-Lyte®/Cl	Tablet	Effervescent tablet¶
K-Lyte DS®	Tablet	Effervescent tablet¶
K-Tab®	Tablet	Slow release†
Levsinex® Timecaps®	Capsule	Slow release
Lexxel®	Tablet	Slow release
Lodrane LD®	Capsule	Slow release•
Mag-Tab® SR	Tablet	Slow release
Mestinon®	Tablet	Slow release†
Mi-Cebrin®	Tablet	Enteric-coated
Mi-Cebrin® T	Tablet	Enteric-coated
Micro-K®	Capsule	Slow release•†
Monafed®	Tablet	Slow release
Monafed® DM	Tablet	Slow release
Motrin®	Tablet	Taste††
MS Contin®	Tablet	Slow release†
Muco-Fen-LA®	Tablet	Slow release♦
Naldecon®	Tablet	Slow release†
Naprelan®	Tablet	Slow release
Nasatab LA®	Tablet	Slow release
Niaspan®	Tablet	Slow release
Nico-400®	Capsule	Slow release
Nicobid®	Capsule	Slow release
Nitro-Bid®	Capsule	Slow release•
Nitroglyn®	Capsule	Slow release•
Nitrong®	Tablet	Sublingual route•
Nitrostat®	Tablet	Sublingual route•
Nolamine®	Tablet	Slow release
Nolex® LA	Tablet	Slow release
Norflex®	Tablet	Slow release
Norpace CR®	Capsule	Slow release form within a special capsule
Novafed® A	Capsule	Slow release
Ondrox®	Tablet	Slow release
Optilets-500®	Tablet	Enteric-coated
Optilets-M-500®	Tablet	Enteric-coated
Oragrafin®	Capsule	**Note:** Product is in liquid form within a special capsule
Ordrine® SR	Capsule	Slow release
Oramorph SR™	Tablet	Slow release†
Ornade® Spansule®	Capsule	Slow release
OxyContin®	Tablet	Slow release
Pabalate®	Tablet	Enteric-coated
Pabalate-SF®	Tablet	Enteric-coated
Pancrease®	Capsule	Enteric-coated•
Pancrease® MT	Capsule	Enteric-coated•
Panmycin®	Capsule	Taste

Drug Product	Dosage Forms	Reasons/Comments
Papaverine Sustained Action	Capsule	Slow release
Pathilon® Sequels®	Capsule	Slow release*
Pavabid® Plateau®	Capsule	Slow release*
PBZ-SR®	Tablet	Slow release†
Pentasa®	Capsule	Slow release
Perdiem®	Granules	Wax coated
Permitil® Chronotab®	Tablet	Slow release†
Phazyme®	Tablet	Slow release
Phazyme® 95	Tablet	Slow release
Phenergan®	Tablet	Taste†††
Phyllocontin®	Tablet	Slow release
Plendil®	Tablet	Slow release
Pneumomist®	Tablet	Slow release♦
Polaramine® Repetabs®	Tablet	Slow release†
Posicor®	Tablet	Mucus membrane irritant
Prelu-2®	Capsule	Slow release
Prevacid®	Capsule	Slow release
Prilosec™	Capsule	Slow release
Pro-Banthine®	Tablet	Taste
Procainamide HCl SR	Tablet	Slow release
Procanbid®	Tablet	Slow release
Procardia®	Capsule	Delays absorption§#
Procardia XL®	Tablet	Slow release **Note:** AUC is unaffected.
Profen® II	Tablet	Slow release♦
Profen LA®	Tablet	Slow release♦
Pronestyl-SR®	Tablet	Slow release
Proscar®	Tablet	**Note:** Crushed tablets should not be handled by women who are pregnant or who may become pregnant
Proventil® Repetabs®	Tablet	Slow release†
Prozac®	Capsule	Slow release*
Quibron-T/ SR®	Tablet	Slow release†
Quinaglute® Dura-Tabs®	Tablet	Slow release
Quinidex® Extentabs®	Tablet	Slow release
Quin-Release®	Tablet	Slow release
Respa-1st®	Tablet	Slow release♦
Respa-DM®	Tablet	Slow release♦
Respa-GF®	Tablet	Slow release♦
Respahist®	Capsule	Slow release*
Respaire® SR	Capsule	Slow release
Respbid®	Tablet	Slow release
Ritalin-SR®	Tablet	Slow release
Robimycin® Robitab®	Tablet	Enteric-coated
Rondec-TR®	Tablet	Slow release†
Roxanol SR™	Tablet	Slow release†
Ru-Tuss® DE	Tablet	Slow release
Sinemet CR®	Tablet	Slow release♦
Singlet for Adults®	Tablet	Slow release
Slo-bid™ Gyrocaps®	Capsule	Slow release*
Slo-Niacin®	Tablet	Slow release
Slo-Phyllin GG®	Capsule	Slow release†
Slo-Phyllin® Gyrocaps®	Capsule	Slow release*†
Slow FE®	Tablet	Slow release†
Slow FE® With Folic Acid	Tablet	Slow release
Slow-K®	Tablet	Slow release†
Slow-Mag®	Tablet	Slow release
Sorbitrate SA®	Tablet	Slow release
Sorbitrate® Sublingual	Tablet	Sublingual route
Sparine®	Tablet	Taste††
S-P-T	Capsule	**Note:** Liquid gelatin thyroid suspension.
Sudafed® 12-Hour	Capsule	Slow release†
Sudal® 60/500	Tablet	Slow release

TABLETS THAT CANNOT BE CRUSHED OR ALTERED
(Continued)

Drug Product	Dosage Forms	Reasons/Comments
Sudal® 120/600	Tablet	Slow release
Sudafed® 12-Hour	Tablet	Slow release
Sudex® 60/500	Tablet	Slow release◆
Sustaire®	Tablet	Slow release†
Syn™-Rx	Tablet	Slow release
Syn™-Rx DM	Tablet	Slow release
Tavist-D®	Tablet	Multiple compressed tablet
Teczam®	Tablet	Slow release
Tegretol XR®	Tablet	Slow release
Teldrin®	Capsule	Slow release*
Tessalon® Perles	Capsule	Slow release
Theo-24®	Tablet	Slow release†
Theobid® Duracaps®	Capsule	Slow release*†
Theoclear® L.A	Capsule	Slow release†
Theochron®	Tablet	Slow release
Theo-Dur®	Tablet	Slow release†◆
Theolair SR®	Tablet	Slow release†
Theo-Sav®	Tablet	Slow release◆
Theo-Time® SR	Tablet	Slow release
Theovent®	Capsule	Slow release†
Theo-X®	Tablet	Slow release
Thorazine® Spansule®	Capsule	Slow release
Toprol XL®	Tablet	Slow release◆
Touro A&H®	Capsule	Slow release*
Touro Ex®	Tablet	Slow release◆
Touro LA®	Tablet	Slow release◆
T-Phyl®	Tablet	Slow release
Trental®	Tablet	Slow release
Triaminic®	Tablet	Enteric-coated†
Triaminic®-12	Tablet	Slow release†
Triaminic® TR	Tablet	Multiple compressed tablet†
Trilafon® Repetabs®	Tablet	Slow release†
Tri-Phen-Chlor® Time Release	Tablet	Slow release
Tri-Phen-Mine® SR	Tablet	Slow release
TripTone® Caplets	Tablet	Slow release
Tuss-LA®	Tablet	Slow release
Tylenol® Extended Relief Caplets	Tablet	Slow release
ULR-LA®	Tablet	Slow release
Uni-Dur®	Tablet	Slow release
Uniphyl®	Tablet	Slow release
Verelan®	Capsule	Slow release*
Volmax®	Tablet	Slow release†
Wellbutrin®	Tablet	Anesthetize mucus membrane
Wygesic®	Tablet	Taste
ZORprin®	Tablet	Slow release
Zyban™	Tablet	Slow release
Zymase®	Capsule	Enteric-coated

*Capsule may be opened and the contents taken without crushing or chewing; soft food such as applesauce or pudding may facilitate administration; contents may generally be administered via nasogastric tube using an appropriate fluid, provided entire contents are washed down the tube.

†Liquid dosage forms of the product are available; however, dose, frequency of administration, and manufacturers may differ from that of the solid dosage form.

‡Antacids and/or milk may prematurely dissolve the coating of the tablet.

§Capsule may be opened and the liquid contents removed for administration.

††The taste of this product in a liquid form would likely be unacceptable to the patient; administration via nasogastric tube should be acceptable.

¶Effervescent tablets must be dissolved in the amount of diluent recommended by the manufacturer.

#If the liquid capsule is crushed or the contents expressed, the active ingredient will be, in part, absorbed sublingually.

•Tablets are made to disintegrate under the tongue.

◆Tablet is scored and may be broken in half without affecting release characteristics.

Adapted from Mitchell JF and Pawlicki KS, "Oral Solid Dosage Forms That Should Not Be Crushed: 1998 Revision," *Hosp Pharm*, 1994, 29(7):666-75.

TRANSFER OF DRUGS INTO HUMAN MILK

Adapted from "American Academy of Pediatrics Committee on Drugs: Transfer of Drugs and Other Chemicals Into Human Milk," *Pediatrics*, 1994, 93:137-50.

The following questions and options should be considered when prescribing drug therapy to lactating women. (1) Is the drug therapy really necessary? Consultation between the pediatrician and the mother's physician can be most useful. (2) Use the safest drug, for example, acetaminophen rather than aspirin for analgesia. (3) If there is a possibility that a drug may present a risk to the infant, consideration should be given to measurement of blood concentrations in the nursing infant. (4) Drug exposure to the nursing infant may be minimized by having the mother take the medication just after she has breast-fed the infant and/or just before the infant is due to have a lengthy sleep period.

Table 1. Drugs That Are Contraindicated During Breast-Feeding

Drug	Reason for Concern, Reported Sign or Symptom in Infant, or Effect on Lactation
Bromocriptine	Suppresses lactation; may be hazardous to the mother
Cocaine	Cocaine intoxication
Cyclophosphamide	Possible immune suppression; unknown effect on growth or association with carcinogenesis; neutropenia
Cyclosporine	Possible immune suppression; unknown effect on growth or association with carcinogenesis
Doxorubicin*	Possible immune suppression; unknown effect on growth or association with carcinogenesis
Ergotamine	Vomiting, diarrhea, convulsions (doses used in migraine medications)
Lithium	One-third to one-half therapeutic blood concentration in infants
Methotrexate	Possible immune suppression; unknown effect on growth or association with carcinogenesis; neutropenia
Phencyclidine (PCP)	Potent hallucinogen
Phenindione	Anticoagulant: increased prothrombin and partial thromboplastin time in one infant; not used in the United States

*Drug is concentrated in human milk.

Table 2. Drugs of Abuse: Contraindicated During Breast-Feeding*

Drug Reference	Reported Effect or Reasons for Concern
Amphetamine†	Irritability, poor sleeping pattern
Cocaine	Cocaine intoxication
Heroin	Tremors, restlessness, vomiting, poor feeding
Marijuana	Only one report in literature; no effect mentioned
Nicotine (smoking)	Shock, vomiting, diarrhea, rapid heart rate, restlessness; decreased milk production
Phencyclidine	Potent hallucinogen

*The Committee on Drugs strongly believes that nursing mothers should not ingest any compounds listed in Table 2. Not only are they hazardous to the nursing infant, but they are also detrimental to the physical and emotional health of the mother. This list is obviously not complete; no drug of abuse should be ingested by nursing mothers even though adverse reports are not in the literature.

†Drug is concentrated in human milk.

TRANSFER OF DRUGS INTO HUMAN MILK (Continued)

Table 3. Radioactive Compounds That Require Temporary Cessation of Breast-Feeding*

Drug	Recommended Time for Cessation of Breast-Feeding
Copper 64 (^{64}Cu)	Radioactivity in milk present at 50 h
Gallium 67 (^{67}Ga)	Radioactivity in milk present for 2 wk
Indium 111 (^{111}In)	Very small amount present at 20 h
Iodine 123 (^{123}I)	Radioactivity in milk present up to 36 h
Iodine 125 (^{125}I)	Radioactivity in milk present for 12 d
Iodine 131 (^{131}I)	Radioactivity in milk present 2-14 d, depending on study
Radioactive sodium	Radioactivity in milk present 96 h
Technetium-99m (^{99m}Tc), ^{99m}Rc macroaggregates, ^{99m}Tc O4	Radioactivity in milk present 15 h to 3 d

*Consult nuclear medicine physician before performing diagnostic study so that radionuclide that has shortest excretion time in breast milk can be used. Before study, the mother should pump her breast and store enough milk in freezer for feeding the infant; after study, the mother should pump her breast to maintain milk production but discard all milk pumped for the required time that radioactivity is present in milk. Milk samples can be screened by radiology departments for radioactivity before resumption of nursing.

Table 4. Drugs Whose Effect on Nursing Infants Is Unknown But May Be of Concern

Psychotropic drugs, the compounds listed under antianxiety, antidepressant, and antipsychotic categories, are of special concern when given to nursing mothers for long periods. Although there are no case reports of adverse effects in breast-feeding infants, these drugs do appear in human milk and thus conceivably alter short-term and long-term central nervous system function.

Drug	Reported or Possible Effect
Antianxiety	
Diazepam	None
Lorazepam	None
Midazolam	...
Perphenazine	None
Prazepam*	None
Quazepam	None
Temazepam	...
Antidepressants	
Amitriptyline	None
Amoxapine	None
Desipramine	None
Dothiepin	None
Doxepin	None
Fluoxetine	...
Fluvoxamine	...
Imipramine	None
Trazodone	None
Antipsychotic	
Chlorpromazine	Galactorrhea in adult; drowsiness and lethargy in infant
Chlorprothixene	None
Haloperidol	None
Mesoridazine	None
Chloramphenicol	Possible idiosyncratic bone marrow suppression
Metoclopramide*	None described; dopaminergic blocking agent
Metronidazole	In vitro mutagen; may discontinue breast-feeding 12-24 h to allow excretion of dose when single-dose therapy given to mother
Tinidazole	See metronidazole

*Drug is concentrated in human milk.

Table 5. Drugs That Have Been Associated With Significant Effects on Some Nursing Infants and Should Be Given to Nursing Mothers With Caution*

Drug	Reported Effect
5-Aminosalicylic acid	Diarrhea (one case)
Aspirin (salicylates)	Metabolic acidosis (one case)
Clemastine	Drowsiness, irritability, refusal to feed, high-pitched cry, neck stiffness (one case)
Phenobarbital	Sedation; infantile spasms after weaning from milk-containing phenobarbital, methemoglobinemia (one case)
Primidone	Sedation, feeding problems
Sulfasalazine (salicylazosulfapyridine)	Bloody diarrhea (one case)

*Measure blood concentration in the infant when possible.

Table 6. Maternal Medication Usually Compatible With Breast-Feeding*

Drug	Reported Sign or Symptom in Infant or Effect on Lactation
Acebutolol	None
Acetaminophen	None
Acetazolamide	None
Acitretin	...
Acyclovir†	None
Alcohol (ethanol)	With large amounts of drowsiness, diaphoresis, deep sleep, weakness, decrease in linear growth, abnormal weight gain, maternal ingestion of 1 g/kg daily decreases milk ejection reflex
Allopurinol	...
Amoxicillin	None
Antimony	...
Atenolol	None
Atropine	None
Azapropazone (apazone)	...
Aztreonam	None
B_1 (thiamine)	None
B_6 (pyridoxine)	None
B_{12}	None
Baclofen	None
Barbiturate	See Table 5.
Bendroflumethiazide	Suppresses lactation
Bishydroxycoumarin (Dicumarol®)	None
Bromide	Rash, weakness, absence of cry with maternal intake of 5.4 g/d
Butorphanol	None
Caffeine	Irritability, poor sleeping pattern, excreted slowly; no effect with usual amount of caffeine beverages
Captopril	None
Carbamazepine	None
Carbimazole	Goiter
Cascara	
None	
Cefadroxil	None
Cefazolin	None
Cefotaxime	None
Cefoxitin	None
Cefprozil	...

TRANSFER OF DRUGS INTO HUMAN MILK *(Continued)*

Table 6. Maternal Medication Usually Compatible With Breast-Feeding* *(continued)*

Drug	Reported Sign or Symptom in Infant or Effect on Lactation
Ceftazidime	None
Ceftriaxone	None
Chloral hydrate	Sleepiness
Chloroform	None
Chloroquine	None
Chlorothiazide	None
Chlorthalidone	Excreted slowly
Cimetidine†	None
Cisapride	None
Cisplatin	Not found in milk
Clindamycin	None
Clogestone	None
Clomipramine	...
Codeine	None
Colchicine	...
Contraceptive pill with estrogen/progesterone	Rare breast enlargement; decrease in milk production and protein content (not confirmed in several studies)
Cycloserine	None
D (vitamin)	None; follow up infant's serum calcium level if mother receives pharmacological doses
Danthron	Increased bowel activity
Dapsone	None; sulfonamide detected in infant's urine
Dexbrompheniramine maleate with d-isoephedrine	Crying, poor sleep patterns, irritability
Digoxin	None
Diltiazem	None
Dipyrone	None
Disopyramide	None
Domperidone	None
Dyphylline†	None
Enalapril	...
Erythromycin†	None
Estradiol	Withdrawal, vaginal bleeding
Ethambutol	None
Ethanol	See Alcohol
Ethosuximide	None; drug appears in infant serum
Fentanyl	...
Flecainide	...
Flufenamic acid	None
Fluorescein	...
Folic acid	None
Gold salts	None
Halothane	None
Hydralazine	None
Hydrochlorothiazide	...
Hydroxychloroquine†	None
Ibuprofen	None
Indomethacin	Seizure (one case)
Iodides	May affect thyroid activity
Iodine	Goiter
Iodine (povidone-iodine/vaginal douche)	Elevated iodine levels in breast milk, odor of iodine on infant's skin

Table 6. Maternal Medication Usually Compatible With Breast-Feeding* *(continued)*

Drug	Reported Sign or Symptom in Infant or Effect on Lactation
Iopanoic acid	None
Isoniazid	None; acetyl metabolite also secreted; ? hepatotoxic
K₁ (vitamin)	None
Kanamycin	None
Ketorolac	...
Labetalol	None
Levonorgestrel	...
Lidocaine	None
Loperamide	...
Magnesium sulfate	None
Medroxyprogesterone	None
Mefenamic acid	None
Methadone	None if mother receiving ≤20 mg/24 h
Methimazole (active metabolite of carbimazole)	None
Methocarbamol	None
Methyldopa	None
Methyprylon	Drowsiness
Metoprolol†	None
Metrizamide	None
Mexiletine	None
Minoxidil	None
Morphine	None; infant may have significant blood concentration
Moxalactam	None
Nadolol†	None
Nalidixic acid	Hemolysis in infant with glucose-6-phosphate dehydrogenase (G-6-PD) deficiency
Naproxen	...
Nefopam	None
Nifedipine	...
Nitrofurantoin	Hemolysis in infant with G-6-PD deficiency
Norethynodrel	None
Norsteroids	None
Noscapine	None
Oxprenolol	None
Phenylbutazone	None
Phenytoin	Methemoglobinemia (one case)
Piroxicam	None
Prednisone	None
Procainamide	None
Progesterone	None
Propoxyphene	None
Propranolol	None
Propylthiouracil	None
Pseudoephedrine†	None
Pyridostigmine	None
Pyrimethamine	None
Quinidine	None
Quinine	None
Riboflavin	None
Rifampin	None
Scopolamine	...
Secobarbital	None
Senna	None

TRANSFER OF DRUGS INTO HUMAN MILK *(Continued)*

Table 6. Maternal Medication Usually Compatible With Breast-Feeding* *(continued)*

Drug	Reported Sign or Symptom in Infant or Effect on Lactation
Sotalol	...
Spironolactone	None
Streptomycin	None
Sulbactam	None
Sulfapyridine	Caution in infant with jaundice or G-6-PD deficiency and ill, stressed, or premature infant; appears in infant's milk
Sulfisoxazole	Caution in infant with jaundice or G-6-PD deficiency and ill, stressed, or premature infant; appears in infant's milk
Suprofen	None
Terbutaline	None
Tetracycline	None; negligible absorption by infant
Theophylline	Irritability
Thiopental	None
Thiouracil	None mentioned; drug not used in U.S.
Ticarcillin	None
Timolol	None
Tolbutamide	Possible jaundice
Tolmetin	None
Trimethoprim and sulfamethoxazole	None
Triprolidine	None
Valproic acid	None
Verapamil	None
Warfarin	None
Zolpidem	None

*Drugs listed have been reported in the literature as having the effects listed or no effect. The word "none" means that no observable change was seen in the nursing infant while the mother was ingesting the compound. It is emphasized that most of the literature citations concern single case reports or small series of infants.

†Drug is concentrated in human milk.

NEW DRUGS INTRODUCED OR APPROVED BY THE FDA IN 1999

Brand Name	Generic Name	Use
Aciphex™	rabeprazole	Reflux ulcer and duodenal ulcer
Actos®	pioglitazone	Type II diabetes
Agenerase™	amprenavir	HIV
Aggrenox®	dipyridamole & aspirin	Reduce risk of nonfatal stroke
Alamast®	pemirolast	Allergic conjunctivitis
Alocril™	nedocromil (ophthalmic)	Allergic conjunctivitis
Antagon™	ganirelix	Prevent premature LH surges
Aromasin®	exemestane	Breast cancer
Avandia®	rosiglitazone	Type II diabetes
Avapro® HCT	irbesartan and hydrochlorothiazide	Hypertension
Busulfex®	busalfan	Chronic myelogenous leukemia
Cenestin®	synthetic conj. estrogens, A	Symptoms of menopause
Chirocaine®	levobupivacaine	Local or regional anesthesia
Comtan®	entacapone	Parkinson's disease
Comvax®	*Haemophilus* B conjugate and hepatitis B vaccine	Vaccination
DepoCyt™	cytarabine (liposomal)	Lymphomatous meningitis
Ellence™	epirubicin	Antineoplastic
Ferrlecit®	sodium ferric gluconate complex	Iron deficiency in dialysis patient
Hectoral™	doxercalciferol	Hyperparathyroidism
Nabi-HB®	hepatitis B immune globulin	Hepatitis B
NovoSeven®	recombinant factor VIIa	Hemophilia A or B
Ontak®	denileukin dititox	Cutaneous T-cell lymphoma (CTCL)
Panretin™	alitretinoin	AIDS-related Kaposi's sarcoma
Pletal®	cilostazol	Intermittent claudication
Preveon®	adefovir	HIV
Rapamune™	sirolimus	Immunosuppressant
Raplan®	rapacuronium	Neuromuscular blocking agent
Relenza®	zanamivir	Influenza
Sonata®	zaleplan	Hypnotic agent
Sucraid™	sacrosidase	Congenital sucrase-isomaltase deficiency
Synercid®	quinupristin/dalfopristin	Antibiotic (vancomycin-resistant bacteria)
Tamiflu™	oseltamivir	Type A & B influenza
Tequin™	gatifloxacin	Antibiotic
Temodar®	temozolomide	Alkylating agent
Thyrogen®	thyrotropin alpha	Diagnostic agent
Tikosyn®	dofetilide	Antiarrhythmic agent
Vioxx®	rofecoxib	Osteoarthritis, pain, dysmenorrhea
Vitravene™	fomivirsen	Cytomegalovirus
Xenical®	orlistat	Obesity
Xopenex®	levalbuterol	Bronchospasm
Zaditor®	ketotifen fumarate	Allergic conjunctivitis
Ziagen™	abacavir	HIV

PENDING DRUGS OR DRUGS IN CLINICAL TRIALS

Brand Name	Generic Name	Use
Alredase®	tolrestat	Controlling late complications of diabetes
Arkin-Z®	vesnarinone	Congestive heart failure agent
Baypress®	nitrendipine	Calcium channel blocker for hypertension
Berotec®	fenoterol	Beta-2 agonist for asthma
Catatrol®	viloxazine	Bicyclic antidepressant
Cipralan®	cifenline succinate	Antiarrhythmic agent
Cytolex®	pexiganan	Diabetic foot ulcers
Decabid®	indecainide hydrochloride	Antiarrhythmic agent
Delaprem®	hexoprenaline sulfate	Tocolytic agent
Dirame®	propiram	Opioid analgesic
Enable®	tenidap sodium	Arthritis
Exelom®	rivastigmine	Alzheimer's disease
Fareston®	toremifene citrate	Antiestrogen for breast cancer
Freedox®	triliazad mesylate	Prevents progressive neuronal degeneration
Frisium®	clobazam	Benzodiazepine
Gastrozepine®	pirenzepine	Antiulcer drug
Inhibace®	cilazapril	ACE inhibitor
Isoprinosine®	inosiplex	Immunomodulating drug
Lacipil®	lacidipine	Hypertension
Malarone®	atavaquone/proguanil	Malaria
Maxicam®	isoxicam	NSAID
Mentane®	velnacrine	Alzheimer's disease agent
Micturin®	terodiline hydrochloride	Agent for urinary incontinence
Mogadon®	nitrazepam	Benzodiazepine
Motilium®	domperidone	Antiemetic
Napa®	acecainide	Antiarrhythmic agent
Natrecor®	nesiritide	Congestive heart failure
Pindac®	pinacidil	Antihypertensive
Prothiaden®	dothiepin hydrochloride	Tricyclic antidepressant
Protonix®	pantopraxole	Proton pump inhibitor
Rimadyl®	caprofen	NSAID
Roxiam®	remoxipride	Antipsychotic agent
Selecor®	celiprolol hydrochloride	Beta-adrenergic blocker
Spexil®	trospectomycin	Antibiotic, a spectinomycin analog
Targocoid®	teicoplanin	Antibiotic, similar to vancomycin
Unicard®	dilevalol	Beta-adrenergic blocker

DRUG PRODUCTS NO LONGER AVAILABLE IN THE U.S.

Brand Name	Generic Name
Achromycin® Parenteral	tetracycline
Achromycin® V Capsule	tetracycline
Achromycin® V Oral Suspension	tetracycline
ACTH-40®	corticotropin
Actidil®	triprolidine
Actifed® Syrup	triprolidine and pseudoephedrine
Actifed® With Codeine	triprolidine, pseudoephedrine, and codeine
Adipex-P®	phentermine (all products)
Adipost®	phendimetrazine tartrate
Adphen®	phendimetrazine tartrate
Adrin®	nylidrin hydrochloride
Aerolate® Oral Solution	theophylline
Aerosporin® Injection	polymyxin B
Agoral® Plain	mineral oil
Akoline® C.B. Tablet	vitamin
Ak-Zol®	acetazolamide
Ala-Tet®	tetracycline
Amin-Aid®	amino acid
Amonidrin® Tablet	guaifenesin
Anacin-3® (all products)	acetaminophen
Anaids® Tablet	alginic acid and sodium bicarbonate
Anergan® 25 Injection	promethazine hydrochloride
Anoxine-AM® Capsule	phentermine hydrochloride
Antinea® Cream	benzoic acid and salicylic acid
Antivert® Chewable Tablet	meclizine hydrochloride
Antrocol® Capsule & Tablet	atropine and belladonna
Apomorphine	apomorphine (now available as an orphan drug only)
Arcotinic® Tablet	iron and liver combination
Argyrol® S.S.	silver protein, mild
Arlidin®	nylidrin (all products)
Arthritis Foundation® Ibuprofen	ibuprofen
Arthritis Foundation® Nighttime	acetaminophen and diphenhydramine
Arthritis Foundation® Pain Reliever, Aspirin Free	acetaminophen
Arthritis Strength Bufferin®	aspirin (buffered)
Articulose-50® Injection	prednisolone
Asbron-G® Elixir	theophylline and guaifenesin
Asbron-G® Tablet	theophylline and guaifenesin
Asproject®	sodium thiosalicylate
Atabrine® Tablet	quinacrine hydrochloride
Atropine Soluble Tablet	atropine soluble tablet
Aureomycin®	chlortetracycline
Axotal®	butalbital compound and aspirin
Azlin® Injection	azlocillin
Azo Gantanol®	sulfamethoxazole and phenazopyridine
Azo Gantrisin®	sulfisoxazole and phenazopyridine
Azulfidine® Suspension	sulfasalazine
B-A-C®	butalbital compound with aspirin
Bactocill®	oxacillin
Bancap®	butalbital compound with acetaminophen
Banesin®	acetaminophen
Bantron®	lobeline (all products)

DRUG PRODUCTS NO LONGER AVAILABLE IN THE U.S.
(Continued)

Brand Name	Generic Name
Baypress®	nitrendipine
Becomject-100®	vitamin B complex
Beesix®	pyridoxine hydrochloride
Bellafoline®	levorotatory alkaloids of belladonna (all products)
Bemote®	dicyclomine
Bena-D®	diphenhydramine
Benadryl® 50 mg Capsule	diphenhydramine hydrochloride
Benadryl® Cold/Flu	acetaminophen, diphenhydramine, and pseudoephedrine
Benahist® Injection	diphenhydramine hydrochloride
Benoject®	diphenhydramine hydrochloride
Betapen-VK®	penicillin V potassium
Beta-Val® Ointment	betamethasone
Biamine® Injection	thiamine hydrochloride
Bilezyme® Tablet	pancrelipase
Biomox®	amoxicillin
Biphetamine®	amphetamine and dextroamphetamine
Blanex® Capsule	chloroxazone and acetaminophen
Bretylol®	bretylium
Bronkephrine®	ethylnorepinephrine hydrochloride
Buffered®, Tri-buffered	aspirin
Bufferin® Arthritis Strength	aspirin
Bufferin® Extra Strength	aspirin
Buf-Puf® Acne Cleansing Bar	salicylic acid
Butace®	butalbital compound
Caladryl® Spray	diphenhydramine and calamine
Calciparine® Injection	heparin calcium
Camalox® Suspension & Tablet	aluminum hydroxide, calcium carbonate, and magnesium hydroxide
Cantharone®	cantharidin
Cantharone Plus®	cantharidin
Caroid®	cascara sagrada and phenolphthalein
Catarase® 1:5000	chymotrypsin (all products)
Cedilanid-D® Injection	deslanoside
Cenocort® A-40	triamcinolone
Cenocort® Forte	triamcinolone
Centrax® Capsule & Tablet	prazepam
Cerespan®	papaverine hydrochloride
Cetane®	ascorbic acid
Chenix® Tablet	chenodiol
Chlorgest-HD® Elixir	chlorpheniramine, phenylephrine, and hydrocodone
Chlorofon-A® Tablet	chlorzoxazone
Chloromycetin® Cream	chloramphenicol
Chloromycetin® Kapseals®	chloramphenicol
Chloromycetin® Ophthalmic	chloramphenicol
Chloromycetin® Otic	chloramphenicol
Chloromycetin® Palmitate Oral Suspension	chloramphenicol
Chloroserpine®	reserpine and hydrochorothiazide
Chlortab®	chlorpheniramine maleate
Choledyl®	oxtriphylline
Chymex®	bentiromide (all products)
Cipralan®	cifenline

Brand Name	Generic Name
Cithalith-S® Syrup	lithium citrate
Citro-Nesia® Solution	magnesium citrate
Clistin® Tablet	carbinoxamine maleate
Clorpactin® XCB Powder	oxychlorosene sodium
Cobalasine® Injection	adenosine phosphate
Codimal-A® Injection	brompheniramine maleate
Codimal® Expectorant	guaifenesin and phenylpropanolamine
Coly-Mycin® S Oral	colistin sulfate
Constant-T® Tablet	theophylline
Control-L®	pyrethrins
Cortaid® Ointment	hydrocortisone
Cortrophin-Zinc®	corticotropin
Crysticillin® 300 A.S.	penicillin G procaine
Crysticillin® 600 A.S.	penicillin G procaine
Crystodigin® 0.05 mg & 0.15 mg Tablet	digitoxin
Cyclospasmol®	cyclandelate (all products)
Cycrin® 10 mg Tablet	medroxyprogesterone acetate
D-Amp®	ampicillin
Danex® Shampoo	pyrithione zinc
Dapex-37.5®	phentermine hydrochloride
Darbid® Tablet	isopropamide iodide (all products)
Daricon®	oxyphencyclimine (all products)
Darvon® 32 mg Capsule	propoxyphene hydrochloride
Darvon-N® Oral Suspension	propoxyphene napsylate
Datril® Extra Strength	acetaminophen
Decadron® 0.25 mg and 6 mg Tablets	dexamethasone
Decaspray®	dexamethasone
Dehist®	brompheniramine maleate
Deltalin® Capsule	ergocalciferol
Depo-Provera® 100 mg/mL	medroxyprogesterone
Deprol®	meprobamate and benactyzine hydrochloride
Dermoxyl® Gel	benzoyl peroxide
Despec® Liquid	guaifenesin, phenylpropanolamine, and phenylephrine
Dexacen-4®	dexamethasone
Dexacen® LA-8	dexamethasone
Dexedrine® Elixir	dextroamphetamine sulfate
Dialose® Capsule	docusate sodium
Diaparene® Cradol®	methylbenzethonium
Dilantin-30® Pediatric Suspension	phenytoin
Dilantin® With Phenobarbital	phenytoin with phenobarbital
Dilaudid® 1 mg & 3 mg Tablet	hydromorphone hydrochloride
Dimetane®	brompheniramine maleate
Dispos-a-Med® Isoproterenol	isoproterenol
Diupress®	chlorothiazide and reserpine
Dizymes® Tablet	pancreatin
Dommanate® Injection	dimenhydrinate
Donphen® Tablet	hyoscyamine, atropine, scopolamine, and phenobarbital
Dopastat® Injection	dopamine hydrochloride
Doriden® Tablet	glutethimide
Doxinate® Capsule	docusate sodium
Dramamine® Injection	dimenhydrinate
Dramocen®	dimenhydrinate
Dramoject®	dimenhydramine
D-S-S Plus®	docusate and casanthranol

DRUG PRODUCTS NO LONGER AVAILABLE IN THE U.S.
(Continued)

Brand Name	Generic Name
Duo-Medihaler®	isoproterenol and phenylephrine
Duracid®	aluminum hydroxide, magnesium carbonate, and calcium carbonate
Duract®	bromfenac (all products)
Dyflex-400® Tablet	dyphylline
Elase® Ointment	fibrinolysin and desoxyribonuclease (all products)
Elase®-Chloromycetin® Ointment	fibrinolysin and desoxyribonuclease
Eldepryl® Tablet	selegiline
Eldoquin® Lotion	hydroquinone
Elixophyllin SR®	theophylline
E-Lor® Tablet	propoxyphene and acetaminophen
Emete-Con® Injection	benzquinamide
Emetine Hydrochloride	emetine hydrochloride
Endep®	amitriptyline hydrochloride
Enduron® 2.5 mg Tablet	methyclothiazide
Enkaid®	encainide
Enovid®	mestranol and norethynodrel
E.N.T.®	brompheniramine and phenylpropanolamine
Entozyme®	pancreatin
E.P. Mycin® Capsule	oxytetracycline
Ergostat®	ergotamine
Ergotrate® Maleate	ergonovine maleate
Eridium®	phenazopyridine hydrochloride
Ery-Sol® Topical Solution	erythromycin, topical
Esidrix® 100 mg Tablet	hydrochlorothiazide
Estradurin® Injection	polyestradiol phosphate
Estroject-2® Injection	estradiol
Estroject-L.A.® Injection	estradiol
Estronol® Injection	estrone
Estrovis®	quinestrol
Ethaquin®	ethaverine hydrochloride
Ethatab®	ethaverine hydrochloride
Ethavex-100®	ethaverine hydrochloride
Euthroid® Tablet	liotrix
Fansidar®	sulfadoxine and pyrimethamine
Fastin®	phentermine (all products)
FemCare®	clotrimazole
Femstat®	butoconazole nitrate
Fergon Plus®	iron with vitamin B
Fer-In-Sol® Capsule	ferrous sulfate
Fermalox®	ferrous sulfate, magnesium hydroxide, and docusate
Ferndex®	dextroamphetamine sulfate
Flonase® 9 g	fluticasone
Folex® Injection	methotrexate
Gamastan®	immune globulin, intramuscular
Gammagard® Injection	immune globulin, intravenous
Gammar®	immune globulin, intramuscular
Gantrisin® Ophthalmic	sulfisoxazole
Gantrisin® Tablet	sulfisoxazole
Gelusil® Liquid	aluminum hydroxide, magnesium hydroxide, and simethicone
Gen-D-phen®	diphenhydramine hydrochloride

Brand Name	Generic Name
Grisactin®	griseofulvin
Gynogen® Injection	estradiol
Halazone Tablet	halazone
Halenol® Tablet	acetaminophen
Harmonyl®	deserpidine
HemFe®	iron with vitamins
Hep-B-Gammagee®	hepatitis B immune globulin
Herplex®	idoxuridine
Hetrazan®	diethylcarbamazine citrate
Hismanal®	astemizole
Histaject®	brompheniramine maleate
Histamine Phosphate Injection	histamine phosphate
Hydeltra-T.B.A.®	prednisolone
Hydramine®	diphenhydramine hydrochloride
Hydrobexan® Injection	hydroxocobalamin
Hydropres® 25 mg Tablet	hydrochlorothiazide and reserpine
Hydroxacen®	hydroxyzine
Intal® Inhalation Capsule	cromolyn sodium
Intercept®	nonoxynol 9
Iodo-Niacin® Tablet	potassium iodide and niacinamide hydroiodide
Ionamin®	phentermine (all products)
Iophen®	iodinated glycerol
Iophen-C®	iodinated glycerol and codeine
Iophen-DM®	iodinated glycerol and dextromethorphan (all products)
Iophylline®	iodinated glycerol and theophylline
Iotuss®	iodinated glycerol and codeine
Iotuss-DM®	iodinated glycerol and dextromethorphan (all products)
Iso-Bid®	isosorbide dinitrate
Isopto® P-ES	pilocarpine and physostigmine
Isovex®	ethaverine hydrochloride
Isuprel® Glossets®	isoproterenol
Kaopectate® Children's Tablet	attapulgite
Kato® Powder	potassium chloride
Keflin®	cephalothin sodium
Kestrin® Injection	estrone
Koate®-HS Injection	antihemophilic factor (human)
Koate®-HT Injection	antihemophilic factor (human)
Kolyum® Powder	potassium chloride and potassium gluconate
Konyne-HT® Injection	factor IX complex (human)
Kwell®	lindane
Lamprene® 100 mg	clofazimine
Laniazid® Tablet	isoniazid
Lasan® Topical	anthralin
Lasan® HP-1 Topical	anthralin
Ledercillin VK®	penicillin V potassium
Libritabs® 5 mg	chlordiazepoxide
Listerex® Scrub	salicylic acid
Lorcet®	hydrocodone and acetaminophen
Lorelco®	probucol
Malatal®	hyoscyamine, atropine, scopolamine, and phenobarbital
Malotuss® Syrup	guaifenesin
Mandelamine® Tablet	methenamine
Mantadil® Cream	chlorcyclizine

DRUG PRODUCTS NO LONGER AVAILABLE IN THE U.S.
(Continued)

Brand Name	Generic Name
Marezine® Injection	cyclizine hydrochloride
Marplan®	isocarboxazid
Max-Caro®	beta-carotene
Meclomen®	meclofenamate sodium
Medihaler-Epi®	epinephrine
Medihaler Ergotamine®	ergotamine
Medrapred®	prednisolone and atropine
Medrol® Acetate Topical	methylprednisolone
Melfiat® Tablet	phendimetrazine tartrate
Meprospan®	meprobamate
Metaprel® Aerosol	metaproterenol sulfate
Metaprel® Inhalation Solution	metaproterenol sulfate
Metaprel® Tablet	metaproterenol sulfate
Metizol® Tablet	metronidazole
Metopirone® Tablet	metyrapone tartrate
Metra®	phendimetrazine tartrate
Miflex® Tablet	chlorzoxazone and acetaminophen
Milprem®	meprobamate and conjugated estrogens
Minocin® Tablet	minocycline
Miochol®	acetylcholine
Moisturel® Lotion	dimethicone
Monocete® Topical Liquid	monochloroacetic acid
Moxam® Injection	moxalactam
Mus-Lax®	chlorzoxazone
Mylaxen® Injection	hexafluorenium bromide
Myochrysine®	gold sodium thiomalate
Nafcil®	nafcillin
Nalfon® Tablet	fenoprofen calcium
Nandrobolic® Injection	nandrolone phenpropionate
Narcan® 1 mg/mL Injection	naloxone hydrochloride
Navane® Concentrate & Injection	thiothixene
N-B-P® Ointment	bacitracin, neomycin, and polymyxin B
Neo-Castaderm®	resorcinol, boric acid, acetone
Neo-Cortef® Topical	neomycin and hydrocortisone
NeoDecadron® Topical	neomycin and dexamethasone
Neo-Medrol® Acetate Topical	methylprednisolone and neomycin
Neoquess® Injection	dicyclomine hydrochloride
Neoquess® Tablet	hyoscyamine sulfate
Neo-Synalar® Topical	neomycin and fluocinolone
Neo-Synephrine® 12 Hour Nasal Solution	oxymetazoline hydrochloride
Neutra-Phos® Capsule	potassium phosphate and sodium phosphate
Niac®	niacin
Niacels®	niacin
Niclocide®	niclosamide
Nidryl®	diphenhydramine hydrochloride
Niferex Forte®	iron with vitamins
Niloric®	ergoloid mesylates
Nipride® Injection	nitroprusside sodium
Nisaval®	pyrilamine maleate
Nitro-Bid® Oral	nitroglycerin
Nitrocine® Oral	nitroglycerin
Nitrostat® 0.15 mg Tablet	nitroglycerin
Noctec®	chloral hydrate

Brand Name	Generic Name
Noludar®	methyprylon
Norlutate®	norethindrone
Norlutin®	norethindrone
Novafed®	pseudoephedrine
Novahistine DH® Liquid	chlorpheniramine, pseudoephedrine, and codeine
Novahistine DMX® Liquid	guaifenesin, pseudoephedrine, and dextromethorphan
Novahistine® Elixir	chlorpheniramine and phenylephrine
Novahistine® Expectorant	guaifenesin, pseudoephedrine, and codeine
Nursoy®	enteral nutritional therapy
Nydrazid® Injection	isoniazid
Obe-Nix® 30	phentermine (all products)
Obephen®	phentermine (all products)
Obermine®	phentermine (all products)
Obestin-30®	phentermine (all products)
Ophthaine®	proparacaine
Ophthocort®	chloramphenicol, polymyxin B, and hydrocortisone
Oradex-C®	dyclonine
Oratect®	benzocaine
Oreticyl®	deserpidine and hydrochlorothiazide
Organidin®	iodinated glycerol
Otic Tridesilon®	desonide and acetic acid
Oxsoralen® Oral	methoxsalen
Panwarfin®	warfarin sodium
Paplex®	salicylic acid
Paradione®	paramethadione
Para-Hist AT®	promethazine, phenylephrine, and codeine
Pargen Fortified®	chlorzoxazone
Par Glycerol®	iodinated glycerol
Parmine®	phentermine hydrochloride
Parsidol®	ethopropazine (all products)
Pavabid HP®	papaverine hydrochloride
Pavasule®	papaverine hydrochloride
Pavatym®	papaverine hydrochloride
Pavesed®	papaverine hydrochloride
PBZ® Elixir	tripelennamine
Pentids®	penicillin G potassium, oral (all products)
Pfizerpen-AS®	penicillin G procaine
Phenaphen®	acetaminophen
Phenaphen®/Codeine #4	acetaminophen and codeine
Phenaseptic®	phenol
Phencen-50®	promethazine
Phenetron®	chlorpheniramine
Phentrol®	phentermine (all products)
Phenurone®	phenacemide
Phos-Ex® 62.5	calcium acetate
Phos-Ex® 125	calcium acetate
Phos-Ex® 167	calcium acetate
Phos-Ex® 250	calcium acetate
pHos-pHaid®	ammonium biphosphate, sodium biphosphate, and sodium acid pyrophosphate
Phosphaljel®	aluminum phosphate
Pindac®	pinacidil

DRUG PRODUCTS NO LONGER AVAILABLE IN THE U.S.
(Continued)

Brand Name	Generic Name
Polargen®	dexchlorpheniramine maleate
Poliovax® Injection	poliovirus vaccine, inactivated
Polycillin® Oral	ampicillin
Polycillin-N® Injection	ampicillin
Polycillin-PRB®	ampicillin and probenecid (all products)
Polyflex® Tablet	chlorzoxazone
Polygam® Injection	immune globulin, intravenous
Polymox®	amoxicillin
Pondimin®	fenfluramine
Posicor®	mibefradil (all products)
Predaject-50®	prednisolone
Predalone®	prednisolone
Predicort-50®	prednisolone
Preludin®	phenmetrazine hydrochloride
Premarin® Vaginal Cream	conjugated estrogens
Proampacin®	ampicillin and probenecid (all products)
Procan SR®	procainamide
Profilate-HP®	antihemophilic factor (human)
Projestaject® Injection	progesterone
Prokine® Injection	sargramostim
Prolamine®	phenylpropanolamine
Proloid®	thyroglobulin
Prometh®	promethazine
Proplex® SX-T Injection	factor IX complex (human)
Pro-Sof®	docusate sodium
Prostaphlin®	oxacillin
Protopam® Tablet	pralidoxime chloride
Provatene®	beta-carotene
Pyridium Plus®	phenazopyridine, hyoscyamine, and butabarbital
Questran® Tablet	cholestyramine resin
Quinamm®	quinine sulfate
Quiphile®	quinine sulfate
Q-vel®	quinine sulfate
Rectacort® suppository	hydrocortisone
Redux®	dexfenfluramine
Regutol®	docusate
Rep-Pred®	methylprednisolone
R-Gen®	iodinated glycerol
Rhesonativ® Injection	Rh_o(D) immune globulin
Rhindecon®	phenylpropanolamine
Rhinolar®	chlorpheniramine, phenylpropanolamine, and methscopolamine
Rhuli® Cream	benzocaine, calamine, and camphor
Robicillin® Tablet	penicillin V potassium
Robitet®	tetracycline
Romycin® Solution	erythromycin, topical
Rondomycin® Capsule	methacycline hydrochloride (all products)
Rufen®	ibuprofen
Scabene®	lindane
Sclavo - PPD® Solution	tuberculin purified protein derivative
Sclavo Test-PPD®	tuberculin purified protein derivative
Sebulex®	sulfur and salicylic acid
Sebulon®	pyrithione zinc
Seconal™ Oral	secobarbital sodium

Brand Name	Generic Name
Seldane®	terfenadine
Seldane-D®	terfenadine and pseudoephedrine
Selecor®	celiprolol
Selestoject®	betamethasone
Senolax®	senna
Serpasil®	reserpine
Siblin®	psyllium
Skelex®	chlorzoxazone
Slo-Salt®	salt substitute
Sodium P.A.S.®	aminosalicylate sodium
Sofarin®	warfarin sodium
Solatene®	beta-carotene
Spasmoject®	dicyclomine
Spectrobid® Oral Suspension	bacampicillin
Staphcillin®	methicillin (all products)
Statobex®	phendimetrazine tartrate
Sterapred®	prednisone
Streptomycin	streptomycin
Sucostrin®	succinylcholine chloride
Sudafed® Children	pseudoephedrine
Sudafed® Cough	guaifenesin, pseudoephedrine, and dextromethorphan
Sudafed® Plus Liquid	chlorpheniramine and pseudoephedrine
Superchar®	charcoal
Superchar® With Sorbitol	charcoal
Surital®	thiamylal sodium
Symmetrel® Capsule	amantadine hydrochloride
Synkayvite®	menadiol sodium
Syntocinon® Nasal	oxytocin
Tabron®	vitamins, multiple
Tacaryl®	methdilazine hydrochloride (all products)
Taractan®	chlorprothixene
T-Caine® Lozenge	benzocaine
Tegopen®	cloxacillin
Teline®	tetracycline
Temaril®	trimeprazine tartrate
Tepanil®	diethylpropion hydrochloride
Tepanil® TenTabs®	diethylpropion hydrochloride
Tes-Tape®	diagnostic aids (*in vitro*), urine
Tetralan®	tetracycline
Tetram®	tetracycline
Theelin® Aqueous Injection	estrone
Theobid® Jr Duracaps®	theophylline
Theo-Dur® Sprinkle®	theophylline
Theo-Organidin®	iodinated glycerol and theophylline
Theramin® Expectorant	guaifenesin and phenylpropanolamine
Thiacide®	methenamine and potassium acid phosphate
Tiject-20®	trimethobenzamide
Tindal®	acetophenazine maleate
Torecan® Suppository	thiethylperazine
Totacillin-N®	ampicillin
Tral®	hexocyclium methylsulfate
Travase®	sutilains
Tridione® Suppository	trimethadione
Trimox® 500 mg	amoxicillin
Trofan®	L-tryptophan

DRUG PRODUCTS NO LONGER AVAILABLE IN THE U.S.
(Continued)

Brand Name	Generic Name
Trofan DS®	L-tryptophan
Tryptacin®	L-tryptophan
Tucks® Cream	witch hazel
Tusal®	sodium thiosalicylate
Tussi-Organidin®	iodinated glycerol and codeine
Tussi-Organidin® DM	iodinated glycerol and dextromethorphan (all products)
Tusso-DM®	iodinated glycerol and dextromethorphan (all products)
Tuss-Ornade®	caramiphen and phenylpropanolamine
Ultralente® U	insulin zinc suspension, extended
Ultrase® MT24	pancrelipase
Unipen®	nafcillin
Unipres®	hydralazine, hydrochlorothiazide, and reserpine
Ureacin®-40 Topical	urea
Uri-Tet®	oxytetracycline
Urobiotic-25®	oxytetracycline and sulfamethizole
Uticort®	betamethasone (all products)
Valadol®	acetaminophen
Valergen® Injection	estradiol
Valmid® Capsule	ethinamate
Valpin® 50	anisotropine methylbromide
Valrelease®	diazepam
Vanex-LA®	guaifenesin and phenylpropanolamine
Vanseb-T® Shampoo	coal tar, sulfur, and salicylic acid
V-Cillin K®	penicillin V potassium
Velsar® Injection	vinblastine sulfate
Vercyte®	pipobroman
Verr-Canth®	cantharidin
Verrex®	podophyllin and salicylic acid
Verrusol®	salicylic acid, podophyllin, and cantharidin
V-Gan® Injection	promethazine hydrochloride
Vicks® Vatronol®	ephedrine
Vioform®-Hydrocortisone Topical	clioquinol and hydrocortisone
Visine®	tetrahydrozoline hydrochloride
Vistaject-25®	hydroxyzine
Vistaject-50®	hydroxyzine
Vontrol®	diphenidol
Wehamine® Injection	dimenhydrinate
Wehdryl®	diphenhydramine
Wesprin® Buffered	aspirin
Wyamycin S®	erythromycin
Zebrax®	clidinium and chlordiazepoxide
Zetran®	diazepam
Zolyse®	chymotrypsin alpha (all products)
Zyban® 100 mg	bupropion

PHARMACEUTICAL MANUFACTURERS DIRECTORY

Abbott Laboratories
(Abbott Diagnostic Division)
One Abbott Park Road
Abbott Park, IL 60064-3500
www.abbott.com

Abbott Laboratories
(Hospital Products Division)
200 Abbott Park Road
Abbott Park, IL 60064-3537

Abbott Laboratories
(Pharmaceutical Product Division)
100 Abbott Park Road
Abbott Park, IL 60064-3500
www.abbott.com

Able Laboratories
6 Hollywood Court
South Plainfield, NJ 07080

Adams (see Medeva)

Adria (see Pharmacia)

Agouron Pharmaceuticals, Inc
10350 N Torrey Pines Road
La Jolla, CA 92037
www.agouron.com

Akorn, Inc
2500 Millbrook Drive
Buffalo Grove, IL 60089
www.akorn.com

Alcon Laboratories, Inc
6201 South Freeway
Ft Worth, TX 76134-2099
www.alconlabs.com

Allerderm Laboratories
PO Box 2070
Petaluma, CA 94953-2070

Allergan Herbert (see Allergan)

Allergan Pharmaceuticals
PO Box 19534
Irvine, CA 92623-9534
www.allergan.com

Alpha Therapeutic Corp
5555 Valley Boulevard
Los Angeles, CA 90032

Alpharma
(U.S. Pharmaceuticals Division)
7205 Windsor Boulevard
Baltimore, MD 21244

Alra Labs, Inc
3850 Clearview Court
Gurnee, IL 60031

Alto Pharmaceuticals, Inc
PO Box 1910
Land O'Lakes, FL 34639-1910
altopharm@aol.com

Alza Pharmaceuticals
950 Page Mill Road
Palo Alto, CA 94303-0802
www.alza.com

Ambix Labs, Inc
210 Orchard Street
East Rutherford, NJ 07073

American Drug Industries, Inc
5810 South Perry Avenue
Chicago, IL 60621

American Pharmaceutical, Co
12 Dwight Place
Fairfield, NJ 07004-3434

American Regent Laboratories Inc
1 Luitpold Drive
Shirley, NY 11967

Ames (see Miles Biological Products)

Amgen Inc
One Amgen Center Drive
Thousand Oaks, CA 91320-1789
www.ext.amgen.com

Amide Pharmaceuticals, Inc
101 East Main Street
Little Falls, NJ 07424

Anaquest (see Ohmeda)

ANDRX Pharmaceuticals, Inc
4001 South West 47th Avenue
Fort Lauderdale, FL 33314

Angelini Pharmaceuticals, Inc
70 Grand Avenue
River Edge, NJ 07661
dapp@nac.net

Apotex Corp
50 Lakeview Parkway
Suite 127
Vernon Hills, IL 60061

Apothecary Products, Inc
11531 Rupp Drive
Burnsville, MN 55337-1295
pillminder@aol.com

Apothecon Products
(A Bristol-Myers Squibb Company)
PO Box 4500
Princeton, NJ 08543-4500
www.apothecon.com

Applied Genetics Inc
205 Buffalo Avenue
Freeport, NY 11520
www.agiderm.com

Arcola Laboratories
500 Arcola Road
Collegeville, PA 19426-0107
www.rpr.rpna.com

Astra Pharmaceuticals, L.P.
725 Chesterbrook Blvd
Wayne, PA 19087-5677
information.center@astramerck.com
www.astramerck.com

Baker Norton Pharmaceuticals, Inc
4400 Biscayne Boulevard
Miami, FL 33137

Banner Pharmacaps, Inc
PO Box 2210
4125 Premier Drive
High Point, NC 27261-2210

PHARMACEUTICAL MANUFACTURERS DIRECTORY
(Continued)

Barr Laboratories, Inc
Box 2900
Pomona, NY 10970-0519
www.barrlabs.com

Bausch & Lomb Pharmaceuticals, Inc
8500 Hidden River Parkway
Tampa, FL 33637
www.bausch.com

Bausch & Lomb Surgical
555 W Arrow Highway
Claremont, CA 91711
www.blsurgical.com

Baxter Healthcare Corporation
Corporate Headquarters
One Baxter Parkway
Deerfield, IL 60015-4833
www.baxter.com

Baxter Healthcare Corporation
(I.V. Systems Division)
One Baxter Parkway
Deerfield, IL 60015
www.baxter.com

Bayer Corporation
N 3525 Regal Street
Box 3145
Spokane, WA 99220

Bayer Corporation
(Diagnostic Division)
430 South Beiger Street
PO Box 2004
Mishawaka, IN 46544-2004
www.bayerdiag.com

Bayer Corporation
(Pharmaceutical Division)
400 Morgan Lane
West Haven, CT 06516-4175
www.bayer.com

Bayer, Inc
77 Belfield Road
Toronto, Ontario, Canada M9W 1G6
www.bayerdiag.com

Becton Dickinson Microbiology
Systems
(Division of Becton Dickinson and Company)
PO Box 999
7 Loveton Circle
Sparks, MD 21152
www.ms.bd.com

Bedford Laboratories
(Division of Ben Venue Laboratories)
300 Northfield Road
PO Box 46568
Bedford, OH 44146
www.boehringer-ingelheim.com

Beecham (see SmithKline Beecham)

Beiersdorf
PO Box 5529
Norwalk, CT 06856-5529

Beiersdorf Inc
187 Danbury Road
Wilton, CT 06897

Berlex Laboratories
15049 San Pablo Avenue
Richmond, CA 94804-0099
www.betaseron.com
www.fludara.com

Berna Products, Corp
4216 Ponce de Leon Blvd
Coral Gables, FL 33146
www.bernaproducts.com

Beta Dermaceuticals, Inc
PO Box 691106
San Antonio, TX 78216-1106

Beutlich Pharmaceuticals
1541 Shields Drive
Waukegan, IL 60085-8304
www.beutlich.com

Biocraft (see Teva USA)

Biogen Inc
14 Cambridge Center
Cambridge, MA 02142
www.biogen.com

Biopharmaceutics, Inc
990 Station Road
Bellport, NY 11713
www.feminique.com

Bio-Technology General Corp
70 Wood Avenue South
Iselin, NJ 08830

Blaine Company, Inc
1515 Production Drive
Burlington, KY 41005
www.blainepharma.com

Bock (see Sanofi Winthrop)

Boehringer Ingelheim
Pharmaceuticals, Inc
900 Ridgebury Road
PO Box 368
Ridgefield, CT 06877-0368
www.boehringer-ingelheim.com

Boots (see Knoll)

Braintree Laboratories, Inc
PO Box 850929
Braintree, MA 02185-0929

Brightstone Pharma
109 MacKenan Drive
Cary, NC 27511
www.brightstonepharma.com

Bristol-Myers Squibb
(Oncology/Immunology Division)
PO Box 4500
Princeton, NJ 08543-4500
www.bms.com

Bristol-Myers Squibb
(OTC Products)
225 High Ridge Road
Stanford, CT 06905
www.bms.com

Bristol-Myers Squibb Company
(Pharmaceutical Division)
PO Box 4500
Princeton, NJ 08543-4500

BTG (see Bio-Technology General Corp)

Burroughs Wellcome
(see Glaxo Wellcome)

C&M Pharmacal, Inc
1721 Maple Lane Avenue
Hazel Park, MI 48030-2696
www.glytone.com

**Caraco Pharmaceutical
Laboratories Ltd**
1150 Elijah McCoy Drive
Detroit, MI 48202
www.caraco.com

Celgene Corporation
7 Powder Horn Drive
Warren, NJ 07059

Centeon
1020 First Avenue
King of Prussia, PA 19406-1310
www.centeon.com/na

Center Labs
35 Channel Drive
Port Washington, NY 11050
www.centerpharm.com

Century Pharmaceuticals, Inc
10377 Hague Road
Indianapolis, IN 46256

Chemrich Laboratories
5211 Telegraph Road
Los Angeles, CA 90022

Cheshire Drugs
6225 Shiloh Road, Suite D
Alpharetta, GA 30005
www.cpsrx.com

Circa Pharmaceuticals, Inc
33 Ralph Avenue
PO Box 30
Copiague, NY 11726-0030
www.circapharm.com

Clay-Park Labs, Inc
Bathgate Industrial Park
1700 Bathgate Avenue
Bronx, NY 10457

Coast Labs, Inc
521 West 17th Street
Long Beach, CA 90813-1513

Copley Labs, Inc
25 John Road
Canton, MA 02021

Danbury Pharmacal, Inc
131 West Street
Danbury, CT 06810

Del-Ray Laboratories, Inc
22-20th Avenue North West
Birmingham, AL 35215

Denison Pharmaceuticals, Inc
60 Dunnell Lane
PO Box 1305
Pawtucket, RI 02862

Dermik Labs, Inc
500 Arcola Road
PO Box 1200
Collegeville, PA 19426-0107
www.rpr.rpna.com

Déy Laboratories
2751 Napa Valley Corporate Drive
Napa, CA 94558
www.deyinc.com

Duramed Pharmaceuticals, Inc
5040 Duramed Drive
Cincinnati, OH 45213
www.duramed.com

**Emrex/Economed Pharmaceuticals,
Inc**
4305 Sartin Road
PO Box 3303
Burlington, NC 27217

Endo Generic Products
223 Wilmington West Chester Pike
Chadds Ford, PA 19317
www.endo.com

Eon Labs Manufacturing, Inc
227-15 North Conduit Avenue
Laurelton, NY 11413

ESI Lederle
PO Box 41502
Philadelphia, PA 19101
www.AHP.com

Ethex Corp
10888 Metro Court
St Louis, MO 63043-2413
www.ethex.com

Falcon Opthalmics, Inc
6201 South Freeway
Fort Worth, TX 76134
Parent Company: Alcon Laboratories
www.alconlabs.com

**Faulding/Purepac Pharmaceutical
Co**
200 Elmora Avenue
Elizabeth, NJ 07207
www.faulding.com.au

Ferndale Laboratories, Inc
780 West Eight Mile Road
Ferndale, MI 48220

Fisons (see Medeva)

Fisons (see Rhone-Poulenc Rorer)

C.B. Fleet Co, Inc
4615 Murray Place
P0 Box 11349
Lynchburg, VA 24506-1349

Forest/Inwood Laboratories, Inc
500 Commack Road
Commack, NY 11725-5000

Forest Pharmaceuticals, Inc
13600 Shoreline Drive
St Louis, MO 63045
www.tiazac.com

**Fougera
(Division of Altana Inc)**
60 Baylis Road
Melville, NY 11747
www.fougera.com

**Fujisawa Healthcare, Inc
Parkway North Center**
Three Parkway North
Deerfield, IL 60015-2548
www.fujisawa.com

Galderma Laboratories, Inc
PO Box 331329
Fort Worth, TX 76163-1329
www.galderma.com

PHARMACEUTICAL MANUFACTURERS DIRECTORY
(Continued)

Gebauer Company
9410 St Catherine Avenue
Cleveland, OH 44104
www.gebauerco.com

GenDerm Corporation
600 Knightsbridge Parkway
Lincolnshire, IL 60069
www.genderm.com

Genentech, Inc
1 DNA Way
South San Francisco, CA 94080
www.gene.com

Genetco, Inc
711 Union Parkway
Ronkonkoma, NY 11779

Geneva Pharmaceuticals, Inc
2655 W Midway Boulevard
PO Box 446
Broomfield, CO 80038-0446
www.genevarx.com

Gensia Automedics, Inc
9360 Town Center Drive
San Diego, CA 92121
www.gensia.com

GensiaSicor Pharmaceuticals, Inc
19 Hughes
Irvine, CA 92618-1902
www.gensiasicor.com

Genzyme Corp
One Kendall Square
Cambridge, MA 02139
www.genzyme.com

Genzyme Genetics
5 Mountain Road
Framingham, MA 01701

Genzyme Tissue Repair
64 Sidney Street
Cambridge, MA 02139

Genzyme Transgenics
5 Mountain Road
Framingham, MA 01701

Gilead Sciences, Inc
333 Lakeside Drive
Foster City, CA 94404
www.gilead.com

Glades Pharmaceuticals, Inc
500 Satellite Boulevard
Suwanee, GA 30024
www.glades.com

Glaxo Wellcome, Inc
Five Moore Drive
Research Triangle Park, NC 27709
www.glaxowellcome.com

Glenwood, LLC
83 North Summit Street
Tenafly, NJ 07670
www.glenwood-llc.com

Glenwood-Palisades
One New England Avenue
Piscataway, NJ 08855

Global Pharmaceutical Corp
Castor & Kensington Avenues
Philadelphia, PA 19124
www.globalphar.com

Gray Pharmaceutical Company
100 Connecticut Avenue
Norwalk, CT 06856

Great Southern Laboratories
10863 Rockley Road
Houston, TX 77099

Guardian Drug Co
72 Prince Street
Trenton, NJ 08638

G&W Laboratories, Inc
111 Coolidge Street
South Plainfield, NJ 07080-3895

Gynex (see BTG)

Halsey Drug Company, Inc
695 North Perryville Road
Rockford, IL 61107
www.halseydrug.com

The Harvard Drug Group
31778 Enterprise Drive
Lovonia, MI 48150

Healthpoint
2600 Airport Freeway
Forth Worth, TX 76111
www.healthpoint.com

Heartland Healthcare Services
4755 South Avenue
Toledo, OH 43615

H&H Laboratories
4701 25 Mile Road
Shelby Township, MI 48316

Hi-Tech Pharmacal Co, Inc
369 Bayview Avenue
Amityville, NY 11701
www.diabeticproducts.com

Hoechst Marion Roussel, Inc
PO Box 9627
Kansas City, MO 64134-0627
www.hmri.com

Hoechst-Roussel
(see Hoechst Marion Roussel)

ICI Pharma (see Zeneca)

ICN Pharmaceuticals, Inc
3300 Hyland Avenue
Costa Mesa, CA 92626

Immunex Corporation
51 University Street
Seattle, WA 98101
www.immunex.com

ImmunoGen, Inc
148 Sidney Street
Cambridge, MA 02139

Immuno-U.S., Inc
1200 Parkdale Road
Rochester, MI 48307-1744

International Ethical Labs
Avenue America Miranda #1021
Reparto Metropolitano
Rio Piedras, Puerto Rico 00921

International Medication Systems, Ltd (IMS)
1886 Santa Anita Avenue
S El Monte, CA 91733

Interpharm, Inc
3 Fairchild Avenue
Plainview, NY 11803

Invamed, Inc
2400 Route 130 North
Dayton, NJ 08810

Ion Laboratories
7431 Pebble Drive
Fort Worth, TX 76118-6416

Janssen Pharmaceutica
1125 Trenton-Harbourton Road
PO Box 200
Titusville, NJ 08560-0200

Jerome Stevens Pharmaceuticals, Inc
60 Da Vinci Drive
Bohemia, NY 11716

Jones Pharma
1945 Craig Road
PO Box 46903
St Louis, MO 63146
www.jmedpharma.com

Kabi (see Pharmacia)

Kenwood Laboratories
383 Route 46 West
Fairfield, NJ 07004-2402
www.bradpharm.com

Key Pharmaceutical
2000 Galloping Hill Road
Kenilworth, NJ 07033

King Pharmaceuticals, Inc
501 Fifth Street
Bristol, TN 37620
www.kingpharm.com

The Knoll Pharmaceutical Company
30 North Jefferson Road
Whippany, NJ 07981

Konsyl Pharmaceuticals, Inc
4200 South Hulen
Fort Worth, TX 76109
www.konsyl.com

Kremers Urban
PO Box 427
Mequon, WI 53092

Lannett Co, Inc
9000 State Road
Philadelphia, PA 19136-1615
www.lannett.com

Lederle (see Wyeth-Ayerst)

Lemmon (see Teva USA)

Eli Lilly and Company
Lilly Corporate Center
Indianapolis, IN 46285
www.lilly.com

The Liposome Company, Inc
One Research Way
Princeton, NJ 08540-6619
www.lipo.com

Liquipharm, Inc
PO Box D-3700
Pomona, NY 10970
www.liquipharm.com

L. Perrigo Company
515 Eastern Avenue
Allegan, MI 49010
www.perrigo.com

Lyphomed (see Fujisawa)

3M Pharmaceuticals
3M Center, 275-2E-13
PO Box 33275
St Paul, MN 55133-3275
www.mmm.com/pharma/

Mallinckrodt
675 McDonnell Boulevard
PO Box 5840
St Louis, MO 63134
www.mkg.com
www.mallinckrodt.com

Marion Merrell Dow
(see Hoechst Marion Roussel)

Marlop Pharmaceuticals, Inc
5704 Mosholu Avenue
Bronx, NY 10471-0536

Marsam Pharmaceuticals Inc (Subsidiary of Schein Pharmaceutical, Inc)
PO Box 1022
24 Olney Avenue, Bldg 31
Cherry Hill, NJ 08003
www.schein-rx.com

Martec Pharmaceutical, Inc
1800 North Topping Avenue
PO Box 33510
Kansas City, MO 64120-3510
Parent Company: Ratiopharm, GmbH
www.martec-kc.com

Mason Pharmaceuticals, Inc
4425 Jamboree Road
Suite 250
Newport Beach, CA 92660

McGaw, Inc
PO Box 19791
Irvine, CA 92713-9791

McNeil Pharmaceutical
Route 202, PO Box 300
Raritan, NJ 08869-0602
www.ortho-mcneil.com

Mead Johnson (see Bristol-Myers Squibb)

Med-Derm Pharmaceuticals
PO Box 5193
Kingsport, TN 37663

Medeva Pharmaceuticals, Inc
PO Box 1710
755 Jefferson Road
Rochester, NY 14603-1710
www.medeva.com

Medirex, Inc
20 Chapin Road
PO Box 731
Pine Brook, NJ 07058
Parent Company: Sidmak Laboratories

PHARMACEUTICAL MANUFACTURERS DIRECTORY
(Continued)

Merck Human Health Division
PO Box 4, WP39-207
West Point, PA 19486-0004
www.merck.com

Meridian Medical Technologies, Inc
10240 Old Columbia Road
Columbia, MD 21046
info@meridianmt.com
www.meridianmeds.com

Merrell Dow
(see Hoechst Marion Roussel)

Merz Pharmaceuticals, Inc
4215 Tudor Lane
Greensboro, NC 27410

MGI Pharma, Inc
9900 Bren Road East
Suite 300E, Opus Center
Minnetonka, MN 55343-9667

Mikart, Inc
1750 Chattahoochee Avenue
Atlanta, GA 30318
www.mikart.com

Miles (see Bayer)

Miles Allergy (see Bayer)

Monarch (see King Pharm)

Monarch Pharmaceuticals, Inc
355 Beecham Street
Bristol, TN 37620
www.monarchpharm.com

Moore Medical
389 John Downey Drive
New Britain, CT 06050
www.mooremedical.com

Morton Grove Pharmaceuticals, Inc
6451 West Main Street
Morton Grove, IL 60053
www.mgp-online.com

Mova Pharmaceutical Corp
214 Carnegie Center
Suite 106
Princeton, NJ 08540

Muro Pharmaceuticals, Inc
890 East Street
Tewksbury, MA 01876

**Mutual Pharmaceutical Co, Inc/
United Research Laboratories**
1100 Orthodox Street
Philadelphia, PA 19124
www.mutual.com

Mylan Pharmaceuticals, Inc
781 Chestnut Ridge Rd
PO Box 4310
Morgantown, WV 26504-4310
www.mylan.com

**Nephron Pharmaceuticals
Corporation**
4121 - 34th Street SW
Orlando, FL 32811-6458
www.hephronpharm.com
rwilburn@pharmacy.com

Nestle Clinical Nutrition
3 Parkway North, Suite 500
PO Box 760
Deerfield, IL 60015

Norwich Eaton (see Proctor &
Gamble)

Novartis Pharmaceuticals
59 Route 10
East Hanover, NJ 07939
www.novartis.com

Novo Nordisk Pharmaceuticals Inc
100 Overlook Center
Suite 200
Princeton, NJ 08540
www.novo-nordisk.com

Novopharm USA, Inc
165 East Commerce Drive
Schaumburg, IL 60173-5326
www.novopharmusa.com

Ohm Laboratories, Inc
PO Box 7397
North Brunswick, NJ 08902
Parent Company: Ranbaxy
Pharmaceuticals
www.ranbaxy.com

Ohmeda
(see Baxter Pharmaceutical Products)

OMJ Pharmaceuticals, Inc
PO Box 367
San German, Puerto Rico 00683

Organon Inc
375 Mt Pleasant Avenue
West Orange, NJ 07052
shapsed@am.father.umc.akzonobel.nl

Ortho Biotech Inc
700 Route 202 South
PO Box 670
Raritan, NJ 08869-0670
www.procrit.com

Ortho-McNeil Pharmaceutical, Inc
PO Box 300
Route 202
Raritan, NJ 08869-06O2
www.ortho-mcneil.com

Otsuka America Pharmaceutical Inc
2440 Research Boulevard
Rockville, MD 20850

Paddock Laboratories
PO Box 27286
3940 Quebec Avenue North
Minneapolis, MN 55427
www.paddocklabs.com

PAR Pharmaceutical, Inc
One Ram Ridge Road
Spring Valley, NY 10977
Parent Company: Pharmaceutical
Resources, Inc
www.parpharm.com

**Parkedale Pharmaceuticals, Inc
(Subsidiary of King
Pharmaceuticals, Inc)**
501 Fifth Street
Bristol, TN 37620
www.kingpharm.com

Parke-Davis
(Division of Warner-Lambert Company)
201 Tabor Road
Morris Plains, NJ 07950
www.warner-lambert.com

Parmed Pharmaceuticals, Inc
4220 Hyde Park Boulevard
Niagra Falls, NY 14305-6714
Parent Company: Alpharma

Parnell Pharmaceuticals, Inc
1525 Francisco Blvd
San Rafael, CA 94901
www.parnellpharm.com

Pasteur Merieux Connaught
Discovery Drive
Swiftwater, PA 18370-0187
www.us.pmc-vacc.com

PD-RX Pharmaceuticals
72 North Ann Arbor
Oklahoma City, OK 73127
www.pdrx.com

Pecos Pharmaceutical
25301 Cabot Road
Suites 212-213
Laguna Hills, CA 92653

Pedinol Pharmacal Inc
30 Banfi Plaza North
Farmingdale, NY 11735
www.pedinol.com

Person & Covey
616 Allen Avenue
Glendale, CA 91201

Pfizer First Connect Information Network
Pfizer Inc
U.S. Pharmaceuticals Group
235 East 42nd Street
New York, NY 10017-5755
www.pfizer.com

Pharma Tek, Inc
PO Box 1920
Huntington, NY 11743
www.pharma-tek.com

Pharmaceutical Formulations, Inc
460 Plainfield Avenue
Edison, NJ 08818

Pharmaceutical Laboratories
1170 W Corporate Drive
Suite 102
Arlington, TX 76006

Pharmaceutical Specialties, Inc
PO Box 6298
2112 15th Street NW
Rochester, MN 55901
www.psico.com

Pharmacia & Upjohn Company
(Ophthalmics Division)
701 E Milham Road
Kalamazoo, MI 49001
pnu.com

Pharmacia & Upjohn, Inc
7000 Portage Road
Kalamazoo, MI 49001
pnu.com

Pharmacy Division of Bayer
400 Morgan Lane
Westhaven, Conneticut 06516-4175
www.bayer.com

Pharmakon Labs, Inc
6050 Jet Port Industrial Boulevard
Tampa, FL 33634

Pharmics, Inc
PO Box 27554
Salt Lake City, UT 84127
www.pharmics.com

Physician's Total Care
5415 South 125th East Avenue
Suite 205
Tulsa, OK 74146

Plantex USA, Inc
482 Hudson Terrace
Englewood Cliffs, NJ 07632

Pratt Pharmaceuticals Division
Pfizer Inc
U.S. Pharmaceuticals Group
235 East 42nd Street
New York, NY 10017-5755

Procter & Gamble Pharmaceuticals
PO Box 231
Norwich, NY 13815-0231

Procter & Gamble Pharmaceuticals
11450 Grooms Road
Cincinnati, OH 45242-1434

The Purdue Frederick Company
100 Connecticut Avenue
Norwalk, CT 06850-3590

PUREPAC Pharmaceutical Co
200 Elmora Avenue
Elizabeth, NJ 07207
Parent Company: F.H. Faulding and Company
www.Faulding.com

Qualitest Pharmaceuticals, Inc
1236 Jordan Road
Huntsville, AL 35811

Quality Research Pharmaceuticals, Inc
1117 Third Avenue South West
Carmel, IN 46032

Ranbaxy Pharmaceuticals, Inc
600 College Road East
Princeton, NJ 08540

Reed & Carnrick (see Schwarz Pharma)

Rhone-Poulenc Rorer Pharmaceuticals, Inc
500 Arcola Road
PO Box 5094
Collegeville, PA 19426-0998
www.rp-rorer.com

Richwood Pharmaceutical Company, Inc
7900 Tanners Gate Drive
Suite 200
Florence, KY 41042

R.I.D. Inc
609 North Mednik Avenue
Los Angeles, CA 90022

PHARMACEUTICAL MANUFACTURERS DIRECTORY
(Continued)

Roberts Pharmaceutical Corp
4 Industrial Way West
Eatontown, NJ 07724
www.robertspharm.com

Robins (see Wyeth-Ayerst)

Roche Laboratories
340 Kingsland Street
Nutley, NJ 07110
www.roche.com

Roerig Division
Pfizer Inc
U.S. Pharmaceuticals Group
235 East 42nd Street
New York, NY 10017-5755

Rorer (see Rhone-Poulenc Rorer)

Rosemont Pharmaceutical Corp
301 South Cherokee Street
Denver, CO 80223
Parent Company: Akzo Nobel

Roxane Laboratories, Inc
1809 Wilson Road
Columbus, OH 43228
PO Box 16532
Columbus, OH 43216
www.roxane.com

Rugby Laboratories, Inc
2725 Northwoods Parkway
Norcross, GA 30071
Parent Company: Watson Laboratories

Sandoz Pharmaceuticals Corp
59 Route 10
East Hanover, NJ 07936
www.sandoz.com

Sanofi Pharmaceuticals
90 Park Avenue
New York, NY 10016

Savage Laboratories
(Division of Altana Inc)
60 Baylis Road
Melville, NY 11747
www.savagelabs.com

Scandipharm, Inc
22 Inverness Center Parkway
Suite 310
Birmingham, AL 35242
www.scandipharm.com

Schaffer Laboratories
1058 North Allen Avenue
Pasadina, CA 91104

Schein Pharmaceutical, Inc
100 Campus Drive
Florham Park, NJ 07932
www.schein-rx.com

Schering Laboratories
2000 Galloping Hill Road
Kenilworth, NJ 07033
www.myhealth.com

Schwarz Pharma
5600 West County Line Road
Mequon, WI 53092
www.schwarzusa.com
www.schwarzpharma.com

G.D. Searle & Company
5200 Old Orchard Road
Skokie, IL 60077
www.searlehealthnet.com

Seneca Pharmaceutical, Inc
PO Box 25021
8621 Barefoot Industrial Road
Raleigh, NC 27613

Sequus Pharmaceuticals, Inc
980 Hamilton Court
Mento Park, CA 94025
www.sequus.com

Serono Laboratories, Inc
100 Longwater Circle
Norwell, MA 02061
www.seronousa.com

Sheffield Laboratories
170 Broad Street
New London, CT 06320
www.sheffield-labs.com

Shire Richwood, Inc
7900 Tanners Gate Drive
Suite 200
Florence, KY 41042
www.shiregroup.com

Sidmak Laboratories, Inc
17 West Street
PO Box 371
East Hanover, NJ 07936-0371
www.sidmaklab.com

Sigma-Tau Pharmaceuticals, Inc
800 South Frederick Avenue
Suite 300
Gaithersburg, MD 20877
www.sigmatau.com/na

SmithKline Beecham
PO Box 7929
One Franklin Plaza
Philadelphia, PA 19101-7920
charles.depew@sb.com
www.sb.com

SmithKline Beecham Consumer
Healthcare
PO Box 1467
Pittsburgh, PA 15230
www.sb.com

Sola/Barnes (see Pilkington Barnes
Hind)

SoloPak Pharmaceuticals Inc
6001 Broken Sound Parkway
Suite 600
Boca Raton, FL 33487

Solvay Pharmaceuticals, Inc
901 Sawyer Road
Marietta, GA 30062
www.solvay.com

Somerset Pharmaceuticals, Inc
PO Box 30706
Tampa, FL 33630-3706

Southward Pharmaceuticals, Inc
33 Hammond Street
Suite 201
Irvine, CA 92718

Squibb (see Bristol-Myers Squibb)

Steris Laboratories, Inc
620 N 51st Avenue
Phoenix, AZ 85043-4705
Parent Company: Schein Pharmaceutical
www.schein-rx.com

Sterling (see Sanofi Winthrop)

Stratus Pharmaceuticals
14377 South West 142nd Street
Miami, FL 33186
www.stratuspharmaceuticals.com

Stuart (see Zeneca)

Superior Pharmaceutical Co
1385 Kemper Meadow Drive
Cincinnati, OH 45240-1635
www.superiorpharm.com

Survival (see Meridian Medical)

Syncor Pharmaceuticals, Inc
1313 Washington Avenue
Golden, CO 80401

Syntex (see Roche)

TAP Pharmaceuticals, Inc
2355 Waukegan Road
Deerfield, IL 60015

Taro Pharmaceuticals USA, Inc
5 Skyline Drive
Hawthorne, NY 10532
www.taropharma.com

Taylor Pharmaceuticals
1222 West Grand
Decatur, IL 62526

Teva Pharmaceuticals USA
151 Domorah Drive
Montgomeryville, PA 18936
www.tevapharmusa.com

Teva Pharmaceuticals USA
650 Cathill Road
Sellersville, PA 18960
www.tevapharmusa.com

Thames Pharmacal Co
2100 Fifth Avenue
Ronkonkoma, NY 11779

Triton (see Berlex)

UCB Pharma, Inc
1950 Lake Park Drive
Smyrna, GA 30080
suzan.leake@ucb-group.com

UDL Laboratories, Inc
PO Box 2629
Loves Park, IL 61132-2629

Upjohn (see Pharmacia & Upjohn)

Upsher-Smith Laboratories, Inc
14905 23rd Avenue North
Minneapolis, MN 55447
www.upsher-smith.com

U.S. Pharmaceutical Corp
2401 Mellon Court
Suite C
Decatur, GA 30035

Value in Pharmaceuticals (VIP)
3000 Alt Boulevard
Grand Island, NY 14702
www.vippharm.com

Wallace Laboratories
(Division of Carter-Wallace, Inc)
Half Acre Road
Cranbury, NJ 08512-0181

Warner Chilcott Laboratories
Rockaway 80 Corporate Center
100 Enterprise Drive
Suite 280
Rockaway, NJ 07866
www.wclabs.com

Warrick Pharmaceuticals
1095 Morris Avenue
Union, NJ 07083-7137

Watson Laboratories, Inc
311 Bonnie Circle
Corona, CA 91720
www.watsonpharm.com

West-Ward
465 Industrial Way West
Eatontown, NJ 07724
Parent Company: Hikma Pharmaceuticals

Westwood-Squibb
(Dermatologic Division)
100 Forest Avenue
Buffalo, NY 14213
www.westwood-squibb.com

Whitby (see UCB Pharma)

Winthrop (see Sanofi Winthrop)

Wyeth-Ayerst Laboratories
PO Box 8299
Philadelphia, PA 19101-1245
www.ahp.com

Zeneca Pharmaceuticals
1800 Concord Pike
Wilmington, DE 19803
www.zeneca.com

Zenith Goldline Pharmaceuticals
4400 Biscayne Boulevard
Miami, FL 33137
Parent Company: Ivax Corp
www.ivax.com

Zila Pharmaceuticals, Inc
5227 North 7th Street
Phoenix, AZ 85014-2800
www.zila.com

INDICATION/THERAPEUTIC CATEGORY
INDEX

ABDOMINAL DISTENTION (POSTOPERATIVE)

Hormone, Posterior Pituitary

ABETALIPOPROTEINEMIA

Vitamin, Fat Soluble

ABORTION

Electrolyte Supplement, Oral

Oxytocic Agent

Prostaglandin

ACETAMINOPHEN POISONING

Mucolytic Agent

ACHALASIA

Adrenergic Agonist Agent

Calcium Channel Blocker

Vasodilator

ACHLORHYDRIA

Gastrointestinal Agent, Miscellaneous

ACIDOSIS (METABOLIC)

Alkalinizing Agent

Electrolyte Supplement, Oral

ACNE

Acne Products

Antibiotic, Topical

Antiseborrheic Agent, Topical

Keratolytic Agent

Retinoic Acid Derivative

Tetracycline Derivative

ANESTHESIA (OPHTHALMIC)

Local Anesthetic

ANGINA

Beta-Adrenergic Blocker

Calcium Channel Blocker

Vasodilator

ANGIOEDEMA (HEREDITARY)

Anabolic Steroid

Androgen

ANGIOGRAPHY (OPHTHALMIC)

Diagnostic Agent

ANTHRAX

Vaccine

ANTICHOLINERGIC DRUG POISONING

Cholinesterase Inhibitor

ANTIFREEZE POISONING

Antidote

ANTITHROMBIN III DEFICIENCY (HEREDITARY)

Blood Product Derivative

ANXIETY

Antianxiety Agent

Antianxiety Agent, Miscellaneous

Antidepressant/Phenothiazine

Antidepressant, Tetracyclic

Antidepressant, Tricyclic (Secondary Amine)

Antidepressant, Tricyclic (Tertiary Amine)

Antihistamine

Barbiturate

Benzodiazepine

General Anesthetic

Phenothiazine Derivative

Sedative

APNEA (NEONATAL IDIOPATHIC)

Theophylline Derivative

ARIBOFLAVINOSIS

Vitamin, Water Soluble

ARRHYTHMIAS

Adrenergic Agonist Agent

Antiarrhythmic Agent, Class I

Antiarrhythmic Agent, Class I-A

Antiarrhythmic Agent, Class I-B

Antiarrhythmic Agent, Class I-C

(Continued)

Local Anesthetic

BITES (SNAKE)

Antivenin

BITES (SPIDER)

Antivenin

Electrolyte Supplement, Oral

Skeletal Muscle Relaxant

BLADDER IRRIGATION

Antibacterial, Topical

BLASTOMYCOSIS

Antifungal Agent

BLEPHARITIS

Antifungal Agent

BLEPHAROSPASM

Ophthalmic Agent, Toxin

BOWEL CLEANSING

Laxative

BOWEL STERILIZATION

Aminoglycoside (Antibiotic)

BREAST ENGORGEMENT (POSTPARTUM)

Androgen

Estrogen and Androgen Combination

Estrogen Derivative

BROAD BETA DISEASE

Antihyperlipidemic Agent, Miscellaneous

Antilipemic Agent

BROMIDE INTOXICATION

Diuretic, Loop

BRONCHIECTASIS

Adrenergic Agonist Agent
(Continued)

CARCINOMA

Adrenergic Agonist Agent *(Continued)*

Antihistamine

Antihistamine/Antitussive

Antihistamine/Decongestant/Analgesic

Antihistamine/Decongestant/Anticholinergic

Antihistamine/Decongestant/Antitussive

Antihistamine/Decongestant Combination

Antitussive/Decongestant

(Continued)

(Continued)

ESOTROPIA

Cholinergic Agent
isoflurophate 347

Cholinesterase Inhibitor
demecarium 185
echothiophate iodide 227

ESSENTIAL THROMBOCYTHEMIA (ET)

Platelet Aggregation Inhibitor
anagrelide 48

ETHYLENE GLYCOL POISONING

Pharmaceutical Aid
alcohol, ethyl 26

EXTRAPYRAMIDAL SYMPTOMS

Anticholinergic Agent
benztropine 82
biperiden 87
procyclidine 520
trihexyphenidyl 628

EXTRAVASATION

Alpha-Adrenergic Blocking Agent
phentolamine 487

Antidote
hyaluronidase 315
sodium thiosulfate 576

EYE INFECTION

Antibiotic/Corticosteroid, Ophthalmic
bacitracin, neomycin, polymyxin B, and hydrocortisone 72
chloramphenicol and prednisolone 133
chloramphenicol, polymyxin B, and hydrocortisone 134
neomycin and dexamethasone 435
neomycin and hydrocortisone 435
neomycin, polymyxin B, and dexamethasone 436
neomycin, polymyxin B, and hydrocortisone 437
neomycin, polymyxin B, and prednisolone 438
oxytetracycline and hydrocortisone 465
prednisolone and gentamicin 514
sulfacetamide and prednisolone 585
sulfacetamide sodium and fluorometholone 586
tobramycin and dexamethasone 616

Antibiotic, Ophthalmic
bacitracin 70
bacitracin and polymyxin B 71
bacitracin, neomycin, and polymyxin B 71
chloramphenicol 133
ciprofloxacin 151
erythromycin (ophthalmic/topical) 239
gentamicin 290
neomycin, polymyxin B, and gramicidin 437
ofloxacin 454
oxytetracycline and polymyxin B 465
sulfacetamide 584
sulfacetamide and phenylephrine 585
tetracycline 601
tobramycin 615
trimethoprim and polymyxin B 630

Antibiotic, Topical
silver protein, mild 566

EYE IRRITATION

Adrenergic Agonist Agent
phenylephrine and zinc sulfate 489

EYELID INFECTION

Antibiotic, Ophthalmic
mercuric oxide 395

Pharmaceutical Aid
boric acid 90

FACTOR IX DEFICIENCY

Antihemophilic Agent

FACTOR VIII DEFICIENCY

Blood Product Derivative

Hemophilic Agent

FAMILIAL ADENOMATOUS POLYPOSIS

Nonsteroidal Anti-inflammatory Drug (NSAID), COX-2 Selective

FATTY ACID DEFICIENCY

Intravenous Nutritional Therapy

Nutritional Supplement

FEBRILE NEUTROPENIA

Quinolone

FEVER

Antipyretic

FIBROCYSTIC BREAST DISEASE

Androgen

FIBROCYSTIC DISEASE

Vitamin, Fat Soluble

FIBROMYOSITIS

Antidepressant, Tricyclic (Tertiary Amine)

FOLLICLE STIMULATION

Ovulation Stimulator

FUNGUS (DIAGNOSTIC)

Diagnostic Agent

GAG REFLEX SUPPRESSION

Analgesic, Topical

Local Anesthetic

GALACTORRHEA

Antihistamine

Ergot Alkaloid and Derivative

(Continued)

HERPES SIMPLEX

Antiviral Agent

HERPES ZOSTER

Analgesic, Topical

Antiviral Agent

HIATAL HERNIA

Antacid

HICCUPS

Phenothiazine Derivative

HISTOPLASMOSIS

Antifungal Agent

HODGKIN'S DISEASE

Antineoplastic Agent

HOMOCYSTINURIA

Urinary Tract Product

HOOKWORMS

Anthelmintic

HORMONAL IMBALANCE (FEMALE)

Progestin

H. PYLORI INFECTION

Antidiarrheal

HYPERPROLACTINEMIA

Ergot Alkaloid and Derivative

Ergot-like Derivative

HYPERSENSITIVITY SKIN TESTING (DIAGNOSTIC)

Diagnostic Agent

HYPERTENSION

Adrenergic Agonist Agent

Alpha-Adrenergic Agonist

Alpha-Adrenergic Blocking Agent

Alpha-/Beta- Adrenergic Blocker

Angiotensin-Converting Enzyme (ACE) Inhibitor

Angiotensin II Antagonist

Antihypertensive Agent, Combination
(Continued)

Antihypertensive Agent, Combination *(Continued)*

Beta-Adrenergic Blocker

Calcium Channel Blocker

Diuretic, Combination

Diuretic, Loop

Diuretic, Miscellaneous

Diuretic, Potassium Sparing

Diuretic, Thiazide

Ganglionic Blocking Agent

Miscellaneous Product

Rauwolfia Alkaloid

(Continued)

(Continued)

KERATOSIS (ACTINIC)

Topical Skin Product
masoprocol 385

KIDNEY FUNCTION (DIAGNOSTIC)

Diagnostic Agent
phenolsulfonphthalein 486

KIDNEY STONE

Alkalinizing Agent
potassium citrate 508
sodium citrate and potassium citrate mixture 572

Chelating Agent
penicillamine 473

Electrolyte Supplement, Oral
potassium phosphate 509
potassium phosphate and sodium phosphate 510

Irrigating Solution
citric acid bladder mixture 154

Urinary Tract Product
cellulose sodium phosphate 127
tiopronin 614

Xanthine Oxidase Inhibitor
allopurinol 29

LABOR INDUCTION

Oxytocic Agent
oxytocin 465

Prostaglandin
carboprost tromethamine 115
dinoprostone 207
dinoprost tromethamine 207

LABOR (PREMATURE)

Adrenergic Agonist Agent
ritodrine 551
terbutaline 596

LACTATION (SUPPRESSION)

Ergot Alkaloid and Derivative
bromocriptine 93

LACTOSE INTOLERANCE

Nutritional Supplement
lactase 357

LEAD POISONING

Chelating Agent
dimercaprol 206
edetate calcium disodium 227
penicillamine 473
succimer 582

LEG CRAMPS

Blood Viscosity Reducer Agent
pentoxifylline 480

LEPROSY

Immunosuppressant Agent
thalidomide 602

Leprostatic Agent
clofazimine 158

Sulfone
dapsone 182

LEUKAPHERESIS

Blood Modifiers
pentastarch 478

LEUKEMIA

Antineoplastic Agent
asparaginase 60
(Continued)

(Continued)

MUMPS (DIAGNOSTIC)

Diagnostic Agent

MUSCARINE POISONING

Anticholinergic Agent

MUSCLE SPASM

Skeletal Muscle Relaxant

MYASTHENIA GRAVIS

Cholinergic Agent

Skeletal Muscle Relaxant

MYCOBACTERIUM AVIUM-INTRACELLULARE

Antibiotic, Aminoglycoside

Antibiotic, Miscellaneous

Antimycobacterial Agent

Antitubercular Agent

Carbapenem (Antibiotic)

Leprostatic Agent

Macrolide (Antibiotic)

Quinolone

MYCOSIS (FUNGOIDES)

Psoralen

MYDRIASIS

Adrenergic Agonist Agent

Anticholinergic/Adrenergic Agonist

Anticholinergic Agent

MYELOMA

Antineoplastic Agent

MYOCARDIAL INFARCTION

Anticoagulant

Antiplatelet Agent

Beta-Adrenergic Blocker

Thrombolytic Agent

MYOCARDIAL REINFARCTION

Antiplatelet Agent

Beta-Adrenergic Blocker

NARCOLEPSY

Adrenergic Agonist Agent

Amphetamine

Central Nervous System Stimulant, Nonamphetamine

NARCOTIC DETOXIFICATION

Analgesic, Narcotic

NAUSEA

Anticholinergic Agent

Antiemetic

Antihistamine

Gastrointestinal Agent, Prokinetic

(Continued)

Antidiarrheal

Gastric Acid Secretion Inhibitor

Gastrointestinal Agent, Gastric or Duodenal Ulcer Treatment

Gastrointestinal Agent, Miscellaneous

Histamine H$_2$ Antagonist

Macrolide (Antibiotic)

Penicillin

PERIANAL WART

Immune Response Modifier

PERIPHERAL VASCULAR DISEASE

Vasodilator, Peripheral

PERIPHERAL VASOSPASTIC DISORDERS

Alpha-Adrenergic Blocking Agent

PERSISTENT FETAL CIRCULATION (PFC)

Alpha-Adrenergic Blocking Agent

PERSISTENT PULMONARY HYPERTENSION OF THE NEWBORN (PPHN)

Alpha-Adrenergic Blocking Agent

PERSISTENT PULMONARY VASOCONSTRICTION

Alpha-Adrenergic Blocking Agent

PHARYNGITIS

Antibiotic, Penicillin

Cephalosporin (First Generation)

Cephalosporin (Second Generation)

Cephalosporin (Third Generation)

Macrolide (Antibiotic)

Penicillin
(Continued)

PLATELET AGGREGATION (PROPHYLAXIS)

Antiplatelet Agent

PNEUMOCYSTIS CARINII

Antibiotic, Miscellaneous

Antiprotozoal

Sulfonamide

Sulfone

PNEUMONIA

Aminoglycoside (Antibiotic)

Antibiotic, Miscellaneous

Antibiotic, Penicillin

Antibiotic, Quinolone

Carbapenem (Antibiotic)

Cephalosporin (First Generation)

Cephalosporin (Fourth Generation)

Cephalosporin (Second Generation)

Cephalosporin (Third Generation)

Macrolide (Antibiotic)

Penicillin
(Continued)

PORPHYRIA

Blood Modifiers
hemin 310

Phenothiazine Derivative
chlorpromazine 144

PORTAL-SYSTEMIC ENCEPHALOPATHY (PSE)

Ammonium Detoxicant
lactulose 359

PRE-ECLAMPSIA

Electrolyte Supplement, Oral
magnesium sulfate 382

PREGNANCY (PROPHYLAXIS)

Contraceptive, Implant (Progestin)
levonorgestrel 366

Contraceptive, Oral
ethinyl estradiol and desogestrel 248
ethinyl estradiol and ethynodiol diacetate 249
ethinyl estradiol and levonorgestrel 250
ethinyl estradiol and norethindrone 250
ethinyl estradiol and norgestimate 251
ethinyl estradiol and norgestrel 252
mestranol and norethindrone 396

Contraceptive, Progestin Only
levonorgestrel 366
medroxyprogesterone acetate 389
norethindrone 447
norgestrel 448

Spermicide
nonoxynol 9 446

PREOPERATIVE SEDATION

Analgesic, Narcotic
levorphanol 367
meperidine 392

Antihistamine
hydroxyzine 328

Barbiturate
pentobarbital 479
phenobarbital 485

Benzodiazepine
midazolam 415

General Anesthetic
fentanyl 263

PRIMARY PULMONARY HYPERTENSION (PPH)

Platelet Inhibitor
epoprostenol 236

PROCTITIS

5-Aminosalicylic Acid Derivative
mesalamine 395

PROCTOSIGMOIDITIS

5-Aminosalicylic Acid Derivative
mesalamine 395

PROSTATITIS

Quinolone
ofloxacin 454

Sulfonamide
co-trimoxazole 170

PROTEIN UTILIZATION

Dietary Supplement
l-lysine 373

PROTOZOAL INFECTIONS

Antiprotozoal
furazolidone 285
(Continued)

PURPURA (THROMBOCYTOPENIC)

Antineoplastic Agent
vincristine 648

PYELONEPHRITIS

Antibiotic, Quinolone
gatifloxacin *New Drug* 288

PYRIMETHAMINE POISONING

Folic Acid Derivative
leucovorin 362

RABIES

Serum
antirabies serum (equine) 53

RAT-BITE FEVER

Antibiotic, Aminoglycoside
streptomycin 581

Antitubercular Agent
streptomycin 581

RATTLESNAKE BITE

Antivenin
antivenin (*Crotalidae*) polyvalent 54

RAYNAUD'S DISEASE

Vasodilator
isoxsuprine 350

RENAL ALLOGRAFT REJECTION

Immunosuppressant Agent
antithymocyte globulin (rabbit) *New Drug* 54

RENAL COLIC

Analgesic, Non-narcotic
ketorolac tromethamine 355

Anticholinergic Agent
hyoscyamine, atropine, scopolamine, and phenobarbital 330

RESPIRATORY DISORDERS

Adrenal Corticosteroid
betamethasone (systemic) 84
corticotropin 169
cortisone acetate 169
dexamethasone (oral inhalation) 190
dexamethasone (systemic) 190
hydrocortisone (systemic) 323
methylprednisolone 407
paramethasone acetate 470
prednisolone (systemic) 514
prednisone 515
triamcinolone (inhalation, oral) 623
triamcinolone (systemic) 624

RESPIRATORY DISTRESS SYNDROME

Lung Surfactant
beractant 83
colfosceril palmitate 166

RESPIRATORY DISTRESS SYNDROME (RDS)

Lung Surfactant
calfactant 108

RESPIRATORY SYNCYTIAL VIRUS

Antiviral Agent
ribavirin 547

RESPIRATORY SYNCYTIAL VIRUS (RSV)

Monoclonal Antibody
palivizumab 466

RESPIRATORY TRACT INFECTION

Aminoglycoside (Antibiotic)
gentamicin 290

(Continued)

(Continued)

(Continued)

(Continued)

Antibiotic, Miscellaneous *(Continued)*

Antibiotic, Penicillin

Antibiotic, Quinolone

Cephalosporin (First Generation)

Cephalosporin (Fourth Generation)

Cephalosporin (Second Generation)

Cephalosporin (Third Generation)

Genitourinary Irrigant

Irrigating Solution

Penicillin

Quinolone

(Continued)

Histamine H$_2$ Antagonist *(Continued)*

  Prostaglandin

ZOLLINGER-ELLISON SYNDROME (DIAGNOSTIC)

  Diagnostic Agent

NOTES

Other titles offered by

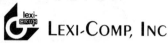
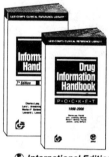
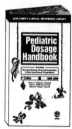
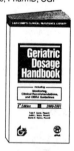

INFECTIOUS DISEASES HANDBOOK 3rd Edition 1999-2000

by Carlos M. Isada MD; Bernard L. Kasten Jr. MD; Morton P. Goldman PharmD; Larry D. Gray PhD; and Judith A. Aberg MD

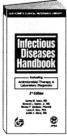

🌐 *International Edition also available*

This four-in-one quick reference is concerned with the identification and treatment of infectious diseases. Each of the four sections of the book (166 disease syndromes, 152 organisms, 238 laboratory tests, and 295 antimicrobials) contain related information and cross-referencing to one or more of the other three sections.

The disease syndrome section provides the clinical presentation, differential diagnosis, diagnostic tests, and drug therapy recommended for treatment of more common infectious diseases. The organism section presents the microbiology, epidemiology, diagnosis, and treatment of each organism. The laboratory diagnosis section describes performance of specific tests and procedures. The antimicrobial therapy section presents important facts and considerations regarding each drug recommended for specific diseases of organisms.

DRUG-INDUCED NUTRIENT DEPLETION HANDBOOK 1999-2000

by Ross Pelton, RPh, PhD, CCN; James B. LaValle, RPh, DHM, NMD, CCN; Ernest B. Hawkins, RPh, MS; Daniel L. Krinsky, RPh, MS

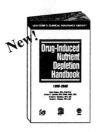

A complete and up-to-date listing of all drugs known to deplete the body of nutritional compounds.

This book is alphabetically organized and provides extensive cross-referencing to related information in the various sections of the book. Nearly 150 generic drugs that cause nutrient depletion are identified and are cross-referenced to more detailed descriptions of the nutrients depleted and their actions. Symptoms of deficiencies, and sources of repletion are also included. This book also contains a Studies and Abstracts section, a valuable Appendix, and Alphabetical & Pharma-cological Indices.

NATURAL THERAPEUTICS POCKET GUIDE 2000-2001

by James B. LaValle, RPh, DHM, NMD, CCN; Daniel L. Krinsky, RPh, MS; Ernest B. Hawkins, RPh, MS; Ross Pelton, RPh, PhD, CCN; Nancy Ashbrook Willis, BA, JD

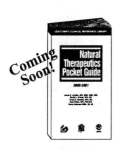

Provides healthcare professionals with condition-specific information on common uses of natural therapies.

Containing information on over 70 conditions, each including the following: Review of Condition, Decision Tree, List Of Commonly Recommended Herbals, Nutritional Supplements, Homeopathic Remedies, Lifestyle Modifications, and Contraindications & Warnings. Provides Herbal/Nutritional/Nutraceutical monographs with over 10 fields including References, Reported Uses, Dosage, Pharmacology, Toxicity, Warnings & Interactions, and Cautions & Contraindications.

Appendix section: Drug-nutrient Depletion, Herb-drug Interactions, Drug-nutrient Interaction, Herbal Medicine Use in Pediatrics, Unsafe Herbs, and Reference of Top Herbals.

To order call toll free: 1-800-837-LEXI (5394)

DRUG INFORMATION HANDBOOK FOR ADVANCED
PRACTICE NURSING 1999/2000
by Beatrice B. Turkoski, RN, PhD; Brenda R. Lance, RN, MSN; Mark F. Bonfiglio, PharmD

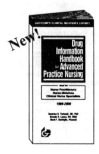

This handbook was designed specifically to meet the needs of Nurse Practitioners, Clinical Nurse Specialists, Nurse Midwives and graduate nursing students. The handbook is a unique resource for detailed, accurate information, which is vital to support the advanced practice nurse's role in patient drug therapy management.

A concise introductory section reviews topics related to Pharmacotherapeutics.

Over 4750 U.S., Canadian, and Mexican medications are covered in the 1055 monographs. Drug data is presented in an easy-to-use, alphabetically organized format covering up to 46 key points of information including Adult, Pediatric and Geriatric Dosing (with adjustments for renal/hepatic impairment), Laboratory Tests used to monitor drug therapy, Pregnancy/Breast-feeding Implications, Physical Assessment/Monitoring Guidelines and Patient Education/Instruction. Monographs are cross-referenced to an Appendix of over 230 pages of valuable comparison tables and additional information. Also included are two indices, Pharmacologic Category and Controlled Substance, which facilitate comparison between agents.

DRUG INFORMATION HANDBOOK FOR NURSING 2nd Edition 1999/2000
by Beatrice B. Turkoski, RN, PhD; Brenda R. Lance, RN, MSN; Mark F. Bonfiglio, PharmD

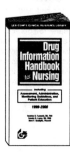

Registered Professional Nurses and upper-division nursing students involved with drug therapy will find this handbook provides quick access to drug data in a concise easy-to-use format.

Over 4750 U.S., Canadian, and Mexican medications are covered with up to 43 key points of information in each monograph. The handbook contains basic pharmacology concepts and nursing issues such as patient factors that influence drug therapy (ie, pregnancy, age, weight, etc) and general nursing issues (ie, assess-ment, administration, monitoring, and patient education). The Appendix contains over 220 pages of valuable information.

DRUG INFORMATION HANDBOOK FOR PHYSICIAN ASSISTANTS
1999-2000 by Michael J. Rudzinski, RPA-C, RPh; J. Fred Bennes, RPA, RPh

This comprehensive and easy-to-use handbook covers over 3600 drugs and also includes monographs on commonly used herbal products. There are up to 24 key fields of information per monograph, such as Pediatric And Adult Dosing With Adjustments for Renal/hepatic Impairment, Labeled And Unlabeled Uses, Pregnancy & Breast-feeding Precautions, and Special PA issues. Brand (U.S. and Canadian) and generic names are listed alphabetically for rapid access. It is fully cross-referenced by page number and includes alphabetical and pharmacologic indices.

To order call toll free: 1-800-837-LEXI (5394)

ANESTHESIOLOGY & CRITICAL CARE DRUG HANDBOOK
2nd Edition 1999-2000
by Andrew J. Donnelly, PharmD; Francesca E. Cunningham, PharmD; and Verna L. Baughman, MD

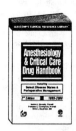

Contains over 512 generic medications with up to 25 fields of information presented in each monograph. It also contains the following Special Issues and Topics: Allergic Reaction, Anesthesia for Cardiac Patients in Noncardiac Surgery, Anesthesia for Obstetric Patients in Nonobstetric Surgery, Anesthesia for Patients With Liver Disease, Chronic Pain Management, Chronic Renal Failure, Conscious Sedation, Perioperative Management of Patients on Antiseizure Medication, Substance Abuse and Anesthesia.

The Appendix includes Abbreviations & Measurements, Anesthesiology Information, Assessment of Liver & Renal Function, Comparative Drug Charts, Infectious Disease-Prophylaxis & Treatment, Laboratory Values, Therapy Recommendation, Toxicology, *and much more . . .*

DRUG INFORMATION HANDBOOK FOR ONCOLOGY 1999-2000
by Dominic A. Solimando, Jr, MA; Linda R. Bressler, PharmD, BCOP; Polly E. Kintzel, PharmD, BCPS, BCOP; Mark C. Geraci, PharmD, BCOP

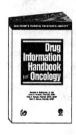

This comprehensive and easy-to-use oncology handbook was designed specifically to meet the needs of anyone who provides, prescribes, or administers therapy to cancer patients.

Presented in a concise and uniform format, this book contains the most comprehensive collection of oncology-related drug information available. Organized like a dictionary for ease of use, drugs can be found by looking up the *brand or generic name*!

This book contains 253 monographs, including over 1100 Antineoplastic Agents and Ancillary Medications.

It also contains up to 33 fields of information per monograph including Use, U.S. Investigational, Bone Marrow/Blood Cell Transplantation, Vesicant, Emetic Potential. A Special Topics Section, Appendix, and Therapeutic Category & Key Word Index are valuable features to this book, as well.

DRUG INFORMATION HANDBOOK FOR CARDIOLOGY 2000
by Bradley G. Phillips, PharmD; Virend K. Somers, MD, Dphi

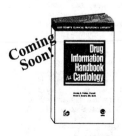

An ideal resource for physicians, pharmacists, nurses, residents, and students. This handbook was designed to provide the most current information on cardio-vascular agents and other ancillary medications.
- Each monograph includes information on Special Cardiovascular Considerations and I.V. to Oral Equivalency
- Alphabetically organized by brand and generic name
- Appendix contains information on Hypertension, Anticoagulation, Cytochrome P-450, Hyperlipidemia, Antiarrhythmia, and Comparative Drug Charts
- Special Topics/Issues include Emerging Risk Factors for Cardiovascular Disease, Treatment of Cardiovascular Disease in the Diabetic, Cardiovascular Stress Testing, and Experimental Cardiovascular Therapeutic Strategies in the New Millenium, and much more . . .

To order call toll free: 1-800-837-LEXI (5394)

DRUG INFORMATION HANDBOOK FOR PSYCHIATRY 2000
by Matthew A. Fuller, PharmD; Martha Sajatovic, MD

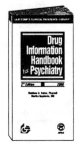

⊕ International Edition also available

As a source for comprehensive and clinically relevant drug information for the mental health professional, this handbook is alphabetically arranged by generic and brand name for ease-of-use. It covers over 4,000 brand names and up to 32 key fields of information including effect on mental status and effect on psychiatric treatment.

A special topics/issues section includes psychiatric assessment, overview of selected major psychiatric disorders, clinical issues in the use of major classes of psychotropic medications, psychiatric emergencies, special populations, diagnostic and statistical manual of mental disorders (DSM-IV), and suggested readings. Also contains a valuable Appendix section, as well as, a Therapeutic Category Index and an Alphabetical Index.

PSYCHOTROPIC DRUG INFORMATION HANDBOOK 2000
by Matthew A. Fuller, PharmD; Martha Sajatovic, MD

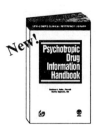

This portable, yet comprehensive guide to psychotropic drugs provides healthcare professionals with detailed information on use, warnings/precautions, drug interactions, pregnancy risk factors, adverse reactions, mechanism of action, and contraindications. Alphabetically organized by brand and generic name this concise handbook provides quick access to the information you need and includes patient education sheets on the psychotropic medications. It is the perfect pocket companion to the *Drug Information Handbook for Psychiatry*.

DRUG INFORMATION HANDBOOK FOR THE CRIMINAL JUSTICE PROFESSIONAL
by Marcelline Burns, PhD; Thomas E. Page, MA; and Jerrold B. Leikin, MD

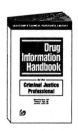

Compiled and designed for police officers, law enforcement officials, and legal professionals who are in need of a reference which relates to information on drugs, chemical substances, and other agents that have abuse and/or impairment potential. This handbook covers over 450 medications, agents, and substances. Each monograph is presented in a consistent format and contains up to 33 fields of information including Scientific Name, Commonly Found In, Abuse Potential, Impairment Potential, Use, When to Admit to Hospital, Mechanism of Toxic Action, Signs & Symptoms of Acute Overdose, Drug Interactions, Warnings/Precautions, and Reference Range. There are many diverse chapter inclusions as well as a glossary of medical terms for the layman along with a slang street drug listing. The Appendix contains Chemical, Bacteriologic, and Radiologic Agents - Effects and Treatment; Controlled Substances - Uses and Effects; Medical Examiner Data; Federal Trafficking Penalties, *and much more*.

To order call toll free: 1-800-837-LEXI (5394)

DENTAL OFFICE MEDICAL EMERGENCIES

by Timothy F. Meiller, DDS, PhD; Richard L. Wynn, BSPharm, PhD; Ann Marie McMullin, MD; Cynthia Biron, RDH, EMT, MA; Harold L. Crossley, DDS, PhD

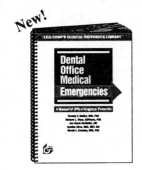

Designed specifically for general dentists during times of emergency. A tabbed paging system allows for quick access to specific crisis events. Created with urgency in mind, it is spiral bound and drilled with a hole for hanging purposes.

- Basic Action Plan for Stabilization
- Loss of Consciousness / Respiratory Distress / Chest Pain
- Allergic / Drug Reactions
- Altered Sensation / Changes in Affect
- Management of Acute Bleeding
- Office Preparedness / Procedures and Protocols

DRUG INFORMATION HANDBOOK FOR DENTISTRY 5th Ed 1999-2000

by Richard L. Wynn, BSPharm, PhD; Timothy F. Meiller, DDS, PhD; and Harold L. Crossley, DDS, PhD

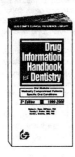

This handbook presents dental management and therapeutic considerations in medically compromised patients. Issues covered include oral manifestations of drugs, pertinent dental drug interactions, and dosing of drugs in dental treatment.

Selected oral medicine topics requiring therapeutic intervention include managing the patient with acute or chronic pain including TMD, managing the patient with oral bacterial or fungal infections, current therapeutics in periodontal patients, managing the patient receiving chemotherapy or radiation for the treatment of cancer, managing the anxious patient, managing dental office emergencies, and treatment of common oral lesions.

CLINICIAN'S ENDODONTIC HANDBOOK 2000

by Thom C. Dumsha, MS, DDS; James L. Gutmann, DDS, FACD, FICD

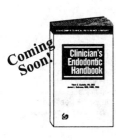

Designed for all general practice dentists.

- Easy to use format
- Latest techniques, procedures, and materials
- Root canal therapy: Why's and Why Nots
- A guide to diagnosis and treatment of endodontic emergencies
- Facts and rationale behind treating endodontically-involved teeth
- Straight-forward dental trauma management information
- Pulpal Histology, Access Openings, Bleaching, Resorption, Radiography, Restoration, and Periodontal / Endodontic Complications
- Each chapter has a Problem Solving / Frequently Asked Questions (FAQ) Section.

POISONING & TOXICOLOGY COMPENDIUM
by Jerrold B. Leikin, MD and Frank P. Paloucek, PharmD

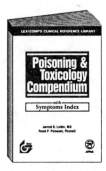

A six-in-one reference wherein each major entry contains information relative to one or more of the other sections. This handbook offers comprehensive concisely-stated monographs covering 645 medicinal agents, 256 nonmedicinal agents, 273 biological agents, 49 herbal agents, 254 laboratory tests, 79 antidotes, and 222 pages of exceptionally useful appendix material.

A truly unique reference that presents signs and symptoms of acute overdose along with considerations for overdose treatment. Ideal reference for emergency situations.

LABORATORY TEST HANDBOOK 4th Edition & CONCISE version
by David S. Jacobs MD, FACP; Wayne R. DeMott, MD, FACP; Harold J. Grady, PhD; Rebecca T. Horvat, PhD; Douglas W. Huestis, MD; and Bernard L. Kasten Jr., MD, FACP

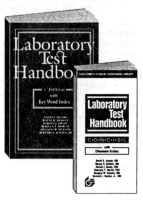

Contains over 900 clinical laboratory tests and is an excellent source of laboratory information for physicians of all specialties, nurses, laboratory professionals, students, medical personnel, or anyone who needs quick access to most the routine and many of the more specialized testing procedures available in today's clinical laboratory.

Including updated AMA CPT coding, each monograph contains test name, synonyms, patient care, specimen requirements, reference ranges, and interpretive information with footnotes and references.

The *Laboratory Test Handbook Concise* is a portable, abridged (800 tests) version and is an ideal, quick reference for anyone requiring information concerning patient preparation, specimen collection and handling, and test result interpretation.

DIAGNOSTIC PROCEDURE HANDBOOK
by Joseph A. Golish, MD

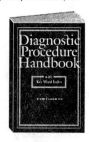

An ideal companion to the Laboratory Test Handbook this publication details 295 diagnostic procedures including Allergy, Immunology/Rheumotology, Infectious Disease, Cardiology, Critical Care, Gastro-enterology, Nephrology, Urology, Hematology, Neurology, Ophthalmology, Pulmonary Function, Pulmonary Medicine, Computed Tomography, Diagnostic Radiology, Invasive Radiology, Magnetic Resonance Imaging, Nuclear Medicine, and Ultra-sound. A great reference handbook for healthcare professionals at any level of training and experience.

To order call toll free: 1-800-837-LEXI (5394)